Nursing Diagnosis

Application to Clinical Practice

LYNDA JUALL CARPENITO-MOYET, R.N., M.S.N., C.R.N.P.

Family Nurse Practitioner
ChesPenn Health Services
Chester, Pennsylvania

Nursing Consultant
Mickleton, New Jersey

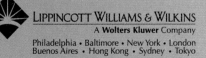

LIPPINCOTT WILLIAMS & WILKINS
A **Wolters Kluwer** Company

Philadelphia • Baltimore • New York • London
Buenos Aires • Hong Kong • Sydney • Tokyo

Senior Acquisitions Editor: Quincy McDonald
Senior Developmental Editor: Michelle Clark
Senior Production Editor: Tom Gibbons
Senior Production Manager: Helen Ewan
Managing Editor/Production: Erika Kors
Art Director: Joan Wendt
Manufacturing Manager: William Alberti
Indexer: Ann Cassar
Compositor: Circle Graphics
Printer: Courier-Kendallville

11th Edition
Copyright © 2006 by Lynda Juall Carpenito-Moyet.
Copyright © 2004 by Lynda Juall Carpenito-Moyet. Copyright © 2002, 2000, 1997, 1995, 1993, 1992 by Lynda Juall Carpenito.

9 8 7 6 5 4 3 2

Library of Congress Cataloging-in Publication Data

Nursing diagnosis : application to clinical practice / [edited by] Lynda Juall Carpenito-Moyet. — 11th ed.
        p. ; cm.
    Includes bibliographical references and index.
    ISBN 0-7817-6131-X (pbk. : alk. paper)
    1. Nursing diagnosis. I. Carpenito-Moyet, Lynda Juall.
    [DNLM: 1. Nursing Diagnosis—Outlines. 2. Patient Care Planning—Outlines. WY 18.2 N9753 2006]
RT48.6.N869 2006
616.07'5—dc22

                                                    2005009807

TO MY EARTH ANGELS

In the eighth edition of this book, I introduced the reader to Earth angels. The dictionary defines "angel" as a "spiritual being . . . an attendant spirit or guardian . . . one who aids or supports." Earth angels can be friends, strangers, adults, or children. Most often, the Earth angel does not even know the profound effects of the angelic encounter.

Seven Earth angels were always there, giving me permission to be imperfect, to grieve, and to heal. These Earth angels—Margo, Ginny, Ros, Jamie, Donna, Heather, and my dear sister Pati—continue to not be afraid of my grief, my anger, or riding the emotional roller-coaster with me, their wings flapping in the wind. Thank you Earth angels, friends and strangers.

Para mi Jorge
   Man meets woman
   Woman wants to run like a rabbit
   She has had her share of sorrow
   But she waits
   She realizes the man has had his share of sorrow too.
   So they both wait,
   And learn to trust and love again.

   Gracias, mi esposo
      Jorge Luis Moyet-Gonzalez

CONTRIBUTORS (Current and Past)

Rosalinda Alfaro-LeFevre, R.N., M.S.N., President, Teaching Smart/Learning Easy, Stuart, Florida
(Risk for Ineffective Respiratory Function; Ineffective Airway Clearance; Ineffective Breathing Patterns; Deficient Diversional Activity; Impaired Verbal Communication; Deficient Fluid Volume; Excess Fluid Volume; Risk for Imbalanced Body Temperature; Hyperthermia and Hypothermia)

Ann H. Barnhouse, R.N., M.S.N., Nurse Educator, Hudson, Ohio
(Relocation Stress)

Christine J. Brugler, R.N., M.S.N., Private Practice, Warren, Ohio
(Relocation Stress)

Judith S. Carscadden, R.N., Head Nurse, London Psychiatric Hospital, London, Ontario, Canada
(Disturbed Self-Concept; Disturbed Body Image; Chronic Low Self-Esteem; Situational Low Self-Esteem, Fifth Edition; Risk for Self-Mutilation)

Deana DeMare, P.T., B.S., Neurobehavioral Specialist, Children's Regional Hospital/Cooper Hospital University Medical Center, Camden, New Jersey
(Disorganized Infant Behavior; Potential for Enhanced Organized Infant Behavior; Risk for Impaired Parent–Infant Attachment)

Rebecca Fairchild, R.N., M.S.N., C.R.N.P., Family Nurse Practitioner, Bethlehem, Pennsylvania
(Collaborative Problems)

Dru Hammell, R.N., M.S.N., Nurse Manager, Newborn Services, Cooper Hospital/University Medical Center, Camden, New Jersey
(Disorganized Infant Behavior; Potential for Enhanced Organized Infant Behavior; Risk for Impaired Parent–Infant Attachment)

Joan T. Harkulich, R.N., M.S.N., Director of Research and Professional Services, Care Services, Beachwood, Ohio
(Relocation Stress)

Eileen Hubler, R.N., M.S., Neonatal Clinical Nurse Specialist, Children's Regional Hospital/Cooper Hospital University Medical Center, Camden, New Jersey
(Disorganized Infant Behavior; Potential for Enhanced Organized Infant Behavior; Risk for Impaired Parent–Infant Attachment)

Jean Jenny, Professor, retired from University of Ottawa, Ottawa Canada
(Dysfunctional Ventilatory Weaning Response; Risk for Dysfunctional Ventilatory Weaning Response)

Jo Logan, R.N., M.Ed., Director of Nursing Research & Professional Development, Ottawa Civic Hospital, Ottawa, Canada
(Dysfunctional Ventilatory Weaning Response; Risk for Dysfunctional Ventilatory Weaning Response)

Morris A. Magnan, R.N., B.S.N., Clinical Nurse Specialist/Case Manager, Harper Hospital, Detroit Medical Center, Detroit, Michigan
(Activity Intolerance)

Jo Ann Maklebust, M.S.N., R.N., C.S., Clinical Nurse Specialist/Wound Care, Nurse Practitioner, Harper Hospital, Detroit Medical Center, Detroit, Michigan
(Impaired Tissue Integrity; Risk for Ineffective Health Maintenance related to lack of knowledge of ostomy care; Impaired Skin Integrity; Impaired Comfort: Pruritus; Impaired Oral Mucous Membrane)

Judy McElvanney, R.N., London Psychiatric Hospital, London, Ontario, Canada
(Disturbed Thought Processes related to effects of dementia)

Amy Meredith, R.N., M.S.N., F.N.P., Private Practice, Chatsworth, New Jersey
(Risk for Imbalanced Body Temperature; Hyperthermia and Hypothermia, Seventh Edition)

Nancy J. Morwessel, R.N., M.S.N., C.P.N.P., Pediatric Nurse Practitioner, Children's Hospital Medical Center, Cincinnati, Ohio
(Impaired Comfort in Children; Ineffective Infant Feeding Pattern)

Mary M. Owen, R.N., B.S.N., P.H.N., Associate Director, Health Outcomes, CalOptima, Orange, California
(Risk for Infection; Risk for Infection Transmission)

Rhonda Panfilli, R.N., M.S.N., Business Manager, Deborah R. Dunison, Ph.D., Bloomfield Hills, Michigan
(Ineffective Health Maintenance related to increased food consumption)

Gayle Vandendool Parker, R.N., B.S.N., C.P.M.H.N.(C.), Program of Assertive Community Treatment, London Psychiatric Hospital, London, Ontario, Canada
(Disturbed Thought Processes; Disturbed Thought Process related to [Specify] as evidenced by inability to evaluate reality; Powerlessness; PC: Neuroleptic Malignant Syndrome)

Mary Sieggreen, M.S.N., R.N., C.S., Nurse Practitioner, Vascular Surgery, Harper Hospital, Detroit Medical Center, Detroit, Michigan
(Ineffective Peripheral Tissue Perfusion; Risk for Injury related to effects secondary to orthostatic hypotension)

Deborah Soholt, R.N., M.S.N., Director, Women & Children Services, Averal McKennan Hospital, Sioux Falls, South Dakota
(Decisional Conflict)

Kristen Switalski, M.S.N., C.R.N.P., Family Nurse Practitioner, Philadelphia, Pennsylvania
(Collaborative Problems)

Julie Waterhouse, R.N., M.S., Assistant Professor, College of Nursing, University of Delaware, Newark, Delaware
(Spiritual Distress; Ineffective Sexuality Patterns, Seventh Edition)

Janet R. Weber, R.N., M.S.N., Ed.D., Associate Professor of Nursing, Southeast Missouri State University, Cape Girardeau, Missouri
(Hopelessness)

Margaret Chamberlain Wilmoth, Assistant Professor, College of Nursing and Health Professions, University of North Carolina, Charlotte, North Carolina
(Ineffective Sexuality Patterns)

PREFACE

Rapid change continues to occur in health care and in the nursing profession. Hospitals continue to trim their nursing staffs, while the acuity of clients continues to rise. Many nurses, and even some faculty, question the usefulness of nursing diagnosis. Unfortunately, nursing diagnosis is still joined at the hip with traditional care planning. It is time to separate these Siamese twins so that both can function separately. Nursing diagnosis defines the science and art of nursing. It is as imperative to nursing as medical diagnoses are to physicians. It serves to organize nursing's knowledge in the literature, in research, and in the clinician's mind. Do not underestimate the importance of this classification. A clinician with expertise with nursing diagnoses can hypothesize several explanations for a client's anger, such as fear, anxiety, powerlessness, or spiritual distress. Without this knowledge, the client is simply angry.

Care planning as it is taught in schools of nursing is an academic exercise. This is not wrong, but as the student progresses into the senior year, this academic care plan must be transformed into a clinically useful product. Nursing diagnosis must be presented as clinically useful. Nurses who are expert in certain nursing diagnoses should be consulted, just as our medical colleagues consult other physicians for their expertise. Health care facilities should publish a list of nursing experts in their facility for consultation.

Faculty, nurse managers, administrators, and clinicians need to do their part. Change is imperative. The documentation requirements are unrealistic. There is little time to think and analyze with these documentation mandates. Nursing must defend its right to determine its documentation requirements just as medicine has.

If nursing continues to do business as usual, nursing as we want it—nursing as clients need it—will cease to exist. Nursing will continue to be defined by what we do and write and not by what we know.

From assessment criteria to specific interventions, the book focuses on nursing. It provides a condensed, organized outline of clinical nursing practice designed to communicate creative clinical nursing. It is not meant to replace textbooks of nursing, but rather to provide nurses in a variety of settings with the information they need without requiring a time-consuming review of the literature. It will assist students in transferring their theoretical knowledge to clinical practice; it can also be used by experienced nurses to recall past learning and to intervene in those clinical situations that previously went ignored or unrecognized.

The author agrees that nursing needs a classification system to organize its functions and define its scope. Use of such a classification system would expedite research activities and facilitate communication between nurses, consumers, and other health care providers. After all, medicine took over 100 years to develop its taxonomy. Our work, at the national level, only began in 1973. It is hoped that the reader will be stimulated to participate at the local, regional, or national level in the utilization and development of these diagnoses.

Since the first edition was published, the use of nursing diagnosis has increased markedly throughout the United States, Canada, and internationally. Practicing nurses vary in experience with nursing diagnosis from just beginning to full practice integration for over 15 years. With such a variance in use, questions posed by the neophyte, such as

- What does the label really mean?
- What kinds of assessment questions will yield nursing diagnoses?
- How do I differentiate one diagnosis from another?
- How do I tailor a diagnosis for a specific individual?
- How should I intervene after I formulate the diagnostic statement?
- How do I care-plan with nursing diagnoses?

differ dramatically from such questions from experts as

- Should nursing diagnoses represent the only diagnoses on the nursing care plan?
- Can medical diagnoses be included in a nursing diagnosis statement?
- What are the ethical issues in using nursing diagnoses?
- What kind of problem statement should I write to describe a person at risk for hemorrhage?

- How can I efficiently use nursing diagnosis?
- What kind of nursing diagnosis should I use to describe a healthy person?
- Do I need nursing diagnoses with critical pathways?

This eleventh edition of *Nursing Diagnosis: Application to Clinical Practice* seeks to continue to answer these questions.

Section One begins with a chapter on the development of nursing diagnosis and the work of the North American Nursing Diagnosis Association (NANDA). The chapter explores the concepts of nursing diagnosis, classification, and taxonomic issues. It discusses the review process of NANDA and describes the evolving taxonomy of NANDA.

Chapter 2 differentiates among actual, risk, and possible nursing diagnoses. It also presents a discussion of wellness and syndrome diagnoses. It outlines guidelines for writing diagnostic statements and avoiding errors. Chapter 2 also covers the use of non–NANDA-approved diagnoses and practice dilemmas associated with nursing diagnoses.

Chapter 3 describes the Bifocal Clinical Practice Model. This chapter includes a more detailed discussion of nursing diagnoses and collaborative problems, covering their relationship to assessment, goals, interventions, and evaluation.

Chapter 4 focuses on assessment and diagnosis, covering data interpretation and assessment format and concluding with a case study to illustrate clinical applications.

Chapter 5 describes the process of care planning and discusses various care planning systems. Topics covered include priority identification, nursing goals versus client goals, case management and nursing accountability. The chapter differentiates interventions for nursing diagnoses and collaborative problems. It also clarifies evaluation, distinguishing evaluation of nursing care from evaluation of the client's condition. It presents a discussion of multidisciplinary care, along with a three-tiered care planning system aimed at increasing the clinical use of care plans without increasing writing. Samples of nursing records appear throughout the chapter.

Chapter 6 addresses issues and controversies. It explores arguments regarding the ethics and cultural implications of nursing diagnoses. It discusses the implications of a consistent language for nurses as members of a multidisciplinary team.

Section Two compiles the nursing diagnoses accepted by NANDA along with additional clinically useful diagnoses. The eleventh edition includes 164 diagnoses (148 NANDA-approved and 13 added by the author). Each nursing diagnosis group is discussed under the following subheads:

- Definition
- Defining Characteristics or Risk Factors
- Related Factors
- Author's Notes
- Errors in Diagnostic Statements
- Focus Assessment
- Key Concepts
- Generic Considerations
- Pediatric Considerations
- Geriatric Considerations
- Transcultural Considerations

Author's Notes and Errors in Diagnostic Statements are designed to help the nurse understand the concept behind the diagnosis, differentiate one diagnosis from another, and avoid diagnostic errors. Maternal, Pediatric, and Geriatric Considerations for all relevant diagnoses provide additional pertinent information. Transcultural Considerations strive to increase the reader's sensitivity to cultural diversity without stereotyping.

Each nursing diagnosis is addressed with generic interventions and rationale. If applicable, Maternal, Pediatric, and Geriatric focus interventions and rationale are included. Each nursing diagnosis is then followed by one or more specific nursing diagnoses that relate to familiar clinical situations. Goals for the diagnosis are provided with the related interventions, which represent activities in the independent domain of nursing derived from the physical and applied sciences, pharmacology, nutrition, mental health, and nursing research.

New to the eleventh edition is the conclusion of the Nursing Outcome Classification (NOC) and Nursing Intervention Classification (NIC). Each nursing diagnosis has NIC major intervention categories and NOC outcome categories. This inclusion was to assist those in the development of electronic care planning. The goals, indicators, and interventions are the work of this author, not NIC or NOC.

Every attempt has been made to provide the reader with the most recent literature and research findings on the subject. Students are frequently instructed not to use references over 5 years old. This is very problematic. Sometimes the original paper or research on a topic remains, even 10 years later, the state of science on that topic. If a subsequent author or researcher uses the original work, often his or her citation is substituted for the older one. I disagree with this practice; both citations should be listed. Therefore, throughout this book, the reader will find citations of various years, many older than 5 years. Web site addresses for diagnoses have been added for the nurse and consumer.

Section Three consists of a Manual of Collaborative Problems. In this section, each of the nine generic collaborative problems is explained under the following subheads:

- Physiologic Overview
- Definition
- Diagnostic Considerations
- Focus Assessment Criteria
- Significant Laboratory Assessment Criteria

Discussed under their appropriate problems are 52 specific collaborative problems, covering:

- Definition
- High-Risk Populations
- Nursing Goals
- Interventions

The author invites comments or suggestions from readers. Correspondence can be directed to the publisher or to the author: e-mail Juall46@bellatlantic.net

Lynda Juall Carpenito-Moyet, R.N., M.S.N., C.R.N.P.

ACKNOWLEDGMENTS

This eleventh edition was made possible with the intensive help of my editors Joe Morita and Quincy McDonald. Again, Tom Gibbons prodded me on as the Senior Production Editor. A special thank you to my daughter-in-law Heather for all her assistance with manuscript preparation. God did not give me a daughter, but gave me a very special daughter-in-law. Thank you, Heather.

The support for this book continues nationally and internationally. It has been translated into 10 languages.

Finally, I would like to thank the group in Detroit (Jo Ann Maklebust, Mary Sieggreen, and Linda Mondoux) for their moral support while I wrote the first edition. Rosalinda Alfaro-LeFevre recognized the need for this book in 1983 and sought me out to make it a reality.

On a personal level, my son Olen Juall Carpenito and his wife Heather have given me a special gift—my grandson Olen, Jr. He lights up my world.

CONTENTS

S E C T I O N   T H R E E
Manual of Collaborative Problems   825

Nursing Diagnosis in the Nursing Process

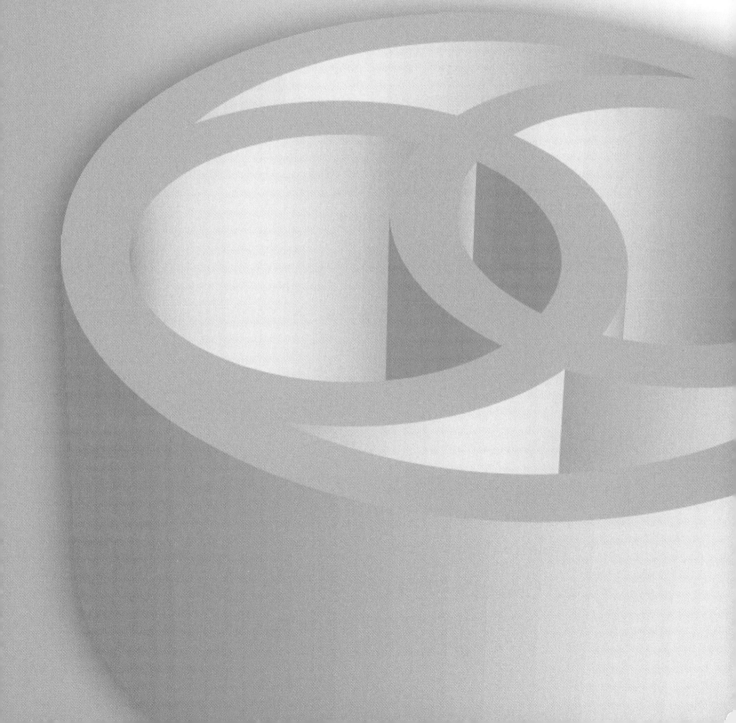

INTRODUCTION

Nursing is primarily assisting individuals (sick or well) with those activities contributing to health or its recovery (or to a peaceful death) that they perform unaided when they have the necessary strength, will, or knowledge; nursing also helps individuals carry out prescribed therapy and to be independent of assistance as soon as possible.*

Individuals are open systems who continually interact with the environment, creating interaction patterns. These patterns are dynamic and also interact with life processes (physiologic, psychological, sociocultural, developmental, and spiritual) to influence the person's behavior and health. *Health* is a dynamic, ever-changing state influenced by past and present interaction patterns. It is the state of wellness as the individual defines it; it is no longer defined as the presence of a biologic disease.

Societal health needs have changed in the last few decades; so must the nurse's view of the consumers of health care (individual, family, community).† An individual becomes a client not only when an actual or potential problem compromises health but also when he or she desires assistance to achieve a higher level of health. The use of *client* in place of *patient* to identify the health care consumer suggests an autonomous person who has freedom of choice in seeking and selecting assistance. The client is no longer a passive recipient of services but an active participant who assumes responsibility for his or her choices and their consequences. He or she is a self-expert responsible for seeking or refusing health care. *Family* is used to describe any persons who serve as support systems to the client. *Group* is used to describe support systems as well as communities, such as senior citizen centers.

The Bifocal Clinical Practice Model describes the unique responsibilities of nursing in two components: nursing diagnoses and collaborative problems. *Nursing diagnoses* address the responses of clients, families, or groups to situations for which the nurse can prescribe interventions for outcome achievement. In contrast, *collaborative problems* describe certain physiologic complications that nurses manage using both nurse-prescribed and physician-prescribed interventions. No other discipline but nursing can treat nursing diagnoses and also manage collaborative problems.

The Bifocal Clinical Practice Model provides nurses with a classification system to describe the health status of a client, family, or community and the risk for complications. Using this system, nurses can describe the health status of individuals or groups concisely and systematically, while also addressing the unique aspects of each situation.

*Henderson, V., & Nite, G. (1960). *Principles and practice of nursing* (5th ed.). New York: Macmillan.
†Carpenito, L. J., & Duespohl, T. A. (1985). *A guide to effective clinical instruction* (2nd ed.). Rockville, MD: Aspen Systems.

DEVELOPMENT OF NURSING DIAGNOSIS

Before the development of a classification or list of nursing diagnoses, nurses used whatever word they wanted to describe client problems. For example, nurses might have described a client recovering from surgery as "the appendectomy," another client as "the diabetic," and another client as "difficult." Clearly, knowing that a person has diabetes brings to mind blood sugar problems and risk for infection, so the focus was on common problems or risk factors derived from medical diagnoses. If the client with diabetes or surgery had another problem that needed nursing attention, this problem would have gone undiagnosed. Before 1972, not only did nurses lack the terms to describe problems (except medical diagnoses), but also they did not have assessment questions to uncover such problems.

The need for a common, consistent language for medicine was identified more than 200 years ago. If physicians chose to use random words to describe their clinical situations, then:

- How could they communicate with one another? With nurses?
- How could they organize research?
- How could they educate new physicians?
- How could they improve quality if they could not retrieve data systematically to determine which interventions improved the client's condition?

For example, before the formal labeling of acquired immunodeficiency syndrome (AIDS), defining or studying the disease was difficult, if not impossible. Often, medical records of affected clients would show various diagnoses or causes of death, such as sepsis, cerebral hemorrhage, or pneumonia, because the AIDS diagnosis did not exist. Every physician in the world uses the same terminology for medical diagnoses. As new diagnoses are discovered, all medical clinicians can access the research using the same words.

A classification system for nursing defines the body of knowledge for which nursing is held accountable. The relationship of nursing diagnosis to accountability and autonomy can be expressed as follows:

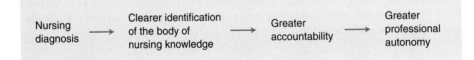

Nursing Diagnosis: Defined

By definition, *diagnosis* is the careful, critical study of something to determine its nature. The question is not *whether* nurses can diagnose, but *what* nurses can diagnose.

In 1953, V. Fry introduced the term *nursing diagnosis* to describe a step necessary in developing a nursing care plan. Over the next 20 years, references to nursing diagnosis appeared sporadically in the literature. From 1973 (the first meeting of the National Group for the Classification of Nursing Diagnosis) to the present, however, references to nursing diagnosis in the literature have increased tenfold.

In 1973, the American Nurses Association (ANA) published its *Standards of Practice;* in 1980, it followed with its *Social Policy Statement,* which defined nursing as "the diagnosis and treatment of human response to actual or potential health problems." Most state nurse practice acts describe nursing in accordance with the ANA definition.

In March 1990, at the Ninth Conference of the North American Nursing Diagnosis Association (NANDA), the General Assembly approved an official definition of nursing diagnosis (NANDA, 1990):

> *Nursing diagnosis is a clinical judgment about individual, family, or community responses to actual or potential health problems/life processes. Nursing diagnosis provides the basis for selection of nursing interventions to achieve outcomes for which the nurse is accountable.*

This definition is very important because it separates one type of judgment that the nurse makes from all other judgments. This judgment, or nursing diagnosis, is the responsibility of nurses to prescribe interventions to achieve outcomes.

It is important also to emphasize that the responses called nursing diagnoses can be to illness and life events. Previously, nurses focused more on responses to medical conditions or treatments. Nurses now diagnose and treat responses to life events such as parenting, aging parents, and school failure.

Nursing Diagnosis: Process or Outcome?

A review of the literature reveals that, over time, the term *nursing diagnosis* has been used in three contexts:

1. *As the second step of the nursing process.* In this step, the nurse analyzes data collected during assessment and evaluates the client's health status. Some conclusions resulting from data analysis lead to nursing diagnoses; others do not. It is important to recognize that the outcome of this process can include problems treated primarily by nurses and problems requiring treatment by professionals from several disciplines. For example, while assessing a particular client, the nurse may record observations that point to the medical problems of seizures, pneumonia, and hypertension, as well as the nursing diagnosis of *Risk for Injury.* Using the term *nursing diagnosis* to designate the second step of the nursing process may be confusing and have the undesirable effect of leading nurses to try to state all conclusions or problems as nursing diagnoses.
2. *As a list of diagnostic labels or titles.* After the first conference on nursing diagnosis in 1973, the term *nursing diagnosis* was applied to specific labels describing health states that nurses could legally diagnose and treat. These labels are concise descriptors of a cluster of signs and symptoms, such as *Anxiety,* or of increased vulnerability, such as *Risk for Injury.*
3. *As a two-part or three-part statement.* Nurses use the term *nursing diagnosis* to describe a two-part or three-part statement about an individual's, a family's, or a group's response to a situation or health problem.

Thus, it has become necessary to indicate clearly whether the term *nursing diagnosis* is being used in the context of problem identification, a classification system of diagnostic labels (such as that developed by NANDA), or an individualized diagnosis. To avoid misuse and confusion, the author recommends using the following terms:

- For the second step of the nursing process: *diagnosis*
- For the list of diagnostic labels or titles: *diagnostic label* or *nursing diagnosis*
- For the diagnostic statement: *nursing diagnosis*

The North American Nursing Diagnosis Association International

In 1973, the first conference on nursing diagnosis was held to identify nursing knowledge and to establish a classification system suitable for computerization. From this conference developed the National Group for the Classification of Nursing Diagnosis, composed of nurses from different regions of the United States and Canada, representing all elements of the profession: practice, education, and research. From 1973 to the present, the National Group has met 15 times. Its most recent list of nursing diagnoses is presented at the end of Section One.

In 2003, the organization was renamed the North American Nursing Diagnosis Association International (NANDA). In addition to reviewing and accepting nursing diagnoses for addition to the list, NANDA also reviews previously accepted nursing diagnoses. For example, in 1994, NANDA revised ten previously accepted diagnoses.

In March 1990, the first issue of *Nursing Diagnosis,* NANDA's official journal, was published. This journal aims to promote the development, refinement, and application of nursing diagnoses and to serve as a forum for issues pertaining to the development and classification of nursing knowledge. The journal is now named *Nursing Diagnosis: The International Journal of Nursing Language and Classification.*

At the International Council of Nursing (ICN) in Seoul in 1989, the Canadian and American Nurses Associations proposed a resolution to the Council of National Representatives. The resolution asked that "ICN encourage member nurses' associations to become involved in developing classification systems for nursing care, nursing information management systems, and nursing data sets to provide tools that nurses in all countries could use to describe nursing and its contributions to health" (Clark & Lang,

1992, p. 110). The resolution passed, and a task force was formed to consider how ICN could best assist member associations.

The International Classification for Nursing Practice (ICNP) is a classification system published in 1993 of nursing diagnoses, interventions, and outcomes. Its purpose is to (Clark & Lang, 1992):

• Capture nursing's contributions to health
• Enable cross-country comparison of nursing practice
• Promote the development of nursing

This initial undertaking strove to compile all terms for nursing diagnoses, interventions, and outcomes in the literature. Since the first draft working paper, the ICN development team has disseminated the classification worldwide. Creating a classification system for nurses in New York City, rural Zimbabwe, Tokyo, and New Guinea is a monumental and exhausting endeavor, but one that is critical to the nursing profession. The ICNP Beta Version, *ICNP: A Unifying Framework,* is available from ICN via requests: FAX: 44-33-908-01-01; e-mail: *ICN@uni2a.uniga.ch.*

NANDA Taxonomy

A *taxonomy* is a type of classification, the theoretical study of systematic classifications including their bases, principles, procedures, and rules. The work of the initial theorist group at the third national conference and subsequently of the NANDA taxonomic committee produced the beginnings of a conceptual framework for the diagnostic classification system. This framework was named NANDA Nursing Diagnosis Taxonomy I, which comprised nine patterns of human response. In 2000, NANDA approved a new Taxonomy II, which has 13 domains, 106 classes, and 155 diagnoses (NANDA, 2001).

Table 1.1 illustrates the 13 domains and associated definitions. The second level, classes, may be useful as assessment criteria. The third level (diagnostic concepts), most useful for clinicians, is the

Table 1.1 Taxonomy II Domains and Definitions

Domain 1	Health Promotion	Awareness of well-being or normality of function and the strategies used to maintain control of and enhance that well-being or normality of function
Domain 2	Nutrition	Activities of taking in, assimilating, and using nutrients for the purposes of tissue maintenance, tissue repair, and production of energy
Domain 3	Elimination	Secretion and excretion of waste products from the body
Domain 4	Activity/Rest	Production, conservation, expenditure, or balance of energy resources
Domain 5	Perception/Cognition	Human information-processing system including attention, orientation, sensation, perception, cognition, and communication
Domain 6	Self-perception	Awareness about the self
Domain 7	Role Relationships	Positive and negative connections or associations between persons or groups of persons and the means by which those connections are demonstrated
Domain 8	Sexuality	Sexual identity, sexual function, and reproduction
Domain 9	Coping/Stress Tolerance	Contending with life events/life processes
Domain 10	Life Principles	Principles underlying conduct, thought, and behavior about acts, customs, or institutions viewed as being true or having intrinsic worth
Domain 11	Safety/Protection	Freedom from danger, physical injury, or immune system damage, preservation from loss, and protection of safety and security
Domain 12	Comfort	Sense of mental, physical, or social well-being or ease
Domain 13	Growth/Development	Age-appropriate increases in physical dimensions, organ systems, and/or attainment of developmental milestones

North American Nursing Diagnosis Association. (2001). *Nursing diagnosis: Definitions and classification 2001–2002.* Philadelphia: NANDA.

nursing diagnosis labels. Changes in terminology were made for consistency; for example, *Altered Nutrition* was changed to *Imbalanced Nutrition.* An example of one domain is:

Domain 4	Activity/Rest	
Class 1	Sleep/Rest	
Diagnostic Concepts	00095	Disturbed Sleep Pattern
	00096	Sleep Deprivation

Summary

A classification system for nursing diagnoses has been in continual development for the past 30 years. During this period, the initial question, "Does nursing really need a classification system?" has been replaced by, "How can such a system be developed in a scientifically sound manner?" The ANA has designated NANDA as the official organization to develop this classification system. Despite problems, through the concerted effort of many fine clinical nurses, nurse researchers, and other nursing professionals and organizations, this evolving classification system increasingly reflects both the art and science of nursing.

TYPES AND COMPONENTS OF NURSING DIAGNOSES

The types of nursing diagnoses are actual, risk, possible, wellness, and syndrome.

Actual Nursing Diagnoses

An *actual nursing diagnosis* represents a problem that has been validated by the presence of major defining characteristics. This type of nursing diagnosis has four components: label, definition, defining characteristics, and related factors.

Label

The label should be in clear, concise terms that convey the meaning of the diagnosis.

Definition

The definition should add clarity to the diagnostic label. It also should help to differentiate a particular diagnosis from similar diagnoses.

Defining Characteristics

For actual nursing diagnoses, defining characteristics are signs and symptoms that, when seen together, represent the nursing diagnosis. Defining characteristics are separated into major and minor designations.

- *Major.* For nonresearched diagnoses, at least one must be present for validation of the diagnosis. For researched diagnoses, at least one must be present under the 80%–100% grouping.
- *Minor.* These characteristics provide supporting evidence but may not be present.

The nursing diagnoses in Section Two will have researched and nonresearched defining characteristics. Table 2.1 represents major and minor defining characteristics for the researched diagnosis *Defensive Coping* (Norris & Kunes-Connell, 1987).

Related Factors

In actual nursing diagnoses, related factors are contributing factors that have influenced the change in health status. Such factors can be grouped into four categories:

- *Pathophysiologic (Biologic or Psychological).* Examples include compromised immune system and inadequate circulation.
- *Treatment-Related.* Examples include medications, diagnostic studies, surgery, and treatments.
- *Situational.* Examples include environmental, home, community, institution, personal, life experiences, and roles.
- *Maturational.* Examples include age-related influences, such as children and the elderly.

TABLE 2.1 Frequency Scores for Defining Characteristics of Defensive Coping

Defining Characteristics	Frequency Scores
Major (80%–100%)	
Denial of obvious problems/weaknesses	88%
Projection of blame/responsibility	87%
Rationalizes failures	86%
Hypersensitive to slight criticism	84%
Minor (50%–79%)	
Grandiosity	79%
Superior attitude toward others	76%
Difficulty in establishing/maintaining relationships	74%
Hostile laughter or ridicule of others	71%
Difficulty in testing perceptions against reality	62%
Lack of follow-through or participation in treatment or therapy	56%

Norris, J., & Kunes-Connell, M. (1987). Self-esteem disturbance: A clinical validation study. In A. McLane (Ed.), *Classification of nursing diagnoses: Proceedings of the seventh NANDA national conference.* St. Louis: CV Mosby.

○○ **INTERACTIVE EXERCISE 2.1**

To determine the presence of an actual diagnosis, ask, "Are major signs and symptoms of the diagnosis in this person?"

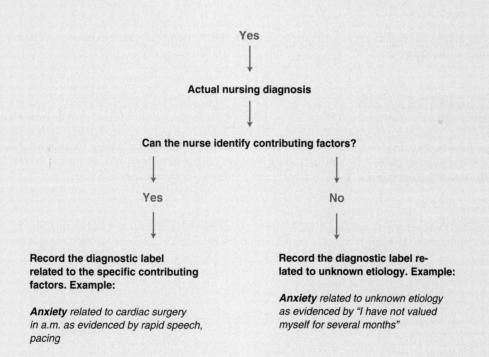

Yes

↓

Actual nursing diagnosis

↓

Can the nurse identify contributing factors?

Yes   No

Record the diagnostic label related to the specific contributing factors. Example:

Anxiety related to cardiac surgery in a.m. as evidenced by rapid speech, pacing

Record the diagnostic label related to unknown etiology. Example:

Anxiety related to unknown etiology as evidenced by "I have not valued myself for several months"

Risk and High-Risk Nursing Diagnoses

NANDA defines a *risk nursing diagnosis* as "a clinical judgment that an individual, family, or community is more vulnerable to develop the problem than others in the same or similar situation." The concept of "at risk" is useful clinically. Nurses routinely prevent problems in people who are not at high risk. For example, all postoperative clients are at risk for infection related to loss of protective barrier secondary to incision. This generic diagnosis for all clients who have undergone surgery is routine; as such, nurses do not need to include it on the client's care plan in the hospital. Instead, this diagnosis is part of the unit's standard of care (see Chapter 5). In contrast, a client with diabetes who has undergone emergency surgery for a perforated gastric ulcer may have a nursing diagnosis of *High Risk for Infection related to surgical incision and impaired healing secondary to diabetes mellitus and blood loss.* Unlike the generic diagnosis, the nurse includes this diagnosis in the client's individualized care plan because the client with diabetes is at *high* risk for infection (the former client is merely at risk). The at-risk concept is also very useful for healthy people who are vulnerable because of age or a condition such as pregnancy. Pregnant women are not at high risk for injury, but they are at risk during the third trimester.

Beginning students will use risk diagnoses initially and gradually should progress to High risk diagnoses. Standards, clinical pathways, or critical paths should contain risk nursing diagnoses. Nurses should reserve high-risk diagnoses for individual problem lists or progress notes. It is not necessary for nurses to include risk diagnoses in individual plans or records. Students, however, should include at-risk diagnoses in their care plans.

Label

In a risk nursing diagnosis, the term *Risk for* precedes the concise description of the client's change in health status. For high-risk populations, the term is *High Risk for.*

Definition

As in an actual nursing diagnosis, the definition in a risk nursing diagnosis expresses a clear, precise meaning of the diagnosis.

Risk Factors

Risk factors for risk and high-risk nursing diagnoses represent those situations that increase the vulnerability of the client or group. These factors differentiate high-risk clients and groups from all others in the same population who are at some risk. The validation to support an actual diagnosis is signs and symptoms (eg, *Impaired Skin Integrity related to immobility secondary to pain as evidenced by 2-cm erythematous sacral lesion*). In contrast, the validation to support a high-risk diagnosis is risk factors (eg, *High Risk for Impaired Skin Integrity related to immobility secondary to pain*).

Related Factors

The related factors for risk nursing diagnoses are the same risk factors previously explained for actual nursing diagnoses. The components of a risk nursing diagnostic statement are discussed later in this chapter.

⊗ INTERACTIVE EXERCISE 2.2

To determine the presence of a risk diagnosis, ask, "Are major signs and symptoms of the diagnosis found in this person?"

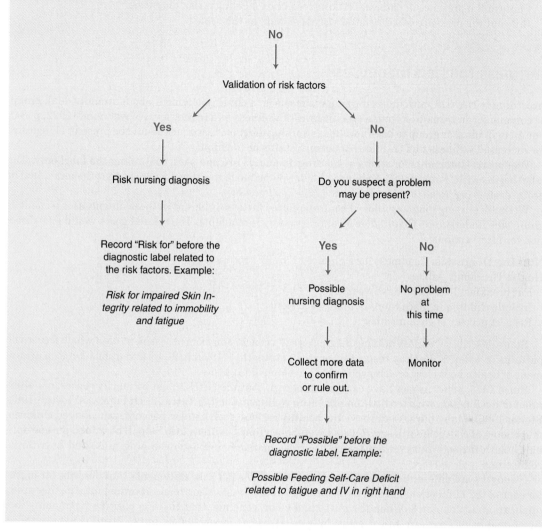

Possible Nursing Diagnoses

Possible nursing diagnoses are statements that describe a suspected problem requiring additional data. It is unfortunate that many nurses have been socialized to avoid appearing tentative. In scientific decision making, a tentative approach is not a sign of weakness or indecision, but an essential part of the process. The nurse should delay a final diagnosis until he or she has gathered and analyzed all necessary information to arrive at a sound scientific conclusion. Physicians demonstrate tentativeness with the statement *rule out (R/O)*. Nurses also should adopt a tentative position until they have completed data collection and evaluation and can confirm or rule out. NANDA does not address possible nursing diagnoses because they are not a classification issue; they are an option for clinical nurses. With a possible nursing diagnosis, the nurse has some, but insufficient, data to support a confirmed diagnosis.

Possible nursing diagnoses are two-part statements consisting of:

- The possible nursing diagnosis
- The "related to" data that lead the nurse to suspect the diagnosis

An example is *Possible Disturbed Self-Concept related to recent loss of role responsibilities secondary to worsening of multiple sclerosis.*

When a nurse records a possible nursing diagnosis, he or she alerts other nurses to assess for more data to support or rule out the tentative diagnosis. After additional data collection, the nurse may take one of three actions:

- Confirm the presence of major signs and symptoms, thus labeling an actual diagnosis.
- Confirm the presence of potential risk factors, thus labeling a risk diagnosis.
- Rule out the presence of a diagnosis (actual or risk) at this time.

Wellness Nursing Diagnoses

According to NANDA, a wellness nursing diagnosis is "a clinical judgment about an individual, group, or community in transition from a specific level of wellness to a higher level of wellness" (1992, p. 84). For an individual or group to have a wellness nursing diagnosis, two cues should be present: (1) a desire for increased wellness and (2) effective present status or function.

Diagnostic statements for wellness nursing diagnoses are one part, containing the label only. The label begins with "Potential for Enhanced," followed by the higher-level wellness that the individual or group desires (eg, *Readiness for Enhanced Family Processes*).

Wellness nursing diagnoses do not contain related factors. Inherent in these diagnoses is a client or group who understands that higher-level functioning is available. The related goals would give direction for interventions:

Nursing Diagnosis: Readiness for Enhanced Family Processes
Goals: The family will:
    Eat breakfast together 5 days/week.
    Include children in discussions of family decisions.
    Respect privacy of each member.

Stolte describes wellness nursing diagnoses as "a conclusion from assessment data which focuses on patterns of wellness, healthy responses, or client strengths" (1996, p. 9). Interventions focus on attainment of health behaviors or achievement of developmental tasks.

Since 1973, many nurses have expressed concern that the NANDA list primarily represents alteration or dysfunction with too little emphasis on wellness (Gleit & Tatro, 1981; Popkess-Vawter, 1984; Stolte, 1996). Many nurses interact with healthy clients, such as new parents, school-aged children, and clients of college health services and well-baby clinics. Nurses also help ill clients to pursue optimal health through interventions such as stress management, exercise programs, and nutritional counseling.

Strengths are different from wellness diagnoses. Table 2.2 lists statements that describe strengths for each of the 11 functional health patterns. These statements also are incorporated into the case study application in Chapter 6. When the nurse and client conclude that there is positive functioning in a functional health pattern, this conclusion is an assessment conclusion, but by itself is not a nursing diagnosis. The nurse uses these data to help the client reach a higher level of functioning or to plan interventions for altered or at risk for altered functioning.

TABLE 2.2 Functional Health Patterns and Associated Positive Functioning Assessment Statements

Functional Health Pattern	Positive Functioning Assessment Statements
1. Health perception–health management pattern	1. Positive health perception Effective health management
2. Nutritional–metabolic pattern	2. Effective nutritional–metabolic pattern
3. Elimination pattern	3. Effective elimination pattern
4. Activity–exercise pattern	4. Effective activity–exercise pattern
5. Sleep–rest pattern	5. Effective sleep–rest pattern
6. Cognitive–perceptual pattern	6. Positive cognitive–perceptual pattern
7. Self-perception pattern	7. Positive self-perception pattern
8. Role–relationship pattern	8. Positive role–relationship pattern
9. Sexuality–reproductive pattern	9. Positive sexuality–reproductive pattern
10. Coping–stress intolerance pattern	10. Effective coping–stress tolerance pattern
11. Value–belief pattern	11. Positive value–belief pattern

One could incorporate positive functioning assessment statements under each functional health pattern on the admission assessment tool, as illustrated by sleep–rest pattern.

Sleep–Rest Pattern

Habits: 8 hr/night _____ <8 hr _X_ >8 hr _____ AM nap _____ PM nap

   Feel rested after sleep _X_ Yes _____ No

Problems: _X_ None _____ Early waking _____ Insomnia _____ Nightmares

   ☒ Effective Sleep–Rest Pattern

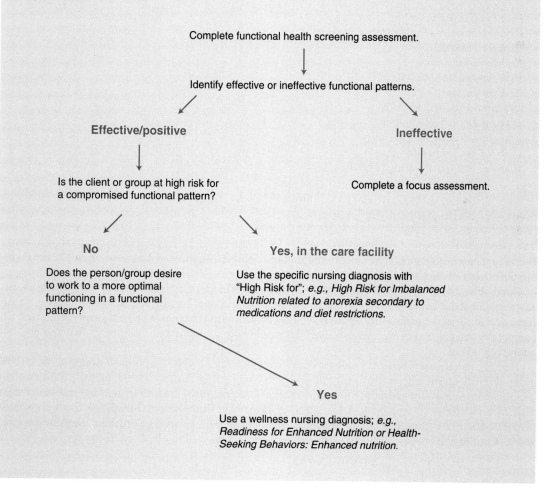

⊗ **INTERACTIVE EXERCISE 2.3**

If you assess a client and find no problems of functioning, ask, "Is the person or group at high risk for a problem?"

Complete functional health screening assessment.

↓

Identify effective or ineffective functional patterns.

↙   ↘

Effective/positive   **Ineffective**

↓   ↓

Is the client or group at high risk for a compromised functional pattern?   Complete a focus assessment.

↙   ↘

No   **Yes, in the care facility**

Does the person/group desire to work to a more optimal functioning in a functional pattern?   Use the specific nursing diagnosis with "High Risk for"; *e.g., High Risk for Imbalanced Nutrition related to anorexia secondary to medications and diet restrictions.*

Yes

Use a wellness nursing diagnosis; *e.g., Readiness for Enhanced Nutrition or Health-Seeking Behaviors: Enhanced nutrition.*

Syndrome Nursing Diagnoses

Syndrome nursing diagnoses are an interesting development in nursing diagnosis. They comprise a cluster of predicted actual or high-risk nursing diagnoses related to a certain event or situation. For example, Carlson-Catalino (1998) used an exploratory qualitative study of post–acute-phase battered women to identify 24 nursing diagnoses in all the subjects. This research supports a diagnosis of *Battered Woman Syndrome*. In medicine, syndromes cluster signs and symptoms, not diagnoses.

Nurses should approach the development of syndrome diagnosis carefully. They also must dialogue with clients to determine other nursing diagnoses indicating the need for client–nurse interventions. The clinical advantage of a syndrome diagnosis is that it alerts the nurse to a "complex clinical condition requiring expert nursing assessments and interventions" (McCourt, 1991).

Syndrome nursing diagnoses usually are one-part diagnostic statements with the etiologic or contributing factors contained in the diagnostic label (eg, *Rape Trauma Syndrome*). NANDA has five syndrome diagnoses: *Rape Trauma Syndrome, Disuse Syndrome, Post-Trauma Syndrome, Relocation Stress Syndrome,* and *Impaired Environmental Interpretation Syndrome.* These syndrome diagnoses cluster signs and symptoms, not actual or risk nursing diagnoses. This author recommends a revision to syndrome diagnoses that reflects a cluster of actual or high-risk nursing diagnoses.

For example, *Rape Trauma Syndrome* could be restructured with a cluster of these nursing diagnoses:

- *Anxiety*
- *Disturbed Sleep Pattern*
- *Fear*
- *High Risk for Ineffective Sexuality Patterns*
- *Grieving*
- *Pain*

Disuse Syndrome has the following cluster of nursing diagnoses:

- *Risk for Constipation*
- *Risk for Impaired Respiratory Function*
- *Risk for Infection*
- *Risk for Thrombosis*
- *Risk for Activity Intolerance*
- *Risk for Injury*
- *Impaired Physical Mobility*
- *Risk for Disturbed Thought Processes*
- *Risk for Disturbed Body Image*
- *Risk for Powerlessness*
- *Risk for Impaired Tissue Integrity*

Non–NANDA-Approved Diagnoses

The issue of whether nurses should use only NANDA-approved diagnoses continues to spark debate. Some agencies and schools of nursing mandate use of NANDA-approved diagnoses only. Others do not support these restrictions.

Several authors, including Alfaro (1990), Gordon (1990), and Carpenito (1990), have made recommendations about using non-NANDA nursing diagnoses. Every agency and school of nursing should have an approved list containing all NANDA-approved nursing diagnoses as well as any other that the agency or school has approved for use. This list would help nurses avoid using unknown and possibly confusing labels.

Nurses, faculty members, or students could submit a non–NANDA-approved diagnosis to be considered for inclusion within the agency or school list for further clinical development. (Of course, any proposed diagnosis should contain all its appropriate components—definition, defining characteristics, risk factors.) Refer to Appendix A for NANDA Diagnosis Submission Guidelines. Including non–NANDA-approved diagnoses on agency or school lists can help encourage orderly, scientific development of nursing diagnoses while avoiding terminologic chaos.

Diagnostic Statements

Nursing diagnostic statements can have one, two, or three parts. One-part statements contain only the diagnostic label, as in wellness and syndrome nursing diagnoses. Two-part statements contain the label and the factors that have contributed or could contribute to a change in health status, as in risk and possible diagnoses. Three-part statements contain the label, contributing factors, and **signs and** symptoms of the diagnosis, as in actual diagnoses. Box 2.1 lists diagnostic statements with examples.

Ⓧ BOX 2.1 TYPES OF DIAGNOSTIC STATEMENTS

One-Part Statement

- Wellness nursing diagnoses (eg, *Readiness for Enhanced Parenting, Readiness for Enhanced Nutrition*)
- Syndrome nursing diagnoses (eg, *Disuse Syndrome, Rape Trauma Syndrome*)

Two-Part Statement

- Risk nursing diagnoses (eg, *Risk for Injury related to lack of awareness of hazards*)
- Possible nursing diagnoses (eg, *Possible Disturbed Body Image related to isolating behaviors postsurgery*)

Three-Part Statement

- Actual nursing diagnoses (eg, *Impaired Skin Integrity related to prolonged immobility secondary to fractured pelvis, as evidenced by a 2-cm lesion on back*)

Writing Diagnostic Statements

Three-part diagnostic statements contain the following elements:

Problem Diagnostic label	*related to*	Etiology Contributing factors	*as evidenced by*	Symptom Signs and symptoms

In two-part and three-part diagnostic statements, *related to* reflects a relationship between the first and second parts of the statement. The more specific that the second part of the statement is, the more specialized the interventions can be. For example, the diagnosis *Noncompliance* stated alone usually conveys the negative implication that the client is not cooperating. When the nurse relates the noncompliance to a factor, however, this diagnosis can transmit a very different message:

- *Noncompliance related to negative side effects of a drug (reduced libido, fatigue), as evidenced by "I stopped my blood pressure medicine."*
- *Noncompliance related to inability to understand the need for weekly blood pressure measurements, as evidenced by "I don't keep my appointments if I'm busy."*

Using "Unknown Etiology" in Diagnostic Statements

If the defining characteristics of a nursing diagnosis are present but the etiologic and contributing factors are unknown, the statement can include the phrase *unknown etiology* (eg, *Fear related to unknown etiology, as evidenced by rapid speech, pacing, and "I'm worried."*). The use of *unknown etiology* alerts the nurse and other members of the nursing staff to assess for contributing factors as they intervene for the current problem.

If the nurse suspects certain factors or a relationship between certain factors and the nursing diagnosis, he or she can use the term *possible* (eg, *Anxiety related to possible marital discord*).

Syndrome diagnoses that may represent exceptions to the need to use the phrase *related to* are *Rape Trauma Syndrome* and *Disuse Syndrome*. As more specific diagnoses evolve, it may become unnecessary for the nurse to write *related to* statements. Instead, many future nursing diagnoses may be one-part statements, such as *Functional Incontinence* or *Death Anxiety*.

Avoiding Errors in Diagnostic Statements

As with any other skill, writing diagnostic statements takes knowledge and practice. To increase the accuracy and usefulness of diagnostic statements (and also to reduce frustration), nurses should avoid several common errors. Nursing diagnoses are *not* new terms for:

- Medical diagnoses (eg, diabetes mellitus)
- Medical pathology (eg, decreased cerebral tissue oxygenation)
- Treatments or equipment (eg, feeding tube)

- Medication side effects
- Diagnostic studies (eg, cardiac catheterization)
- Situations (eg, pregnancy, dying)

Nursing diagnostic statements should not be written in terms of:

- Cues (eg, crying, hemoglobin level)
- Inferences (eg, dyspnea)
- Goals (eg, should perform own colostomy care)
- Client needs (eg, needs to walk every shift; needs to express fears)
- Nursing needs (eg, change dressing, check blood pressure)

Nurses should avoid legally inadvisable or judgmental statements, such as:

- *Fear related to frequent beatings by husband*
- *Ineffective Family Coping related to mother-in-law's continual harassment of daughter-in-law*
- *Risk for Impaired Parenting related to low IQ of mother*

A nursing diagnosis should not be related to a medical diagnosis, such as *Disturbed Self-Concept related to multiple sclerosis* or *Anxiety related to myocardial infarction.* If the use of a medical diagnosis adds clarity to the diagnosis, the nurse can link it to the statement with the phrase *secondary to* (eg, *Disturbed Self-Concept related to recent losses of role responsibilities secondary to multiple sclerosis, as evidenced by, "My mother comes every day to run my house," "I can no longer be the woman in charge of my house."*).

⊛ INTERACTIVE EXERCISE 2.4

Examine the following diagnostic statements and determine whether they are written correctly or incorrectly.

1. *Anxiety related to AIDS*
2. *Chronic Sorrow related to crying and episodes of inability to sleep*
3. *Risk for Injury related to dizziness secondary to high blood pressure*
4. *Impaired Parenting related to frequent screaming at child*
5. *Risk for Constipation related to reports of bowel movements once a week*

Summary

On the surface, nursing diagnosis appears to be a convenient, simple solution to some of professional nursing's problems. This impression has led many nurses to use nursing diagnoses; however, many still do not integrate diagnosis into their nursing practice. Integrating nursing diagnosis into practice is a collective and personal process. Collectively, the nursing profession has developed the structure of nursing diagnosis and continues to identify and refine specific diagnoses. Individually, each nurse struggles with diagnostic reasoning and confirmation as well as with related ethical implications. Collectively and individually, these struggles will continue.

ANSWERS TO INTERACTIVE EXERCISES

Answer 2.4

1. *Incorrect.* The related factor AIDS does not communicate what interventions are needed. Is this diagnosis of AIDS new? Has the disease worsened?
2. *Incorrect.* Crying and inability to sleep are signs and symptoms, not related factors, of a problem. Correct presentation would be *Chronic Sorrow related to ongoing losses as a result of multiple sclerosis as evidenced by crying and inability to sleep.*
3. *Correct.*
4. *Incorrect.* Frequent screaming at a child is a sign of a problem, not a "related to." Correct presentation would be *Impaired Parenting related to unknown etiology as evidenced by frequent screaming at child.*
5. *Incorrect.* Weekly bowel movements are a symptom of constipation, not related to a risk diagnosis. Correct presentation would be *Constipation related to unknown etiology as manifested by weekly bowel movements.*

CHAPTER THREE

NURSING DIAGNOSIS:
WHAT IT IS, WHAT IT IS NOT

As discussed in Chapter 1, the official NANDA definition of nursing diagnosis specifically links nursing diagnosis to nursing interventions. But what about other clinical situations—those that nursing diagnosis does not cover, those that necessitate nursing intervention? Where do they fit within the scope of nursing practice?

Along with nursing diagnoses and interventions, nursing practice also often involves collaborative relationships with other health care disciplines. Frequently, such collaboration provides the nurse with additional interventions. As in any collaborative relationship, functions and activities sometimes overlap.

In 1983, Carpenito introduced a model for practice that describes the clinical focus of professional nurses. This *bifocal clinical practice model* identifies the two clinical situations in which nurses intervene: one as primary prescriber and the other in collaboration with other disciplines. This model not only organizes the focus of nursing practice, but also helps distinguish nursing from other health care disciplines.

Nursing derives its knowledge from various disciplines, including biology, medicine, pharmacology, psychology, nutrition, and physical therapy. Nursing differs from other disciplines in its wide range of knowledge. Figure 3.1 illustrates the varied types of such knowledge as compared with other disciplines. Certainly, the nutritionist has more expertise in the field of nutrition, and the pharmacist in the field of therapeutic pharmacology, than any nurse has. But every nurse brings knowledge of nutrition and pharmacology to client interactions that is sufficient for most clinical situations. (And when a nurse's knowledge is insufficient, nursing practice calls for consultation with appropriate disciplines.)

No other discipline has this wide knowledge base, possibly explaining why past attempts to substitute other disciplines for nursing have proved costly and ultimately unsuccessful. For this reason, any workable model for nursing practice must encompass all the varied situations in which nurses intervene, while also identifying situations in nursing that non-nursing personnel must address. These situations can be organized into five categories:

1. Pathophysiologic (eg, myocardial infarction, borderline personality, burns)
2. Treatment-related (eg, anticoagulant therapy, dialysis, arteriography)
3. Personal (eg, dying, divorce, relocation)
4. Environmental (eg, overcrowded school, no handrails on steps, rodents)
5. Maturational (eg, peer pressure, parenthood, aging)

Nursing prescribes for and treats client and group *responses* to situations. The bifocal clinical practice model, diagrammed in Figure 3.2, identifies these responses as either *nursing diagnoses* or *collaborative problems*. Together, nursing diagnoses and collaborative problems represent the range of conditions that necessitate nursing care. Attempting to attach a nursing diagnosis to every facet of nursing practice would lead to a misuse of nursing diagnoses. The classification of certain situations as collaborative problems has helped minimize such difficulties while further refining the scope of nursing practice.

The major assumptions in the bifocal clinical practice model are as follows:

Client
- Refers to an individual, group, or community
- Has the power for self-healing
- Continually interrelates with the environment
- Makes decisions according to individual priorities
- Is a unified whole, seeking balance
- Has individual worth and dignity
- Is an expert on own health

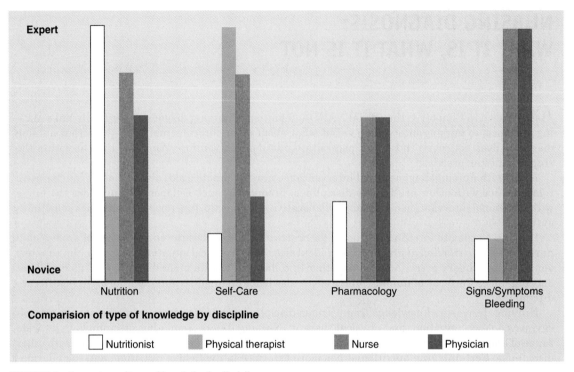

FIGURE 3.1   Comparison of type of knowledge by discipline.

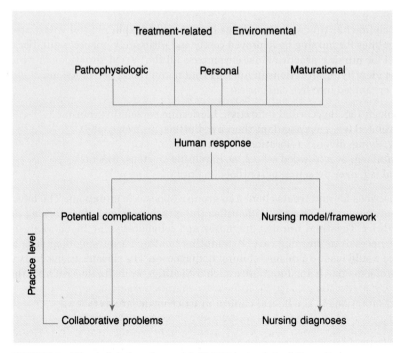

FIGURE 3.2   Bifocal clinical nursing model. (© 1985 by Lynda Juall Carpenito.)

Health
- Is a dynamic, ever-changing state
- Is defined by the client
- Is an expression of optimum well-being
- Is the responsibility of the client

Environment
- Represents external factors, situations, and people who influence or are influenced by the client
- Includes physical and ecologic environments, life events, and treatment modalities

Nursing
- Is accessed by the client when he or she needs assistance to improve, restore, or maintain health or to achieve a peaceful death (Henderson & Nite, 1960)
- Engages the client to assume responsibility in self-healing decisions and practices
- Reduces or eliminates environmental factors that can or do cause compromised functioning

Understanding Collaborative Problems

Carpenito (1999) defines collaborative problems as:

> *Certain physiologic complications that nurses monitor to detect onset or changes in status. Nurses manage collaborative problems using physician-prescribed and nursing-prescribed interventions to minimize the complications of the events.*

The designation *certain* clarifies that all physiologic complications are not collaborative problems. If the nurse can prevent the onset of the complication or provide the primary treatment for it, then the diagnosis is a nursing diagnosis. For example:

Nurses can prevent	**Nursing diagnosis**
Pressure ulcers	Risk for Impaired Skin Integrity
Thrombophlebitis	Risk for Ineffective Peripheral Tissue Perfusion
Complications of immobility	Disuse Syndrome
Aspiration	Risk for Aspiration
Nurses can treat	**Nursing diagnosis**
Stage I or II pressure ulcers	Impaired Skin Integrity
Swallowing problems	Impaired Swallowing
Ineffective cough	Ineffective Airway Clearing
Nurses cannot prevent	**Collaborative problems**
Seizures	Seizures
Bleeding	Bleeding

Unlike medical diagnoses, however, nursing diagnoses represent situations that are the primary responsibility of nurses, who diagnose onset and manage changes in status. When a situation no longer requires nursing management, the client is discharged from nursing care.

For a collaborative problem, nursing focuses on monitoring for onset or change in status of physiologic complications and on responding to any such changes with physician-prescribed and nurse-prescribed nursing interventions. The nurse makes independent decisions for both collaborative problems and nursing diagnoses. The difference is that for nursing diagnoses, nursing prescribes the definitive treatment to achieve the desired outcome; in contrast, for collaborative problems, prescription for definitive treatment comes from both nursing and medicine.

Even though a nurse cannot prevent bleeding, early detection will prevent hemorrhage. So for collaborative problems, nurses can detect onset of a physiologic problem such as urinary bleeding or decreased urine output. The nurse can also monitor for changes in an existing problem such as high blood pressure or pneumonia.

Collaborative Problem Diagnostic Statements

All collaborative problems begin with the diagnostic label *Potential Complication* (or *PC*). For example:

- *Potential Complication: Renal Failure*
- *Potential Complication: Peptic Ulcer*
- *Potential Complication: Asthma*

This label indicates that the nursing focus is to reduce the severity of certain physiologic factors or events. For example, *Potential Complication: Hypertension* alerts the nurse that this client is either experiencing or at high risk for hypertension. In either event, the nurse will receive a report on the status of the collaborative problem or will proceed to evaluate the client's blood pressure. Changing the terminology to distinguish whether the client is actually hypertensive or simply at risk is not necessary or realistic, given the fluctuating condition of most clients. The following illustrates this difference.

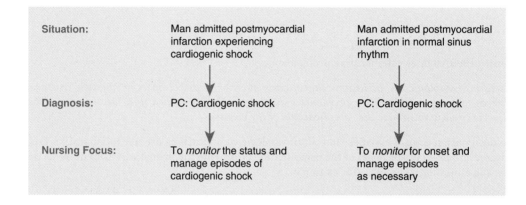

Situation:	Man admitted postmyocardial infarction experiencing cardiogenic shock	Man admitted postmyocardial infarction in normal sinus rhythm
Diagnosis:	PC: Cardiogenic shock	PC: Cardiogenic shock
Nursing Focus:	To *monitor* the status and manage episodes of cardiogenic shock	To *monitor* for onset and manage episodes as necessary

If the nurse is managing a cluster or group of complications, he or she may record the collaborative problems together:

- *Potential Complications: Cardiac*
- *Potential Complications of pacemaker insertion*

The nurse also can word the collaborative problem to reflect a specific cause, as in *Potential Complication: Hyperglycemia related to long-term corticosteroid therapy*. In most cases, however, such a link is unnecessary.

When writing collaborative problem statements, the nurse must make sure not to omit the stem *Potential Complication*. This stem designates that nurse-prescribed interventions are required for treatment. Without the stem, the collaborative problem could be misread as a medical diagnosis, in which case nursing involvement becomes subordinate to medicine, the discipline primarily responsible for the diagnosis and treatment of medical conditions.

Differentiating Nursing Diagnoses From Collaborative Problems

Both nursing diagnoses and collaborative problems involve all steps of the nursing process: assessment, diagnosis, planning, implementation, and evaluation. Each, however, requires a different approach from the nurse.

Assessment and Diagnosis

For nursing diagnoses, assessment involves data collection to identify signs and symptoms of actual nursing diagnoses or risk factors for high-risk nursing diagnoses. For collaborative problems, assessment focuses on determining physiologic stability or risk for instability. The nurse identifies a collaborative problem when certain situations increase the client's vulnerability for or the client has experienced a complication.

Collaborative problems usually are associated with a specific pathology or treatment. For example, all clients who have undergone abdominal surgery are at some risk for such problems as hemorrhage and urinary retention. Expert nursing knowledge is required to assess a particular client's specific risk for these problems and to identify them early to prevent complications and death.

Medical diagnoses are not useful problem statements for nurses. For example, diabetes mellitus is not the problem focus. Instead, hypoglycemia or hyperglycemia is used. Sometimes the medical diagnosis and the collaborative problem use the same terminology, such as seizures or hyperkalcemia. The key is: Can the nurse monitor the condition? The nurse monitors for hyper- or hypoglycemia, not diabetes mellitus.

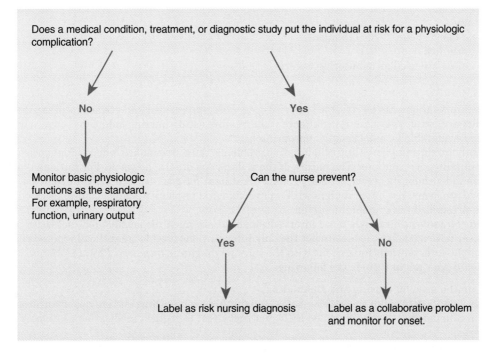

Because of each client's uniqueness, identifying nursing diagnoses is often more difficult than identifying collaborative problems. This does not mean, however, that nursing diagnoses are more important. Each client's situation determines importance.

Goals

Nursing diagnoses and collaborative problems have different implications for goals. Bulechek and McCloskey (1985) define *goals* as "guideposts to the selection of nursing interventions and criteria in the evaluation of nursing interventions." These authors continue by saying that "readily identifiable and logical links should exist between the diagnoses and the plan of care, and the activities prescribed should assist or enable the client to meet the identified expected outcome." Thus, goals and interventions may be critical to differentiating nursing diagnoses from collaborative problems that nurses treat.

⚉ **INTERACTIVE EXERCISE 3.1**

You read on a care plan the following:
Risk for Deficient Fluid Volume related to loss of fluids during surgery and possible hemorrhage postoperatively
Goal: The client will demonstrate BP and pulse within normal limits and no bleeding.
Interventions:

1. Monitor intake of IV fluids.
2. Monitor vital signs every hour.
3. Inspect dressing for s/s of bleeding.
4. Monitor urine output hourly.
5. Notify physician with changes as needed.

During your care of this client, his urine output decreases and his pulse increases. What would you do? (Answer at the end of this chapter)

Client goals are inappropriate for collaborative problems. They represent criteria that nurses cannot use to evaluate the effectiveness or appropriateness of nursing interventions. Collaborative problems have nursing goals. For example,

PC: Hypoglycemia

Nursing Goal

The nurse will monitor for early signs and symptoms of hypoglycemia and collaboratively intervene to stabilize the client.

Indicators

Fasting blood sugar   70–115 mg/dL
Clear, oriented

The indicators are used as monitoring criteria.

Interventions

Nursing interventions can be classified as two types: nurse-prescribed and physician-prescribed (*delegated*). Regardless of type, all nursing interventions require astute nursing judgment because the nurse is legally accountable for intervening appropriately.

For both nursing diagnoses and collaborative problems, the nurse makes independent decisions concerning nursing interventions. The nature of these decisions differs, however. For nursing diagnoses, the nurse independently prescribes the primary treatment for goal achievement. In contrast, for collaborative problems, the nurse confers with a physician and implements physician-prescribed as well as nurse-prescribed nursing interventions.

Primary treatment describes those interventions that are most responsible for successful outcome achievement. Nevertheless, these are not the only interventions used to treat the diagnosed condition. For example, interventions for a client with the nursing diagnosis *Impaired Physical Mobility related to incisional pain* might include the following:

- Explain the need for moving and ambulation.
- Teach client how to splint the incision before coughing, deep breathing, sitting up, or turning in bed.
- If pain relief medication is scheduled PRN, instruct client to request medication as soon as pain returns.
- Evaluate if pain relief is satisfactory; if not, contact the physician for increased dosages or decreased interval between doses.
- Schedule activities, bathing, and ambulation to correspond with times when client's comfort level is highest.
- Discuss and negotiate ambulation goals with client.

All of these are nurse-prescribed interventions. A physician-prescribed intervention for this client might be Demerol 75 mg IM q4h. This medication is important to manage the client's postoperative pain; however, it alone cannot be considered a primary treatment.

The difference between a nursing diagnosis and a collaborative problem is illustrated on page 23.

---

⑩ INTERACTIVE EXERCISE 3.2

Refer to Section Three under collaborative problem PC: GI Bleeding, p. 897. Review the interventions and label each one as nurse-prescribed or physician-prescribed. (Refer to answers at the end of the chapter)

Monitoring Versus Prevention

Is monitoring an intervention? Interventions are directed at improving a person's condition or preventing a problem. *Monitoring* involves continually collecting selected data to evaluate whether the client's condition has changed (improved, deteriorated, not improved, or remained within a normal range). Monitoring does not improve a client's health status or prevent a problem; rather, it provides information necessary to determine *if* or *what type* of interventions are needed. Monitoring detects problems. It is associated with every type of nursing diagnosis and collaborative problem:

- For actual nursing diagnosis—monitor the client's condition for improvement.
- For risk nursing diagnosis—monitor the client for signs of the problem.
- For wellness nursing diagnosis—monitor the client's participation in lifestyle changes.
- For collaborative problems—monitor for onset or change in status of a problem.

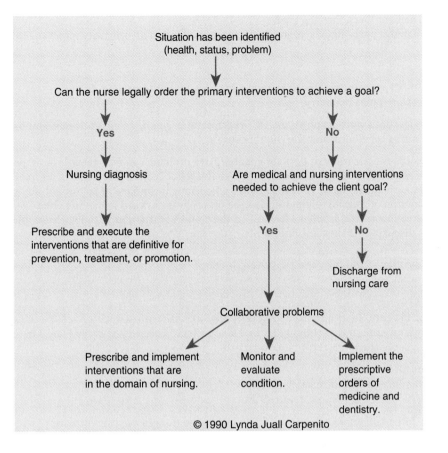

© 1990 Lynda Juall Carpenito

Although monitoring does not qualify as an intervention, it is an activity. For convenience, monitoring is included with the interventions for the diagnoses presented in Sections Two and Three.

Prevention Versus Detection

Nurses can prevent some physiologic complications, such as pressure ulcers and infection from invasive lines. Prevention differs from detection. Nurses do not prevent hemorrhage or seizure; instead, they monitor to detect its presence early to prevent greater severity of complication or even death. Physicians cannot treat collaborative problems without nursing's knowledge, vigilance, and judgment. For collaborative problems, nurses institute orders, such as position changes, client teaching, or specific protocols, in addition to monitoring.

Evaluation

The nurse evaluates a client's status and progress differently for nursing diagnoses and collaborative problems. When evaluating nursing diagnoses, the nurse:

- Assesses the client's status
- Compares this response to the goals
- Concludes whether the client is progressing toward outcome achievement

For example, a client has the goal:
Will walk 25 feet with assistance by 6-18.

Today (6-16) the client walked 20 feet with assistance.
The nurse concludes that he is progressing to goal achievement by 6-18.

The nurse can record this evaluation on a flow record or on a progress note.
In contrast, to evaluate collaborative problems, the nurse:

- Collects selected data
- Compares data with established norms
- Judges whether the data are within an acceptable range

For example, a client has a nursing goal:
The nurse will detect early signs/symptoms of pneumonia and collaboratively intervene to stabilize the client.

Indicators
Respiration 16–20 per minute, breath sounds equal, no adventitious sounds.
Oxygen saturation (pulse oximetry) >95

Today the clinical data were respirations 18, breath sounds equal, no adventitious sounds and a pulse ox of 98. The nurse concludes that the client is stable.

The nurse records the assessment data for collaborative problems on flow records or on progress notes if findings are significant. Nurses evaluate whether the collaborative problem has improved, has worsened, is stable, or is unchanged. They also notify physicians if changes in treatment are indicated.

Thus, evaluation of nursing diagnoses focuses on progress toward achieving client goals, whereas evaluation for collaborative problems focuses on the client's status compared with established norms. Evaluation is discussed further in Chapter 5.

⊚ INTERACTIVE EXERCISE 3.3

Case Study 1
Mr. Smith, 35 years old, is admitted for a possible concussion after a motor vehicle collision, with a physician's order for a clear liquid diet and a neurologic assessment every hour. On admission, the nurse records the following on a flow record:

• Oriented and alert
• Pupils 6 mm, equal, and reactive to light
• BP 120/72, pulse 84, resp 20, temp 99°F

Two hours later, the nurse records the following on the nurse's or progress note:

• Vomiting
• Restlessness
• Pupils 6 mm, equal, with a sluggish response to light
• BP 140/60, pulse 65, resp 12, temp 99°F

Problem: Possible increased intracranial pressure (ICP)
   Now, apply the following criteria questions:
Q: Can the nurse legally order the primary interventions to achieve the client goal (which would be a reversal of the increasing ICP)?
Q: Are medical and nursing interventions needed for goal achievement? (Answers at the end of chapter)

Case Study 2
Mr. Green, 45 years old, has a cholecystectomy incision (10 days postop) that is not healing and has continual purulent drainage. The nursing care consists of:

• Inspecting and cleansing the incision and the surrounding area q8h
• Applying a drainage pouch
• Promoting optimal nutrition and hydration to enhance healing

Problem: Adjacent skin at risk for erosion
   Now apply the criteria questions:
Q: Can the nurse legally order the definitive interventions to achieve the goals (which would be continued intact surrounding tissue)? (Answer at end of chapter)

Summary

According to Wallace and Ivey (1989), "understanding which nursing diagnoses are most effective and the situations in which the term collaborative problem is best applied helps group the mass of data the nurse must consider." The bifocal clinical practice model provides a structure for forming this understanding. In doing so, it uniquely distinguishes nursing from other health care professions, while providing nurses with a logical description of the focus of clinical nursing.

3.1. Call the physician, because the interventions needed are medical treatments. This situation is not a nursing diagnosis, because the nurse does not order the treatment needed. As a collaborative problem, it would be better described as *Potential Complication: Bleeding.* A goal would be "The nurse will monitor for and manage changes in status."

3.2. Of the 11 interventions, the first five are nurse-prescribed, and the remaining six are physician-prescribed. Nursing is responsible for all 11 interventions, although medicine prescribes some.

3.3.

Case Study 1

1. No, nurses do not definitively treat or prevent increased ICP. They collaborate with the physician for definitive treatment.
2. Yes, medical and nursing interventions are needed.

Yes
↓
Collaborative problem
PC: Increased Intracranial Pressure

Prescribes and implements interventions within the domain of nursing	Monitors and evaluates the client's condition	Implements the prescriptive orders of medicine

In this situation, the nurse would monitor to detect increasing ICP. The nurse also prescribes interventions that reduce ICP, but these interventions are not considered primary and must be accompanied by physician-prescribed treatments. This problem is the joint responsibility of medicine and nursing.

Case Study 2

Yes, nurses do prescribe interventions that will prevent skin erosion as a result of wound drainage.

↓
Nursing diagnosis
↓

Risk for Impaired Skin Integrity related to draining purulent wound

In this situation, the nurse would prescribe the interventions to preserve adjacent skin. No collaboration with medicine is warranted.

Because each client is unique, developing exclusive criteria that will always differentiate nursing diagnoses from other client problems is difficult. Ultimately, the decision to use or not to use a nursing diagnosis label rests with the individual nurse until more refined defining characteristics for each diagnosis are developed and tested.

CHAPTER FOUR

NURSING DIAGNOSES:
ASSESSMENT AND DIAGNOSIS

Each client is an autonomous and precious person who interacts uniquely with the environment. Nurses must assess each client within the context of this uniqueness. Because nursing diagnoses derive from assessment findings, and because the client continually interacts with the environment, the nurse must apply the process in a continuous round of assessing, diagnosing, planning, implementing, and evaluating. Nursing diagnosis cannot be taken out of the context of the nursing process. Doing so could result in a misuse of the concept and could lead to incorrect labeling or stereotyping. This, in turn, would interfere with accurate and careful observations and result in inappropriate nursing interventions.

Figure 4.1 illustrates the cyclic relationship of each step of the nursing process to the other steps and to the whole (Alfaro-LeFevre, 1998). Each step depends on the accuracy of the preceding step; assessment and evaluation are related to diagnosis, planning, and implementation. For example, when implementing the plan, the nurse also is assessing the client's current condition and evaluating the client's response to interventions. Thus, the separation into five steps is for explanation purposes only; in reality, the process is continuous, and the steps are interrelated.

Assessment

The first step of the nursing process, *assessment,* is the deliberate and systematic collection of data to determine a client's current and past health status and to evaluate the client's present and past coping patterns. Nurses obtain data by five methods:

1. Interview
2. Physical examination
3. Observation
4. Review of records and diagnostic reports
5. Collaboration with colleagues

Data collection focuses on identifying the client's:

- Current health problems
- Past health status
- Strengths, limitations
- Current and past functional status
- Risk for potential problems
- Desire for a higher level of wellness
- Response to medical and nursing interventions

Nurses collect data to determine the need for nursing service and to assist other professionals (eg, pharmacists, nutritionists, social workers, physicians) in determining their activities. Therefore, health care professionals must freely exchange data about their clients to increase the quality and validity of health care. For example, a nurse assesses the signs of orthostatic hypotension in a client and then refers the client to a physician to investigate the cause and determine the treatment. The nurse plans nursing activities to help the client reduce those factors contributing to the vertigo and also to prevent injury.

The Assessment Process

To perform an accurate assessment, the nurse must be able to communicate effectively, observe systematically, interpret data accurately, and validate data.

Communicating Effectively

All nurse–client interactions are based on communication. The term *therapeutic communication* describes techniques that encourage clients to share views and feelings openly. It incorporates verbal

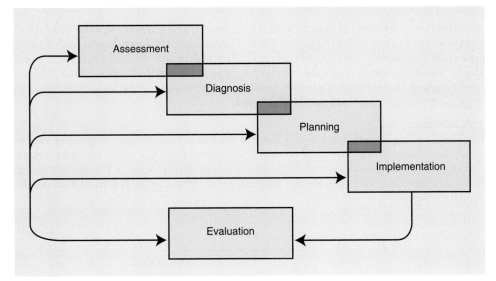

FIGURE 4.1 The nursing process.

and nonverbal skills, as well as respect and a sense of caring. Verbal skills include asking closed-ended and open-ended questions, exploring answers, and validating responses. Nonverbal skills include active listening and using silence, touch, and eye contact. Active listening, vital to data collection, is the most difficult skill to learn. Few people listen objectively; most tend to concentrate on their own responses rather than on what the other person is saying.

Barriers to active listening are always present; the professional nurse must take appropriate measures to eliminate them and their influence. Some barriers to active listening are as follows (Carpenito & Duespohl, 1986):

Internal
- The client's views differ from the nurse's perceptions.
- The client's appearance or accent is different or distracting.
- The client is in pain or anxious.
- The client is saying something that the nurse does not want to hear.
- The nurse dislikes the client.
- The nurse is thinking of something else.
- The nurse is planning the next statement.
- The nurse is anxious or apprehensive.
- The nurse is in a hurry.

External
- Noise from equipment, speakers, television, or radio is interfering.
- Privacy is lacking.
- There are physical hindrances such as desks and equipment.
- Others make verbal remarks such as clichés, trite comments, or interruptions.

Observing Systematically

The ability to observe systematically depends on the nurse's knowledge base. Knowing what contributes to or causes a particular problem enables the nurse to explore these areas with the client. If the nurse does not know what a problem looks like, he or she cannot recognize and diagnose it. For example, if a nurse does not know the signs and symptoms of *Disturbed Self-Concept,* he or she may overlook this response.

Written guidelines can enhance systematic observation. Such guidelines are invaluable because they identify the specific types of data that nurses should collect. Once a nurse is familiar with the guidelines, he or she can gather data without referring to a written guide. An example of an admission assessment tool is found at the end of this chapter.

For each nursing diagnosis in Section Two, a focus assessment is presented to direct the nurse in gathering data to confirm or to rule out the nursing diagnosis. Expanded focus assessment sections for each nursing diagnosis are available on the Connection Web site that accompanies this text.

Interpreting Data Accurately

After data collection, the nurse has many findings to interpret. The nurse must order the data or group cues into chunks or patterns (Alfaro-LeFevre, 1998). For example, the nurse learns to cluster the signs and symptoms of increased heart rate, dilated pupils, irritability, and difficulty concentrating as moderate anxiety. When the nurse recognizes this cluster, he or she infers that the client has moderate anxiety. It is important to note that the nurse must first know what signs and symptoms represent moderate anxiety before it can be clinically diagnosed.

Cues Versus Inferences

A *cue* is information acquired through one or more of the five senses. Primary sources of cues are subjective statements made by the client and objective data observed by the nurse. Secondary sources are family, other health care providers, and diagnostic studies. An *inference* is the nurse's judgment or interpretation of cues. Inferences are always subjective and influenced by the nurse's knowledge base, values, and experiences.

Cue	Corresponding Inference
Hgb 9.1	Abnormal
Crying	Possible fear, sadness
5 ft 1 in, 220 lb	Obesity

Differentiating between cues and inferences is important. Although inferences are subjective judgments, nurses frequently report them as facts or fail to gather sufficient cues to confirm or rule out their inferences. Inferences with few or no supporting cues can result in inappropriate and sometimes dangerous care, especially when nurses pass on invalid inferences to other members of the health care team.

ⓧ **INTERACTIVE EXERCISE 4.1**

After assessing a client focusing on nutrition, the following data are found:

– reports a weak right arm
– weight 202 lb
– height 5'3"
– reports no difficulty swallowing
– decreased oral intake
– obesity

Write a "C" if it is a cue. Write an "I" if it is an inference. Refer to answers at the end of the chapter.

Cognitive Processes in Interpreting Data

Interpreting data involves two cognitive activities:

* Recognizing the cue or inference as significant
* Assigning meaning to the significance

A nurse recognizes the significance of data based on certain knowledge that denotes these data as abnormal or diagnostic. This knowledge can come from memory of similar experiences or from other nurses, nursing faculty, and professional books and journals. Past experiences or knowledge from other sources also can alert the nurse to the significance of certain cues found in pre-encounter data—the information available to the nurse before the initial assessment, such as age, racial or ethnic background, and medical diagnosis.

Consider the following example: When assessing a 45-year-old woman with diabetes mellitus who has been admitted for abdominal surgery, the nurse finds a new lesion on the client's foot. When questioned, the client states, "It must be from my new shoes." Because of prior knowledge of the client's diabetes gained from pre-encounter data, the nurse would assign this assessment finding more significance than it might warrant in another client, because diabetes contributes to foot infections.

Validating Data

As mentioned before, during data collection, the nurse simultaneously interprets and validates data. Validating the data with the client helps the nurse avoid making incorrect inferences. If, for example, the nurse observes a client crying in her room, the nurse familiar with the client's recent medical diagnosis of breast cancer may quite logically connect the crying (cue) with the diagnosis. That the nurse initially makes this inference is not wrong, but problems could result if the nurse does not validate this inference with the client. To validate, the nurse should say something like, "I see that you're crying. Would you like to talk about your feelings?" By doing so, the nurse may, in fact, discover that the client's crying is related to something else, such as missing her loved ones. The client must be an active partner in data validation.

Validation sometimes involves clarifying vague or ambiguous data with the client (Gordon, 1994). For example, a nurse assessing a client who states, "I feel drained," could interpret this statement in various ways, such as evidence of fatigue or stress. For validation, the nurse should ask the client to elaborate on the statement, providing more specific information. In addition, sometimes cues for more than one diagnosis overlap. For example, anger is a cue of several nursing diagnoses (eg, *Ineffective Coping, Anxiety, Interrupted Family Processes*).

To summarize, data to support a nursing diagnosis must be a cluster of cues documented to represent the condition. By carefully validating observations and client complaints, the nurse can avoid or minimize potentially harmful inaccuracies in data interpretation.

Data Collection Formats

Data collection usually consists of two formats: the nursing baseline or screening assessment and the focus or ongoing assessment. The nurse can use each alone or together. As discussed in Chapter 3, nurses encounter, diagnose, and treat two types of responses: nursing diagnoses and collaborative problems. Each type requires a different assessment focus.

Initial, Baseline, or Screening Assessment

An initial, baseline, or screening assessment involves collecting a predetermined set of data during initial contact with the client (eg, on admission, first home visit). This assessment serves as a tool for "narrowing the universe of possibilities" (Gordon, 1994). During this assessment, the nurse interprets data as significant or insignificant. This process is explored later in this chapter.

The nurse should organize the initial assessment to permit systematic, efficient data collection. Figure 4.2 illustrates an assessment form with checking or circling options, which can help save time during documentation. The nurse always can elaborate with additional questions and comments. Open-ended questions are better for assessment of certain functional areas, such as fear or anxiety. Nurses should view printed assessment forms as guides, not mandates. Before requesting information from a client, nurses should ask themselves, "What am I going to do with the data?" If certain information is useless or irrelevant for a particular client, then its collection is unnecessary and potentially distressing. For example, asking a terminally ill client how much he or she smokes is unnecessary unless the nurse has a specific goal. If a client will be NPO, collecting data about eating habits is probably unnecessary. Such assessment will be indicated if the client resumes eating.

If a client is extremely stressed, the nurse should collect only necessary data and defer the assessment of functional patterns to another time. A stressed client is not the best source of data, because stress may cloud the memory.

Functional Health Patterns

As discussed earlier, nursing assessment focuses on collecting data that validate nursing diagnoses. Gordon's system of functional health patterns provides an excellent, relevant format for nursing data collection to determine an individual's or group's health status and functioning (1994). After data collection is complete, the nurse and client can determine positive functioning, altered functioning, or at-risk for altered functioning. Altered functioning is defined as functioning that the client (individual or group) perceives as negative or undesirable.

The functional health patterns include the following:

1. Health Perception–Health Management Pattern
   • Perceived pattern of health, well-being
   • Knowledge of lifestyle and relationship to health

(*continues on page 33*)

NURSING ADMISSION DATA BASE

Date _____ Arrival Time _____ Contact Person _____ Phone _____

ADMITTED FROM: ___ Home alone ___ Home with relative ___ Long-term care
___ Homeless ___ Home with _____ facility
___ ER ___ (Specify) ___ Other _____

MODE OF ARRIVAL: ___ Wheelchair ___ Ambulance ___ Stretcher

REASON FOR HOSPITALIZATION: _____
_____
_____

LAST HOSPITAL ADMISSION: Date _____ Reason _____
_____

PAST MEDICAL HISTORY: _____
_____

MEDICATION (Prescription/Over-the-Counter)	DOSAGE	LAST DOSE	FREQUENCY

HEALTH MAINTENANCE–PERCEPTION PATTERN

USE OF:

Tobacco: ___ None ___ Quit (date) ___ Pipe ___ Cigar ___ <1 pk/day
___ 1–2 pks/day ___ >2 pks/day Pks/year history _____

Alcohol: ___ Date of last drink ___ Amount/type
___ No. of days in a month when alcohol is consumed

Other Drugs: ___ No ___ Yes Type _____ Use _____

Allergies (drugs, food, tape, dyes): _____ Reaction _____
_____

ACTIVITY–EXERCISE PATTERN

SELF-CARE ABILITY:

0 = Independent   1 = Assistive device   2 = Assistance from others
3 = Assistance from person and equipment   4 = Dependent/Unable

	0	1	2	3	4
Eating/Drinking					
Bathing					
Dressing/Grooming					
Toileting					
Bed Mobility					
Transferring					
Ambulating					
Stair Climbing					
Shopping					
Cooking					
Home Maintenance					

ASSISTIVE DEVICES: ___ None ___ Crutches ___ Bedside commode ___ Walker
___ Cane ___ Splint/Brace ___ Wheelchair ___ Other

CODE: (1) Not applicable (2) Unable to acquire
(3) Not a priority at this time (4) Other (specify in notes)

Side One

FIGURE 4.2   Sample nursing admission database.

NUTRITION–METABOLIC PATTERN

Special Diet/Supplements _____

Previous Dietary Instruction: ___ Yes ___ No

Appetite: ___ Normal ___ Increased ___ Decreased ___ Decreased taste sensation
___ Nausea___ Vomiting

Weight Fluctuations Last 6 Months: ___ None _____ lbs. Gained/Lost

Swallowing difficulty: ___ None ___ Solids ___ Liquids

Dentures: ___ Upper (_ Partial _ Full) ___ Lower (_ Partial _ Full)
With Person ___ Yes ___ No

History of Skin/Healing Problems: ___ None ___ Abnormal Healing ___Rash
___ Dryness ___ Excess Perspiration

ELIMINATION PATTERN

Bowel Habits: ___ # BMs/day ___ Date of last BM ___ Within normal limits
___ Constipation ___ Diarrhea ___ Incontinence
___ Ostomy: Type: ___ Appliance ___ Self-care ___ Yes ___ No

Bladder Habits: ___ WNL ___ Frequency ___ Dysuria ___ Nocturia ___ Urgency
___ Hematuria ___Retention

Incontinency: ___ No ___ Yes ___ Total ___ Daytime ___ Nighttime
___ Occasional ___ Difficulty delaying voiding
___ Difficulty reaching toilet

Assistive Devices: ___ Intermittent catheterization
___ Indwelling catheter ___ External catheter
___ Incontinent briefs

SLEEP–REST PATTERN

Habits: ___ hrs/night ___ AM nap ___ PM nap
Feel rested after sleep ___ Yes ___ No

Problems: ___None ___ Early waking ___Insomnia ___ Nightmares

COGNITIVE–PERCEPTUAL PATTERN

Mental Status: ___Alert ___ Receptive aphasia ___ Poor historian
___ Oriented ___ Confused ___ Combative ___ Unresponsive

Speech: ___ Normal ___Slurred ___Garbled ___ Expressive aphasia
Spoken language _____ Interpreter _____

Language Spoken: ___ English ___ Spanish ___ Other _____

Ability to Read English: ___ Yes ___ No _____

Ability to Communicate: ___Yes ___ No _____

Ability to Comprehend: ___ Yes ___ No _____

Level of Anxiety: ___ Mild ___ Moderate ___ Severe ___ Panic

Interactive Skills: ___ Appropriate ___ Other _____

Hearing: ___ WNL ___ Impaired (_ Right _ Left) ___ Deaf (_ Right _ Left)
___ Hearing Aid

Vision: ___ WNL ___ Eyeglasses ___ Contact lens
___ Impaired ___ Right ___ Left
___ Blind ___ Right ___ Left
___ Prosthesis ___ Right ___ Left

Vertigo: ___ Yes ___ No   memory intact ___Yes ___ No

Discomfort/Pain: ___ None ___ Acute ___ Chronic ___ Description _____
_____

Pain Management: _____

COPING–STRESS TOLERANCE/SELF-PERCEPTION/SELF-CONCEPT PATTERN

Major concerns regarding hospitalization or illness (financial, self-care): _____
_____

Major loss/change in past year: ___ No ___ Yes _____

Fear of Violence ___ Yes ___ No Who _____

Outlook on Future _____ (rate 1–poor–to 10–very optimistic)

CODE: (1) Not applicable (2) Unable to acquire
(3) Not a priority at this time (4) Other (specify in notes)

Side Two

FIGURE 4.2 (*Continued*)

SEXUALITY–REPRODUCTIVE PATTERN

LMP: _____ Gravida _____ Para _____ Birth Control _____

Menstrual/Hormonal Problems: ___ Yes ___ No _____

Last Pap Smear: _____ Hx of Abnormal PAP _____

Monthly Self-Breast/Testicular Exam: ___ Yes ___ No Last Mammogram: _____

Sexual Concerns: _____

_____

ROLE–RELATIONSHIP PATTERN

Marital status: _____ Lives with _____

Occupation: _____

Employment Status: ___ Employed ___ Short-term disability
_____ Long-term disability ___ Unemployed

Support System: ___ Spouse ___ Neighbors/Friends ___ None
_____ Family in same residence ___ Family in separate residence
_____ Other _____

Family concerns regarding hospitalization: _____

_____

VALUE–BELIEF PATTERN

Religion: _____

Religious Restrictions: ___ No ___ Yes (Specify) _____

Request Chaplain Visitation at This Time: ___ Yes ___ No

PHYSICAL ASSESSMENT (Objective)

1. CLINICAL DATA

Age _____ Height _____ Weight _____ (Actual/Approximate) BMI _____

Temperature _____

Pulse: ___ Strong ___ Weak ___ Regular ___ Irregular

Blood Pressure: Right Arm ___ Left Arm ___ Sitting ___ Lying ___

2. RESPIRATORY/CIRCULATORY

Rate _____

Quality: ___ WNL ___ Shallow ___ Rapid ___ Labored ___ Other _____

Cough: ___ No ___ Yes/Describe _____

Auscultation:

Upper rt lobes ___ WNL ___ Decreased ___ Absent ___ Abnormal sounds ___

Upper lt lobes ___ WNL ___ Decreased ___ Absent ___ Abnormal sounds ___

Lower rt lobes ___ WNL ___ Decreased ___ Absent ___ Abnormal sounds ___

Lower lt lobes ___ WNL ___ Decreased ___ Absent ___ Abnormal sounds ___

Right Pedal Pulse: ___ Strong ___ Weak ___ Absent

Left Pedal Pulse: ___ Strong ___ Weak ___ Absent

3. METABOLIC–INTEGUMENTARY

SKIN:

Color: ___ WNL ___ Pale ___ Cyanotic ___ Ashen ___ Jaundice ___ Other ___

Temperature: ___ WNL ___ Warm ___ Cool

Edema: ___ No ___ Yes/Description/location _____

Lesions: ___ None ___ Yes/Description/location _____

Bruises: ___ None ___ Yes/Description/location _____

Reddened: ___ No ___ Yes/Description/location _____

Pruritus: ___ No ___ Yes/Description/location _____

Tubes: Specify _____

Changes _____ None, If Yes/Description/location _____

MOUTH:

Gums: ___ WNL ___ White plaque ___ Lesions ___ Other _____

Teeth: ___ WNL ___ Other _____

ABDOMEN:

Bowel Sounds: ___ Present ___ Absent

Side Three

FIGURE 4.2 (*Continued*)

4. NEURO/SENSORY

Pupils: ___ Equal ___ Unequal

Left: • • • • • • • • •

Right: • • • • • • • • •

Reactive to light:

Left: ___ Yes ___ No/Specify _____

Right: ___ Yes ___ No/Specify _____

Eyes: ___ Clear ___ Draining ___ Reddened ___ Other _____

5. MUSCULAR–SKELETAL

Range of Motion: ___ Full ___ Other _____

Balance and Gait: ___ Steady ___ Unsteady

Hand Grasps: ___ Equal ___ Strong ___ Weakness/Paralysis (___ Right ___ Left)

Leg Muscles: ___ Equal ___ Strong ___ Weakness/Paralysis (___ Right ___ Left)

DISCHARGE PLANNING

Lives: Alone ___ With _____ No known residence _____

Intended Destination Post Discharge: ___ Home ___ Undetermined ___ Other ___

Previous Utilization of Community Resources:

___ Home care/Hospice ___ Adult day care ___ Church groups ___ Other _____

___ Meals on Wheels ___ Homemaker/Home health aide ___ Community support group

Post-discharge Transportation:

___ Car ___ Ambulance ___ Bus/Taxi

___ Unable to determine at this time

Anticipated Financial Assistance Post-discharge?: ___ No ___ Yes _____

Anticipated Problems with Self-care Post-discharge?: ___ No ___ Yes _____

Assistive Devices Needed Post-discharge?: ___ No ___ Yes _____

Referrals: (record date)

Discharge Coordinator _____ Home Health _____

Social Service _____

Other Comments: _____

_____

SIGNATURE/TITLE _____ Date _____

Side Four

FIGURE 4.2 (*Continued*)

- Knowledge of preventive health practices
- Adherence to medical, nursing prescriptions

2. Nutritional–Metabolic Pattern
   - Usual pattern of food and fluid intake
   - Types of food and fluid intake
   - Actual weight, weight loss or gain
   - Appetite, preferences

3. Elimination Pattern
   - Bowel elimination pattern, changes
   - Bladder elimination pattern, changes
   - Control problems
   - Use of assistive devices
   - Use of medications

4. Activity–Exercise Pattern
   - Pattern of exercise, activity, leisure, recreation
   - Ability to perform activities of daily living (self-care, home maintenance, work, eating, shopping, cooking)

5. Sleep–Rest Pattern
   - Patterns of sleep, rest
   - Perception of quality, quantity

6. Cognitive–Perceptual Pattern
   - Vision, learning, taste, touch, smell
   - Language adequacy
   - Memory
   - Decision-making ability, patterns
   - Complaints of discomforts

7. Self-Perception–Self-Concept Pattern
   - Attitudes about self, sense of worth
   - Perception of abilities
   - Emotional patterns
   - Body image, identity
8. Role–Relationship Patterns
   - Patterns of relationships
   - Role responsibilities
   - Satisfaction with relationships and responsibilities
9. Sexuality–Reproductive Pattern
   - Menstrual, reproductive history
   - Satisfaction with sexual relationships, sexual identity
   - Premenopausal or postmenopausal problems
   - Accuracy of sex education
10. Coping–Stress Tolerance Patterns
    - Ability to manage stress
    - Knowledge of stress tolerance
    - Sources of support
    - Number of stressful life events in last year
11. Value–Belief Pattern
    - Values, goals, beliefs
    - Spiritual practices
    - Perceived conflicts in values

Figure 4.2 presents a sample initial assessment organized according to functional health patterns. It is designed to assist the nurse in gathering subjective and objective data. Should questions arise concerning a pattern, the nurse would gather more data about the diagnosis by using the focus assessment under the diagnosis.

When collecting data according to the functional health patterns, the nurse questions, observes, and evaluates the client or family. For example, under the Cognitive–Perceptual Pattern, the nurse asks the client if he or she has difficulty hearing, observes if the client is wearing a hearing aid, and evaluates if the client understands English.

Physical Assessment

In addition to functional health pattern assessment, the nurse also collects data related to body system functioning. Physical assessment, the collection of objective data concerning the client's physical status, incorporates head-to-toe examination, with a focus on the body systems. The techniques used include inspection, palpation, percussion, and auscultation.

Figure 4.2 lists those areas of physical assessment in which nurse generalists should be proficient. Physical assessment by nurses should be clearly "nursing" in focus. By examining their philosophy and definition of nursing, nurses should seek to develop expertise in those areas that will enhance nursing practice.

Keep in mind that separation of functional health patterns from physical assessment is done for organizational purposes only. No useful nursing assessment framework can restrict actual data collection in such a manner. Because humans are open systems, a problem in one functional health pattern invariably influences body system functioning or functioning in another functional health pattern.

Ⓧ **INTERACTIVE EXERCISE 4.2**

Mr. Gene, 61 years old, is admitted for neurologic surgery. He has a history of peripheral vascular disease and Parkinson's disease. The nurse's initial assessment reveals the following under the functional health pattern Activity–Exercise and physical assessment of musculoskeletal function:

(continued)

INTERACTIVE EXERCISE 4.2 (*Continued*)

ACTIVITY-EXERCISE PATTERN
SELF-CARE ABILITY:
  0 = Independent   1 = Assistive device   2 = Assistance from others
  3 = Asssistance from person and equipment   4 = Dependent/Unable

	0	1	2	3	4
Eating/Drinking	✓				
Bathing			✓		
Dressing/Grooming			✓		
Toileting			✓		
Bed Mobility			✓		
Transferring			✓		
Ambulating		✓			
Stair Climbing	✓				
Shopping					✓
Cooking					✓
Home Maintenance					✓

ASSISTIVE DEVICES: ____ None ____ Crutches ____ Bedside commode ✓ Walker
____ Cane ____Splint/Brace ____Wheelchair ____ Other ____

PHYSICAL ASSESSMENT
MUSCULAR–SKELETAL
Range of Motion: ✓ Full ____ Other _____
Balance and Gait: ____ Steady ✓ Unsteady
Hand Grasps: ✓ Equal ✓ Strong ____ Weakness/Paralysis (____ Right ____ Left)
Leg Muscles: ____ Equal ____ Strong ✓ Weakness/Paralysis (✓ Right ____ Left)

Examine the above assessment data. What data are significant? (Answers at end of chapter)

Focus Assessment

Focus assessment is the acquisition of selected or specific data as determined by the nurse and the client or family, or by the client's condition. The nurse who assesses the condition of a new postoperative client (vital signs, incision, hydration, comfort) is performing a focus assessment. These are ongoing assessments.

The nurse also can perform a focus assessment during the initial interview if collected data suggest a possible problem that the nurse must validate or rule out. For example, during the baseline interview, the nurse suspects that certain data (S_1, S_2) may represent a nursing diagnosis. The nurse considers a possible or tentative diagnosis. The nurse then collects additional data (focus assessment) to confirm or rule out the tentative diagnosis. This process can be depicted as:

Admission Assessment ──────────────────→ Possible Nursing
S_1 Diagnosis
S_2
Focus Assessment ──────────────────────→ Rule Out or
S_3 Confirm Diagnosis
S_4

Designating data as a diagnostic cue is a complex cognitive activity; grouping a set of cues as a diagnosis is even more difficult (Gordon, 1994). For example, a nurse could cluster a client's unkempt hair, dirty fingernails, and shabby clothes as "poor grooming," an inference that, with other cues, could support a nursing diagnosis of *Self-Care Deficit*. Although a nurse may infer that these assessment data reflect poor grooming, he or she may not understand the possible relation between the client's poor grooming and the inability to perform self-grooming, lack of desire to perform self-grooming, or a lifelong habit of poor grooming. In some cases, apparently significant data may, in fact, have no diagnostic significance, such as if the client stated, "I'm sorry for my appearance. I rushed here from my work at the gas station."

In Section Two, each nursing diagnosis is described in terms of focus assessment criteria to identify specific data that the nurse may need to collect. Some questions confirm or rule out defining characteristics or risk factors. Other questions seek to identify related factors.

Diagnosis

Nurses make judgments concerning various assessment data to determine the need for nursing interventions. Some of these judgments are nursing diagnoses; some are not. When a nurse concludes that a certain electrocardiogram (ECG) pattern is abnormal or labels certain tonic–clonic movements as a seizure, he or she has made a diagnosis. In both situations, the nurse diagnosed something. Nevertheless, neither is a nursing diagnosis. Both situations require nursing and medical interventions for successful outcomes (see Chapter 3).

Identifying Nursing Diagnoses

As mentioned earlier, to cluster or group data for analysis and diagnosis, the nurse must be knowledgeable about the signs and symptoms that represent the diagnosis. Using this knowledge, the nurse then:

- Reviews the data collected during a screening or focus assessment
- Examines each functional health pattern and determines if functioning in the pattern is optimal or if there is a problem
- Identifies risk factors that increase the client's vulnerability to development of a functional pattern problem

---

ⓧ INTERACTIVE EXERCISE 4.3

The following questions may help in analysis of data for Mr. Gene (Interactive Exercise 4.1). Referring to each of the 11 patterns: Does Mr. Gene have a problem with _____, or is he at risk for development of a problem with _____?

1. Health Perception–Health Management
   - Health practices?
   - Compliance?
   - Injuries?
   - Unhealthy lifestyle?
2. Nutritional–Metabolic
   - Nutrition?
   - Fluid intake?
   - Peripheral edema?
   - Infection?
   - Oral cavity health?
3. Elimination
   - Bowel elimination?
   - Incontinence?
4. Activity–Exercise
   - Activities of daily living?
   - Leisure activities?
   - Home care?
   - Respiratory function?
   - Mobility?
5. Sleep–Rest
   - Sleep?

6. Cognitive–Perceptual
   - Decisions?
   - Comfort?
   - Knowledge?
   - Sensory input?
7. Self-Perception–Self-Concept
   - Anxiety/fear?
   - Control?
   - Self-concept?
8. Role–Relationship
   - Communication?
   - Family?
   - Loss?
   - Parenting?
   - Socialization?
   - Violence?
   - Responsibilities?
9. Sexuality–Reproductive
   - Problems?
10. Coping–Stress Tolerance
    - Coping?
11. Value–Belief
    - Spirituality?

Refer to the answers at the end of this chapter.

Identifying Collaborative Problems

During assessment, the nurse acquires data about medical history and treatment. With this information, he or she can identify current physiologic complications or predict those for which the client is at risk. For example, the nurse monitors a client admitted for elective surgery who also has diabetes mellitus for fluctuations in blood glucose level under the collaborative problem *Potential Complication: Hypo/hyperglycemia* (see Chapter 3).

To help identify collaborative problems, the nurse may ask: In any of the following body systems, is a physiologic complication present, or is there a *high* risk for one developing because of a disease, treatment, diagnostic study, or medication that requires monitoring and joint management by a nurse and physician?

- Cardiac, Vascular
- Metabolic, Immune, Hematopoietic
- Respiratory
- Renal, Urinary
- Neurologic, Sensory
- Muscular, Skeletal
- Reproductive
- Gastrointestinal, Hepatic, Biliary

ⓧ INTERACTIVE EXERCISE 4.4

Refer to the case of Mr. Gene in Interactive Exercise 4.1. Does Mr. Gene have a physiologic complication, or does he have a high risk for one because of his peripheral vascular disease?

Summary

Assessment encompasses data collection, clustering, interpretation, and analysis. These complex cognitive activities require knowledge gained from theory, personal experience, and other sources. At some point, assessment data become diagnostic cues that support diagnostic statements: nursing diagnoses and collaborative problems.

The nurse must approach this first step of the nursing process cautiously to reduce erroneous assumptions and interpretations. Errors in assessment result in invalid diagnoses and ineffective interventions, which can be detrimental to clients and lead to inefficient use of nursing resources.

ANSWERS TO INTERACTIVE EXERCISES

4.1.

C reports a weak right arm—this is a cue because the client reported it.
C weight 202 lb—this is a cue because you measured it.
C height 5'3"—this is a cue because you measured it.
C reports no difficulty swallowing—this is a cue because the client reported it.
I decreased oral intake—this is an inference based on the quantity of food eaten.
I obesity—this is an inference based on the client's weight for her height, which is over 20% of ideal.

4.2. Significant data:

Needs assistance for five activities
Could not perform three activities
Walks with walker
Shows unsteady gait
Has right leg weakness

Possible nursing diagnoses:
Self-care Deficit
Risk for Injury
Disuse Syndrome

4.3. Mr. Gene has a problem with activities of daily living (mobility).
Mr. Gene is at risk for a problem with injuries.

4.4. Collaborative problem:

Potential Complication: Deep Vein Thrombosis

PLANNING CARE WITH NURSING DIAGNOSIS

Because clients require nursing care 7 days a week and 24 hours a day, nurses must rely on one another and nonlicensed nursing personnel to help clients achieve outcomes of care. Obviously, some system of communication is necessary. For more than 30 years, this system consisted of handwritten care plans or verbal reports, neither of which was very useful. This chapter addresses the varied methods that nurses use today to communicate a client's care to other caregivers.

Are Care Plans Necessary?

Today, the methods nurses use to communicate client care to other caregivers vary. Critical pathways, automated care planning systems, and preprinted standardized care plans have replaced handwritten care plans. Examples of these systems appear later in this chapter.

Critical pathways and standardized care plans reflect the expected diagnoses and associated goals and interventions commonly related to a client's medical or surgical problem. This type of system frees nurses from the repetitive writing of routine care. The care outlined on the standardized plan or critical pathway should represent the responsible care to which the client is entitled.

The Care Planning Process

Before discussing the care planning process, the nurse must identify the type, as well as the duration, of needed care. People receiving nursing care for less than 8 h, as in the emergency department, short-stay surgery, or recovery room, have a specific medical diagnosis or need a specific procedure. The nursing care must be specific for the condition and length of stay, which can be organized on a standardized care plan or pathway. Additions to this predicted care must be made according to client needs and length of stay. This is also true for hospital admissions for acute illness or surgical procedures.

In nonacute settings such as long-term care, community or home care, or assisted-living and rehabilitation units, nurses usually must supplement critical pathways and standardized plans with personalized care plans. The longer the nurse–client relationship is, the more data are available to individualize the plan.

People with an acute episode of a chronic illness (multiple sclerosis), rehabilitation needs (stroke), or a terminal illness require a different approach. They need care plans and problem lists.

Planning

Care plans represent the planning, not the delivery, of care. This planning phase of the nursing process has three components:

1. Establishing a priority set of diagnoses
2. Designating client goals and nursing goals
3. Prescribing nursing interventions

Establishing a Priority Set of Diagnoses

Realistically, a nurse cannot hope to address all, or even most, of the nursing diagnoses and collaborative problems that can apply to an individual, family, or community. By identifying a priority set—a group of nursing diagnoses and collaborative problems that take precedence over others—the nurse can best direct resources toward goal achievement. Differentiating priority diagnoses from non-priority diagnoses is crucial.

- *Priority diagnoses* are those nursing diagnoses or collaborative problems that, if not managed now, will deter progress to achieve outcomes or will negatively affect functional status.

- **Non-priority diagnoses** are those nursing diagnoses or collaborative problems for which treatment can be delayed without compromising present functional status.

As discussed in Chapter 2, the difference between risk and high-risk nursing diagnoses is relevant in care planning. Risk diagnoses represent vulnerability that all clients in a given situation share, as in *Risk for Infection* for clients who have undergone surgery. Risk diagnoses for postsurgical clients can be found on the critical pathway or standardized care plan.

In an acute care setting, the client enters the hospital for a specific purpose, such as surgery or other treatments for acute illness. In such a situation, certain nursing diagnoses or collaborative problems requiring specific nursing interventions often apply. Carpenito (1995) uses the term *diagnostic cluster* to describe such a group; this cluster can appear in a critical pathway or standardized plan of care.

For example, the following is a diagnostic cluster for a person having abdominal surgery (Carpenito, 2004).

⊙⊙ DIAGNOSTIC CLUSTER

Preoperative

Nursing Diagnosis

- Anxiety/Fear related to surgical experience, loss of control, unpredictable outcome, and insufficient knowledge of preoperative routines, postoperative exercises and activities, and postoperative changes and sensations

Preoperative

Collaborative Problems

PC: Hemorrhage
PC: Hypovolemia/Shock
PC: Evisceration/Dehiscence
PC: Paralytic Ileus
PC: Infection (Peritonitis)
PC: Urinary Retention
PC: Thrombophlebitis

Nursing Diagnosis

- Risk for Ineffective Respiratory Function related to immobility secondary to postanesthesia state and pain
- Risk for Infection related to a site for organism invasion secondary to surgery
- Acute Pain related to surgical interruption of body structures, flatus, and immobility
- Risk for Imbalanced Nutrition: Less Than Body Requirements related to increased protein and vitamin requirements for wound healing and decreased intake secondary to pain, nausea, vomiting, and diet restrictions
- Risk for Constipation related to decreased peristalsis secondary to immobility and the effects of anesthesia and narcotics
- Activity Intolerance related to pain and weakness secondary to anesthesia, tissue hypoxia, and insufficient fluid and nutrient intake
- Risk for Ineffective Therapeutic Regimen Management related to insufficient knowledge of care of operative site, restrictions (diet, activity), medications, signs and symptoms of complications, and follow-up care

---

All of these diagnoses are priority diagnoses.

The following questions can help determine whether the client or family has additional diagnoses (other than in the diagnostic cluster) that need nursing interventions:

- What nursing diagnoses or collaborative problems are associated with the primary condition (eg, surgery)?
- Are there additional collaborative problems associated with coexisting medical conditions that require monitoring (eg, hypoglycemia)?

- Are there additional nursing diagnoses that, if not managed or prevented now, will deter recovery or affect the client's functional status (eg, *High Risk for Constipation*)?
- What problems does the client perceive as priority?

How do nurses select other diagnoses not within the diagnostic cluster for a client's problem list? Limited nursing resources and increasingly reduced time for client care mandate that nurses identify priority nursing diagnoses. They do not need to include such diagnoses on the client's problem list. Non-priority diagnoses that are identified are referred for management after discharge. For example, for a client who is 50 lb overweight and hospitalized after myocardial infarction, the nurse eventually would want to explain the effects of obesity on cardiac function and refer the client to a weight-reduction program after discharge. The discharge summary record would reflect the teaching and referral; a nursing diagnosis related to weight reduction would not need to appear on the problem list.

ⓧ INTERACTIVE EXERCISE 5.1

Mr. Stanley, 76 years old, is admitted for emergency gastric surgery for repair of a bleeding ulcer. He also has diabetes mellitus and peripheral vascular disease. After completing a functional assessment, the nurse identifies the following:

- Compromised gait
- Occasional incontinence
- Wife complaining of many caregiver responsibilities and an unmotivated husband

Examine the data above and begin to formulate nursing diagnoses and collaborative problems that need nursing interventions. Refer to the four questions above to assist with this analysis and to determine whether Mr. Stanley and his family have other diagnoses that require nursing interventions. Mr. Stanley's priority list (diagnostic cluster) follows.

PC: Urinary retention
PC: Hemorrhage
PC: Hypovolemia/shock
PC: Pneumonia (stasis)
PC: Peritonitis
PC: Thrombophlebitis
PC: Paralytic ileus
PC: Evisceration
PC: Dehiscence

Risk for Infection related to destruction of first line of defense against bacterial invasion
Risk for Impaired Respiratory Function related to postanesthesia state, postoperative immobility, and pain
Impaired Physical Mobility related to pain and weakness secondary to anesthesia, tissue hypoxia, and insufficient fluids/nutrients
Risk for Imbalanced Nutrition: Less Than Body Requirements related to increased protein/vitamin requirements for wound healing and decreased intake secondary to pain, nausea, vomiting, and diet restrictions
Risk for Ineffective Therapeutic Regimen Management related to insufficient knowledge of home care, incisional care, signs and symptoms of complications, activity restriction, and follow-up care

> From postoperative standard of care (diagnostic cluster)

PC: Hypo/Hyperglycemia

> From medical history of diabetes mellitus

Possible Functional Incontinence related to reports of occasional incontinence when walking to bathroom

> From nursing admission assessment

(continued)

Mr. and Mrs. Stanley probably have many other important nursing diagnoses; however, because of the limited length of stay, nursing resources must be directed toward those problems that will deter progress at this time. The nurse can discuss important diagnoses with the client and family, with recommendations for future attention (eg, referral to a community agency).

Numbering the diagnoses on a problem list does not indicate priority; rather, it shows the order in which the nurse entered them on the list. Assigning absolute priority to nursing diagnoses or collaborative problems can create the false assumption that number 1 is automatically the first priority. In the clinical setting, priorities can shift rapidly as the client's condition changes. For this reason, the nurse must view the entire problem list as the priority set, with priorities shifting within the list periodically.

Designating Client Goals and Nursing Goals

Client goals (outcome criteria) and nursing goals are standards or measures used to evaluate the client's progress (outcome) or the nurse's performance (process). According to Alfaro (1994), *client goals* are statements describing a measurable behavior of the client, family, or group that denotes a favorable status (changed or maintained) after the delivery of nursing care. *Nursing goals* are statements describing measurable actions that denote the nurse's accountability for the situation or diagnosis. As discussed in Chapter 4, nursing diagnoses have client goals, whereas collaborative problems have nursing goals.

Client goals serve as the criteria for measuring the effectiveness of a care plan. Because these outcome criteria for nursing diagnoses represent favorable statuses that clients can achieve or maintain through nurse-prescribed (independent) interventions, they can help differentiate nursing diagnoses from collaborative problems.

Certain situations may call for involvement from several disciplines. For example, for a client experiencing extreme anxiety, the physician may prescribe an antianxiety medication, an occupational therapist may provide diversional activities, and a nurse may institute nonpharmacologic anxiety-reducing measures, such as relaxation exercises. According to Gordon (1994), "Saying a nursing diagnosis is a health problem a nurse can treat does not mean that non-nursing consultants cannot be used. The critical element is whether the nurse-prescribed interventions can achieve the outcome established with the client."

If a client goal is not achieved or progress toward achievement is not evident, the nurse must reevaluate the attainability of the goal or review the nursing care plan, asking the following questions (Carpenito, 1999):

- Is the diagnosis correct?
- Has the goal been set mutually? Is the client participating?
- Is more time needed for the plan to work?
- Does the goal need to be revised?
- Does the plan need to be revised?
- Are physician-prescribed interventions needed?

Goals for Collaborative Problems

As discussed earlier, identifying client goals for collaborative problems is inappropriate and can imply erroneous accountability for nurses. Rather, collaborative problems involve nursing goals that reflect nursing accountability in situations requiring physician-prescribed and nurse-prescribed interventions. This accountability includes (1) monitoring for physiologic instability, (2) consulting standing orders and protocols or a physician to obtain orders for appropriate interventions, (3) performing specific actions to manage and to reduce the severity of an event or situation, and (4) evaluating client responses.

Nursing goals for collaborative problems can be written as "The nurse will manage and minimize the problem." The following are examples of goals for collaborative problems:

Collaborative Problem	Nursing Goal
Potential Complication: Bleeding *Potential Complication: Fluid/Electrolyte Imbalance*	The nurse will monitor to detect early signs/symptoms of bleeding and fluid/electrolyte imbalances and collaboratively intervene to stabilize the client.

Goals for Nursing Diagnoses

Client goals can represent predicted resolution of a problem, evidence of progress toward resolution of a problem, progress toward improved health status, or continued maintenance of good health or function. Nurses and clients use these goals to direct interventions to achieve desired changes or maintenance and to measure the effectiveness and validity of interventions. Nurses can formulate goals (outcome criteria) to direct and measure positive results or to prevent complications. Goals (outcome criteria) seek to direct interventions to provide the client with:

- Improved health status by increasing comfort (physiologic, psychological, social, spiritual) and coping abilities (eg, The client will discuss relationship between activity and carbohydrate requirements and walk unassisted to end of hall four times a day.)
- Maintenance of present optimal level of health (eg, The client will continue to share fears.)
- Optimal levels of coping with significant others (eg, The client will relate an intent to discuss with her husband her concern about returning to work.)
- Optimal adaptation to deterioration of health status (eg, The client will visually scan the environment to prevent injury while walking.)
- Optimal adaptation to terminal illness (eg, The client will compensate for periods of anorexia and nausea.)
- Collaboration and satisfaction with health care providers (eg, The client will ask questions concerning the care of his colostomy.)

Alternatively, goals (outcome criteria) seek to direct interventions to prevent negative alterations in the client, such as:

- Complications (eg, The client will not experience the complications of imposed bed rest as evidenced by continued intact skin; full range of motion, no calf tenderness, and clear lung fields.)
- Disabilities (eg, The client will elevate left arm on pillow and exercise fingers on sponge ball to reduce edema.)
- Unwarranted death (eg, The infant will be attached to an apnea monitor at night.)

Components of Goals

The essential characteristics of goals are as follows:

- Long-term or short-term
- Measurable behavior
- Specific in content and time
- Attainable

A *long-term goal* is an objective that the client is expected to achieve over weeks or months. A *short-term goal* is an objective that the client is expected to achieve in a few days or as a stepping stone toward a long-term goal (Alfaro, 1998). Long-term goals are appropriate for all clients in long-term care facilities and for some clients in rehabilitation units, mental health units, community nursing settings, and ambulatory services. For a client with a nursing diagnosis of *Risk for Suicide* (Varcarolis, 2003):

Long-term Goal	Client will state that she wants to live.
Short-term Goals	Client will discuss painful feelings. Client will make no-suicide contract with nurse by end of first session.

Measurable behavior is expressed by use of *measurable verbs,* or verbs that describe the exact action that the nurse expects the client to display when he or she has met the goal. The action or behavior must be such that the nurse can validate it through seeing or hearing. (The nurse may occasionally use touch, taste, and smell to measure goal achievement.) If the verb does not describe a result that can be seen or heard (eg, The client *will experience* less anxiety), the nurse can change it to a behaviorally measurable one (eg, The client *will report* less anxiety).

ⓧ INTERACTIVE EXERCISE 5.3

Examine the following goals:
The client will

- Accept the death of his wife
- State the signs and symptoms of high blood glucose
- Know the signs and symptoms of low blood glucose
- Administer insulin correctly
- Understand the importance of a low-fat diet

Which goals can you evaluate by seeing or hearing? (Answer at end of chapter)

Nurses can make the measurement of goal achievement easier by:

- Using the phrase *as evidenced by* to introduce measurable evidence of reduced signs and symptoms (eg, The client will experience less anxiety, as evidenced by reduced pacing; The client will demonstrate tolerance to activity, as evidenced by a return to resting pulse (76) 3 min after activity)
- Adding the phrase *within normal limits* (WNL) (eg, The client will demonstrate healing WNL.)

A student may be asked to define what WNL is. For example, the client will demonstrate healing WNL as evidenced by intact, approximate wound edges and no or little abnormal drainage.
The process of writing measurable goals is diagrammed on page 44.

Goals should be *specific in content and time.* Three elements add to the specificity of a goal: (1) content, (2) modifiers, and (3) achievement time. The *content* indicates what the client is to do, experience, or learn (eg, drink, walk, cough, verbalize). *Modifiers* add individual preferences to the goal and are usually adjectives or adverbs explaining what, where, when, and how. Nurses can add the *time for achievement* to a goal using one of three options:

1. By discharge (eg, The client will relate intent to discuss fears regarding diagnosis with wife at home.)
2. Continued (eg, The client will demonstrate continued intact skin.)
3. By date (eg, The client will walk half the length of the hallway with assistance by Friday morning.)

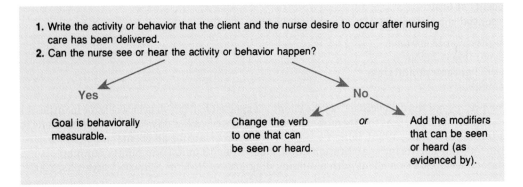

1. Write the activity or behavior that the client and the nurse desire to occur after nursing care has been delivered.

2. Can the nurse see or hear the activity or behavior happen?

Yes

No

Goal is behaviorally measurable.

Change the verb to one that can be seen or heard.

or

Add the modifiers that can be seen or heard (as evidenced by).

Finally, a goal must be *attainable,* meaning that the client must be able to achieve the goal based on his or her age, condition, mental status, and motivation.

Individualized Goals

For each nursing diagnosis in Section Two, goals are stated in measurable terms. Nurses, however, must make goals *specific* to each client by adding modifiers that highlight areas to observe and measure. In the following example, a goal for the diagnosis *Pain* has been rewritten to reflect goals for particular clients on a rehabilitation unit:

Goal: The client will report reduced pain and improved mobility by discharge.

Individualized Goals:

1. The client will complete his bath without assistance.
2. The client will report reduced pain (<5 on 0 to 10 scale).
3. The client will remain out of bed from 11 AM to 2 PM and from 5 PM to 9 PM.

Goals for Possible Nursing Diagnoses

Because goals refer to changes expected in a client's status after the delivery of nursing care, it is inappropriate for nurses to formulate client goals for collaborative problems and possible nursing diagnoses. Consider the following possible nursing diagnosis and associated goal:

• **Nursing diagnosis:** *Possible Feeding Self-Care Deficit related to IV in right hand*
• **Goal:** The client will feed himself.

As one can easily see, this goal is problematic. How can the nurse write a client goal for a possible nursing diagnosis if the nurse does not know whether the client actually has the problem? Thus, nurses omit goals for possible nursing diagnoses because they are not indicated.

Prescribing Nursing Interventions

As previously discussed (see Chapter 3), the two types of nursing interventions are nurse prescribed and physician prescribed (delegated). *Nurse-prescribed interventions* are those that nurses formulate for themselves or other nursing staff to implement. *Physician-prescribed (delegated) interventions* are prescriptions for clients that physicians formulate for nursing staff to implement. Physicians' orders are not orders for nurses; rather, they are orders for clients that nurses implement if indicated.

Both types of interventions require independent nursing judgment, because legally the nurse must determine whether it is appropriate to initiate the action, regardless of whether it is independent or delegated. Box 5.1 shows a sample nursing care plan with both types of interventions.

Note that nurses can and should consult with other disciplines, such as social workers, nutritionists, and physical therapists, as appropriate. Nevertheless, doing so is consultative only; if interventions for nursing diagnoses result from such consultation, the nurse writes these orders on the nursing care plan for other nursing staff to implement. (A discussion of other disciplines and their role in nursing care plans is included later in this chapter.)

Bulechek and McCloskey (1989) define nursing interventions as "any direct care treatment that a nurse performs on behalf of a client. These treatments include nurse-initiated treatments resulting from nursing diagnoses, physician-initiated treatments resulting from medical diagnoses, and performance of essential daily functions for the client who cannot do these." Their definition links all nursing interventions with nursing diagnoses. This author links all nursing interventions with nursing diagnoses and collaborative problems. Figure 5.1 lists the six basic types of nursing interventions identified by Bulechek and McCloskey (1989), with this author's changes.

⊗ BOX 5.1 NURSE-PRESCRIBED AND DELEGATED INTERVENTIONS

Standard of Care

Potential Complication: Increased Intracranial Pressure

NP   1. Monitor for signs and symptoms of increased intracranial pressure.
- Pulse changes: slowing rate to 60 or below; increasing rate to 100 or above
- Respiratory irregularities: slowing rate with lengthening periods of apnea
- Rising blood pressure or widening pulse pressure with moderately elevated temperature
- Temperature rising
- Level of responsiveness: variable change from baseline (alert, lethargic, comatose)
- Pupillary changes (size, equality, reaction to light, movements)
- Eye movements (doll's eyes, nystagmus)
- Vomiting
- Headache: constant, increasing in intensity; aggravated by movement/standing
- Subtle changes: restlessness, forced breathing, purposeless movements, and mental cloudiness
- Paresthesia, paralysis

NP   2. Avoid:
- Carotid massage
- Prone position
- Neck flexion
- Extreme neck rotation
- Valsalva maneuver
- Isometric exercises
- Digital stimulation (anal)

NP   3. Maintain a position with slight head elevation.

NP   4. Avoid rapidly changing positions.

NP   5. Maintain a quiet, calm environment (soft lighting).

NP   6. Plan activities to reduce interruptions.

NP   7. Intake and output; use infusion pump to ensure accuracy.

NP   8. Consult for stool softeners.

Del   9. Maintain fluid restrictions as ordered (may be restricted to 1000 mL/day for a few days).

Del   10. Administer fluids at an even rate as prescribed.

Del   11. Administer medications (osmotic diuretics [eg, mannitol]; and corticosteroids [eg, dexamethasone, methylprednisolone if administered]).

(Del = Delegated; NP = Nurse-prescribed)

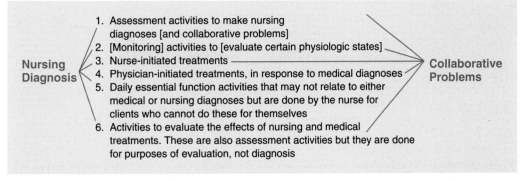

FIGURE 5.1 Relationship of nursing interventions to nursing diagnosis and collaborative problems. (Bulechek, G., & McCloskey, J. Nursing interventions: Treatments for potential nursing diagnoses. In Carroll-Johnson, M. [Ed.]. *Classification of nursing diagnoses: Proceedings of the eighth national conference.* Philadelphia: J.B. Lippincott. Brackets indicate changes made by author.)

Focus of Nursing Interventions

As discussed in Chapter 3, the major focus of interventions differs for actual, risk, and possible nursing diagnoses and collaborative problems.

For *actual nursing diagnoses,* interventions seek to:

- Reduce or eliminate contributing factors or the diagnosis
- Promote higher-level wellness
- Monitor and evaluate status

For *risk nursing diagnoses,* interventions seek to:

- Reduce or eliminate risk factors
- Prevent the problem
- Monitor and evaluate status

For *possible nursing diagnoses,* interventions seek to:

- Collect additional data to rule out or confirm the diagnosis

For *collaborative problems,* interventions seek to:

- Monitor for changes in status
- Manage changes in status with nurse-prescribed and physician-prescribed interventions
- Evaluate response

Nursing Orders

The specific directions for nursing—*nursing orders*—consist of the following:

- Date
- Directive verb
- What, when, how often, how long, where
- Signature

What If the Nurse Cannot Treat the Contributing Factors?

Sometimes, nursing interventions cannot reduce or eliminate the related factors for the nursing diagnosis. The literature has specified that nurses direct interventions toward reducing or eliminating etiologic or contributing factors. Specifically, if the nurse cannot treat the contributing factors, then the nursing diagnosis is considered incorrect. This is problematic. As the diagnostic labels evolve into more specific labels, nurses may encounter nursing diagnoses with contributing factors that nursing cannot treat. Consider, for example, *Risk for Infection related to compromised immune system.* The nurse does not prescribe for a compromised immune system but can prevent infection in some clients with this problem. In some instances, the label directs the interventions, and the etiologic or contributing factors are not involved. Examples of such categories include the following:

- *Impaired Swallowing*
- *Functional Incontinence*
- *Risk for Infection*

The following illustrates this relationship:

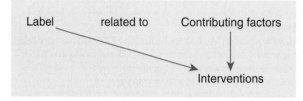

The nurse should be able to prescribe the definite therapy for the nursing diagnosis label or related factors. Consider the diagnosis *Disturbed Sensory Perception related to progressive loss of vision.* The nurse cannot prescribe interventions for either part of this diagnosis. When this happens, write the interventions that are indicated for this problem. Examine the interventions and decide what problems they are treating.

For example,
Disturbed Sensory Perception related to progressive loss of vision.

Interventions

Allow person to share his feelings.
Explain strategies to prevent injury.

The diagnosis that would relate to these interventions is *Fear related to progressive loss of vision.*

Implementation

The implementation component of the nursing process involves applying the skills that nurses need to implement the nursing interventions. The skills and knowledge necessary for implementation usually focus on:

- Performing the activity for or assisting the client
- Performing nursing assessments to identify new problems or to monitor the status of existing problems
- Teaching to help clients gain new knowledge concerning their own health or the management of a disorder
- Assisting clients to make decisions about their own health care
- Consulting with and referring to other health care professionals to obtain appropriate direction
- Providing specific treatment actions to remove, reduce, or resolve health problems
- Assisting clients to perform activities themselves
- Assisting clients to identify risks or problems and to explore options available
  (Alfaro-LeFevre, 1998)

Nurses not only must possess these skills, but they also must assess, teach, and evaluate them in all nursing personnel that they manage. Often, the nurse is responsible for planning, but not actually implementing, care. This requires the management skills of delegation, assertion, evaluation, and knowledge of change and motivational theory. Nurses should consult the appropriate literature on these topics.

Evaluation

Evaluation involves three different considerations:

- Evaluation of the client's status
- Evaluation of the client's progress toward goal achievement
- Evaluation of the care plan's status and currency

The nurse is responsible for evaluating the client's status regularly. Some clients require daily evaluation; others, such as those with neurologic problems, need hourly or continuous evaluation. The nurse approaches evaluation differently for nursing diagnoses and collaborative problems.

Evaluating Nursing Diagnoses

Nurses need client goals (outcome criteria) to evaluate a nursing diagnosis. After the nurse and client mutually set client goals, the nurse will (1) assess the client's status, (2) compare this response to the outcome criteria, and (3) conclude whether the client is progressing toward outcome achievement. The example on page 48 illustrates this evaluation process:

If a goal is "The client will walk unassisted half the length of the hall by 6/5," the nurse would observe the client's response to interventions, asking, "How far did the client walk?" and "Did he or she need assistance?" The nurse then would compare the client's response after interventions with the established goals.

The nurse can record the client's response on flow charts or progress notes. Flow charts record clinical data, such as vital signs, skin condition, any side effects, and wound assessments. Progress notes record specific responses that are not appropriate for flow charts, such as response to counseling, response of family members to the client, and any unusual responses.

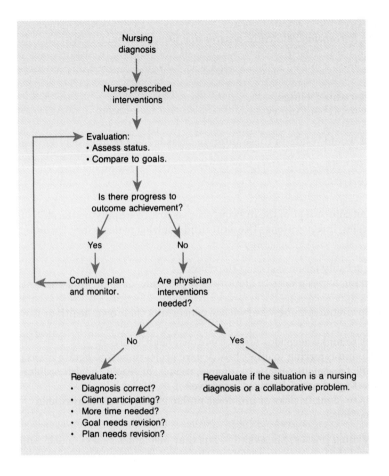

Evaluating Collaborative Problems

Because collaborative problems do not have client goals, the nurse evaluates them differently than nursing diagnoses. For collaborative problems, the nurse will (1) assess the client's status, (2) compare the data to established norms, (3) judge whether the data fall within acceptable ranges, and (4) conclude if the client's condition is stable, improved, unimproved, or worse.

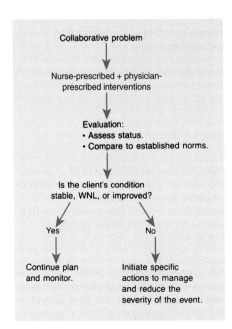

For example, for *Potential Complication: Hypertension,* the nurse takes a blood pressure reading and compares the finding against the normal range. If it falls within the range, the nurse concludes that the client exhibits normal blood pressure. If the blood pressure is outside the normal range, the nurse checks the client's previous blood pressure readings. If this is a recent change, consult with a physician or nurse-practitioner.

The nurse can record the assessment data for collaborative problems on flow records and use progress notes for significant or unusual findings, along with nursing interventions for the situation.

Evaluating the Care Plan

This type of evaluation depends on the conclusions derived from the evaluation of the client's progress or condition. After examining the client's response, the nurse should ask the following questions:

Nursing Diagnosis
- Does the diagnosis still exist?
- Does a risk or high-risk diagnosis still exist?
- Has the possible diagnosis been confirmed or ruled out?
- Does a new diagnosis need to be added?

Goals
- Have they been achieved?
- Do they reflect the present focus of care?
- Can more specific modifiers be added?
- Are they acceptable to the client?

Interventions
- Are they acceptable to the client?
- Are they specific to the client?
- Do they provide clear instructions to the nursing staff?

Collaborative Problems
- Is continuing monitoring indicated?

In reviewing the problems and interventions, the nurse records one of the following decisions in the evaluation column or in the progress notes at the time prescribed for evaluation:

- ***Continue.*** The diagnosis is still present, and the goals and interventions are appropriate.
- ***Revised.*** The diagnosis is still present, but the goals or nursing orders require revision. The revisions are then recorded.
- ***Ruled Out/Confirmed.*** Additional data collection has confirmed or ruled out a possible diagnosis. Goals and nursing orders are written.
- ***Achieved.*** The goals have been achieved, and that portion of the care plan is discontinued.
- ***Reinstate.*** A diagnosis that had been resolved returns.

The nurse caring for or directing the client's care can make minor revisions on a care plan daily. He or she can use a yellow felt-tip marker (Hi-Liter) to mark those areas no longer in use. Because it is still possible to read through the yellow marking, the nurse can refer to previous planning. In addition, the marking will not interfere with photocopying. Examples of evaluation documentation are presented later in this chapter.

Multidisciplinary Care Planning

Commonly, at least two disciplines (sometimes more) provide the care of individuals, families, or groups. Good coordination of this care is critical for optimal use of resources and to prevent duplication. Given overall knowledge level and time spent with clients, nurses typically are in the best position to coordinate this care. The case management model subscribes to this philosophy.

Agencies take various steps to promote coordinated multidisciplinary planning:

- Conducting regular multidisciplinary planning conferences
- Creating multidisciplinary problem lists
- Creating multidisciplinary care plans

Some of these strategies, however, can be problematic for nurses. As discussed in this chapter, care plans serve as directions for nursing staff in providing client care. Should staff from other disciplines— physical therapy, social services, nutrition—write on nursing care plans? If so, should they write interventions for nurses to follow or specific to their discipline?

When a client requires services other than nursing, the physician orders a consultation of the services. Staff members from the needed discipline then create a plan of care with goals and interventions relating specifically to their discipline, not to nursing. Should this plan be part of a multidisciplinary care plan? Yes, but only if the plan clearly designates which sections apply only to specific disciplines.

Physician-prescribed interventions are transferred from the chart to appropriate documents, such as medication administration records, treatment records, and Kardexes. It is not necessary to enter physician-prescribed interventions on nursing care plans.

A nurse is accountable for following the interventions that other professional nurses prescribe. If a nurse disagrees with another nurse's care plan, the two nurses should consult and discuss the problem. If doing so is impossible, then the disagreeing nurse can delete or revise the existing nursing orders. Professional courtesy dictates that the nurse should leave a note to the previous nurse explaining the change, if it could be problematic.

Should other disciplines add interventions for nursing staff to the nursing care plan? When a discipline other than nursing or medicine has suggestions for nursing management of a nursing diagnosis, the nurse should view these suggestions as expert advice. The nurse may or may not incorporate such advice into the nursing care plan. This situation is similar to that of a consulting physician, who may make recommendations but does not write medical orders for another physician's client.

When a nurse enters an intervention on the care plan based on a suggestion from another discipline, professional courtesy mandates that the nurse credit the order to that discipline. For example:

Gently perform passive ROM to arms after meals and at 8–9 pm, as suggested by C. Levy, RPT.

Historically, nurses exclusively have used nursing diagnoses and collaborative problems to describe the focus of nursing care. But nursing diagnoses and collaborative problems also can describe the focus of care for other nonphysician disciplines, such as physical therapy, respiratory therapy, social service, occupational therapy, nutritional therapy, and speech therapy. Other disciplines could add their discipline-specific interventions to standardized care plans with the designation that the interventions are prescribed and provided by that discipline (not nursing). These disciplines also would be encouraged to revise or add to care plans for their interventions. Box 5.2 illustrates a multidisciplinary care plan. Note that all nursing diagnoses or collaborative problems do not have non–nurse-prescribed interventions.

Multidisciplinary conferencing provides an excellent way to review and evaluate a client's, family's, or group's status and progress. In some facilities, such conferencing is required for all applicable clients.

Care Planning Systems

Standards of care are detailed guidelines that represent the predicted care for specific situations. They do not direct nurses to provide medical interventions; rather, they provide an efficient method for retrieving predicted generic nursing interventions. Standards of care identify a set of problems (actual or at risk) that typically occur in a particular situation—a diagnostic cluster. An efficient, professional, and useful care planning system encompasses standards of care, client problem lists, and standardized and addendum care plans.

○○ **BOX 5.2 SAMPLE MULTIDISCIPLINARY CARE PLAN FOR A CLIENT AFTER TOTAL HIP REPLACEMENT**

Nursing Diagnosis:

Impaired Physical Mobility related to pain, stiffness, fatigue, restrictive equipment, and prescribed activity restrictions

Goal:

The client will increase activity to a level consistent with abilities.

Interventions:

PT	1. Establish an exercise program tailored to the client's ability.
	2. Implement exercises at regular intervals.
PT/Nsg	3. Teach body mechanics and transfer techniques.
	4. Encourage independence.
PT/Nsg	5. Teach and supervise use of ambulatory aids.

Standardization

Like any concept or system, standardized care planning forms have both advantages and disadvantages. Advantages include the following:

- Eliminate the need to write routine nursing interventions
- Illustrate to new or part-time employees the unit standard of care
- Direct nursing staff to selected documentation requirements
- Provide the criteria for a quality improvement program and resource management
- Allow the nurse to spend more time delivering than documenting care

Disadvantages are as follows:

- May replace a needed individualized intervention
- May encourage nurses to focus on predictable instead of additional problems

Some nurses experienced these disadvantages when standardized care plans were introduced into their clinical setting. In such cases, the solution was to eliminate standardized care plans. Follow-up care plan audits revealed that the nurses were writing what previously was contained on the standard of care (eg, *turn q2h, administer pain relief medication*).

Nurses also have been socialized to view standardization as mediocre and unprofessional care. Standards of care or standardized care plans should represent responsible nursing care predicted for certain situations. Nurses should view these predictions as scientific. When problems arise with the use of standardized forms, the solution is not to change the forms but to address their misuse.

The documentation of implementation does not take place on a care plan but on flow charts, graphic charts, or nursing progress notes, depending on the types of data being recorded. Figure 5.2 illustrates the nursing process with the related documentation.

Flow charts are excellent formats for recording treatments, activities of daily living, selected teaching, and observations. Figure 5.3 is an example of a flow chart. Nurses should use flow charts cautiously to record interactions in the spiritual, cultural, social, and psychological domains. They may need to record these responses in the progress notes, as in explanations and counseling given to clients and families and unusual or unexpected situations (eg, injuries, clinical emergencies). If the nurses are

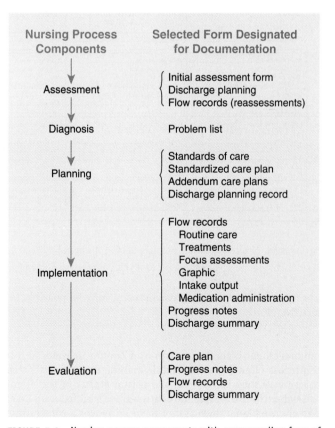

FIGURE 5.2 Nursing process components with corresponding form of documentation.

Harper·Grace Hospitals
Detroit, Michigan
☐ Harper Hospital Division (48201)

NURSING SHIFT ASSESSMENT

CODE: LOC = LEVEL OF CONSCIOUSNESS; NA = NOT APPLICABLE; NP = NO PROBLEM; + = POSITIVE; - = NEGATIVE; x = TIMES

INITIAL ASSESSMENT	2300-0700	0700-1500	1500-2300
NUTRITION/ METABOLIC PATTERN	Skin: ☐ NP ☐ Edema ☐ Pressure Areas: ____ Other: ____	Skin: ☐ NP ☐ Edema ☐ Pressure Areas: ____ Other: ____	Skin: ☐ NP ☐ Edema ☐ Pressure Areas: ____ Other: ____
RESPIRATION/ CIRCULATION PATTERN	Breath Sounds: ☐ Normal ☐ Abnormal ____ ☐ NA Cough: ☐ YES ☐ NO ☐ Productive ☐ Non-productive Peripheral Pulses: ☐ NA ☐ + ☐ - Other: ____	Breath Sounds: ☐ Normal ☐ Abnormal ____ ☐ NA Cough: ☐ YES ☐ NO ☐ Productive ☐ Non-productive Peripheral Pulses: ☐ NA ☐ + ☐ - Other: ____	Breath Sounds: ☐ Normal ☐ Abnormal ____ ☐ NA Cough: ☐ YES ☐ NO ☐ Productive ☐ Non-productive Peripheral Pulses: ☐ NA ☐ + ☐ - Other: ____
ELIMINATION PATTERN	☐ Nausea ☐ Vomiting ☐ Diarrhea ☐ NP Abdomen: ☐ Distended ☐ Non-Distended Bowel Sounds: ☐ + ☐ - ☐ NA Other: ____	☐ Nausea ☐ Vomiting ☐ Diarrhea ☐ NP Abdomen: ☐ Distended ☐ Non-Distended Bowel Sounds: ☐ + ☐ - ☐ NA Other: ____	☐ Nausea ☐ Vomiting ☐ Diarrhea ☐ NP Abdomen: ☐ Distended ☐ Non-Distended Bowel Sounds: ☐ + ☐ - ☐ NA Other: ____
COGNITIVE/ PERCEPTUAL PATTERN	LOC: ☐ Person ☐ Place ☐ Time Responds appropriately to questions: ☐ Yes ☐ No Discomfort: ☐ + ☐ - Type: ____ Location: ____ Other: ____	LOC: ☐ Person ☐ Place ☐ Time Responds appropriately to questions: ☐ Yes ☐ No Discomfort: ☐ + ☐ - Type: ____ Location: ____ Other: ____	LOC: ☐ Person ☐ Place ☐ Time Responds appropriately to questions: ☐ Yes ☐ No Discomfort: ☐ + ☐ - Type: ____ Location: ____ Other: ____
ONGOING ASSESSMENT	Time:	Time:	Time:
HEALTH PERCEPTION/ HEALTH MANAGEMENT PATTERN	Safety: Siderails x ____ ☐ Equipment ____ ☐ Restraints ____ ☐ Special Precautions ____ Other ____	Safety: Siderails x ____ ☐ Equipment ____ ☐ Restraints ____ ☐ Special Precautions ____ Other ____	Safety: Siderails x ____ ☐ Equipment ____ ☐ Restraints ____ ☐ Special Precautions ____ Other ____
NUTRITION/ METABOLIC PATTERN	Supplement/Tube Feeding ____ ☐ NPO Other ____	Diet ____ Breakfast ☐ 100% ☐ 75% ☐ 50% ☐ 25% ☐ Refused ☐ NPO Lunch: ☐ 100% ☐ 75% ☐ 50% ☐ 25% ☐ Refused ☐ NPO Supplement ____ Other ____	Diet ____ Dinner ☐ 100% ☐ 75% ☐ 50% ☐ 25% ☐ Refused ☐ NPO Supplement ____ Other ____
ELIMINATION PATTERN	Bowel Movement X ____ ☐ Incontinent of stool Urine ☐ NP ☐ Incontinent of Urine Devices ____ Other ____	Bowel Movement X ____ ☐ Incontinent of stool Urine ☐ NP ☐ Incontinent of Urine Devices ____ Other ____	Bowel Movement X ____ ☐ Incontinent of stool Urine ☐ NP ☐ Incontinent of Urine Devices ____ Other ____
ACTIVITY/EXERCISE PATTERN	Hygiene ☐ Complete ☐ Partial ☐ Self-Care ☐ NA Skin Products ____ Mouth Care ____ Ambulated x ____ Chair x ____ ☐ Bedrest Positioned x ____ Other ____	Hygiene ☐ Complete ☐ Partial ☐ Self-Care ☐ NA Skin Products ____ Mouth Care ____ Ambulated x ____ Chair x ____ ☐ Bedrest Positioned x ____ Other ____	Hygiene ☐ Complete ☐ Partial ☐ Self-Care ☐ NA Skin Products ____ Mouth Care ____ Ambulated x ____ Chair x ____ ☐ Bedrest Positioned x ____ Other ____
SLEEP/REST PATTERN	☐ Restless ☐ Sleeping at Intervals ☐ Awake ☐ None Other ____	☐ Restless ☐ Sleeping at Intervals ☐ Awake ☐ None Other ____	☐ Restless ☐ Sleeping at Intervals ☐ Awake ☐ None Other ____
SIGNATURE & TITLE			

300955 (3/90)

FIGURE 5.3 Sample flow chart. (Courtesy of Harper Hospital, Detroit, Michigan.)

recording the same data repeatedly in the progress notes, it may be possible to adapt a flow chart to accommodate them more frequently.

Critical Pathways

Critical pathways are management tools that Bower and Zander introduced into health care in 1985. They "are based on the process of anticipating and describing *in advance* the care clients, within the specific case types, require and then comparing the actual status of the client to that anticipated" (Bower, 1993, p. 10). Critical paths are simple, direct timelines that focus on an episode of illness. They are not standards of care or care plans; they cannot focus care over a continuum.

Critical pathways should represent an at-a-glance reminder of the standard of care. In other words, they should be drawn from the standard of care. Box 5.3 represents a portion of a critical pathway for clients undergoing a total hip replacement. On this pathway, nursing diagnoses and collaborative prob-

Harper·Grace Hospitals
Detroit, Michigan
☐ Harper Hospital Division (48201)

NURSING TREATMENTS/PROCEDURES

		Time/Initials			Time/Initials			Time/Initials		
		Date:			Date:			Date:		
Start Date	TREATMENTS	2300-0700	0700-1500	1500-2300	2300-0700	0700-1500	1500-2300	2300-0700	0700-1500	1500-2300
Date	SPECIMENS									

Initials	Date	PROCEDURES: TO OTHER DEPARTMENTS	Department	Mode of Transportation	Time

Initials	Signature & Title	Initials	Signature & Title	Initials	Signature & Title

FIGURE 5.3 *(Continued)*

lems are linked with outcomes and intermediate goals. A corresponding standard of care would provide the nurse with specific, detailed interventions for nursing care.

As discussed, critical paths offer an at-a-glance timeline to evaluate the progression of a client in a population. They cannot accommodate additional nursing diagnoses or collaborative problems (addendum diagnoses) that need nursing interventions. These addendum diagnoses, if not addressed, can delay client progress. For example, a woman scheduled for a hip replacement also has been taking steroids for 2 years. This would necessitate monitoring for the collaborative problem—*PC: Hypo/Hyperglycemia and Adrenal Insufficiency.* How will the nurse communicate this problem to other nurses with a critical path? One option is to write this additional problem under the problem list in the critical pathway and to insert the monitoring of blood glucose levels under the assessment section. This would work if the interventions were brief, such as "monitor blood glucose levels." What if this woman also is confused before surgery? This would necessitate the addition of *Chronic Confusion* to the problem list. The interventions for this addendum diagnosis are not brief. A problem list/care plan can provide the solution. A detailed explanation of problem lists is found later in this chapter.

Levels of Care

Keep in mind that standards of care should represent the care that nurses are responsible for providing, not an ideal level of care. As discussed earlier, the nurse cannot hope to address all—or, usually, even most—of a client's problems. Rather, the nurse must focus on the client's most serious, or priority, problems. The nurse should refer problems that will not be addressed in the health care facility to both the client and family for interventions after discharge. Referrals to community agencies, such as weight loss or smoking cessation programs and psychological counseling, may be indicated after discharge. Nurses must create realistic standards based on client acuity, length of stay, and available resources. Unrealistic, ideal standards merely frustrate nurses and hold them legally accountable for care that they cannot provide.

A care planning system can be structured with three tiers or levels of care:

1. Level I—generic unit standard of care
2. Level II—diagnostic cluster or single-diagnosis standardized care plan
3. Level III—addendum care plans

⊗ BOX 5.3 CRITICAL PATHWAYS—TOTAL HIP REPLACEMENT

Nsg Dx/Coll Prob	Intermediate Goals		Outcomes
	Day 1	**Day 2**	**Day 8**
PC • Fat emboli • Compartmental syndrome • Hemorrhage • Joint displacement • Sepsis • Thrombosis	Nurse will monitor for early signs and symptoms of vascular and joint complications.	→	Client will state signs and symptoms that must be reported to health care professional.
Risk for Infection		Client will exhibit wound healing free of infection.	Client will demonstrate healing with approximated wound edges.
Impaired Physical Mobility	Client will relate the purpose of strengthening exercises.	Client will do strengthening exercises.	Client will regain mobility while adhering to weight-bearing restrictions using walker.
Acute Pain	Client will report satisfactory relief of pain.	→	Client will report progressive reduction of pain and increased activity.
Risk for Injury	Client will identify factors that increase risk of injury; describe appropriate safety measures.	→	Client will describe risk factors for injury in home.
Risk for Impaired Skin Integrity	Client will demonstrate skin integrity free of pressure ulcers.	→	Client will demonstrate skin integrity free of pressure ulcers.
Risk for Ineffective Therapeutic Regimen Management	Client will communicate questions and concerns.	→	Client will describe activity restrictions. Client will describe a plan for resuming activities of daily living (ADLs).

	/OR DAY	**/POD #1**	**/POD #2**	**/POD #3**
Consults		OT PT Home care		
Tests	Postop x-ray Hct; Chem Panel PT/PTT	→	→	
Treatments	Hemovac drain	→	D/C Hemovac	D/C staples
Medication	IV Antibiotic preop	Antibiotic IM pain meds Anticoagulant	po pain meds	Prescription D/C anticoagulant
Diet				
Activity	As ordered Bed rest with abduction pillow; maintain alignment	→ OOB/Chair	→ Weight bear as tolerated; transfer/assist	→

(continued)

BOX 5.3 CRITICAL PATHWAYS—TOTAL HIP REPLACEMENT (*Continued*)

	/OR DAY	/POD #1	/POD #2	/POD #3
Assessments			Ambulate/walker	
	Postop assessments	Assess Ace Wrap Monitor neuro-vascular status Monitor tissue integrity	→	→
Teaching				
	S/S neurovascular compromise; rein-force activity and safety measures	Postop exercises	→	Written instructions
Discharge Planning			Social work prn Home care prn	Written instructions

Carpenito, L. J. (2003). *Nursing care plans and documentation* (4th ed.). Philadelphia: Lippincott Williams & Wilkins; used with permission.

Level I—Unit Standards of Care

Level I standards of care represent the predicted generic care required for all or most clients on a unit. These standards contain nursing diagnoses or collaborative problems (the diagnostic cluster) applicable to the specific situation. Box 5.4 presents a sample diagnostic cluster for standards of care in a general medical unit. Each unit—orthopedics, oncology, pediatrics, surgical, postanesthesia, neonatal, emergency, mental health, and so on—should have a generic unit standard of care.

Level I standards can be laminated and placed in each client care area as a reference for nurses. Because these standards apply to all clients, the nurse does not have to write the associated nursing diagnoses or collaborative problems on an individual client's care plan. Instead, institutional policy can specify that the generic standard will be implemented for all clients if indicated.

BOX 5.4 GENERIC DIAGNOSTIC CLUSTER FOR HOSPITALIZED ADULTS WITH MEDICAL CONDITIONS

Collaborative Problems

- *Potential Complication: Cardiovascular*
- *Potential Complication: Respiratory*

Nursing Diagnosis

- *Anxiety* related to unfamiliar environment, routines, diagnostic tests and treatments, and loss of control
- *Risk for Injury* related to unfamiliar environment and physical/mental limitations secondary to condition, medications, therapies, and diagnostic tests
- *Risk for Infection* related to increased microorganisms in environment, the risk of person-to-person transmission, and invasive tests and therapies
- *Self-Care Deficit* related to sensory, cognitive, mobility, endurance, or motivation problems
- *Risk for Imbalanced Nutrition: Less Than Body Requirements* related to decreased appetite secondary to treatments, fatigue, environment, and changes in usual diet, and increased protein/vitamin requirements for healing
- *Risk for Constipation* related to change in fluid/food intake, routine and activity level, effects of medications, and emotional stress
- *Disturbed Sleep Pattern* related to unfamiliar, noisy environment, change in bedtime ritual, emotional stress, and change in circadian rhythm
- *Risk for Spiritual Distress* related to separation from religious support system, lack of privacy, or inability to practice spiritual rituals
- *Interrupted Family Process* related to disruption of routines, change in role responsibilities, and fatigue associated with increased workload and visiting hour requirements

The concept of high risk is not useful at the unit standard level. At this level, all or most clients are at risk, but not at *high* risk. For example, after surgery all individuals are at risk for infection, but not all are at high risk.

To document Level I standards of care, the nurse should use flow chart notations unless he or she finds unusual data or significant incidents occur. Although standards of care do not have to be part of the client's record, the record should specify what standards have been selected for the client. The problem list, representing the priority nursing diagnoses and collaborative problems for an individual client, can serve this purpose.

Level II—Standardized Care Plans

Preprinted care plans that represent care to provide for a client, family, or group in addition to the Level I unit standards of care, Level II standardized care plans are supplements to the generic unit standard. Thus, a client admitted to a medical unit will receive nursing care based on both Level I unit standards and the Level II standardized care plan for the specific condition that led to admission.

A Level II standardized care plan contains either a diagnostic cluster or a single nursing diagnosis or collaborative problem, such as *High Risk for Impaired Skin Integrity* or *PC: Fluid / Electrolyte Imbalances.* Figure 5.4 presents a Level II standardized care plan for the collaborative problem *PC: Hypo / Hyperglycemia.*

A diagnostic cluster Level II standard would contain additional nursing diagnoses and collaborative problems that are predicted to be present and prior because of a medical condition, surgical intervention, or therapy. For example, the following presents a problem list of the client who is 1 day after total hip replacement surgery, and the source of the care.

> *PC: Dislocation of Joint*
> *PC: Neurovascular Compromise*
> *PC: Emboli (fat, blood)*
> *Impaired Physical Mobility*
> *High Risk for Impaired Skin Integrity*
> *High Risk for Injury*
> *High Risk for Ineffective Therapeutic Regimen Management*
>
> } Client's problem list from Level II Standard—Post Total Hip Replacement

If this client also had diabetes mellitus, the nurse would add the following single diagnosis standard to the problem list: *PC: Hypo / Hyperglycemia.*

POTENTIAL COMPLICATION: HYPO/HYPERGLYCEMIA

Nursing Goal: The nurse will manage and minimize hypo- or hyperglycemia episodes.

1. Monitor for signs and symptoms of hypoglycemia:
   - Blood glucose <70 mg/dL
   - Pale, moist, cool skin
   - Tachycardia, diaphoresis
   - Jitteriness, irritability
   - Headache, slurred speech
   - Incoordination
   - Drowsiness
   - Visual changes
   - Hunger, nausea, abdominal pain
2. Follow protocols when indicated, *e.g.,* concentrated glucose (oral, IV).
3. Monitor for signs and symptoms of ketoacidosis:
   - Blood glucose >300 mg/dL
   - Positive plasma ketone, acetone breath
   - Headache, tachycardia
   - Kussmaul's respirations, decreased BP
   - Anorexia, nausea, vomiting
   - Polyuria, polydipsia
4. If ketoacidosis occurs, follow protocols, *e.g.,* initiation of IV fluids, insulin IV.
5. If episode is severe, monitor vital signs, urine output, specific gravity, ketones, blood glucose electrolytes q 30 mins or PRN.
6. Document blood glucose findings and other assessment data on flow record. Document unusual events or responses on progress notes.

FIGURE 5.4 Level II standardized care plan for *Potential Complication: Hypo/hyperglycemia.*

After the nursing staff are well oriented to the details of the unit standard, the diagnoses on the Level I unit standard can be omitted from individual client problem lists or care plans. Policy would indicate that this standard would apply to all the clients on the unit.

Level III—Addendum Care Plans

An addendum care plan lists additional interventions beyond the Level I and II standards that an individual client requires. These specific interventions may be added to a standardized care plan or may be associated with additional priority nursing diagnoses or collaborative problems not included on the Level II standardized care plan or Level I unit standards.

For many hospitalized clients, the nurse can direct initial care responsibility using standards of care. Assessment information obtained during subsequent nurse–client interactions may warrant specific additions to the client's care plan to ensure outcome achievement. The nurse can add or delete from standardized plans or handwrite or free-text (by computer) an addendum diagnosis with its applicable goals and interventions.

Problem List/Care Plan

As discussed earlier, a problem list represents the priority set of nursing diagnoses and collaborative problems that the nursing staff will manage for a particular client. When appropriate, the term *diagnostic* can be used in place of *problem* (ie, diagnostic list/care plan) to accommodate wellness diagnoses.

The problem list is a permanent chart record that identifies both the nursing diagnoses and collaborative problems receiving nursing management and also the source for interventions: standard of care, standardized care plan, or addendum care plan. Figure 5.5 illustrates a sample nursing problem list/care

NURSING PROBLEM LIST/CARE PLAN

NURSING DIAGNOSIS/ COLLABORATIVE PROBLEM	STATUS	STANDARD	ADDENDUM	EVALUATION OF PROGRESS					
Med Unit Standard	9/20 A	✔		9/21 P/LJC	9/22 P/Pw	9/23 P-GA			
PC: Hyperthermia	9/20			S/LJC	S/Iw	S-GA			
PC: Hyper/Hypoglycemia	9/20 A	✔							
Acute Pain	9/20 A	✔	✔						

STATUS CODE: A = Active   R = Resolved   RO = Ruled-out
EVALUATION CODE: S = Stable, I = Improved, *W = Worsened, U = Unchanged, *P = Not Progressing, P = Progressing

Reviewed With Client/Family ___9/21 LJC___ , _____ , _____ , (Date)

ADDENDUM CARE PLAN

Nsg Dx/ Coll Prob	Client/ Nursing Goals	Date/ Initials	Interventions
Acute Pain	—	9/23 LJC	1. Provide a gentle back rub in evening.
			2. Leave blanket at foot of bed for easy access.

Initials/Signature
1. LJC Lynda J. Carpenito   3.   5.   7.
2. Pw Poti Wychoff   4. G. Arcangelo   6.   8.

FIGURE 5.5   Sample problem list/care plan.

plan for a client with a history of type 1 diabetes mellitus who is admitted to a medical unit for treatment of pneumonia. This sample includes the client's priority set of diagnoses as well as the addendum interventions that the nurse has added to the standardized care plan under the diagnosis *Acute Pain*.

Case Study Applications of Care Planning

The following two case studies and related documentation illustrate care planning for the clients discussed. Functional health patterns are used in organizing the assessment and the analysis of the data.

CASE STUDY 1
Mrs. Gates, 42 years old, was recently diagnosed with metastatic carcinoma of the breast.

Medical History
Mrs. Gates went to see her medical doctor because of a lump under her left arm. After a biopsy confirmed a diagnosis of metastatic carcinoma of the breast, a mammogram revealed a lesion in the left breast. Mrs. Gates is scheduled for a left lower quadrant resection of the breast and node dissection today.

Medical Plan
Present
Schedule for surgery on Thursday 9/20
Schedule bone scan, liver scan, chest x-ray
Complete blood count and urinalysis
Blood studies
ECG

Future
Dr. Drong discussed with Mrs. Gates that approximately 3 weeks after surgery she will begin a course of chemotherapy to last 8 months.

Assessment Data	Assessment Conclusions
Health History	• Nursing Diagnoses (actual, risk, possible)
Appendectomy at age 21	• Positive Functioning
Menarche at age 13 with a 28-day cycle	• Collaborative Problems
Health Perception–Health Management Pattern	
Does not smoke	
Drinks 1 glass of wine with dinner	
*Nutritional–Metabolic Pattern**	
Elimination Pattern	*Colonic Constipation related to inadequate water intake, insufficient exercise* as evidenced by reports of BM q 3–4 days
Chronic constipation, which she treats with over-the-counter laxatives	
Bowel movement q 3–4 days	
*Activity–Exercise Pattern**	
Sleep–Rest Pattern	Effective sleep–rest pattern
Sleeps 7–8 h a night	
Retires at 11 PM, awakens at 6 AM	
Falls asleep easily	
Cognitive–Perceptual Pattern	Effective cognitive–perceptual pattern
Master's degree	
*Self-Perception Pattern**	
Role–Relationship Pattern	Positive role–relationship pattern
Married 22 years	
Relies on husband for daily support	
Married sister with 2 children (ages 12 and 14) lives 20 min away; they talk qod (every other day) on telephone and usually have Saturday or Sunday dinner together	

(continued)

CASE STUDY 1 (*Continued*)
*Sexuality–Reproductive Pattern**

Coping–Stress Management Pattern
Is worried what her husband will do without her at home (eg, meals)
Expressed concern about getting sick with chemotherapy
Related that her cousin, who had chemotherapy for leukemia, vomited all the time and lost all her hair but has been doing well for 5 years now

Value–Belief Pattern
Is active in her church (Lutheran)
Teaches Sunday school each week

Present Medical Status
Left lower quadrant resection of left breast and node dissection surgery 9/20

Fear related to cancer diagnosis, uncertainty about treatments and future

Positive Value–Belief Pattern
Postoperative Potential Complications:
  Bleeding
  Paralytic ileus

Below is the problem list for Mrs. Gates 1 day after surgery. It contains the priority nursing diagnoses and collaborative problems for this client and the status of each. The two diagnoses, *Chronic Constipation* and *Fear*, have both standardized and addendum interventions, as indicated by a check in each column (Standard, ACP).

Nursing Diagnosis/ Collaborative Problem	Status	Standard of Care	ACP (Addendum Care Plan)
1. Surgical Unit Standard	A 9/20	✓	
2. High Risk for Excess Fluid Volume: left arm related to effects of mastectomy and dependent positions	A 9/20	✓	
3. Colonic Constipation related to possible inadequate water intake, insufficient exercise as evidenced by reports of bowel movements q 3–4 days	A 9/20	✓	✓
4. Fear related to cancer diagnosis, uncertainty about treatments and future as evidenced by expressions of concern about chemotherapy and its success	A 9/21	✓	✓
5. High Risk for Ineffective Therapeutic Regimen Management related to lack of knowledge of arm exercises, self-breast exams, hazards to affected arm, community services	A 9/20	✓	

*Deferred. Because Mrs. Gates will be a 24-hour stay, with a morning admission, the nurse may defer some data collection.

CASE STUDY 2
J. S. is a 32-year-old admitted with bronchitis with an exacerbation of her asthma. She has not taken her medications for 1 month. You are assigned to her the first day after her evening admission through the E.R.

Medical History
Asthma, moderate
One–4 episodes of upper respiratory infection each year with E.R. visit, no known drug allergies.

Medical Diagnosis
Asthma Moderate
Bronchitis

(continued)

CASE STUDY 2 (*Continued*)
Medical Plan

Prednisone, refer to medical orders for dosage
Biaxin 500 mg bid 10 days
Advair inhaler 100/50 2 puffs bid
Proventyl inhaler 2 puffs

Admission Database

Health Perception–Health Maintenance Pattern

Up to date on immunizations, annual PAP, dental care yearly

Nutritional–Metabolic Pattern

Reports a usual daily intake of fruits, vegetables, meat, dairy and starches
Reports intake of water and diet soda

Elimination Pattern

Reports soft, formed BM

Activity–Exercise Pattern

Works as accountant
Aeorobic exercises at class 2–3 x week

Sleep–Rest Pattern

Retires at 10–11 PM
Arises at 6:30 AM

Cognitive–Perceptual Pattern

College degree
Wears glasses to read
Alert

Self-Perception Pattern

Rates outlook for future—7
(rate 0—poor, 10—very optimistic)

Role–Relationship Pattern

Divorced 7 years
Sees mother and sister weekly; has no children

Sexuality–Reproduction Pattern

Deferred Coping–Stress Management Pattern

No major losses in past year
Seeks advice from sister; when needed has two good friends she confides in

Value–Belief Pattern

Attends church 1–2 x month—Methodist

⊗ INTERACTIVE EXERCISE 5.4

You are a part-time nurse caring for JS today.

1. Examine the preceding data. For each of the following functional patterns, are there data to support:
   Positive functioning?
   Altered functioning?
   High risk for altered functioning?*
   A. Health Perception–Health Management Pattern
      Health practices
      Compliance?
      Injuries?
      Unhealthy lifestyle?
   B. Nutritional–Metabolic Pattern
      Nutrition?
      Fluid intake?
      Peripheral edema?
      Infection?
      Oral cavity health?
   C. Elimination Pattern
      Bowel elimination?
      Incontinence?
   D. Activity–Exercise Pattern
      Activities of daily living?
      Leisure activities?
      Home care?
      Respiratory function?
   E. Sleep–Rest Pattern
      Sleep?
   F. Cognitive–Perceptual Pattern
      Comfort?
      Knowledge?
      Sensory input?
   G. Self-Perception Pattern
      Anxiety/fear?
      Control?
      Self-concept?
   H. Role–Relationship Pattern
      Communication?
      Family?
      Loss?
      Parenting?
      Socialization?
      Violence?
   I. Sexuality–Reproductive Pattern
      Knowledge of?
      Sexuality?
   J. Coping–Stress Tolerance Pattern
      Coping?
   K. Value–Belief Pattern
      Spirituality?
2. Is there a physiologic complication present, or is there a *high* risk for one developing because of a disease, treatment, diagnostic study, or medication, that requires monitoring and joint management by you and a physician?
   Cardiac, circulatory
   Immune, hematopoietic
   Respiratory

*Copyright 1985, Lynda Juall Carpenito.

(continued)

INTERACTIVE EXERCISE 5.4 (*Continued*)

Renal
Neurologic
Muscular, skeletal
Reproductive
Endocrine, metabolic
Gastrointestinal, hepatic, biliary

3. After you have determined which functional patterns are altered or at risk for altered functioning, review the list of nursing diagnoses under that pattern and select the appropriate diagnosis.*
    A. If you select an actual diagnosis:
        Are there signs and symptoms to support its presence? (Refer to Section Two under the selected diagnosis.)
        Write the actual diagnosis in three parts: (1) label, (2) related to contributing factors, (3) as evidenced by signs and symptoms.
    B. If you select a risk or high-risk diagnosis:
        Do you have risk factors present?
        Write the diagnosis in two parts: (1) High Risk (label), (2) related to risk factors.
    C. Check each nursing diagnosis with the following review questions:*
        (1) Is the statement clearly stated?
        (2) Is the terminology correct?
        (3) Is there a two-part statement?
        (4) Does the second part of the statement reflect the specific factors that have contributed or may contribute to the development of the nursing diagnosis?
        (5) Is there documentation of validation (signs and symptoms) for actual diagnoses?
        (6) Does the nursing diagnosis statement reflect a situation for which a nurse can order the definitive interventions to treat or prevent?
        (7) Do you need additional client contact to individualize the diagnostic statement?
4. After you have identified which physiologic complications to monitor for, list them as:
    Potential Complications: (list here)
5. Write short-term outcome (client goals) for each actual and high-risk nursing diagnosis. Write nursing goals for collaborative problems.
6. Check each client goal with the following review questions:*
    A. Is the goal a client goal or a nursing goal?
    B. Is the goal realistic and attainable?
    C. Is it measurable? (Can the nurse validate it by seeing or hearing?)
    D. Are the verbs measurable (states, demonstrates) or not measurable (knows, understands, experiences)?
    E. Has the content been clearly specified (how much, when, where)?
    F. Can a time for achievement be realistically identified?
    G. Do you need additional client contact to individualize the goals?
7. Write interventions for both the nursing diagnoses and the collaborative problems.
8. Check each intervention with the following review questions:*
    A. Are the nursing orders clear (what, when, how often, how long, and where)?
    B. Do the nursing orders reflect creativity (and current practice)?
    C. Do you need additional client contact to individualize the interventions?

Refer to the end of the chapter for answers.

ANSWERS TO INTERACTIVE EXERCISES

5.2. The only appropriate choice is the fourth. If physician-prescribed interventions are needed when goals are not achieved, then the problem is a collaborative problem. The goals would be nursing goals, not client goals. The goals listed on page 41 should be replaced with "The nurse should monitor for changes in physiologic states and minimize complications."

5.3. You can see or hear goals 2 and 4. You cannot see or hear "accept," "know," or "understand." To measure knowledge or understanding, the person has to tell (hear) you what he or she knows or demonstrate (see) how to do something.

5.4. Priority Problem List with Goals

PC: Respiratory Insufficiency

Nursing Goals

The nurse will monitor to detect early signs and symptoms of respiratory insufficiency.

Indicators

> Respirations 16–20 breaths per minute
> Respirations even and no abnormal breath sounds

Ineffective therapeutic regimen management related to unknown etiology as evident by failure to take medications for asthma.

Outcome Criteria

Before discharge, the client will
1. Describe how often each inhaler is needed and why.
2. Describe when to contact her primary care office and why.

Discussion
Since J.S. has asthma, an assessment of her respiratory status is needed at least every 8 hours. This assessment would include peak flow respiratory rate and rhythm and evidence of wheezing.

J.S. reports she has not taken her medications for 1 month. The reason is not evident yet, so the related factor is unknown etiology. The nurse will seeks reasons and intervene with teaching.

TEN STEPS TO PUTTING IT ALL TOGETHER

Now you have learned the five steps in the nursing process. You will have the tools to create a plan of care (or care plan) for your assigned client.

Step 1: Assessment

If you interview your assigned client before you write your care plan, complete your assessment using the form recommended by your faculty. If you need to write a care plan before you can interview the client, go to Step 2 now. After you complete your assessment, you will now need to identify:

- Strengths
- Risk factors
- Problems in functioning

Strengths are qualities or factors that will help the person to recover, cope with stressors, and progress to his or her original health or as close as possible prior to hospitalization, illness, or surgery. The client's strengths can be used to motivate him or her to perform some difficult activities. Examples of strengths are:

- Positive spiritual framework
- Positive support system
- Ability to perform self-care
- No eating difficulties
- Effective sleep habits
- Alertness and good memory
- Financial stability
- Ability to relax most of the time
- Motivation

Write a list of your assigned client's strengths.

Risk factors are situations, personal characteristics, disabilities, or medical conditions that can hinder the person's ability to heal, cope with stressors, and progress to his or her original health prior to hospitalization, illness, or surgery. Examples of risk factors are as follows:

- No or ineffective support system
- No or little regular exercise
- Inadequate or poor nutritional habits
- Learning difficulties
- Denial
- Poor coping skills
- Communication problems
- Obesity
- Fatigue
- Limited ability to speak or understand English
- Memory problems
- Hearing problems
- Self-care problems before hospitalization
- Difficulty walking
- Financial problems

Write a list of risk factors for your assigned client.

Step 2: Same Day Assessment

If you have not completed a screening assessment of your assigned client, determine the following as soon as you can by asking the client, family, or nurse assigned to your client the following questions.

- Before hospitalization:
  — Could the client perform self-care?
  — Did the client need assistance?
  — Could the client walk unassisted?
  — Did the client have memory problems?
  — Did the client have hearing problems?
  — Did the client smoke cigarettes?
- What conditions or diseases does the client have that make him or her more vulnerable to:
  — Falling
  — Infection
  — Nutrition/fluid imbalance
  — Pressure ulcers
  — Severe or panic anxiety
  — Physiological instability (e.g., electrolytes, blood glucose, blood pressure, respiratory function, healing problems)
- When you meet the assigned client, determine if any of the risk factors are present:
  — Obesity
  — Impaired ability to speak/understand English
  — Movement difficulties
  — High anxiety

Write significant data on index card. Go to Step 3.

Step 3: Create Your Initial Care Plan

If your client is in the hospital for a medical problem, refer to the generic medical care plan in Appendix I (or online). If your client is in the hospital for a surgical condition, refer to the generic surgical care plan in Appendix II (or online). These generic care plans reflect the usual predicted care a client needs. Ask your instructor how you can use them to prevent excessive writing.

Step 4: Review the Collaborative Problems on the Generic Plan

- Review the collaborative problems listed. These are the physiological complications that you need to monitor. Do not delete any because they all relate to the condition or procedure that your client has had. You will need to add how often you should take vital signs, record intake and output, change dressings, etc. Ask the nurse you are assigned with for these times and review the Kardex, which also may have the time frames.
- Review each intervention for collaborative problems. Are any interventions unsafe or contra-indicated for your client? For example, if your client has edema and renal problems, the fluid requirements may be too high for him or her. Ask a nurse or instructor for help here.
- Review the collaborative problems on the standard plan. Also review all additional collaborative problems that you found that are related to any medical or treatment problems. For example, if your client has diabetes mellitus, you need to add:

PC: hypoglycemia/hyperglycemia

Step 5: Review the Nursing Diagnoses on the Standard Plan

Review each nursing diagnosis on the plan.

- Does it apply to your assigned client?
- Does your client have any risk factors (see your index card) that could make this diagnosis worse?

An example on the Generic Medical Care Plan is *Risk for Injury related to unfamiliar environment and physical or mental limitations secondary to condition, medication, therapies, or diagnostic tests.*

Now look at your list of risk factors for your assigned client. Can any factors listed contribute to the client's sustaining an injury? For example, is he or she having problems walking or seeing? Is he or she experiencing dizziness?

If your client has an unstable gait related to peripheral vascular disease (PVD), you would add the following diagnosis: *Risk for Injury related to unfamiliar environment and unstable gait secondary to peripheral vascular disease.*

Review each intervention for each nursing diagnosis:

- Are they relevant for your client?
- Will you have time to provide them?
- Are any interventions not appropriate or contraindicated for your assigned client?
- Can you add any specific interventions?
- Do you need to modify any interventions because of risk factors (see index card)?

Review the goals listed for the nursing diagnosis:

- Are they pertinent to your client?
- Can the client demonstrate achievement of the goal on the day you provide care?
- Do you need more time?

Delete goals that are inappropriate for your client. If your client will need more time to meet the goal, add "by discharge." If the client can accomplish the goal this day, write, "by (insert date)" after the goal.

Using the same diagnosis *Risk for injury related to unfamiliar environment and physical and mental limitations secondary to the condition, therapies, and diagnostic tests,* consider this goal:

The client will request assistance with ADLs.

Indicators
- Identify factors that increase risk of injury.
- Describe appropriate safety measures.

If it is realistic for your client to achieve all the goals on the day of your care, you should add the date to all of them. If your client is confused, you can add the date to the main goal, but you would delete all the indicators because the person is confused. Or you could modify the goal by writing:

Family member will identify factors that increase the client's risk of injury.

Remember that you cannot individualize a care plan for a client until you spend time with him or her, but you can add or delete interventions based on your preclinical knowledge of this client (e.g., medical diagnosis, coexisting medical conditions).

Step 6: Prepare the Care Plan (Written or Printed)

You can prepare the care plan by:

- Typing a generic care plan from this book into your word processor, then deleting or adding specifics for your client (use another color for additions/deletions or a different type font)
- Photocopying a care plan from this book, then adding or deleting specifics for your client
- Writing the care plan

Ask your faculty person what options are acceptable. Using different colors or fonts allows him or her to clearly see your analysis. Be prepared to provide rationales for why you added or deleted items.

Step 7: Initial Care Plan Completed

Now that you have a care plan of the collaborative problems and nursing diagnoses, which are associated with the primary condition for which your client was admitted? If your assigned client is a healthy adult undergoing surgery or was admitted for an acute medical problem and you have not assessed any significant factors in Step 1, you have completed the initial care plan. Go to Step 10.

Step 8: Additional Risk Factors

If your client has risk factors (on the index card) that you identified in Steps 1 and 2, evaluate if these risk factors make your assigned client more vulnerable to develop a problem. The following questions can help to determine if the client or family has additional diagnoses that need nursing interventions:

- Are additional collaborative problems associated with coexisting medical conditions that require monitoring (e.g., hypoglycemia)?
- Are there additional nursing diagnoses that, if not managed or prevented now, will deter recovery or affect the client's functional status (e.g., *High Risk for Constipation*)?
- What problems does the client perceive as priority?
- What nursing diagnoses are important but treatment for them can be delayed without compromising functional status?

You can address nursing diagnoses not on the priority list by referring the client for assistance after discharge (e.g., counseling, weight loss program).

Priority identification is a very important but difficult concept. Because of shortened hospital stays and because many clients have several chronic diseases at once, nurses cannot address all nursing diagnoses for every client. Nurses must focus on those for which the client would be harmed or not make progress if they were not addressed. Ask your clinical faculty to review your list. Be prepared to provide rationales for your selections.

Step 9: Evaluate the Status of Your Client (After You Provide Care)

Collaborative Problems

Review the nursing goals for the collaborative problems:

- Assess the client's status.
- Compare the data to established norms (indicators).
- Judge if the data fall within acceptable ranges.
- Conclude if the client is stable, improved, unimproved, or worse.

Is your client stable or improved?

- If yes, continue to monitor the client and to provide interventions indicated.
- If not, has there been a dramatic change (e.g., elevated blood pressure and decreased urinary output)? Have you notified the physician or advanced practice nurse? Have you increased your monitoring of the client? Communicate your evaluations of the status of collaborative problems to your clinical faculty and to the nurse assigned to your client.

Nursing Diagnosis

Review the goals or outcome criteria for each nursing diagnosis. Did the client demonstrate or state the activity defined in the goal? If yes, then communicate (document) the achievement on your plan. If not and the client needs more time, change the target date. If time is not the issue, evaluate why the client did not achieve the goal. Was the goal:

- Not realistic because of other priorities?
- Not acceptable to the client?

Step 10: Document the Care on the Agency's Forms, Flow Records, and Progress Notes

NURSING DIAGNOSES: ISSUES AND CONTROVERSIES

Nursing diagnosis arouses some emotion in almost every nurse. Responses range from apathy to excitement, from rejection to enthusiasm for scientific investigation. Although nursing diagnoses have been an accepted part of professional nursing practice for more than 25 years, some nurses continue to resist using them. This chapter explores some of the most commonly cited reasons for doing so, including the following:

- Why can't we just use the words we've always used?
- Other disciplines will not understand our diagnoses.
- Clients will not understand our diagnoses.
- Nurse practitioners, nurse anesthetists, and nurse midwives do not need nursing diagnoses.
- Nursing diagnoses are not culturally sensitive.
- Labeling behaviors is unethical.
- Nursing diagnoses can violate confidentiality.

Why Can't We Just Use the Words We've Always Used?

What words have nurses always used? Diabetes mellitus? Prematurity? Pneumonia? Difficult? Cystic fibrosis? For many years, nurses used only medical diagnoses to describe the client problems that they addressed. Gradually, however, nurses have learned that medical diagnoses do not describe many client problems in sufficient detail to enable other nurses to provide continuing care for clients with special needs.

Early on, Abdellah and Levine (1965, p. 25) pointed to the need for a specialized nursing language to describe nursing practice:

> Crucial to the development of nursing science is the nurse's ability to make a nursing diagnosis and prescribe nursing actions that will result in specific responses in the client. Nursing diagnosis is a determination of the nature and extent of nursing problems presented by individual clients or families receiving nursing care. The position is taken that it is an independent function of the professional nurse to make a nursing diagnosis and to decide upon a course of action to be followed for the solution of the problem.

Until 1973, when the first Conference for the Classification of Nursing Diagnosis convened, some attempts at classifying nursing actions were made but were not sustained (eg, Henderson's needs, Abdellah's 21 nursing problems).

The fact is that nurses always have shared with other disciplines, such as medicine, respiratory therapy, and physical therapy, a common language for certain client problems. Examples of terms from this language include *hypokalemia, hypovolemic shock, hyperglycemia,* and *increased intracranial pressure.* Any attempt to rename labels such as these should be viewed as foolhardy and unnecessary. For instance, *dysrhythmias* should not be renamed *decreased cardiac output,* nor should *hyperglycemia* be relabeled as *altered carbohydrate metabolism.*

This author takes the position that nurses should use pre-established terminology when appropriate, whether as a collaborative problem (eg, *Potential Complication: Hyperglycemia*) or as a nursing diagnosis (eg, *Risk for Pressure Ulcer*). Nursing should continue to use the terminology that clearly communicates a client situation or problem to other nurses and other disciplines.

Having said this, let us now examine the discipline-specific language of nurses. Have nurses had a common language or set of labels for client problems that they diagnose and treat in addition to the shared language previously discussed? Before the advent of nursing diagnoses, how did nurses describe client problems such as

- Inability to dress self
- Difficulty selecting among treatment options

- Risk for infection
- Breast-feeding problems
- Ineffective cough
- Spiritual dilemmas

Sometimes a nurse would use the terms listed above, but sometimes not. Often, the nurse had many options available to describe a problem. For example, a nurse could use any of the following terms to describe a client at risk for pressure ulcers:

- Immobility
- Comatose
- Decubitus ulcers
- Reddened skin
- Incontinence
- Inability to turn in bed
- Bed sores
- Paralysis

An examination of this list reveals the inconsistency of the terms. Some are signs and symptoms. Some are causative factors. Some are risk factors. Some are problems.

Some nurses, particularly those with much experience, want to be able to describe client problems in any way they wish. Although an experienced nurse may be able to decipher inconsistent terminology, how can the nursing profession teach its science to its students if each instructor, textbook, and staff nurse uses different words to describe the same situation? Consider medicine: How could medical students learn the difference between cirrhosis and cancer of the liver if "impaired liver function" was used to describe both situations? Medicine relies on a standardized classification system to teach its science and to communicate client problems to other disciplines. Nursing needs to do likewise.

So, although nurses traditionally have had a common language for certain problems, this language has been incomplete to describe all the client responses that nurses diagnose and treat. It also is important to emphasize that some responses labeled as nursing diagnoses (eg, *Decisional Conflict, Powerlessness*) were nonexistent in the nursing literature as recently as 15 years ago. The official classification of these responses as nursing diagnoses has advanced their investigation and increased their presence in the nursing literature. For example, whereas in 1982 there were two citations in the literature on powerlessness, the number increased to 113 by 1994.

Other Disciplines Will Not Understand Our Diagnoses

According to Seahill (1991), the use of nursing diagnosis in a multidisciplinary inpatient child psychiatry setting proved problematic because this setting emphasized the "whole patient" and the importance of effective information sharing among disciplines. Let us examine the validity of this assertion. For the purposes of this discussion, health care disciplines are separated into three groups: medicine, licensed health care disciplines, and nonlicensed health care personnel.

Medicine

Because it is important for nurses to understand certain aspects of medical diagnoses, nurses have committed to learning them and to be knowledgeable about current changes in conditions and treatments. But as physicians originally defined these conditions, how often did they say, "Do you think that nurses will understand (for example) disseminated intravascular coagulation?" Most likely never.

If it is important for a physician to understand such nursing diagnoses as *Spiritual Distress* or *Decisional Conflict,* then the physician can seek the pertinent knowledge as a nurse does. The nurse also should share information with the physician concerning nursing diagnoses that the client and nurse have identified as priorities. Multidisciplinary conferences provide an opportunity for this sharing. Some nursing diagnoses may prove useful to some physicians, such as those in primary care.

Licensed Health Care Disciplines

In addition to nursing, licensed health care disciplines include physical, occupational, speech, nutritional, respiratory, and recreational therapies and social service. Each of these disciplines is involved in care planning for clients—some in their individual departments and some as part of multidisciplinary teams. These disciplines should be introduced to the language of nursing diagnosis and encouraged to use any applicable diagnoses. Box 6-1 lists examples of nursing diagnoses that are often useful to other disciplines.

Sharing nursing diagnosis terminology with other disciplines can only strengthen the role of nursing and emphasize a multidisciplinary approach. Keep in mind, however, that other disciplines should not use nursing diagnoses to determine interventions that nurses should perform. For example, a physical therapist using the nursing diagnosis *Impaired Physical Mobility* will write interventions only for physical therapy, not for nursing. Refer to Chapter 5 for a discussion of multidisciplinary care planning.

Nonlicensed Health Care Personnel

In most acute, long-term, and community health care settings in the United States and Canada, registered nurses, licensed practical nurses, and registered nurse assistants, nursing aides, or technicians provide nursing care. It is not important that all nursing team members understand nursing diagnoses, but it is important for each team member to understand the interventions for which he or she is responsible. For example, an aide may be expected to explain why a client needs to be repositioned every 2 h and given assistance to the bathroom after eating, but may not be expected to explain the difference between functional and total incontinence.

Clients Will Not Understand Our Diagnoses

It is important for the client and family to understand and agree with nursing diagnoses and the associated goals and interventions. The nurse should emphasize to the client and family that nursing diagnosis terminology is designed primarily to give nurses consistent language for communicating this information. The nurse also can explain why a medical diagnosis does not describe the client's problems or concerns from a nurse–client perspective. Keep in mind that, regardless of the specific terminology used, the nurse must tailor all explanations to the client's and family's ability and readiness to learn, cultural background, educational level, and so forth. This will help promote understanding and decision making.

⦿ BOX 7.1 EXAMPLES OF NURSING DIAGNOSES USEFUL FOR OTHER DISCIPLINES

Physical Therapy

Self-Care Deficit
High Risk for Injury
Impaired Physical Mobility
Noncompliance
Unilateral Neglect
Fatigue

Occupational Therapy

Deficient Diversional Activity
Fatigue
Impaired Home Maintenance
Instrumental Self-Care Deficit

Social Service

Caregiver Role Strain
Ineffective Family Coping
Decisional Conflict
Interrupted Family Processes
Impaired Home Maintenance
Instrumental Self-Care Deficit
Social Isolation

Speech Therapy

Impaired Communication
Impaired Swallowing
Disturbed Thought Processes

Nutritional Therapy

Imbalanced Nutrition: More Than Body Requirements
Imbalanced Nutrition: Less Than Body Requirements
Impaired Swallowing
Feeding Self-Care Deficit

Respiratory Therapy

High Risk for Aspiration
High Risk for Impaired Respiratory Function
Ineffective Airway Clearance
Dysfunctional Weaning Response

Nurse Practitioners, Nurse Anesthetists, and Nurse Midwives Do Not Need Nursing Diagnoses*

Advanced nursing practice has been a hot topic of discussion in nursing circles and legislative forums. Many state boards of nursing have defined or are in the process of defining advanced practice. For example, the Florida Board of Nursing defines an advanced registered nurse practitioner as "educated to perform in the monitoring and altering of drug therapies and initiation of appropriate therapies according to the established protocol and consistent with the practice setting" (1988, p. 16). The 2002 annual update in the journal *Nurse Practitioner* presented the legislation for reimbursement and prescriptive authority and the source of the legal authority for nurses in advanced practice. All states grant nurse practitioners some form of prescriptive authority; in 12 states, nurse practitioners can prescribe independently (Pearson, 2002). In the last 10 years, prescriptive and protocol authority for certain nurses has come to be equated with advanced practice.

In reality, nurse practitioners are responsible for diagnosing medical problems and initiating treatment. For some acute conditions (eg, respiratory infection), this diagnosis may be all that is needed. If, however, a client returns with repeated infections, then the nurse practitioner needs to obtain more data to ensure that another medical diagnosis is not present or to identify poor client health habits (eg, inadequate rest or nutrition) that may be contributing to the problem.

An editorial in the *Journal of Pediatric Nurse Practitioners* described nursing diagnoses as "a separate language that is often burdensome and has the potential to be misunderstood by those not educated in the use of the language" (Nelms, 1991). The writer went on to state, "as editor of this journal, I find few [pediatric nurse practitioners] submit articles that include nursing diagnoses. Is that because we do not use them?" (Nelms, 1991).

Advanced nurses demonstrate expert nursing practice by diagnosing client responses to varied situations (eg, medical diagnoses, personal or maturational crises), which are nursing diagnoses. An advanced nurse would explore such questions as:

• How has the client's ability to function changed since his cerebrovascular accident?
• How has a family system changed, or how is it vulnerable because of an ill newborn who required several months of hospitalization?

Compared with nursing, medicine has little to offer clients and families experiencing chronic disease such as multiple sclerosis or diabetes. Clients' most common complaints do not involve the medical care they receive, but rather focus on dissatisfaction with how their other problems are addressed. Nurses are in the optimum position to address such problems and increase client satisfaction with health care.

Certain complex nursing diagnoses may be beyond the scope of practice of the average registered nurse. Examples of such advanced nursing diagnoses include the following:

• *Risk for Caregiver Stress*
• *Powerlessness*
• *Risk for Ineffective Coping*
• *Risk for Altered Parenting*

A nurse cannot learn the diagnosis and treatment of advanced nursing diagnoses on the job. Rather, he or she must study the theory and concepts behind them to learn how to put them into practice. Nursing science is no less rigorous, less scientific, or less difficult to learn than medical science. If nurses in advanced practice do not use nursing diagnosis terminology, but only treat the nursing diagnosis concept, they fail to define their practice as nursing.

Nurse practitioners, nurse anesthetists, or nurse midwives who do not formulate or treat nursing diagnoses may be too focused on medicine. To evaluate this practice, a nurse in advanced practice should ask: Do I consult with physician colleagues for complex medical problems? Do physicians consult with me for complex nursing diagnoses? If the answer is no, the nurse should explore why. Does the problem lie with the physician's attitude, or is the nurse not overtly demonstrating diagnosis and treatment of nursing diagnoses? Or is the nurse not practicing nursing?

If nurse practitioners, nurse anesthetists, and nurse midwives do not define their practice as advanced nurses, as diagnosing and treating selected medical diagnoses using protocols, and as formulating and

---

*Excerpted from Carpenito, L. J. (1992, February). *Are nurse practitioners expert nurses?* Paper presented at the 11th Annual National Nursing Symposium, Advanced Practice Within a Restructured Health Care Environment, Los Angeles.

treating nursing diagnoses, 5 years from now these nurses may still be struggling to define their roles. Carpenito (1995) uses nursing diagnoses to differentiate the discipline-specific expertise of nurse practitioners and physicians in primary care. Figure 7.1 illustrates this relationship.

Nursing Diagnoses Are Not Culturally Sensitive

Nursing diagnoses, specifically the NANDA classifications, have been accused of being insensitive to cultural considerations. According to Leininger (1990), major concerns with the NANDA classifications are the "problems of using, promoting, and implementing the taxonomy with such limited international or transcultural data, including theoretical cultural ideas, conditions, and practices in diverse cultures." Leininger (1990) also states that there are "a host of culture-specific illnesses and culture-bound syndromes that need to be documented and understood by nurses," because expressions of health care, wellness, and illness are different in different cultures.

NANDA is the clearinghouse for nursing diagnosis work from nurses in the United States, Canada, Europe, Asia, and South America. Nursing diagnoses accepted by NANDA are based primarily on the dominant Anglo-American cultural values, norms, and standards. Never has this work been portrayed or disseminated as relevant to other cultures. Clearly, North America is home to hundreds of distinctly diverse ethnic groups, but the NANDA classifications do not address this cultural diversity.

How can nursing diagnosis represent the wide cultural diversity in North America? Only those nurses who deeply understand a particular culture can develop the culture-specific defining characteristics and risk factors to make a nursing diagnosis relevant. For example, Native American nurses

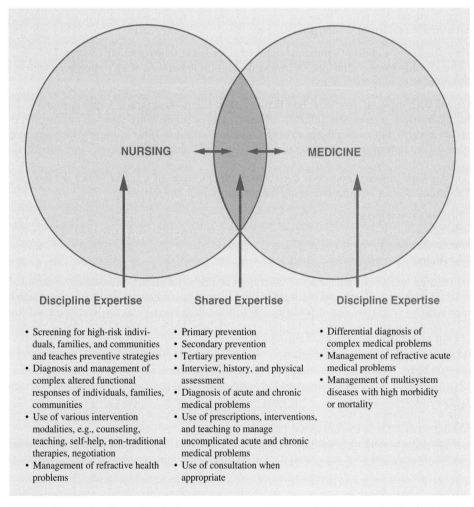

FIGURE 7.1 Domains of expertise of primary care nurse practitioners and primary care physicians. (© 1995, by Lynda Juall Carpenito; written permission needed to duplicate.)

and non–Native American nurses who care for Native American clients can examine NANDA's work and determine its relevance to Native American culture. They can promote necessary additions and revisions to the NANDA classifications and also can develop and submit culturally specific responses currently not on the NANDA list.

Many texts on nursing diagnosis have been translated for use outside North America. Although nurses from different cultures do these translations, all too often they do not address important cultural differences. If nursing diagnosis is determined to be useful as a concept, then nurses in other countries will need to develop diagnoses relevant to their particular cultures. The following two books specifically address nursing diagnoses from different cultural perspectives: *Planification des Soins Infirmiers* (Grondin, Lussier, Phaneuf & Riopelle, 1990) from a French-Canadian perspective, and *Diagnostico de Enfermeria* (Luis, 2002) from a Spanish perspective.

Keep in mind that a nursing diagnosis is not a judgment that nurses make about a client's or family's responses, values, or health based on *their own* cultural perspectives. Rather, it represents a response that the client or family finds problematic according to the cultural perspective. For example, some cultures believe in fatalism (ie, outside forces control one's fate and health). The nurse unfamiliar with this belief may incorrectly diagnose the problem as *Powerlessness.*

Transcultural Considerations are incorporated into Section Two to increase the nurse's appreciation of cultural diversity.

Nursing Diagnosis Is Unethical

Some have criticized nursing diagnosis as emphasizing problem-based practice, encouraging professional arrogance, and requiring "value judgments by nurses about another's way of living, viewing self, being or relating with others" (Mitchell, 1991, p. 102). Case studies cited in the literature (Mitchell, 1991) of nursing diagnosis causing poor or unethical nursing care are interesting. Close examination of these cases reveals that the origin of the unacceptable nursing care rested in the nurse, not in the nursing diagnosis. Obviously, unsatisfactory, irresponsible, and unethical nursing care existed before the advent of nursing diagnosis.

According to Mitchell (1991), "when an individual's definition of health is not consistent with the nurse's, the person's health value is judged as ineffective, maladaptive, or dysfunctional" (p. 100). The nurse's determination of a client's response as ineffective, maladaptive, or dysfunctional should be based on the client's perspective of the problem and on the nurse's knowledge and expertise. A client's ineffective response is not ineffective for the nurse, but rather is ineffective for the client.

To illustrate, let us examine the diagnosis *Dysfunctional Grieving,* with the defining characteristics of unsuccessful adaptation to loss, prolonged denial, depression, and delayed emotional reaction. How can a nurse diagnose dysfunctional grieving? What may be a sign or symptom of dysfunctional grieving in one person may not be such in another. The question is: For whom is the grieving dysfunctional? The client? The family? Or the nurse? For grieving to be dysfunctional, it must be dysfunctional for the person experiencing the grief. For example, if a mother visits the gravesite of her deceased child every day for 1 year after the child's death, is this dysfunctional? To determine if it is, the nurse should explore with this client whether these visits interfere with other necessary or enjoyable activities. What does she do when she is not visiting the gravesite? What would happen if she decreased the visits? Only through such a dialogue could the nurse and client be able to identify whether the client's grieving is dysfunctional or whether, perhaps, the client finds the visits comforting and an effective coping mechanism.

Nursing Diagnoses Can Violate Confidentiality

Nurses and other health professionals commonly are privy to significant personal concerns of clients under their care. According to the American Nurses Association Code of Ethics, "the nurse safeguards the client's right to privacy by judiciously protecting information of a confidential nature." The professional mandate to apply the nursing process for all clients, however, sometimes places the nurse in a position of conflict. Certain information recorded in assessments and diagnostic statements may compromise a client's right to privacy, choice, or confidentiality. Nurses should never use nursing diagnostic statements to influence others to view or treat an individual, family, or group negatively. They must take great caution to ensure that a nursing diagnosis does no harm!

Nurses have a responsibility to make nursing diagnoses and to prescribe nursing treatments. Inherent in the diagnostic process and planning of care is the responsibility to ascertain that there is permission to write, treat, or refer the diagnosis as appropriate.

When a client shares personal information or emotions with the nurse, does this information automatically become part of the client's record or care plan? The nurse has two basic obligations to a client: (1) to address applicable nursing diagnoses and (2) to protect the client's confidentiality. The nurse is *not* obligated to pass on all of a client's nursing diagnoses to other nurses, as long as the nurse can ensure that all diagnoses are addressed.

Consider the following example: Ms. Jackson, 45 years old, is hospitalized for treatment of ovarian cancer. At one point, she states to the nurse, "the God I worship did this to me, and I hate Him for it." Further discussion validates that Ms. Jackson is disturbed about her feelings and changes in her previous beliefs. From these assessment data, the nurse develops the nursing diagnosis *Spiritual Distress related to conflict between disease occurrence and religious faith.* But what should the nurse do with the information, which Ms. Jackson makes clear she considers confidential? The nurse can assist Ms. Jackson with this nursing diagnosis through several different avenues:

1. Apprising her of available community resources for follow-up assistance in dealing with her spiritual distress
2. Continuing to assist her to explore her feelings and using the nurse's notes to reflect discussions (without using quotation marks to denote her actual words)
3. Recording the nursing diagnosis *Spiritual Distress* on the care plan and developing appropriate interventions
4. Referring her to an appropriate spiritual advisor

Option 1 returns the problem to the client for management after discharge. Sometimes the nature of a problem and its priority among the client's other problems make providing the client or family with information on available resources for use after discharge the most appropriate option. The nurse should, however, be cautioned against using this option merely to "wash one's hands" of a problem.

Option 2 allows the nurse to continue a dialogue with the client about the issue, but without divulging it specifically. The problem with this option is that the client's care plan will not reflect this problem as a nursing diagnosis on the active list. As a result, should the client's nurse become unable to care for the client, this diagnosis likely would not be addressed.

Option 3 incorporates the problem, as a nursing diagnosis, into the client's care plan, where the entire nursing staff can address it. To help protect the confidentiality of very sensitive disclosed information, the nurse should make a few modifications, such as not quoting the client's statements exactly.

Documentation of the nursing diagnosis on the care plan raises another possible dilemma. What if the primary nurse in whom the client or family has confided cannot follow the diagnosis full-time? How can the primary nurse involve others in addressing this diagnosis without violating the client's confidentiality? The primary nurse should encourage the client to allow another nurse to intervene in his or her absence. If the client refuses referral or another nurse, the nurse should document this in the progress notes, continuing to protect the client's confidentiality. For example:

> *Discussed with Ms. Jackson the feasibility of another nurse intervening with her regarding her spiritual concerns in my absence. Ms. Jackson declined involvement of another nurse. Instructed her on whom to contact if she changes her mind.*

This note documents the nurse's responsibility to the client as well as the nurse's accountability.

It is also important to note that, in most cases, the nurse should not share confidential information with family members without the client's permission. Exceptions to preserving confidentiality, however, "may be necessary if the information the client shares with the nurse contains indications of a threat to the lives of the patient or others" (Curtin & Flaherty, 1982).

Option 4 is a commonly chosen action for clients with spiritual conflicts. Before referring a client, however, the nurse should ascertain the client's receptivity to such a referral. To assume receptivity without first consulting the client can be problematic. The client chose to share very personal information with a particular nurse, who then is obligated to assist the client with the problem. If the nurse believes that a religious leader or another professional would be beneficial to the client, the nurse should approach the client with the option. An example of such a dialogue follows:

> *Ms. Jackson, we've been discussing your concerns about your illness and how it has changed your spiritual beliefs. I know someone who has been very helpful for people with concerns similar to yours. I'd like to ask her to visit you. What do you think about this?*

Such a dialogue clearly designates the choice as Ms. Jackson's. Just as nurses have an obligation to inform clients and families of available resources, clients have the right to accept or reject these resources.

Summary

Nursing diagnosis has sparked much debate. Too often, those opposed to nursing diagnosis practice in isolation as primary providers and see no need for diagnoses in their nurse–client relationships. If they engage in therapeutic interventions, they are engaged in treating phenomena. They see no need for diagnoses, yet they must analyze responses, which directs them to future interventions. If intervening is not part of a nurse–client relationship, then perhaps there is no nurse–client relationship. Nursing actively assists clients, families, or communities to reduce or eliminate problems, reduce risk factors, prevent problems, and promote healthier lifestyles.

Nursing diagnosis provides nursing with a framework within which to organize its science. It is, however, each individual nurse's responsibility to apply nursing diagnoses with caution and care.

Manual of Nursing Diagnoses

INTRODUCTION

The *Manual of Nursing Diagnoses* consists of nursing diagnoses. They are described with the three NANDA-required elements first:

- Definition
- Defining characteristics, signs and symptoms, or risk factors of the diagnosis
- Related factors, organized according to pathophysiologic, treatment-related, situational, and maturational, that may contribute to or cause the actual diagnosis

Additional components include the following:

- *Author's Note,* which clarifies the concept and clinical use of the diagnosis
- *Errors in Diagnostic Statements,* which explain common mistakes in formulating diagnoses and ways to correct them
- *Key Concepts,* which list scientific explanations about the diagnosis and interventions, categorized as *Generic, Pediatric, Maternal, Geriatric,* and *Transcultural Considerations*
- *Focus Assessment Criteria,* subjective and objective, which serve to guide specific data collection to help confirm or rule out the diagnosis

Each diagnosis has one group of interventions that focuses on the treatment associated with the diagnostic label, regardless of the etiologic and contributing factors, with outcome criteria. Interventions specifically direct the nurse to:

- Clarify causative and contributing factors
- Reduce or eliminate the factors
- Promote selected activities
- Teach healthy choices and make referrals

Some diagnoses are further explained by one or more specific nursing diagnoses, which were selected because of their frequency in nursing. They do not in any way represent exclusive categories. For example, *Activity Intolerance* has specific contributing factors:

- Related to insufficient knowledge of adaptive techniques needed secondary to *chronic obstructive pulmonary disease*
- Related to insufficient knowledge of adaptive techniques needed secondary to *impaired cardiac function*
- Related to bed rest *deconditioning*

Some diagnoses have population-specific interventions for children, pregnant women, and older adults.

A bibliography organized by Nursing Diagnoses is found at the end of Section Two. Internet sites are cited when useful.

Activity Intolerance
   Related to Insufficient Knowledge of Adaptive Techniques Needed Secondary to COPD
   Related to Insufficient Knowledge of Adaptive Techniques Needed Secondary to Impaired
      Cardiac Function
   Related to Bed Rest Deconditioning

ACTIVITY INTOLERANCE

DEFINITION

Activity Intolerance: A reduction in one's physiologic capacity to endure activities to the degree desired or required (Magnan, 1987)

DEFINING CHARACTERISTICS
Major (Must Be Present)

An altered physiologic response to activity

Respiratory
Dyspnea   Excessively increased rate
Shortness of breath   Decreased rate

Pulse
Weak   Decreased
Excessively increased   Failure to return to pre-
Rhythm change   activity level after 3 min

Blood Pressure
Failure to increase with   Increased diastolic pressure
   activity   >15 mm Hg

Minor (May Be Present)

Weakness   Fatigue
Pallor or cyanosis   Confusion
Vertigo

RELATED FACTORS

Any factors that compromise oxygen transport, physical conditioning, or create excessive energy demands that outstrip the person's physical and psychological abilities can cause activity intolerance. Some common factors are listed below.

Pathophysiologic

Related to compromised oxygen transport system secondary to:
Cardiac
Cardiomyopathies   Congestive heart failure
Dysrhythmias   Angina
Myocardial infarction   Valvular disease
Congenital heart disease

Respiratory
Chronic obstructive   Bronchopulmonary dysplasia
   pulmonary disease (COPD)   Atelectasis

Circulatory

Anemia	Peripheral arterial disease
Hypovolemia	

Related to increased metabolic demands secondary to:
Acute or chronic infections

Viral infection	Mononucleosis
Endocrine or metabolic disorders	Hepatitis

Chronic diseases

Renal	Hepatic
Inflammatory	Musculoskeletal
Neurologic	

Related to inadequate energy sources secondary to:

Obesity	Inadequate diet
Malnourishment	

Treatment-Related

Related to increased metabolic demands secondary to:

Malignancies	Surgery
Diagnostic studies	Treatment schedule/frequency

Related to compromised oxygen transport secondary to:

Hypovolemia	Prolonged bed rest

Situational (Personal, Environmental)

Related to inactivity secondary to:

Depression	Sedentary lifestyle
Lack of motivation	

Related to increased metabolic demands secondary to:
Assistive equipment (walkers, crutches, braces)
Extreme stress
Pain
Environmental barriers (eg, stairs)
Climate extremes (especially hot, humid climates)
Air pollution (eg, smog)
Atmospheric pressure (eg, recent relocation to high-altitude living)

Maturational

Older adults may have decreased muscle strength and flexibility, as well as sensory deficits. These factors can undermine body confidence and may contribute directly or indirectly to activity intolerance.

ⓧ **AUTHOR'S NOTE**

Activity Intolerance is a diagnostic judgment that describes a person with compromised physical conditioning. This person can engage in therapies to increase strength and endurance. Moreover, in *Activity Intolerance,* the goal is to increase tolerance to activity; in *Fatigue,* the goal is to assist the person to adapt to the fatigue, not to increase endurance.

ⓧ **ERRORS IN DIAGNOSTIC STATEMENTS**

1. *Activity Intolerance related to dysrhythmic episodes in response to increased activity secondary to recent MI*

   The current goals would be to monitor cardiac response to activity and to prevent decreased cardiac output, not to increase tolerance to activity. This situation would be labeled more appropriately as a collaborative problem: *PC: Decreased Cardiac Output.*

2. *Activity Intolerance related to fatigue secondary to chemotherapy*

   Rest does not relieve fatigue associated with chemotherapy, nor is such fatigue amenable to interventions to increase endurance. The correction would be: *Fatigue related to anemia and chemical changes secondary to toxic effects of chemotherapy.*

KEY CONCEPTS
Generic Considerations

- *Endurance* is the ability to continue a specified task; *fatigue* is the inability to continue a specified task. Conceptually, endurance and fatigue are opposites. Nursing interventions, such as work simplification, aim to delay task-related fatigue by maximizing efficient use of the muscles that control motion, movement, and locomotion.
- The ability to maintain a given level of performance depends on *personal factors:* strength, coordination, reaction time, alertness, and motivation; and on *activity-related factors:* frequency, duration, and intensity.
- In normal people, the work of breathing is very limited. In those with COPD, however, it may increase five to ten times above normal. Under such conditions, the oxygen required *just for breathing* may be a large fraction of total oxygen consumption.
- The effects of bed rest deconditioning develop rapidly and may take weeks or months to reverse. All people confined to bed are at risk for activity intolerance as a result of bed rest–induced deconditioning.

Pediatric Considerations

- Children at special risk for activity intolerance include those with respiratory conditions, cardiovascular conditions, anemia, and chronic illnesses (Wong, 2003).
- Research shows that supervised exercise training at moderate intensity is safe and produces significant beneficial changes in hemodynamics and exercise time in children with cardiac disease (Balfour, 1991).

Geriatric Considerations

- Decreased cardiac output in older adults has been attributed to disease-related, not age-related, processes (Miller, 2004). Fleg (1986) found no age-related changes in resting cardiac output in a study of healthy people between 30 and 80 years of age.
- Studies have demonstrated an average decline of 5% to 10% per decade in maximum oxygen consumption (VO_2max) from 25 to 75 years of age. Very athletic people have declines in VO_2max; however, it is only half of the 10% per decade decline that less athletic people exhibit. There seems to be either decreased efficiency in mobilizing blood to exercising muscles or increased difficulty for muscles to extract and use oxygen because of decreased muscle mass.
- By 75 years of age, only 10% of the pacemaker cells in the SA node remain, which could account for slowed conduction during exercise.
- Prolonged immobility and inactivity through self-imposed restrictions, mental status changes, or pathophysiologic changes can contribute to decreased activity tolerance (Cohen et al., 2000).
- Decreased muscle mass leads to decreased strength, which, in turn, leads to decreased endurance. Muscle strength, which is maximal between 20 to 30 years of age, drops to 80% of that value by 65 years of age (Cohen, Gorenberg & Schader, 2000).
- Increased chest wall rigidity with aging leads to decreased lung expansion, resulting in decreased tissue oxygenation. This immediately affects activity tolerance.

Focus Assessment Criteria

Assessing for activity intolerance is a dynamic process that starts before activity, proceeds continuously throughout, and terminates in postactivity evaluation. During preactivity assessment, the nurse establishes baseline "at rest" measurements of blood pressure, pulse, and respiration. If pathology is known in a particular organ system, then assessment during activity focuses on signs and symptoms indicating intolerance in that system (eg, exertional dyspnea in pulmonary disease, angina in cardiac disease, increased spasticity in neuromuscular disease). During postactivity evaluation, the nurse assesses recovery time, the time required for blood pressure, pulse, and respiration to return to preactivity levels, which reflects physiologic tolerance for activity.

Subjective Data

Assess for Defining Characteristics.

Weakness   Fatigue
Dyspnea

Assess for Related Factors.

Lack of incentive
Lack of confidence in ability to perform activity
Pain that interferes with performance of activities
Fear of injury or aggravating disease as a result of participation in activity

Objective Data

Assess for Defining Characteristics.

Assess strength and balance; evaluate person's ability to:

Reposition self in bed   Maintain erect posture
Rise to standing position   Perform activities of daily
Ambulate   living (ADLs)
Assume and maintain
  sitting position

Assess response to activity:

1. Take resting vital signs (Table II.1): pulse (rate, rhythm, quality); respirations (rate, depth, effort); and blood pressure.
2. Have person perform the activity.
3. Take vital signs immediately after the activity.
4. Have person rest for 3 min; take vital signs again. Compare finding with resting vital signs (Table II.1).
5. Assess for pallor, cyanosis, confusion, and vertigo.

Assess for Related Factors.

Situational
Personal
Coping strategies focusing   Inadequate social support
  on avoidance

TABLE II.1 Physiology Response to Activity (Expected and Abnormal)

	Pulse	Blood Pressure	Respiration
Resting			
Normal	60–90	<140/90	<20
Abnormal	>100	>140/90	>20
Immediately After Activity			
Normal	↑Rate ↑Strength	↑Systolic	↑Rate ↑Depth
Abnormal	↑Rate ↑Strength Irregular rhythm	Decrease or no change in systolic	Excessive ↓Rate or ↑Rate
3 Minutes After Activity			
Normal	Within 6 beats of resting pulse		
Abnormal	>7 beats of resting pulse		

Environmental

Social isolation

Sensory overload

Insufficient rest and sleep

Sensory deprivation

Climatic extremes

Disease-Related

Cardiopulmonary disorders

Nutritional deficiencies

Musculoskeletal disorders

Neurologic disorders

Fluid/electrolyte imbalances

Chronic diseases

Treatment-Related

Bed rest/imposed immobility

Diagnostic studies

Medications

Treatment schedule

Diet

Surgery

Caregivers' expectations

Assistive equipment that
   requires strength

For more information on Focus Assessment Criteria, visit http://connection.lww.com.

Goal

NOC   Activity Tolerance

The person will progress activity to (specify level of activity desired).

Indicators
- Identify factors that aggravate activity intolerance.
- Identify methods to reduce activity intolerance.
- Maintain blood pressure within normal limits 3 min after activity.

General Interventions

NIC   Activity Tolerance, Energy Management,
Exercise Promotion, Sleep Enhancement,
Mutual Goal Setting

Monitor the Person's Response to Activity.

1. Take resting pulse, blood pressure, and respirations.
2. Consider rate, rhythm, and quality (if signs are abnormal—eg, pulse above 100—consult with physician about advisability of increasing activity).
3. Have person perform the activity.
4. Take vital signs immediately after activity. (Strenuous activity may increase the pulse by 50 beats. This rate is still satisfactory as long as it returns to resting pulse within 3 min.)
5. Have person rest for 3 min; take vital signs again.
6. Discontinue the activity if the person responds with:
   - Complaints of chest pain, vertigo, or confusion
   - Decreased pulse rate
   - Failure of systolic blood pressure to increase
   - Decreased systolic blood pressure
   - Increased diastolic blood pressure by 15 mm Hg
   - Decreased respiratory response
7. Reduce the intensity or duration of the activity if:
   - The pulse takes longer than 3 to 4 min to return to within six beats of the resting pulse.
   - The respiratory rate increase is excessive after the activity.

Increase the Activity Gradually.

Increase tolerance for activity by having the person perform the activity more slowly, for a shorter time with more rest pauses, or with more assistance.

Minimize the deconditioning effects of prolonged bed rest and imposed immobility:
- Begin active range of motion (ROM) at least twice a day. For the person who is unable, the nurse should perform passive ROM.
- Encourage isometric exercise.
- Encourage the person to turn and lift self actively unless contraindicated.
- Promote optimal sitting balance and tolerance by increasing muscle strength.
- Gradually increase tolerance by starting with 15 min the first time out of bed.

- Have the person get out of bed three times a day, increasing the time out of bed by 15 min each day.
- Practice transfers. Have the person do as much active movement as possible during transfers.
- Promote ambulation with or without assistive devices.
- Provide support when the person begins to stand.
- If the person cannot stand without buckling the knees, he or she is not ready for ambulation; help the person to practice standing in place with assistance.
- Choose a safe gait. (If the gait appears awkward but stable, continue; stay close by and give clear coaching messages, eg, "Look straight ahead, not down.")
- Allow the person to gauge the rate of ambulation.
- Provide sufficient support to ensure safety and prevent falling.
- Encourage the person to wear comfortable walking shoes (slippers do not support the feet properly).

Discuss Effects of Condition on Role Responsibilities, Occupation, and Finances.

Determine Adequacy of Sleep (See Disturbed Sleep Pattern for More Information).

Plan rest periods according to the person's daily schedule. (They should occur throughout the day and between activities.)

Encourage person to rest during the first hour after meals. (Rest can take many forms: napping, watching TV, or sitting with legs elevated.)

Promote a Sincere "Can-do" Attitude.

Identify factors that undermine person's confidence, such as fear of falling, perceived weakness, and visual impairment.

Explore possible incentives with the person and the family; consider what the person values:

Playing with grandchildren	Going fishing
Returning to work	Performing a task, such as a craft

Allow person to set activity schedule and functional activity goals. If the goal is too low, negotiate (eg, "Walking 25 feet seems low. Let's increase it to 50 feet. I'll walk with you.").

Plan a purpose for the activity, such as sitting up in a chair to eat lunch, walking to a window to see the view, or walking to the kitchen to get some juice.

Help person to identify progress. Do not underestimate the value of praise and encouragement as effective motivational techniques. In selected cases, assisting the client to keep a written record of activities may help to demonstrate progress.

Encourage the Family to Share Concerns.

Assess their knowledge of the condition, treatment, and prognosis.

Encourage them to share their concerns about the future and about role responsibilities.

Rationales

- Response to activity can be evaluated by comparing preactivity blood pressure, pulse, and respiration with postactivity results. These, in turn, are compared with recovery time.
- Activity tolerance develops cyclically through adjusting frequency, duration, and intensity of activity until the desired level is achieved. Increasing activity frequency precedes increasing duration and intensity (work demand). Increased intensity is offset by reduced duration and frequency. As tolerance for more intensive activity of short duration develops, frequency is once again increased.
- The reliability of self-reports of activity has been questioned (Klesges et al., 1989). Keeping a record of actual activities and responses provides a more reliable means of demonstrating progress.
- Rest relieves the symptoms of activity intolerance. The daily schedule is planned to allow for alternating periods of activity and rest and coordinated to reduce excess energy expenditure.
- Nursing interventions for activity intolerance promote participation in activities to achieve a level of activity desired by the person for the therapeutic regimen.
- Knowledge, values, beliefs, and perceived capability for action influence a person's decision to engage in a particular activity (Magnan, 1987).

ACTIVITY INTOLERANCE

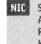 **RELATED TO INSUFFICIENT KNOWLEDGE OF ADAPTIVE TECHNIQUES NEEDED SECONDARY TO COPD**

Goal

NOC	Activity Tolerance

The person will progress activity to (specify level of activity desired).

Indicators
- Demonstrate methods of controlled breathing to conserve energy.
- Demonstrate ability to coordinate controlled breathing with activity.

General Interventions

NIC	Same as for Generic, Smoking Cessation Assistance, Nutrition Management, Respiratory Status: Airway Patency, Knowledge: Illness Care

The following interventions apply to people experiencing *Activity Intolerance* resulting from a known cause: COPD. Nurses use these interventions in conjunction with the interventions identified for general cases of *Activity Intolerance* (see pp. 84–86).

Assess Adequacy of:

Knowledge of therapeutic regimen
Breathing techniques
Nutritional intake
Pulmonary hygiene
Activity level
Health-related behaviors

Eliminate or Reduce Contributing Factors.

Lack of Knowledge

Assess understanding of prescribed therapeutic regimen; proceed with health teaching using simple, clear instructions; include family members.

Specifically assess knowledge of pulmonary hygiene and adaptive breathing techniques.

Inadequate Pulmonary Hygiene Routine

Explain the importance of adhering to daily coughing schedule for clearing the lungs and that doing so is a lifetime commitment.

Teach the proper method of controlled coughing:
1. Breathe deeply and slowly while sitting up as upright as possible.
2. Use diaphragmatic breathing.
3. Hold the breath for 3 to 5 s; then slowly exhale as much of this breath as possible through the mouth. (Lower rib cage and abdomen should sink down with exhaling.)
4. Take a second deep breath, hold, and cough forcefully from deep in the chest (not from the back of the mouth or throat); use two short, forceful coughs.
5. Rest after coughing sessions.

Instruct person to practice controlled coughing four times a day: 30 min before meals and at bedtime. Allow 15 to 30 min of rest after coughing session and before meals.

Consider use of inhaled humidity, postural drainage, and chest clapping before coughing session. Assess for use of prescribed aerosol bronchodilators to dilate airways and thin secretions.

Suboptimal Breathing Techniques

Encourage conscious controlled breathing techniques (pursed-lip and diaphragmatic breathing) for use during increased activity and emotional and physical stress.

Beginning instruction in physical and mental relaxation techniques is helpful before teaching controlled breathing.

Instruct client by demonstrating the desired breathing technique, then directing him or her to mimic your breathing pattern.

For pursed-lip breathing, the person should breathe in through the nose, then breathe out slowly through partially closed lips while counting to 7 and making a "pu" sound. (Often, people with progressive lung disease learn this naturally.)

For diaphragmatic breathing:

1. Place your hands on the person's abdomen below the base of the ribs and keep them there while he or she inhales.
2. To inhale, the person relaxes the shoulders, breathes in through the nose, and pushes the stomach outward against your hands. The person holds the breath for 1 to 2 s to keep the alveoli open, then exhales.
3. To exhale, the person breathes out slowly through the mouth while you apply slight pressure at the base of the ribs.
4. Have the person practice this breathing technique several times with you; then, the person should place his or her own hands at the base of the ribs to practice alone.
5. Once the person has learned the technique, have him or her practice it a few times each hour.

Insufficient Activity Level

Assess current activity level. Consider:

- Current pattern of activity/rest
- Distribution of energy demand over course of day
- Perceptions of most demanding required activities
- Perceptions of areas for which the client desires or requires increased participation
- Efficacy of current adaptive techniques

Identify physical barriers at home and work (eg, number of stairs) that seem insurmountable or limit participation in activities.

Identify ways to reduce the work demand of frequently performed tasks (eg, sitting, rather than standing, to prepare vegetables; keeping frequently used utensils on a counter top to avoid unnecessary overhead reaching or bending).

Identify ways of alternating periods of exertion with periods of rest to overcome barriers (eg, place a chair in the bathroom near the sink so the person can rest during daily hygiene).

Keep in mind that a plan including frequent short rest periods during an activity is less demanding and more conducive to completing the activity than a plan that calls for a burst of energy followed by a long period of rest.

Inadequate Nutritional Intake

Recommend that the person brush teeth and use mouthwash before meals and especially after coughing session, because there is frequently an associated bad taste in the mouth, causing decreased appetite and sense of taste.

Encourage smaller, more frequent meals. (Large portions require more oxygen/energy to digest and also limit the downward movement of the diaphragm during inspiration.)

Choose foods that are easy to chew and swallow. (Food that needs extensive chewing requires more work, causing fatigue.)

Assist in food preparation (eg, cutting meat) if person is prone to fatigue easily.

Avoid gas-producing foods or liquids.

Discourage talking while eating; encourage thorough chewing and slow eating.

Encourage drinking 2 to 3 quarts of liquid a day (minimum) if fluids are unrestricted. (Consult physician for desired daily fluid intake.)

Poor Health-Related Behaviors

Teach person to avoid factors that aggravate symptoms and advance disease (eg, excessive allergens, pollution).

Discourage smoking. Smoking cessation should be considered of highest priority in any program of comprehensive care of clients with COPD.

If person chooses to smoke, discourage smoking before meals and activity.

If person wishes to reduce or stop smoking, see further interventions under *Ineffective Health Maintenance related to tobacco use.*

Monitor Client's Response to Activity.

See General Interventions, pp. 84–86.

While monitoring response, observe for signs and symptoms of respiratory intolerance:

Aggravated dyspnea	Markedly increased respiratory rate
Pallor	Cyanosis
Use of accessory muscles	Inability to maintain rhythmic, controlled breathing

Increase Activity Gradually.

Reassure person that some increase in daily activity is possible.

Instruct person in controlled breathing techniques.

Encourage person to use controlled breathing techniques to decrease work of breathing during activities.

After the person masters controlled breathing in relaxed positions, begin to increase activity.

Teach person to maintain controlled breathing pattern while sitting or standing.

Progress person to maintaining controlled breathing during bed-to-chair transfers and walking.

Many clients can learn to maintain rhythmic breathing during walking by using a simple 2:4 ratio: two steps during inspiration and four steps during expiration.

Do not progress the person to more demanding activity until breathing is well controlled during less demanding activities.

Encourage Discussion of Sexuality.

Encourage client to discuss effects of the condition on sexuality.

Refer to *Ineffective Sexuality Patterns*.

Initiate Health Teaching.

Teach client to observe sputum; note changes in color, amount, and odor; and seek professional advice if sputum changes.

Explain that the person with COPD is susceptible to infection and must detect symptoms early and consult with physician for treatment (frequently, early antibiotic therapy is necessary).

Discuss the need for annual influenza immunizations. (The usefulness of one-time-only pneumococcal vaccinations has recently been questioned; therefore, administration should be on an individual basis.)

Instruct person to wear warm, dry clothing; avoid crowds, heavy smoke, fumes, and irritants; avoid exertion in cold, hot, or humid weather; and balance work, rest, and recreation to regulate energy expenditure.

Emphasize the importance of maintaining a nutritious diet (high calorie, high vitamin C, high protein, and 2 to 3 quarts of liquid a day, unless on fluid restriction).

Evaluate the person's knowledge of the care, cleansing, and use of inhalator equipment.

If using oxygen therapy, especially at home, evaluate awareness of fire hazards; explain need for home extinguisher.

Teach the importance of supporting arm weight to reduce the need for respiratory muscles to stabilize the chest wall (Bauldoff et al., 1996; Breslin, 1992).

Teach how to increase unsupported arm endurance with lower extremity exercises performed during the exhalation phase of respiration (Bauldoff et al., 1996; Breslin, 1992).

Make Referrals as Indicated.

Refer to community nurse for follow-up.

Consult physical therapist for a comprehensive exercise program especially for people with COPD.

Refer to community support groups (eg, Better Breathers) and pertinent literature for people with lung disorders.

Rationales

- An integrated program that incorporates the principles of physical relaxation, pulmonary hygiene, controlled breathing, and adequate nutrition and hydration; energy conservation through work simplification; and smoking cessation maximizes activity tolerance.
- Techniques of physical relaxation minimize muscle tension. Relaxation is an essential preliminary step in teaching controlled breathing to eliminate wasteful and unproductive motions of the upper chest, shoulders, and neck.

- Clearing and defense of the airways are of utmost importance in meeting tissue demands for increased oxygen during periods of rest and periods of increased activity.
- People with COPD can benefit from specific breathing exercises, which involve retraining of breathing patterns, and from general exercise programs that support normal daily activities (Bauldoff et al., 1996).
- Therapeutic efforts to improve respiratory muscle function need to be tailored to each person, according to the muscle group most likely to benefit. In early stages of COPD, treatment should focus on the diaphragm, whereas for more advanced disease, the focus must shift to the inspiratory muscles of the rib cage and of exhalation.
- Symptom-limited endurance training has been shown effective for improving performance and reducing perceived breathlessness (Punzal, Ries, Kaplan & Prewitt, 1991). The minimal duration and frequency of exercise required to improve performance appear to be 20 to 30 min three to five times per week. Not all people, however, are candidates for exercise reconditioning. A pulmonologist should be consulted.
- The physiologic demands of unsupported arm tasks lead to both exercise-induced increases in respiratory muscle work and nonventilatory recruitment of respiratory muscles to maintain chest wall position (Breslin, 1992). Research has shown that arm support during performance of arm tasks reduces diaphragmatic recruitment (Martinez, Couser & Celli, 1989), increases respiratory endurance (Bauldoff et al., 1996), and increases arm exercise endurance (Celli, Criner & Rassulo, 1988). Providing arm support (eg, resting elbows on a table top while shaving or eating) may enhance independence and improve functional capacity (Bauldoff et al., 1996).
- Pulmonary rehabilitation can decrease anxiety and depression associated with severe COPD.

ACTIVITY INTOLERANCE

⊗ RELATED TO INSUFFICIENT KNOWLEDGE OF ADAPTIVE TECHNIQUES NEEDED SECONDARY TO IMPAIRED CARDIAC FUNCTION

Goal

NOC Activity Tolerance

The person will demonstrate tolerance for increased activity by maintaining pulse, respirations, and blood pressure within predetermined ranges.

Indicators
- Identify factors that increase cardiac workload.
- Describe adaptive techniques needed to perform ADLs.
- Identify cues for stopping activity: fatigue, shortness of breath, chest pain.

General Interventions

NIC Same as for Generic, Smoking Cessation Assistance, Weight Reduction Assistance, Knowledge: Illness Care, Nutrition Management

Assess for Causative/ Contributing Factors.

Knowledge of therapeutic regimen
Smoking

Activity level
Overweight/obesity

Eliminate or Reduce Contributing Factors.

Assess Knowledge and Behavior Related to the Four "E's": Eating, Exertion, Exposure, and Emotional Stress (Adapted from Day, 1984).

Eating
Assess knowledge of restricted diet.
Explain importance of adhering to prescribed salt-restricted diet.
Explore alternatives for seasoning foods to taste using natural herbs and spices.
Encourage a light meal in the evening to promote a more comfortable night's rest.
Initially provide easily digestible and chewable foods.
Schedule meals to avoid interfering with other activities.
Offer food preferences, avoiding dislikes.
Consider sociocultural influences.

Exertion
Teach person to modify approaches to activities to regulate energy expenditure and reduce cardiac workload (eg, take rest periods during activities, at intervals during the day, and for 1 h after meals; sit rather than stand when performing activities; when performing a task, rest every 3 min for 5 min to allow the heart to recover; stop an activity if exertional fatigue or signs of cardiac hypoxia, such as markedly increased pulse rate, dyspnea, or chest pain, occur).
Instruct person to avoid certain types of exertion: isometric exercises (eg, using arms to lift self, carry objects) and Valsalva maneuver (eg, bending at the waist in a sit-up fashion to rise from bed, straining during a bowel movement).

Exposure
Instruct person to avoid unnecessary exposure to environmental extremes and exertion during hot, humid weather or extreme cold weather, which places additional demands on the heart.
Instruct person to dress warmly during cold weather (eg, create a barrier to cold weather by wearing layers of clothing).

Emotional Stress
Assist person to identify emotional stressors (eg, at home, at work, social).
Discuss usual response to emotional stress (eg, anger, depression, avoidance, discussion).
Explain the effects of emotional stress on the cardiovascular system (increased heart rate, blood pressure, respirations).
Discuss various methods for stress management/reduction (eg, deliberate problem solving, relaxation techniques, yoga or meditation, biofeedback, regular exercise).

Assess Current Activity Level. Consider:
- Current pattern of activity/rest
- Distribution of energy demand over course of day
- Perceptions of most demanding required activities
- Perceptions of areas for which increased participation is desired or required

Identify Symptoms of Cardiac Intolerance.
Evaluate effectiveness of adaptive techniques to manage symptoms (eg, pacing activities, frequent rest pauses, use of nitrates before planned exertion).
Organize in-hospital care to allow periods of undisturbed rest.

Discuss Smoking.
Discuss effects of smoking on the cardiovascular system (eg, vasoconstriction increases workload of the heart).
Teach person when not to smoke: before and immediately after an activity.
Discuss methods that can help reduce cigarettes smoked (see *Ineffective Health Maintenance related to tobacco use*).
Advise that at least several attempts may be needed to be successful.

Address Overweight/Obesity.
Assess whether person is overweight or obese by measuring height and weight and comparing findings with a standardized height–weight chart, or use anthropometric measurements (see *Imbalanced Nutrition: More Than Body Requirements* for charts of weight for height and anthropometric norms).

Monitor Response to Activity (See General Interventions, pp. 84–86) and Teach Self-monitoring Techniques.

Take resting pulse.

Take pulse during or immediately after activity.

Take pulse 3 min after cessation of activity.

Instruct person to stop activity and report:

- Decreased pulse rate during activity
- Pulse rate >112 beats/min
- Irregular pulse
- Pulse rate that does not return to within six beats of resting pulse after 3 min
- Dyspnea
- Chest pain
- Palpitations
- Perceptions of exertional fatigue

Increase the Activity Gradually.

Allow for periods of rest before and after planned periods of exertion, such as treatments, ambulation, meals.

Encourage gradual increases in activity and ambulation to prevent a sudden increase in cardiac workload.

Assess person's perceived capability for increased activity.

Assist person in setting short-term activity goals that are realistic and achievable.

Reassure person that even small increases in activity will lift spirits and restore self-confidence.

Encourage the Person to Discuss the Effects of Condition on Sexuality.

Refer to *Ineffective Sexuality Patterns.*

Encourage Family to Share Concerns.

See General Interventions, pp. 84–86.

Initiate Health Teaching and Referrals as Indicated.

Instruct person to consult his or her physician and physiatrist for a long-term exercise program or to contact the American Heart Association for available local cardiac rehabilitation programs.

Explain dietary restrictions to client and family. Give them written instructions or refer them to pertinent literature on preparation of food for restricted diets.

Explain dosage, side effects, administration, and storage of prescribed drug therapy (eg, diuretics, vasodilators).

Rationales

- People with impaired cardiac function often can increase both activity level and tolerance through adaptations in lifestyle, modifications in approach to activities, and careful monitoring of responses.
- An integrated program of medically supervised exercise, dietary restriction, stress management, and limited exposure to environmental extremes maximizes activity tolerance.
- People with impaired cardiac function can achieve some immediate gains in activity tolerance by modifying their approach (eg, pacing activities, avoiding isometric work, limiting the duration of dynamic work by taking frequent rests).
- Required reduction in the level of personal activity may result in role identification conflict and disruption of divisions of labor within the family unit.
- Response to activity can be evaluated by comparing preactivity blood pressure, pulse, and respiration with postactivity blood pressure, pulse, and respiration. These, in turn, are compared with recovery time.
- Tolerance for activity develops cyclically through adjusting frequency, duration, and intensity of activity until the desired level is achieved. Increasing activity frequency precedes increasing duration and intensity (work demand). Increased intensity is offset by reduced duration and frequency. As tolerance for more intensive activity of short duration develops, frequency is once again increased.
- Tobacco is the leading cause of preventable death in women (Sarna & Bialous, 2004).

ACTIVITY INTOLERANCE

RELATED TO BED REST DECONDITIONING

Goal

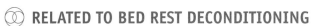

NOC Activity Tolerance

The person will participate in planned therapies to minimize or reverse the effects of deconditioning.

Indicators
- Identify factors that contribute to deconditioning.
- Demonstrate sufficient energy and strength to participate in and complete desired or required activities.

General Interventions

NIC Exercise Therapy: Joint Mobility, Teaching: Prescribed Activity Exercise

Nursing interventions focus on overcoming the deleterious effects of bed rest deconditioning through a planned program of reconditioning. They are used in conjunction with the interventions identified for general *Activity Intolerance* (see pp. 84–86).

Assess for Causative/Contributing Factors.

Prolonged or recurrent confinement to bed rest
Adequacy of positioning, repositioning, and ROM regimens
Adequacy of nutritional intake

Disturbances of motor function
Orthostatic intolerance

Eliminate or Reduce Contributing Factors.

Assess Prolonged or Recurrent Confinement to Bed Rest.
Assess history of bed or bed–chair confinement (eg, short-term, long-term, repeated). Is bed or chair confinement prescribed by the medical plan of care, self-imposed, or imposed by expectations/limitations of caregivers?
Evaluate bed mobility. (People without independent bed mobility may be more accurately diagnosed with *Disuse Syndrome*.)

Assess for Motor Function Disturbances.
Muscle Atrophy and Strength
When assessing for muscle atrophy, inspect the pelvic and shoulder girdles, hands, and extremities. Muscle wasting in the extremities may give the appearance of excessively large joints. Measuring the circumference of an extremity does not provide reliable information about muscle atrophy because it is unclear what is being measured. Comparable body parts can be compared for symmetry; however, the dominant extremities are often larger than their nondominant counterparts.

Assess muscle strength around each major joint. Strength is conventionally expressed using the Lovett 6-grade scale:

0 (Zero)	No contraction
1 (Trace)	Some contraction; no motion
2 (Poor)	Cannot move against gravity
3 (Fair)	Can move against gravity only
4 (Good)	Moves against moderate resistance
5 (Normal)	Moves against full resistance

Spasticity
Determine the degree of spasticity or abnormally increased muscle tone.
Spasticity increases the energy costs of activities, can seriously limit functional independence, and interferes with gait training, orthotic prescription, and contracture prevention.

The extent and severity of spasticity often vary in a given person, depending on time of day, previous activity, posture, and tactile and kinesthetic stimuli.

Designate spasticity as mild, moderate, or severe.

Relating spasticity to functional aspects of the client's activities (eg, mild spasticity of lower extremities that progresses to severe spasticity after walking 20 ft on a level grade) can be helpful.

Coordination

Impaired motor coordination may interfere with completion of many tasks (eg, feeding or sitting and standing) as a result of poor balance.

By convention, two tests of coordination are usually performed: rapid alternating movements and point-to-point testing.

Assess coordination of both upper and lower extremities.

The most effective therapy for improving coordination is repeated practice, beginning with simple exercises and progressing to more complex tasks. Clients who are confused, inattentive, or who have poor memory may have considerable difficulty in acquiring coordination skills necessary for completion of therapeutic and self-care activities.

Assess Adequacy of Positioning, Repositioning, and ROM Regimens.

Positioning for comfort and pressure relief should be done at least every 2 h.

If not contraindicated, the repositioning regimen should include periods of upright positioning (eg, high Fowler's position or up in chair).

Periods of therapeutic positioning where muscles are fully stretched should be included in the repositioning regimen to prevent muscle shortening (shortened muscles atrophy more quickly).

Prolonged stretching for 20 min using moderate force is much more effective than application of brief, vigorous stretches to prevent muscle shortening and contractures.

Evaluate need for dorsiflexion orthotics to protect plantar flexors of lower extremities from shortening and accelerated atrophy.

Evaluate ROM of all major joints; express ROM in degrees.

Assess adequacy of ROM exercises. Consider thoroughness, frequency, and resistance (eg, passive or active).

Assess for Orthostatic Intolerance.

Refer to *Risk for Injury related to vertigo secondary to postural hypotension.*

Assess Adequacy of Nutritional Intake.

Evaluate calorie–nitrogen intake. Nitrogen intake must be sufficient for protein synthesis. Enough non-nitrogen calories must also be taken in to ensure that protein calories are not metabolized to meet energy needs. A malnourished or stressed client requires almost double the nitrogen as a healthy individual.

If inadequate nutritional intake is suspected, keep a daily record of foods eaten and consult a dietitian.

See *Imbalanced Nutrition: Less Than Body Requirements* for specific interventions.

Monitor Response to Activity.

See General Interventions, pp. 84–86.

Rapid onset of task-related fatigue is an early indicator of intolerance in deconditioned clients.

While monitoring the response to activity, assess for signs and symptoms of orthostatic intolerance (tachycardia, nausea, diaphoresis, and syncope). (See *Risk for Injury related to orthostatic hypotension* for specific interventions.)

Gradually Increase Activity.

Plan strategies to increase bed mobility (eg, use of overhead trapeze).

Implement a planned exercise program that includes lower extremity exercises against resistance.

Progress client to exercise in upright positions against gravitational strain as early as possible.

Begin weight bearing as early as possible to minimize atrophy of plantar flexors in lower legs.

Promote independence in ADLs. The client should perform as many such activities independently as possible.

Initiate Health Teaching and Referrals.

Instruct client and caregivers in ROM and therapeutic exercises.

Consult physical therapist for an exercise program tailored to the client's needs.

Consult dietitian for dietary evaluation and nutritional counseling.

Rationales

- Repeated confinement to bed rest and age older than 65 years are thought to compound deconditioning, which may predispose the chronically ill and older adults to activity intolerance from bed rest deconditioning.
- Loss of skeletal muscle mass, changes in neurohumoral mechanisms, and associated general decreases in metabolic needs contribute to bed rest deconditioning.
- Bed rest deconditioning leads to decreased physical capacity for work in the supine position from changes in the cardiac, circulatory, and musculoskeletal systems. The lack of exposure to orthostatic stress during bed rest leads to further decreases in the physical capacity for work in the upright position.
- Some muscle groups seem more vulnerable to bed rest deconditioning than others, resulting in differences in the rate and degree of muscle atrophy. During bed rest, leg muscles tend to lose strength about twice as fast as arm muscles (Greenleaf, Wade & Leftheriotis, 1989).
- A onefold loss of muscle mass in plantar flexors of the lower legs (eg, gastrocnemius and soleus muscles) is associated with a twofold loss in muscle strength.
- Exercises targeted at muscle groups that are more susceptible to bed rest deconditioning may be a more effective countermeasure for deconditioning than general exercise regimens (Corcoran, 1991).
- Exercises performed in an upright position, against gravitational strain, are of greater value in overcoming the effects of bed rest deconditioning than exercises performed in a supine position.
- A person's response to activity can be evaluated by comparing preactivity blood pressure, pulse, and respiration with postactivity blood pressure, pulse, and respiration. These, in turn, are compared with recovery time.

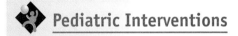 ## Pediatric Interventions

Provide age-appropriate games and activities that are quiet and challenging (Wong, 2002), such as sensory adventures (what does the hospital smell, sound, or look like?), story telling, story writing, collages, puppets, and play acting.

Rationales

- A child's response to activity can be evaluated through physiologic parameters and engagement in age-appropriate activities. For example, assess the infant's sleep–rest cycle, motor activities, and eating behavior. Assess these parameters in a toddler, preschooler, and school-aged child, as well as the child's involvement in play activities.
- Play activities are important, even for the hospitalized child with activity intolerance. Play normalizes the child's experience in the hospital and reduces stress. Continually assess the child's fatigue or readiness to engage in more vigorous activity (Wong, 2003).

Maternal Interventions

Explain the causes of fatigue and dyspnea in middle to late pregnancy.
Teach energy conservation methods (see General Interventions, pp. 84–86).

Rationales

- Changes in center of gravity and increased weight and pressure of the enlarging uterus on the diaphragm contribute to fatigue and breathlessness.

DECREASED INTRACRANIAL ADAPTIVE CAPACITY

DEFINITION

Decreased Intracranial Adaptive Capacity: A clinical state in which intracranial fluid dynamic mechanisms that normally compensate for increases in intracranial volumes are compromised, resulting in repeated disproportionate increases in intracranial pressure (ICP) in response to a variety of noxious and nonnoxious stimuli

DEFINING CHARACTERISTICS
Major (Must Be Present)

Repeated increases in ICP of >10 mm Hg for more than 5 min after any of a variety of external stimuli

Minor (May Be Present)

Disproportionate increase in ICP after a single environmental or nursing maneuver stimulus
Elevated P2 ICP waveform
Volume-pressure response test variation (volume-pressure ratio >2; pressure-volume index <10)
Baseline ICP ≥10 mm Hg
Wide-amplitude ICP waveform

AUTHOR'S NOTE

This diagnosis represents increased intracranial pressure. It is a collaborative problem because it requires treatment from both nursing and medicine. In addition, it requires invasive monitoring. *Potential Complication: Increased Intracranial Pressure* represents this clinical situation. Refer to Section Three for interventions for which nurses are responsible.

IMPAIRED ADJUSTMENT

DEFINITION

Impaired Adjustment: The state in which the individual is unwilling to modify his or her lifestyle/behavior in a manner consistent with a change in health status

DEFINING CHARACTERISTICS
Major (Must Be Present)

Verbalization of nonacceptance of health status change or inadequate capacity to be involved in problem solving or goal setting

Minor (May Be Present)

Lack of movement toward independence; extended period of shock, disbelief, or anger regarding health status change; lack of future-oriented thinking

---

 AUTHOR'S NOTE

This diagnosis has presented problems in clinical use because of its lack of specificity. Generally speaking, are not most diagnoses problems with adjustment? Such a general diagnosis is not clinically useful. Responses to illness and disabilities vary, and it is important that the nurse clarify the response so it will be most helpful with treatment. Responses can be *Grieving, Anxiety, Fear,* and *Ineffective Coping.*

If a client is attempting to manage the changes the illness or disability has caused, but is having difficulty, *Ineffective Therapeutic Regimen Management* would be more useful.

This author recommends not using this diagnosis.

Anxiety
Related to Insufficient Knowledge of Preoperative Routines, Postoperative Exercises/
Activities, Postoperative Alteration/Sensations
Death Anxiety

ANXIETY

DEFINITION

Anxiety: A state in which the individual/group experiences feelings of uneasiness (apprehension) and activation of the autonomic nervous system in response to a vague, nonspecific threat

DEFINING CHARACTERISTICS
Major (Must Be Present)

Manifested by symptoms from each category—physiologic, emotional, and cognitive; symptoms vary according to level of anxiety (Whitley, 1994)

Physiologic

Increased heart and respiratory rates	Elevated blood pressure
Diaphoresis	Dilated pupils
Voice tremors/pitch changes	Trembling, twitching
Palpitations	Nausea or vomiting
Frequent urination	Diarrhea
Insomnia	Fatigue and weakness
Flushing or pallor	Dry mouth
Body aches and pains (especially chest, back, neck)	Restlessness
	Faintness/dizziness
Paresthesias	Hot and cold flashes
	Anorexia

Emotional
Person states feelings of

Apprehension	Helplessness
Nervousness	Lack of self-confidence
Loss of control	Tension or being "keyed up"
Inability to relax	Anticipation of misfortune

Person exhibits

Irritability/impatience	Angry outbursts
Crying	Tendency to blame others
Startle reaction	Criticism of self and others
Withdrawal	Lack of initiative
Self-deprecation	Poor eye contact

Cognitive

Inability to concentrate	Lack of awareness of surroundings
Forgetfulness	Rumination
Orientation to past	Blocking of thoughts (inability to remember)
Hyperattentiveness	Preoccupation
Diminished learning ability	Confusion

RELATED FACTORS
Pathophysiologic
Any factor that interferes with the basic human needs for food, air, comfort, and security

Situational (Personal, Environmental)
Related to actual or perceived threat to self-concept secondary to:

Change in status and prestige	Lack of recognition from others
Failure (or success)	Loss of valued possessions
Ethical dilemma	

Related to actual or perceived loss of significant others secondary to:

Death	Divorce
Cultural pressures	Moving
Temporary or permanent separation	

Related to actual or perceived threat to biologic integrity secondary to:

Dying	Assault
Invasive procedures	Disease

Related to actual or perceived change in environment secondary to:

Hospitalization	Moving
Retirement	Safety hazards
Environmental pollutants	

Related to actual or perceived change in socioeconomic status secondary to:

Unemployment	New job
Promotion	

Related to idealistic expectations of self and unrealistic goals

Maturational
Infant/Child
Related to separation
Related to unfamiliar environment, people
Related to changes in peer relationships

Adolescent
Related to threat to self-concept secondary to:

Sexual development	Peer relationships changes

Adult
Related to threat to self-concept secondary to:

Pregnancy	Parenting
Career changes	Effects of aging

Older Adult
Related to threat to self-concept secondary to:

Sensory losses	Motor losses
Financial problems	Retirement changes

AUTHOR'S NOTE

Several researchers have examined the nursing diagnoses of *Anxiety* and *Fear* (Jones & Jacob, 1984; Taylor-Loughran, O'Brien, LaChapelle & Rangel, 1989; Whitley, 1994; Yokom, 1984). Differentiation of these diagnoses focuses on whether the threat can be identified. If so, the diagnosis is *Fear;* if not, it is *Anxiety* (NANDA, 2001). This differentiation, however, has not proved useful for clinicians (Taylor-Loughran et al., 1989).

Anxiety is a vague feeling of apprehension and uneasiness in response to a threat to one's value system or security pattern (May, 1977). The person may be able to identify the situation

(continued)

> **AUTHOR'S NOTE** (*Continued*)
>
> (eg, surgery, cancer), but actually the threat to self relates to the enmeshed uneasiness and apprehension. In other words, the situation is the source of, but is not itself, the threat. In contrast, fear is feelings of apprehension related to a specific threat or danger to which one's security patterns respond (eg, flying, heights, snakes). When the threat is removed, fear dissipates (May, 1977).
>
> Anxiety and fear produce a similar sympathetic response: cardiovascular excitation, pupillary dilation, sweating, tremors, and dry mouth. Anxiety also involves a parasympathetic response of increased gastrointestinal (GI) activity; in contrast, fear is associated with decreased GI activity. Behaviorally, the fearful person exhibits increased alertness and concentration, with avoidance, attack, or decreasing the risk of threat. Conversely, the anxious person experiences increased tension, general restlessness, insomnia, worry, and helplessness and vagueness concerning a situation that cannot be easily avoided or attacked.
>
> Clinically, both anxiety and fear may coexist in a response to a situation. For example, a person facing surgery may be fearful of pain and anxious about possible cancer. According to Yokom (1984), "Fear can be allayed by withdrawal from the situation, removal of the offending object, or by reassurance. Anxiety is reduced by admitting its presence and by being convinced that the values to be gained by moving ahead are greater than those to be gained by escape."

> **ERRORS IN DIAGNOSTIC STATEMENTS**
>
> 1. *Fear related to upcoming surgery*
> Anticipated surgery can be a source of many threats, including threats to security patterns, health, values, self-concept, role functioning, goal achievement, and relationships. These threats can produce vague feelings ranging from mild uneasiness to panic. Identifying a threat as merely surgery is too simplistic; personal threats also are involved. Moreover, although some uneasiness may be attributed to fear (which teaching can eliminate), the remaining feelings relate to anxiety. Because this situation is inescapable, the nurse must assist the person with coping mechanisms for managing anxiety and fear.

KEY CONCEPTS
Generic Considerations
- Anxiety refers to feelings aroused by a nonspecific threat to a person's self-concept that impinges on health, assets, values, environment, role functioning, needs fulfillment, goal achievement, personal relationships, and sense of security (Miller, 2004). It varies in intensity depending on the severity of the perceived threat and the success or failure of efforts to cope with the feelings.
- Anxiety attacks at a deeper level than fear (Varcarolis, 2002). Anxiety affects the central core of personality. It erodes feelings of self-esteem and personal worth.
- A person uses both interpersonal and intrapsychic mechanisms to reduce or relieve anxiety. The effectiveness of coping strategies depends on the person and situation, not on the behavior itself.
- *Interpersonal patterns* of coping include the following:
  Acting out: converting anxiety into anger (either overtly or covertly expressed)
  Paralysis or retreating behaviors: withdrawing or being immobilized by anxiety
  Somatizing: converting anxiety into physical symptoms
  Constructive action: using anxiety to learn and to solve problems (includes goal setting, learning new skills, and seeking information)
- *Intrapsychic mechanisms,* often called defense mechanisms, lower anxiety and protect self-esteem. Examples include repression, sublimation, regression, displacement, projection, denial, conversion, rationalization, suppression, and identification.
- People develop a range of coping behaviors, both maladaptive and adaptive. Maladaptive coping mechanisms are characterized by the inability to make choices, conflict, repetition, rigidity, alienation, and secondary gains.
- Anxiety can be classified as normal, acute (state), and chronic (trait) (Varcarolis, 2002).
  Normal anxiety is necessary for survival. It prompts constructive behaviors, such as being on time or studying for a test.
- Acute, or state, anxiety is the response to an imminent loss or change that disrupts one's sense of security. Examples include apprehension before a speech or the death of a close relative or friend.

- Chronic, or trait, anxiety is anxiety that one lives with daily. In children, chronic anxiety may manifest as permanent apprehension or overreaction to unexpected stimuli. In adults, chronic anxiety may manifest as poor concentration, insomnia, relationship problems, and chronic fatigue.
- The anxious person tends to overgeneralize, assume, and anticipate catastrophe. Resulting cognitive problems include difficulty with attention and concentration, loss of objectivity, and vigilance.
- The effects of anxiety on a person's abilities vary with degree:

Mild
Heightened perception and attention; alertness
Ability to deal with problems
Ability to integrate past, present, and future experiences
Use of learning and consensual validation
Mild tension-relieving behaviors (nail biting, hair twisting)
Sleeplessness

Moderate
Slightly narrowed perception; selective inattention, which can be directed
Slight difficulty concentrating; learning requires more effort
View of present experiences in terms of past
Possible failure to notice what is happening in a peripheral situation; some difficulty adapting and analyzing
Voice/pitch changes
Increased respiratory and heart rates
Tremors, shakiness

Severe
Distorted perception; focus on scattered details; inability to attend to more even when instructed
Severely impaired learning; high distractibility and inability to concentrate
View of present experiences in terms of past; almost cannot understand current situation
Poor function; communication difficult to understand
Hyperventilation, tachycardia, headache, dizziness, nausea
Complete self-absorption

Panic
Irrational reasoning; focuses on blown-up detail
Inability to learn
Inability to integrate experiences; focus only on present; inability to see or understand situation; lapses in recall of thoughts
Inability to function; usually increased motor activity or unpredictable responses to minor stimuli; communication not understandable
Feelings of impending doom (dyspnea, dizziness/faintness, palpitations, trembling, choking, paresthesia, hot/cold flashes, sweating)
Thoughts related to loss of control, death, illness

- Lyons (2002) has identified five factors that contribute to stressful lifestyles as idealistic expectations of self, unrealistic goals, toxic thoughts, negative self-talk, and procrastination.

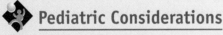 **Pediatric Considerations**

- Signs of anxiety in children vary greatly depending on developmental stage, temperament, past experience, and parental involvement (Wong, 2003). The most common sign in children and adolescents is increased motor activity. Signs of anxiety can be viewed developmentally and may be reflected in the following ways:
  - *Birth to 9 months:* Disruption in physiologic functioning (eg, sleep disorders, colic)
  - *9 months to 4 years:* Major source is loss of significant others and loss of love; therefore, anxiety may be seen as anger when parents leave, somatic illnesses, motor restlessness, regressive behaviors (thumb sucking, rocking), regression in toilet training
  - *4 to 6 years:* Major source is fear of body damage; belief that bad behavior causes bad things (eg, illness); somatic complaints of headache, stomachache   *(continued)*

Pediatric Considerations (continued)

- *6 to 12 years:* Excessive verbalization, compulsive behavior (eg, repeating tasks)
- *Adolescence:* Similar to 6 to 12 years plus negativistic behavior
- Separation from parents, change in usual routines, strange environments, painful procedures, and parental anxiety may heighten anxiety (Wong, 2003). Assess for alterations in the functional health patterns to detect anxiety.
- Sources of anxiety for children and adolescents are related to school (eg, performance, peer pressure), separation, social situations, and family (Oski, 2001).
- Refer children who manifest disorders of avoidance, overanxiousness, separation anxiety, and school phobia to mental health experts.

Maternal Considerations

- Expectant mothers experience some emotional lability.
- Multiple sources of anxiety are fear for personal or fetal well-being, anticipated labor, responsibilities of parenthood, and relationship with partner (Pillitteri, 2003).

Geriatric Considerations

- Older adults may manifest anxiety with complaints of nervousness, "nerve trouble," or feelings of uneasiness (Mohr, 2003).
- Additional signs and symptoms of anxiety are pacing, fidgeting, changes in sleeping or eating patterns, and complaints of fatigue, pain, insomnia, or GI upsets (Miller, 2004).

Transcultural Considerations

- Clients and families from different cultures face many challenges when they seek health care in the dominant culture's health care delivery systems. In addition to usual sources of anxiety (eg, unfamiliar people, unknown prognosis), they may be anxious about language difficulties, privacy, separation from support systems, and cost (Andrews & Boyle, 2003).
- Members of cultures that depend on kin for caring will expect more humanistic kinds of nursing care and less scientific–technologic care (Andrews & Boyle, 2003).

Focus Assessment Criteria

Subjective Data
Assess for Defining Characteristics.
Palpitations, Dyspnea, Dry Mouth, Nausea, Diaphoresis
Precipitating factors
Frequency
Duration

Feelings: extreme sadness and worthlessness, guilt, apprehension, rejection or isolation, inability to cope, falling apart, racing thoughts

Assess for Related Factors.
History of individual from client and significant others
Lifestyle
Support system (availability, quality of support)
History of medical problems/treatments

Usual coping behavior

"How do you usually handle a particular situation (ie, anger, disappointment, loss, rejection)?"

"What did you usually do when you faced similar situations in the past?"

"What happens when you do that?" (relevant coping mechanism)

Subjective and Objective Data
Assess for Defining Characteristics.

General appearance

Facial expression (eg, sad, hostile, expressionless)

Dress (eg, meticulous, disheveled, seductive, eccentric)

Behavior during interview

Communication Pattern

Rambling	Appropriate
Denial of problem	Suspicious
Hallucinations	Delusions

Flow of Thought (eg, appropriate, difficulty concentrating)

Nonverbal Behavior

Affect appropriate/inappropriate to verbal content

Gestures, mannerisms, facial grimaces

Posture

Interaction skills

With Nurse

Shows dependency	Relates well
Demanding/pleading	Withdrawn/preoccupied with self
Hostile	

With Significant Others

Relates with all family members or with some

Hostile toward one member/all members

Present coping behavior

"Acting-out" Behaviors

Derogating	Manipulating others to do tasks he or she can perform
Arguing	Restlessness
Intimidating	Pacing
Ritualistic behavior	
Smoking, alcohol, drugs	

Paralysis and Retreating Behaviors

Withdrawing	Avoiding talking about self
Showing signs of depression	Minimizing signs and symptoms
Engaging in denial	Developing dissociation
Diverting attention	Engaging in ritualistic behavior
Sleeping	Blocking

Somatizing

Headache	Anorexia
Dyspnea	Colitis
Multiple complaints	Syncope
Hives, eczema	Menstrual disturbance

For more information on Focus Assessment Criteria, visit http://connection.lww.com.

Goal

NOC	Anxiety Reduction, Coping, Impulse Control

The person will relate increased psychological and physiologic comfort.

Indicators

• Describe own anxiety and coping patterns.

• Use effective coping mechanisms.

General Interventions

 NIC Anxiety Reduction, Impulse Control Training, Anticipatory Guidance

Nursing interventions for *Anxiety* can apply to anyone with anxiety regardless of etiologic and contributing factors.

Assist Person to Reduce Present Level of Anxiety.

Assess Level of Anxiety (See Key Concepts): Mild, Moderate, Severe, or Panic.

Provide reassurance and comfort.

Stay with the person.

Do not make demands or ask person to make decisions.

Support present coping mechanisms (eg, allow client to talk, cry); do not confront or argue with defenses or rationalizations.

Speak slowly and calmly.

Be aware of your own concern and avoid reciprocal anxiety.

Convey empathic understanding (eg, quiet presence, touch, allowing crying, talking).

Provide reassurance that a solution can be found.

Remind person that feelings are not harmful.

Respect personal space.

If Anxiety is at Severe or Panic Level:

Provide a quiet, nonstimulating environment with soft lighting.

Use short, simple sentences; speak slowly.

Give concise directions.

Focus on the present.

Remove excess stimulation (eg, take person to quieter room); limit contact with others (eg, other clients, family) who are also anxious.

Provide physical measures that will aid in relaxation such as warm baths, back massage, aromatherapy, and music.

Consult physician for possible pharmacologic therapy, if indicated.

Provide opportunity to exercise (eg, walk fast).

If Person is Hyperventilating or Experiencing Dyspnea (DeVito, 1990):

Demonstrate breathing techniques; ask client to practice the technique with you.

Acknowledge client's fear and give positive reinforcement for efforts.

Acknowledge when dyspnea is worse than usual.

Acknowledge feelings of helplessness. Avoid suggesting that client "relax." Do not leave alone.

Provide assistance with all tasks during acute episodes of dyspnea.

During acute episode, do not discuss preventive measures.

During nonacute episodes, teach relaxation techniques (eg, tapes, guided imagery).

When Anxiety Diminishes, Assist Person to Recognize Anxiety and Causes.

Request validation of your assessment of anxiety (eg, "Are you uncomfortable now?").

If person says yes, continue with learning process; if client cannot acknowledge anxiety, continue supportive measures until he or she can.

When client can learn, determine usual coping mechanisms: "What do you usually do when you get upset?" (eg, read, discuss problems, distance, use substances, seek social support).

Assess for unmet needs or expectations; encourage recall and description of what person experienced immediately before feeling anxious.

Assist in reevaluation of perceived threat by discussing the following:

• Were expectations realistic? Too idealistic?
• Was it possible to meet expectations?
• Where in the sequence of events was change possible?

Encourage to recall and to analyze similar instances of anxiety.

Explore alternatives the client might have used to replace maladaptive coping mechanisms, such as procrastination and toxic thoughts.

Teach anxiety interrupters to use when client cannot avoid stressful situations:

• Look up.
• Control breathing.
• Lower shoulders.
• Slow thoughts.
• Alter voice.

- Give self directions (out loud, if possible).
- Exercise.
- "Scruff your face"—change facial expression.
- Change perspective: imagine watching situation from a distance (Grainger, 1990).

Reduce or Eliminate Problematic Coping Mechanisms.

Depression, withdrawal (see *Ineffective Coping*)

Violent behavior (see *Risk for Violence*)

Denial*

- Develop an atmosphere of empathic understanding.
- Assist in lowering level of anxiety.
- Focus on present situation.
- Give feedback about current reality; identify positive achievements.
- Have person describe events in detail; focus on specifics of who, what, when, and where.

Numerous physical complaints with no known organic base (Maynard, 2004)

- Encourage expression of feelings.
- Give positive feedback when person is symptom free.
- Acknowledge that symptoms must be burdensome.
- Encourage interest in external environment (eg, volunteering, helping others).
- Listen to complaints.
- Evaluate secondary gains the person receives and attempt to interrupt cycle; see person regularly, not simply in response to somatic complaints.
- Engage in discussions not related to symptoms.
- Avoid "doing something" to each complaint; set limits consistently.

Anger† (eg, demanding behavior, manipulation; with adults, see *Ineffective Coping*)

Unrealistic expectations of self (Lyon, 2002)

- Help to set realistic goals and subgoals.
- Allow for setbacks.
- Use positive self-talk.
- Practice "thought stopping" with toxic thinking.
- Organize time.

Toxic thoughts (Lyon, 2002)

- Avoid assigning negative meaning to an event.
- Avoid "reading someones else's mind."
- Avoid all-or-nothing, black-or-white thinking.
- Avoid making the worst of a situation.
- Attempt to fix the problem; avoid assigning blame.
- Avoid minimizing positive experiences.
- Resilience is a combination of abilities and characteristics that interact to allow an individual to bounce back, cope successfully and function above the norm is spite of significant stress or adversity (Tusaie & Dyer 2004).
- Characteristics of Resilient persons are optimism, intelligence, creativity humor, an existential belief system. And an appreciation of the uniqueness of oneself (Tusaie & Dyer 2004).
- Environmental factors that favor resilience are perceived social support or a sense of connectiveness (Tusaie & Dyer 2004).

Initiate Health Teaching and Referrals as Indicated.

For people identified as having chronic anxiety and maladaptive coping mechanisms, refer for ongoing psychiatric treatment.

Instruct in nontechnical, understandable terms regarding illness and associated treatments.

Repeat explanations, because anxiety may interfere with learning.

Instruct in maintenance of physical well-being (ie, nutrition, exercise, elimination).

Instruct (or refer) person for assertiveness training.

Instruct in use of relaxation techniques (eg, aromatherapy, hydrotherapy, music therapy, massage).

Explain the benefits of foot massage and reflexology (Grealish et al., 2000; Stephenson et al., 2000).

Instruct in constructive problem solving.

Provide telephone numbers for emergency intervention: hotlines, psychiatric emergency room, on-call staff if available.

---

*Denial serves a protective function and is not always maladaptive.

†Anger is a response to frustration and anxiety. Not all anger is problematic. It can be used for problem solving.

Rationales

- Nursing strategies differ depending on the level of anxiety (Tarsitano, 1992).
- Participating in decision making can give a client a sense of control, which enhances coping ability. Perception of loss of control can result in a sense of powerlessness, then hopelessness (Courts, Barba & Tesh, 2001).
- Providing emotional support and encouraging sharing may help a client clarify and verbalize fears, allowing the nurse to give realistic feedback and reassurance.
- An anxious client has a narrowed perceptual field with a diminished ability to learn. The client may experience symptoms caused by increased muscle tension and disrupted sleep. Anxiety tends to feed on itself, trapping the client in a spiral of increasing anxiety, tension, and emotional and physical pain.
- Some fears are based on inaccurate information, which accurate data can relieve. A client with severe anxiety or panic does not retain learning.
- Verbalization allows sharing and provides an opportunity to correct misconceptions.
- Praising the client for effective coping can reinforce future positive coping responses.
- Relaxation techniques enhance the client's sense of control over the body's response to stress (DeMarco-Sinatra, 2000).
- Research has shown that involving family members in care increases client cooperation and positive adjustment to the experience (Leske, 1993).
- Helping the client to understand anxiety and its sources provides an opportunity to work through it
- The conversion of emotional distress into physical symptoms is called somatization.
- Psychological concepts that may underlie somatization are amplification of body sensations, the need to be sick, the need for one family member to be the identified client, and sensory experiences in the Absence of Stimulation (Maynard, 2004).
- Complementary therapies such as massage, aromatherapy, and hydrotherapy are useful in managing stress and anxiety (Keegan, 2000; Wong, Lopez-Wahas & Molassiotis, 2001).
- Exercise can effectively reduce anxiety (Blanchard, Courneya & Laing, 2001).
- Music therapy is an effective nursing intervention in decreasing anxiety (Wong, Lopez-Nahas & Molassiotis, 2001).
- Exercise is an effective method for reducing state anxiety in breast cancer survivors (Blanchard, Courneya & Laing, 2001).

❖ Pediatric Interventions

Actions

Explain events using simple, age-appropriate terms and illustrations, puppets, dolls, and sample equipment.

Allow child to wear underwear and have familiar toys or objects.

Assist parents/caregivers to manage their anxiety when with child.

Assist child to cope with anxiety (Wong, 2003):
- Establish a trusting relationship.
- Minimize separation from parents.
- Encourage expression of feelings.
- Involve child in play.
- Prepare child for new experiences (eg, procedures, surgery).
- Provide comfort measures.
- Allow for regression.
- Encourage parental involvement in care.
- Allay parental apprehension and provide them information.

Assist a child with anger.
- Encourage child to share anger (eg, "How did you feel when you had your injection?").
- Tell child that being angry is okay (eg, "I sometimes get angry when I can't have what I want.").
- Encourage and allow child to express anger in acceptable ways (eg, loud talking, running outside around the house).

Rationales

- Children need opportunities and encouragement to express anger in a controlled, acceptable way (eg, choosing not to play a particular game or with a particular person, slamming a door, voicing anger). Unacceptable expressions of anger include throwing or breaking objects and hitting others. Children who are not permitted to express anger may develop hostility and perceive the world as unfriendly.
- The presence of parents provides a familiar, stabilizing support.
- Parental anxiety influences the child's anxiety.

Maternal Interventions

Actions

Discuss expectations and concerns regarding pregnancy and parenthood with the woman alone, her partner alone, and then together as indicated.

Help identify unrealistic expectations.

Acknowledge anxieties and their normality (Lugina et al., 2001):

- 1 week postpartum: worried about feeling tired and nervous about breasts, perineum, infection
- 1 week postpartum: worried about baby's eyes, respirations, temperature, safety, crying
- 6 weeks postpartum: worried about partner's reaction to her and baby

Rationales

- Providing emotional support and encouraging sharing may help a client clarify and verbalize fears, allowing the nurse to give realistic feedback and reassurance.
- Some fears are based on inaccurate information, which accurate data can relieve.

⊙ Geriatric Interventions

Actions

Use consistent caregivers when possible.

Maintain a calm, unhurried manner by allowing person to set pace.

Evaluate effects of medical conditions, medications, and caffeine intake on anxiety level.

Rationales

- Pathologic processes (eg, decreased cerebral oxygen, hyperthyroidism) can precipitate or exacerbate anxiety (Miller, 2004).
- Medications or chemicals that stimulate the central nervous system (CNS) can cause or increase anxiety.

ANXIETY

 RELATED TO INSUFFICIENT KNOWLEDGE OF PREOPERATIVE ROUTINES, POSTOPERATIVE EXERCISES/ACTIVITIES, POSTOPERATIVE ALTERATIONS/SENSATIONS

Goals

NOC	Knowledge: Treatment Procedures

The person will:

- Verbalize, if asked, what to expect (routines, environment)
- Demonstrate postoperative exercises, splinting, and respiratory regimen
- Relate less anxiety after teaching

General Interventions

NIC	Preparatory Sensory Information, Teaching: Procedure/Treatment, Anxiety Reduction

Before Surgery, the Physician Should Explain:

Nature of surgery needed   Reason for and anticipated outcomes of surgery
Risks   Type of anesthesia
Expectations for length and limitations imposed during recovery

Determine Level of Understanding of Surgical Procedure.

Reinforce physician's explanation. Notify physician if additional explanations are indicated.

Evaluate Anxiety Level of Client and Family.

Low (expected)
Moderate (narrowed perception, difficulty concentrating, some difficulty analyzing, shakiness)
High (perception greatly reduced, high distraction, poor concentration, severe learning impairment)

Notify Physician if Client Exhibits Severe Anxiety or Panic.

If Anxiety is Moderate:

- Assist person to gain insight into anxiety and reason.
- Help client reappraise the threat and learn a new way to deal with it (Tarsitano, 1992).

For Clients with Morning Admissions or Same-day Surgery:

Provide access to general information pertaining to need for active participation, routines, equipment, environment, personnel, postoperative sensations, and care before day of surgery.

Group classes   Printed materials
Audio or videotapes

Establish a system of follow-up to educational program (eg, telephone call day before).

For Hospitalized Individual:

Give bedside instruction concerning specific type of surgery, sensations, and appearances (eg, machines, tubes) that client and family may encounter postoperatively.

Explain all procedures, the reasons for them, and their importance: *preoperative:* NPO, medications, laboratory tests; *postoperative:* parenteral fluids, vital signs, dressings, nasogastric and other tubes, indwelling bladder catheter, pain and availability of medications.

Explain the Importance of and Teach Using Return Demonstration:
Turn, cough, and deep breathe, depending on surgical procedure.
Support incision during coughing.
Deep breathe hourly postoperatively.
Exercise actively (show how passive range-of-motion (ROM) exercises will be done).
Sit up, get up, and ambulate—avoid sitting in a chair.
Importance of progressive care
Early ambulation
Self-care, as soon as able

Explain Rationale for Leg Exercises, Demonstrate, and Have Client Return Demonstration (Tarsitano, 1992).
1. With heels on bed, push toes of both feet toward the foot of the bed until the calf muscles of the leg tighten. Relax both feet. Pull toes toward the chin, until calf muscles tighten. Relax feet.
2. With heels on bed, circle both ankles, first to the right and then to the left. Repeat three times. Relax.
3. Bend each knee alternately, sliding foot up along the bed. Relax.
4. Explain the rationale of deep breathing, demonstrate, and have client return demonstrate
5. Place one hand over abdomen and other where incision will be.
6. Inspire and expand abdomen.
7. Expire slowly and deeply.

Explain the Rationale of Coughing, Demonstrate, and Have Client Return Demonstrate.
Cough on Expiration Only to Prevent Elevation of Pleural Pressure.

Discuss Purpose of Recovery Room with Patient and Family.

Visiting policies	Type of care
Length of stay, if applicable	Placement in intensive care unit if needed or indicated

Explain other Hospital Policies as Indicated.

Visiting hours	Number of visitors
Location of waiting rooms	How physician will contact them after operation

Evaluate:
Person's/family's ability to meet preset, mutually planned learning goals (behaviors)
Need for further teaching and support

Rationales

- Preoperative teaching provides client with information, which can help decrease anxiety and fear associated with the unknown and enhance sense of control.
- Explaining the importance and purpose of all preoperative procedures helps relieve anxiety and fear associated with lack of knowledge of necessary preoperative activities and routines.
- Explaining postoperative routines and sensations helps reduce fears associated with the unknown and unexpected (Christman & Kirchhoff, 1992).
- Exercises and movement promote lung expansion and mobilization of secretions. Incentive spirometry promotes deep breathing by providing a visual indicator of the effectiveness of the breathing effort.
- Leg exercises increase venous return and prevent stasis.

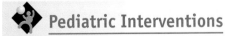 **Pediatric Interventions**

Actions
Create an Information Packet for Home Use (Lancaster, 1997).
Schedule tours of operating room (OR) and post-anesthesia recovery (PAR) units.
Give information for preoperative preparation, surgical day, and discharge.
Follow oral guidelines: no solids or milk after midnight; clear liquids or breast milk until 2 h before surgery for premature babies and infants younger than 6 months; clear liquids until 3 h before surgery for children 6 months to 18 years.
Give instructions to call if the child's health changes.

Include an age-appropriate story booklet.

Organize tours for children about 5 to 7 days before surgery.

Group together children with similar problems.

Encourage participation of parents and siblings to provide added security for the child.

Involve as many senses as possible. Explain how it feels and smells and whether it will hurt.

Using a doll, demonstrate the OR garments and blood sample acquisition.

Using a volunteer child, demonstrate taking blood pressure, temperature, and heart and respiration rates.

Take children on OR cart to show them where their parents will wait during surgery.

Have an OR nurse (fully dressed) explain:

  Reasons for OR attire

  Anesthesia machine

  Anesthesia as "hospital air" or "hospital sleep" to avoid confusion

  Postanesthesia recovery room

Explain/demonstrate on doll or child:

  Straps on OR table

  Monitoring devices (electrocardiogram [ECG], pulse)

  Anesthesia mask (on each child, or on parent if child is frightened)

  Intravenous lines (inserted after induction; removed after child is eating and drinking)

Increase effectiveness of the teaching program and promote security by:

  Using name tags so children can be addressed by name

  Involving children in discussion (eg, ask them the colors of objects)

  Not forcing any child to do anything (if a child resists, have parent perform the activity and encourage child to help)

  Allowing child to handle equipment

  Avoiding calling anesthesia "gas," which the child may confuse with gas in a car or used in euthanasia of animals

  Explaining that anesthesia does not affect memory

  Allowing children to take home masks, hats, and ECG buttons

  Encouraging child to bring a favorite toy when returning for surgery

Talk with Child Regarding Previous Experiences and Current Concerns (Pillitteri, 2003).

Clarify misinformation.

Offer choices when possible.

Telephone Family.

Before surgery to review instructions and answer questions

Day after surgery to evaluate status

Rationales

- Tours of the facilities with opportunities to see and handle some equipment and meet with personnel can help lessen anxiety (Wong, 2003).
- Playing with equipment allows the child to act out feelings, establish familiarity, and question procedures.
- Preschool children experience higher levels of emotional distress during surgery than any other age group.

DEATH ANXIETY

DEFINITION

Death Anxiety: The state in which an individual experiences apprehension, worry, or fear related to death or dying.

DEFINING CHARACTERISTICS

Worrying about the effects of one's own death on significant others
Powerless over issues related to dying
Fear of loss of physical and/or mental abilities when dying
Anticipated pain related to dying
Deep sadness
Fear of the process of dying
Concerns of overworking the caregiver as terminal illness incapacitates self
Concern about meeting one's creator or feeling doubtful about the existence of a god or higher being
Total loss of control over any aspect of one's own death
Negative death images or unpleasant thoughts about any event related to death or dying
Fear of delayed demise
Fear of premature death because it prevents the accomplishment of important life goals

RELATED FACTORS

Impending death causes this diagnosis. Additional factors can contribute to death anxiety.

Situational (Personal, Environmental)

Related to situational factors (anxiety)
Related to fear of being a burden
Related to fear of unmanageable pain
Related to fear of abandonment
Related to unresolved conflict (family, friends)
Related to fear that one's life lacked meaning
Related to social disengagement
Related to powerlessness and vulnerability

AUTHOR'S NOTE

The inclusion of *Death Anxiety* in the NANDA classification creates a diagnostic category with the etiology in the label. This opens the NANDA list to thousands of diagnostic labels with etiology (eg, separation anxiety, failure anxiety, travel anxiety). Many diagnostic labels can take this same path: fear as claustrophobic fear, diarrhea as traveler's diarrhea, decisional conflict as end-of-life decisional conflict.

This author recommends deleting the etiology in the diagnostic label except for syndrome diagnoses, which require etiology in the label. Syndrome diagnoses have no "related to" factors.

ERRORS IN DIAGNOSTIC STATEMENTS

See *Anxiety*.

KEY CONCEPTS

In a research study of the reactions of 153 rehabilitation counselors to possible client death, 22% reported they preferred not to work with clients with life-threatening illnesses. Death anxiety scores were higher in younger respondents (< 44 years of age). Educational programs and support groups help reduce death anxiety in health care workers (Hunt, 2000).

Focus Assessment Criteria

See *Anxiety* and *Grieving*.

For more information on Focus Assessment Criteria, visit http://connection.lww.com.

Goal

NOC Dignified Dying, Fear Control

The person will report diminished anxiety or fear.

Indicators

- Share feelings regarding dying.
- Identify two activities that increase control and self-knowledge.

General Interventions

NIC Coping Enhancement, Emotional Support, Spiritual Support

Encourage the person to reconstruct his or her world view (Taylor, 2000).
  Allow client to verbalize feelings about the meaning of death.
  Advise that there are no right or wrong feelings.
  Advise client that responses are his or her choice.
  Acknowledge struggles.
Encourage the person to share conflicts and concerns.
  Explore possible resolutions to conflicts (eg, letter, phone call).
  Encourage dialogue with a spiritual mentor or soul friend.
Explore the person's interpretation of suffering: punishment, bad luck, nature's course, will of Greater Other, denial.
Encourage telling life stories and reminiscing.
Discuss leaving a legacy: donation, personal articles, or taped messages.
Encourage reflective activities, such as personal prayer, meditation, and journal writing.
If possible, encourage a return to a previously pleasurable activity. Examples include painting, music, woodworking, and quilting.
Encourage return of the gift of love to others by listening, praying for others, sharing personal wisdom gained from illness, and creating legacy gifts.
Aggressively manage unrelieved symptoms.

Nausea	Vomiting
Pruritus	Fatigue
Pain	

Encourage friends and families to be emotionally and spiritually honest.
Explain advance directives and assist in process if desired.

Rationales

- Every attempt should be made to encourage family and friends to talk to, not about, the person (Brant, 1998).
- Strategies that help the person find meaning in failures and successes can reduce anxiety.
- Promoting and restoring interests, imagination, and creativity enhance quality of life (Brant, 1998).
- When a person is facing death, reconstructing a world view involves balancing thoughts about the painful subject with avoiding painful thoughts (Taylor, 2000).
- Serious unrelieved symptoms can cause a distressing death and needless added suffering for families (Nelson et al., 2000).

Risk for Imbalanced Body Temperature
Hyperthermia
Hypothermia
Ineffective Thermoregulation
  Related to Newborn Transition to Extrauterine Environment

RISK FOR IMBALANCED BODY TEMPERATURE

DEFINITION

Risk for Imbalanced Body Temperature: The state in which the individual is at risk for failing to maintain body temperature within normal range (36°C to 37.5°C or 98°F to 99.5°F) (Smeltzer & Bare, 2004)

RISK FACTORS

Presence of risk factors (see Related Factors)

RELATED FACTORS
Treatment-Related

Related to cooling effects of:

Parenteral fluid infusion/
  blood transfusion
Cooling blanket

Dialysis
Operating suite

Situational (Personal, Environmental)

Related to:

Exposure to cold, rain, snow,
  wind/exposure to heat, sun,
  and humidity extremes
Inappropriate clothing for climate

Inability to pay for shelter, heat, or air conditioning
Extremes of weight
Consumption of alcohol
Dehydration/malnutrition

Maturational

Related to ineffective temperature regulation secondary to extremes of age (eg, newborn, older adult)

⊙⊙ AUTHOR'S NOTE

Risk for Imbalanced Body Temperature includes those at risk for *Hyperthermia, Hypothermia, Ineffective Thermoregulation,* or all of these. If the person is at risk for only one (eg, *Hypothermia* but not *Hyperthermia*), then it is more useful to label the problem with the specific diagnosis (*Risk for Hypothermia*). If the person is at risk for two or more, then *Risk for Imbalanced Body Temperature* is more appropriate. The focus of nursing care is preventing abnormal body temperatures by identifying and treating those with normal temperature who demonstrate risk factors that nurse-prescribed interventions (eg, removing blankets, adjusting environmental temperature) can control. If the imbalance is related to a pathophysiologic complication that requires nursing and medical interventions, then the problem should be labeled as a collaborative problem (eg, *PC: Severe Hypothermia related to hypothalamus injury*). The focus of concern then becomes monitoring to detect and report significant temperature fluctuations and implementing collaborative interventions (eg, a warming or cooling blanket) as ordered. See also Author's Notes for *Hyperthermia* and *Hypothermia.*

KEY CONCEPTS
Generic Considerations

- The body has two major compartments: the *shell* (skin and subcutaneous tissue) and the *core* (vital internal organs, intestinal tract, and large muscle groups). Heat transfer involves shell and core; it is possible for the shell to be warm while the core is cold, and vice versa.
- Regulation of body temperature is a dynamic process involving four mechanisms (Porth, 2002):

   Conduction: Direct transfer of heat from the body to cooler objects without motion (eg, from cells and capillaries to skin and onto clothing)

   Convection: Transfer of heat by circulation (eg, from warmer core areas to peripheral areas and from air movement next to the skin)

   Radiation: Transfer of heat between the skin and the environment

   Evaporation: Transfer of heat when skin or clothing is wet and heat is lost through moisture into the environment

- Heat production occurs in the core, which is innervated by thermoreceptor stimulation from the hypothalamus.
- Normothermia is defined as a core temperature of 36.6° to 37.5°C or 98° to 99.5°F (Smeltzer & Bare, 2004).
- Heat loss and gain vary in individuals and are influenced by body surface area, peripheral vasomotor tone, and quantity of subcutaneous tissue.
- Shivering, the body's physiologic attempt to create more heat, produces profound physiologic responses:

   Increased oxygen consumption to two to five times the normal rate

   Increased metabolic demand to as much as 400% to 500%

   Increased myocardial work, carbon dioxide production, cutaneous vasoconstriction, and eventual lactic acid production

   The reliability of temperature depends on accurate temperature-taking technique, minimization of variables affecting the temperature measurement device, and the site chosen for measurement.

- Oral temperature readings may be unreliable (from such variables as poor contact between the thermometer and mucosa, air movement, and smoking or drinking before temperature taking); oral temperatures measure 0.5° below core temperature (Giuliano et al., 2000).
- Rectal temperature readings, which have fewer affecting variables and are more reliable than oral readings, measure 0.5°C above core temperature at normothermia, and at temperatures less than 36.5°C measure *peripheral* temperature rather than *core* temperature. Rectal temperatures measure 1° *higher* than oral temperature readings.
- Axillary temperature readings are reliable only for skin temperature; they measure 1° *lower* than oral temperature readings.

Hyperthermia

- The body responds to hot environments by increasing heat dissipation through increased sweat production and dilation of peripheral blood vessels.
- Increased metabolic rate increases body temperature, and vice versa (increased body temperature increases metabolic rate).
- Fever is a major sign of onset of infection, inflammation, and disease: treatment with aspirin or acetaminophen without medical consultation may mask important symptoms that should receive medical attention.
- Blood is the body's cooling fluid: low blood volume from dehydration predisposes to fever.

Hypothermia

- The body responds to cold environments with mechanisms aimed at preventing heat loss and increasing heat production:

   Muscle contraction

   Increased heart rate

   Shivering and vasodilation

   Peripheral vasoconstriction

   Dilation of blood vessels in muscles

   Release of thyroxine and corticosteroids

- Severe hypothermia can cause life-threatening dysrhythmias and must be referred to a physician.
- Without safe and effective rewarming, hypothermia (a core temperature <35°C [95°F]) in the postoperative period has many profound negative effects (decreased myocardial and cerebral functions, respiratory acidosis, impaired hematologic and immunologic functions, and cold diuresis; Howell, Macrae, Sanjines, Burke & DeStefano, 1992). Hypothermia also reduces blood pressure and contributes to shock.
- Vasodilation promotes heat loss and predisposes to hypothermia.

Pediatric Considerations

- Almost every child experiences a fever of 100° to 104°F at some time. It usually does not harm normal children; only approximately 4% of febrile children are susceptible to convulsions (Hunsberger, 1989). Children younger than 18 years with fever accompanied by symptoms of influenza should never be medicated with aspirin or products containing aspirin because of the risk of development of potentially fatal Reye's syndrome.
- Newborns are vulnerable to heat loss because of the following (Varda & Behnke, 2000). The following sequence illustrates this mechanism:

Large body surface area relative to body mass	Increased basal metabolism rate
Less adipose tissue for insulation	Environment (delivery room, nursery)

- Nonshivering thermogenesis is a heat production mechanism located in brown fat (highly vascular adipose tissue), found only in infants. When skin temperature begins to drop, thermal receptors transmit impulses to the central nervous system (May & Mahlmeister, 1994). The following sequence illustrates this mechanism:

  CNS → Stimulates sympathetic nervous system → Release of norepinephrine from adrenal gland and at nerve endings in brown fat → Heat production

- Treating all fevers in children is unnecessary. Fevers related to heat stroke can be treated with tepid or cold sponging. Fevers (<104°F or 40°C) in previously well children with no history of febrile convulsions and without a threatening illness can be left untreated or, if desired, treated with acetaminophen. Sponging increases the child's discomfort.
- Tepid sponging instead of antipyretic drugs is indicated for very young infants and children with severe liver disease or a history of hypersensitivity to antipyretic drugs.

Geriatric Considerations

Older adults can become hypothermic or hyperthermic in moderately cold or hot environments, compared with younger adults, who require exposure to severe cold or hot temperatures (Miller, 2004).

- Age-related changes that interfere with the body's ability to adapt to cold temperature include inefficient vasoconstriction, decreased cardiac output, decreased subcutaneous tissue, and delayed and diminished sweating (Miller, 2004).
- Older adults have a higher threshold for onset and decreased efficiency of sweating.
- Older adults have a dulled perception of cold and warmth and thus may lack the stimulus to initiate protective actions.
- The thirst mechanism becomes less efficient with aging, as does the kidney's ability to concentrate urine, increasing the risk of heat-related dehydration.
- Inactivity and immobility increase susceptibility to hypothermia by suppressing shivering and reducing heat-generating muscle activity.
- Seventy percent of all victims of heat stroke are older than 60 years.

Focus Assessment Criteria

Subjective Data
Assess for Defining Characteristics.

History of symptoms (abnormal skin temperature, altered mentation, headaches, nausea, lethargy, vertigo)

Onset

Assess for Related Factors.

Hyperthermia

Dehydration

Recent exposure to communicable disease without known immunity (eg, measles without vaccine or previous illness)

Recent overexposure to sun, heat, humidity
Recent overactivity
Radiation/chemotherapy/immunosuppression
Alcohol use
Impaired judgment
Home environment
    Adequate ventilation?   Air conditioning?   Room temperature?
Medications
    Diuretics   Anticholinergics   CNS Depressants
    Antidepressants   Vasoconstrictors
    How often taken? Last
       dose taken when?

Hypothermia
Recent exposure to cold/dampness
Inactivity
Impaired judgment
Medications
    Vasodilators   CNS depressants
Home environment
    Heating, blankets   Clothing (eg, socks, hat, gloves)   Shelter

Problems That May Contribute to Hyperthermia or Hypothermia
Smoking   Circulatory problems (specify)   History of frostbite
Diabetes   Mobility problems   Cardiovascular disorders/
Repeated infections   Neurologic disorders   peripheral vascular disease

Objective Data
Assess for Defining Characteristics.
Vital signs
Normal baseline temperature   Present temperature   Abnormal respiratory rate
Abnormal heart rate, rhythm   Abnormal blood pressure
Mental status
Skin and circulation
Signs of dehydration
Parched mouth/furrowed   Increased urine specific gravity
   tongue/dry lips

For more information on Focus Assessment Criteria, visit http://connection.lww.com.

HYPERTHERMIA

DEFINITION

Hyperthermia: The state in which an individual has or is at risk of having a sustained elevation of body temperature greater than 37.8°C (100°F) orally or 38.8°C (101°F) rectally due to external factors

DEFINING CHARACTERISTICS
Major (Must Be Present)

Temperature higher than 37.8°C (100°F) orally or 38.8°C (101°F) rectally

Minor (May Be Present)

Flushed skin

Warm to touch

Increased respiratory rate

Tachycardia

Shivering/goose pimples

Dehydration

Specific or generalized aches
  and pains (eg, headache)

Malaise/fatigue/weakness

Loss of appetite

RELATED FACTORS
Treatment-Related

Decreased ability to sweat secondary to (specify medication)

Situational (Personal, Environmental)

Related to:

Exposure to heat, sun

Inappropriate clothing for climate

No access to air conditioning

Related to decreased circulation secondary to:

Extremes of weight

Dehydration

Related to insufficient hydration for vigorous activity

Maturational

Related to ineffective temperature regulation secondary to age (refer to *Ineffective Thermoregulation*)

 AUTHOR'S NOTE

The nursing diagnoses *Hypothermia* and *Hyperthermia* represent people with temperature below and above normal, respectively. Some of these states are treatable by nursing interventions, such as correcting external causes (eg, inappropriate clothing, exposure to elements [heat or cold], dehydration). Nursing care centers on preventing or treating mild hypothermia and hyperthermia. As life-threatening situations that require medical and nursing interventions, severe hypothermia and hyperthermia represent collaborative problems and should be labeled *PC: Hypothermia* or *PC: Hyperthermia*.

Temperature elevation from infections, other disorders (eg, hypothalamic), or treatments (eg, hypothermia units) requires collaborative treatment. If desired, the nurse could use the nursing diagnosis *Impaired Comfort* and the collaborative problem *PC: Hypothermia* or *PC: Hyperthermia*.

 ERRORS IN DIAGNOSTIC STATEMENTS

1. *Hyperthermia related to intraoperative pharmacogenic hypermetabolism*
    This situation describes malignant hyperthermia, a life-threatening, inherited disorder resulting in a hypermetabolic state related to use of anesthetic agents and depolarizing muscle relaxants. *PC: Malignant Hypertension* would more appropriately describe this situation, which necessitates rapid detection and treatment by both nursing and medicine.
2. *Hyperthermia related to effect of circulating endotoxins on hypothalamus secondary to sepsis*
    Nursing for people with elevated temperature in acute care focuses on monitoring and managing the fever with nursing and physician orders or promoting comfort through nursing orders. *Impaired Comfort* would more appropriately describe a situation that nurses treat, with *PC: Sepsis* representing the physiologic complication that nurses monitor for and manage with nurse-prescribed and physician-prescribed interventions.

Focus Assessment Criteria

See *Risk for Imbalanced Body Temperature.*
    For more information on Focus Assessment Criteria, visit http://connection.lww.com.

Goal

NOC Thermoregulation

The person will maintain body temperature.

Indicators
- Identify risk factors for hyperthermia.
- Reduce risk factors for hyperthermia.

General Interventions

NIC Fever Treatment, Temperature Regulation, Environmental Management, Fluid Management

Assess Body and Environmental Temperature.

Assess for Contributing Risk Factors.

Dehydration   Environmental warmth/exercise

Remove or Reduce Contributing Risk Factors.

Dehydration

Monitor intake and output and provide favorite fluids to maintain a balance between intake and output.

Teach importance of maintaining adequate fluid intake (at least 2000 mL a day of cool liquids unless contraindicated by heart or kidney disease) to prevent dehydration. Explain importance of not relying on thirst sensation as an indication of the need for fluid.

Recommended fluid replacement for moderate activities in hot weather (DeFabio, 2000) is as follows:
- 78°F to 84.9°F   16 oz/h
- 85°F to 89.9°F   24 oz/h
- >90°F   32 oz/h

See also *Deficient Fluid Volume.*

Environmental Warmth/Exercise

Assess whether clothing or bedcovers are too warm for the environment or planned activity.

Remove excess clothing or blankets (remove hat, gloves, or socks, as appropriate) to promote heat loss. Encourage wearing loose cotton clothing.

Provide air conditioning, dehumidifiers, fans, or cool baths or compresses as appropriate.

Teach the importance of increasing fluid intake during warm weather and exercise. Advise against exercising in hot weather.

Teach the need to wear a hat or use an umbrella during sun exposure.

Initiate Health Teaching as Indicated.

Explain that children and older adults are more at risk for hyperthermia.

Teach the early signs of hyperthermia or heat stroke:

Flushed skin	Headache/confusion
Fatigue	Loss of appetite

Teach to take cool baths several times a day in hot temperatures, avoiding soap to prevent skin drying.

Teach to apply ice packs or cool, wet towels to the body, especially on the axillae and groin.

Explain the need to avoid alcohol, caffeine, and large, heavy meals during hot weather.

Stress the need to report persistent elevated temperature.

Rationales

- Activity level and environmental temperature greatly affect body temperature; high humidity increases the effect of cold or heat on the body.
- Exposure of the head, face, hands, and feet can affect body temperature greatly. Heat is conducted from blood vessels of these vascular areas to the skin and from the skin to the air, and where cold is conducted from the air to the skin and from the skin to the blood vessels.
- Cooling of a person with hyperthermia and rewarming of a person with hypothermia must be done with great care to avoid overcooling or overwarming; in acute care settings, cooling and rewarming often require close collaboration with the physician.
- Adding clothes or blankets inhibits the body's natural ability to reduce body temperature; removing clothes or blankets enhances the body's natural ability to reduce body temperature.
- Increased calories and fluids are required to maintain metabolic functions during fever.
- Axillary temperatures should be measured for 5 min.
- Electronic or tympanic thermometers give rapid, accurate readings in neonates, children, and adults.

HYPOTHERMIA

DEFINITION

Hypothermia: The state in which an individual has or is at risk of having a sustained reduction of body temperature of below 35.5°C (96°F) rectally because of increased vulnerability to external factors*

DEFINING CHARACTERISTICS†
Major (80% to 100%)

Reduction in body temperature below 35.5°C (96°F) rectally*

Cool skin
Pallor (moderate)
Shivering (mild)

Minor (50% to 79%)

Mental confusion/drowsiness/restlessness
Decreased pulse and respiration
Cachexia/malnutrition

---

*Temperatures below 35°C (95°F) rectally should be reported to the physician for collaborative management of rewarming.

†Adapted from Carroll, S. M. (1989). Nursing diagnosis: Hypothermia. In R. M. Carroll-Johnson (Ed.). *Classification of nursing diagnosis: Proceedings of the eighth conference.* Philadelphia: J. B. Lippincott.

RELATED FACTORS
Situational (Personal, Environmental)
Related to:
Exposure to cold, rain, snow, wind
Inappropriate clothing for climate
Inability to pay for shelter or heat

Related to decreased circulation secondary to:
Extremes of weight   Dehydration
Consumption of alcohol   Inactivity

Maturational
Related to ineffective temperature regulation secondary to age (eg, neonate, older adult)

Ⓧ **AUTHOR'S NOTE**

Because more serious hypothermia (temperatures below 35°C or 95°F rectally) can cause severe pathophysiologic consequences, such as decreased myocardial and respiratory function, the nurse is cautioned to report these low readings to the physician. Nurses most often initiate nurse-prescribed interventions for mild hypothermia (temperatures between 35°C [95°F] and 36°C [97°F] rectally) to prevent more serious hypothermia. Nurses are commonly responsible for identifying and treating *Risk for Hypothermia*. See also diagnostic considerations for *Risk for Imbalanced Body Temperature*.

Ⓧ **ERRORS IN DIAGNOSTIC STATEMENTS**

See *Risk for Imbalanced Body Temperature* and *Hyperthermia*.

FOCUS ASSESSMENT CRITERIA
See *Risk for Imbalanced Body Temperature*.
For more information on Focus Assessment Criteria, visit http://connection.lww.com.

Goal
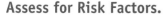

NOC Thermoregulation

The person will maintain body temperature within normal limits.

Indicators
• Identify risk factors for hypothermia.
• Reduce risk factors for hypothermia.

General Interventions

NIC Hypothermia Treatment,
Temperature Regulation,
Temperature Regulation: Intraoperative,
Environmental Management

Assess for Risk Factors.
Prolonged exposure to cold environment
  (either home or outside)
Poverty/inability to pay for adequate heat/shelter
Extremes of age (eg, newborn, older adult)
Neurovascular/peripheral vascular disease
Malnutrition/cachexia
Perioperative experience

Monitor Body and Environmental Temperatures.

Reduce or Eliminate Causative or Contributing Factors, if Possible.

Prolonged Exposure to Cold Environment

Assess room temperatures at home.

Teach to keep room temperatures at 70°F to 75°F or to layer clothing with sweaters.

Explain the importance of wearing a hat, gloves, and warm socks and shoes to prevent heat loss.

Encourage limiting going outside when temperatures are very cold.

Acquire an electric blanket, warm blankets, or down comforter and flannel sheets for bed.

Provide a hot bath before the person is cold.

Teach to wear close-knit undergarments to prevent heat loss.

Explain that more clothes may be needed in the morning, when body metabolism is lowest.

Poverty/Inability to Pay for Heat

Consult with social service to identify sources of financial assistance/warm clothing/blankets, shelter.

Teach the importance of preventing heat loss before body temperature is actually lowered.

Acquire warm socks, sweaters, gloves, and hats.

Neurovascular/Peripheral Vascular Disease

Keep room temperature at 70°F to 74°F.

Assess for adequate circulation to extremities (ie, satisfactory peripheral pulses).

Instruct to wear warm gloves and socks to reduce heat loss.

Teach the person to take a warm bath if he or she cannot get warm.

Initiate Health Teaching if Indicated.

Explain the relationship of age as a risk for hypothermia.

Teach the early signs of hypothermia: cool skin, pallor, blanching, and redness.

Explain the need to drink 8 to 10 glasses of water daily and to consume frequent, small meals with warm liquids.

Explain the need to avoid alcohol during periods of very cold weather.

Reduce Heat Loss during Surgery.

Warmed blankets

Limit exposed areas

Warmed fluids (intravenous, irrigating)

Heating and humidifying inhaled gases

Rationales

- Minimizing evaporation, convection, conduction, and radiation can prevent significant heat losses (Puterbough, 1991).
- People whose temperatures are maintained at normal levels during the intraoperative period experience fewer adverse outcomes; hospital costs also are lower (Mahoney & Odom, 1999).
- Greatest reduction in temperature is during the first hour of surgery (Bernthal, 1999).

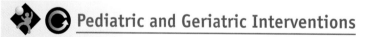 **Pediatric and Geriatric Interventions**

For Extremes of Age (Newborns, Older Adults):

Maintain room temperature at 70°F to 74°F.

Instruct to wear hat, gloves, and socks if necessary to prevent heat loss.

Explain to family members that newborns, infants, and older adults are more susceptible to heat loss (see also *Ineffective Thermoregulation*).

During Intraoperative Experience:

For children and older adults, unless hypothermia is desired to reduce blood loss, consider the following interventions (Puterbough, 1991):

Increase ambient temperature of operating room (OR) before case.

Use a portable radiant heating lamp to provide additional heat during surgery.
Cover with warm blankets when arriving in OR.
When possible, use a warming mattress.
During prepping and surgery, keep as much of body surface covered as possible.
Warm prep set, blood, fluids, anesthesia, irrigants.
Replace wet gowns and drapes with dry ones.
Keep head well covered.
Continue heat-conserving interventions postoperatively.

Rationales

- Children and older adults can become hypothermic in moderately cold OR environments (Miller, 2004; Wong, 2003).
- During the immediate postoperative period, clients are prone to hypothermia related to prolonged exposure to cold in the OR and the infusion of large quantities of cool intravenous fluids.

INEFFECTIVE THERMOREGULATION

DEFINITION
Ineffective Thermoregulation: The state in which an individual experiences or is at risk of experiencing an inability to maintain a stable core normal body temperature in the presence of adverse or changing external factors

DEFINING CHARACTERISTICS
Temperature fluctuations related to limited metabolic compensatory regulation in response to environmental factors

RELATED FACTORS
Situational (Personal, Environmental)
Related to:
Fluctuating environmental temperatures
Cold or wet articles (clothes, cribs, equipment)
Inadequate housing
Wet body surface
Inadequate clothing for weather (excessive, insufficient)

Maturational
Related to limited metabolic compensatory regulation secondary to age (eg, neonate, older adult)

(X) **AUTHOR'S NOTE**

Ineffective Thermoregulation is a useful diagnosis for people with difficulty maintaining a stable core body temperature over a wide range of environmental temperatures. This diagnosis most commonly applies to older adults and newborns. Thermoregulation involves balancing heat production and heat loss. Nursing care focuses on manipulating external factors (eg, clothing and environmental conditions) to maintain body temperature within normal limits, and on teaching prevention strategies.

(X) **ERRORS IN DIAGNOSTIC STATEMENTS**

1. *Ineffective Thermoregulation related to effects of a hypothalamic tumor*
   Hypothalamic tumors can affect the temperature-regulating centers, resulting in body temperature shifts. This situation requires constant surveillance and rapid response to changes with appropriate nursing and medical treatments. Thus, this situation would be better described as a collaborative problem: *PC: Hypo/Hyperthermia.*
2. *Ineffective Thermoregulation related to temperature fluctuations*
   Temperature fluctuations represent a manifestation of the diagnosis, not a related factor. If the fluctuations result from age-related limited compensatory regulation, the diagnosis would be written: *Ineffective Thermoregulation related to decreased ability to acclimatize to heat or cold secondary to age,* as evidenced by temperature fluctuations.

Focus Assessment Criteria

Objective Data
Assess for Defining Characteristics.

Skin

Color	Nailbeds
Temperature	Rashes

Temperature
Environment (home, infant [ambient, radiant, Isolette])
Body (adult, child [rectal, oral], newborn [axillary])

Respiration

Rate	Rhythm
Any retractions	Breath sounds

Heart rate

For more information on Focus Assessment Criteria, visit http://connection.lww.com.

INEFFECTIVE THERMOREGULATION

 RELATED TO NEWBORN TRANSITION TO EXTRAUTERINE ENVIRONMENT

Goals

NOC Thermoregulation

The infant will have a temperature between 36.4°C and 37°C.
The parent will explain techniques to avoid heat loss at home.

Indicators

- List situations that increase heat loss.
- Demonstrate how to conserve heat during bathing.
- Demonstrate how to take infant's temperature.

General Interventions

NIC Temperature Regulation, Environmental Management, Newborn Monitoring, Vital Sign Monitoring

Assess for Contributing Factors.

Environmental sources of heat loss
Lack of knowledge (caregivers, parents)

Reduce or Eliminate Sources of Heat Loss.

Evaporation
In the delivery room, quickly dry skin and hair with a heated towel and place infant in a heated environment.
When bathing, provide a warm environment.
Wash and dry infant in sections to reduce evaporation.
Limit time in contact with wet diapers or blankets.

Convection
Reduce drafts in delivery room.
Avoid drafts on infant (air conditioning, fans, windows, open portholes on Isolette).

Conduction
Warm all articles for care (stethoscopes, scales, hands of caregivers, clothes, bed linens, cribs).
Place infant very close to mother to conserve heat (and foster bonding).

Radiation
Place infant next to mother in the delivery room.
Reduce objects in the room that absorb heat (metal).
Place crib or Isolette as far away from walls (outside) or windows as possible.
Preheat incubator.

Monitor Temperature of Newborn (Pillitteri, 2003).
Assess Axillary Temperature Initially Every 30 Min until Stable, then Every 4 to 8 h.
If temperature is less than 36.3°C

1. Wrap infant in two blankets.
2. Put stockinette cap on.
3. Assess for environmental sources of heat loss.

    4. If hypothermia persists over 1 h, notify physician.
    5. Assess for complications of cold stress: hypoxia, respiratory acidosis, hypoglycemia, fluid and electrolyte imbalances, weight loss.

If temperature is greater than 37°C

    1. Loosen blanket.
    2. Remove cap, if on.
    3. Assess environment for thermal gain.
    4. If hyperthermia persists over 1 h, notify physician.

Assess for Signs and Symptoms of Sepsis Every Shift.

Respiratory function (rate, rhythm, pattern)
Poor feeding

Signs of localized infections (skin, umbilicus, circumcision, eyes, birth lacerations)

Skin (tone, color, perfusion)
Irritability

Initiate Health Teaching.

Teach caregiver why infant is vulnerable to temperature fluctuations (cold and heat).
Explain sources of environmental heat loss.
Demonstrate how to conserve heat during bathing.
Instruct that it is not necessary routinely to check temperature at home.
Teach to check temperature if infant is hot, sick, or irritable, as follows:

    1. Shake down the thermometer.
    2. Place in femoral fold.
    3. Hold in place for 11 min.
    4. Read at eye level.
    5. Report temperature greater than 37.5°C to health care professional.

Rationales

- The newborn loses heat through (Wong, 2003)
  - Evaporation (loss of heat when water on skin changes to vapor)
  - Convection (loss of heat when cool air flows over skin)
  - Conduction (transfer of heat when skin surface is in direct contact with a cool surface)
  - Radiation (transfer of heat from infant to cooler surfaces without direct contact)
- Caloric requirements are high for newborns (approximately 117 cal/kg body weight/day).
- An increased metabolic rate for heat production results in increased demands for oxygen and glucose. With prolonged cold stress or in compromised neonates, acidosis can result.
- Premature or low–birth-weight infants are more susceptible to heat loss because of the reduced metabolic reserves available (eg, glycogen).
- The newborn also can experience overheating from excessive clothing in hot weather. The full-term infant can sweat in response to overheating, but the premature infant cannot.
- Significant heat losses the first few moments after birth can drop the newborn's temperature 1°C to 3°C. Drying, heated blankets, and swaddling can reduce these losses (Varda et al., 2000).

BOWEL INCONTINENCE

DEFINITION

Bowel Incontinence: A state in which an individual experiences a change in normal bowel habits characterized by involuntary passage of stool

DEFINING CHARACTERISTICS

Involuntary passage of stool

RELATED FACTORS
Pathophysiologic

Related to impaired rectal sphincter secondary to:

Anal or rectal surgery   Obstetric injuries
Anal or rectal injury   Peripheral neuropathy

Related to cognitive impairment

Related to overdistention of rectum secondary to chronic constipation

Related to lack of voluntary sphincter control secondary to:

Progressive neuromuscular   Cerebral vascular accident
  disorder   Spinal cord injury
Spinal cord compression   Multiple sclerosis

Related to impaired reservoir capacity secondary to:

Inflammatory bowel disease   Chronic rectal ischemia

Treatment-Related

Related to impaired reservoir capacity secondary to:

Colectomy   Radiation proctitis

Situational (Personal, Environmental)

Related to inability to recognize, interpret, or respond to rectal cues secondary to:

Depression   Cognitive impairment

⊕ ERRORS IN DIAGNOSTIC STATEMENTS

Bowel Incontinence related to oozing of stool
Oozing of stool does not cause bowel incontinence; rather, it is evidence. If the etiology is unknown, the diagnosis should be written: *Bowel Incontinence related to unknown etiology,* as evidenced by oozing of stool. When the etiology is known, the diagnosis should reflect this (eg, *Bowel Incontinence related to relaxed anal sphincter secondary to S4 lesion*).

KEY CONCEPTS
Generic Considerations

- Bowel incontinence has three major causes: underlying disease of the colon, rectum, or anus; long-standing constipation or fecal impaction; and neurogenic rectal changes.
- Complete spinal cord injury, spinal cord lesions, neurologic disease, or congenital defects that interrupt the sacral reflex arc (at the sacral segments S2, S3, S4) result in an areflexic (autonomous) or flaccid bowel. Flaccid paralysis at this level, known as an LMN lesion, results in

loss of the defecation reflex, loss of sphincter control (flaccid anal sphincter), and no bulbocaver-nosus reflex (Demata, 2000).

- Because of an interrupted sacral reflex arc and a flaccid anal sphincter, bowel incontinence can occur without rectal stimulation whenever stool is in the rectal vault. The stool may leak out if too soft or remain (if not extracted), predisposing the person to fecal impaction or constipation. Some intrinsic contractile abilities of the colon remain, but peristalsis is sluggish, leading to stool reten-tion with contents in the rectal vault (Demata, 2000).
- Complete central nervous system (CNS) lesions or trauma above sacral cord segments S2, S3, S4 (T12–L1–L2 vertebral level) result in a reflexic neurogenic bowel. They interrupt the ascending sensory signals between the sacral reflex center and the brain, resulting in the inability to feel the urge to defecate. They also interrupt descending motor signals from the brain, causing loss of vol-untary control over the anal sphincter. Because the sacral reflex center is preserved, it is possible to develop a stimulation–response bowel evacuation program using digital stimulation or digital stimulation devices (Demata, 2000).

Geriatric Considerations

The sensation of rectal fullness, which produces the urge to defecate, may be diminished in older adults (Demata, 2000).

Focus Assessment Criteria

See *Constipation* (Hickey, 2002).

For more information on Focus Assessment Criteria, visit http://connection.lww.com.

Goal

> **NOC** Bowel Continence, Tissue Integrity, Bowel Elimination

The person will evacuate a soft, formed stool every other day or every third day.

Indicators

- Relate bowel elimination techniques.
- Describe fluid and dietary requirements.

General Interventions

> **NIC** Bowel Incontinence Care, Bowel Training, Bowel Management, Skin Surveillance

Assess Contributing Factors.

Lack of routine evacuation schedule
Insufficient fluid and fiber intake

Constipation
Lack of knowledge of bowel elimination techniques
Insufficient physical activity

Use of elimination aids (eg, laxatives)

Assess Person's Ability to Participate.

Neurologic status

Functional ability

Plan a Consistent, Appropriate Time for Elimination.

Institute a daily bowel program for 5 days or until a pattern develops, then move to an alternate-day program (morning or evening).
Provide privacy and a nonstressful environment.
Give reassurance and protect from embarrassment while establishing the bowel program.

Teach Effective Bowel Elimination Techniques.

Position a functionally able person upright or sitting. If he or she is not functionally able (eg, quadri-plegic), place in left side-lying position.
For a functionally able person, use assistive devices (eg, dil stick, digital stimulator, raised commode seat, lubricant and gloves), as appropriate.

For a person with upper extremity mobility and abdominal musculature innervation, teach bowel elimination facilitation techniques as appropriate:

Valsalva maneuver   Forward bends
Sitting push-ups   Abdominal massage
Pelvic floor exercises

Assist with or provide equipment needed for hygiene measures, as necessary.

Maintain an elimination record or a flow sheet of the bowel schedule that includes time, stool characteristics, assistive methods used, and number of involuntary stools, if any.

Explain Fluid and Dietary Requirements for Good Bowel Movements.

Ensure client drinks 8 to 10 glasses of water daily.
Design a diet high in bulk and fiber.
Refer to *Colonic Constipation* for specific dietary instructions.

Explain Effects of Activity on Peristalsis.

Assist in determining the appropriate exercises for person's functional ability.

Initiate Health Teaching, as Indicated.

Explain the hazards of using stool softeners, laxatives, suppositories, and enemas.

Explain the signs and symptoms of fecal impaction and constipation. (Refer to *Dysreflexia* for additional information.)

Initiate teaching of a bowel program before discharge. If the client is functionally able, encourage independence with bowel program; if not, incorporate assistive devices or attendant care, as needed.

Explain effects of stool on skin and prevention techniques (refer to *Diarrhea* for interventions).

Rationales

- To maintain bowel continence, a person must be motivated, have intact anorectal sensation, be able to store feces consciously, be able to contract puborectalis and external anal sphincter muscles, and have access to a toileting facility.
- Stool consistency and volume are important for continence. Large volumes of loose stool overwhelm the continence mechanism. Small, hard stools that do not distend or stimulate the rectum do not alert the person to the need to defecate.
- Exercise increases gastrointestinal motility and hastens bowel function.
- Pelvic floor exercises can increase the strength of the puborectalis and external anal sphincter muscles.
- Digital stimulation results in reflex peristalsis and evacuation.
- Laxatives cause unscheduled bowel movements, loss of colon tone, and inconsistent stool consistency. Enemas can overstretch the bowel and decrease tone. Stool softeners are not needed with adequate food or fluid intake.
- Techniques that facilitate gravity and increase intraabdominal pressure to pass stool enhance bowel elimination.
- Long-standing constipation or fecal impaction causes overdistention of the rectum by feces. Subsequent continuous reflex stimulation reduces sphincter tone. Incontinence will be either diarrhea leaking around the impaction or leaking of feces from a full rectum (Chassagne et al., 2000).
- Bowel incontinence is common in institutionalized older adults and those with chronic illnesses. Cognitive impairments can impede recognition of bowel cues. Long-standing constipation can cause leaking around the impaction. Another cause of bowel incontinence is rectal sphincter abnormalities.

EFFECTIVE BREAST-FEEDING

DEFINITION

Effective Breast-feeding: The state in which a mother–infant dyad exhibits adequate proficiency and satisfaction with the breast-feeding process

DEFINING CHARACTERISTICS
Major (Must Be Present)

Mother's ability to position infant at breast to promote a successful latch-on response
Infant content after feeding
Regular and sustained suckling/swallowing at the breast
Infant weight patterns appropriate for age
Effective mother–infant communication patterns (infant cues, maternal interpretation and response)

Minor (May Be Present)

Signs or symptoms of oxytocin release (let-down or milk ejection reflex)
Adequate infant elimination patterns for age
Eagerness of infant to nurse
Maternal verbalization of satisfaction with breast-feeding

AUTHOR'S NOTE

This diagnosis reportedly represents a newly proposed NANDA wellness diagnosis, defined as "a clinical judgment about an individual, family, or community in transition from a specific level of wellness to a higher level of wellness." The definition does not describe a mother–infant dyad seeking higher-level breast-feeding, but "adequate proficiency and satisfaction with the breast-feeding process."

In the management of breast-feeding, nurses will encounter three situations covered by the following nursing diagnoses:

- *Ineffective Breast-feeding*
- *Risk for Ineffective Breast-feeding*
- *Potential for Enhanced Breast-feeding*

The nurse would use *Ineffective Breast-feeding* to describe an evaluation judgment of a mother's and infant's breast-feeding session for both ineffective and potentially ineffective breast-feeding. This evaluation results from the nurse observing or the mother reporting those signs and symptoms listed as defining characteristics. These signs and symptoms do not describe higher-level breast-feeding.

If the nurse cares for a mother reporting proficiency and satisfaction with breast-feeding and desiring additional teaching to achieve even greater proficiency and satisfaction, *Potential for Enhanced Breast-feeding* would be appropriate. The focus of this teaching and continued support would not be on preventing ineffective breast-feeding or maintaining adequate proficiency and satisfaction, but on promoting higher-quality breast-feeding.

This diagnosis is not useful in its present form; instead, the nurse should use *Ineffective Breast-feeding* or *Risk for Ineffective Breast-feeding*. Nurses desiring to use a wellness nursing diagnosis could use *Potential for Enhanced Breast-feeding*. Because this diagnosis is not on the NANDA list, nurses using it should send their experiences to NANDA.

INEFFECTIVE BREAST-FEEDING

DEFINITION

Ineffective Breast-feeding: The state in which a mother, infant, or child experiences or is at risk of experiencing dissatisfaction or difficulty with the breast-feeding process

DEFINING CHARACTERISTICS

Unsatisfactory breast-feeding process:

- Actual or perceived inadequate milk supply
- Inability of infant to attach onto maternal breast correctly
- No observable signs of oxytocin release
- Observable signs of inadequate infant intake
- Nonsustained suckling at the breast
- Persistence of sore nipples beyond the first week of breast-feeding
- Fussiness and crying of infant within the first hour after breast-feeding; lack of response to other comfort measures
- Infant arching and crying at the breast, resisting latching on

RELATED FACTORS
Physiologic

Related to difficulty of neonate to attach or suck secondary to:

Cleft lip/palate   Prematurity
Previous breast surgery   Inverted nipples, inadequate let-down reflex

Situational (Personal, Environmental)

Related to maternal fatigue
Related to maternal anxiety
Related to maternal ambivalence
Related to multiple birth
Related to inadequate nutrition intake
Related to inadequate fluid intake
Related to history of unsuccessful breast-feeding
Related to nonsupportive partner/family
Related to lack of knowledge
Related to interruption in breast-feeding secondary to ill mother, ill infant
Related to work schedule and/or barriers in the work environment

---

> ⓪⓪ **AUTHOR'S NOTE**
>
> In managing breast-feeding, nurses strive to reduce or eliminate factors that contribute to *Ineffective Breast-feeding* or factors that can increase vulnerability for a problem using the diagnosis *Risk for Ineffective Breast-feeding*.
>
> In the acute setting after delivery, too little time will have elapsed for the nurse to conclude that there is no problem in breast-feeding, unless the mother is experienced. For many mother–infant dyads, *Risk for Ineffective Breast-feeding related to inexperience with the breast-feeding process* would represent a nursing focus on preventing problems in breast-feeding. *Risk* would not be indicated for all mothers.

> ⊙⊙ **ERRORS IN DIAGNOSTIC STATEMENTS**
>
> 1. *Ineffective Breast-feeding related to reports of no symptoms of let-down reflex*
>   When a mother reports or the nurse observes no signs of let-down reflex, *Ineffective Breast-feeding* is validated. If contributing factors are unknown, the diagnosis could be written as *Ineffective Breast-feeding related to unknown etiology,* as evidenced by reports of no signs of let-down reflex and mother's anxiety regarding feeding.
>   If the nurse has validated contributing factors, he or she can add them. The nurse should assess for various possible contributing factors, rather than prematurely focusing on a common etiology that may be incorrect for the specific situation.

KEY CONCEPTS
Generic Considerations

- Lactation results from complex interactions among the mother's health and nutrition status, the infant's health status, and breast tissue development under the influence of estrogen and progesterone.
- Prolactin and oxytocin are pituitary hormones that control milk production and are stimulated by infant sucking and maternal emotions.
- Many medications are excreted in breast milk. Some are harmful to the infant. Advise the mother to consult with a health care professional (nurse, physician, pharmacist) before taking a medication (prescribed or over-the-counter).
- The advantages of breast-feeding for the infant are as follows:
  - Is easier to digest
  - Meets nutritional needs
  - Reduces allergies, asthma
  - Provides antibodies and macrophages for early immunization
  - Causes fewer gastrointestinal infections and almost no constipation
  - Improves tooth alignment
  - Reduces childhood infections throughout childhood if nursing continues for 1 year (respiratory, ear)
  - In juvenile diabetes, can significantly stall the onset of diabetes, perhaps even into adulthood
  - Results in fewer incidents of sudden infant death syndrome
  - Gives bowel movements a pleasant odor
  - Does not smell sour or stain clothing in vomitus
- The advantages of breast-feeding for the mother are as follows:
  - Hastens uterine involution and postpartum resolution
  - Reduces risks for breast cancer
  - Allows more time to rest during feedings
  - Requires less preparation and decreased costs
  - Promotes faster bonding
- The disadvantages of breast-feeding are:
  - Someone cannot substitute.
  - Breast-feeding is a learned process for mother and baby. It requires about 2 to 3 weeks of commitment to adjust to and learn the skills of breast-feeding.
  - Breast milk is nearly completely digested—intestinal emptying is faster and newborn may need to feed more often than with formula.

> ❖ **Pediatric Consideration**
>
> Physical and psychosocial pressure influence an adolescent's eating habits, which may put the teenage mother and her infant at risk during the breast-feeding period (National Academy of Sciences, 1991).

Focus Assessment Criteria

Subjective Data
Assess for Related Factors.

History of breast-feeding (self, sibling, friend)
Supportive people (partner, friend, sibling, parent)
Daily intake

Calories	Basic food groups
Calcium	Fluids
Vitamin supplements	Medications

History of breast surgery

Objective Data
Assess for Defining Characteristics.

Breast condition (soft, firm, engorged)
Nipples (cracked, sore, inverted)

For more information on Focus Assessment Criteria, visit http://connection.lww.com.

Goals

NOC Breastfeeding Establishment: Infant, Breastfeeding Establishment: Maternal, Breastfeeding Management, Knowledge: Breastfeeding

The mother will report confidence in
  establishing satisfying, effective breast-feeding.
The mother will demonstrate effective breast-feeding independently.

Indicators
- Identify factors that deter breast-feeding.
- Identify factors that promote breast-feeding.
- Demonstrate effective positioning.
- Have a relaxed, feeding infant.

General Interventions

NIC Breastfeeding Assistance, Lactation Counseling

Assess for Causative or Contributing Factors.

Lack of knowledge
Lack of role model
Lack of support (partner, physician, family)
Discomfort

Leaking	Engorgement
Loss of control of bodily fluid	Nipple soreness

Embarrassment
Attitudes and misconceptions of mother
Social pressure against breast-feeding
Change in body image
Change in sexuality
Feelings of being tied down
Stress
Lack of conviction regarding decision to breast-feed
Sleepy, unresponsive infant
Fatigue
Separation from infant (premature or sick infant, sick mother)
Barriers in workplace

Promote Open Dialogue.

Assess Knowledge.
Has woman taken a class in breast-feeding?
Has she read anything on the subject?
Does she have friends who are breast-feeding their babies?
Did her mother breast-feed?

Explain Myths and Misconceptions.
Ask her to list anticipated difficulties. Common myths include the following:

- My breasts are too small.
- My breasts are too large.
- My mother couldn't breast-feed.
- How do I know my milk is good?
- How do I know the baby is getting enough?
- The baby will know that I'm nervous.
- I have to go back to work, so what's the point of breast-feeding for a short time?
- I'll never have any freedom.
- Breast-feeding will cause my breasts to sag.
- My nipples are inverted, so I can't breast-feed.
- My husband won't like my breasts anymore.
- I'll have to stay fat if I breast-feed.
- I can't breast-feed if I have a cesarean section.

Build on Mother's Knowledge.
Clarify misconceptions.
Explain process of breast-feeding.
Offer literature.
Show video.
Discuss advantages and disadvantages.
Bring breast-feeding mothers together to talk about breast-feeding and their concerns.

Support Mother's Decision to Breast- or Bottle-feed.

Assist Mother during First Feedings.

Promote Relaxation.
Position comfortably, using pillows (especially cesarean-section mothers).
Use foot stool or phone book to bring knees up while sitting.
Use relaxation breathing techniques.

Demonstrate Different Positions.
Sitting
Lying
Cradle hold—Instruct woman to place supporting hand on baby's bottom and turn body toward mother's (promotes security in infant). Cradle hold stabilizes head and reduces force.

Demonstrate and Explain Rooting Reflex.
Show how mother can use it to help infant latch on.
Show how to grasp breast with fingers under breast and thumbs on top; this way she can point nipple directly at baby's mouth (avoid scissors hold, which constricts milk flow).
Make sure baby grasps a good portion of areola, not just the nipple.
Observe gliding action of jaw, which indicates proper latch-on and suck.
Infant should not be chewing or simply sucking with lips.
Observe for bruising after feeding.

Advise to Increase Feeding Times Gradually.
Start at 10 min per side.
Build up over next 3 to 5 days.

Instruct to Offer both Breasts at Each Feeding.
Alternate the beginning side each time.

Demonstrate:
How to use a finger to keep breast tissue from obstructing infant's nose
Use of finger in infant's mouth to break seal before removing from breast
Ways to awaken infant (may be necessary before offering the second breast)

Discuss Burping.
Inform that burping may be unnecessary with breast-fed infants.
If infant grunts and seems full between breasts, mother should attempt to burp infant, then continue feeding.

Provide Follow-up Support during Hospital Stay.

Develop care plan so other health team members are aware of any problems or needs. Try to establish a consistent plan so the breast-feeding mother does not receive mixed and opposing opinions from her health care providers.

Allow for flexibility of feeding schedule; avoid scheduling feedings. Strive for 10 to 12 feedings/24 h according to the infant's size and need. (Frequent feedings help prevent or reduce breast engorgement.)

Promote rooming in.

Allow for privacy during feedings.

Be available for questions.

Be positive even if experience is difficult.

Reassure mother that this is a learning time for her and the infant. They will develop together as the days pass.

Teach Ways to Control Specific Nursing Problems (May Need Assistance of Lactation Consultant).

Engorgement

Wear well-fitting support brassiere day and night.

Apply warm compresses for 15 to 20 min before breast-feeding.

Nurse frequently.

Use hand expression, hand pump, or electric pump to tap off some of the tension before putting infant to breast.

Massage breasts and apply warm washcloth before expression.

Sore Nipples

Apply warm, moist compress for 5 to 10 min after breast-feeding.

Decrease breast-feeding time to 5 to 10 min per side. Start baby on nontender side first. Allow for more frequent, short feedings. Suggest alternate positions to rotate infant's grasps. Allow breasts to dry after each feeding.

Keep nursing pads dry.

Coat nipples with breast milk (which has healing properties) and allow to air-dry.

Use breast shield as last measure and remove after milk has let down.

Explain that nipple soreness usually resolves within 7 to 10 days.

Bacterial and Fungal Infections (Bell & Rawlings, 1998)

For bacterial infections: Apply a topical antibiotic against *Staphylococcus aureus* sparingly three times a day after the feeding.

For candidiasis:
- Apply a topical antifungal cream two to four times daily, depending on medication.
- Rinse nipples with warm water and air-dry before applying the cream.
- An alternative to medication is to bathe the nipples with a solution of 1 tablespoon of vinegar in 1 cup of water or 1 teaspoon of baking soda in 1 cup of water.
- The infant requires treatment also.

Stasis, Mastitis

If one area of breast is sore or tender, apply moist heat before each breast-feeding session.

Gently massage from the base of breast toward the nipple before beginning to breast-feed and during feeding.

Breast-feed frequently and change position during feeding.

Rest frequently.

If stasis lasts more than 48 h, consult with nurse practitioner, midwife, or physician for antibiotic therapy.

Monitor for signs and symptoms of mastitis: chills, body aches, fatigue, fever >100.4°F.

Difficulty with Baby Grasping Nipple

Cup breast with fingers underneath.

Position baby for mother's and infant's comfort (turn baby's abdomen toward mother's body).

Stroke infant's cheek for rooting reflex.

Hand-express some milk into infant's mouth.

Roll nipples to bring them out before feeding.

Use a nipple shell between feedings to help extend inverted nipples. Remove shield after let-down.

Assess infant's suck—the baby may need assistance in development of suck. Use lactation consultant if indicated.

Separation

After cesarean section for stressed infants, premature infants, and jaundiced infants, nurses:

Encourage visits and bonding as much as possible.

Provide comfortable, private location for breast-feeding during visit.

Provide supportive atmosphere (eg, freedom to ask questions).

Provide breast pump or make patient aware of availability.

Rental of electric pump	Cylinder-type hand pump
Battery-operated pump	(do not use bicycle horn pump)

Provide instruction in use of pump and assist mother to integrate breast-feeding into lifestyle. Many hospitals have a lactation educator or consultant on hand to assist with instruction and support.

Encourage Verbal Expression of Feelings Regarding Changes in Body.

Many women dislike leaking and lack of control. Explain that this is temporary.

Demonstrate use of nursing pad. With a disposable pad, client should not use waterproof backing, to prevent irritation; cotton (washable) seems to reduce irritation.

Breasts change from "sexual objects" to implements of nutrition, which can affect sexual relationship. Sexual partners will get milk if they suck on woman's nipples. Orgasm releases milk. Infant suckling is "sensual"—this may cause guilt or confusion in woman. Encourage discussion with other mothers. Include partner in at least one discussion to assess his or her feelings and how they most affect the breast-feeding experience.

Explore woman's feelings about self-consciousness during feedings.
Where?
Around whom?
What is partner's reaction to when and where she breast-feeds?

Demonstrate use of shawl for modesty, allowing breast-feeding in public.

Remind her that what she is doing is normal and natural.

Assist the Family with:

Sibling Reaction

Explore feelings and anticipation of problems. Older child may be jealous of contact with baby. Mother can use this time to read to older child.

Older child may want to breast-feed. Allow him or her to try; usually, the child will not like it.

Stress older child's attributes: freedom, movement, and choices.

Fatigue and Stress

Explore situation.

Encourage mother to make herself and infant a priority.

Encourage her to limit visits from relatives for first 4 weeks.

Emphasize than she will need support and assistance during first 4 weeks. Encourage support person to help as much as possible.

Explain to mother not to try to be "superwoman," but to ask directly for help from friends or relations, or to hire someone.

Feelings of Being Enslaved

Allow mother to express feelings.

Encourage her to seek assistance and to pump milk to allow others to feed baby.

Advise her that she can store harvested breast milk for 8 h at room temperature, 3 days in refrigerator, 6 months in freezer. (*Note:* Alert woman never to microwave frozen breast milk, as doing so will destroy its immune properties.)

Remember that time between feedings will get longer (every 2 h for 4 weeks, then every 3 to 4 h by 3 months).

Initiate Referrals, as Indicated.

Refer to lactation consultant if indicated by:
- Lack of confidence
- Ambivalence
- Problems with infant suck and latch-on
- Infant weight drop or lack of urination
- Barriers in workplace
- Prolonged soreness
- Hot, tender spots on breast

Refer to La Leche League.

Refer to childbirth educator and childbirth class members.

Refer to other breast-feeding mothers.

Rationales

- Listening to mother's and partner's concerns can help prioritize concerns.
- The decision to breast-feed is very personal and should not be made without adequate information (Pillitteri, 2003).

- Successful breast-feeding depends on both physical and emotional support. Physical support includes promotion of comfort and proper technique (Pillitteri, 2003).
- Constant positive feedback is essential for an inexperienced mother (Pillitteri, 2003).
- Lactation has two mechanisms: secretion of milk and milk-ejection reflex. Mothers learn techniques to increase milk production (eg, sufficient emptying).
- Inadequate let-down reflex can result from a tense or nervous mother, pain, insufficient milk, engorgement, or inadequate sucking position or motions (Reeder et al., 1997).
- Nipple shields diminish milk supply and should not be recommended routinely. The newborn may develop a nipple shield preference (Auerbach, 1990).
- Providing enough time for adequate milk removal and not limiting feeding time can prevent engorgement (Moon & Humernick, 1989).
- The infant at the breast must be in relaxed, correct alignment, have correct tongue and areolar placement, have sufficient motion for areolar compression, and demonstrate audible swallowing (Shirago & Bocar, 1990).
- Referrals to community resources can provide continued support and information.
- Company-sponsored lactation programs enable employed mothers to continue breastfeeding as long as they desire (Ortiz, McGilligan, & Kelly, 2004).

INTERRUPTED BREAST-FEEDING

DEFINITION

Interrupted Breast-feeding: A break in the continuity of the breast-feeding process as a result of inability or inadvisability to put baby to breast for feeding

DEFINING CHARACTERISTICS
Major (Must Be Present)

Infant does not receive nourishment at the breast for some or all feedings

Minor (May Be Present)

Maternal desire to maintain lactation and provide (or eventually provide) her breast milk for her infant's nutritional needs
Separation of mother and infant
Lack of knowledge regarding expression and storage of breast milk

RELATED FACTORS

Maternal or infant illness	Prematurity
Maternal employment	Contraindications (eg, drugs,
Need to wean infant abruptly	true breast milk jaundice)

AUTHOR'S NOTE

This diagnosis represents a situation, not a response. Nursing interventions do not treat the interruption but, instead, its effects. The situation is interrupted breast-feeding; the responses can vary. For example, if continued breast-feeding or use of a breast pump is contraindicated, the nurse focuses on the loss of this breast-feeding experience using the nursing diagnosis *Grieving*.

If breast-feeding continues with expression and storage of breast milk, teaching, and support, the diagnosis will be *Risk for Ineffective Breast-feeding related to continuity problems secondary to (eg, maternal employment)*. If difficulty is experienced, the diagnosis would be *Ineffective Breast-feeding related to interruption secondary to (specify) and lack of knowledge*.

DECREASED CARDIAC OUTPUT

DEFINITION

Decreased Cardiac Output: A state in which the individual experiences a reduction in the amount of blood pumped by the heart, resulting in compromised cardiac function

DEFINING CHARACTERISTICS

Low blood pressure	Dyspnea	Fatigability
Rapid pulse	Angina	Vertigo
Restlessness	Dysrhythmia	Edema (peripheral, sacral)
Cyanosis	Oliguria	

AUTHOR'S NOTE

This nursing diagnosis represents a situation in which nurses have multiple responsibilities. People experiencing decreased cardiac output may display various responses that disrupt functioning (eg, activity intolerance, disturbed sleep–rest, anxiety, fear). Or they may be at risk for developing such physiologic complications as dysrhythmias, cardiogenic shock, and congestive heart failure.

   When *Decreased Cardiac Output* is used clinically, associated goals usually are written:

Systolic blood pressure   Cardiac output is >5
  is >100   Cardiac rate, rhythm are
Urine output is >30 mL/h   within normal limits

These goals do not represent parameters for evaluating nursing care, but for evaluating the person's status. Because they are monitoring criteria that the nurse uses to guide implementation of nurse-prescribed and physician-prescribed interventions, *Decreased Cardiac Output* is not appropriate as a nursing diagnosis. Not using it allows the nurse to describe more specifically the related situations that nurses treat as nursing diagnoses or co-treat as collaborative problems. (Refer to *Activity Intolerance related to insufficient knowledge of adaptive techniques needed secondary to impaired cardiac function* and to *PC: Cardiac/Vascular* [Section Three] for more information.)

ERRORS IN DIAGNOSTIC STATEMENTS

1. *Decreased Cardiac Output related to dysrhythmias*
   This diagnosis necessitates continuous monitoring, early detection of changes in physiologic status, rapid initiation of medical and nursing interventions, and evaluation of response. Because the nurse manages this situation with nurse-prescribed and physician-prescribed interventions, it is a collaborative problem: *PC: Decreased Cardiac Output related to dysrhythmias.*
2. *Decreased Cardiac Output related to vasodilation and bradycardia secondary to spinal shock*
   As with the previous example, this is a situation for which nurses cannot write outcomes that can be used to measure the effectiveness of nursing interventions. Thus, this situation should be written as a collaborative problem: *PC: Spinal Shock.* A nurse reading this knows that the client either is experiencing or is at risk for spinal shock. Shift reports or initial assessment will determine present status.

CAREGIVER ROLE STRAIN

DEFINITION

Caregiver Role Strain: A state in which a person is experiencing physical, emotional, social, and/or financial burden(s) in the process of giving care to another

DEFINING CHARACTERISTICS

Expressed or observed

Insufficient time or physical energy

Difficulty performing required caregiving activities

Conflicts between caregiving responsibilities and other important roles (eg, work, relationships)

Apprehension about the future for the care receiver's health and ability to provide care

Apprehension about care receiver's care when caregiver is ill or deceased

Feelings of depression or anger

RELATED FACTORS
Pathophysiologic

Related to unrelenting or complex care requirements secondary to:

Debilitating conditions (acute, progressive)

Addiction

Unpredictable illness course

Progressive dementia

Chronic mental illness

Disability

Treatment-Related

Related to 24-hour care responsibilities
Related to time-consuming activities (eg, dialysis, transportation)

Situational (Personal, Environmental)

Related to unrealistic expectations of caregiver by care receiver
Related to pattern of ineffective coping
Related to compromised physical health
Related to unrealistic expectations of self
Related to history of poor relationship
Related to history of family dysfunction
Related to unrealistic expectations for caregiver by others (society, other family members)
Related to duration of caregiving required
Related to isolation
Related to insufficient respite
Related to insufficient recreation
Related to insufficient finances
Related to no or unavailable support

Maturational

Infant, child, adolescent related to unrelenting care requirements secondary to:

Mental disabilities (specify)   Physical disabilities (specify)

137

⊛ AUTHOR'S NOTE

More than 2.2 million unpaid home caregivers are in the United States (Stone et al., 1987). They provide care for people of all ages, some across the entire life span (eg, children with permanent disabilities). The care receivers have physical and/or mental disabilities, which can be temporary or permanent. Some disabilities are permanent but stable (eg, blindness); others signal progressive deterioration (eg, Alzheimer's disease).

Caring and caregiving are intrinsic to all close relationships. They are "found in the context of established roles such as wife–husband, child–parent" (Pearlin, Mullan, Semple & Skaff, 1990, p. 583). Under some circumstances, caregiving is "transformed from the ordinary exchange of assistance among people standing in close relationship to one another to an extraordinary and unequally distributed burden" (ibid.). It becomes a dominant, overriding component occupying the entire situation (ibid.).

Chronic sorrow has been associated with caregivers of people with mental illness and children with chronic illness. See *Chronic Sorrow* for more information.

Caregiver Role Strain represents the burden of caregiving on the physical and emotional health of the caregiver and its effects on the family and social system of the caregiver and care receiver. *Risk for Caregiver Role Strain* can be a very significant nursing diagnosis because nurses can identify those at high risk and assist them to prevent this grave situation.

⊛ ERROR IN DIAGNOSTIC STATEMENTS

Caregiver Role Strain related to depression and anger at family, as evidenced by unrealistic expectations of caregiver for self and by others

Too often, caregivers with multiple, unrelenting responsibilities are reluctant to admit they need help. Others may interpret this reluctance as not needing help. The caregiver is further isolated, feeling no one really cares or appreciates the work involved, which can contribute to depression and anger. Thus, this diagnosis must be rewritten to reflect the unrealistic expectations as the related factors and the resulting symptoms as evidence. It is helpful to quote the data if relevant: *Caregiver Role Strain related to unrealistic expectations of caregiver for self and by others, as evidenced by depressed feelings and anger at family who "don't understand my burden."*

KEY CONCEPTS
Generic Considerations

- In the United States, 110,000,000 people require some form of home care, 1,000,000 of whom are children (O'Connor, Vander Plaats & Betz, 1992).
- Caring for people at home results in substantial cost savings. For example, Wong (1991) found that caring for a ventilator-dependent child at home cost $40,000 less per month than hospital care.
- With the growing aging population and advances in medicine increasing the longevity of chronically ill people, the need for health care escalates. Of 4 million Americans with Alzheimer's disease, more than 70% live at home (Winslow & Carter, 1999). One family member largely provides such home health care. Women (eg, wife, daughter, daughter-in-law) represent 70% of these caregivers.
- Burden is related to caregiver's gender, age, social support, income, and resources and care receiver's cognitive and functional limitations (Winslow & Carter, 1999).
- Smith, Smith, and Toseland (1991) reported the following problems (by priority) identified by family caregivers:
  1. Improving coping skills (eg, time management, stress management)
  2. Family issues (sibling conflict, other role conflicts)
  3. Responding to care receiver's needs (emotional, physical, financial)
  4. Eliciting formal, informal support
  5. Guilt and feelings of inadequacy
  6. Long-term planning
  7. Quality of relationship with care receiver
- Caregiving to a chronically ill family member or friend with many behavioral problems is the most stressful situation one can encounter.

- Social support can be described as:
  - Emotional (concern, trust)
  - Appraisal (affirms self-worth)
  - Informational (useful advice, information for problem solving)
  - Instrumental (caregiving) or tangible assistance (money, help with chores)
- The stress process related to caregiver role strain arises from four domains (Box II-1) (Pearlin et al., 1990).
- Caregiver stress is not an event but "a mix of circumstances, experiences, responses and resources that vary considerably among caregivers and that consequently vary in their impact on caregivers' health and behavior" (Pearlin et al., 1990, p. 584). A change in one component in Box II-1 results in a change in the other components.
- The number of people in a household influences how many secondary, informal caregivers assist the primary caregiver. Spouse primary caregivers are less likely to have secondary caregivers to help them with care activities. Older people cared for by spouses received "about 15%–20% fewer person-days of help than those cared for by adult children" (Miller & McFall, 1991).
- "Health care policies that rely on caregiver sacrifice can be made to appear cost effective only if the emotional, social, physical, and financial costs incurred by the caregiver are ignored" (Winslow & Carter, 1999, p. 285).

⊗ BOX II.1. DOMAINS OF THE STRESS PROCESS OF CAREGIVING

Background/Content of Stress

Caregiver characteristics (age, education, financial, and social status)
Caregiving history
Networks
Resources available

Stressors (Primary, Secondary)

Primary (Directly Related to Needs of Care Receiver)

Impaired cognitive status
Problematic behavior (*eg,* verbal abuse, wandering)
Extent of dependency
Resistance to caregiver's help
Fatigue of caregiver
Relational deprivation (spouse, parent)

Secondary (Derived from Primary Stressors)

Family conflicts about care receiver's condition or care
Economic strain
Constriction of social life
Intrapsychic strain (loss of self, loss of control, feelings of inadequacy)

Mediators of Stressors

Efficacy of coping
Social support

Outcomes of Stressors

Depression
Anxiety
Cognitive disruptions
Physical problems
Yielding of role

Adapted from Pearlin, L., Mullan, J., Semple, S., & Skaff, M. (1990). Caregiving and the stress process: An overview of concepts and their measures. *The Gerontologist, 45*(5), 192–195.

◈ Pediatric Considerations

- Children considered candidates for home care services are those:
  - Dependent on mechanical ventilation
  - Needing prolonged intravenous nutritional or drug therapy
  - With terminal illness
  - Requiring nutritional (eg, tube feedings) or respiratory support (eg, tracheostomy, suctioning)
  - Needing daily or near-daily nursing care for apnea monitoring, dialysis, urinary catheters, or colostomy pouches
- The child and family provide the basis for home care and collaborate with the nurse to provide its direction.
- Caregivers of preterm infants on apnea monitors experienced more fatigue than caregivers of preterm infants not on apnea monitors. This fatigue increased in the caregivers of monitored infants over 1 month and decreased in caregivers of nonmonitored infants. This fatigue interfered with activities of daily living (ADLs), socialization, and leisure.

Focus Assessment Criteria

Subjective Data

Assess for Defining Characteristics.

How well do you manage your
Caregiving responsibilities? Household responsibilities?
Work responsibilities? Family responsibilities?

On a scale from 0 to 10 (0 = not tired, peppy, to 10 = total exhaustion), rate the fatigue you usually feel. Does it change during the day or week? If so, why?

Do you feel stressed between caring for your _____ and trying to meet other responsibilities?

How would you describe your usual emotional state? (Calm, stressed, angry, anxious, depressed, exhausted, guilty)

What do you do when you are very stressed?

What are you most concerned about?
For present For future

When was the last time you went out to eat?

What have you done for fun lately?

Assess for Related Factors.

Caregiver history

Lifestyle
Typical day Work history
Weekly hobbies Leisure activities

Health
Ability to perform ADLs Chronic conditions

Family members
Parents, spouse Children, siblings
In-laws

Economic resources
Sources Adequacy (present, future)

Care receiver characteristics

Cognitive status (eg, memory, speech)
Problematic behaviors (Pearlin et al., 1990)
Wanders Cries easily
Threatens Repeats questions and
Uses foul language   requests
Incontinence Clings

Suspicious
Sexually inappropriate

Depressed
Up at night

Activities with which the care receiver needs assistance

Bathing
Dressing, grooming
Eating
Toileting
Mobility

Medicines
Transportation
Laundry
Shopping

Caregiver–care receiver relationship

Support system
Who? (family, friends, clergy, agency, group)
What? (visits, respite, chores, empathy)
How often?
What have you lost because of your caregiver responsibilities?

Care issues related to chronically ill child

Parenting issues
Discipline of ill child

Discipline of well siblings

Family adaptations
Living arrangements
Vacations

Day-to-day management

Support systems
School issues

Goal

NOC	Caregiver Well-Being, Role Performance, Caregiver Endurance Potential, Family Coping, Family Integrity

The caregiver will report a plan to decrease caregiver's burden.

Indicators

- Share frustrations regarding caregiving responsibilities.
- Identify one source of support.
- Identify two changes that, if made, would improve daily life.

The family will establish a plan for weekly support or help.

Indicators

- Relate an intent to listen without giving advice,
- Convey empathy to caregiver regarding daily responsibilities.

General Interventions

NIC	Caregiver Support, Respite Care, Coping Enhancement, Family Mobilization, Mutual Goal Setting, Support System Enhancement, Anticipatory Guidance

Assess for Causative or Contributing Factors.

Poor insight into situation
Reluctance or inability
  to access help
Insufficient resources
  (eg, help, financial)
Insufficient leisure

Unrealistic expectations
  (caregiver, family)
Unsatisfactory relationship
Social isolation
Competing roles (spouse,
  parenting, work)

Provide Empathy and Promote a Sense of Competency.

Allow caregiver to share feelings.
Emphasize the difficulties of the caregiving responsibilities.
Convey admiration of the caregiver's competency.
Evaluate effects of caregiving periodically (depression, burnout).

Promote Realistic Appraisal of the Situation.

Determine how long the caregiving has been (Winslow & Carter, 1999).

Ask caregiver to describe future life in 3 months, 6 months, and 1 year.

Discuss the effects of present schedule and responsibilities on physical health, emotional status, and relationships.

Discuss positive outcomes of caregiving responsibilities (for self, care receiver, family).

Evaluate if behavior is getting worse.

Promote Insight into the Situation.

Ask caregiver to describe "a typical day":

Caregiving tasks	Household tasks
Work outside the home	Role responsibilities

Ask to describe:

At-home leisure activities (daily, weekly)

Outside-the-home social activities (weekly)

Engage other family members in discussion, as appropriate.

Discuss the danger of viewing helpers as less competent or less essential.

Explain that dementia causes memory loss, which results in (Young, 2001):

Repetitive questions	Denial of memory loss
Forgetting	Fluctuations in memory

Explain resilience (see Key Concepts) and qualities to promote to family and caregiver (Tusaie & Dyer, 2004).

Optimism	Humor
Creativity	Spiritual beliefs

Assist Caregiver to Identify Activities for which He or She Desires Assistance.

Care receiver's needs (hygiene, food, treatments, mobility; refer to Self-Care Deficits)

Laundry	House cleaning
Meals	Shopping, errands
Transportation	Appointments (doctor, hairdresser)
Yard work	House repairs
Respite (hours per week)	Money management

Engage Family (Apart from Caregiver) to Appraise Situation (Shields, 1992).

Allow to share frustrations.

Share the need for the caregiver to feel appreciated.

Discuss importance of regularly acknowledging the burden of the situation for the caregiver.

Discuss the benefits of listening without giving advice.

Differentiate the types of social support (emotional, appraisal, informational, instrumental).

Emphasize the importance of emotional and appraisal support.

Regular phone calls	Cards, letters
Visits	

Stress "that in many situations, there are no problems to be solved, only pain to be shared" (Shields, 1992, p. 31).

Discuss the need to give caregiver "permission" to enjoy self (eg, vacations, day trips).

Allow caregiver opportunities to respond to "How can I help you?"

Assist with Accessing Informational and Instrumental Support.

Role play how to ask for help with activities (eg, "I have three appointments this week, could you drive me to one?" "I could watch your children once or twice a week in exchange for you watching my husband.").

Identify all possible sources of volunteer help: family (siblings, cousins), friends, neighbors, church, and community groups.

Discuss how most people feel good when they provide a "little help."

If Appropriate, Discuss If and When an Alternative Source of Care (eg, Nursing Home) May be Indicated.

Evaluate for factors that reduce the stress of decision making of nursing home placement (Hagen, 2001):

- Low level of guilt
- Independence in the relationship
- Availability of support from others

- Low fear of loneliness
- Positive or neutral nursing home attitudes
- Positive sense of life without care burden

Initiate Health Teaching and Referrals, if Indicated.

Emphasize the need for caregiver to protect health, with a balance of work, sleep, leisure, and good nutrition.

Explain the benefits of sharing with other caregivers.

Support group

Telephone buddy system with another caregiver

Identify community resources available.

Counseling   Social service

Day care

Arrange a home visit by a physical or occupational therapist to evaluate the environment (safety, assistive devices, home alterations).

Arrange a home visit by professional nurse or physical therapy to provide strategies to improve communication, time management, and caregiving (Corcaran & Gitlin, 2001).

Engage others to work actively to increase state, federal, and private agencies' financial support for resources to enhance caregiving in the home.

Rationales

- Coping with the burdens of caregiving requires "constantly changing cognitive and behavioral efforts to manage specific external and/or internal demands that are appraised as taxing or exceeding the resources of the person" (Lazarus & Folkman, 1984).
- Lazarus and Folkman (1984) have identified the resources needed for successful coping as energy, beliefs, commitments, health, social skills, social support, and material resources.
- Lindgren (1990) reported that burnout in caregivers was related to emotional exhaustion and a low sense of accomplishment. Caregivers who were commended for their accomplishments reported lower levels of burnout.
- Numerous researchers have identified consistent social supports as the single most significant factor that reduces or prevents caregiver role strain (Clipp & George, 1990; Pearlin et al., 1990; Shields, 1992).
- Shields (1992) reported a primary source of conflict among family members and the caregiver as unsatisfied needs. The caregiver wishes for others to affirm the burden, when, in fact, the family responds to the caregiver's complaints with problem-solving techniques. The caregiver appears to reject suggestions, which annoys the family. The results are a "caregiver feeling unappreciated, unsupported and depressed and family members feeling angry and rejecting toward the caregiver" (Shields, 1992).
- Pruchno, Kleban, Michaels, and Dempsey (1990) reported that in female caregiving spouses, depression predicts a decline in physical health over 6 months. The amount of care provided had few effects on levels of depression, feelings of burden, or health.
- Institutionalization of a family member has many admission-related stressors (eg, financial constraints, transferring belongings, emotional strain, feelings of failure [Hagan, 2001]).
- The most critical period for caregiver stress is the 2- to 4-year period (Gaynor, 1990).
- Respite and the sharing of care responsibilities are vital to prevent the caregiver–care recipient dyad from becoming the center of the universe, with all others viewed as less competent or less essential (Flaskerud et al., 2001).
- Guilt, negative attitudes about nursing homes, sense of existential self, independence in the relationship, fear of loneliness, and perceived presence of support affect the decision-making process for nursing home placement (Hagan, 2001).

◆ Pediatric Interventions

Determine Parents' Understanding of and Concerns About Child's Illness, Course, Prognosis, and Related Care Needs.

Discuss Parenting Skills and Issues for Ill Child.

Elicit the Effects of Caregiving Responsibility on

Personal life (work, rest, leisure)

Marriage (time alone, communication, decisions, attention)

Assist Parents to Meet the Well Siblings' Needs for
Knowledge of sibling's illness and relationship to own health
Sharing feelings of anger, unfairness, embarrassment
Discussions of future of ill sibling and self (eg, family planning, care responsibilities)

Discuss Strategies to Help Siblings Adapt.
Include in family decisions when appropriate.
Keep informed about ill child's condition.
Maintain routines (eg, meals, vacations).
Prepare for changes in home life.
Promote activities with peers.
Avoid making the ill child the center of the family.
Determine what daily assistance in caregiving is realistic.
Plan for time alone.
Advise teachers of home situation.
Address developmental needs. See *Delayed Growth and Development.*

Advise that Caregiving Activities Produce Fatigue that Can Increase Over Time (Williams, 2000).
Discuss Strategies to Reduce Caregiver Fatigue (Williams, 2000).
Partner support   Household help
Child care for siblings   Provisions to ensure adequacy of caregiver's sleep

Rationales

- Helping the family identify predictable stressors can assist them to plan coping strategies.
- Addressing the developmental tasks of the ill child and the well siblings provides opportunities to grow, develop, gain independence, and master effective coping skills.
- Strategies to promote family cohesiveness and individual family needs can enhance effective stress management (Williams, 2000).
- All family members are encouraged to learn specific skills to balance the responsibilities.
- Strategies to promote family cohesiveness reduce isolation or aloneness.

RISK FOR CAREGIVER ROLE STRAIN

DEFINITION
Risk for Caregiver Role Strain: A state in which a person is at high risk to experience physical, emotional, social, and/or financial burden(s) in the process of giving care to another

RISK FACTORS
Presence of Risk Factors (refer to Related Factors)

RELATED FACTORS
Primary caregiver responsibilities for a recipient who requires regular assistance with self-care or supervision because of physical or mental disabilities in addition to one or more of the following:

Related to unrelenting or complex care requirements secondary to:

Care receiver characteristics

Inability to perform self-care	Lack of motivation to
Cognitive problems	perform self-care
Unrealistic expectations	Psychological problems

Caregiver/spouse characteristics

Pattern of ineffective coping	Compromised physical health
Unrealistic expectations of self	

Related to history of poor relationship
Related to history of family dysfunction
Related to unrealistic expectations for caregiver by others (society, other family members)
Related to duration of caregiving required
Related to isolation
Related to insufficient respite
Related to insufficient recreation
Related to insufficient finances
Related to no or unavailable support

○○ **AUTHOR'S NOTE**

See *Caregiver Role Strain.*

○○ **ERRORS IN DIAGNOSTIC STATEMENTS**

See *Caregiver Role Strain.*

KEY CONCEPTS
See *Caregiver Role Strain.*

Focus Assessment Criteria

See *Caregiver Role Strain.*

Goal

NOC Refer to *Caregiver Role Strain*

The person will relate a plan on how to continue social activities despite caregiving responsibilities.

Indicators
- Identify activities that are important for self.
- Relate intent to enlist the help of at least two people.

General Interventions

NIC Refer to Caregiver Role Strain

Explain Causes of Caregiver Role Strain.
See Box II-1.

Explain the Four Types of Social Support to All Involved: Emotional, Appraisal, Informational, and Instrumental.

Discuss the Implications of Daily Responsibilities with the Primary Caregiver (Irvin & Acton, 1997).

Emphasize that the caregiver also has needs.

Encourage caregiver to set realistic goals for self and care recipient.

Discuss the need for respite and short-term relief.

Encourage caregiver to accept offers of help.

Practice asking for help; avoid "they should know I need help" thinking and martyrdom behavior.

Caution on viewing others as not "competent enough."

Discuss that past conflicts will not disappear. Try to work on resolution and emphasize today.

Stress importance of daily health promotion activities (see *Health-Seeking Behaviors*):
- Rest–exercise balance
- Effective stress management
- Low-fat, high–complex carbohydrate diet
- Supportive social networks
- Appropriate screening practices for age

Maintain a good sense of humor; associate with others who laugh.

Caution against excessive complaining, which is depressing for all involved and may lead to avoidance.

Advise to initiate phone contacts or visits with friends or relatives rather than waiting for others to do it.

Assist those Involved to Appraise the Situation.

What is at stake? Provide accurate information and answers to encourage a realistic perspective.

What are the choices? Assist family to reorganize roles at home and set priorities to maintain family integrity and reduce stress.

Initiate discussions concerning stressors of home care (physical, emotional, environmental, financial).

Emphasize importance of respites to prevent isolating behaviors that foster depression.

Discuss with nonprimary caregivers their responsibilities in caring for the primary caregiver.

Where is there help? Direct family to community agencies, home health care organizations, and sources of financial assistance as needed. (See *Impaired Home Maintenance Management*.)

Discuss with all Household Members the Implications of Caring for Ill Family Member.

Available resources (finances, environmental)

24-hour responsibility

Effects on other household members

Likelihood of progressive deterioration

Sharing of responsibilities (with other household members, siblings, neighbors)

Likelihood of exacerbation of long-standing conflicts

Effects on lifestyle

Alternative or assistive options (eg, community-based providers, group living, nursing home)

Assist Caregiver to Identify Activities for which He or She Desires Assistance.

See *Caregiver Role Strain* (p. 141).

Assist with Accessing Informational and Instrumental Support.

See *Caregiver Role Strain* (p. 141).

Initiate Health Teaching and Referrals, if Indicated.

See *Caregiver Role Strain*.

Rationales

See *Caregiver Role Strain*.

Impaired Comfort*
Acute Pain
Chronic Pain
Nausea

IMPAIRED COMFORT

DEFINITION
Impaired Comfort: The state in which a person experiences an uncomfortable sensation in response to a noxious stimulus

DEFINING CHARACTERISTICS
Major (Must Be Present)
The person reports or demonstrates discomfort.

Minor (May Be Present)
Autonomic response in acute pain
    Increased blood pressure   Diaphoresis
    Increased pulse   Dilated pupils
    Increased respirations
Guarded position
Facial mask of pain
Crying, moaning
Abdominal heaviness
Nausea
Vomiting
Malaise
Pruritus

RELATED FACTORS
Any factor can contribute to impaired comfort. The most common are listed below.

Biopathophysiologic
Related to uterine contractions during labor
Related to trauma to perineum during labor and delivery
Related to involution of uterus and engorged breasts
Related to tissue trauma and reflex muscle spasms secondary to:

Musculoskeletal disorders
Fractures   Arthritis
Contractures   Spinal cord disorders
Spasms

Visceral disorders
Cardiac   Intestinal
Renal   Pulmonary
Hepatic

---

*This diagnosis is not currently on the NANDA list but has been included for clarity and usefulness.

Cancer
Vascular disorders
Vasospasm   Phlebitis
Occlusion   Vasodilation (headache)

Related to inflammation of:
Nerve   Joint
Tendon   Muscle
Bursa   Juxta-articular structures

Related to fatigue, malaise, or pruritus secondary to contagious diseases:
Rubella   Chicken pox
Hepatitis   Mononucleosis
Pancreatitis

Related to effects of cancer on (specify)
Related to abdominal cramps, diarrhea, and vomiting secondary to:
Gastroenteritis   Influenza
Gastric ulcers

Related to inflammation and smooth muscle spasms secondary to:
Renal calculi   Gastrointestinal infections

Treatment-Related
Related to tissue trauma and reflex muscle spasms secondary to:
Surgery   Diagnostic tests
Burns   (venipuncture, invasive
Accidents   scanning, biopsy)

Related to nausea and vomiting secondary to:
Chemotherapy   Anesthesia
Side effects of (specify)

Situational (Personal, Environmental)
Related to fever
Related to immobility/improper positioning
Related to overactivity
Related to pressure points (tight cast, elastic bandages)
Related to allergic response
Related to chemical irritants
Related to unmet dependency needs
Related to severe repressed anxiety

Maturational
Related to tissue trauma and reflex muscle spasms secondary to:
Infancy: Colic
Infancy and early childhood: Teething, ear pain
Middle childhood: Recurrent abdominal pain, growing pains
Adolescence: Headaches, chest pain, dysmenorrhea

○○ AUTHOR'S NOTE

A diagnosis not on the current NANDA list, *Impaired Comfort* can represent various uncomfortable sensations (eg, pruritus, immobility, NPO status). For a person experiencing nausea and vomiting, the nurse should assess whether *Impaired Comfort, Risk for Impaired Comfort,* or *Risk for Imbalanced Nutrition: Less Than Body Requirements* is appropriate. Short-lived episodes of nausea, vomiting, or both (*eg,* postoperatively) is best described with *Impaired Comfort related to effects of anesthesia or analgesics.* When nausea/vomiting may compromise nutritional intake, the appropriate diagnosis may be *Risk for Imbalanced Nutrition: Less Than Body Requirements related to nausea and vomiting secondary to (specify). Impaired Comfort* also can be used to describe a cluster of discomforts related to a condition or treatment, such as radiation therapy.

⊗ **ERRORS IN DIAGNOSTIC STATEMENTS**

1. *Impaired Comfort related to immobility*

Although immobility can contribute to impaired comfort, the nursing diagnosis *Disuse Syndrome* describes a cluster of nursing diagnoses that apply or are at high risk to apply as a result of immobility. *Impaired Comfort* can be included in *Disuse Syndrome;* thus, the diagnosis should be written as *Disuse Syndrome.*

2. *Impaired Comfort related to nausea and vomiting secondary to chemotherapy*

Nausea and vomiting represent signs and symptoms, not contributing factors, of impaired comfort. *Impaired Comfort* can be used to describe a cluster of discomforts associated with chemotherapy, such as *Impaired Comfort related to the effects of chemotherapy on bone marrow production and irritation of emetic center, as evidenced by complaints of nausea, vomiting, anorexia, and fatigue.*

KEY CONCEPTS
Generic Considerations

- Pruritus (itching) is the most common skin alteration. It can be a response to an allergen or a sign or symptom of a systemic disease, such as cancer, renal dysfunction, or diabetes.
- Pruritus, described as a tickling or tormenting sensation, originates exclusively in the skin and provokes the urge to scratch.
- Although the same neurons are likely to transmit signals for itching as for pressure, pain, and touch, each sensation is perceived and mediated differently (Branov et al., 1989b).
- Pruritus arises from subepidermal nerve stimulation by proteolytic enzymes, which the epidermis releases as a result of either primary irritation or secondary allergic responses (Porth, 2002).
- The same unmyelinated nerves that act for burning pain also serve for pruritus. As a pruritic sensation increases in intensity, it may become burning (Porth, 2002).
- Areas that immediately surround body openings are most susceptible to itching. This apparently is related to a concentration of sensory nerve endings and vulnerability to external contamination (Porth, 2002).

◉ Geriatric Considerations

Asteatosis (excessive skin dryness) is the most common cause of pruritus in older adults. Its incidence ranges from 40% to 80%, as a result of varying criteria and climate differences. With scratching, small breaks in the epidermis can increase the risk of infection owing to age-related changes in the immune system (Miller, 2004).

◉ Transcultural Considerations

- Pain is a universally recognized "private experience that is greatly influenced by cultural heritage" (Ludwig-Beymer, 1989, p. 283).
- US nurses are preponderantly white, middle-class women socialized to believe "that in any situation self-control is better than open displays of strong feelings" (Ludwig-Beymer, 1989, p. 294). Nurses should not stereotype members of a particular culture, but instead accept a wide range of pain expressions (Ludwig-Beymer, 1989).
- Families transmit to their children cultural norms related to pain (Ludwig-Beymer, 1989).
- Zborowski (1952), in his classic studies on the influence of culture on the pain experience, found that the pain event, its meaning, and responses are culturally learned and culturally specific. He reported the following cultural variations in interpretation and responses to pain:
  - *Third-generation Americans:* Unexpressive; concerned with implications; controlled emotional response

(continued)

> ### 🌐 Transcultural Considerations (continued)
>
> - *Jewish:* Concerned about the implication of the pain; readily seek relief; frequently express pain to others
> - *Irish:* See pain as private; unexpressive; unemotional
> - *Italian:* Concerned with immediate pain relief; present oriented
> - *Japanese:* Value self-control; will not express pain or ask for relief
> - *Hispanic:* Present oriented; use folk medicine frequently; view suffering as a positive spiritual experience
> - *Chinese:* May ignore symptoms; use alternative health practices
> - *Black Americans:* May respond stoically because of dominant culture pressure or belief that pain is God's will
> - Chinese women believe they will dishonor themselves and their family if they are loud during labor (Weber, 1996).
> - Women from many South and Central American cultures believe the more intense the expression of pain during labor, the stronger the love toward the infant (Weber, 1996).

Focus Assessment Criteria

This nursing assessment of pain is designed to acquire data for assessing a person's adaptation to pain, not for determining the cause or existence of pain.

Subjective Data

Assess for Defining Characteristics.

Pain

"Where is your discomfort located; does it radiate?" (Ask child to point to place).

"When did it begin?"

"Can you relate the cause of this discomfort?" or "What do you think has caused your discomfort?"

"Describe the discomfort and its pattern."

Time of day	Frequency (constant, inter-
Duration	mittent, transient)
Quality/intensity	

Ask person to rate the pain: at its best, after pain-relief measures, and at its worst. Use consistent scale, language, or set of behaviors to assess pain.

For adults, use an oral or visual analogue scale of 0 to 10 (0 = no pain, 10 = worst pain ever).

For children, select a scale appropriate for *developmental* age: can use scale for assessed age or younger; include child in selection.

- 3 years and older: Use drawings or photographs of faces (Oucher scale) ranging from smiling to frowning to crying with numeric scale (Beyer, 1984).
- 4 years and older: Use four white poker chips to ask child how many pieces of hurt he or she feels (no hurt = no chips; Hester, 1979).
- 6 years and older: Use a numeric scale, 0 to 5 or 0 to 10 (verbally or visually); use blank drawing of body, front and back, asking child to use three different crayons to color places with a little pain, medium pain, and a lot of pain (Eland Color Tool).

"How do you usually react to pain (crying, anger, silence)?"

"Are any other symptoms associated with your discomfort (nausea, vomiting, numbness)?"

Effects of pain

"Do you talk to others about your discomfort (spouse, friends, nurse)?" "To whom do you talk?" Ask client to indicate if each of the following increases, decreases, or has no effect on discomfort.*

Liquor	Vibration	Defecation
Stimulants (eg, caffeine)	Pressure	Tension
Eating	No movement	Bright lights
Heat	Movement/activity	Loud noises
Cold	Sleep, rest	Going to work

---

*Adapted from the McGill Pain Questionnaire.

Damp	Lying down	Intercourse
Weather changes	Distraction (eg, TV)	Mild exercise
Massage	Urination	Fatigue

Ask person what effect pain has had or is anticipated to have on the following patterns:

Work/activity (work/home activities, leisure/play)
Relationships/relating (wanting to be alone, with people)
Sleep (difficulty falling asleep/staying asleep)
Eating (appetite, weight gain/loss)
Elimination (bowel, constipation/diarrhea, bladder)
Menses
Sex (libido, function)

Cultural effects on pain (Weber, 1996)

Country of origin	Religious practices (blood
Time in United States	transfusion, specific
Native language	clothing, male attendants)
Ability to understand/speak	Food, beverage preferences
Availability of interpreter	Hygiene practices

Pruritus

Onset	Relieved by what
Precipitated by what	History of allergy
Site(s)	(individual, family)

Nausea/vomiting

| Onset, duration | Frequency, severity |
| Vomitus (amount, appearance) | Relief measures |

Objective Data (Acute/Chronic Pain)
Assess for Defining Characteristics.

Behavioral manifestations

Mood	Eye movements
Calmness	Fixed
Moaning	Searching
Crying	Open
Grimacing	Closed
Pacing	Perceptions
Restlessness	Oriented to time and place
Withdrawn	

Musculoskeletal manifestations

Mobility of painful part	Muscle tone
Full	Spasm
Limited/guarded	Tenderness
No movement	Tremors (in effort to hide pain)

Dermatologic manifestations

| Color (redness) | Moisture/diaphoresis |
| Temperature | Edema |

Cardiorespiratory manifestations

Cardiac	Respiratory
Rate	Rate
Blood pressure	Rhythm
Palpitations present	Depth

Sensory alterations

| Paresthesia | Dysesthesias |

Developmental manifestations

Infant

| Irritability | Changes in eating or sleeping |
| Inconsolability | Generalized body movements |

Toddler

Irritability	Changes in eating or sleeping
Aggression (kicking, biting)	Rocking
Sucking	Clenched teeth

Preschool

Irritability	Changes in eating or sleeping
Aggression	Verbal expressions of pain

School-aged

Changes in eating or sleeping	Change in play patterns
Verbal expressions of pain	Denial of pain

Adolescent

Mood changes	Behavior extremes ("acting out")
Verbal expressions when asked	Changes in eating or sleeping

For more information on Focus Assessment Criteria, visit http://connection.lww.com.

Goal

 NOC Symptom Control

The client will report acceptable control of symptoms.

Indicators

- Describe factors that increase symptoms.
- Describe measures to improve comfort.

General Interventions

NIC Pruritus Management, Fever Treatment, Environmental Management: Comfort

Assess for Sources of Discomfort.

Pruritus	Prolonged bed rest
Fever	

Reduce Pruritus and Promote Comfort.

Maintain Hygiene without Producing Dry Skin.
Encourage frequent baths.
  Use cool water when acceptable.
  Use mild soap (Castile, lanolin) or a soap substitute.
  Blot skin dry; do not rub.
Apply cornstarch lightly to skin folds by first sprinkling on hand (to avoid caking of powder); for fungal conditions, use antifungal or antiyeast powder preparations [Mycostatin (nystatin)], or miconazole cream.
Massage pruritic scar tissue with cocoa butter daily (Field et al., 2000).

Prevent Excessive Dryness.
Lubricate skin with a moisturizer unless contraindicated; pat on with hand or gauze.
Apply lubrication after bath, before skin is dry, to encourage moisture retention.
Apply wet dressings continuously or intermittently to relieve itching and remove crusts and exudate.
Provide 20- to 30-min tub soaks of 32°F to 38°F; water can contain oatmeal powder, Aveeno, cornstarch, or baking soda.

Promote Comfort and Prevent further Injury.
Advise against scratching; explain the scratch–itch–scratch cycle.
Secure order for topical corticosteroid cream for local inflamed pruritic areas; apply sparingly and occlude area with plastic wrap at night to increase effectiveness of cream and prevent further scratching.
Secure an antihistamine order if itching is unrelieved.
Use mitts (or cotton socks), if necessary, on children and confused adults.
Maintained trimmed nails to prevent injury; file after trimming.
Remove particles from bed (food crumbs, caked powder).

Use old, soft sheets and avoid wrinkles in bed; if bed protector pads are used, place draw sheet over them to eliminate direct contact with skin.

Avoid using perfumes and scented lotions.

Avoid contact with chemical irritants/solutions.

Wash clothes in a mild detergent and put through a second rinse cycle to reduce residue; avoid use of fabric softeners.

Prevent excessive warmth by use of cool room temperatures and low humidity, light covers with bed cradle; avoid overdressing.

Apply ointments with gloved or bare hand, depending on type, to lightly cover skin; rub creams into skin.

Use frequent, thin applications of ointment, rather than one thick application.

Proceed with Health Teaching, when Indicated.

Explain causes of pruritus and possible prevention methods.

Explain factors that increase symptoms (eg, low humidity, heat).

Explain interventions that relieve symptoms (eg, fluid intake of 3,000 mL/day unless contraindicated).

Advise about exposure to sun and heat and protective products.

Teach person to avoid fabrics that irritate skin (wool, coarse textures).

Teach person to wear protective clothing (rubber gloves, apron) when using chemical irritants.

Refer for allergy testing, if indicated.

Provide opportunity to discuss frustrations.

For further interventions, refer to *Ineffective Coping* if pruritus is stress related.

For Excessive Warmth, Provide Comfort Measures as Indicated.

Keep the room cool; remove blankets as needed.

Offer a cool washcloth for forehead; change frequently to maintain coolness.

Provide tepid sponge baths or alcohol rubs; finish with powder to minimize moisture.

Monitor bed linens (especially pillowcase) for dampness; change linens whenever moist.

Encourage wearing absorbent cotton bedclothes rather than silk or nylon.

Flip pillows and straighten linens frequently; assist with frequent repositioning.

Provide for periods of uninterrupted rest.

If requested, provide distractions (eg, TV, magazines, visitors).

Consult with physician about the use of aspirin and acetaminophen on an alternating basis (aspirin q 4 h with acetaminophen q 4 h in between).

For Coldness, Provide Comfort Measures as Indicated.

Apply socks, gloves, or head covering as needed.

Monitor room temperature; keep thermostat at 75°F to 80°F and monitor client's temperature for response.

If possible, encourage taking a warm tub bath; offer hot liquids.

Provide warmed blankets.

Consult with a physician for use of a rewarming device.

For a Person on Bed Rest:

Vary position at least every 2 h unless other variables necessitate more frequent changes.

Use small pillows or folded towels to support limbs.

Vary positions with flexion and extension, abduction, or adduction.

Use prone position if tolerable.

Rationales

- Excessive warmth or dryness, rough fabrics, fatigue, stress, and monotony (lack of distractions) aggravate pruritus (Thorns & Edmonds, 2000).
- Methods that interrupt pain also will interrupt pruritus. Examples include local anesthetics, cold, and peripheral nerve resection.
- Coolness reduces vasodilatation.
- Dryness increases skin sensitivity by stimulating nerve endings.
- Scratching stimulates histamine release, increasing pruritus.
- Massaging pruritic scars decreases itching, pain, and anxiety (Field et al., 2000).

Pediatric Interventions

Explain to children why they should not scratch.
Dress child in long sleeves, long pants, or a one-piece outfit to prevent scratching.
Avoid overdressing child, which will increase warmth.
Give child a tepid bath before bedtime; add two cups of cornstarch to bath water.
Apply Caladryl lotion to weeping pruritic lesions; apply with small paintbrush.
Use cotton blankets or sheets next to skin.
Remove furry toys that may increase lint and pruritus.
Teach child to press or (if permitted) put a cool cloth on the area that itches, but not to scratch.

Rationales

See Rationales for General Interventions.

Maternal Interventions

Teach the following to prevent strain on back muscles.

- Avoid heavy lifting; use leg muscles, not back muscles.
- Place one foot higher than the other when standing for prolonged periods.
- Wear heels lower than 1 inch.
- Wear maternity girdle and exercise daily (eg, walk, stretch).
- Apply heat or cold to back two or three times daily.

If leg cramps occur and are not caused by thrombophlebitis, teach client to flex or bend foot and not massage. Instruct client to stretch calf muscles before going to bed.

Rationales

- Approximately 50% of all pregnant women report backache; causes include postural changes, relaxation of pelvic ligaments, and movement of symphysis pubis (Davis, 1996).
- Lowered serum calcium and increased phosphate levels are thought to increase neuromuscular irritability.

ACUTE PAIN

DEFINITION

Acute Pain: The state in which a person experiences and reports the presence of severe discomfort or an uncomfortable sensation, lasting from 1 s to less than 6 months

DEFINING CHARACTERISTICS
Subjective Data

Communication (verbal or coded) of pain descriptors

Objective Data

Guarding, protective behavior
Self-focusing

Narrowed focus (altered time perception, withdrawal from social contact, impaired thought processes)

Distraction behavior (moaning, crying, pacing, seeking out other people or activities, restlessness)

Facial mask of pain (lackluster eyes, "beaten look," fixed or scattered movement, grimace)

Altered muscle tone (may span from listless to rigid)

Autonomic responses not seen in chronic stable pain (diaphoresis, changes in blood pressure and pulse, pupillary dilation, increased or decreased respiratory rate)

RELATED FACTORS

See *Impaired Comfort.*

ⓧ AUTHOR'S NOTE

Nursing management of pain presents specific challenges. Is acute pain a response that nurses treat as a nursing diagnosis or collaborative problem? Is acute pain the etiology of another response that better describes the condition that nurses treat? Does some cluster of nursing diagnoses represent a pain syndrome or chronic pain syndrome (eg, *Fear, Risk for Ineffective Family Coping, Impaired Physical Mobility, Social Isolation, Ineffective Sexuality Patterns, Risk for Colonic Constipation, Fatigue*)? McCafferty and Beebe (1989) cite 18 nursing diagnoses that can apply to people experiencing pain. Viewing pain as a syndrome diagnosis can provide nurses with a comprehensive nursing diagnosis for people in pain to whom many related nursing diagnoses could apply.

ⓧ ERRORS IN DIAGNOSTIC STATEMENTS

1. *Pain related to surgical incision*

Viewing incisional pain as an etiology rather than a response may better relate to nursing's focus. For a client who has undergone surgery, the nurse focuses on reducing pain to permit increased participation in activities and to reduce anxiety, as described by the nursing diagnosis *Impaired Physical Mobility related to fear of pain and weakness secondary to anesthesia and insufficient fluids and nutrients.*

2. *Pain related to cardiac tissue ischemia*

The nurse has several responsibilities for a person experiencing chest pain: evaluating cardiac status, reducing activity, administering PRN medication, and reducing anxiety. Before discharge, the nurse teaches self-monitoring, self-medication, signs and symptoms of complications, follow-up care, and necessary lifestyle modifications. Because nursing management of chest pain involves nurse-prescribed and physician-prescribed interventions, this situation should be described as the collaborative problem *PC: Cardiac.* This collaborative problem encompasses various cardiac complications (eg, dysrhythmias, decreased cardiac output, angina). In addition, two nursing diagnoses would apply: *Anxiety related to present situation, unknown future, and perceived effects on self and significant others,* and *Ineffective Health Maintenance related to insufficient knowledge of condition, signs and symptoms of complications, risk factors, activity restrictions, and follow-up care.*

KEY CONCEPTS
Generic Considerations

- "Pain has been described as an experience that overwhelms the individual and consumes every aspect of life" (Ferrell, 1995, p. 609).
- All pain is real, regardless of its cause. Pure psychogenic pain is probably rare, as is pure organic pain. Most bodily pain is a combination of mental events (psychogenic) and physical stimuli (organic).
- Pain has two components: sensory, which is neurophysiologic, and perceptual or experiential, which has cognitive and emotional origins. The interaction of these two components determines the amount of suffering.

- Pain tolerance means the duration and intensity of pain that a person is willing to endure. It differs among people and may vary in one person in different situations.
- Personal factors that influence pain tolerance are as follows:

Knowledge of pain and its cause	Ability to control pain
	Energy level (fatigue)
Meaning of pain	Stress level

- Social and environmental factors that influence pain tolerance are as follows:

Interactions with others	Secondary gains
Response of others (family, friends)	Sensory overload or deprivation
	Stressors

- Pain threshold is the point at which a person reports that a stimulus is painful (McCafferty & Beebe, 1989).
- Studies have shown that diagnosed physiologic pain does respond to placebos, so a positive response to placebo cannot be used to diagnose pain as psychogenic.
- Pain can be classified as acute or chronic, according to cause and duration, not intensity.
  - *Acute pain* has a duration of 1 s to less than 6 months. The cause is usually organic disease or injury. With healing, the pain subsides and eventually disappears.
  - *Chronic pain* lasts for 6 months or longer. It can be described as limited, intermittent, or persistent.
  - *Limited pain* results from a known physical lesion, and an end of the pain will come (eg, burns).
  - *Intermittent pain* provides the person with pain-free periods. The cause may or may not be known (eg, headaches).
  - *Persistent pain* usually occurs daily. The cause may or may not be known and is usually not a threat to life (eg, low back pain).
- The visible signs of pain (physical and behavioral) are determined by the person's pain tolerance and the duration of the pain, not the pain intensity.
- The person may respond to acute pain physiologically by diaphoresis and increased blood pressure and heart and respiratory rates and behaviorally by crying, moaning, or showing anger.
- The person with chronic pain usually has adapted to it, both physiologically and behaviorally. Thus, he or she may not show visible signs of the pain.
- Nurses' fear of precipitating addiction often makes them reluctant to administer narcotics. Porter and Jick (1980) identified that 4 addicts of 11,000 reported they received Demerol in the hospital.
- *Drug tolerance* is a physiologic phenomenon in which, after repeated doses, the prescribed dose begins to lose its effectiveness.
- *Drug dependence* is a physiologic state that results from repeated administration of a drug.
- *Withdrawal* occurs if a drug is discontinued abruptly. Tapering down the drug dosage manages the withdrawal symptoms.

Pediatric Considerations

- Studies have shown that, when adults and children undergo the same surgery, children are undermedicated (Beyer, 1984; Eland & Anderson, 1977; Wong, 2003). In one study, 52% of the children received no analgesic postoperatively, whereas the remaining 48% received preponderantly aspirin or acetaminophen.
- Maturational and chronologic age, cause of pain, coping style, parental response, culture, past pain experiences, and whether pain is acute or chronic influence the child's response to pain.

Infant
- Associates environment with painful experience
- Cries loudly and makes verbal protests long after the stimulus is withdrawn

Toddler
- Fears body intrusion
- Does not understand rationale for pain or have ability to conceptualize the duration of the experience, even if told
- Seeks out parental figures as a source of comfort

(continued)

Pediatric Considerations (continued)

Preschooler
- Engages in magical thinking or fantasies (eg, believes something they thought or did caused the pain)
- Uses increased verbal skills to communicate pain
- Has limited understanding of time
- After pain passes, talks to toys or other children about the pain experience
- Denies pain, especially if he or she associates it with adverse consequences (eg, injection, ridicule if not brave)

School-Aged
- Fears body injury
- Can describe the cause, type, quality, and severity of pain
- Can rate the severity of pain
- Attempts to relate the pain experience to previous events and gain control over actions
- Denies pain, especially if he or she associates it with adverse consequences
- May be influenced by presence of parents in expressing pain

Adolescent
- Considers body image as very important
- May use overconfidence to compensate for fear
- May use more "socially acceptable" behavioral responses to pain than do younger children, but fear and anxiety are *not* decreased
- May be influenced by presence of parents in expressing pain

Maternal Considerations

- The discomforts of labor vary: backaches, leg cramps, imposed immobility, and contractions.
- Chapman (1991) reported that expectant fathers assumed that their roles during labor are to act as coach, teammate, or witness.
- Prolonged latent phase of labor (>20 h for primigravida or 14 h for multipara) usually results from an unripe cervix. Other causes are abnormal fetal position, dysfunctional labor, cephalopelvic disproportion, or sedation or analgesia used too early.

Geriatric Considerations

- Pain is omnipresent in older adults and may be accepted by them and professionals as a normal and unavoidable accompaniment to aging. Unfortunately, many chronic diseases that are common in older adults, such as osteoarthritis and rheumatoid arthritis, may not receive adequate pain management.
- Older adults may not demonstrate objective signs and symptoms of pain because of years of adaptation and increased pain tolerance. They may eventually accept the pain, thereby lowering expectations for comfort and mobility. Pain-coping mechanisms cultivated throughout life are important to identify and reinforce in pain management. Effective pain management can greatly improve overall physical functioning and emotional well-being.
- The effects of narcotic analgesics are prolonged in older adults because of decreased metabolism and clearance of the drug. Also, side effects seem to be more frequent and pronounced, especially anticholinergic effects, extrapyramidal effects, and sedation. For older adults, it is advised that drugs be started at a lower dosage. Because older adults often take multiple drugs, drug interactions should be monitored (Malseed, 1995).

Focus Assessment Criteria

See *Impaired Comfort.*

Goal

NOC Comfort Level, Pain Control

The person will experience a satisfactory relief measure as evidenced by (specify).

Indicators

- Relate factors that increase pain.
- Relate interventions that are effective.
- Convey that others validate that the pain exists.

General Interventions

NIC Pain Management, Medication Management, Emotional Support, Teaching: Individual, Hot/Cold Application, Simple Massage

Assess for Factors that Decrease Pain Tolerance.

Disbelief from others	Lack of knowledge
Fear (eg, of addiction or loss of control)	Fatigue
Monotony	

Reduce or Eliminate Factors that Increase Pain.

Disbelief from others

Relate your acceptance of the client's response to pain.

  Acknowledge the pain.

  Listen attentively to client's discussion of pain.

  Convey that you are assessing pain because you want to understand it better (not determine if it really exists).

Assess the family for any misconceptions about pain or its treatment.

  Explain the concept of pain as an individual experience.

  Discuss why a person may experience increased or decreased pain (eg, fatigue [increased], distractions [decreased]).

  Encourage family members to share their concerns privately (eg, fear that the person will use pain for secondary gains if he or she receives too much attention).

  Assess whether family members doubt the pain; discuss the effects of doubting on the person's pain and on the relationship.

  Encourage the family to give attention also when the client does not exhibit pain.

Lack of knowledge

Explain the cause of the pain, if known.

Relate the severity of the pain and how long it will last, if known.

Explain diagnostic tests and procedures in detail by relating the discomforts and sensations that the client will feel; approximate the duration (eg, "During the intravenous pyelogram, you might feel a momentary hot flash through your entire body").

Allow person to see and handle equipment if possible.

Fear

Provide accurate information to reduce fear of addiction.

  Explore reasons for the fear.

  Explain the difference between drug tolerance and drug addiction (see Key Concepts).

Assist in reducing fear of losing control.

  Provide privacy for the client's pain experience.

  Attempt to limit the number of health care providers who provide care.

  Allow client to share intensity of pain; express to client how well he or she tolerated it.

Provide information to reduce fear that the medication will gradually lose its effectiveness.

  Discuss drug tolerance.

  Discuss interventions for drug tolerance with the physician (eg, changing the medication, increasing the dose, decreasing the interval).

  Discuss the effect of relaxation techniques on medication effects.

Fatigue

Determine the cause of fatigue (sedatives, analgesics, sleep deprivation).

Explain that pain contributes to stress, which increases fatigue.

Assess present sleep pattern and the influence of pain on sleep.

Provide opportunities to rest during the day and with periods of uninterrupted sleep at night (must rest when pain is decreased).

Consult with physician for an increased dose of pain medication at bedtime.

Refer to *Disturbed Sleep Pattern* for specific interventions to enhance sleep.

Monotony

Discuss with client and family the therapeutic uses of distraction, along with other methods of pain relief.

Emphasize that the degree to which a person can be distracted from the pain is not at all related to the existence or intensity of the pain.

Explain that distraction usually increases pain tolerance and decreases pain intensity; however, after the distraction ceases, the person may have an increased awareness of pain and fatigue.

Vary the environment if possible.

If the client is on bed rest:
- Encourage personnel to wear seasonal pins and bright-colored apparel.
- Encourage family to decorate the room with flowers, plants, and pictures.
- Provide music.
- Consult with a recreational therapist for appropriate tasks.

If the client is at home:
- Encourage person to plan an activity for each day, preferably outside the home.
- Discuss the possibility of learning a new skill (eg, a craft, a musical instrument).
- Teach a method of distraction during acute pain that is not a burden (eg, count items in a picture, count anything in the room, such as patterns on wallpaper, count silently to self); breathe rhythmically; listen to music and increase the volume as pain increases.

Collaborate with Client about Possible Methods to Reduce Pain Intensity.

Consider the Following before Selecting a Specific Pain-relief Method:

Client's willingness (motivation) and ability to participate

Preference

Support of significant others for method

Contraindications (allergy, health problem)

Method's cost, complexity, precautions, and convenience

Explain the Various Noninvasive Pain-relief Methods to the Client and Family and Why they are Effective.

Discuss the Use of Heat Applications,* their Therapeutic Effects, Indications, and Related Precautions.

Hot water bottle	Moist heat pack
Warm tub	Thin plastic wrap over
Hot summer sun	painful area to retain body
Electric heating pad	heat (eg, knee, elbow)

Discuss the Use of Cold Applications,* their Therapeutic Effects, Indications, and Related Precautions.

Cold towels (wrung out)	Cold water immersion for
Ice bag	small body parts
Ice massage	Cold gel pack

Explain the Therapeutic Uses of Menthol Preparations, Massage, and Vibration.

Teach Client to Avoid Negative Thoughts about Ability to Cope with Pain (Gaston-Johnson et al., 2000).

Practice Distraction (eg, Guided Imagery, Music).

---

*May require a primary care provider's order.

Provide Optimal Pain Relief with Prescribed Analgesics.

Determine preferred route of administration: oral, intramuscular (IM), intravenous (IV), rectal (see Key Concepts).

Assess vital signs, especially respiratory rate, before administration.

Consult with pharmacist for possible adverse interactions with other medications (eg, muscle relaxants, tranquilizers).

Use a preventive approach.

1. Medicate before an activity (eg, ambulation) to increase participation, but evaluate the hazard of sedation.
2. Instruct client to request PRN pain medication before the pain is severe.
3. Collaborate with physician to order medications on a 24-h basis rather than PRN.

Assess Client's Response to the Pain-relief Medication.

After administration, return in 30 min to assess effectiveness.

Ask client to rate severity of pain before the medication and amount of relief received.

Ask person to indicate when the pain began to increase.

Consult with physician if a dosage or interval change is needed; the dose may be increased by 50% until effective (Agency for Health Care Policy and Research [AHCPR], 1992).

Reduce or Eliminate Common Side Effects of Narcotics.

Sedation

Assess whether the cause is the narcotic, fatigue, sleep deprivation, or other drugs (sedatives, antiemetics).

Inform person that drowsiness usually occurs the first 2 to 3 days, then subsides.

If drowsiness is excessive, consult with physician to slightly reduce the dose.

Constipation

Explain the effects of narcotics on peristalsis.

For long-term drug use, consult with physician on the use of a stool softener.

Refer to *Constipation* for additional interventions.

Nausea and Vomiting (see also Nausea/Vomiting)

Instruct person that nausea usually subsides after a few doses.

Refrain from withholding narcotic doses because of nausea; rather, secure an order for an antiemetic.

If nausea persists, consult with physician for the appropriate antiemetic or for a change of narcotic that produces less nausea (eg, morphine).

Dry mouth

Explain that narcotics decrease saliva production.

Instruct person to rinse mouth often, suck on sugarless sour candies, eat pineapple chunks or watermelon (if permissible), and drink liquids often.

Explain the necessity of good oral hygiene and dental care.

Assist Family to Respond Optimally to Client's Pain Experience.

Assess family's knowledge of pain and response to it.

Give accurate information to correct misconceptions (eg, addiction, doubt about pain).

Provide each family member with opportunities to discuss fears, anger, and frustrations privately; acknowledge the difficulty of the situation.

Incorporate family members in the pain-relief modality, if possible (eg, stroking, massage) (Grealish et al., 2000).

Praise their participation and concern.

Assist with the Aftermath of Pain.

Inform person when the cause of the pain has been removed or decreased (eg, spinal tap).

Encourage person to discuss the pain experience.

Praise client for his or her endurance and convey that he or she handled the pain well, regardless of actual behavior.

Allow person to keep souvenir of pain, if desired (eg, gallstones), or a record of repeated procedures (eg, venipunctures).

Assist with Phantom Limb Pain.

Advise that 80% of amputees experience phantom limb sensations during the first year after surgery (Sherman, 1989).

Explain that no one knows the exact cause of phantom limb pain. One possible cause is stimulus of peripheral nerves proximal to the amputation. Another explanation is that severed nerves may send impulses that the brain perceives as abnormal (Rounseville, 1992).

Explain the sensations that may be present, including feeling limb is still present; limb is floating; tight band below amputation; warm, tingling feeling (Rounseville, 1992).

Explain that psychological stress does not cause phantom pain but can trigger or increase it (Sherman, 1989).

Explain measures that have been effective in alleviating phantom limb pain (Williamson, 1998):
- Applying heat to stump
- Applying pressure to stump (eg, elastic bandages)
- Distraction, diversion techniques, relaxation exercises
- Massage therapy (after 2 weeks postoperatively)
- Applying capsaicin cream to stump, but not wound, for pain

Explain that narcotics are ineffective for phantom limb pain but are effective for surgical stump pain (Sherman, 1989).

Consult for pharmacologic treatment of phantom limb pain (eg, beta blockers, anticonvulsants, tricyclic antidepressants.

Initiate Health Teaching, as Indicated.

Discuss with client and family noninvasive pain-relief measures (relaxation, distraction, massage). Teach the techniques of choice to the person and family.

Explain the expected course of the pain (resolution) if known (eg, fractured arm, surgical incision).

Rationales

- Trying to convince health care providers that he or she is experiencing pain will cause the client anxiety, which compounds the pain. Both are energy depleting.
- People who are prepared for painful procedures by explanations of the actual sensations experience less stress than those who receive vague explanations.
- Studies have shown that the human brain secretes endorphins, which have opiatelike properties that relieve pain. The release of endorphins may be responsible for the positive effects of placebos and noninvasive pain-relief measures.
- Studies have shown that diagnosed physiologic pain does respond to placebos, so a positive response to placebos cannot be used to diagnose pain as psychogenic.
- The use of noninvasive pain-relief measures (eg, relaxation, massage, distraction) can enhance the therapeutic effects of pain-relief medications.
- Adults and children who are experiencing pain feel their bodies and their lives are out of control. Attempts must be made to provide some choice or control during their day.
- Inadequate sleep decreases the ability to tolerate pain and depletes the energy needed to participate in social activities.
- Pain management should be aggressive and individualized to eliminate any unnecessary pain, with drugs administered on a regular schedule rather than PRN in the early postoperative period (AHCPR, 1992).
- The preventive approach may reduce the total 24-h dose compared with the PRN approach; it provides a constant blood level of the drug, it reduces craving for the drug, and it reduces the anxiety of having to ask and wait for PRN relief (AHCPR, 1992).
- Oral administration is preferred when possible. Liquid medications can be given to those who have difficulty swallowing (AHCPR, 1992).
- If frequent injections are necessary, the IV route is preferred because it is not painful and absorption is guaranteed. Side effects (decreased respirations and blood pressure), however, may be more profound.
- Addiction is a psychological syndrome characterized by compulsive drug-seeking behavior generally associated with a desire for drug administration to produce euphoria or other effects, not pain relief. Addiction is believed to be rare, and there is no evidence that adequate administration of opioids for pain produces addiction.
- Nonpharmacologic interventions provide a major treatment approach for pain, specifically chronic pain (McGuire, Sheidler & Polomano, 2000). They provide clients with an increased sense of control, promote active involvement, reduce stress and anxiety, elevate mood, and raise the pain threshold (McGuire, Sheidler & Polomano, 2000).

- Cognitive pain interventions try to modify thought processes to relieve pain. Examples are distraction (eg, counting, word games, conversation, breathing exercises), imagery, and educational programs about pain management (McGuire, Sheidler & Polomano, 2000).
- Behavioral methods attempt to modify physiologic reactions to pain. Examples are relaxation, meditation, music therapy, hypnosis, and biofeedback (McGuire, Sheidler & Polomano, 2000).
- Information given before a potentially stressful event reduces fear of the unknown and assists the person to adapt.
- Relaxation and guided imagery effectively manage pain by increasing sense of control, reducing feelings of helplessness and hopelessness, providing a calming diversion, and disrupting the pain–anxiety–tension cycle (Sloman, 1995).

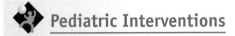 ## Pediatric Interventions

Assess for Pain.

Assess the Child's Pain Experience.

Determine the child's concept of the cause of pain, if feasible.

Ask child to point to the area that hurts. See Focus Assessment under *Impaired Comfort.*

Determine the intensity of the pain at its worst and best. Use a pain assessment scale appropriate for the child's developmental age. Use the same scale the same way each time, and encourage its use by parents and other health care professionals. Indicate on the care plan which scale to use and how (introduction of scale, language specific for child); attach copy if visual scale. (See p. 149 for a description of pain scales.)

Ask the child what makes the pain better and what makes it worse.

Include the parents' rating of their child's pain in assessment. Parents and nurses can rate a child's pain differently. The parents' observation is often more accurate.

Assess whether fear, loneliness, or anxiety is contributing to pain.

Assess effect of pain on sleep and play. *Note:* A child who sleeps, plays, or both can still be in pain (sleep and play can serve as distractions) or adequately medicated for pain.

With infants, assess crying, facial expressions, body postures, and movements. Infants exhibit distress from environmental stimuli (light, sound) as well as from touch and treatments. Use tactile and vocal stimuli to comfort infants, but assess the effect of comfort measures (does it increase or decrease distress?) and individualized intervention.

Assess the Child and Family for Misconceptions about Pain or its Treatment.

Explain the pain source to the child using verbal and sensory (visual, tactile) explanations (eg, allow child to handle equipment, perform treatment on doll).

Explicitly explain and reinforce to the child that he or she is not being punished.

Explain to the parents the necessity of good explanations to promote trust.

Explain to the parents that the child may cry more openly when they are present, but that their presence is important for promoting trust.

Parents and older children may have misconceptions about analgesia and may fear narcotic use/abuse. Emphasize that narcotic use for moderate or severe pain does not lead to addiction. Discuss with parents and older children that "say no to drugs" does not apply to analgesia for pain prescribed by physicians and monitored by physicians and nurses.

Promote Security with Honest Explanations and Opportunities for Choice.

Promote Open, Honest Communication.

Tell the truth; explain:

- How much it will hurt
- How long it will last
- What will help the pain

Do not threaten (eg, *do not* tell the child, "If you don't hold still, you won't go home").

Explain to the child that the procedure is necessary so he or she can get better and that holding still is important so it can be done quickly.

Discuss with parents the importance of truth-telling. Instruct them to:

Tell child when they are leaving and when they will return.

Relate to the child that they cannot take away pain, but that they will be with him or her (except in circumstances when parents are not permitted to remain).

Allow parents opportunities to share their feelings about witnessing their child's pain and their help-lessness.

Prepare the Child for a Painful Procedure.
Discuss the procedure with the parents; determine what they have told the child.
Explain the procedure in words suited to the child's age and developmental level (see *Delayed Growth and Development* for age-related needs).
    Allow a 2-year-old child to watch you take out sutures from a doll or stuffed animal.
    Permit the child to hold instruments.
Relate the likely discomforts (eg, what the child will feel, taste, see, or smell).
    "You will get an injection that will hurt for a little while and then it will stop."
    Be sure to explain when an injection will cause two discomforts: the prick of the needle and the absorption of the drug.
Encourage the child to ask questions before and during the procedure; ask the child to share what he or she thinks will happen and why.
Share with the child older than 3½ years that:
    You expect the child to hold still and that it will please you if he or she can.
    It is all right to cry or squeeze your hand if it hurts.
Find something to praise after the procedure, even if child could not hold still.
Arrange to have parents present for procedures (especially for children younger than 10 years); describe what to expect to parents before procedure, and give them a role during procedure (eg, hold the child's hand, talk to the child).

Reduce the Pain during Treatments when Possible.
If restraints must be used, have sufficient personnel available so the procedure is not delayed.
If injections are ordered, try to obtain an order for oral or IV analgesics instead. If injections must be used:
    1. Expect the child (older than 2½ or 3 years) to hold still.
    2. Have the child participate by holding the Band-Aid for you.
    3. Tell the child how pleased you are that he or she helped.
    4. Pull the skin surface as taut as possible (for IM).
    5. Comfort the child after the procedure.
    6. Tell child step-by-step what is going to happen right before it is done.
Offer the child the option of learning distraction techniques for use during the procedure. (The use of distraction without the child's knowledge of the impending discomfort is not advocated because the child will learn to mistrust.)
    Tell a story with a puppet.
    Blow a party noisemaker.
    Ask the child to name or count objects in a picture.
    Ask the child to look at the picture and to locate certain objects ("Where is the dog?").
    Ask child to tell you about his or her pet.
    Ask child to count your blinks.
Avoid rectal thermometers in preschoolers; if possible, use electronic oral or ear probes.
Provide the child with privacy during the painful procedure; use a treatment room rather than the child's bed.
    The child's bed should be a "safe" place.
    No procedures should be done in the playroom or schoolroom.

Provide the Child Optimal Pain Relief with Prescribed Analgesics.
Medicate child before painful procedure or activity (eg, ambulation).
Consult with physician for a change of the IM route to the IV route.
Assess appropriateness of medication, dose, and schedule for cause of pain, child's weight, and child's response.
Along with using pain assessment scales, observe for behavioral signs of pain (because the child may deny pain); if possible, identify specific behaviors that indicate pain in an individual child.
Assess the potential for use of patient-controlled analgesia (PCA), which provides intermittent controlled doses of IV analgesia (with/without continuous infusion) as determined by the child's need. Children as young as 5 years of age can use PCA. Parents of children physically unable can administer it to them. PCA has been found safe and to provide superior pain relief compared with conventional-demand analgesia.
Consult with physician about the use of epidural infusion of morphine for treatment of postoperative pain. Epidural morphine infusion has been used safely in both adults and children in nonintensive care settings.

Reduce or Eliminate the Common Side Effects of Narcotics.

Sedation

Assess whether the cause is the narcotic, fatigue, sleep deprivation, or other drugs (sedatives, antiemetics).

If drowsiness is excessive, consult with physician to slightly reduce the dose.

Constipation

Explain to older children why pain medications cause constipation.

Increase roughage in diet (eg, fruits; 1 teaspoon of bran on cereal).

Encourage child to drink 8 to 10 glasses of liquid each day.

Teach child how to do abdominal isometric exercises if activity is restricted (eg, "Pull in your tummy; now relax your tummy; do this ten times each hour during the day").

Instruct child to keep a record of exercises (eg, make a chart with a star sticker placed on it whenever the exercises are done).

Refer to *Constipation* for additional interventions.

Dry mouth

Explain to older children that narcotics decrease saliva production.

Instruct child to rinse mouth often, suck on sugarless sour candies, eat pineapple chunks and watermelon, and drink liquids often.

Explain the necessity of brushing teeth after every meal.

Assist Child with the Aftermath of Pain.

Tell the child when the painful procedure is over. Pick up the small child to indicate it is over.

Encourage child to discuss pain experience (draw or act out with dolls).

Encourage child to perform the painful procedure using the same equipment on a doll under supervision.

Praise the child for his or her endurance and convey that he or she handled the pain well regardless of actual behavior (unless the child was violent to others).

Give the child a souvenir of the pain (Band-Aid, badge for bravery).

Teach child to keep a record of painful experiences and to plan a reward each time he or she achieves a behavioral goal, such as a gold star (reward) for each time the child holds still (goal) during an injection. Encourage achievable goals; holding still during an injection may not be possible for every child, but counting or blowing may be.

Collaborate with Child to Initiate Appropriate Noninvasive Pain-relief Modalities.

Encourage mobility as much as indicated, especially when pain is lowest.

Discuss with child and parents activities that they like, and incorporate them in daily schedule (eg, clay modeling, painting).

Discuss with the child older than 7 years that thinking about something else can decrease the pain, and demonstrate the effects.

1. Ask child to count to 100 (or count your eye blinks).
2. As child is counting, apply gentle pressure to Achilles tendon (pinch back of heel).
3. Gradually increase the pressure.
4. Ask child to stop counting but keep pressure on heel.
5. Ask if the child can feel the discomfort in his or her heel now and if the child felt it during counting.

Consider the use of transcutaneous electrical nerve stimulation (TENS) for procedural, acute, and chronic pain. TENS has been studied and used effectively in children with postoperative pain, headache, and procedural pain, without adverse effects.

Refer to guidelines for noninvasive pain-relief measures.

Assist Family to Respond Optimally to Child's Pain Experience.

Assess family's knowledge of and response to pain (eg, do parents support the child who has pain?).

Assure parents that they can touch or hold their child, if feasible (eg, demonstrate that touching is possible even with tubes and equipment).

Give accurate information to correct misconceptions (eg, the necessity of the treatment even though it causes pain).

Provide parents opportunities to discuss privately their fears, anger, and frustrations.

Acknowledge the difficulty of the situation.

Incorporate parents in the pain-relief modality if possible (eg, stroking, massage, distraction).

Praise their participation and concern.

Negotiate goals of pain management plan; reevaluate regularly (eg, pain-free, decreased pain).

Promote Coping Behaviors.

Observe for coping behaviors that assist the child to prepare for and recover from pain.

Tension reduction strategies (keep as still as possible, think about other things, sing, talk, listen to others talk)

Self-talk (tell themselves that they are OK, that the procedure is going well, that they are getting better; rephrase the experience in terms of its benefits)

Information-seeking behaviors (ask questions about both detailed and broad aspects of the experience, immediate and future data)

Controlling behaviors (use verbal suggestions, rules, who does what when, how things are done)

Hand-holding, comforting touch

Stalling strategies (drink water, TV program, time)

Body stiffening or muscle relaxation

Silent or audible cursing

Laughter (usually after pain is relieved)

Along with child and parents, identify and promote coping behaviors that are effective for that child. Children cope more effectively with pain when they use their preferred coping behaviors.

Initiate Health Teaching and Referrals, if Indicated.

Provide child and family with ongoing explanations.

Use the care plan to promote continuity of care for hospitalized child.

Use available mental health professionals, if needed, for assistance with guided imagery, progressive relaxation, and hypnosis.

Use available pain service (pain team) at pediatric health care centers for an interdisciplinary and comprehensive approach to pain management in children.

Refer parents to pertinent literature for themselves and children (see Bibliography).

Rationales

- Assessment of pain in children consists of three parts: the nature of the pain-producing pathology, the autonomic responses of acute pain, and the child's behaviors. It never should be based only on behavior.
- Toddlers in pain may be hyperactive in an attempt to escape the pain. Screams are ways to express their outrage.
- School-aged children can understand why a procedure needs to be done. Assessment tools can be used.
- Anxiety, fear, and separation can increase pain.
- Pharmacologic measures combined with noninvasive techniques provide the most effective means of treating pain in children.
- Nurses, physicians, and parents should identify and use consistent pain assessment criteria (eg, assessment scale, specific behaviors) to assess pain in a child.
- Verbal communication usually is not sufficient or reliable to explain pain or painful procedures with children younger than 7 years. The nurse can explain by demonstrating with pictures or dolls. The more senses that are stimulated in explanations to children, the greater the communication. When possible, parents should be included in preparation.
- Because a child may respond more openly to pain when they are near, parents' presence should be encouraged to facilitate pain assessment, provide support, and promote trust.
- The child's weight, not age, should be considered when calculating analgesic relief.
- Children and adolescents often deny pain to avoid injections. Although oral administration of analgesia is the route of choice for children, followed by IV administration, O'Brien and Konsler (1988) found that 40% of medications for postoperative pain were administered IM.

Maternal Interventions

Advise the woman that she will be assisted in managing her labor. Explore her wishes.

Determine the role the expectant father chooses for the labor and birth experience: coach, teammate, or witness (Chapman, 1991), or support the doula or coach.

Explain all procedures before initiation.

Provide comfort techniques as desired (eg, walking, music, massage, acupressure, shower, baths, hot or cold applications, hypnosis, imagery; Pillitteri, 2003).

Instruct woman not to use breathing techniques too early.

Engage the woman in pleasant dialogue and thoughts about specific subjects (eg, other children, favorite friends, new baby, memorable vacation).

As labor progresses to active stage:

1. Evaluate effectiveness of breathing techniques.
2. If pain or anxiety is not reduced, consult with midwife or physician for a new plan.
3. Evaluate fatigue level.
4. Assess how well labor partner is anticipating the woman's needs.
5. Encourage ambulation and position changes every 20 to 30 min.
6. Approach the woman in an unhurried, gentle manner.
7. Experiment with rhythmic chanting or moaning with contractions.

Rationales

- Labor pain belongs to the woman experiencing it (Lowe, 1996).
- Lowe (1996) found that women who engage in positive dialogue and thinking experience less pain.
- Depending on the choice of roles by the expectant father, the nurse supplements, supervises, or provides the supportive care.
- Calm explanations can reduce fear and anxiety.
- Sensory overload can contribute to anxiety and fear.
- Walking promotes less frequent, more efficient contractions.
- Position changes can prevent or correct malposition of the fetus, promote rotation and labor progress, and reduce lower back pain.
- If prolonged latent labor is expected, a new plan of care is needed to prevent sleep deprivation, maternal exhaustion, and increased anxiety.
- Maternal exhaustion can occur if breathing techniques are used too early.

CHRONIC PAIN

DEFINITION

Chronic Pain: The state in which a person experiences pain that is persistent or intermittent and lasts for more than 6 months

DEFINING CHARACTERISTICS
Major (Must Be Present)

The person reports that pain has existed for more than 6 months (may be the only assessment data present).

Minor (May Be Present)

Discomfort

Anger, frustration, depression because of situation

Facial mask of pain

Anorexia, weight loss

Insomnia

Guarded movement

Muscle spasms

Redness, swelling, heat

Color changes in affected area

Reflex abnormalities

RELATED FACTORS

See *Impaired Comfort.*

 AUTHOR'S NOTE

Semon (1977) and Crez and Pimenta (2001) have debated chronic pain as a single nursing diagnosis. It is well known that chronic pain affects coping, sleep, sexual activity, socialization, family processes, nutrition, spirituality, and activity tolerance. Cruz and Pimenta reported possible components of *Chronic Pain Syndrome* as *Risk for Constipation, Disturbed Sleep Pattern, Deficient Knowledge, Impaired Physical Mobility, Anxiety/Fear, Activity Intolerance,* and *Imbalanced Nutrition.* This author proposes that *Chronic Pain Syndrome* could represent only the effects of chronic pain on the psychosocial domain. When chronic pain affects sleep, self-care, nutrition, elimination, activity tolerance, or sexual activity, individual diagnoses may be more useful clinically.

ERRORS IN DIAGNOSTIC STATEMENTS

See *Impaired Comfort.*

KEY CONCEPTS
Refer to *Acute Pain.*

Focus Assessment Criteria

See *Impaired Comfort.*

Goal

NOC Comfort Level, Pain: Disruptive Effects, Pain Control, Depression Control

The person will relate improvement of pain and increased daily activities as evidenced by (specify).

Indicators
• Relate that others validate that their pain exists.
• Practice selected noninvasive pain-relief measures.

The child will demonstrate coping mechanism for pain, methods to control pain, and the pain cause/ disease, as evidenced by increased play and usual activities of childhood, and (specify).

Indicators
• Communicate improvement in pain verbally, by pain assessment scale, or by behavior (specify).
• Maintain usual family role and relationships throughout pain experience, as evidenced by (specify).

General Interventions

NIC Pain Management, Medication Management, Exercise Promotion, Mood Management, Coping Enhancement

Assess the Person's Pain Experience.
Determine the intensity of the pain at its worst and best.
Ask person to rate pain using a scale of 0 to 10 (0 = no pain; 10 = worst pain) or 0 to 5.
   1. Rate it at its best.
   2. Rate it after a pain-relief measure.
   3. Rate it at its worst.
   4. Collaborate to determine what methods could be used to reduce the intensity.

Assess for Factors that Decrease Pain Tolerance.
See *Acute Pain.*

Reduce or Eliminate Factors that Increase Pain.

See *Acute Pain*.

Determine with Client and Family the Effects of Chronic Pain on the Person's Life (Ferrell, 1995).

Physical well-being (fatigue, strength, appetite, sleep, function, constipation, nausea)

Psychological well-being (anxiety, depression, coping, control, concentration, sense of usefulness, fear, enjoyment)

Spiritual well-being (religiosity, uncertainty, positive changes, sense of purpose, hopefulness, suffering, meaning of pain, transcendence)

Social well-being (family support, family distress, sexuality, affection, employment, isolation, financial burden, appearance, roles, relationships)

Assist Client and Family to Reduce the Effects of Depression on Lifestyle.

Explain the relationship between chronic pain and depression.

Encourage verbalization concerning difficult situations.

Listen carefully.

See *Ineffective Coping* for additional interventions.

Collaborate with Client about Possible Methods to Reduce Pain Intensity.

See *Acute Pain*.

Collaborate with Client to Initiate Appropriate Non-pharmaceutical Pain-Relief Measures.

See *Acute Pain*.

Provide Pain Relief with Prescribed Analgesics.*

Determine preferred route of administration: oral, IM, IV, rectal (refer to Key Concepts).

Assess client's response to the medication. For those admitted to acute care settings:

After administration, return in 30 min to assess effectiveness.

Ask person to rate severity of pain before the medication and amount of relief received.

Ask client to indicate when the pain began to increase.

Consult with the physician if a dosage or interval change is needed.

For outpatients:

Ask person to keep a record of when he or she takes medication and kind of relief received.

Instruct person to consult physician with questions concerning medication dosage.

Encourage the use of oral medications as soon as possible.

Consult with physician for a schedule to change from IM to oral.

Explain to client and family that oral medications can be as effective as IM.

Explain how the transition will occur:

1. Begin oral medication at a larger dose than necessary (loading dose).
2. Continue PRN IM medication.
3. Gradually reduce IM medication dose.
4. Use the person's account of pain to regulate oral doses.

Consult with physician about possibly adding aspirin or acetaminophen to medication regimen.

Reduce or Eliminate Common Side Effects of Narcotics.

See *Acute Pain*.

Assist Family to Respond Optimally to the Client's Pain Experience.

See *Acute Pain*.

Encourage family to seek assistance if needed for specific problems, such as coping with chronic pain: family counselor; financial and service agencies (eg, American Cancer Society).

---

*May require a primary care provider's order.

Promote Optimal Mobility.

Discuss the value of exercise to strengthen and stretch muscles, decrease stress, and promote sleep. Plan daily activities when pain is at its lowest level.

Initiate Health Teaching and Referrals as Indicated.

Discuss with client and family the various treatment modalities available:

Family therapy	Group therapy
Behavior modification	Biofeedback
Hypnosis	Acupuncture
Exercise program	

Rationales

- See Rationales for *Acute Pain.*
- Ferrell (1995) validated that pain affects quality of life. Assessment of the specific effects is essential.
- Nursing care that improves pain also improves well-being (Ferrell, 1995).
- Pain is an intense experience for the client and family members. Interventions focus on helping families understand pain's effects on roles and relationships.
- Nonpharmacologic interventions provide a major treatment approach for pain, specifically chronic pain (McGuire, Sheidler & Polomano, 2000).
- The person with chronic pain may respond with withdrawal, depression, anger, frustration, and dependency, all of which can affect the family in the same way.

Pediatric Interventions

Assess pain experiences by using developmentally appropriate assessment scales and by assessing behavior. Incorporate child and family in ongoing assessment. Identify potential for secondary gain for reporting pain (eg, companionship, attention, concern, caring, distraction); include strategies for meeting identified needs in plan of care.

Set short-term and long-term goals for pain management with child and family and evaluate regularly (eg, totally or partially relieve pain, control behavior or anxiety associated with pain).

Promote normal growth and development; involve family and available resources, such as occupational, physical, and child life therapists.

Promote the "normal" aspects of the child's life: play, school, family relationships, physical activity.

Promote a trusting environment for child and family.

Believe the child's pain.

Encourage child's perception that interventions are attempts to help.

Provide continuity of care and pain management by health care providers (nurse, physician, pain team) and in different settings (inpatient, outpatient, emergency department, home).

Use interdisciplinary team for pain management as necessary (eg, nurse, physician, child life therapist, mental health therapist, occupational therapist, physical therapist, nutritionist).

Identify myths and misconceptions about pediatric pain management (eg, IM analgesia, narcotic use and dosing, assessment) in attitudes of health care professionals, child, and family; provide accurate information and opportunities for effective communication.

Provide parents and siblings with opportunities to share their experiences and fears.

Rationales

- See Rationales for *Acute Pain.*
- Parents of a child with pain report unendurable pain, helplessness, total commitment, feeling the pain physically, being unprepared, agony, terror, and wishing for death in cases of terminal illness (Ferrell, 1995). Interventions attempt to elicit these feelings and experiences.
- Assessing the child's cognitive level and age is important to provide appropriate explanations.
- Preschoolers assume their pain has resulted from bad deeds. Nurses must attempt to reduce their sense of personal blame.

NAUSEA

DEFINITION

Nausea: The state in which a person experiences an unpleasant, wavelike sensation in the back of the throat, epigastrium, or throughout the abdomen that may or may not lead to vomiting

DEFINING CHARACTERISTICS
Major

A vague, unpleasant, subjective sensation of being "sick to stomach"
Can be accompanied by watery salivation, pallor, sweating, tachycardia
May precede vomiting

RELATED FACTORS
Biopathophysiologic

Related to tissue trauma and reflex muscle spasms secondary to:
Acute gastroenteritis
Peptic ulcer disease
Irritable bowel syndrome
Pancreatitis
Infections (eg, food poisoning)
Drug overdose
Renal calculi
Uterine cramps associated with menses
Motion sickness
Stress

Treatment-Related

Related to effects of chemotherapy, theophylline, digitalis, antibiotics
Related to effects of anesthesia

ⓧ **ERRORS IN DIAGNOSTIC STATEMENTS**

Refer to *Impaired Comfort.*

KEY CONCEPTS
Generic Considerations

Nausea results from stimulation of the medullary vomiting center in the brain (Porth, 2002).

Nausea and vomiting, when determined to have emotional origins, may result from developmental adjustment and adaptation. A child learns that vomiting is unacceptable and thus learns to control it. He or she receives approval for not vomiting. Should childhood situations or conflicts resurface, the adult may experience nausea and vomiting.

Nausea is the third most common side effect of chemotherapy after alopecia and fatigue (Foltz et al., 1996).

Inadequate management of previous nausea causes anticipatory nausea before chemotherapy (Eckert, 2001).

Maternal Considerations

The etiology of nausea during pregnancy is unknown. Contributing factors include fatigue and hormonal, neurologic, and psychological changes (Davis, 1996).

Focus Assessment Criteria

Subjective Data

Onset/duration
  Time of day, pattern
Frequency
Vomitus (amount, time of day)
Associated with
  Medications   Activity
  Specific foods   Pain
  Position
Relief measures

For more information on Focus Assessment Criteria, visit http://connection.lww.com.

Goal

NOC Comfort Level, Nutrition Status, Hydration

The client will report decreased nausea.

Indicators

- Name foods or beverages that do not increase nausea.
- Describe factors that increase nausea.

General Interventions

NIC Medication Management, Nausea Management, Fluid/Electrolyte Management, Nutrition Management

Explain the Cause of the Nausea and the Duration, if Known.

Teach how to Use Antiemetic Medications Before and After Chemotherapy.

Promote Comfort during Nausea and Vomiting.

Protect people at risk for aspiration (immobile clients, children).
Address the cleanliness of the person and environment.
Provide an opportunity for oral care after each episode.
Apply a cool, damp cloth to the person's forehead, neck, and wrists.

Reduce or Eliminate Noxious Stimuli.

Pain
Plan care to avoid unpleasant or painful procedures before meals.
Medicate clients for pain 30 min before meals according to physician's orders.
Provide a pleasant, relaxed atmosphere for eating (no bedpans in sight; do not rush); try a "surprise" (eg, flowers with meal).
Arrange the plan of care to decrease or eliminate nauseating odors or procedures near mealtimes.

Fatigue
Teach or assist client to rest before meals.
Teach client to spend minimal energy preparing food (cook large quantities and freeze several meals at a time; request assistance from others).

Odor of food
Teach client to avoid cooking odors—frying food, brewing coffee—if possible (take a walk; select foods that can be eaten cold).

Suggest using foods that require little cooking during periods of nausea.
Suggest trying sour foods.

Decrease Stimulation of the Vomiting Center.

Reduce unpleasant sights and odors. Restrict activity.
Provide good mouth care after vomiting.
Teach client to practice deep breathing and voluntary swallowing to suppress the vomiting reflex.
Instruct the person to sit down after eating, but not to lie down.
Encourage the person to eat smaller meals and to eat slowly.
Restrict liquids with meals to avoid overdistending the stomach; also, avoid fluids 1 h before and after meals.
Loosen clothing.
Encourage client to sit in fresh air or use a fan to circulate air.
Advise client to avoid lying flat for at least 2 h after eating (a person who must rest should sit or recline so the head is at least 4 inches higher than the feet).
Advise client to listen to music.

Rationales

- Vomiting is a first-line defense against injurious agents ingested. Nausea may precede it. Both may signal disease, injury, or normal physiologic adjustment to pregnancy.
- Unpleasant sights or odors can stimulate the vomiting center.
- Music can serve as a diversional adjunct to antiemetic therapy (Ezzone et al., 1998).
- Aggressive management before, during, and after chemotherapy can prevent nausea (Eckert, 2002).

Maternal Interventions

Teach that Various Interventions Have Been Reported to Help Control Nausea during Pregnancy.

Avoid fatigue; greasy, high-fat foods; and strong odors.
Eat high-protein meals and a snack before retiring.
Eat carbohydrates (crackers) on arising; eat immediately when hungry.
Consume carbonated beverages, Coke syrup, orange juice, ginger ale, and herbal teas.
Lie down to relieve symptoms.

Instruct the Pregnant Woman to Try One Food or Beverage Type at a Time (eg, High-protein Meals/Bedtime Snack); if Nausea is not Relieved, Try Another Measure.

Rationales

- From 50% to 80% of all pregnant women experience "morning sickness" (Davis, 1996). Fatigue has been reported to precipitate such nausea/vomiting (Voda & Randall, 1982).
- Voda and Randall (1982) reported that eating a high-protein snack before going to bed at night decreases morning nausea in some pregnant women.

Impaired Communication
    Related to Effects of Hearing Loss
    Related to Effects of Aphasia on Expression or Interpretation
    Related to Foreign Language Barrier
Impaired Verbal Communication

IMPAIRED COMMUNICATION*

DEFINITION

Impaired Communication: The state in which a person experiences, or is at risk to experience, difficulty exchanging thoughts, ideas, wants, or needs with others

DEFINING CHARACTERISTICS
Major (Must Be Present)

Inappropriate or absent speech or response
Impaired ability to speak or hear

Minor (May Be Present)

Incongruence between verbal and nonverbal messages
Stuttering
Slurring
Word-finding problems
Weak or absent voice
Statements of being misunderstood or not understanding
Dysarthria
Aphasia
Language barrier

RELATED FACTORS
Pathophysiologic

Related to disordered, unrealistic thinking secondary to:

Schizophrenic disorder   Psychotic disorder
Delusional disorder   Paranoid disorder

Related to impaired motor function of muscles of speech:
or

to ischemia of temporal frontal lobe secondary to:
Cerebrovascular accident
Oral or facial trauma
Brain damage (eg, birth/head trauma)
Central nervous system (CNS) depression/increased intracranial pressure
Tumor (of the head, neck, or spinal cord)
Chronic hypoxia/decreased cerebral blood flow
Nervous system diseases (eg, myasthenia gravis, multiple sclerosis, muscular dystrophy, Alzheimer's
    disease)
Vocal cord paralysis/quadriplegia

*Note: This diagnosis was developed by Rosalinda Alfaro-LeFevre and is not currently on the NANDA list, but is included here for clarity and usefulness.

Related to impaired ability to produce speech secondary to:
Respiratory impairment (eg, shortness of breath)
Laryngeal edema/infection
Oral deformities
    Cleft lip or palate   Missing teeth
    Malocclusion or fractured jaw   Dysarthria

Related to auditory impairment

Treatment-Related

Related to impaired ability to produce speech secondary to:
Endotracheal intubation   Tracheostomy/tracheotomy/
Surgery of the head, face,   laryngectomy
  neck, or mouth   Pain (especially of the mouth
CNS depressants, anesthesia   or throat)

Situational (Personal, Environmental)

Related to decreased attention secondary to fatigue, anger, anxiety, or pain
Related to no access to or malfunction of hearing aid
Related to psychological barrier (eg, fear, shyness)
Related to lack of privacy
Related to unavailable interpreter

Maturational

Infant/Child
Related to inadequate sensory stimulation

Older Adult (Auditory Losses)
Related to hearing impairment
Related to cognitive impairments secondary to (specify):

⊚ AUTHOR'S NOTE

Impaired Communication may not be useful to describe communication problems that are a manifestation of psychiatric illness or coping problems. If nursing interventions focus on reducing hallucinations, fear, or anxiety, *Disturbed Thought Processes, Fear,* or *Anxiety* would be more appropriate.

⊚ ERRORS IN DIAGNOSTIC STATEMENTS

Impaired Communication related to failure of staff to use effective communication techniques
    The diagnostic statement should not be used as a vehicle to reveal a problem resulting from incorrect or insufficient nursing intervention. Instead, the diagnosis should be *Impaired Verbal Communication related to effects of tracheotomy on ability to talk.* The care plan should specify the communication techniques to use.

KEY CONCEPTS
Generic Considerations

- Effective communication is an interactive process involving the *mutual exchange* of information (thoughts, ideas, feelings, and perceptions) between two or more people. Problems with *sending* or *receiving* messages (or both) can hamper this process.
- Messages are sent more by body language and tone of voice than by words.
- After survival, perhaps the most basic human need is to communicate with others. Communication provides security by reinforcing that clients are not alone and that others will listen. Poor communication can cause frustration, anger, hostility, depression, fear, confusion, and isolation.
- Speech represents the fundamental way for humans to express needs, desires, and feelings. If only one person expresses information without any feedback from a listener, effective communication cannot be said to have happened.

- Any of the following can cause problems with *sending* information:
  - Inability or failure to send messages that the listener can clearly understand (eg, language or word-meaning problems, failure to speak when listener is ready)
  - Fear of being overheard, judged, or misunderstood (eg, lack of privacy, confidentiality, trust, or nonjudgmental attitude)
  - Concern over response (eg, "I don't want to hurt or anger anyone.")
  - Use of words that "talk down" to the receiver (eg, talking to an elderly or handicapped person as if he or she were a child)
  - Failure to allow sufficient time for listening or providing feedback
  - Physical problems that interfere with the ability to see, talk, or move
- Any of the following can cause problems with *receiving* information:
  - Language or vocabulary problems
  - Fatigue, pain, fear, anxiety, distractions, attention span problems
  - Not realizing the importance of the information
  - Problems that interfere with the ability to see or hear
- Good communicators are also good listeners, who listen for both facts and feelings.
- "Presencing," or just being present and available, even if one says or does little, can effectively communicate caring to another (Benner, 1984).
- Therapeutic communication begins with:
  - Offering *unconditional positive regard,* or genuine warmth for the person being helped
  - Caring about the other person and being free of judgment of what he or she thinks or feels
- Ongoing therapeutic communication requires:
  - A capacity for empathic understanding of the client's *internal frame of reference*
  - This means working to understand how the person really feels and remaining unbiased
  - The ability to be genuine, human, and *authentic*
- Knowledge of a foreign language depends on four elements: how to speak, understand, read, and write the language.
- Dysarthria is a disturbance in the voluntary muscular control of speech. It is caused by conditions such as Parkinson's disease, multiple sclerosis, myasthenia gravis, cerebral palsy, and CNS damage. The same muscles are used in eating and swallowing. People with dysarthria usually do not have problems with comprehension.
- *Expressive aphasia* is a disturbance in the ability to speak, write, or gesture understandably.
- *Receptive aphasia* is a disturbance in the ability to comprehend written and spoken language. Those with receptive aphasia may have intact hearing, but cannot process or are unaware of their own sounds.
- Emotional lability (swings between crying and laughing) is common in people with aphasia. This behavior is not intentional and declines with recovery.
- Ten percent of deaf people have the skill and language level to read lips. Only 40% of the English language is visible.
- Successful interaction with deaf or hearing-impaired clients requires knowing background issues, including age of onset, choice of language, cultural background, education level, and type of hearing loss.
- Understanding of and respect for differences in personality and thinking styles are essential for communicating in ways that enhance interpersonal relations.

Pediatric Considerations

- Communication with children must be based on developmental stage, language abilities, and cognitive level.
- Although most verbal communication occurs between the nurse and parents, the adults should not ignore the child's input. Nurses should assess writing, drawing, play, and body language (facial expressions, gestures).
- Play therapy can be invaluable to establishing rapport and communicating true feelings.
- In children, receptive language is always more advanced than expressive language; children understand more than they can articulate. (See Table II.12 in the diagnostic category *Growth and Development, Delayed,* under Language/Cognition.)

(continued)

Pediatric Considerations (continued)

- The child with hearing loss may exhibit alterations in the following responses:
  - Orientation (eg, lack of startle reflex to a loud sound)
  - Vocalizations and sound production (eg, lack of babbling by 7 months of age)
  - Visual attention (eg, responding more to facial expression than verbal explanation)
  - Social/emotional behavior (eg, becomes irritable at inability to make self understood)
- For deaf infants, visual and tactile modalities are particularly important for communicating, interacting, and gaining information about the environment (Koester et al., 1998).

Geriatric Considerations

- Hearing loss is the third most prevalent condition affecting institutionalized older adults, exceeded only by arthritis and hypertension (Lindblade & McDonald, 1995). Only 18% of older adults with hearing loss own hearing aids. Many deny hearing loss because of fear of pressure to buy a hearing aid.
- Table II.2 illustrates age-related changes affecting hearing (Miller, 2004).
- About 40% of people older than 65 years have a significant hearing impairment that interferes with communication.
- Reduced auditory acuity correlates positively with social isolation. Understanding speech in group conversation has been identified as a prime area of difficulty for older adults. Some withdraw from social gatherings because they feel frustrated asking people to repeat things. Friends and family may refrain from entertaining hearing-impaired people because they misperceive their turning their heads away during conversation or failure to participate as disinterest. They may also misperceive hearing impairments as mental impairments because of inappropriate comments during conversation, irritability, and inattention.
- Older adults have a high prevalence of chronic conditions that can interfere with speech or understanding of speech.

TABLE II.2 Age-Related Changes Affecting Hearing

Change	Consequence
External Canal	
• Longer, thicker hair • Thinner, drier skin • Increased keratin	Potential for impacted cerumen with impaired sound conduction
Middle Ear	
• Diminished resiliency of tympanic membrane • Calcified, hardened ossicles • Weakened and stiff muscles and ligaments	Impaired sound conduction
Inner Ear and Nervous System	**Presbycusis**
• Diminished neurons, endolymph, hair cells, and blood supply • Degeneration of spiral ganglion and arterial blood vessels • Decreased flexibility of basilar membrane • Narrowing of auditory meatus • Degeneration of central processing systems	Diminished ability to hear high-pitched sounds, especially in the presence of background noise

Miller, C. A. (2004). *Nursing care of older adults* (4th ed.). Philadelphia: Lippincott Williams & Wilkins.

🌐 Transcultural Considerations

- The dominant US culture tends to conceal feelings and is considered low touch (Giger & Davidhizar, 2003). Difficulties can occur if the person or family does not communicate in a way that the nurse expects.
- In some cultures, a nod is a polite response meaning "I heard you, but I do not necessarily understand or agree" (Giger & Davidhizar, 2003).
- Touch is a strong form of communication with many meanings and interpretations.
  - Cultural uses of touch vary, with touch between same-sex people as taboo in some cultures but expected in others (Giger & Davidhizar, 2003).
  - English and German cultures do not encourage touching.
  - Some highly tactile cultures are Spanish, Italian, French, Jewish, and South American.
  - All cultures have rules about who touches whom, when, and where.
- The dominant US culture views eye contact as an indication of a positive self-concept, openness, and honesty. It views lack of eye contact as low self-esteem, guilt, or lack of interest. Some cultures are not accustomed to eye contact, including Filipino, Native American, and Vietnamese (Giger & Davidhizar, 2003).
- The client and family should be encouraged to communicate their interpretations of health, illness, and health care (Giger & Davidhizar, 2003) within the context of their specific culture.
- African Americans speak English with varied geographic dialects. Some African Americans pronounce certain syllables or consonants differently (eg, they may pronounce *th* as *d*, as in "*des*" for "these"). These different pronunciations should not be viewed as substandard or ungrammatical. In addition, some slang words may have different meanings—for example, "the birth of my daughter was a real bad experience." The person may mean it was unique and positive (Giger & Davidhizar, 2003).
- Mexican Americans speak Spanish, which has more than 50 dialects; thus, a nurse who speaks Spanish may have difficulty understanding a different dialect. Both men and women are very modest and restrict self-disclosure to those whom they know well. They consider direct confrontation and arguments rude; thus, agreeing may be a courtesy, not a commitment. A folk illness called *malojo* (evil eye) is thought to harm a child when the child is admired, but not touched, by a person thought to have special powers. When interacting with children, touch them lightly to avoid *malojo*. These clients may view kidding as rude and deprecating.
- Chinese Americans value silence and avoid disagreeing or criticizing. Whereas many Americans of other cultural backgrounds naturally raise the voice to make a point, Chinese Americans associate raising the voice with anger and loss of control. They rarely use "no," and "yes" can mean "perhaps" or "no." Touching the head is a serious breach of etiquette. Hesitation, ambiguity, and subtlety dominate Chinese speech (Giger & Davidhizar, 2003).

Focus Assessment Criteria

Subjective Data

Assess for Defining Characteristics.

Note the usual pattern of communication as described by the person or family.

Very verbal	Responds inappropriately
Sometimes verbal	Does not speak/respond
Uses sign language	Speaks only when spoken to
Writes only	Gestures only

Does the person feel he or she is communicating normally today?

If not, what does the client feel may help him or her to communicate better?

Would the client like to talk with or have present a specific person to help express ideas?

Does the client have trouble hearing?

Hearing problem	Use of a hearing aid
Both ears or one	Family history of hearing loss
How long? gradual? sudden?	History of exposure to loud noises

Ask person/caregiver to:

Rate ability to communicate on a scale of 0 to 10, with 0 signifying "completely unable to communicate" and 10 signifying "communicates well."

Describe factors that aid communication.

Assess for Related Factors.

Does the person feel that barriers hinder his or her ability to communicate?

Lack of privacy

Fear of uncertain origin

Fear of being inappropriate or "stupid"

Not enough time to gather thoughts and ask questions

Need for significant other or familiar face

Language, dialect, or cultural barrier (specify)

Lack of knowledge of subject being discussed

Pain, stress, or fatigue

Objective Data

Assess for Defining Characteristics.

Describe Ability to Form Words.

Not able	Fair	Good

Speech Pattern

Slurred speech	Voice weakness (whisper)
Lisping	Language barrier
Stuttering	

Ability to Comprehend

Follows simple commands or ideas

Can follow complex instructions or ideas

Sometimes can follow instructions or ideas

Can follow simple instructions or ideas

Follows commands and ideas only if hearing aid is working

Follows commands and ideas only if he or she can see speaker's mouth (lip-reads)

What is the Developmental Age?

Describe Ability to Form Sentences.

Good	Nonsensical or confused
Slow	Can make short,
Not able	simple sentences
Unclear ideas	Language barrier

Is Eye Contact Maintained?

Yes	Rarely
No	Blind/impaired vision
Occasionally	

Hearing Loss (Check Each Ear Separately)

External ear

Deformities	Lesions
Lumps or tenderness	

Middle and inner ear

Cerumen	Discharge
Redness	Swelling

Auditory acuity

Can hear ticking watch or whispered words

With decreased hearing

Weber and Rinne test results

Hearing aid?

Left ear	Right ear

Assess for Related Factors.

Barriers
Tracheostomy
Endotracheal tube

Affect or Manner

Nervous	Flat	Anxious
Angry	Attentive	Uncomfortable
Fearful	Comfortable	Withdrawn

Contributing Factors
Do contributing factors inhibit ability to communicate (see Related Factors)?
For more information on Focus Assessment Criteria, visit http://connection.lww.com.

Goal

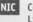 **NOC** Communication Ability

The person will report improved satisfaction with ability to communicate.

Indicators

- Demonstrate increased ability to understand.
- Demonstrate improved ability to express self.
- Use alternative methods of communication, as indicated.

General Interventions

NIC Communication Enhancement, Active Listening, Socialization Enhancement

Identify a Method to Communicate Basic Needs.

Assess Ability to Comprehend, Speak, Read, and Write.
Provide Alternative Methods of Communication.
Use computer, pad and pencil, hand signals, eye blinks, head nods, and bell signals.
Make flash cards with pictures or words depicting frequently used phrases (eg, "Wet my lips," "Move my foot," "I need a glass of water" or "I need a bedpan").
Encourage person to point, use gestures, and pantomime.

Identify Factors that Promote Communication.

Create Atmosphere of Acceptance and Privacy.
Provide a Nonrushed Environment.
Use normal loudness level and speak slowly in short phrases.
Encourage client to take time talking and to enunciate words carefully with good lip movement.
Decrease external distractions.
Delay conversation when the person is tired.

Assess Client's Frustration Level; Do not Push Beyond It.
Estimate 30 s of passed time before providing client with the word he or she may be trying to find (except when person is frustrated or needs the request immediately [eg, bedpan]).
Provide cues through pictures or gestures.

Use Techniques to Increase Understanding.
Face client and establish eye contact if possible.
Use uncomplicated one-step commands and directives.
Have only one person talk (following a conversation with multiple parties can be difficult).
Encourage the use of gestures and pantomime.
Match words with actions; use pictures.
Terminate conversation on a note of success (eg, move back to an easier item).
Validate that client understands message.
Give information in writing to reinforce.

Initiate Health Teaching and Referrals, if Needed.

Seek consultation with a speech or audiology specialist.

Rationales

- Using alternative forms of communication can help decrease anxiety, isolation, and alienation; promote a sense of control; and enhance safety (Iezzoni et al., 2004).
- Communication is the core of all human relations. Impaired ability to communicate spontaneously is frustrating and embarrassing. Nursing actions should focus on decreasing tension and conveying understanding of how difficult the situation must be for the client (Underwood, 2004).
- The nurse should make every attempt to understand the client. Each success, regardless of how minor, decreases frustration and increases motivation.

 ## Pediatric Interventions

Use age-appropriate words and gestures (see *Delayed Growth and Development,* Table II.12).
Initially talk to parent and allow child to observe. Gradually include child.
1. Approach the child slowly and speak in a quiet, unhurried, confident voice.
2. Assume an eye-level position.
3. Use simple words and short sentences.
4. Talk about something not related to present situation (eg, school, toy, hair, clothes).
Offer choices as much as possible.
Encourage child to share concerns and fears.
Allow child an opportunity to touch and use articles (eg, stethoscope, tongue blade).
Do not use analogies with small children (eg, "The injection will feel like a stick in your arm.").
For deaf infants, enhance messages by using increased visual and tactile cues.

Rationales

- Listening carefully will allow you to pick up cues about issues for the child or adolescent.
- The initial interaction sets the tone for future interactions with the child and family.
- Use of open-ended, nonjudgmental style can reduce suspicions.
- Criticizing or lecturing does not promote an understanding of risk behaviors.
- Successful communication depends on the nurse's ability to involve the adolescent in discussions.
- Adolescents need opportunities to demonstrate their independence and to appraise options accurately (Wong, 2003).
- For deaf infants, visual and tactile modalities are particularly important for communicating, interacting, and gaining information about their environment (Koester, Karkowski & Traci, 1998).

IMPAIRED COMMUNICATION

 ## RELATED TO EFFECTS OF HEARING LOSS

Goal

NOC Communication Ability,
Communication: Receptance Ability

The person will relate/demonstrate an improved ability to communicate.

Indicators
- Wear functioning hearing aid if appropriate.
- Communicate through alternative methods.

Interventions

> **NIC** Active Listening, Communication Enhancement: Hearing Deficit

Ask the Person What Mode of Communication He or She Desires.

Record on Care Plan the Method to Use (May be Combination of the Following):

Writing
Speaking
Gesturing
Speech-reading
(or lip-reading)
Sign language

Assess Ability to Receive Verbal Messages.

If Client Can Hear With a Hearing Aid, Make Sure that it is on and Functioning.

Check batteries by turning volume all the way up until it whistles. (If it does not whistle, insert new batteries.)

Make sure volume is at a level that enhances hearing. (Many people with hearing aids turn the volume down occasionally for peace and quiet.)

Make a special effort to ensure client wears the hearing aid during off-the-unit visits (eg, special studies, the operating room [OR]).

If Client Can Hear With Only One Ear, Speak Slowly and Clearly Directly into the Good Ear. It is More Important to Speak Distinctly than Loudly.

Place bed in a position so the person's good ear faces the door.

Stand or sit on the side on which client hears best (eg, if left ear is better, sit on the left).

If the Person Can Speech-Read:

Look directly at the person and talk slowly and clearly.

Avoid standing in front of light—have the light on your face so the person can see your lips.

Minimize distractions that may inhibit the person's concentration.

Minimize conversations if the person is fatigued or use written communication.

Reinforce important communications by writing them down.

If Client Can Read and Write, Provide Pad and Pencil at All Times.

If Client Can Understand Only Sign Language, Have an Interpreter With Him or Her as Much as Possible.

Address all communication to the person, not to the interpreter (eg, do not say, "ask Mrs. Jones . . .").

Record name and phone number of interpreter(s) on the care plan.

If in a group setting (eg, diabetes class), place client at front of the room near the instructor or send interpreter with him or her.

Carefully evaluate the person's understanding of required knowledge.

Give information in writing.

Use Factors that Promote Hearing and Understanding.

Talk distinctly and clearly, facing the person.

Minimize unnecessary sounds in the room:

Have only one person talk.

Be aware of background noises (eg, close the door, turn off the television or radio).

Repeat, then rephrase a thought, if the person does not seem to understand the whole meaning.

Use gestures to enhance communication.

Encourage the person to maintain contact with other deaf people to minimize feelings of social isolation.

Write as well as speak all important messages.

Validate the person's understanding by asking questions that require more than "yes" or "no" answers. Avoid asking, "Do you understand?"

Initiate Referrals as Needed.

Seek consultation with a speech or audiology specialist.

Rationales

- Under the Rehabilitation Act of 1973 and the Americans with Disabilities Act (ADA) of 1990, hospitals must offer reasonable accommodations for hearing-impaired clients. For example, they must provide qualified interpreters and auxiliary tools such as teletype machines, unless doing so imposes an undue financial or other burden.*

---

*Accessed from: *http://www.mweb.com/legal/legal1a.html#2*

- When using an interpreter, some things may be omitted or misunderstood. Whenever possible, give information in writing as well as through the interpreter.
- Hearing aids magnify *all* sounds. Therefore, extraneous sounds (eg, rustling of papers, minor squeaks) can inhibit understanding of voiced messages.
- Deafness can disrupt the reciprocal relationship necessary in the health care process.
- Speech-reading is difficult and fatiguing in the hospital. Unfamiliar terminology, anxiety, and poor lighting all can contribute to errors.
- Writing messages is slow, causing a tendency to abbreviate content. Moreover, expressing emotions in writing is difficult.
- The following are available to assist clients with hearing impairment:
  - DEAFNET, a computer system that allows clients to type messages to a computer at the phone company, which a voice synthesizer translates verbally
  - Telecommunication devices for the deaf (know as TDD) that operate by communicating electronically messages that are typed, infrared systems, computers, voice amplifiers, amplified telephones, low-frequency doorbells and telephone ringers, closed-caption TV decoders, flashing alarm clocks, flashing smoke detectors, hearing aids, and lip reading and signing instruction
  - Deaf service centers available in most communities to help with housing, job seeking, travel arrangements, recreation, and adult education opportunities
- Many older adults with hearing impairments don't wear hearing aids. Those who wear them must be encouraged to use them consistently, clean and maintain them, and replace batteries. They should be assertive in letting significant others know about situations and environmental areas in which they experience difficulty because of background noise.

IMPAIRED COMMUNICATION

⊗ RELATED TO EFFECTS OF APHASIA ON EXPRESSION OR INTERPRETATION

Aphasia is a communication impairment—a difficulty in expressing, a difficulty in understanding, or a combination of both—resulting from cerebral impairments.

Goal

NOC Communication: Expressive Ability

The person will report decreased frustration with communication.

Indicators

- Demonstrate increased ability to understand.
- Demonstrate improved ability to express ideas, thoughts, needs.

Interventions

NIC Communication Enhancement: Speech Deficit, Active Listening, Anxiety Reduction

Use Techniques that Enhance Verbal Expression.

Make a Concerted Effort to Understand the Person.

Allow enough time to listen.

Rephrase messages aloud to validate what was said.

Acknowledge when you understand, and do not be concerned with imperfect pronunciation at first.
Ignore mistakes and profanity.
Do not pretend you understand if you do not.
Observe nonverbal cues for validation (eg, answers yes and shakes head no).
Allow person time to respond; do not interrupt; supply words only occasionally.

Teach Techniques to Improve Speech.
Ask to slow speech down and say each word clearly, while providing the example.
Encourage client to speak in short phrases.
Explain that client's words are not clearly understood (eg, "I can't understand what you're saying.").
Suggest a slower rate of talking, or taking a breath before beginning to speak.
Ask client to write down message, or to draw a picture, if verbal communication is difficult.
Focus on the present; avoid controversial, emotional, abstract, or lengthy topics.

Explain the Benefits of Daily Speech Practice. Consult with Speech Therapist for Specific Exercises.

Acknowledge Client's Frustration and Improvements.

Verbally address frustration over inability to communicate, and explain that both nurse and client need to use patience.
Maintain a calm, positive attitude (eg, "I can understand you if we work at it.").
Use reassurance (eg, "I know it's difficult, but you'll get it."); use touch if acceptable.
Maintain a sense of humor.
Allow tears (eg, "It's OK. I know it's frustrating. Crying can let it all out.").
Give the person opportunities to make care-related decisions (eg, "Would you rather have orange juice or prune juice?").
Provide alternative methods of self-expression
    Humming/singing
    Dancing/exercising/walking
    Writing/drawing/painting/coloring
    Helping (tasks such as opening mail, choosing meals)

Identify Factors that Promote Comprehension.

Assess Hearing Ability and Use of Functioning Hearing Aids.
Assess Ability to See, and Encourage the Person to Wear Glasses if Indicated.
Explain that seeing better will increase understanding of what is happening in the environment.
Even if the person is blind, look at him or her when talking to "throw" voice in that direction.

Provide Sufficient Light and Remove Distractions (see *Disturbed Sensory Perception*).
Speak When the Person is Ready to Listen.
Achieve eye contact, if possible.
Gain the person's attention by a gentle touch on the arm and a verbal message of "Listen to me" or "I want to talk to you."

Modify your Speech.
Speak slowly; enunciate distinctly.
Use common adult words.
Do not change subjects or ask multiple questions in succession.
Repeat or rephrase requests.
Do not increase volume of voice unless person has a hearing deficit.
Match your nonverbal behavior with your verbal actions to avoid misinterpretation (eg, do not laugh with a coworker while performing a task).
Try to use the same words with the same task (eg, bathroom vs toilet, pill vs medication).
Keep a record at bedside of the words to maintain continuity.
As the person improves, allow him or her to complete your sentences (eg, "This is a . . . [pill]").

Use Multiple Methods of Communication.
Use pantomime.
Point.
Use flash cards.
Show what you mean (eg, pick up a glass).
Write key words on a card, so client can practice them while you show the object (eg, paper).

Show Respect when Providing Care.

Avoid discussing the person's condition in his or her presence; assume client can understand despite deficits.

Monitor other health care providers for adherence to plan of care.

Talk to the person whenever you are with him or her.

Initiate Health Teaching and Referrals, if Indicated.

Teach communication techniques and repetitive approaches to significant others.

Encourage family to share feelings concerning communication problems.

Explain the reasons for labile emotions and profanity.

Explain the need to include the person in family decision making.

Seek consultation with a speech pathologist early in treatment regimen.

Rationales

- See Rationales for *Impaired Communication.*
- Deliberate actions can improve speech. As speech improves, confidence increases and the client will make more attempts at speaking.
- Improving the client's comprehension can help decrease frustration and increase trust. Clients with aphasia can correctly interpret tone of voice.
- Daily exercises help improve the efficiency of speech musculature and increase rate, volume, and articulation.

IMPAIRED COMMUNICATION

RELATED TO FOREIGN LANGUAGE BARRIER

Goal

NOC Communication Ability

The person will communicate needs and concerns (through interpreter if needed).

Indicators

- Demonstrate ability to understand information.
- Relate feelings of reduced frustration and isolation.

Interventions

NIC Culture Brokerage, Active Listening, Communication Enhancement

Assess Ability to Communicate in English.*

Assess language the client speaks best.

Assess client's ability to read, write, speak, and comprehend English.

Do not evaluate understanding based on "yes" or "no" responses.

---

*English is used as an example of the dominant language.

Identify Factors that Promote Communication Without a Translator.

Face the person and give a pleasant greeting, in a normal tone of voice.

Talk clearly and somewhat slower than normal (do not overdo it).

If the person does not understand or speak (respond), use an alternative communication method.

Write message.

Use gestures or actions.

Use pictures or drawings.

Make flash cards that translate words or phrases.

Encourage client to teach others some words or greetings of his or her own language (helps to promote acceptance and willingness to learn).

Do not correct a client's or family's pronunciation.

Clarify the exact meaning of an unclear word.

Use medical terms and the slang word when indicated (eg, vomiting/throwing up).

Be Cognizant of Possible Cultural Barriers.

Be careful when touching the person; some cultures may consider touch inappropriate.

Be aware of different ways the culture expects men and women to be treated (cultural attitudes may influence whether a man speaks to a woman about certain matters, or vice versa).

Make a conscious effort to be nonjudgmental about cultural differences.

Make note of what seems to be a comfortable distance from which to speak.

Initiate Referrals, When Needed.

Use a *fluent* translator when discussing important matters (eg, taking a health history, signing an operation permit). Reinforce communications through the translator with written information.

If possible, allow the translator to spend as much time as the person wishes (be flexible with visitors' rules and regulations).

If a translator is unavailable, plan a daily visit from someone who has some knowledge of the person's language (many hospitals and social welfare offices keep a "language" bank with names and phone numbers of people who are willing to translate).

Use AT&T telephone translating system when necessary.

Rationales

- An answer of "yes" may be an effort to please, rather than a sign of understanding.
- Although the nurse cannot speak another's language, he or she can convey acceptance by talking in a pleasant tone of voice and using actions to demonstrate meaning (eg, smiling and motioning to sit down, while saying, "Sit down, please.").
- Usually language comprehension is far greater than the ability to speak or write language.
- An attempt on the nurse's part to communicate over a language barrier encourages the client to do the same.
- People should overcome the human tendency either to ignore or to shout at people who do not speak the dominant language.
- Be aware that, when one learns a language, one usually learns only one meaning for a word. Some words have more than one meaning, such as "discharge" and "pupil."
- During the initial assessment, start with general questions. Allow time for the person to talk even if it is not related. Use nondirect, open-ended questions when possible. Delay asking very personal questions, if possible.
- Nurses must have transcultural sensitivity, understand how to impart knowledge, and know how to advocate to represent the client's needs. Interpreting with cultural sensitivity is much more complex than simply putting words in another language (Giger & Davidhizar, 2003).
- Appropriate distance between communicators varies across cultures. Some normally stand face to face, whereas others stand several feet apart to be comfortable.
- Communicating through touch or holding varies among cultures. Some cultures view touch as an extremely familiar gesture, some shy away from touching a given part of the body (a pat on the head may be offensive), and some consider it appropriate for men to kiss one another and for women to hold hands.

IMPAIRED VERBAL COMMUNICATION

DEFINITION

Impaired Verbal Communication: The state in which a person experiences, or is at high risk to experience, a decreased ability to speak but can understand others

DEFINING CHARACTERISTICS
Major (One Must Be Present)

Inability to speak words but can understand others
Articulation or motor planning deficits

Minor (May Be Present)

Shortness of breath

RELATED FACTORS

See *Impaired Communication*.

KEY CONCEPTS

See *Impaired Communication*.

Focus Assessment Criteria

See *Impaired Communication*.

Goal

 NOC Communication : Expressive Ability

The person will demonstrate improved ability to express self.

Indicators

- Relate decreased frustration with communication.
- Use alternative methods as indicated.

General Interventions

NIC Active Listening, Communication
Enhancement: Speech Deficit

Identify a Method for Communicating Basic Needs.

See *Impaired Communication*.

Identify Factors that Promote Communication.

For Clients with Dysarthria:

Reduce environmental noise (eg, radio, TV) to increase caregiver's ability to listen to words.

Do not alter your speech or messages, because the client's comprehension is not affected; speak on an adult level.

Encourage client to make a conscious effort to slow down speech and to speak louder (eg, "Take a deep breath between sentences.").

Ask client to repeat unclear words; observe for nonverbal cues to help understanding.

If client is tired, ask questions that require only short answers.

If speech is unintelligible, teach use of gestures, written messages, and communication cards.

For Those Who Cannot Speak (eg, Endotracheal Intubation, Tracheostomy):

Reassure that speech will return, if it will. If not, explain available alternatives (eg, esophageal speech, sign language).

Do not alter your speech, tone, or type of message, because the person's ability to understand is not affected; speak on an adult level.

Read lips for cues.

Promote Continuity of Care to Reduce Frustration.

Observe for Signs of Frustration or Withdrawal.

Verbally address frustration over inability to communicate, and explain that both nurse and client must use patience.

Maintain a calm, positive attitude (eg, "I can understand you if we work at it.").

Use reassurance (eg, "I know it's difficult, but you'll get it").

Maintain a sense of humor.

Allow tears (eg, "It's OK. I know it's frustrating. Crying can let it all out.").

For the client with limited speaking ability (eg, can make simple requests, but not lengthy statements), encourage letter writing or keeping a diary to express feelings and share concerns.

Anticipate needs and ask questions that need a simple yes or no answer.

Maintain a Specific Care Plan.

Write the method of communication that is used (eg, "Uses word cards," "Points for bedpan").

Record directions for specific measures to reduce communication problems (eg, allow him to keep urinal in bed).

Initiate Health Teaching and Referrals, as Indicated.

Teach communication techniques and repetitive approaches to significant others.

Encourage family to share feelings concerning communication problems.

Seek consultation with a speech pathologist early in the treatment regimen.

Rationales

See *Impaired Communication*.

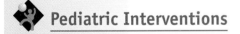 ## Pediatric Interventions

Establish a method of communication appropriate for age.

If a young child is deprived of vocalization, teach basic language gestures (time, food, family relationships, emotions, animals, numbers, frequent requests).

Consult with a speech pathologist for ongoing assistance.

Discuss with parents or caregivers the importance of providing the child with a method of communication.

Rationales

- Children who cannot vocalize are at risk for delays in receptive and expressive language development (ie, vocal speech, voice production.
- Communication promotes bonding and attachment with the child's caregiver as the primary social reinforcer.
- The ability to communicate with people in the environment increases the child's independence, self-esteem, and self-actualization.

CONFUSION*

DEFINITION

Confusion: The state in which a person experiences or is at risk of experiencing a disturbance in cognition, attention, memory, and orientation, of an undetermined origin or onset

DEFINING CHARACTERISTICS

Major (Must Be Present)

Disturbances of:

Consciousness

Attention

Perception

Sleep–wake cycle

Memory

Orientation

Thinking

Psychomotor behavior (reaction time, speed of movement, flow of speech, involuntary movements, handwriting)

Minor (May Be Present)

Misperceptions

Hypervigilance

Agitation

> **AUTHOR'S NOTE**
>
> This author has added *Confusion* to the diagnostic list to provide an option when the origin, onset, or duration of the confusion is unknown. With this option, the nurse can refrain from too quickly labeling confusion as acute or chronic. Careful assessment is indicated. Until data collection is complete, the diagnosis can be written as *Confusion related to unknown etiology as evidenced by* (specify supporting data).
>
> "The terms delirium and confusion are not interchangeable" (Anderson, 1999, p. 497). Confusion is a symptom of irreversible organic mental disorder; delirium is acute confusion of short duration and reversible when the underlying cause is treated (Anderson, 1999; Foreman et al., 1999). Refer to Key Concepts for descriptions of chronic confusion and acute confusion (delirium).

---

*This diagnosis is not currently on the NANDA list but has been included for clarity and usefulness.

ACUTE CONFUSION

DEFINITION

Acute Confusion: The state in which there is an abrupt onset of a cluster of global, fluctuating disturbances in consciousness, attention, perception, memory, orientation, thinking, sleep–wake cycle, and psychomotor behavior (American Psychiatric Association [APA], 2000)

DEFINING CHARACTERISTICS
Major (Some Must Be Present)

Abrupt onset of:

Reduced ability to focus	Confusion
Disorientation	Restlessness
Incoherence	Fear
Anxiety	Excitement
Hypervigilance	

Symptoms worse at nights or when fatigued

Minor (May Be Present)

Illusions	Hallucinations
Delusions	Misperception of stimuli

RISK FACTORS

Presence of risk factors (see Related Factors)

RELATED FACTORS

Related to abrupt onset of cerebral hypoxia or disturbance in cerebral metabolism secondary to (Miller, 2004):

Fluid and Electrolyte Disturbances

Dehydration	Hypokalemia
Volume depletion	Hyponatremia/hypernatremia
Acidosis/alkalosis	Hypoglycemia/hyperglycemia
Hypercalcemia	

Nutritional Deficiencies

Folate or vitamin B_{12} deficiency	Niacin deficiency
Anemia	Magnesium deficiency

Cardiovascular Disturbances

Myocardial infarction	Heart block
Congestive heart failure	Temporal arteritis
Dysrhythmias	

Respiratory Disorders

Chronic obstructive pulmonary disease	Tuberculosis
Pulmonary embolism	Pneumonia

Infections

Sepsis	Urinary tract infection
Meningitis, encephalitis	

Metabolic and Endocrine Disorders

Hypothyroidism/hyperthyroidism	Hypoadrenocorticism/hyperadrenocorticism

Hypopituitarism/
  hyperpituitarism
Parathyroid disorders

Postural hypotension
Hypothermia/hyperthermia
Hepatic or renal failure

Central Nervous System (CNS) Disorders
Multiple infarctions
Tumors
Normal-pressure hydrocephalus

Head trauma
Seizures and postconvulsive states

Treatment-Related

Related to a disturbance in cerebral metabolism secondary to:
Surgery
Therapeutic drug intoxication
    Neuroleptics   Narcotics
General anesthesia
Side effects of medication

Diuretics	Barbiturates	Sulfa drugs
Digitalis	Methyldopa	Ciprofloxin
Propranolol	Disulfiram	Metronidazole
Atropine	Lithium	Acyclovir
Oral hypoglycemics	Phenytoin	H2 receptor antagonists
Antiinflammatories	Over-the-counter cold, cough,	Anticholinergics
Antianxiety agents	and sleeping preparations	
Phenothiazines		

Situational (Personal, Environmental)

Related to disturbance in cerebral metabolism secondary to:
Withdrawal from alcohol, sedatives, hypnotics
Heavy metal or carbon monoxide intoxication

Related to:
Pain
Bowel impaction

Immobility
Depression

Related to chemical intoxications or medications (specify):
Alcohol
Cocaine
Amphetamines
Anticholinergics

Opiates
Barbiturates
Hallucinogens

○○ **AUTHOR'S NOTE**

The addition of *Acute Confusion* and *Chronic Confusion* to the NANDA list provides the nurse with more diagnostic clarity than *Disturbed Thought Processes. Acute Confusion* has an abrupt onset with fluctuating symptoms; *Chronic Confusion* describes long-standing or progressive degeneration. *Disturbed Thought Processes* is also a disruption of cognitive processes; however, the causes are coping problems or personality disorders.

○○ **ERRORS IN DIAGNOSTIC STATEMENT**

1. *Acute Confusion related to advanced age*
   This diagnosis does not represent an understanding of confusion, aging, and its effects on cognition. An aged person who is confused could have various reasons for confusion (eg, electrolytic imbalance, fever, cerebral infarctions, Alzheimer's disease). He or she needs a medical and nursing assessment. Before the causes are known, this diagnosis can be stated as *Chronic Confusion related to unknown etiology.*

KEY CONCEPTS
Generic Considerations

- "Confusion" is a term nurses use frequently to describe an array of cognitive impairments. "Identifying a person as confused is just an initial step" (Rasin, 1990; Roberts, 2001). Confusion is a biopsychological concept that indicates a disturbance in cerebral metabolism. Reduced cerebral metabolism decreases neurotransmitter levels in the brain, especially acetylcholine and epinephrine. Acetylcholine is necessary for attention, learning, memory, and information processing (Rasin, 1990; Roberts, 2001).
- *Acute confusion* or delirium results from transient biochemical disruptions caused by medications, infections, dehydration, electrolyte imbalances, and metabolic disturbances (Foreman et al., 1999). It usually lasts less than 5 days when the underlying causes are treated. Early detection and treatment can prevent unnecessarily long hospital stays (Foreman et al., 1999).
- Chronic confusion results from progressive degeneration of the cerebral cortex. Diseases that cause such degeneration vary but manifest similar behavioral disturbances. Alzheimer's disease causes about 60% of cases of chronic confusion, whereas multiple infarctions or strokes cause about 10% of the pathology labeled multiinfarct disease (MID). A combination of senile dementia of Alzheimer's type (SDAT) and MID cause another 17%. Rare and occasionally reversible conditions such as Pick's disease, Creutzfeldt-Jakob disease, and chronic chemical intoxication (eg, alcohol, lead, opioids, cocaine) cause the remaining 13% (Hall, 1991). People with chronic confusion can experience delirium, also.

⊙ Geriatric Considerations

- Moderate to severe cognitive impairment in older adults can result from dementia, delirium, or depression. Nurses must approach their assessment carefully and cautiously; they should not base diagnosis on a single symptom or physical finding.
- Thinking and arithmetic abilities, memory, judgment, and problem solving are measured in older adults to give a general index of overall cognitive ability. Short-term memory may decline somewhat, but long-term memory often remains intact (Miller, 2004).
- With age, intelligence does not alter (perhaps until the very later years), but the person needs more time to process information. Reaction time increases as well. There may be some difficulty in learning new information because of increased distractibility, decreased concrete thinking, and difficulty solving new problems. Older adults usually compensate for these deficiencies by taking more time to process the information, screening out distractions, and using extreme care in making decisions. Marked cognitive decline usually is attributed to disease processes such as atherosclerosis, loss of neurons, and other pathologic changes (Miller, 2004).
- Most older adults exhibit no cognitive impairment. Severe cognitive impairment, a consequence of disease process, occurs in only 1% of people older than 65 years and 20% of people older than 85 years (Katzman, 1988).
- Age-related changes can influence medication actions and produce negative consequences. See Table II.3.
- Dementia describes impairments of intellectual, not behavioral, functioning. It refers to a group of symptoms, not a disease (Miller, 2004). Alzheimer's disease, the fourth leading case of death in adults, is one type of dementia.
- Blazer (1986) reported depressive symptoms in 27% of community-living older adults. According to Parmelee, Katz, and Lawton (1989), 12% of older adults living in nursing homes met the criteria for major depression, whereas 30% were identified with minor depressive symptoms.
- Blazer (1986) describes a multiple causation theory for late-life depression, which emphasizes the complex interactions of several etiologic factors. Examples identified include poor economic resources, decreased social support, and decreased physical health functioning. These factors negatively affect self-esteem and motivation, which increases guilt and anger. The resulting negative emotions depress affect and increase ruminations. The person reduces social contact or is shunned, which starts the cycle again.
- Suicide is always a possibility, especially in the early stage of dementia, for numerous reasons: depression, loss of self-worth, and impaired judgment.

Focus Assessment Criteria

Acquire data from client and significant others.

Subjective Data
History of the Individual
Lifestyle

Interests	Strengths and limitations	Work history
Past and present coping	Education	Use of alcohol/drugs
Previous functioning	Previous handling of stress	

Support system (availability)
History of medical problems and treatments (medications)
Activities of daily living (ADLs; ability and desire to perform)

History of Symptoms (Onset and Duration)

Acute or chronic	Time of day	Sudden or gradual
Downward progression	Continuous or intermittent	

Assess for Feelings of

Extreme sadness	Worthlessness	Mistrust or suspicion
Guilt for past actions	Excessive self-importance	Apprehension
Being rejected or isolated	Depersonalization	Living in an unreal world
Others controlling client		

Assess for Fears.

Harm from others	Thoughts racing	External agents control mind
Being held prisoner	Being unable to cope	Falling apart

Assess for Hallucinations.

Visual	Tactile (includes objective	Gustatory
Olfactory	component)	
Auditory		

Assess for Behaviors Associated with Depression, Dementia, and Delirium (Dellasega, 1998).

Depression	*Dementia*	*Delirium*
Sudden or gradual onset	Gradual, insidious onset	Sudden, acute onset
Sleep difficulties	May sleep less; restlessness	Behavior worsens at night
Slowed motor behavior	Wandering behavior	Hypo/hyperarousal
Sadness, loss of interest and pleasure	Defensiveness	Hallucinations and illusions in attention
Memory intact	Gradual loss of ability to remember	Fluctuating performance

TABLE II.3 Age-Related Changes That May Influence Medications

Age-Related Change	Effect on Some Medications
Decreased body water, decreased lean tissue, increased body fat	Increased or decreased serum concentration
Decreased serum albumin	Increased amount of the active portion of protein-bound medications
Decreased renal and liver functioning	Increased serum concentration
Decreased gastric acid, increased gastric pH	Altered absorption of medications that are sensitive to stomach pH
Altered homeostatic mechanisms	Increased potential for adverse effects
Altered receptor sensitivity	Increased or decreased therapeutic effect

Miller, C. (2004). *Nursing care of older adults* (4th ed.). Philadelphia: Lippincott Williams & Wilkins.

Objective Data (Includes a Subjective Component)

General Appearance
Facial expression (alert, sad, hostile, expressionless)
Dress (meticulous, disheveled, seductive, eccentric)

Behavior During Interview

Withdrawn	Level of anxiety	Hostile
Cooperative	Apathetic	Quiet
Attention/concentration	Negativism	

Communication Pattern

Appropriate	Obsessions	Rambling
Sexual preoccupations	Suspicious	Homicidal plans
Denying problem	Suicidal ideas	Worthlessness
Delusions		

Speech Pattern

Appropriate	Loose connections	Blocking (can't finish idea)
Topic jumping	Circumstantial	Cannot reach a conclusion

Rate of Speech

Appropriate	Reduced	Excessive
Pressured		

Affect

Blunted	Congruent with content	Bright
Appropriate to content	Flat	Inappropriate to content
Sad		

Interaction Skills
With nurse

Inappropriate	Demanding/pleading	Relates well
Hostile	Withdrawn/preoccupied	

With significant others

Relates with all (some) family members	Hostile toward one (all) members	Does not seek interaction
		Does not have visitors

Activities of Daily Living
Capable of self-care (observed, reported)

Nutrition–hydration Status

Appetite	Weight	Eating patterns

Sleep–Rest Pattern

Sleeps too much or too little	Early wakefulness	Cycle reversed
Insomnia	Fragmented sleep	

Personal Hygiene

Cleanliness	Clothes	Grooming

Motor Activity

Within normal limits	Agitated	Decreased/stuporous

For more information on Focus Assessment Criteria, visit http://connection.lww.com.

Goal

NOC	Cognitive Orientation, Safety Behavior: Personal, Distorted Thought Control, Information Processing

The person will have diminished episodes of delirium.

Indicators

- Be less agitated.
- Participate in ADLs.
- Be less combative.

General Interventions

NIC Delirium Management, Cognitive Stimulation, Calming Technique, Reality Orientation, Environmental Management: Safety

Assess for Causative and Contributing Factors.

Ensure that a thorough diagnostic workup has been completed.

Laboratory

CBC and electrolytes

Vitamin B_{12} and folate, thiamine

Rapid plasma reagin (RPR)

NA and K

SGOT, SGPT, and bilirubin

Urinalysis

TSH, T_4

Serum thyroxine and serum-free thyroxine

Calcium and phosphate

Creatinine, BUN

Serum glucose and fasting blood sugar

Diagnostic

EEG

Chest x-ray

CT scan

ECG

Psychiatric Evaluation

Evaluate for depression. (See Focus Assessment Criteria in *Ineffective Coping*.)

Promote Client's Sense of Integrity.

Examine Attitudes About Confusion (In Self, Caregivers, Significant Others).

Educate family, significant others, and caregivers about the situation and coping methods.

Maintain Standards of Empathic, Respectful Care.

Be an advocate when other caregivers are insensitive to the client's needs.

Function as a role model with coworkers.

Provide other caregivers with up-to-date information on confusion.

Expect empathic, respectful care and monitor its administration.

Attempt to Obtain Information that Provides Useful and Meaningful Topics for Conversation (Likes, Dislikes; Interests, Hobbies; Work History). Interview Early in Day.

Encourage Significant Others and Caregivers to Speak Slowly with a Low Voice Pitch and at an Average Volume (Unless Hearing Deficits are Present), as One Adult to Another, with Eye Contact, and as if Expecting Person to Understand.

Provide Respect and Promote Sharing.

Pay attention to what person says.

Pick out meaningful comments and continue talking.

Call person by name and introduce yourself each time you make contact; use touch if welcomed.

Use name the person prefers; avoid "Pops" or "Mom," which can increase confusion and is unacceptable.

Convey to person that you are concerned and friendly (through smiles, an unhurried pace, humor, and praise; do not argue).

Focus on feeling behind the spoken word or action.

Reduce Abrupt Changes in Schedule or Relocation.

Provide Sufficient and Meaningful Sensory Input.

Keep Person Oriented to Time and Place.

Refer to time of day and place each morning.

Provide person with a clock and calendar large enough to see.

If dementia is severe, remove all visible mirrors.

Use nightlights or dim lights at night.

Use indirect lighting.

Turn lights on before it gets dark.

Provide person with opportunity to see daylight and dark through a window, or take person outdoors.

Single out holidays with cards or pins (eg, wear a red heart for Valentine's Day).

Use Adaptive Devices to Diminish Sensory Impediments (eg, Lighting, Glasses, Hearing Aids).

Encourage Family to Bring in Familiar Objects from Home (eg, Photographs with Nonglare Glass, Afghan).

Ask person to tell you about the picture.

Focus on familiar topics.

Discuss Current Events, Seasonal Events (Snow, Water Activities); Share Your Interests (Travel, Crafts).

Assess if Person Can Perform an Activity with His Hands (Eg, Latch Rugs, Wood Crafts).
Provide reading materials, audio tapes, puzzles (manual, computer, crossword).
Encourage person to keep his own records if possible (eg, intake and output).
Provide tasks to perform (addressing envelopes, occupational therapy).

In Teaching a Task or Activity—for Example, Eating—Break it into Small, Brief Steps by Giving Only One Instruction at a Time.
Remove covers from food plate and cups.
Locate napkin and utensils.
Add sugar and milk to coffee.
Add condiments to food (sugar, salt, pepper).
Cut foods.
Proceed with eating.

Explain All Activities.
Offer simple explanations of tasks.
Allow individual to handle equipment related to each task.
Allow individual to participate in task, such as washing his face.
Acknowledge that you are leaving and say when you will return.

Increase Person's Self-Esteem.

Allow former habits (eg, reading in the bathroom).
Encourage the wearing of dentures.
Assist with removal of facial hair.
Ask family to provide spending money.
Ask person/significant others his usual grooming routine and encourage him to follow it.
Provide privacy at all times; when it is necessary to expose a body surface, take precautions to cover all other areas (eg, if washing a back, use towels or blankets to cover legs and front torso).
Provide for personal hygiene according to person's preferences (hair grooming, showers or bath, nail care, cosmetics, deodorants and fragrances).

Promote a Well Role.

Discourage the use of nightclothes during the day; have person wear shoes, not slippers.
Promote mobility as much as possible.
Have person eat meals out of bed, unless contraindicated.
Promote socialization during meals (eg, set up lunch for four individuals in lounge).
Plan an activity each day to look forward to (eg, bingo, ice cream sundae gathering).
Encourage participation in decision making (eg, selecting what he wishes to wear).

Do Not Endorse Confusion.

Do not argue with person.
Never agree with confused statements.
Direct person back to reality; do not allow him to ramble.
Adhere to the schedule; if changes are necessary, advise person of them.
Avoid talking to coworkers about other topics in person's presence.
Provide simple explanations that cannot be misinterpreted.
Remember to acknowledge your entrance with a greeting and your exit with a closure ("I will be back in 10 min.").
Avoid open-ended questions.
Replace five- or six-step tasks with two- or three-step tasks.

Prevent Injury to the Individual.

Discourage the use of restraints; explore other alternatives (Rateau, 2000).
    Put person in a room with others who can help watch him.
    Enlist aid of family or friends to watch person during confused periods.
    If person is pulling out tubes, use mitts instead of wrist restraints.
Refer to *Risk for Injury* for strategies for assessing and manipulating the environment for hazards.
Register with an emergency medical system, including "wanderers' list" with local police department.

Assist Family with Effective Coping (Young, 2001).

Explain cause of confusion.
Explain person does not realize situation.

Explain the need to remain patient, flexible, and calm.
Stress to respond to person as an adult.
Explain behavior is part of a disorder and is not voluntary.

Rationales

- Differentiating between acute (reversible) and chronic (irreversible) confusion is important for nurses and physicians (Miller, 2004).
- Unconditional positive regard communicates acceptance and affection to a person who has difficulty interpreting the environment.
- Careful listening is critical to evaluate responses to prevent escalation of anxiety and to detect physiologic discomforts (Miller, 2004).
- Memory loss and diminished intellectual functioning create a need for consistency.
- Sensory input is carefully planned to reduce excess stimuli, which increase confusion (Miller, 2004).
- Structured rest periods prevent fatigue and allow for lower-stress periods.
- Restraints are a violation of a person's rights and increase anxiety. All attempts to protect the person should be used before selecting restraints.
- "Functional or baseline behavior is likely to occur when the external demands (stressors) on the individual are adjusted to the level to which the person has adapted" (Hall, 1991).
- Four biologic mechanisms are required for coping: movement, energy production, sensing, and cerebral integrating. "As competence decreases, external environmental factors become increasingly important determinants of behavior and affect" (Hall, 1991).
- People with dementia can be assisted to maximize their function level by reducing or eliminating certain factors. These factors include:
  - Fatigue
  - Change in routine, environment, or caregiver
  - High-stimulus activity (eg, crowds) or images (eg, frightening pictures or movies)
  - Frustration from trying to function beyond capabilities or from being restrained
  - Pain, discomforts, illness, or side effects from medications
  - Competing or misleading stimuli (eg, mirrors, television, costumes)
- Anxiety influences cognitive abilities through excessive self-focusing and worrying. Depression causes decreased concentration, attention deficits, and negative expectations (Miller, 2004).
- Restrained elderly have increased levels of confusion, especially at night (Rateau, 2000).

CHRONIC CONFUSION

DEFINITION
Chronic Confusion: A state in which a person experiences an irreversible, long-standing, and/or progressive deterioration of intellect and personality

DEFINING CHARACTERISTICS
Major (Must Be Present)
Cognitive or intellectual losses
Loss of memory   Inability to make choices, decisions
Loss of time sense

Inability to solve problems, reason
    Altered perceptions   Poor judgment
    Loss of language abilities
Affective or personality losses
    Loss of affect   Increasing self-preoccupation
    Diminished inhibition   Psychotic features
    Loss of tact, control of temper   Antisocial behavior
    Loss of recognition (others,   Loss of energy reserve
      environment, self)
Cognitive or planning losses
    Loss of general ability to plan   Impaired ability to set goals, plan
Progressively lowered stress threshold
    Purposeful wandering   Purposeless behavior
    Violent, agitated, or   Withdrawal or avoidance behavior
      anxious behavior   Compulsive repetitive behavior

RELATED FACTORS
Pathophysiologic (Hall, 1991)
Related to progressive degeneration of the cerebral cortex secondary to:

Alzheimer's disease   Multiinfarct disease (MID)
Combination

Related to disturbance in cerebral metabolism, structure, or integrity secondary to:

Pick's disease   Creutzfeldt-Jakob disease
Toxic substance injection   Degenerative neurologic disease
Brain tumors   Huntington's chorea
End-stage diseases   Psychiatric disorders
  (AIDS, cirrhosis, cancer,
  renal failure, cardiac failure,
  chronic obstructive
  pulmonary disease)

⊕ **AUTHOR'S NOTE**

Refer to *Acute Confusion.*

⊕ **ERRORS IN DIAGNOSTIC CONSIDERATIONS**

Refer to *Acute Confusion.*

KEY CONCEPTS
- See *Acute Confusion.*
- Progressive dementing illnesses have four clusters of symptoms (Hall, 1991):

Intellectual Losses
Loss of memory   Inability to make choices
  (recent initially)   Altered ability to identify visual or auditory stimuli
Loss of sense of time   Loss of expressive and receptive language
Inability to solve problems
  and reason

Affective Personality Losses
Loss of affect   Emotional lability
Decreased attention span   Loss of tact
Decreased inhibitions   Increased self-preoccupation

Cognitive or Planning Losses

Loss of ability to plan

Loss of instrumental
  functions (eg, money
  management, mail,
  shopping)

Functional losses (eg, bathing, choosing clothes)

Loss of energy reserves

Motor apraxia

Frustration, refusal to participate

Progressively Lowered Stress Threshold

Confused or agitated night
  awakening

Purposeful wandering

Violent, agitated, anxious behavior

Compulsive repetitive behavior

Both depression and dementia cause cognitive impairments. Differentiating the underlying cause is critical, because depression is treatable (Miller, 2004).

Focus Assessment Criteria

Refer to *Acute Confusion.*

Goal

 NOC Cognitive Ability, Cognitive Orientation, Distorted Thought Control, Surveillance: Safety, Emotional Support, Environmental Management, Fall Prevention, Calming Technique

The person will participate to maximum level of independence in a therapeutic milieu.

Indicators

- Decreased frustration
- Diminished episodes of combativeness
- Decreased use of restraints
- Increased hours of sleep at night
- Stabilized or increased weight

General Interventions

NIC Cognitive Stimulation, Calming Technique, Reality Orientation, Environmental Management: Safety

Refer to Interventions Under
Acute Confusion.

Assess Who the Person Was Before the Onset of Confusion.

Educational level, career
Coping styles

Hobbies, lifestyle

Observe Client to Determine Baseline Behaviors.

Best time of day

Amount of distraction
  tolerated

Insight into disability

Routine

Response time to a simple question

Judgment

Signs/symptoms of depression

Promote Client's Sense of Integrity (Miller, 2004).

Adapt communication to client's level.
    Avoid "baby talk" and a condescending tone of voice.
    Use simple sentences and present one idea at a time.
    If person does not understand, repeat sentence using the same words.
Use positive statements; avoid "don'ts."
Unless a safety issue is involved, do not argue.
Avoid general questions, such as, "What would you like to do?" Instead, ask, "Do you want to go for a walk or work on your rug?"
Be sensitive to the feelings the person is trying to express.
Avoid questions you know the client cannot answer.
If possible, demonstrate to reinforce verbal communication.
Use touch to gain attention or show concern unless a negative response is elicited.

Maintain good eye contact and pleasant facial expressions.

Determine which sense dominates the client's perception of the world (auditory, kinesthetic, olfactory, or gustatory). Communicate through the preferred sense (Feil, 1992).

Promote the Client's Safety.

Ensure that client carries identification.

Adapt the environment so the client can pace or walk if desired.

Keep the environment uncluttered.

Keep medications, cleaning solutions, and other toxic chemicals in inaccessible places.

If person cannot manipulate call button, use another method (eg, bell, extension from bed call system).

Reduce abrupt relocations.

Discourage Use of Restraints; Explore Other Alternatives.

If client's behavior disrupts treatment (eg, nasogastric tube, urinary catheter, intravenous [IV] line), reevaluate whether treatment is appropriate.

Intravenous therapy

Camouflage tubing with loose gauze.

Consider an intermittent access device instead of continuous IV therapy.

If dehydration is a problem, institute a regular schedule for offering oral fluids.

Use the least restrictive sites.

Urinary Catheters

Evaluate causes of incontinence.

Institute specific treatment depending on type. Refer to *Impaired Urinary Elimination.*

Place urinary collection bag at end of bed with catheter between rather than draped over legs. Velcro bands can hold catheter against leg.

Gastrointestinal Tubes

Check frequently for pressure against nares.

Camouflage gastrostomy tube with a loosely applied abdominal binder.

If person is pulling out tubes, use mitts instead of wrist restraints.

Evaluate if restlessness is associated with pain. If analgesics are used, adjust dosage to reduce side effects.

Put person in a room with others who can help watch him or her.

Enlist aid of family or friends to watch person during confused periods.

Give person something to hold (eg, stuffed animal).

If Combative, Determine Source of the Fear and Frustration.

Fatigue

Change in routine, environment, caregiver

Physical stress, pain, infection, acute illness, discomfort

Misleading or inappropriate stimuli

Pressure to exceed functional capacity

If a Dysfunctional Episode or Sudden Functional Loss Has Occurred:

Address person by surname.

Assume a dependent position to the client.

Distract client with cues that require automatic social behavior (eg, "Mrs. Smith, would you like some juice now?").

After the episode has passed, discuss the episode with the client.

Document antecedents, behavior observed, and consequences.

Ensure Physical Comfort and Maintenance of Basic Health Needs.

Refer to Self-Care Deficits.

Select Modalities That Provide Favorable Stimuli for the Client.

Music Therapy

Determine client's preferences. Play this music before usual level of agitation for at least 30 min; **assess response.**

Provide soft, familiar music during meals.
Arrange group songfests with consideration to cultural/ethical orientation.
Play music during other therapies (physical, occupational, and speech).
Have person exercise to music.
Organize guest entertainment.
Use client-developed songbooks (large print and decorative covers).

Recreation Therapy

Encourage arts and crafts.   Suggest creative writing.
Provide puzzles.   Organize group games.

Remotivation Therapy

Organize group sessions into five steps (Dennis, 1984):

   Step 1: Create a climate of acceptance (approx. 5 min).

   • Maintain a relaxed atmosphere; introduce leaders and participants.
   • Provide large-letter nametags and names on chairs.
   • Maintain assigned places for every session.

   Step 2: Creating a bridge to reality (approx. 15 min).

   • Use a prop (visual, audio, song, picture, object, poem) to introduce theme of session.

   Step 3: Share the world we live in (approx. 15 min).

   • Discuss the topic as a group.
   • Promote stimulation of senses.

   Step 4: Appreciate the work of the world (approx. 20 min).

   • Discuss how the topic relates to their past experiences (work, leisure).

   Step 5: Create a climate of appreciation (approx. 5 min).

   • Thank each member individually.
   • Announce the next session's topic and meeting date.
   • Use associations and analogies (eg, "If ice is cold, then fire is . . . ?" "If day is light, then night is . . . ?").

Choose topics for remotivation sessions based on suggestions from group leaders and group interests. Examples are pets, bodies of water, canning fruits and vegetables, transportation, holidays (Janssen & Giberson, 1988).

Sensory Training

Stimulate vision (with brightly colored items of different shape, pictures, colored decorations, kaleidoscopes).
Stimulate smell (with flowers, coffee, cologne).
Stimulate hearing (ring a bell, play music).
Stimulate touch (sandpaper, velvet, steel wool pads, silk, stuffed animals).
Stimulate taste (spices, salt, sugar, sour substances).

Reminiscence Therapy (Burnside & Haight, 1994; Smith, 1990)

Consider instituting on a one-to-one or group basis. Discuss purpose and goals with client care team. Prepare well before initiating. Refer to Burnside and Haight (1994) for specific protocols.

Implement Techniques to Lower the Stress Threshold (Hall & Buckwalter, 1987; Miller, 2004).

Reduce Competing or Excessive Stimuli.

Keep environment simple and uncluttered.
Use simple written cues to clarify directions for use of radio and television.
Eliminate or minimize unnecessary noise.

Plan and Maintain a Consistent Routine.

Attempt to assign same caregivers.
Elicit from family members specific methods that help or hinder care.
Arrange personal care items in order of use (clothes, toothbrush, mouthwash, and so forth).
Determine a daily routine with client and family.

Write down sequence for all caregivers.
Reduce the stress when change is anticipated.
 Keep the change as simple as possible (eg, minimal holiday decorations).
 Ensure person is well rested.
 Institute change during person's best time of day if possible.

Focus on the Client's Ability Level.
Do not request performance of function beyond ability.
Express unconditional positive regard for the person.
Modify environment to compensate for ability (eg, use of Velcro fasteners, loose clothing, elastic
 waistbands).
Use simple sentences; demonstrate activity.
Do not ask questions that the person cannot answer.
Avoid open-ended questions (eg, "What do you want to eat?" "When do you want to take a bath?").
Avoid using pronouns; name objects.
Offer simple choices (eg, "Do you want a cookie or crackers?").
Use finger foods (eg, sandwiches) to encourage self-feeding.

Minimize Fatigue (Hall, 1994).
Provide rest periods twice daily.
Determine with client a rest activity, such as reading or listening to music.
Encourage napping in recliner chairs, not bed.
Plan high-stress or fatiguing activities during best time for the client.
Allow the person to cease an activity at any time.
Incorporate regular exercise in daily plan.
Allow for wandering.
Be alert to expressions of fatigue and increased anxiety; immediately reduce stimuli.

Rationales

* Assessing the client's personal history can provide insight into current behavior patterns and communicates the nurse's interest (Hall, 1994).
* Specific personal data can improve individualization of care (Hall, 1994).
* Baseline behavior can be used to develop a plan for activities and daily care routines (Hall, 1994).
* Alzheimer's disease-related dementia affects communication abilities (ie, receptive and expressive; Hall, 1994).
* Clients with dementia compensate for conative (ability to plan and sequence activities) losses by developing a daily routine.
* Dysfunctional episodes are transient changes characterized by cognitive and social inaccessibility (eg, inability to recognize familiar faces, belligerence, stubbornness; Hall, 1994; Miller, 2004).
* Fatigue is the most frequent cause of dysfunctional episodes.
* Daytime rest periods help prevent night wakenings.
* Overstimulation, understimulation, or misleading stimuli can cause dysfunctional episodes because of impaired sensory interpretation (Hall, 1994).
* Attempting to perform functions that exceed cognitive capacity will result in fear, anger, and frustration (Hall, 1994).
* Physical stressors can precipitate a dysfunctional episode (eg, urinary tract infections, caffeine, constipation).
* Dysfunctional episodes are manifestations of fear; the goals of management are to prevent injury, provide a sense of serenity, and promote self-mastery (Hall, 1994).
* Music therapy at least 30 min before the person's usual peak level of agitation can reduce agitation (Gerdner, 1999).
* Confused clients cannot remember asking questions or that there is memory loss (Young, 2001).

CONSTIPATION

DEFINITION

Constipation: The state in which a person experiences or is at high risk of experiencing stasis of the large intestine resulting in infrequent (two or less weekly) elimination and/or hard, dry feces

DEFINING CHARACTERISTICS
Major (Must Be Present)

Hard, formed stool
Prolonged and difficult
  evacuation

Defecation fewer than two times a week

Minor (May Be Present)

Decreased bowel sounds
Reported feeling of rectal
  fullness
Reported feeling of pressure
  in rectum

Straining on defecation
Palpable impaction
Feeling of inadequate emptying

RELATED FACTORS
Pathophysiologic

Related to defective nerve stimulation, weak pelvic floor muscles, and immobility secondary to:

Spinal cord lesions
Spinal cord injury
Spina bifida

Cerebrovascular accident (CVA, stroke)
Neurologic diseases (multiple sclerosis, Parkinson's)
Dementia

Related to decreased metabolic rate secondary to:

Obesity
Pheochromocytoma
Hypothyroidism

Hyperparathyroidism
Uremia

Hypopituitarism
Diabetic neuropathy

Related to decreased response to urge to defecate secondary to:
Affective disorders

Related to pain (on defecation):
Hemorrhoids

Back injury

Related to decreased peristalsis secondary to hypoxia (cardiac, pulmonary)
Related to motility disturbances secondary to irritable bowel syndrome
Related to failure to relax anal sphincter or high resting pressure in the anal canal secondary to:

Multiple vaginal deliveries

Chronic straining

Treatment-Related

Related to side effects of (specify):

Antidepressants
Antacids (calcium, aluminum)

Calcium channel blockers
Calcium

Iron   Anticholinergics
Barium   Anesthetics
Aluminum   Narcotics (codeine, morphine)
Aspirin   Diuretics
Phenothiazines   Anti-Parkinson agents

Related to effects of anesthesia and surgical manipulation on peristalsis
Related to habitual laxative use
Related to mucositis secondary to radiation

Situational (Personal, Environmental)
Related to decreased peristalsis secondary to:
Immobility   Stress
Pregnancy   Lack of exercise

Related to irregular evacuation patterns
Related to cultural/health beliefs
Related to lack of privacy
Related to inadequate diet (lack of roughage, fiber, thiamine)
Related to inadequate fluid intake
Related to fear of rectal or cardiac pain
Related to faulty appraisal
Related to inability to perceive bowel cues

⊛ AUTHOR'S NOTE

Constipation results from delayed passage of food residue in the bowel because of factors that the nurse can treat (eg, dehydration, insufficient dietary roughage, immobility). Perceived constipation refers to a faulty perception of constipation with self-prescribed overuse of laxatives, enemas, and/or suppositories.

When constipation stems from factors amenable to nursing interventions other than those related to colonic or perceived constipation, the nursing diagnosis *Constipation* can apply.

⊛ ERRORS IN DIAGNOSTIC STATEMENTS

1. *Constipation related to reports of infrequent hard, dry feces*
   A report of infrequent hard, dry feces validates constipation—it is not a contributing factor. If the nurse does not know the cause, he or she can write: *Constipation related to unknown etiology, as evidenced by reports of infrequent hard, dry feces.*

KEY CONCEPTS
Generic Considerations

- Bowel elimination is controlled primarily by muscular and neurologic activity. Undigested food or feces passes through the large intestine propelled by involuntary muscles within the intestinal walls. At the same time, water that was needed for digestion is reabsorbed. The feces pass through the sigmoid colon, which empties into the rectum. At some point, the amount of stool in the rectum stimulates a defecation reflex, which causes the anal sphincter to relax and defecation to occur (Shua-Haim et al., 1999). Table II.4 illustrates the components needed for normal bowel elimination and the conditions that impede them.
- Bowel patterns are culturally or familially determined. Range of normal is wide, from three times a day to once every 3 days (Shua-Haim et al., 1999).
- Some medical conditions, such as brain disorders or spinal cord injuries, interfere with neurotransmission. Others, such as diabetes mellitus or rectal or anal trauma, cause rectal sphincter abnormalities. Inflammatory bowel disease, radiation proctitis, chronic constipation, and ileoanal

TABLE II.4 Components for Normal Bowel Elimination and Corresponding Barriers

Components	Barriers
Daily diet of fiber (15–25 g)	Lack of access to fresh foods
	Financial constraints
	Insufficient knowledge*
8–10 glasses of water a day	Mobility problems
	Fear of incontinence
	Impaired thought process*
	Low motivation
Daily exercise	Minimal activity level
	Pain, fatigue
	Fear of falling
Cognitive appraisal	Impaired thought process
	Faulty appraisal
Toileting routine	Low motivation
	Change in routine
	Stress
Response to rectal cues	Mobility problems
	Decreased awareness
	Environmental constraints
	Self-care deficits

*These barriers can impede all the components.

surgery can decrease the fecal reservoir capacity and cause leaking (Shua-Haim et al., 1999).

- Three tablespoons of bran daily increases dietary fiber by 25% to 40% and eliminates constipation in 60% of individuals (Shua-Haim et al., 1999).
- Diets high in unrefined fibrous food produce large, soft stools that decrease the colon's susceptibility to disease. Diets low in fiber and high in concentrated refined foods produce small, hard stools that increase the colon's susceptibility to disease.
- Undigested fiber absorbs water, which adds bulk and softness to the stool, speeding its passage through the intestines. Fiber without adequate fluid can aggravate, not facilitate, bowel function.
- Laxatives and enemas are not components of a bowel management program. They are for emergency use only.
- Chronic use of stool softeners can cause fecal incontinence and is not recommended for treatment of chronic constipation in nonambulatory individuals (Shua-Haim et al., 1999).

 Pediatric Considerations

- Unlike in adults, constipation in children is not defined by frequency, but by the character of stool. Passage of firm or hard stool with symptoms of difficulty in expulsion, blood-streaked bowel movements, and abdominal discomfort characterize constipation in children.
- As the infant ages, the stomach enlarges to hold more food, and the peristaltic activity of the gastrointestinal (GI) tract slows. Thus, stools change in color, consistency, and frequency (Wong, 2003).
- Voluntary withholding (functional constipation) is the most common cause of constipation beyond the neonatal period. Conflicts in toilet training or pain on defecation may lead to stool retention (Wong, 2003).
- Encopresis is fecal soiling or incontinence secondary to constipation. Previously toilet-trained children with encopresis should be evaluated psychologically.
- Children with functional constipation associate defecation with discomfort. When the sensation of relaxation of the internal anal sphincter occurs, the child contracts the external sphincter to prevent the expulsion of stools. Eventually the rectum dilates, resulting in more stool retention and diminished sensory response.

⚘ Maternal Considerations

- Constipation in pregnancy results from:
  - Displacement of the intestines
  - Increased water absorption from colon
  - Hormonal influences
  - Prolonged intestinal time
  - Use of iron supplements
- Postpartum causes of constipation are:
  - Relaxed abdominal tone
  - Decreased peristalsis
  - Food and fluid restrictions during labor

Ⓒ Geriatric Considerations

- Older adults experience reduced mucus secretion in the large intestines and decreased elasticity of the rectal wall (Miller, 2004).
- Sensory dysfunction in the anorectal area of older adults can reduce sensing rectal distention (Shua-Haim et al., 1999).
- Some older adults are prone to constipation owing to such factors as decreased activity, insufficient dietary fiber and bulk, insufficient fluid intake, side effects of medications, laxative abuse, and inattention to defecation cues (Miller, 2004).
- Thirty percent of older adults complain of constipation compared to 2% of the general population (Shaefer & Cheskin, 1998).

🌐 Transcultural Considerations

Some cultures have folk medicine for elimination problems. For example, Mexican Americans differentiate diarrhea as hot or cold. If the stool is green or yellow, it is hot and treated with cold tea. If white, the stool is cold and treated with hot tea (Giger & Davidhizar, 2003).

Focus Assessment Criteria

Subjective Data

Assess for Defining Characteristics.

Elimination pattern
  Usual   Present
What frequency is considered normal?
Laxative/enema use
  Type   How often
Episodes of diarrhea
  How often?   Frequency?   Duration?
  Precipitated by what?
Associated symptoms/complaints of
  Headache   Thirst   Weakness
  Pain   Lethargy   Cramping
  Anorexia   Weight loss/gain   Awareness of bowel cues

Assess for Related Factors.

Lifestyle
Activity level
Occupation
Exercise (what? how often?)
Nutrition

24-hour recall of foods and liquids taken	Protein
	Usual 24-hour intake
Carbohydrates	Fiber
Fat	Liquids

Current drug therapy

Antibiotics	Antacids
Iron	Central nervous system (CNS) depressants
Steroids	

Medical–surgical history

Present conditions	Past conditions
Surgical history (colostomy? ileostomy?)	Awareness of bowel cues

Objective Data
Assess for Defining Characteristics.

Stool
Color
Odor
Consistency
Components

Blood	Undigested food
Parasites	Pus
Mucus	

Gastrointestinal motility (auscultation, light palpation)

Bowel Sounds

High-pitched, gurgling (5/min)	High-pitched, frequent, loud, pushing
	Absent
Weak and infrequent	

Assess for Related Factors.

Nutrition

Food intake	Fluid intake
Type	Type
Amounts	Amounts

Perianal Area/Rectal Examination

Hemorrhoids	Irritation
Fissures	Impaction
Control of rectal sphincter (presence of anal wink, bulbocavernosus reflex)	Stool in rectum

For more information on Focus Assessment Criteria, visit http://connection.lww.com.

Goal

NOC | Bowel Elimination, Hydration, Symptom Control

The person will report on bowel movements at least every 2 to 3 days.

Indicators

- Describe components for effective bowel movements.
- Explain rationale for lifestyle change(s).

General Interventions

 NIC Bowel Management, Fluid Management, Constipation/Impaction Management

Assess Contributing Factors.

Irregular schedule

Side effects of medical
  regimen

Stress

Inadequate exercise

Imbalanced diet

Promote Corrective Measures.

Regular Time for Elimination

Review daily routine.

Advise client to include time for defecation as part of daily routine.

Discuss suitable time (based on responsibilities, availability of facilities, and so forth).

Provide stimulus to defecation (eg, coffee, prune juice).

Advise client to attempt to defecate about 1 h or so after meals and that remaining in the bathroom for a suitable length of time may be necessary.

Use bathroom instead of bedpan if possible.

Provide privacy (close door, draw curtains around bed, play television or radio to mask sounds, have room deodorizer available).

Provide comfort (reading material as diversion) and safety (call bell available).

Allow suitable position (sitting, if not contraindicated).

Adequate Exercise

Review current exercise pattern.

Provide for frequent moderate physical exercise (if not contraindicated).

Provide frequent ambulation of hospitalized client when tolerable.

Perform range-of-motion exercises for person who is bedridden.

Teach exercises for increased abdominal muscle tone (unless contraindicated; Weeks et al., 2000).

- Contract abdominal muscles several times throughout day.
- Do sit-ups, keeping heels on floor with knees slightly flexed.
- While supine, raise lower limbs, keeping knees straight.

Turn and change positions in bed, lifting hips.

Lift knees alternately to the chest, stretching arms out to side and up over the head.

Balanced Diet

Review list of foods high in bulk:

Fresh fruits and vegetables
  with skins

Bran

Nuts and seeds

Beans (navy, kidney, lima)

Whole-grain breads and cereal

Cooked fruits and vegetables

Fruit juices

Discuss dietary preferences.

Consider any food intolerances or allergies.

Include approximately 800 g of fruits and vegetables (about four pieces of fresh fruit and large salad) for normal daily bowel movement.

Suggest moderate use of bran at first (may irritate GI tract, produce flatulence, cause diarrhea or blockage).

Gradually increase bran as tolerated (may add to cereals, baked goods, and the like). Explain the need for fluid intake with bran.

Suggest 30 to 60 mL daily of a recipe of 2 cups All Bran cereal, 2 cups applesauce, and 1 cup prune juice.

Consider financial limitations (encourage the use of fruits and vegetables in season).

Adequate Fluid Intake

Encourage intake of at least 2 L (8 to 10 glasses) unless contraindicated.

Discuss fluid preferences.

Set up regular schedule for fluid intake.

Recommend drinking a glass of hot water 30 min before breakfast, which may stimulate bowel evacuation.

Advise avoiding grapefruit juice, coffee, tea, cola, and chocolate drinks as daily fluid intake.

Optimal Position

Assist client to normal semisquatting position to allow optimum use of abdominal muscles and effect of force of gravity.

Assist client onto bedpan if necessary; elevate head of bed to high Fowler's position or elevation permitted.
Use fracture bedpan for comfort, if preferred.
Stress the avoidance of straining.
Encourage exhaling during straining.
Chart results (color, consistency, amount).
Elevate legs on footstool when on toilet.

Eliminate or Reduce Contributing Factors.

Administer mild laxative after oral administration of barium sulfate.*
Assess elimination status while on antacid therapy (may be necessary to alternate magnesium-type antacid with other types).*
Encourage increased intake of high-roughage foods and increased fluid intake as adjunct to iron therapy (eg, fresh fruits and vegetables with skins; bran, nuts, and seeds; whole-wheat bread).
Encourage early ambulation, with assistance if necessary, to counter effects of anesthetic agents.
Assess elimination status while client receives certain narcotic analgesics (morphine, codeine) and alert physician if client experiences difficulty with defecation.
Advise client about medications that cause constipation (eg, antacids, bismuth, calcium channel blockers, clonidine, levodopa, iron, nonsteroidal antiinflammatories, opiates, sucralfate; Shua-Haim et al., 1999).
Discuss laxative abuse (see *Perceived Constipation*).

Conduct Health Teaching, as Indicated.

Explain the relationship of lifestyle changes to constipation.
Explain interventions that relieve symptoms.
Explain techniques to reduce the effects of stress and immobility.

Rationales

- A daily diet of fiber, 6 to 8 glasses of water, and exercise maintain a normal bowel elimination pattern. In addition, the person must be able to appraise the need to evacuate and establish a toileting routine.
- Regular physical activity promotes muscle tonicity needed for fecal expulsion. It also increases circulation to the digestive system, which promotes peristalsis and easier feces evacuation.
- Sufficient fluid intake, at least 2 L daily, is necessary to maintain bowel patterns and to promote proper stool consistency.
- Certain fluids act as diuretics: caffeine-containing drinks and grapefruit juice (Weeks et al., 2000).
- A well-balanced high-fiber diet stimulates peristalsis. Foods high in fiber should be avoided during episodes of diarrhea:
  - Whole grains and nuts (bran, shredded wheat, brown rice, whole-wheat bread)
  - Raw and coarse vegetables (broccoli, cauliflower, cucumbers, lettuce, cabbage, turnips, Brussels sprouts)
  - Fresh fruits, with skins
- The gastrocolic and duodenocolic reflexes stimulate mass peristalsis two or three times a day, most often after meals.
- Voluntary contraction of the abdominal muscles aids in the expulsion of feces.
- Frequency and consistency of stool are related to fluid and food intake. Fiber increases fecal bulk and enhances water absorption into stool. Adequate dietary fiber and fluid promote firm, but soft, well-formed stools and decrease hard, dry, constipated stools. Physical activity promotes peristalsis, aids digestion, and facilitates elimination (Shua-Haim et al., 1999).
- Laxatives upset a bowel program, because they cause much of the bowel to empty and can cause unscheduled bowel movements. With constant use, the colon loses tone and stool retention becomes difficult. Chronic use of bowel aids can lead to problems in stool consistency, which interferes with the scheduled bowel program and bowel management. Stool softeners may not be necessary if diet and fluid intake are adequate. Enemas lead to an overstretched bowel and loss of bowel tone, contributing to further constipation.
- Elevating the legs can increase intraabdominal pressure (Shua-Haim et al., 1999).

---

*May require a primary care provider's order.

🧩 Pediatric Considerations

Discuss some causes of constipation in infants and children (eg, underfeeding; high-protein, low-carbohydrate diet; lack of roughage; dehydration).

If bowel movements are infrequent with hard stools:
- With infants, add corn syrup to feeding or fruit to diet. Avoid apple juice or sauce.
- With children, add bran cereal, prune juice, and fruits and vegetables high in bulk.

Refer cases of persistent constipation for medical evaluation.

If child has functional constipation, consult with primary care provider for a laxative regimen.

Explain to adolescents the effects of fluids, fiber, and exercise on bowel function.

Rationales

- Several factors contribute to constipation:
  - Insufficient roughage or bulk
  - A bland diet, too high in dairy products, which results in reduced colonic motility
  - Insufficient oral intake of fluids, which allows the normal resorption of water from the colon to dehydrate the feces too much, or dehydration stemming from any activities that increase fluid loss from sweating
  - Fecal retention by the child
  - Medications (eg, narcotics or anticonvulsants)
  - The child's emotional state
- Children with long-standing functional constipation need a program of daily laxatives to allow the rectum to return to normal.

👤 Maternal Considerations

Explain the risks of constipation in pregnancy and postpartum:
- Decreased gastric motility
- Prolonged intestinal time
- Pressure of enlarging uterus
- Distended abdominal muscles (post)
- Relaxation of intestines (post)

Explain aggravating factors for hemorrhoid development (straining at defecation, constipation, prolonged standing, wearing constrictive clothing).

If woman has a history of constipation, discuss use of bulk-producing laxatives to soften stool.

Postdelivery

Assess abdomen (bowel sounds, distention, presence of flatus).

Assess for hemorrhoids and perineal swelling.

Provide relief of rectal or perineal pain.

Instruct client to take sitz baths and use cool, astringent compresses for hemorrhoids.

Rationales

Explaining the causes of constipation during pregnancy and the postpartum period can increase participation in behaviors that decrease or prevent constipation.

CONSTIPATION

 RELATED TO EFFECTS OF IMMOBILITY ON PERISTALSIS

Goal

NOC	Bowel Elimination, Hydration, Mobility Level

The person will report improved bowel movements every 2 to 3 days.

Indicators

- Describe components for effective bowel movements.
- Explain rationale for lifestyle change(s).

Interventions

NIC	Activity Therapy, Bowel Management, Fluid Management, Health Education, Nutrition Management

Assess Causative Factors of Immobility.

Musculoskeletal
(eg, fractures, hip
replacement)
Chronic or acute illness
Physical handicap
Bed rest
Degenerative joint changes
(arthritis)

Minimal activity
Reliance on life-support systems
Trauma (eg, burns, head injury)
Inappropriate coping mechanisms
Psychosomatic illness
Surgery

Eliminate or Reduce Contributing Factors

Fecal Impaction

If fecal impaction is suspected, perform digital rectal examination (DRE).
1. Client should assume position lying on left side.
2. Don glove, lubricate forefinger, and insert; attempt to break up any hardened fecal mass and remove pieces.
3. If impaction is out of reach of gloved finger:
   a. Administer oil retention enema to aid in removal of mass.*
   b. Instruct person to retain enema at least 1 h or possibly overnight.
   c. Follow with cleansing enema* (both enemas may need to be repeated; may need to follow with repeated attempt to break up mass digitally).

Make client comfortable and allow rest.
Client may require temporary use of stool softener or mild cathartic.*
Maintain accurate bowel elimination record.

Severe Constipation

First day, insert glycerin suppository and have client attempt bowel movement through intermittent straining efforts.
If ineffective, on second day, insert glycerin suppository and follow same routine.
If no results, on third day, request prescription for suppository, which if not effective should be followed by enema.*
To aid in stimulation of reflex emptying, a suppository may be followed in 20 to 30 min by digital stimulation of anal sphincter.
Return to first-day routine and follow until pattern is established (may be every 2 to 3 days).

---

*May require a primary care provider's order.

Conduct Health Teaching, as Indicated.

Explain interventions to prevent (eg, diet, exercise) versus those to treat constipation.

Refer to Constipation for Additional Interventions.

Rationales

- Defecation involves the simultaneous relaxation of the puborectalis and external anal sphincter muscles coordinated with increased intraabdominal pressure, forcing stool toward the rectum.
- Immobility can interfere with bowel elimination through loss of muscle tone, decreased GI motility, and decreased gravity filling of lower rectum with a resulting diminished defecation reflex.

PERCEIVED CONSTIPATION

DEFINITION

Perceived Constipation: The state in which an individual self-prescribes the daily use of laxatives, enemas, and/or suppositories to ensure a daily bowel movement

DEFINING CHARACTERISTICS*

Expectation of a daily bowel movement with the resulting overuse of laxatives, enemas, and suppositories
Expected passage of stool at same time, every day

RELATED FACTORS
Pathophysiologic

Related to faulty appraisal secondary to:
Obsessive–compulsive disorders   Depression
Deterioration of the CNS

Situational (Personal, Environmental)

Related to inaccurate information secondary to:
Cultural beliefs   Family beliefs

⊛ **AUTHOR'S NOTE**

Refer to Author's Note under *Constipation*.

KEY CONCEPTS

Refer to Key Concepts under *Constipation*.

---

*Adapted from McLane, A. M., & McShane, R. E. (1986). Empirical validation of defining characteristics of constipation: A study of bowel elimination practices of healthy adults. In M. E. Hurley (Ed.). *Classification of nursing diagnosis: Proceedings of the sixth conference*. St. Louis: C. V. Mosby.

Focus Assessment Criteria

Refer to Focus Assessment Criteria under *Constipation*.

Goal

NOC Bowel Elimination,
Health Beliefs: Perceived Threat

The person will verbalize acceptance of bowel movement every 2 to 3 days.

Indicators

- Not use laxatives regularly.
- Relate the causes of constipation.
- Describe the hazards of laxative use.
- Relate an intent to increase fiber, fluid, and exercise in daily life as instructed.

General Interventions

NIC Bowel Management, Health Education,
Behavior Modification,
Nutrition Management

Assess Causative or Contributing Factors.

Cultural/familial belief   Faulty appraisal

Explain that Bowel Movements Are Needed Every 2 to 3 Days, Not Daily.

Be sensitive to person's beliefs.
Be patient.

Explain the Hazards of Regular Laxative Use.

They provide only temporary relief.
They promote constipation by interfering with peristalsis.
They can interfere with absorption of vitamins A, D, E, and K.
They can cause diarrhea.

If a Laxative is Desired, Teach Client How to Use Bulk-Forming Agents, such as Psyllium Seed or Bran.

Start slowly with one half the recommended dose.
Increase dose gradually over weeks.

Refer to Constipation for Interventions to Promote Optimal Elimination.

Rationales

- Stimulant laxatives purge the bowel of stool so effectively that a bowel movement may not occur normally for a few days. The person's response is to take the laxative again. This begins a cycle of laxative dependence (DiPiro, Talbert, Hayes, Yee, Matzke & Posey, 2001).
- The chronic laxative user must learn dietary modifications and use of bulk-forming laxatives, with the elimination of stimulant laxatives.

Ineffective Coping
Defensive Coping
Ineffective Denial
Related to Impaired Ability to Accept Consequences of Own Behavior as Evidenced by
Lack of Acknowledgment of Substance Abuse/Dependency

INEFFECTIVE COPING

DEFINITION

Ineffective Coping: A state in which a person experiences, or is at risk to experience, an inability to manage internal or environmental stressors adequately due to inadequate resources (physical, psychological, behavioral, and/or cognitive)

DEFINING CHARACTERISTICS*
Major (One Must Be Present)

Verbalization of inability to cope or ask for help
or
Inappropriate use of defense mechanisms
or
Inability to meet role expectations

Minor (May Be Present)

Chronic worry, anxiety
Reported difficulty with life
  stressors
Impaired social participation
Destructive behavior toward
  self or others
High incidence of accidents

Frequent illnesses
Verbal manipulation
Inability to meet basic needs
Nonassertive response patterns
Change in usual
  communication pattern
Substance abuse

RELATED FACTORS
Pathophysiologic

Related to chronicity of condition or complex self-care regimens
Related to changes in body integrity secondary to:
Loss of body part   Disfigurement secondary to trauma

Related to altered affect caused by changes secondary to:
Body chemistry   Intake of mood-altering substance
Tumor (brain)   Mental retardation

Treatment-Related

Related to separation from family and home (eg, hospitalization, nursing home)
Related to disfigurement caused by surgery
Related to altered appearance from drugs, radiation, or other treatment

---

*Adapted from Vincent, K. G. (1985). The validation of a nursing diagnosis. *Nursing Clinics of North America, 20,* 631–639.

Situational (Personal, Environmental)

Related to increased food consumption in response to stressors
Related to changes in physical environment secondary to:

War	Poverty	Natural disaster
Homelessness	Relocation	Inadequate finances
Seasonal work		

Related to disruption of emotional bonds secondary to:

Death	Institutionalization	Relocation
Desertion	Separation or divorce	Orphanage/foster care
Jail	Educational institution	

Related to unsatisfactory support system

Related to sensory overload secondary to:

Factory environment	Urbanization: crowding, noise pollution, excessive activity

Related to inadequate psychological resources secondary to:

Poor self-esteem	Helplessness
Excessive negative beliefs about self	Lack of motivation to respond
Negative role modeling	

Related to culturally related conflicts with (specify):

Premarital sex	Abortion

Maturational

Child/Adolescent

Related to:

Poor impulse control	Panic	Peer rejection
Parental substance abuse	Childhood trauma	Parental rejection
Inconsistent methods of discipline	Poor social skills	Fear of failure
	Repressed anxiety	

Adolescent

Related to inadequate psychological resources to adapt to:

Physical and emotional changes	Sexual awareness	Independence from family
	Sexual relationships	Career choices
Educational demands		

Young Adult

Related to inadequate psychological resources to adapt to:

Career choices	Marriage	Educational demands
Parenthood	Leaving home	

Middle Adult

Related to inadequate psychological resources to adapt to:

Physical signs of aging	Problems with relatives	Career pressures
Social status needs	Child-rearing problems	Aging parents

Older Adult

Related to inadequate psychological resources to adapt to:

Physical changes	Retirement	Changes in financial status
Response of others	Changes in residence	

Ⓧ **AUTHOR'S NOTE**

Ineffective Coping describes a person experiencing difficulty adapting to stressful event(s). Usual effective coping mechanisms may be inappropriate or ineffective, or the person may have a poor history of coping with stressors.   *(continued)*

> ⊚ **AUTHOR'S NOTE** (*Continued*)
>
> If the event is recent, *Ineffective Coping* may be a premature judgment. For example, a person may respond to overwhelming stress with a grief response such as denial, anger, or sadness, making a *Grieving* diagnosis appropriate.
>
> *Impaired Adjustment* may be more useful than *Ineffective Coping* in the initial period after a stressful event. *Ineffective Coping* and its related diagnoses may be more applicable to prolonged or chronic coping problems, such as *Defensive Coping* for a person with a long-standing pattern of ineffective coping.

> ⊚ **ERRORS IN DIAGNOSTIC STATEMENTS**
>
> 1. *Ineffective Coping related to perceived effects of breast cancer on life goals, as evidenced by crying and refusal to talk*
>   If the diagnosis of breast cancer was recent, the person's response of crying and refusal to talk would be normal. Thus, the proper diagnosis would be *Grieving related to perceived effects of breast cancer on life goals*. If this response was prolonged with no evidence of "moving on" (eg, initiation of social activities), *Ineffective Coping* may be appropriate.
> 2. *Ineffective Coping related to reports of substance abuse*
>   Substance abuse is a reportable or observable cue validating a diagnosis. If the person acknowledged the abuse and desires assistance, the diagnosis would be *Ineffective Coping related to inability to manage stressors without drugs*. If the substance abuse was observed but the person denied it or that it was a problem, the diagnosis would be *Ineffective Denial related to unknown etiology, as evidenced by lack of acknowledgment of drug dependency*.

KEY CONCEPTS
Generic Considerations

- Lazarus (1985) defines coping as "constantly changing cognitive and behavioral efforts to manage specific external and/or internal demands that are taxing or exceeding the resources of the person."
- Expectations of mastery encourage maturation and persistence. Expectations of failure induce avoidance behaviors.
- Coping behaviors fall into two broad categories (Lazarus & Folkman, 1984):
  - *Problem-focused.* These are behaviors that attempt to improve the situation through change or taking action. Examples include making an appointment with one's boss to discuss a pay raise, creating and following a schedule for homework, and seeking help.
  - *Emotion-focused:* These are thoughts or actions that relieve emotional distress. They do not alter the situation, but they help the person feel better. Examples include playing basketball, denying anything is wrong, using food to relax, and joking.
    - *Minimization* is when the person minimizes the seriousness of a problem. This may be useful as a way to provide needed time for appraisal, but it may become dysfunctional when it precludes appraisal.
    - *Projection, displacement,* and *suppression of anger* is when a person attributes anger to or expresses it toward a less threatening person or thing. Doing so may reduce the threat enough to allow the person to deal with it. Distortion of reality and disturbance of relationships may result, which further compound the problem. Suppressed anger may result in stress-related physical symptoms.
    - *Anticipatory preparation* is the mental rehearsal of possible consequences or outcomes of behavior or stressful situations. It provides an opportunity to develop perspective as well as to prepare for the worst. It becomes dysfunctional when it creates unmanageable stress, as, for example, in anticipatory mourning.
    - *Attribution* is finding personal meaning in the problem. Examples include religious faith, individual belief, fate, and luck. Attribution may offer consolation but becomes maladaptive when a person loses all sense of self-responsibility.
- Addictive behavior is a habitual maladaptive way of coping with stress.

TABLE II.5 Reactive vs Endogenous Depression

Element	Reactive Depression	Endogenous Depression
Precipitating event	Identifiable	Unclear
Family history	Unrelated	Familial tendency
Symptoms	Related to grief and anxiety; worse at night	Seemingly unrelated to events; worse in morning
Activity	Diminished motor and cognitive behavior	Agitated, restless
Emotion	Client feels sad	Alternates between sadness and manic gaiety
Cognitive abilities	May be slightly diminished	Retarded psychomotor performance
Orientation	Oriented and responsive to environment	May not be oriented or responsive
Treatment	Responds well to counseling and environmental change	May require somatic treatment in addition to counseling

- According to Miller (2004), people "who have a rigid set or narrow range of coping skills are at more risk for impaired coping because different types of coping strategies are effective in different situations."
- Miller (1983) defines crisis as "the experiencing of an acute situation where one's repertoire of coping responses is inadequate in effecting a resolution of the stress." It usually represents a turning point and a reorganization of some important aspects of a person's psychological structure.
- An individual crisis can be described in four sequential stages: shock, defensive retreat, acknowledgment, and adaptation.
- Selye (1974) defined stress as the nonspecific response of the body to any demand. Responses to stress vary according to personal perceptions. Both positive and negative life events may initiate a stress response.
- Personal and environmental factors influence how a person copes with a disability. Research findings have supported that social support, self-concept, locus of control, and hardiness affect motivation and morale (Miller, 2004).
- Responses to illness, disability, or treatments are influenced by:
  - Attitude toward event (eg, punishment, weakness, challenge)
  - Developmental level or age
  - Extent disability interferes with goal-directed activity and significance of the goal
- Beck's cognitive theory of depression holds that those with depression process information negatively, even when there is evidence to the contrary. They filter information through a view of the world that is negatively toned, thus leading to thought distortions (Calarco & Krone, 1991). See Table II.5.
- People with chronic mental illness experience low self-esteem and a lack of confidence, competence, and sense of efficacy. Altered perceptions, attention deficits, cognitive confusion, and labile emotions interfere with decision making, problem solving, and interpersonal relationships (Finkelman, 2000).
- Taylor et al. (2000) have found that the fight-or-flight response is more characteristic of males. Females respond to stress with the tend-and-befriend theory.
- The fight-or-flight response is mediated by catecholamines. The tend-and-befriend response is mediated by oxytocin and endogenous opioids (Taylor et al., 2000).

Pediatric Considerations

- Inborn traits, social support, and family coping affect a child's ability to cope (Wong, 2002).
- As children mature, they develop and expand their coping strategies.
- In the United States, 3% to 5% of children have attention deficit-hyperactivity disorder (ADHD), with boys outnumbering girls nine to one (American Psychiatric Association [APA], 2000). The symptoms of this developmental disorder change over time. The diagnosis is made when symptoms of inattention or hyperactivity–impulsivity persist for at least 6 months and are maladaptive and inconsistent with developmental level (APA, 2000).

⊙ Geriatric Considerations

- Miller (2004) identifies six major psychosocial challenges for older adults: (1) retirement, (2) death of friends, (3) chronic illness, (4) relocation of family, (5) disruption of household, and (6) stereotypes associated with the 65th birthday.
- Folkman, Lazarus, Pimley, and Novacek (1987) found that younger subjects reported more stress related to finances and work, whereas older subjects reported stress related to health, home maintenance, and social and environmental issues.
- Anticipation and perceived control over circumstances are predictors of the effects of stress on older adults (Willis, Thomas, Garry & Goodwin, 1987).
- In older adults, coping is facilitated in those with higher incomes, occupational status, and feelings of self-efficacy. When significant life changes are necessary, however, higher occupational status and feelings of self-efficacy are liabilities, because these people hold an unrealistic view of what is controllable (Simons & West, 1984).
- No one life event has consistently negative effects on an older adult; rather, several events in a short period represent the greatest challenge (Miller, 2004).

⊕ Transcultural Considerations

- Three major components of cultural systems influence responses to illness or chronic disease and a person's ability to make healthful changes in lifestyle: (1) family support systems, (2) coping behaviors, and (3) health beliefs and practices (Andrews & Boyle, 2004).
- In certain cultures, the family plays a critical role in all aspects of the client's life, including rejection or reinforcement of healthy lifestyle changes (Andrews & Boyle, 2004).
- Asian cultures emphasize maintaining harmony and respect. It is not unusual for an Asian client, who sees the nurse as an authority, to agree with all he or she suggests. Agreeing does not mean intended compliance, only good manners. This behavior is opposite to the assertive, questioning behavior emphasized in the dominant US culture (Andrews & Boyle, 2004).
- Some cultures do not have a vocabulary for expressing emotional distress. There may be strong sanctions or taboos against complaining about one's fate (Mechanic, 1972).
- Some symptoms that Western medicine would interpret as mental illness are considered normal in other cultures. Visions, hexes, and hearing voices are acceptable in some US subcultures: Appalachian, Asian, African American, Hispanic, and Native American (Flaskerud, 1984).
- East Indian Hindu Americans believe in internal and external forces of control. Uncontrolled psychological factors, such as anger, shame, and envy, make a person more susceptible to disease. They also believe external events or misfortune, such as the wrath of a disease goddess, malevolent spirits of dead ancestors, sins committed in previous lives, or jealous living relatives, cause illness. Hindus wear charms to ward off evil intentions.
- The Chinese culture views mental illness as shameful. Chinese families may wait until a relative's mental illness is unmanageable before seeking Western medicine.

Focus Assessment Criteria

Ineffective coping can be manifested in various ways. A person or family may respond with a disturbance in another functional pattern (eg, spirituality, parenting). The nurse should be aware of this and use assessment data to ascertain the dimensions affected.

Subjective Data
Assess for Defining Characteristics.

Physiologic Stress-Related Symptoms
Cardiovascular
Headache
Chest pain
Increased pulse

Fainting (blackouts, spells)
Palpitations
Increased blood pressure

Respiratory
Shortness of breath
Smoking history

Increased rate and depth of breathing
Chest discomfort (pain, tightness, ache)

Gastrointestinal
Nausea
Vomiting
Abdominal pain

Change in stool
Change in appetite
Obesity/frequent weight changes

Musculoskeletal
Pain
Fatigue

Weakness

Genitourinary
Menstrual changes
Sexual difficulty

Urinary discomforts (pain, burning, urgency, hesitancy)

Dermatologic
Itching
Rash

"Sweats"
Eczema

Perception of Stressor
How have these stressors affected you?
How are the problems working out?

Obtain History of Drinking Pattern from Client or Significant Others (Kappas-Larson & Lathrop, 1993)
What was the day of last drink?
How much was consumed on that day?
On how many days of the last 30 was alcohol consumed?
What was the average intake?
What was the most you drank?

Determine Attitude Toward Drinking by Asking CAGE Questions:
Have you ever thought you should *C*ut down your drinking?
Have you ever been *A*nnoyed by criticism of your drinking?
Have you ever felt *G*uilty about your drinking?
Do you drink in the morning (ie, *E*yeopener; Ewing, 1984)?

Symptoms of Depression (Depression Guideline Panel, 1993)*
Depressed mood most of day, nearly every day
Markedly diminished interest or pleasure in almost all activities most of the day, nearly every day
Significant weight loss/gain
Insomnia/hypersomnia
Psychomotor agitation/retardation
Fatigue (loss of energy)
Impaired concentration (indecisiveness)
Recurrent thoughts of death or suicide

Coping–Self-Awareness (Finkelman, 2000)
What motivates you to get up in the morning?
If 1 is the worst your problem can be and 10 is your problem solved, where are you today?

---

*Diagnostic criteria for a major depressive disorder include that at least five of the eight symptoms and at least one of the first two symptoms must be present most of the day nearly daily for at least 2 weeks.

What would it take to raise the number?
How would you know it was higher than a 6?

Assess for Related Factors.

Current/recent stressors (number, type, duration)
Major life events and everyday stresses
Social—financial change, job pressure, marital/family conflicts, role changes, retirement, pregnancy, marriage, divorce, aging, school, death
Psychological—anxiety, depression, low self-esteem, lack of interpersonal skills, loneliness
Environmental—moving, hospitalization, loss of privacy, sensory deprivation/overload

Objective Data
Assess for Defining Characteristics.

Appearance

Altered affect ("poker" face)	Poor grooming
Appropriate	Inappropriate dress

Behavior

Calm	Sudden mood swings
Hostile	Withdrawn
Tearful	

Cognitive Function

Impaired orientation to time, place, person	Impaired memory
	Impaired judgment
Impaired concentration	
Altered ability to solve problems	

Abusive Behaviors
To Self

Excessive smoking	Reckless driving
Excessive alcohol intake	Suicide attempts
Excessive food intake	Unsafe sexual practices
Drug abuse	

To Others

Does not care	Does not communicate
Is unwilling to listen	Imposes physical harm on family member (bruises, burns, broken bones)
Unsafe sexual practices	
Neglects needs of family members	

In Children, Attention Difficulties (Johnson, 1995)

Difficulty listening	Speech problems
Easily distracted	Reading problems
Difficulty concentrating	Oppositional, stubborn
Impulsivity	Low frustration
Poor judgment	Labile mood
Motor hyperactivity	

For more information on Focus Assessment Criteria, visit http://connection.lww.com.

Goals

NOC Coping, Self-Esteem, Social Interaction Skills

The person will make decisions and follow through with appropriate actions to change provocative situations in personal environment.

Indicators

- Verbalize feelings related to emotional state.
- Focus on the present.

- Identify response patterns and the consequences of resulting behavior.
- Identify personal strengths and accept support through the nursing relationship.

General Interventions

> **NIC** Coping Enhancement, Counseling, Emotional Support, Active Listening, Assertiveness Training, Behavior Modification

Assess Causative and Contributing Factors (Lyon, 2002).

Idealistic expectations of self
Unrealistic goals
Toxic thoughts
Negative self-talk
Clinging to unrealistic expectations of others
Procrastination, poor time management

Establish Rapport.

Spend time with client. Provide supportive companionship.
Avoid being overly cheerful and clichés such as, "Things will get better."
Convey honesty and empathy.
Offer support. Encourage expression of feelings. Let client know you understand his or her feelings. Don't argue with expressions of worthlessness by saying things such as, "How can you say that? Look at all you accomplished in life."
Offer matter-of-fact appraisals. Be realistic.
Allow extra time for the person to respond.

Assess Present Coping Status.

Determine onset of feelings and symptoms and their correlation with events and life changes.
Assess ability to relate facts.
Listen carefully as client speaks to collect facts; observe facial expressions, gestures, eye contact, body positioning, and tone and intensity of voice.
Determine risk of client's inflicting self-harm; intervene appropriately.
   Assess for signs of potential suicide:
   - History of previous attempts or threats (overt and covert)
   - Changes in personality, behavior, sex life, appetite, sleep habits
   - Preparations for death (putting things in order, making a will, giving away personal possessions, acquiring a weapon)
   - Sudden elevation in mood

   See *Risk for Suicide* for additional information on suicide prevention.

Assess Level of Depression.

Severely depressed or suicidal people need environmental controls, usually hospitalization.
Severely depressed people need assistance with decision making, grooming and hygiene, and nutrition.
As depression lifts, people can solve problems and increase their coping behaviors. Involve client in activities. Do not allow social withdrawal.
Teach self-care and stress-reducing skills (Lyon, 2002).

Assist Client to Develop Appropriate Problem-Solving Strategies.

Ask client to describe previous encounters with conflict and how he or she resolved them.
Evaluate whether his or her stress response is "fight or flight" or "tend and befriend" (Taylor et al., 2000).
Encourage client to evaluate his or her behavior: "Did that work for you?" "How did it help?" "What did you learn from that experience?"
Discuss possible alternatives (ie, talk over the problem with those involved, try to change the situation, or do nothing and accept the consequences).
Assist to identify problems that the client cannot control directly; help client to practice stress-reducing activities for control (eg, exercise, yoga).
Be supportive of functional coping behaviors.
   "The way you handled this situation 2 years ago worked well then. Can you do it now?"
   Give options; however, leave the decision making to the client.

Mobilize client to gradually increase activity.

    Identify activities that were previously gratifying but have been neglected: personal grooming or dress habits, shopping, hobbies, athletic endeavors, arts and crafts.

    Encourage client to include these activities in daily routine for a set time span (eg, "I will play the piano for 30 minutes every afternoon.").

    Stress importance of activity in helping client to recover from depression; state that depression is immobilizing and that client must make a conscious effort to fight it to recover.

Explore outlets that foster feelings of personal achievement and self-esteem.

    Make time for relaxing activities (eg, dancing, exercising, sewing, woodworking).

    Find a helper to take over responsibilities occasionally (eg, sitter).

    Learn to compartmentalize (do not carry problems around with you always; enjoy free time).

    Encourage longer vacations (not just a few days here and there).

    Provide opportunities to learn and use stress management techniques (eg, jogging, yoga).

Facilitate emotional support from others.

    Seek out people who share a common challenge: establish telephone contact, initiate friendships within the clinical setting, develop and institute educational and support groups.

    Establish a network of people who understand your situation.

    Decide who can best act as a support system (do not expect empathy from people who themselves are overwhelmed with their own problems).

    Make time to share personal feelings and concern with coworkers (encourage expression; frequently people who share the same circumstances help one another).

    Maintain a sense of humor.

    Allow tears.

Teach self-monitoring tools (Finkelman, 2000).

    Develop a daily schedule to monitor for signs of improvement or worsening.

    Discuss reasonable goals for present relationships.

    Write down what is done when in control, depressed, confused, angry, happy.

    Identify activities tried, would like to try, or should do more.

    Create a warning sign checklist that indicates worsening and how to access help.

Initiate Health Teaching and Referrals, as Indicated.

Prepare for problems that may occur after discharge.

- Medications—schedule, cost, misuse, side effects
- Increased anxiety
- Sleep problems
- Eating problems—access, decreased appetite
- Inability to structure time
- Family/significant other conflicts
- Follow-up—forgetting, access, difficulty organizing time

For depression-related problems beyond the scope of nurse generalists, refer to appropriate professional (marriage counselor, psychiatric nurse therapist, psychologist, psychiatrist).

Instruct client in relaxation techniques; emphasize the importance of setting 15 to 20 min aside each day to practice relaxation.

1. Find a comfortable position in chair or on floor.
2. Close eyes.
3. Keep noise to a minimum (only very soft music, if desired).
4. Concentrate on breathing slowly and deeply.
5. Feel the heaviness of all extremities.
6. If muscles are tense, tighten, then relax, each one from toes to scalp.

Teach assertiveness skills.

Teach use of cognitive therapy techniques.

Rationales

- The person with a chronic mental illness "must be helped to give up the role of being sick for that of being different" (Finkelman, 2000, p. 99).
- Self-monitoring can help the client to learn how to observe symptoms and recognize when he or she needs more intensive help (Finkelman, 2000).
- Coping effectively requires successful maintenance of many tasks: self-concept, satisfying relationships with others, emotional balance, and stress.

- Clients can learn problem-solving techniques:
  - *Goal setting* is consciously setting time limits on behaviors, which is useful when goals are attainable and manageable. It may become stress-inducing if unrealistic or short-sighted.
  - *Information seeking* is learning about all aspects of a problem, which provides perspective and, in some cases, reinforces self-control.
  - *Mastery* is learning new procedures or skills, which facilitates self-esteem and self-control (eg, self-care of colostomies, insulin injection, or catheter care).
  - *Help seeking* is reaching out to others for support. Sharing feelings provides an emotional release, reassurance, and comfort (eg, self-help and support groups).
- Everyone has implicit or explicit goals. Experience develops patterns of successful behavior in achieving these individual goals. A person then regularly uses this behavior to achieve goals. Goals are established to maintain:
  - Physical well-being
  - Self-esteem
  - Productive satisfying interactions with others
- Behavior is such that:
  - People act to meet needs and achieve goals.
  - They develop relatively stable patterns of behavior.
  - Behavior is disrupted when both needs and goals are threatened.
- People who work through the anticipated event (eg, retirement, surgery) are more likely to cope effectively than those who avoid thinking about the upcoming event.
- Optimal intervention can occur only when the defensive attempts have failed and the person has begun to examine the current situation.
- Adaptation is the process by which a person strives to achieve comfortable and effective functioning in the environment. It is not static, but ongoing.
- Cognitive interventions help the person regain control over his or her life. They include identifying automatic thoughts and replacing them with positive thoughts (Finkelman, 2000).

Pediatric Interventions

If attention disorders are present, explain their etiology and behavioral manifestations to child and caregivers.

Help child to understand he or she is not "bad" or "dumb."

Establish target behaviors with child and caregivers.

Work with parents and teachers to learn more effective behavioral strategies to support success.
- Establish eye contact before giving instructions.
- Set firm, responsible limits.
- Avoid lectures, simply state rules.
- Maintain routines as much as possible.
- Attempt to keep a calm and simple environment.
- Reinforce appropriate behavior with a positive reinforcer (eg, praise, hug).

Assist to improve play with peers (Johnson, 1995).
1. Start with short play periods.
2. Use simple, concrete games.
3. Begin with sympathetic siblings or family members.
4. Initially, select a quieter and less demanding peer as playmate.
5. Provide immediate and instant feedback (eg, "I see you are being distracted"; "You are playing nicely").

Initiate health teaching and referrals as needed.

Provide information about medication therapy if indicated.

Consult with specialists as needed (eg, psychological, learning specialists).

Rationales

- Interventions focus on helping the child develop self-control and self-respect.
- Children with attention disorders are often very intelligent and do not need repetitive lectures.

- Routine helps to reduce stress for caregivers and child.
- Children with attention disorders cannot filter extraneous stimuli and, therefore, respond to everything, thus losing focus.
- Success with peers in play is critical for positive reinforcement and self-esteem.

● Geriatric Interventions

Assess for risk factors for ineffective coping in older adults (Miller, 2004):
- Inadequate economic resources
- Immature developmental level
- Unanticipated stressful events
- Several major events in short period
- Unrealistic goals

Rationale

Miller (2004) identifies the following as risk factors for increased stress and poor coping in older adults: diminished economic resources, immature developmental level, unanticipated events, several daily hassles at the same time, several major life events in a short period, high social status, and high feelings of self-efficacy in situations that cannot change.

DEFENSIVE COPING

DEFINITION
Defensive Coping: The state in which a person repeatedly presents falsely positive self-evaluation as a defense against underlying perceived threats to positive self-regard

DEFINING CHARACTERISTICS*
Major (80%–100%)
Denial of obvious problems/weaknesses
Rationalization of failures
Grandiosity

Projection of blame/responsibility
Hypersensitivity to slight criticism

Minor (50%–79%)
Superior attitude toward others
Hostile laughter or ridicule of others
Lack of follow-through or participation in treatment or therapy

Difficulty establishing/maintaining relationships
Difficulty testing perceptions against reality

RELATED FACTORS
See *Chronic Low Self-Esteem, Powerlessness,* and *Impaired Social Interaction.*

---

*Source: Norris, J., & Kunes-Connell, M. (1987). Self-esteem disturbance: A clinical validation study. In A. McLane (Ed.). *Classification of nursing diagnoses: Proceedings of the seventh conference.* St. Louis: C. V. Mosby.

AUTHOR'S NOTE

In selecting this diagnosis, it is important to consider the potentially related diagnoses of *Chronic Low Self-Esteem, Powerlessness,* and *Impaired Social Interaction.* They may express how the person established, or why he or she maintains, the defensive pattern.

Defensive Coping is defined by the person's dysfunction and inability to cope over time. It is reinforced if the nurse can establish a correlation between exacerbations and identified stressors. When a defensive pattern is a barrier to effective relationships, *Defensive Coping* is a useful diagnosis.

KEY CONCEPTS
- Defensive functioning is the ability to use defense mechanisms to protect the ego from overwhelming anxiety. If defensive mechanisms are overused, they become ineffective or ego-defeating (Mohr, 2003).
- See Key Concepts under *Ineffective Coping.*

Focus Assessment Criteria

See *Ineffective Coping.*

Goal

| NOC | Acceptance: Health Status, Coping, Self-Esteem, Social Interaction Skills |

The person will report or demonstrate less defensive behavior.

Indicators
- Identify defensive responses.
- Establish realistic goals in concert with caregivers.
- Work effectively toward achieving these goals.

General Interventions

| NIC | Coping Enhancement, Emotional Support, Self-Awareness Enhancement, Environment Management, Presence, Active Listening |

Reduce Demands on the Client If Stress Levels Increase.

Environmental—Modify the level of or remove environmental stimuli (eg, noise, activity).
Interpersonal—Decrease (or limit) contacts with others (eg, visitors, other clients, staff) as required.
Task—Clearly articulate minimal expectations for activities. Decrease or increase as tolerated.
Therapeutic—Structure interactions with staff so the client knows to whom he or she is to talk, when, for how long, and on what topics.
Strategic—Identify stressors placing demands on the client's coping resources; develop plans to deal with them. The general goal is to freeze, reduce, or eliminate stress; more specifically, it is to target and deal with those stressors most exacerbating the defensive pattern.

Establish a Therapeutic Relationship.

Maintain a neutral, matter-of-fact tone with a consistent positive regard. Ensure that all staff relate in a consistent fashion, with consistent expectations.
Focus on simple, here-and-now, goal-directed topics when encountering the client's defenses.
Encourage client to express goals, and then establish agreement with the client in at least one or two areas. (Note that "reflecting-in" statements, such as, "It sounds like you are saying 'x' " *can* produce declarative statements from the client such as, "No, I'm saying '–x'," which can then be agreed with.)
Do not react to, defend, or dwell on client's negative projections or displacements; also do not challenge distortions or unrealistic/grandiose self-expressions. Try instead to shift to more neutral, positive, or goal-directed topics.
Disengage or allow the client to disengage from disagreement.
Avoid directive statements. Encourage client-initiated activities.
Avoid control issues, or attempt to present positive options to the client, which allows a measure of choice.
Avoid evaluative statements (negative *or* positive). Encourage client to evaluate self-progress.

To limit maladaptive behaviors, identify for client those actions that compromise the achievement of established goals.

To promote learning from the client's own actions (ie, "natural consequences"), identify those actions that have interfered with the achievement of established goals.

Reinforce more adaptive coping patterns (eg, sublimation, formal problem solving, rationalization) that are assisting the person in achieving established goals.

Evaluate interactions, progress, and approach with other team members to ensure consistency within the treatment milieu.

Promote Dialogue to Decrease the Need to Defend and Permit a More Direct Addressing of Underlying, Related Factors (see *Chronic Low Self-Esteem*).

Validate client's reluctance to trust in the beginning. Over time, reinforce the consistency of your statements, responses, and actions. Give special attention to your meeting of (reasonable) requests or your following through with plans and agreements.

Engage client in diversional, non–goal-directed, noncompetitive activities (eg, relaxation therapy, games, outings).

Encourage self-expression of neutral themes, positive reminiscences, and so forth.

Encourage other means for self-expression (eg, writing, art) if verbal interaction is difficult or if this is an area of personal strength.

Listen passively to *some* grandiose or negative self-expression to reinforce your positive regard. If this does not lead to more positive self-expression or activity, then such listening may prove counterproductive.

Establish an ego-support role for yourself by assisting the client to review and examine his interactive patterns with others.

Rationales

- Diversional, supportive interactions must be balanced with goal-directed/problem-focused inter-actions according to client's tolerance.
- Increased stress increases defensive coping (Mohr, 2003).
- Interventions should help put the client at ease and focus on self-evaluation (Mohr, 2003).
- Interventions that increase trust may provide an opportunity to use cognitive appraisal that could reduce the perceived threat.
- If an ego-support role can be established, it is then possible for the client to begin to learn new, more effective coping strategies. Active stressors continue to elicit and reinforce the established defensive pattern, however, so this effort can be limited by the degree to which the client remains stressed or threatened.

INEFFECTIVE DENIAL

DEFINITION

Ineffective Denial: The state in which a person minimizes or disavows symptoms or a situation to the detriment of his health

DEFINING CHARACTERISTICS*
Major (Must Be Present)

Delays seeking or refuses health care attention to the detriment of health
Does not perceive personal relevance of symptoms or danger

*Source: Lynch, C. S., & Phillips, M. W. (1989). Nursing diagnosis: Ineffective denial. In R. M. Carroll-Johnson (Ed.). *Classification of nursing diagnosis: Proceedings of the eighth conference.* Philadelphia: J. B. Lippincott.

Minor (May Be Present)

Uses home remedies (self-treatment) to relieve symptoms
Does not admit fear of death or invalidism
Minimizes symptoms
Displaces source of symptoms to other areas of the body
Cannot admit effects of disease on life pattern
Makes dismissive gestures or comments when speaking of distressing events
Displaces fear of effects of the condition
Displays inappropriate affect

RELATED FACTORS
Pathophysiologic
Related to inability to tolerate consciously the consequences of any chronic or terminal illness

Treatment-Related
Related to prolonged treatment with no positive results

Situational/Psychological
Related to inability to tolerate consciously the consequences of:

Loss of job	Negative self-concept, inadequacy,
Financial crisis	guilt, loneliness, despair,
Substance abuse	sense of failure
Smoking	Alcohol use
Loss of spouse/significant	Obesity
other	Domestic abuse

Related to feelings of increased anxiety/stress, need to escape personal problems, anger, and frustration
Related to feelings of omnipotence
Related to culturally permissive attitudes toward alcohol/drug use

Biologic/Genetic
Related to family history of alcoholism

⚭ **AUTHOR'S NOTE**

Ineffective Denial differs from denial in response to loss. Denial in response to illness or loss is necessary and beneficial to maintain psychological equilibrium. *Ineffective Denial* is not beneficial when the person will not participate in regimens to improve health or the situation (eg, denies substance abuse). If the cause is not known, *Ineffective Denial related to unknown etiology* can be used, such as *Ineffective Denial related to unknown etiology as evidenced by repetitive refusal to admit barbiturate use is a problem.*

⚭ **ERRORS IN DIAGNOSTIC STATEMENTS**

See *Ineffective Coping.*

KEY CONCEPTS
- Denial is a set of dynamic processes that protect the person from threats to self-esteem. It is common in the grieving process.
- When action is essential to change a threatening or damaging situation, denial is maladaptive; however, when no action is needed or when the outcome cannot be changed, denial can be positive and can help reduce stress (Lazarus, 1985).

- A strong, intact denial system interferes with the person's realistic perceptions of the consequences (eg, loss, violence, substance abuse; Boyd, 2002; Tweed, 1989).
- Denial can take several forms:

  Denial of relevance to the person   Denial of immediacy of the threat

  Denial of responsibility   Denial that threat is anxiety-provoking

  Denial of threatening information   Denial of any information

- Denial is a major response in people with addictions. It is the inability to accept one's loss of control over the addictive behavior or severity of the associated consequences (Boyd, 2002).

Focus Assessment Criteria

See *Ineffective Coping* for general assessment.

If substance abuse is suspected:

Subjective Data

Assess for Defining Characteristics.

The person will:

Deny that alcohol/drug use is problematic

Justify use of alcohol/drugs

Blame others for use of alcohol/drugs

Objective Data

The person will demonstrate interference in:

Occupational Functioning

Absenteeism	Daytime fatigue
Frequent unexplained brief absences	Failed assignments
Elaborate excuses	Loss of job

Social Functioning

Mood swings	Isolation (avoidance of others)
Arguments with mate/friends	Violence while intoxicated
Traffic accidents/citations	

Legal Difficulties

Physical Complications

Alcohol Abuse

Blackout	Liver dysfunction
Memory impairment	Gout symptoms
Lower extremity paresthesias	Anemia
Malnutrition	Gastritis/gastric ulcers
Pancreatitis	Cardiomyopathy

Withdrawal symptoms (eg, tremors, nausea, vomiting, increased blood pressure and pulse, sleep disturbances, disorientation, hallucinations, agitation, seizures)

Opiate Abuse

Drowsiness	Impaired memory
Slurred speech	Slowed motor movements
Pupillary constriction	Malnutrition
Skin infections	Respiratory depression
Liver disease	Constipation
Low testosterone levels	Respiratory infections
Gastric ulcers	Decreased response to pain

Withdrawal symptoms (eg, tearing, runny nose, gooseflesh, yawning, dilated pupils, mild hypertension, tachycardia, nausea, vomiting, restlessness, abdominal cramps, joint pain)

Amphetamine and Cocaine Abuse

Hyperactivity	Increased alertness
Skin infections	Decreased appetite/weight loss
Cerebrovascular accident	Increased heart rate
Hallucinations	Dilated pupils
Cardiac dysrhythmias	Chills
Seizures	Nausea and vomiting
Respiratory depression	Hepatitis

Hallucinogen Abuse

Increased heart rate	
Sweating	Tremors
Hallucinations	Incoordination
Flashbacks	Blurred vision

Cannabis Abuse

Dry mouth	Increased appetite
Increased heart rate	Impaired lung structure
Conjunctival infection	Sinusitis

Barbiturate/Sedative–Hypnotic Abuse

Drowsiness	Endocarditis
Impaired memory	Pneumonia
Cellulitis	Respiratory depression
Hepatitis	Signs of intoxication and withdrawal

For more information on Focus Assessment Criteria, visit http://connection.lww.com .

Goal

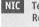 **NOC** Acceptance: Health Status, Anxiety Control, Fear Control, Health Beliefs: Perceived Threat, Active Listening

The person will use alternative coping mechanism instead of denial.

Indicators

- Acknowledge the source of anxiety or stress.
- Use problem-focused coping skills.

General Interventions

NIC Teaching: Disease Process, Anxiety Reduction, Counseling, Active Listening

Initiate a Therapeutic Relationship.
Assess effectiveness of denial.
Avoid confronting client that he or she is using denial.
Approach client directly, matter-of-factly, and nonjudgmentally.

Encourage Client to Share Perceptions of the Situation (eg, Fears, Anxieties).
Focus on the feelings shared.
Use reflection to encourage more sharing.

When Appropriate, Help Client with Problem Solving.
Attempt to elicit from the person a description of the problem.

Rationales

- Partial, tentative, or minimal denial allows the client to use problem-focused coping skills while reducing distress (an emotion-focused coping skill; Lazarus, 1985).
- Denial may be valuable in the early stages of coping, when resources are not sufficient to manage more problem-focused approaches (Lazarus, 1985).
- As denial is reduced, interventions must focus on emerging strong feelings of anxiety and fear.

INEFFECTIVE DENIAL

RELATED TO IMPAIRED ABILITY TO ACCEPT CONSEQUENCES OF OWN BEHAVIOR AS EVIDENCED BY LACK OF ACKNOWLEDGMENT OF SUBSTANCE ABUSE/DEPENDENCY

Goals

> **NOC** Anxiety Control, Coping, Social Support, Substance Addiction Consequences, Knowledge: Substance Use Control, Knowledge: Disease Process

The person will abstain from alcohol/drug use and state recognition of the need for continued treatment.

Indicators

- Acknowledge an alcohol/drug abuse problem.
- Explain the psychological and physiologic effects of alcohol or drug use.
- Abstain from alcohol/drug use.
- State recognition of the need for continued treatment.
- Express a sense of hope.
- Use alternative coping mechanisms to cope with stress.
- Have a plan for high-risk situations for relapse.

Interventions

> **NIC** Coping Enhancement, Anxiety Reduction, Counseling, Mutual Goal Setting, Substance Use Treatment, Support System Enhancement, Support Group

Assist client to improve self-esteem.

Be nonjudgmental.
Assist person to gain an intellectual understanding that this is an illness, not a moral problem.
Provide opportunities to perform successfully; gradually increase responsibility.
Provide educational information about the progressive nature of substance abuse and its effects on the body and interpersonal relationships.
Explain why women are more affected by alcohol (see Key Concepts)

Refer to *Disturbed Self-Esteem* for further interventions.

Instill a Sense of Hope.

Maintain a positive attitude.
Communicate the expectation that the client can overcome problems.
Promote the setting of realistic, short-term goals.
Facilitate interactions with people who have recovered or are recovering.
Discuss the reality of relapse and that several attempts may be necessary.

Provide Interventions Appropriate with the Phase of Addictive Behavior Change.

Precontemplation Phase (Unaware of Problems Related to Addictive Behaviors)
Attempt to raise awareness of problem and its consequences (eg, relationships, job, finances).
Discuss the possibility of change.
Explore feelings about making changes.

Contemplation Phase (Aware of Addiction-Related Problems and Considering Change, but Ambivalent)
Allow client to express past successful attempts.
List the advantages and disadvantages for changing and continuing to use.

Preparation Phase (Intending to take Action within the Next Month or Unsuccessful in the Past Year)
Initiate referrals to the next most acceptable, appropriate, and effective resource for the client.
Assist client to make a specific, detailed plan for change and identify barriers.

Action Phase (Overtly Involved in Behavioral Changes for at least 1 Day)
Reaffirm decision to change.
Emphasize successful actions.
Help client anticipate and prepare for situations that may challenge decisions.

Maintenance Phase (Free of Addictive Behavior for more than 6 Months)
Help client identify strategies to prevent relapse.
Review reasons why change was made.
Review benefits gained from change.

Openly Discuss the Reality of Relapse; Emphasize That Relapse Does Not Mean Failure.

After relapse, help to identify triggers.
Plan an alternative action if triggers are present, eg, call sponsor, take a walk.
Encourage discussions of relapse with other recovering substance abusers.
Emphasize a "one day at a time" philosophy.

Assist Client to Identify and Alter Patterns of Substance Abuse.

Explore situations in which the person is expected to use substance (eg, after work with friends).
Encourage avoidance of situations in which alcohol/drugs are being used.
Assist client to replace drinking/smoking buddies with nonusers. (Alcoholics Anonymous and Narcotics Anonymous are helpful. Each AA/NA group is unique; encourage person to find a comfortable group for him or her.)
Assist client to organize and adhere to a daily routine.
Have client chart (amount, time, situation) alcohol/drug use (useful with early-stage substance abusers resistant to treatment; Metzger, 1988).

Assist Client to Meet Physiologic and Safety Needs.

Observe for signs of withdrawal. See collaborative problem, *PC: Alcohol Withdrawal.*
Provide supportive care throughout detoxification.
Prevent access to abused substances. Monitor visitors and belongings as appropriate.
Assess for any medical consequences of alcohol/drug use:
- Prostatitis
- Fetal alcohol syndrome (mental retardation, malformations, hyperactivity, growth deficiency, cardiac problems)
- White blood cell, red blood cell, platelet deficiencies
- Bleeding tendencies (decreased vitamin K production)
- Peripheral neuropathy, myopathy
- Hypertension
- Cardiac tissue damage, cardiomyopathy
- Gastritis, pancreatitis
- Hepatitis (alcoholic) cirrhosis
- Vitamin metabolism defects
- Esophageal varices, hemorrhoids, ascites
- HIV-positive status or AIDS (high-risk sexual behavior or sharing of needles)

Assess potential for violence; refer to *Risk for Violence* for further interventions.
Assess for suicide potential; refer to *Risk for Self-Harm* for further interventions.
Teach side effects and appropriate interventions associated with medications (eg, disulfiram [Antabuse], methadone, antianxiety drugs [Librium]).

Discuss Alternative Coping Strategies.

Teach relaxation techniques and meditation. Encourage use when client recognizes anxiety.
Teach thought-stopping techniques to use during thoughts about drinking/substance use. Instruct client to say vocally or subvocally, "STOP, STOP" and to replace that thought with a positive one. The client must practice the technique and may need assistance in identifying replacements.
Assist client to anticipate stressful events (eg, job, family, social situations) in which alcohol/drug use is expected; role-play alternative strategies and teach assertiveness skills.
Teach client how to handle anger constructively.

Assist Client to Achieve Abstinence.

Assist client to set short-term goals (eg, stopping one day at a time).

Assist client in structured planning:

- Discard supplies.
- Break contact with dealers/users.
- Avoid high-risk places.
- Structure free time.
- Avoid large blocks of time without activities.
- Plan leisure activities not associated with alcohol/drug use.

Assist client to recognize stressors that lead to substance abuse (eg, boredom, interpersonal situations).

Assist client to evaluate the negative consequences of the behavior. Visualization may be helpful.

When he or she denies alcohol/drug use, look for nonverbal clues to substantiate facts (eg, deteriorating appearance, job performance, social skills).

After you have established a trusting relationship, confront the client's denial.

Discourage client from trying to correct other problems (eg, obesity, smoking) during this time.

Do not attempt to probe past history in early abstinence.

Assist with Resocialization.

Involve client in groups and in establishing an alcohol/drug-free network.

Establish a trusting relationship.

Involve family in the treatment process.

Initiate Health Teaching and Referral, as Indicated.

Refer client to AA, Alanon, AlaTeen.

Refer client to treatment facility.

Teach side effects of drug use.

Provide nutritional counseling.

Rationales

- The client probably has been reprimanded by many and is distrustful. The nurse's personal experiences with alcohol may increase or decrease empathy for the client.
- Historically, alcoholics have been viewed as immoral and degenerate. Acknowledgment of alcoholism as a disease can increase the client's sense of trust.
- Confrontation with family and peers may help break down the client's denial.
- The client may try to focus on the reasons for using alcohol in an attempt to minimize the problem's significance.
- Participation in a structured treatment program greatly increases the chance of successful recovery from alcoholism.
- Recovering alcoholics provide honest, direct confrontation with the realities of the disease.
- Affording the client direct contact with an expert who can help promotes a sense of hope.
- The client's family needs assistance to identify enabling behaviors and strategies for dealing with a recovering or existing alcoholic.
- Denial in alcoholism may include denial of loss of control, family pain, or the alcoholic's part in the family problem. Relatives and colleagues also may exhibit such denial, because acceptance of the problem is difficult.
- Alcohol and drug abuse is reinforced by the drug itself (eg, feelings of being high, increased congeniality, gaining attention) or avoiding unpleasant situations. Treatment approaches must aim at removing identified reinforcers (Smith-DiJulio, 1998).
- The purpose of the interventions is to assist the client to recognize and affirm the negative relationship between denial and resulting adverse consequences (health or social; Smith-DiJulio, 1998).
- "Sobriety in the alcoholic represents a major change and necessitates a redefinition of family member relationships if this change is to be maintained" (Captain, 1989, p. 57).
- Helping families work through manageable changes is critical.
- A substance-dependent person sees the substance as a solution to every problem. He or she needs new problem-solving techniques (Smith-DiJulio, 1998).

Disabled Family Coping
   Related to (Specify), as Evidenced by Domestic Abuse
   Related to (Specify), as Evidenced by Child Abuse/Neglect
High Risk for Disabled Family Coping
   Related to Multiple Stressors Associated With Elder Care

DISABLED FAMILY COPING

DEFINITION

Disabled Family Coping: The state in which a family demonstrates, or is at risk to demonstrate, destructive behavior in response to an inability to manage internal or external stressors due to inadequate resources (physical, psychological, cognitive)

DEFINING CHARACTERISTICS
Major (One Must Be Present)

Abusive or neglectful care of individual(s)
Decisions/actions that are detrimental to family well-being
Abusive or neglectful relationships with other family members

Minor (May Be Present)

Distortion of reality regarding the health problem
Rejection
Agitation
Aggression
Impaired restructuring of a family unit
Intolerance
Abandonment
Depression
Hostility

RELATED FACTORS
Biopathophysiologic

Related to impaired ability to fulfill role responsibilities secondary to:
   Any acute or chronic illness

Situational (Personal, Environmental)

Related to impaired ability to constructively manage stressors secondary to:
Substance Abuse
Alcoholism
Negative role modeling
History of ineffective relationship with own parents
History of abusive relationship with parents

Related to unrealistic expectations of child by parent
Related to unrealistic expectations of parent by child
Related to unmet psychosocial needs of child by parent
Related to unmet psychosocial needs of parent by child

AUTHOR'S NOTE

Disabled Family Coping describes a family with a history of overt or covert destructive behavior or responses to stressors. This diagnosis necessitates long-term care from a nurse therapist with advanced specialization in family systems and abuse.

The use of this diagnosis in this book focuses on nursing interventions appropriate for a nurse generalist in a short-term relationship (eg, emergency unit, nonpsychiatric in-house unit) and for any nurse in the position to prevent *Disabled Family Coping* through teaching, counseling, or referrals.

ERRORS IN DIAGNOSTIC STATEMENTS

1. *Disabled Family Coping related to reports of beatings by alcoholic husband*

This diagnostic statement is formulated incorrectly and legally inadvisable for a nurse to write. Reported beating by a husband with alcoholism is not the contributing factor, but rather a diagnostic cue. This diagnosis should be written as *Disabled Family Coping related to unknown etiology, as evidenced by wife reporting,* "My husband is an alcoholic and beats me frequently." The quoted statement represents the data as reported by the wife, rather than the nurse's judgment.

KEY CONCEPTS
Generic Considerations

- See *Interrupted Family Processes* for Key Concepts of the family.
- Abuse is "willful infliction of physical injury or mental anguish and the deprivation by the caregiver of essential services" (Verwoerdt, 1976, as cited in Smith-DiJulio & Holzapfel, 1998) and nurturing. Patterns of family maltreatment can take many forms, including physical abuse, endangerment, sexual abuse, emotional abuse, neglect, and economic abuse (Smith-DiJulio & Holzapfel, 1998).
- "Battering is a discordant, disrespectful and violent behavior exercised by people to attack or injure another person physically, psychologically and sexuality" (Willis & Porche, 2004, p. 271).
- It is a criminal activity; no matter the reason, battering is an unacceptable response. Never ask a victim of battering why he or she stays; instead, focus on the criminal behavior and protection for the victim.
- Violence and abuse are choices batterers make.
- People involved in family violence have higher levels of depression, suicidal feelings, self-contempt, inability to trust, and inability to develop intimate relationships in later life (Smith-DiJulio & Holzapfel, 1998).
- Children who witness abuse in their homes after 5 or 6 years of age begin to identify with the aggressor and lose respect for the victim (Smith-DiJulio & Holzapfel, 1998).
- The following are characteristics of abusive families:
  - Poor differentiation of individuals within the family
  - Lack of autonomy
  - Insulation from the influence of others; social isolation
  - Desperate competition for affection and nurturance among members
  - Feelings of helplessness and hopelessness
  - Abuse/violence learned as a way to reduce tension
  - Low tolerance for frustration; poor impulse control
  - Closeness and caring confused with abuse/violence
  - Communication patterns characterized by mixed and double messages
  - High level of conflict surrounding family tasks
  - Nonexistent parental coalition
- The role of the victim is a critical factor in child and spouse abuse. It is socially learned and characterized by helplessness. This occurs when victims learn over time that they cannot control their lives.
- Guilt reactions are common among victims; they frequently feel responsible for the incident. This helps to protect them against feelings of powerlessness.

Spouse Abuse

- "Domestic violence is a behavior that is chosen by a batterer in order to exercise power and control over another person. The batterer, and only the batterer, decides to use abusive and violent behavior. A battered partner cannot make the abuser stop being violent and/or abusive, as the batterer chooses to use this behavior as a form of control. A battered partner does not ask for, invite or provoke the abuser to be violent. The batterer does not become violent because of the use or abuse of alcohol and/or drugs." (AWARE, 1994, p. 1)
- The sociologic-cultural factors linked to battering are gender and power dynamics, criminal deviance, structural and institutional hierarchies of male dominance, patriarchy, entitlement, family structure, aggressive behaviors, stereotypical views of women, and the intergenerational transmission of violence as a learned behavior (Willis & Porche, 2004).
- Spouse abuse in the form of beatings occurs in 1% of all families. Some form of violence disrupts 50% of US families. About 20% to 35% of all women presenting at the emergency room or primary

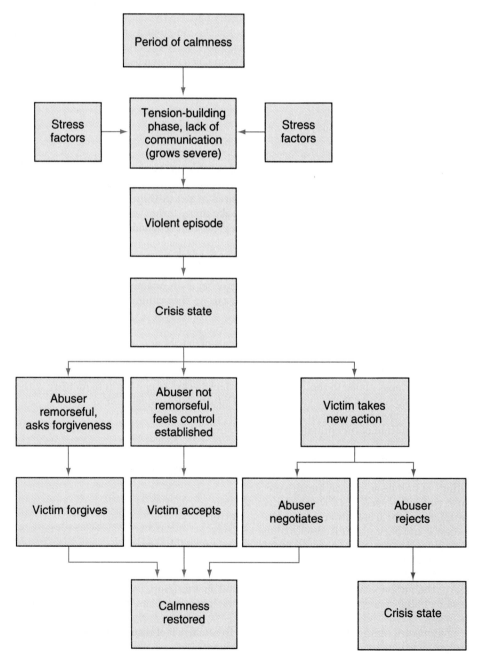

FIGURE II.1 Escalation of violence.

care setting are battered (Chescheir, 1996). Three out of every 100 males severely batter their intimate partners within a 1-year period (CDC, 2003). Fifteen percent of all homicides are spouse killings; 50% of the victims are women. Women usually kill their husbands with guns and knives, whereas husbands usually beat wives to death (Chescheir, 1996; Novello & Soto-Torres, 1992).

- The battered wife syndrome has three major concepts: cycle of violence (Figure II.1), learned helplessness, and anticipatory fear (Blair, 1986).
- Learned helplessness can result from childhood experiences, witnessing or receiving abuse, or the outcome of the battering relationship (Blair, 1986).
- Victims of abuse are "brainwashed by terror." They use denial and rationalization when they remain in the battering relationship (Blair, 1986).
- Battered women rarely report incidents to health care providers; rather, they seek assistance for psychosomatic conditions (chest pain, choking sensations, abdominal pain, fatigue, gastrointestinal disorders, and pelvic pain) or with injuries with inappropriate explanations (Greany, 1984). Victims seldom report abuse because of (Blair, 1986):
  - Feelings of guilt and shame
  - Fear of social stigmatization
  - Fear of the abuser
  - View of violence as normal
  - Lack of alternative resources
- Violent episodes
  - Escalate in frequency and severity over time
  - Require less and less provocation to trigger them
  - Include verbal as well as physical abuse
  - Are made more brutal by alcohol use
- Carlson-Catalano (1998) found that of the battered women in her study, all reported they left to protect another loved one (child or pet). None of the women reported that she left because of her own safety or discomfort.
- Women who attempt to defend themselves during the tension-building phase often succeed in preventing the beating, whereas women who attempt to defend themselves during the assaultive phase often sustain a more brutal beating.
- The abuser's ability to control his spouse directly increases his feelings of autonomy and esteem. Therefore, the fear of loss (and loss of control) of his spouse directly influences his feelings about himself.
- Factors contributing to a battered woman's remaining in the relationship follow:
  - Belief that children need a two-parent family
  - Lack of financial support
  - Lack of a place to go
  - Belief that the abuse will stop
  - Fear for her life or her children's lives
  - Fear of unknown future
- Personal characteristics of the abuser include the following (Else et al., 1993; Smith-DiJulio & Holzapfel, 1998):
  - History of a family devoid of love, affection, and security
  - Unfulfilled, overwhelming need for love and security
  - Unrealistic expectations about others (usually spouse or child) as being able to fill void from childhood, resulting in feelings of rejection, anger, and abuse
  - Blaming of outside factors for everything that goes wrong; blaming of wife for causing him to get angry
  - Denial of the violence or minimizing its severity
  - Impulsiveness
  - Excessive dependence on and jealousy of spouse (usually the only significant relationship he has)
  - Fear of losing her, which can contribute to suicide, homicide, depression, or anger
  - Belief in male supremacy
- Personal characteristics of the battered woman include the following:
  - Low self-esteem, defining of self in terms of partner
  - Unrealistic hopes for change
  - Belief that she has incited her husband to beat her and is to blame
  - Raised in a family that restricted emotional expression (eg, anger, hugging)
  - Subscribing to the feminine sex-role stereotype
  - History of marrying to escape restrictive, confining family

- Extreme resourcefulness and self-sufficiency to survive
- Usually not abused as a child and did not witness abuse
- View of herself as a victim with no option but to appease her spouse
- Gradually increased social isolation
- Belief that partner "can't help it"
- The likelihood of a woman seeking and using assistance for abuse increases if (Sammons, 1981):
  - She has been in the relationship less than 5 years.
  - She is employed.
  - She has friends or relatives who live nearby (within a few miles).
  - She discussed the abuse with others.
  - The abuse is frequent (daily, weekly), severe (requires medical treatment/hospitalization), or increasing in frequency.

❖ Pediatric Considerations

- About 3 million cases of suspected child abuse and neglect were reported in 1994, with 2022 deaths (National Center on Child Abuse and Neglect, 1995). Westat, Inc., conducted a federally funded study in 1986 and estimated that the professionals surveyed failed to report almost 40% of sexually abused children, 30% of fatal or serious physical abuse cases, almost 50% of moderate physical abuse cases, and 70% of neglect cases. At the same time, an equally serious problem is a high number of "unfounded" (not indicated) reports of child maltreatment (Besharov, 1990).
- The discrepancy between the reported cases of child abuse and neglect and the estimated number is related to differences in laws defining abuse/neglect, professionals' failure to recognize the signs, ignorance of the law, fear of court involvement, and lack of faith in child protective services. Professionals report only about one third of cases they recognize (Wissow, 1994).
- The nurse may come in contact with an abused child in an emergency room, school, or physician's office or in her personal life (Kauffman, Neill & Thomas, 1986).
- "Child neglect is defined as the failure of the child's parents or caretaker to provide the child with the basic necessities of life, when financially able to do so or when offered reasonable means to do so" (Cowen, 1999, p. 401). Basic necessities are shelter, nutrition, health care, supervision, education, affection, and protection (Cowen, 1999).
- Family interactions in neglectful families are "more chaotic, less able to resolve conflict, less cohesive, less verbally expressive and less warm and empathetic (Cowen, 1999, p. 409).
- In one study, 85% of cases of neglected children had a parent who was indifferent, intolerant, or overanxious (Browne, 1989).
- Child abuse is a symptom of a family in crisis or a family dysfunction. The crisis can be illness, financial difficulties, or any recent change in the family unit (eg, new members, loss of a member, relocation; Cowen, 1999; Kauffman et al., 1986).
- Separation of the infant from its parents, as in the case of prematurity, can reduce the attachment and nurturing behaviors of the mother toward her child. A disproportionate number of abused children were premature or ill at birth (Kauffman et al., 1986).
- Children usually are abused by someone they know: parent, babysitter, relative, or friend of the family.
- Factors that contribute to child abuse include the following (Wong, 2003):
  - Lack or unavailability of extended family
  - Economic conditions (eg, inflation, unemployment)
  - Lack of role model as a child
  - High-risk children (eg, unwanted, undesired sex or appearance, physically or mentally handicapped, hyperactive, terminally ill)
  - High-risk parents (eg, single, adolescent, emotionally disturbed, alcoholic, drug addicted, physically ill)
- Characteristic personal patterns of abusers include the following (Kauffman et al., 1986):
  - No dominant ethnic or socioeconomic characteristics
  - History of abuse by and lack of warmth and affection from parents
  - Social isolation (few friends or outlets for tensions)
  - Marked lack of self-esteem, with low tolerance for criticism
  - Emotional immaturity and dependency

(continued)

Pediatric Considerations (continued)

- Distrust of others
- Inability to admit the need for help
- Unrealistic expectations for/of child
- Desire for the child to give them pleasure
- The nonabusing parent, who is usually passive and compliant in the abuse, must be included in the treatment plan (Kauffman et al., 1986).
- The effects of abuse on the parent include termination of parental rights, angry reactions from professionals, court proceedings and court-ordered treatment, reactions of family members and community, and financial obligations (from medical and legal expenses).

Maternal Considerations

- Studies have shown that 3.9% to 8% of women are battered during pregnancy (Campbell, Poland, Waller & Ager, 1992).
- Low birth weight correlates with trauma to the fetus and battering.

Geriatric Considerations

- Elder mistreatment is defined as maltreatment, intentional or unintentional, resulting from actions or inactions of others, within the context of a relationship. Types include physical and psychological mistreatment, neglect, misuse of property, and violation of personal rights (Miller, 2004). Older adults are increasingly vulnerable to mistreatment as they become economically, physically, socially, and emotionally more dependent and resources of caretakers are limited.
- Estimates are that 1.2 million elders are abused or mistreated each year (Fulmer & Paveza, 1998). Theories of causation include intrafamily violence, learned behavior (cycle of family violence), psychopathology of the abuser, dependency of the elder, dependency of the caregiver, lack of social support, caregiver burden, and poor health of the elder or caregiver (Fulmer & Paveza, 1998).
- According to Miller (2004), mandatory reporting laws do not require reporters to know that abuse or neglect has occurred, but merely to report it if they suspect it.

Transcultural Considerations

- Domestic violence is cross-cultural. It exists in every culture and is a sign of individual and family dysfunction.
- Traditional Native American life did not include spouse or child abuse. Unfortunately, domestic violence has evolved and is frequently alcohol-related.

Focus Assessment Criteria

Owing to the complexity and variability of this nursing diagnosis, the nurse must determine the type and extent of the assessment each family needs.

Individual Coping Patterns of Adult Members

Refer to assessment criteria for *Ineffective Coping*.

Family Coping Patterns

Refer to assessment criteria for *Interrupted Family Processes.*

Parenting Patterns

Refer to assessment criteria for *Interrupted Parenting.*

Violence Potential

Refer to assessment criteria for *Risk for Violence.*

Subjective Data
Assess for Defining Characteristics.

*Domestic Abuse**

Have you ever been emotionally or physically abused by your partner or someone important to you?

In the last year, have you been hit, slapped, kicked, or otherwise physically hurt by someone?

Are you or have you ever been pregnant? If yes, have you been hit, slapped, kicked, or otherwise physically hurt by someone? If yes, by whom? How many times?

Within the last year, has anyone forced you to have sexual activities? If yes, who? Number of times?

Are you afraid of your partner or anyone else you listed above?

Has your partner:

Tried to choke you?	Been violent to your children?
Threatened you with a weapon?	Been violent outside the home?
Threatened to try suicide?	Threatened to kill you?

Does your partner:

Drink to excess?	Control all the money?
Use drugs?	Destroy possessions?
Try to control your daily activities?	Try to control who your friends are?
Have a gun?	Exhibit violent jealousy?

Subjective/Objective Data
Assess for Defining Characteristics.

Child Abuse Suspicion

Trauma (fractures, lacerations, bruises, welts, burns, dislocations)

Unexplained or unwitnessed injuries

Nature and extent of injury not consistent with explanation

Injuries in various stages of healing

Injuries to face

Abdominal injuries

Multiple bruises (trunk, buttocks, wrists, ankles, ears, neck, around mouth)

Fractures (rib, metaphyseal, scapular, distal clavicle, all humerus fractures [except supracondylar] in children younger than 3 years, vertebral fractures or subluxations, midshaft ulnar fractures, bilateral fractures)

Bruises of varied colors:

Red, black, or blue	Immediate to 5 days
Green	5 to 7 days
Yellow	7 to 10 days
Brown	10 to 14 days

Physical indicators of sexual abuse

Vaginal or penile discharges	Venereal diseases
Genital or anal injuries or swelling	Pain or itching in genital area
Pain while urinating	Difficulty walking

Behavioral indicators

Wary of adult contact	Afraid to go home
Fearful of parents	High pain threshold
Excessive effort to please	Excessive seeking of affection

---

*Source: Nursing Research Consortium on Violence and Abuse, 1989.

Indicators of neglect (subjective, objective; Cowen, 1999; Heindl 1979)

Hunger	Abandonment
Inappropriate dress for weather	Poor growth patterns
	Delinquency
Consistent lack of supervision	Assumes adult responsibilities
	Constant fatigue or listlessness
Unattended medical or dental needs	

How soon was medical care sought? Immediately after injury? Day or more later?

Is medical care sought at the same place or are different places used? Why?

Caregiver–sibling interaction

Is child afraid of adult?	Are they interacting with each other?
Is adult concerned?	Does child report problem with sibling?
What happens during fights?	

Assess for Related Factors.

Employment status

Unemployed	Job satisfaction

Housing

Physical space: adequate, crowded	Privacy
	Cleanliness

Transportation

Car	Proximity to work/school/shopping
Bus	Shared
Dependency on other	

Financial

Resources	Medical expenses
Additional expenses	

Caregiver (Cowen, 1999)

Poor coping skills	Psychological problems
Substance abuse	Poor impulse control
Depression	Limited household management skills
Limited finances	Inadequate support system

Child/elder care provisions

Who shares burden	Legal history
Change in job/school status	History of criminal/delinquent offenses

For more information on Focus Assessment Criteria, visit http://connection.lww.com.

Goals

NOC Caregiver Emotional Support, Family Coping, Family Normalization

The person will set short-term and long-term goals for change.

Indicators

- Appraise unhealthy coping behaviors for family members.
- Relate expectations for self and family.
- Relate community resources available.

General Interventions

NIC Caregiver Support, Referral, Emotional Support, Family Therapy, Family Involvement Promotion

Assist Members to Appraise Family Behaviors.

Discuss the Effects of Behaviors on Individuals and Family Unit.

Emotions	Roles
Support	Performance

Assist family to Set Short-Term and Long-Term Goals.
Promote Family Stabilization.
Ask each family member to identify one activity he or she would like to add to their family.
Identify stressors that can be reduced or eliminated. Ask each family member to identify one behavior he or she could control.
Begin to help members to work through resentments of the past.

Improve Family Cohesiveness.
Determine family recreational activities that include all members and are enjoyable.

Initiate Referrals as Needed.
Support groups   Family therapy

Rationales

- Interventions focus on helping the family renegotiate roles and patterns of interacting and functioning.
- Each family member is provided an opportunity to share feelings about the present and past (Smith-DiJulio & Holzapfel, 1998).
- Families with a dysfunctional member (eg, an alcoholic) are assisted to see that the entire family is dysfunctional, not just the individual.
- Short-term goals focus on stabilizing the family as much as possible. Long-term goals focus on changes needed in functioning and establishing patterns to foster lasting change.
- Dysfunctional families have a history of isolation. Interventions focus on increasing their socialization and use of community resources.
- Family recreational activities foster family cohesion with positive experiences.

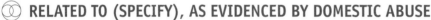

DISABLED FAMILY COPING

 RELATED TO (SPECIFY), AS EVIDENCED BY DOMESTIC ABUSE

Domestic abuse is defined as any action intended to harm another person (physical, emotional, financial, social, sexual).

Goal

NOC Family Coping, Family Normalization, Family Functioning, Abuse Protection, Abuse Cessation

The person will seek assistance for abusive behaviors.

Indicators
- Discuss the physical assaults.
- Identify factors that contribute to violence.
- Seek assistance for abusive behavior; legally and emotionally.
- Relate community resources available when help is desired.

Interventions

NIC Caregiver Support, Emotional Support, Referral, Counseling, Decision-Making Support, Support Group, Anger Control Assistance, Abuse Protection Support: Domestic Partner, Conflict Mediation

Interventions to address the complexity and magnitude of the problems inherent in domestic violence usually are beyond the scope of a nurse generalist. Those provided here are to assist the nurse who has a short-term interaction with a client.

Develop Rapport.

Interview in private. Be empathic.
Don't assume you know what the person needs.
Ask, "How can I help you?"
Avoid displaying shock or surprise at the details.
If contact is made by phone, find out how to get in touch with the victim.

Evaluate Potential Danger to Victim and Others.

Assess Actual Physical Abuse:
Current and past physical/sexual abuse
When did it happen last?
Are you hurt now?
Are the children hurt?
Assess danger to children.

Assess Support System:
Does she have a safe place to go?
Does she want police called?
Does she need an ambulance?

Assess Drug and Alcohol Use:
Is victim using drugs/alcohol?
Is abuser using drugs/alcohol?

Assess for Factors that Inhibit Victims from Seeking Aid.

Personal Beliefs

Fear for safety of self or
  children
Low self-esteem
Myths ("It is normal" or
  "It will stop")

Fear of embarrassment
Guilt (punishment justified)

Lack of Knowledge of

The severity of the problem
Legal rights

Community resources

Lack of Financial Independence

Lack of Support System

Encourage Decision Making.

Provide an opportunity to validate abuse and talk about feelings; if the acutely injured person is accompanied by spouse/caregiver who is persistent about staying, make an attempt to see the person alone (eg, tell her you need a urine specimen and accompany her to the bathroom).
Be direct and nonjudgmental.
  How do you handle stress?
  How does your partner or caregiver handle stress?
  How do you and your partner argue?
  Are you afraid of him?
  Have you ever been hit, pushed, or injured by your partner?
Provide options but allow client to make a decision at her own pace.
Encourage a realistic appraisal of the situation; dispel guilt and myths.
  Violence is not normal for most families.
  Violence may stop, but it usually becomes increasingly worse.
  The victim is not responsible for the violence.
Establish a safety and/or escape plan (refer to abuse specialists).

Assess for Risk Factors Associated with Murder and Suicide.

Discuss Factors with Individual:

Increased frequency or severity of violence	Violence outside home
	Use of weapon or threat with weapon
Choking	Gun in house
Forced sex	Drug use
Death threats	Drunk every day or almost every day
Control of most or all of client's activities	Violent jealousy
	Violence toward children
Suicide threat or attempt	

Provide Referral Information.

Discreetly inform of community agencies available to victim and abuser (emergency and long-term).

Hotlines	Legal services
Shelters	Counseling agencies

Discuss the availability of the social service department for assistance.

Consult with legal resources in the community and familiarize the victim with state laws regarding:

Eviction of abuser	Counseling
Temporary support	Protection orders
Criminal law	Types of police interventions

Refer for individual, group, or couples counseling.

Explore strategies to reduce stress and more constructively manage stressors (eg, relaxation exercises, walking, assertiveness training).

Document Findings and Dialogue for Possible Future Court Use (Blair, 1986).

Occurrence, frequency

Type of injury

Record suspect injuries when "the pattern of injuries is inconsistent with the history."

Initiate Health Teaching if Indicated.

Teach the community (eg, parent–school organizations, women's clubs, programs for schoolchildren) about the problem of spouse/elder abuse.

Instruct caregivers in how properly to manage an elderly client at home (eg, transferring to chair, modified appliances, how to maintain orientation).

Refer for financial assistance and transportation arrangements.

Refer for assertiveness training.

Inform family of senior citizen centers or day care programs.

Refer the abuser to the appropriate community service (only refer men who have asked for assistance or admitted their abuse, because revealing the wife's confidential disclosure may trigger more abuse).

To secure additional information, contact National Clearinghouse on Domestic Violence, P.O. Box 2309, Rockville, MD 20852; www.ncodv.org.

Rationales

- Nursing interventions should focus on safety and protection.
- Nurses must be cautious not to pressure the victim into a premature decision.
- Strategies to address domestic violence must be carefully planned with experts.
- Consequences of rash decisions can be fatal.
- The nurse must openly dispel myths that offer explanations and tolerance for battering and give an illusion of control and rationality (Smith-DiJulio & Holzapfel, 1998).
- Information and referrals are provided to encourage decision making.
- A safety plan is a specific plan for a fast escape if the victim identifies "now is the time to leave" (eg, destination, money, articles of clothing, insurance information, essential items, medications).
- Battering interventions must take place in the context of a coordinated community and criminal justice response to battering.

DISABLED FAMILY COPING

RELATED TO (SPECIFY), AS EVIDENCED BY CHILD ABUSE/NEGLECT

Child abuse is an action or inaction that brings injury to a child, including physical and psychological injury, neglect, and sexual abuse.

Goal

NOC Family Coping, Family Normalization, Family Functioning, Abuse Protection, Abuse Cessation

The child will be free from injury or neglect.

Indicators

Receive comfort from another caretaker.
The parent will receive assistance for abusive behavior.

Indicators

Acknowledge abusive behaviors.

General Interventions

NIC Caregiver Support, Emotional Support, Counseling, Decision-Making Support, Support Group, Anger Control Assistance, Abuse Protection Support: Child, Conflict Mediation, Referral

Identify Families at Risk for Child Abuse.

Refer to Key Concepts.

Intervene with Families at Risk.

Establish a relationship with parents that encourages them to share difficulties ("Being a parent is sure difficult [frustrating] work, isn't it?").
Provide parents with access to information about parenting and child development (see *Delayed Growth and Development*).
Provide anticipatory guidance relative to growth and development (eg, the need to cry in early months; toilet training).
Stress the importance of support systems (eg, encourage parents to exchange experiences with other parents).
Encourage parents to allow time for their own needs (eg, exercise three times a week).
Discuss with parents how they respond to parental frustrations (share feelings with other parents) and instruct them not to discipline children when very angry.
Explore other methods of discipline aside from physical punishment.
Refer parents to expert help.
Inform parents of community services (telephone hotlines, clergy).

Identify Suspected Cases of Child Abuse.

Assess for and evaluate:

Evidence of maltreatment (refer to Focus Assessment Criteria)
History of incident or injury
- Conflicting stories
- Story improbable for child's age
- Story not consistent with injury
Parental behaviors
- Seeks care for a minor complaint (eg, cold) when other injuries are visible

- Shows exaggerated or no emotional response to the injury
- Is unavailable for questioning
- Fails to show empathy for child
- Expresses anger or criticism of child for being injured
- Demands to take child home if pressured for answers

Child behaviors

- Does not expect to be comforted
- Adjusts inappropriately to hospitalization
- Defends parents
- Blames self for inciting parents to rage

Report Suspected Cases of Child Abuse.

Know your state's child abuse laws and procedures for reporting child abuse (eg, Bureau of Child Welfare, Department of Social Services, Child Protective Services).

Maintain an objective record (Cowen, 1999):

Health history, including accidental or environmental injuries

Detailed description of physical examination (nutritional status, hygiene, growth and development, cognitive and functional status)

Environmental assessment of home (if in community)

Description of injuries

Verbal conversations with parents and child in quotes

Description of behaviors, not interpretation (eg, avoid "angry father," instead, "Father screamed at child, 'If you weren't so bad this wouldn't have happened.' ")

Description of parent–child interactions (eg, shies away from mother's touch)

Promote a Therapeutic Environment.

Provide the Child with Acceptance and Affection.

Show child attention without reinforcing inappropriate behavior.

Use play therapy to allow child self-expression.

Provide consistent caregivers and reasonable limits on behavior; avoid pity.

Avoid asking too many questions and criticizing parent's actions.

Ensure that play and educational needs are met.

Explain in detail all routines and procedures in age-appropriate language.

Assist Child with Grieving if Foster Home Placement is Necessary.

Acknowledge that child will not want to leave parents despite severity of abuse.

Allow opportunities for child to express feelings.

Explain reasons for not allowing child to return home; dispel belief it is a punishment.

Encourage foster parents to visit child in hospital.

Provide Interventions that Promote Parent's Self-Esteem and Sense of Trust.

Tell them it was good that they brought the child to the hospital.

Welcome parents to the unit and orient them to activities.

Promote their confidence by presenting a warm, helpful attitude and acknowledging any competent parenting activities.

Provide opportunities for parents to participate in child's care (eg, feeding, bathing).

Promote Comfort and Reduce Fear for Child (Smith-DiJulio & Holzapfel, 1998).

Do not display anger, horror, or shock.

Do not blame abuser.

Reassure child that he or she was not "bad" or at fault.

Do not pressure child to give answers.

Do not force child to undress.

Initiate Health Teaching and Referrals, as Indicated.

Provide Anticipatory Guidance for Families at Risk.

Assist individuals to recognize stress and to practice management techniques (eg, plan for time alone away from child).

Discuss the need for realistic expectations of the child's capabilities.

Teach about child development and constructive methods for handling developmental problems (enuresis, toilet training, temper tantrums); refer to Bibliography.

Discuss methods of discipline other than physical (eg, deprive the child of favorite pastime: "May not ride your bike for a whole day"; "May not play your stereo").

Emphasize rewarding positive behavior.

Report Abusive Parents to Community Agencies and Refer to Professionals for Counseling.

Disseminate Information to the Community About Child Abuse
(eg, Parent–School Organizations, Radio, Television, Newspaper).

Discuss with parents and parents-to-be the problems of parenting.

Teach those who are at risk of being future abusers.

Discuss constructive stress management.

Teach the signs and symptoms of abuse and the method for reporting.

Focus on abuse as a problem resulting from child-rearing difficulties, not parental deficiencies.

Relay your understanding of stresses, but do not condone abuse.

Focus on the parent's needs; avoid an authoritative approach.

Take opportunities to demonstrate constructive methods for working with children (give the child choices; listen carefully to the child).

Consider developing parenting classes for parents (preventive, corrective) to increase their skills as nurturers and teachers. Weekly topic examples:

What is parenting?	Child development and play
Discipline and toilet training	Play and nutrition
Safety and health	Discipline and common problems
Parental needs	Expectations vs realities (Seditus & Mock, 1988)

Rationales

- Identification of child abuse depends on recognizing the physical signs, specific parent behavior, specific child behavior, inconsistencies in injury history, and contributing factors (eg, familial, environmental; Boyd, 2002; Kauffman et al., 1986).
- The nurse should consult the legislation mandating the reporting of child abuse for the specifics of legal definition, penalties for failure to report, reporting procedure, and legal immunity for reporting (Kauffman et al., 1986).
- The first priority of care for the abused child is preventing further injury (Wong, 2003).
- Successful interactions with abusing parents must be provided in the context of acceptance and approval to compensate for their low self-esteem and fear of rejection (Wissow, 1994).
- Strong negative feelings can interfere with the nurse's judgment and effectiveness (Smith-DiJulio & Holzapfel, 1998).
- Parents' involvement in the treatment plan may help stop abuse.
- Children, being egocentric, assume they are responsible for the maltreatment or neglect (Wong, 2003).
- Programs that teach parents to interpret and understand their children's behaviors and to give appropriate responses can reduce child maltreatment (Wissow, 1994).
- The color of a bruise can determine when it occurred (Patterson, 1998).
- Primary prevention (public awareness, community education, parenting classes, nutrition programs) is directed at the general population. Secondary prevention is directed at high-risk groups. Home-based and center-based programs have had positive outcomes (eg, home visitation programs, substance abuse/mental health referrals, crisis intervention; Cowan, 1999).

HIGH RISK FOR DISABLED FAMILY COPING

RELATED TO MULTIPLE STRESSORS ASSOCIATED WITH ELDER CARE

Goal

The caregiver will acknowledge the need for assistance with abusive behavior.

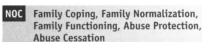

NOC Family Coping, Family Normalization, Family Functioning, Abuse Protection, Abuse Cessation

Indicators

- Discuss the stressors of elder care.
- Relate strategies to reduce stressors.
- Identify community resources available.

The older adult will be free of abusive behavior.
- Describe methods to increase socialization beyond caregiver.
- Identify resources available for assistance.

Interventions

NIC Caregiver Support, Emotional Support, Counseling, Support Group, Decision-Making Support, Anger Control Assistance, Abuse Protection Support: Elder, Conflict Mediation, Referral

Identify Individuals (Caregiver, Older Adult) at High Risk for Abuse or Neglect.

Caregiver
Social isolation
Dependency on elder (financial, emotional); coresidency
Health problems (physical, mental)
Substance abuse
Poor relationship history with elder
Financial problems
Transgenerational violence
Relationship problems

Older Adult
Dependent on others for activities of daily living
Isolation
Financial insecurity
Impaired cognitive functioning
Depressive personality
History of abuse to caregiver
Incontinence

Assist Caregivers to Reduce Stressors.

Establish a relationship with caregivers that encourages them to share difficulties.
Encourage them to share experiences with others in same situation.
Evaluate caregiver's ability to provide long-term in-home care.
Explore sources of help (eg, housekeeping, home-delivered meals, day care, respite care, transportation assistance).

Encourage caregiver to discuss sharing responsibilities with other family members.

Discuss alternative sources of care (eg, nursing home, senior housing).

Discuss how caregiver can allow time for personal needs.

Discuss community resources available for help (eg, crisis hotline, social service, voluntary emergency caregivers).

Refer also to *Caregiver Role Strain.*

Assist Older Adults to Reduce Risks of Abuse.

Encourage contact with old friends and neighbors if living with relative.

Plan a weekly contact in person with friend, neighbor.

Encourage client to participate in community activities as much as possible.

Help client take care of own personal needs.

Encourage client to have his or her own telephone.

Assist client to acquire legal advice for possible future disability.

Ensure client is not accepting personal care in exchange for transfer of assets or property without legal advice.

Ensure client is not living with someone who has a history of violence or substance abuse.

Identify Suspected Cases of Elder Abuse (Fulmer & Paveza, 1998).

Signs include the following:

   Failure to adhere to therapeutic regimens, which can pose threats to life (eg, insulin administration, ulcerated conditions)

   Evidence of malnutrition, dehydration, elimination problems

   Bruises, swelling, lacerations, burns, bites

   Pressure ulcers

   Caregiver not allowing nurse to be alone with elder

Consult with home health nurse to plan a home visit for assessment of signs of abuse or neglect (Smith-DiJulio & Holzapfel, 1998):

   House in poor repair

   Inadequate heat, lighting, furniture, or cooking utensils

   Unpleasant odors

   Inaccessible food

   Old food

   Older adult lying on soiled materials (eg, urine, food)

   Medication not being taken

   Garbage

Report Suspected Cases.

Consult with supervisor for procedures for reporting suspected cases of abuse.

Maintain an objective record, including:

   Description of injuries   Conversations with elder and caregivers

   Description of behaviors   Nutritional, hydration status

Consider the elder's right to choose to live at risk of harm, providing he or she is capable of making that choice.

Do not initiate an action that could increase the elder's risk of harm or antagonize the abuser.

Respect the elder's right to secrecy and the right for self-determination.

Initiate Health Teaching and Referrals, as Indicated.

Refer high-risk caregivers for counseling.

Refer elder for counseling to explore choices.

Explore support services (eg, respite, home health aide, homemaker services).

Disseminate information to community regarding prevention.

   Publicize support services.

   Seek to assist caregiving families (eg, companions, respite care, day care centers).

   Seek to establish weekly contact with dependent elderly.

   Attempt to reduce isolation of caregivers and elders.

   Develop procedures for investigation, public education.

Rationales

- Strategies for management of abuse include identification, access and assessment, intervention, follow-up, and prevention.
- Multiple, interrelated variables seem responsible for elder abuse. Invisibility of the problem and vulnerability of the older person are common to all cases (Miller, 2004).
- Steinmetz (1988) reported that caregivers' perceptions of stress and feelings of burden are strong predictors of elder abuse.
- Abused elders usually do not report abuse because of fear of reprisal or abandonment. Rather, elder abuse must be detected.
- Interventions focus on assisting caregivers to reduce stress and select constructive coping responses (Miller, 2004).
- Educational programs serve to advocate for elders and to raise the consciousness of the community.
- Each state has specific guidelines for reporting suspected cases of elder abuse.
- Caregivers need an opportunity to share their feelings of frustration and stress.

COMPROMISED FAMILY COPING

DEFINITION

Compromised Family Coping: That state in which a usually supportive primary person (family member or close friend) is providing insufficient, ineffective, or compromised support, comfort, assistance, or encouragement that may be needed by the client to manage or master adaptive tasks related to his or her health challenge

DEFINING CHARACTERISTICS
Subjective Data

Client expresses or confirms a concern or complaint about significant other's response to his or her health problem.

Significant person describes preoccupation with personal reactions (eg, fear, anticipatory grief, guilt, anxiety) to client's illness, disability, or to other situational or developmental crises.

Significant person describes or confirms an inadequate understanding or knowledge base, which interferes with effective assistive or supportive behaviors.

Objective Data

Significant person attempts assistive or supportive behaviors with less than satisfactory results.

Significant person withdraws or enters into limited or temporary personal communication with the client at time of need.

Significant person displays protective behavior disproportionate (too little or too much) to the client's abilities or need for autonomy.

RELATED FACTORS

See *Interrupted Family Processes.*

> ⊗ AUTHOR'S NOTE
>
> This nursing diagnosis describes situations similar to the diagnosis *Interrupted Family Processes.* Until clinical research differentiates this diagnosis from the aforementioned diagnosis, use *Interrupted Family Processes.*

READINESS FOR ENHANCED FAMILY COPING

DEFINITION

Readiness for Enhanced Family Coping: Effective managing of adaptive tasks by family member involved with the client's health challenge, who now is exhibiting desire and readiness for enhanced health and growth in regard to self and in relation to the client

DEFINING CHARACTERISTICS

Family member attempting to describe growth impact of crisis on his or her own values, priorities, goals, or relationships

Family member moving in direction of health-promoting and enriching lifestyle that supports and monitors maturational processes, audits and negotiates treatment programs, and generally chooses experiences that optimize wellness

Individual expressing interest in making contact on a one-to-one basis or on a mutual-aid group basis with another person who has experienced a similar situation

RELATED FACTORS

See *Health-Seeking Behaviors* and *Interrupted Family Processes*.

> ⓒ **AUTHOR'S NOTE**
>
> This nursing diagnosis describes components found in *Interrupted Family Processes* and *Health-Seeking Behaviors*. Until clinical research differentiates the category from the aforementioned categories, use *Interrupted Family Processes* or *Health-Seeking Behaviors*, depending on the data presented.

INEFFECTIVE COMMUNITY COPING

DEFINITION

Ineffective Community Coping: The state in which a community's pattern of activities for adaptation and problem solving is unsatisfactory for meeting the demands or needs of the community

DEFINING CHARACTERISTICS
Major (Must Be Present)

Community does not meet its own expectations
Unresolved community conflicts
Expressed difficulty in meeting demands for change
Expressed vulnerability

Minor (May Be Present)

Angry   Bitter   Indifferent
Apathetic   Helpless   Hopeless
Overwhelmed

RISK FACTORS

Presence of risk factors (see Related Factors)

RELATED FACTORS
Situational

Related to lack of knowledge of resources
Related to inadequate communication patterns
Related to inadequate community cohesiveness
Related to inadequate problem solving
Related to inadequate community resources
Related to inadequate law-enforcement services
Related to overwhelming community destruction secondary to:
Flood   Hurricane
Earthquake   Epidemic
Avalanche

Related to traumatic effects of:
Airplane crash   Industrial disaster
Large fire   Environmental accident

Related to threat to community safety (eg, murder, rape, kidnapping, robberies)
Related to sudden rise in community employment

Maturational

Related to inadequate resources for:
Children   Working parents
Adolescents   Older adult

⊗ AUTHOR'S NOTE

This diagnosis is useful for nurses who practice with aggregates. An *aggregate* is a group of people "who have in common one or more personal or environmental characteristics" (Williams, 1977). Thus, an aggregate can be the population of a small town, high-school girls, or Hispanic men with hypertension in Philadelphia.

This diagnosis may be used more frequently as a risk than an actual diagnosis. Nurses practicing with community aggregates would identify risk factors for *Ineffective Community Coping.* The focus would be on prevention.

⊗ ERRORS IN DIAGNOSTIC STATEMENTS

1. *Ineffective Community Coping related to unresolved community conflicts*
Unresolved community conflicts are a sign of *Ineffective Community Coping,* not a contributing factor. The nurse needs to assess the community for causes of unresolved conflicts, such as lack of knowledge or insufficient resources.

TABLE II.6 Differences Between Community and Home Health Care

Community Health Care: Continuous	Home Health Care: Episodic
Targets populations	Targets individuals, families
Focuses on groups that do not seek care	Focuses on individuals who seek care
Emphasizes wellness and primary prevention	Emphasizes restoring health after an acute episode

KEY CONCEPTS

- "In community settings, there is a generally broader focus on both physical and mental health than on the disease per se and on the variables that affect health directly or indirectly, such as life style, family interaction patterns and community resources (public transportation and adequate housing)" (Aroskar, 1979, p. 36).
- Community health care differs from home health care. See Table II.6.
- The goal of epidemiology is to identify populations at risk to institute programs and services that prevent or halt progression of disease (Clemen-Stone, Eigasti & McGuire, 2002).
- Community competence describes the collective functioning of the total community unit.
- A competent community has four important characteristics (Allender & Spradley, 2001):
  - It collaborates effectively to identify community needs and problems.
  - It achieves a working consensus on goals and priorities.
  - It agrees on ways and means to implement the agreed-on goals.
  - It collaborates effectively in the required actions.
- Interventions with communities are categorized the same way as with individuals: primary, secondary, and tertiary prevention.
  - Primary prevention means interventions that seek to strengthen the normal line of defense. Examples include immunization programs and classes for adults to prevent osteoporosis.
  - Secondary prevention means interventions that seek to detect and treat existing health problems at the earliest stage possible. Examples include hypertension-screening programs and teaching breast or testicular self-examinations to high-school students.
  - Tertiary prevention means interventions that attempt to reduce the extent and severity of a health problem and to reestablish system equilibrium. An example would be posters to warn children playing in vacant lots about rats. Another example is Alcoholics Anonymous.
- Community health nursing interventions can be grouped under the categories of educative, engineering, and enforcement.
  - Educative interventions provide knowledge to foster preventive health behaviors.
  - Engineering focuses on environmental modification to reduce or eliminate barriers to healthy living (eg, unsafe walkways).
  - Enforcement involves using regulatory agencies to promote health and to protect the community (Clemen-Stone et al., 1997).

Focus Assessment Criteria

Assess for Defining Characteristics.

Expressed vulnerability
History of unresolved conflicts
Response to present situation

Angry	Indifferent	Bitter
Apathetic	Helpless	Overwhelmed
Hopeless		

Assess for Related Factors.

Support Available

Financial	Housing	Counseling
Food	Clothing	

Problem-Solving Ability

Past	Present

Adequacy of Community Resources

Emergency relief (funds, food, shelter)?	Law enforcement?
	Counseling?
Required health services?	Community meeting place?

Community Limitations

Lack of cohesiveness	Inadequate communication system
Isolating patterns	Inadequate information

Channels of Communication
Closed   Disregards subgroups
Top-down style

For more information on Focus Assessment Criteria, visit http://connection.lww.com.

Goal

NOC Community Competence, Community Health Status, Community Risk Control

The community will engage in effective problem solving.

Indicators

- Identify problem.
- Access information to improve coping.
- Use communication channels to access assistance.

General Interventions

NIC Community Health Development, Environmental Risk Protection, Program Development, Risk Identification

Assess for Causative or Contributing Factors.

Lack of knowledge of available resources
Inadequate problem solving
Inadequate communication links
Value conflicts
Threat to community safety

Provide Opportunities for Community Members to Meet and Discuss the Situation (eg, Schools, Churches, Synagogues, Town Hall).

Demonstrate acceptance of their anger, withdrawal, or denial.
Correct misinformation as needed.
Discourage blaming.

Promote Community Competence in Coping.

Focus on community goals, not individuals.
Engage subgroups into group discussions and planning.
Ensure resource access for all members (eg, flexible hours for working members).
Devise a method for formal disagreements.
Evaluate each decision's impact on all community members.

Explore Techniques that May Improve Coping; Elicit Suggestions from the Group.

Discuss Resources that Can Be Accessed; Prepare the Group to Accept Outside Help.

Emergency shelter, funds, food, clothes
Counseling
Transportation
Health care

Plan How to Access Isolated People in Community.

Establish a Method to Access Information and Support (eg, Local Health Department, Hospital, Churches, Synagogues, Community Center).

Initiate Referrals as Indicated.

Counseling
Public assistance

Rationales

- Assessment of the community involves studying the interacting variables that influence its health (Spradley, 1996).
- Certain behaviors or beliefs (eg, anxiety, fear, value conflicts) can interfere with problem solving. They should be explored in discussions (Clemen-Stone et al., 2002).
- Community-oriented nursing addresses the health needs of aggregates at risk and ways to organize the community to meet the identified needs.
- Spradley described essential conditions for community competence (1996):
  - A high degree of awareness that "we are a community"
  - Use of natural resources while taking steps to conserve them for future generations
  - Open recognition of subgroups and encouragement of their participation in community affairs
  - Ready to meet crises
  - Problem solving: community identifies, analyzes, and organizes to meet its own needs
  - Open channels of communication that allow information to flow among all subgroups of citizens in all directions
  - Desire to make each resource available to all members of the community
  - Legitimate and effective ways to settle disputes
  - Encouragement of maximum citizen participation in decision making
  - Promotion of high-level wellness among all its members

The interventions for *Ineffective Community Coping* ideally would be secondary, not tertiary, prevention. Interventions to treat early community disequilibrium can prevent serious problems.

READINESS FOR ENHANCED COMMUNITY COPING

DEFINITION

Readiness for Enhanced Community Coping: A state in which a community's pattern for adaptation and problem solving is satisfactory for meeting the demands or needs of the community, but the community desires to improve management of current and future problems/stressors

DEFINING CHARACTERISTICS
Major (Must Be Present)

Successful coping with a previous crisis

Minor (May Be Present)

Active planning by community for predicted stressors
Active problem solving by community when faced with issues
Agreement that community is responsible for stress management
Positive communication among community members
Positive communication between community/aggregates and larger community
Programs available for recreation and relaxation
Resources sufficient for managing stressors

RISK FACTORS

Presence of risk factors (see Related Factors)

RELATED FACTORS
Situational

Related to availability of community programs to augment (specify)

Nutritional status	Exercise program	Weight control
Self-actualization	Stress management	Social support

Maturational

Related to availability of community programs to augment coping with life cycle events, such as

Aging	Parenting	Adolescence
Retirement	Pregnancy	"Empty nest"

ⓒ AUTHOR'S NOTE

This diagnosis can be used to describe a community that wishes to improve an already effective pattern of coping. For a community to be able to be assisted to a higher level of functioning, its basic needs for food, shelter, safety, a clean environment, and a supportive network must first be addressed. When these needs are met, programs can focus on higher functioning, such as wellness and self-actualization. Community programs can be designed after a community assessment and because of community requests. They can focus on enhancing health promotion with topics related to optimal nutrition, weight control, regular exercise programs, constructive stress management, social support, role responsibilities, and preparing for and coping with life cycle events such as retirement, parenting, and pregnancy.

> ⊕ **ERRORS IN DIAGNOSTIC STATEMENTS**
>
> *Readiness for Enhanced Coping related to present destructive response to the flood disaster*
>   When a community is assessed as having a destructive response to a disaster, *Readiness for Enhanced Coping* is incorrect. The diagnosis should be *Ineffective Community Coping*. Interventions would focus on problem solving and accessing resources to promote effective coping.

KEY CONCEPTS

- A community has five major elements: goals, needs, environment, service system, and boundaries (Clemen-Stone, Eigasti & McGuire, 1997). Communities are a social unit "of people living in an environment that has the ability to meet their life goals and needs" (Clemen-Stone et al., 2002, p. 97).
- Communities have six common components (Clemen-Stone et al., 2002):
  - *People.* People are the most important resource or core of the community. Functional, cohesive communities have shared values.
  - *Goals/needs:* Goals and needs of individuals and groups in the community reflect the community goals and needs. As in Maslow's hierarchy, a community must have fulfilled needs in physiology, safety, and social affiliation before meeting higher needs of esteem and self-actualization.
  - *Community environment:* The environment (climate, natural resources, buildings, food, water supply, flora, animals, insects, economics, health and welfare services, leadership, social networks, recreation, and religion) has major effects on health.
  - *Service systems:* These are a network of agencies and organizations in the community that help to meet the basic needs (social welfare, education, economic) and the health needs of the community.
  - *Boundaries:* These define communities. Some boundaries are concrete, such as geographic, political (eg, cities, states), or situational (eg, home, school, work). Interests define conceptual boundaries (eg, book clubs).
- Communities have functions to achieve life goals and needs of the population:
  - *Production/distribution/consumption:* Goods and services that are essential for community well-being and functioning are available. Tax funds are used to fund this system.
  - *Socialization:* This is the process of relating in a social environment. Knowledge, values, beliefs, customs, and behaviors are transmitted to community members.
  - *Social control:* Norms and rules of social control provide safety and order. Law agencies, courts, and government enforce social order.
  - *Social participation:* Interactions with others meet basic needs for self-expression and self-fulfillment.
  - *Mutual support:* Communities provide networks of people helping each other as individuals, religious groups, and official agencies.
- Rural communities have fewer than 2500 residents. Rural people are more self-reliant and reluctant to seek assistance from others (Bushy, 1990). Researchers have found that rural people "define health as the ability to work and to do what needs to be done" (Bushy, 1990, p. 89). They do not value comfort, cosmetic issues, and health promotion. They access health care services when they cannot work (Bushy, 1990).
- Rural communities often resist outsiders' ideas and prefer health care professionals who live in their community. Because people all know one another, however, they are reluctant to ask for help or share problems for fear neighbors will find out (Bushy, 1990).
- For a community with a history of effective coping with problems and stressors, the community nurse can offer programs and services to promote high-level wellness. These programs would focus on:
  - Optimal nutrition
  - Weight control
  - Stress management
  - Exercise programs
  - Self-actualization
  - Social support
  - Coping with life cycle events
- Life cycle events are predictable developmental tasks of young adults, middle-aged adults, and older adults. These events include (Clemen-Stone et al., 1997):

Young Adult (18 to 35 Years)
- Gaining autonomy from parents
- Selecting and choosing a career

- Developing an intimate relationship
- Developing parenting skills
- Developing personal lifestyle
- Accepting one's citizen's role

Middle-Aged Adult (35 to 65 Years)
- Evaluating one's career
- Helping children become autonomous
- Sustaining a few deep friendships
- Supporting aging parents
- Participating in civic or social activities
- Maintaining home property
- Having satisfying leisure time
- Adapting to changes associated with aging

Older Adult (65 Years and Older)
- Being flexible in views
- Seeking to update knowledge
- Seeking to develop mutually supportive relationships with children and the younger generation
- Nurturing partner relationships
- Adjusting to personal losses
- Helping aged parents
- Using increased leisure time pleasurably
- Preparing for retirement or another career
- Adapting to losses associated with aging
- Involving community leaders in planning can increase community commitment and participation with their personal influence (Clemen-Stone et al., 2002).
- Effective community functioning can be promoted when service systems are functioning to reduce community member stressors (Clemen-Stone et al., 2002).
- Programs to reduce developmental-related stressors can reduce tension-producing stimuli that can disrupt a community (Clemen-Stone et al., 2002).
- Health care program planning provides an orderly structure for organizing large quantities of data to achieve community health goals successfully (Clemen-Stone et al., 2002).

Focus Assessment Criteria

Community Screening Assessment (Clemen-Stone et al., 2002)

When assessing each area, consider the community's major strengths and needs.

Population
Density
Composition

Gender ratio	Ethnic origins
Age distribution	Race distribution

Characteristics

Mobility	Educational level
Socioeconomic status	Level of employment

Mortality rates

Overall rate	Age-specific rates
Leading causes of death	Maternal mortality

Morbidity rates
Specific disease incidence rates
Community norms
Values, attitudes
Family composition

Environmental

Climate	Types and frequency of natural disasters
Housing types	Air quality
Water supply, quality	Industrial pollutants, toxins
Types of animals, insects, reptiles	

Health Systems
Emergency
Hospitals
Long-term care
Preventive services

Hospice, respite
Home care
School health services
Ambulatory services

Public Assistance
Type available
Transportation
Meals

Housing
Special services

Public Safety
Police
Ambulance

Fire

Education
Public
Libraries
Educational level of
  members

Private
Special educational services (eg, health)

Economic
Major industry
Banks, credit unions
Sources of income
Percentage of retired
  people

Major occupations
Median income
Percentage of population below

poverty level

Government
Official leadership
Accessibility

Town, city offices

Recreation
Public
Private
Recreational activities
  (frequently used)

Leisure activities (frequently used)
Programs for special populations

Religion
Types

Community programs, services

Communication Ability
TV, radio
Local newspaper

Community groups

For more information on Focus Assessment Criteria, visit http://connection.lww.com.

READINESS FOR ENHANCED COMMUNITY COPING

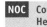 **RELATED TO AVAILABILITY OF COMMUNITY PROGRAMS TO AUGMENT (SPECIFY)**

Goal

NOC Community Competence, Community Health Status, Community Risk Control

The community will provide programs to improve well-being.

Indicators

- Identify health promotion needs.
- Access resources needed.
- Develop programs based on needs assessment.

Interventions

| NIC | Program Development, Risk Identification, Community Health Development, Environmental Risk Protection |

Meet with Influential Community Members to Determine Health Promotion Needs (Archer, 1983).

For what needs of members could the nursing agency develop services?
How can the agency promote or market the services to motivate people to use them?
Will enough members of the targeted population use the service?
Based on past programming, what improvements can be made for the future?
Are similar services provided by another agency or organization (hospital, religious)?

Plan Programs Targeted for a Specific Population.

Adolescents (13 to 18 years)
Career planning   Stress management

Pregnant Women
Adolescent   Adult

Young Adults (18 to 35 years)
Career selection   Constructive relationships
Balancing one's life   Parenting issues

Middle Age (35 to 65 years)
Launching children   Reciprocal relationships
Aging parents

Older Adults (65 Years and Older)
Aging parents   Balancing one's life
Retirement issues   Facts and myths of aging

All Ages
Civic planning   Meeting needs of all community members
Crisis intervention   Grieving

Define the Target Health Promotion Needs.

Analyze assessment of community (eg, risk groups, health problems). Prioritize the needs:
  Severity of the risk
  Probability of success
  Cost–benefit ratio (eg, resources available)
Select a health promotion program.
Identify target population (eg, entire community, older adults, adolescents).
Delineate a timetable for the planning and implementation stages.

Develop Detailed Program Objectives and the Evaluation Framework to be Used.

Content   Time needed
Ideal teaching method for   Teaching aids (eg, large-print materials)
  targeting group

Establish Resources Needed and Sources.

Space   Transportation facilities
Optimal day of week   Optimal time of year
Supplies, audiovisual   Financial (budgeted, donations)
  equipment

Market the Program.

Media (eg, newspaper, TV,   Posters (food market, train station)
  radio)   Word of mouth (religious organizations,
Flyers (distribute via   community clubs, schools)
  school to home)

Guest speaker (community
clubs, schools)

**Provide Program and Evaluate Whether Desired Results (Objectives)
Were Achieved.**

Number of participants	Negative feedback
Objectives achieved	Actual expenditures vs budgeted
Statistics (eg, bicycle accidents)	Participant evaluations
	Revisions for future planning
Adequate planning	Shared responsibility

Rationales

- In population-based planning, assessment involves conducting a needs assessment, analyzing data, prioritizing needs, and setting objectives (Clemen-Stone et al., 2002).
- Life cycle events are predictable developmental tasks of young adults, middle-aged adults, and older adults. (Refer to Key Concepts for specifics.) Programs in the community can be planned to assist persons with adapting successfully to life cycle events (Clemen-Stone et al., 2002).
- Programs focusing on strategies to promote high-level wellness can also target specific age groups.

DECISIONAL CONFLICT

DEFINITION

Decisional Conflict: The state in which a person/group experiences uncertainty about a course of action when the choice of options involves risk, loss, or challenge to personal life values

DEFINING CHARACTERISTICS
Major (80% to 100%)

Verbalized uncertainty about choices
Verbalization of undesired consequences of alternatives being considered
Vacillation between alternatives
Delayed decision making

Minor (50% to 79%)

Verbalized feeling of distress while attempting a decision
Self-focusing
Physical signs of distress or tension (eg, increased heart rate, increased muscle tension, restlessness) whenever the decision comes within focus of attention
Questioning of personal values and beliefs while attempting to make a decision

RELATED FACTORS

Many situations can contribute to decisional conflict, particularly those that involve complex medical interventions of great risk. Any decisional situation can precipitate conflict for a person; thus, the examples listed below are not exhaustive, but reflective of situations that may be problematic and possess factors that increase the difficulty.

Treatment-Related

Related to risks versus the benefits of (specify test, treatment):
Surgery

Tumor removal	Orchiectomy	Mastectomy

Cosmetic surgery
Amputation
Transplant
Diagnostics
Amniocentesis
Chemotherapy
Radiation
Dialysis
Mechanical ventilation
Enteral feedings
Intravenous hydration
Use of preterm labor medications
Participation in treatment study trials
HIV antiviral therapy

Prostatectomy
Hysterectomy
Laminectomy

X-rays

Joint replacement
Cataract removal
Cesarean section

Ultrasound

Situational

Related to risks versus the benefits of:
Personal
Marriage
Breast vs bottle feeding
Parenthood
Sterilization
In vitro fertilization
Transport from rural facilities
Work / Task
Career change
Professional ethics

Circumcision
Divorce
Abortion
Artificial insemination
Adoption
Separation

Business investments

Institutionalization
  (child, parent)
Contraception
Nursing home placement
Foster home placement

Relocation

Related to
Lack of relevant information

Confusing information

Related to
Disagreement within support systems
Inexperience with decision making
Unclear personal values/beliefs
Conflict with personal values/beliefs
Resignation
Family history of poor prognosis
Hospital paternalism—loss of control
Ethical dilemmas of:
  Quality of life
  Cessation of life-support
    systems
  "Do not resuscitate" orders

Termination of pregnancy
Organ transplant
Selective termination with multiple-
  gestation pregnancies

Maturational

Related to risks versus benefits of:
Adolescent
Peer pressure
Alcohol/drug use
Career choice
Use of birth control
Adult
Career change
Older adult
Retirement

College
Whether to continue a
  relationship

Relocation

Nursing home placement

Sexual activity
Illegal/dangerous situations

Retirement

○○ **AUTHOR'S NOTE**

The nurse has an important role in assisting clients and families with making decisions. Because nurses usually do not benefit financially from decisions made regarding treatments and trans-
(continued)

> ⊚⊚ **AUTHOR'S NOTE** (*Continued*)
>
> fers, they are in an ideal position to assist with decisions. Although, according to Davis (1989), "nursing or medical expertise does not enable health care professionals to know the values of patients or what patients think is best for themselves," nursing expertise does enable nurses to facilitate systematic decision making that considers all possible alternatives and possible outcomes, as well as individual beliefs and values. The focus is on assisting with logical decision making, not on promoting a certain decision.
>
> *When people are making a treatment decision of considerable risk, they do not necessarily experience conflict. In situations where the treatment option is "choosing life," individual perception may be one of submitting to fate and be relatively unconflicted. Because of this, nurses must be cautious in labeling patients with the nursing diagnosis of 'Decisional Conflict' without sufficient validating cues (Soholt, 1990).*

> ⊚⊚ **ERRORS IN DIAGNOSTIC STATEMENTS**
>
> 1. *Decisional Conflict related to failure of physician to gain permission for mechanical ventilation from family*
>   In such a situation, this statement represents an unprofessional and legally problematic approach. Failure of the physician to gain permission for mechanical ventilation would be a practice dilemma necessitating formal reporting to the appropriate parties. Should the family have evidence that the client did not desire this treatment (ie, a living will), this situation would not be described as *Decisional Conflict,* because there is no uncertainty about a course of action. The nurse should further assess the family for responses fitting other nursing diagnoses, such as *Grieving.*
> 2. *Decisional Conflict related to uncertainty about choices*
>   Uncertainty about choices validates *Decisional Conflict;* it is not a causative or contributing factor. If the person needed more information, the diagnosis would be *Decisional Conflict related to insufficient knowledge about choices and effects.*

KEY CONCEPTS
Generic Considerations

- An antecedent condition of decision making is a problem. Problems exist when goals are to be attained and there is uncertainty about an appropriate solution. A problem suggests more than one alternative solution.
- Making a decision is a systematic process—a means, rather than an end. Decision making is sequential—each step builds on the previous one. Optimal decision making is more likely when done systematically, but it does not necessarily have to be a rigid, step-by-step process.
- The logical steps of decision making are well identified in clinical practice. They can be summarized in the following steps:
    1. Defining the problem
    2. Listing the possible alternatives or options
    3. Identifying the probable outcomes of the various alternatives
    4. Evaluating the alternatives based on actual or potential threats to beliefs/values
    5. Making a decision
- People usually are not taught a systematic method for making a decision, so they rely frequently on past experiences and intuition. The intuitive mode of decision making is characterized by interaction and association among ideas that seem to coexist simultaneously (Soholt, 1990).
- Soholt (1990) identified that the following factors may influence a person when making a health care treatment decision:
    - Reliance on the truth of medical advice
    - Submission to fate when the treatment option is "choosing life"
    - Consideration of values
    - Regard for public opinion

- The decision-making process is complicated when there is a need for a rapid decision. Making an intelligent decision during acute stress is difficult, if not impossible. The stress can be enormous if a sense of urgency compounds the decision.
- Decisional conflict occurs when a person has simultaneous opposing tendencies to accept or reject a course of action (Janis & Mann, 1977).
- Decisional conflict becomes more intense when it involves a threat to status and self-esteem.
- Decisional conflict is greater when none of the alternatives is good.
- Jezewski (1993) reported that both intrapersonal and interpersonal conflict occurs when do-not-resuscitate decisions are being made. Intrapersonal conflict results from discord with individual values and life events. The most common interpersonal conflict arises between staff and family members and among family members.
- There are essentially three decision-making models in health care:

Paternalism
- Health care providers make all the decisions regarding client care.
- Decisions are based on a perceived need to protect the client.
- Locus of control is external to the client and significant others.

Consumerism
- Health care providers give the client and significant others only the information they request.
- Decisions are based on the premise that the client knows best.
- Locus of control is internal for the client and significant others.

Humanism/Advocacy
- Health care providers collaborate with the client and significant others to arrive at a decision.
- Decisions are based on mutual respect for individual dignity and worth.
- Locus of control is shared; all participants have an equal role in decision making.
- The most important right that a person possesses is the right of self-determination, or the right to make the ultimate decision concerning what will or will not be done to his or her body. Choice is facilitated when a person is free to make it.
- Not all clients desire the same degree of control over treatment decision making. The need to play an active, collaborative, or passive role is very individualized and must be assessed carefully.
- Perception of the effect of a treatment on a client's life may be more important in his or her decision than considerations of the medical effectiveness (Kelly-Powell, 1997).
- Value conflicts often lead to confusion, indecision, and inconsistency. Decision making is more complicated when a client's goals conflict with those of significant others. People may decide against their values if the need to please others is greater than the need to please themselves.
- One study found that older adults' end-of-life decisions were strongly related to their religiosity and values regarding preservation of life and quality of life (Cicirelli & MacLean, 2000). Those who preferred "to hasten death were less religious and place a higher value on quality of life" (Cicirelli & MacLean, 2000, p. 414). Most of the study group favored hastening death if terminally ill, regardless of religious beliefs (Cicirelli & MacLean, 2000).

Pediatric Considerations

- In most cases, children do not make major decisions for themselves. A surrogate, usually a parent, must make the decision on the child's behalf.
- A child's ability to understand a situation and make a decision depends on age, developmental level, and past experience. Understanding, however, should not be confused with legal competence.
- As adolescents mature, their ability to analyze problems and make decisions increases.
- Researchers working with children should seek assent from children with a mental age of 7 years or older. Parents must give written, informed consent for the child to participate in the study (Wong, 2003).

⊙ Geriatric Considerations

- Decisions are often made for, not with, older adults.
- Barriers to decision making for older adults include dementia, depression, long-term passivity, and hearing or other communication problems (Miller, 2004).
- Reasons why decision makers exclude older adults from involvement in decisions that profoundly affect their lives include beliefs that older adults are incompetent, not qualified, or not interested, and the desire to avoid discussion of sensitive topics (eg, finances, relocation; Miller, 2004).
- Family members making a decision to place an older family member in a long-term facility found information from health care professionals inadequate. Friends who validated the situation were most helpful.

🌐 Transcultural Considerations

- Fatalism is a belief that little can be done to change life events and the best response is submission and acceptance. Americans of Latin, Irish, Appalachian, Filipino, Puerto Rican, and Russian Orthodox origins frequently have this external focus of control (Giger & Davidhizar, 1999).
- Northern European and African Americans have been found to have both internal and external foci of control (Giger & Davidhizar, 2003).
- One study indicated that Mexican-American and Korean-American elders referred end-of-life decisions to family members (Blackhall et al., 1995).

Focus Assessment Criteria

Decisional conflict is a subjective state that the nurse must validate with the client. The nurse should assess each person to determine his or her level of decision making within the conflict situation. Some of the same cues may be seen in people with *Hopelessness, Powerlessness,* and *Spiritual Distress.*

Subjective Data
Assess for Defining Characteristics.

Decision-making patterns
"Tell me about the decision you need to make."
"How would you describe your usual method of making decisions?"
"How involved would you like to be in making the decision?"

Perception of the conflict
"How do you feel when you think about the decision you have to make?"
"Has there been a change in your sleep patterns, appetite, activity level?"

Assess for Related Factors.
"Why is this a stressful decision for you?"
"What things make you uncomfortable about deciding?"
"In the past, how did you arrive at decisions that had a positive outcome?"
"What decisions have you made that you felt confident about?"
"When you make a decision, do you do it alone or do you like to involve other people? If so, whom do you consult for advice?"

Objective Data
Assess for Defining Characteristics.

Body language
Posture (rigid)   Facial expression (annoyed, tense)
Hands (rigid, wringing)   Eye contact (darting)

Motor activity
Immobile   Pacing
Increased   Agitation

Affect
Labile   Flat
Inappropriate

For more information on Focus Assessment Criteria, visit http://connection.lww.com.

Goal

 NOC Decision Making, Information Processing, Participation: Health Care Decisions

The individual/group will make an informed choice.

Indicators

- Relate the advantages and disadvantages of choices.
- Share fears and concerns regarding choices and responses of others.
- Define what would be most helpful to support the decision-making process.
- Make an informed choice.

General Interventions

NIC Decision-Making Support, Mutual Goal Setting, Learning Facilitation, Health System Guidance, Anticipatory Guidance, Patient Right Protection, Values Clarification, Anxiety Reduction

Assess Causative/Contributing Factors.

Lack of experience with or ineffective decision making
Value conflict
Fear of outcome/response of others
Insufficient/inconsistent information
Controversy with support system
Unsatisfactory health care environment

Reduce or Eliminate Causative or Contributing Factors.

Internal
Lack of experience with or ineffective decision making
Review past decisions and what steps were taken to help the person decide.
Facilitate logical decision making.
1. Assist the person to recognize the problem and to clearly identify the needed decision.
2. Generate a list of all possible alternatives or options.
3. Help identify the probable outcomes of the various alternatives.
4. Aid in evaluating the alternatives based on actual or potential threats to beliefs/values.
5. Encourage the person to make a decision.
Encourage significant others to be involved in the entire decision-making process.
Suggest the person use significant others as a sounding board when considering alternatives.
Respect and support the role that the person desires in the decision, whether it is active, collaborative, or passive.
Be available to review the needed decision and the various alternatives.
Facilitate refocusing on the needed decision when the person experiences fragmented thinking during high anxiety.
Encourage the person to take time in deciding.
With adolescents, focus on the present—what will happen versus what will not. Help identify the important things, because they do not have extensive past experiences on which to base decisions.
Value conflict (also refer to Spiritual Distress*)*
Assist client to explore personal values and relationships that may affect the decision.
Explore obtaining a referral with the person's spiritual leader.
Use values clarification techniques to assist client to review the parts of his or her life that reflect his or her beliefs.
1. Help client to identify his or her most prized and cherished activities.
2. Ask reflective statements that lead to further clarification.
3. Review past decisions in which the person needed to publicly affirm opinions and beliefs.
4. Evaluate stands the person has taken on controversial subjects. Does he or she view them in black-and-white terms, or various shades of gray?
5. Identify values the person is proud of. Rank them in order of importance.
Encourage the person to base decision on the most important values.

Support the decision—even if decision conflicts with your own values.
Fear of outcome / response of others (also refer to Fear*)*
Provide clarification regarding potential outcomes and correct misconceptions.
Explore with the person what the risks of not deciding would be.
Encourage expression of feelings.
Promote self-worth.
Encourage the person to face fears.
Encourage the person to share fears with significant others.
Actively reassure the client that the decision is his or hers to make and that he or she has the right to do so.
Assist client to recognize that it is his or her life; if he or she is comfortable with the decision, others will respect the conviction.
Reassure the person that individuality is acceptable.

External
Insufficient or inconsistent information
Provide information comprehensively and sensitively.
Correct misinformation.
Give concise information that covers the major points when the decision must be made quickly.
Inform the person of his or her right to know.
Enable client to determine the amount of information that he or she desires.
Encourage verbalization to determine the person's perception of choices.
Ensure that the person clearly understands what is involved in the decision and the various alternatives (ie, informed choice).
Encourage the person to seek second professional opinions regarding health.
Collaborate with other health care members/significant others to determine appropriate timing for truthfulness.
Controversy with support system
Reassure client that he or she does not have to give in to pressure from others, whether family, friends, or health professionals.
Advocate for client's wishes if others attempt to undermine his or her ability to make the decision personally.
Identify leaders within the support system and provide information.
Advocate for the client if the family/significant others are excluding him or her from decision making.
Recognize that the person may become ambivalent about "choosing" when putting the needs of the support system above his or her own.
Unsatisfactory health care environment
Establish a trusting and meaningful relationship that promotes mutual understanding and caring.
Provide a quiet environment for thought; reduce sensory stimulation.
Allow uninterrupted periods with significant others.
Promote accepting, nonjudgmental attitudes.
Reduce the number of small decisions that the person must make to facilitate focusing on the decision in conflict.

Explore End-of-Life Decisions.
Explore with client and family whether they have discussed and recorded their end-of-life decisions.
Describe the possible future dilemmas when these discussions are avoided.
Instruct client and family to provide directives in the following areas:
> Person to contact in emergency
> Person individual trusts most with personal decisions
> Decision to be kept alive if client will be mentally incompetent or terminally ill
> Preference to die at home, hospital, no preference
> Desire to sign a living will
> Decision regarding organ donation
> Funeral arrangements, burial, cremation
> Circumstances (if any) when information should be withheld from individual

Document these decisions and make two copies (retain one and give one to the person who is designated to be the decision maker in an emergency).
Discuss the purpose of a living will. Provide information when requested. To obtain a copy of your state's living will, write to the Society for the Right to Die, 250 West 57th Street, New York, NY 10107.

Rationales

- Physical and mental fatigue limits the ability to concentrate or to make a rational decision (Pinch & Spielman, 1990).
- Mastering content for effective decision making requires time. Time allows a person to choose the option that provides the most benefit with the least risk.
- Difficult decisions create stress and conflict, because values and actions are not congruent. Conflict may lead to fear and anxiety that negatively affect decision making. External resources become very important for the person in decisional conflict with a low level of self-confidence in making autonomous decisions.
- Sims, Boland, and O'Neill (1992) interviewed families involved in caregiving and concluded that the process by which a person "frames" a problem is key to understanding decision making. They observed that values, feelings, and previous experiences significantly influenced caregivers' decision making. Information caregivers lack to make a decision is balanced by their intimate "person-specific" knowledge about the client.
- Resolution of decisional conflict may be impossible in settings such as critical care (Hiltunen, 1994). Decision making may be delayed until physiologic stressors have lessened.
- Roberts, Krouse, and Michaud (1995) involved students with upper respiratory symptoms in a study to determine differences in client perceptions of two types of nurse–client interactive styles. Results demonstrate that clients involved in an actively negotiated process of decision making have stronger feelings of control.
- The roles of individual values greatly influence the resolution of ethical decision-making dilemmas.
- The role of nurses in situations of interpersonal/intrapersonal conflict reflects a culture broker framework incorporating advocacy, negotiation, mediation, and sensitivity to clients' and families' needs.
- Health care providers' own values and attitudes shape their interaction with clients and families facing ethical decisions (Minogue & Reedy, 1988; Taylor, 1993).
- Geary (1987) reported decision conflict for clients in critical care facing life-and-death decisions. Conflicts in client and family religious beliefs and personal values precipitated the difficult decision making. Taylor (1993) also found conflict in discussions about death and related issues when the client thought his or her wishes differed from those of the family.
- Every decision is based on consciously or unconsciously held beliefs, attitudes, and values.
- People are the experts about their life goals and values; therefore, health care professionals need to use a participatory decision-making model.
- Personal characteristics influence the desire to maintain control over decision making.
- People who are strongly self-directed and have taken past responsibility for health practices are more likely to assume an active role in decision making.

DIARRHEA

DEFINITION

Diarrhea: The state in which a person experiences or is at risk of experiencing frequent passage of liquid stool or unformed stool

DEFINING CHARACTERISTICS
Major (Must Be Present)

Loose, liquid stools and/or
Increased frequency (more than three times a day)

Minor (May Be Present)

Urgency

Increased frequency of bowel
sounds

Cramping/abdominal pain

Increased fluidity or volume of stools

RELATED FACTORS
Pathophysiologic

Related to malabsorption or inflammation secondary to:

Colon cancer	Crohn's disease	Gastritis
Diverticulitis	Peptic ulcer	Spastic colon
Irritable bowel	Celiac disease (sprue)	Ulcerative colitis

Related to lactose deficiency
Related to increased peristalsis secondary to increased metabolic rate (hyperthyroidism)
Related to dumping syndrome
Related to infectious process secondary to:

Trichinosis	Shigellosis	Dysentery
Typhoid fever	Cholera	Infectious hepatitis
Malaria	Microsporidia	Cryptosporidium

Related to excessive secretion of fats in stool secondary to liver dysfunction
*Related to inflammation and ulceration of gastrointestinal mucosa secondary to high levels
of nitrogenous wastes (renal failure)*

Treatment-Related

Related to malabsorption or inflammation secondary to surgical intervention of the bowel
Related to side effects of (specify):

Thyroid agents	Chemotherapy	Antacids
Analgesics	Laxatives	Cimetidine
Stool softeners	Iron sulfate	Antibiotics

Related to solute tube feedings

Situational (Personal, Environmental)

Related to stress or anxiety
Related to irritating foods (fruits, bran cereals)
Related to changes in water and food secondary to travel
Related to change in bacteria in water
Related to bacteria, virus, parasite to which no immunity is present
Related to increased caffeine consumption

Maturational

Infant: Related to breast milk

○○ **AUTHOR'S NOTE**

See *Constipation.*

○○ **ERRORS IN DIAGNOSTIC STATEMENTS**

1. *Diarrhea related to opportunistic enteric pathogens secondary to AIDS*
   Diarrhea, sometimes chronic, occurs in 60% to 90% of people with AIDS. Prolonged diarrhea
represents a collaborative problem: *PC: Fluid/electrolyte/nutritional imbalances related to
diarrhea.* Besides cotreating with a physician, the nurse treats other responses to chronic diarrhea (eg, *Risk for Impaired Skin Integrity, Risk for Social Isolation*).

KEY CONCEPTS
Generic Considerations

- Diarrhea can be acute or chronic. Causes of acute diarrhea include infection, drug reactions,
heavy metal poisoning, fecal impaction, and dietary changes. Causes of chronic diarrhea include

irritable bowel syndrome, lactose deficiency, colon cancer, inflammatory bowel disease, mal-absorption disorders, alcohol, medication side effects, and laxatives.
- Drugs that can induce diarrhea are laxatives, antacids, certain antibiotics (eg, tetracyclines), certain hypertensives (eg, reserpine), cholinergics, certain antivirals, and select cardiac agents.
- Rapid transit of feces through the large intestine results in decreased water absorption and unformed, liquid stool. Ongoing diarrhea leads to dehydration and electrolyte imbalance.
- Hyperperistalsis is the motor response to intestinal irritants.
- Diarrhea may be related to an inflammatory process in which the intestinal mucosal wall becomes irritated, resulting in increased moisture content in the fecal masses.

Pediatric Considerations

- Acute gastroenteritis and related diarrhea cause dehydration and are responsible for 300 to 500 annual deaths of US children younger than 5 years (Goepp & Santosham, 1994).
- Oral rehydration therapy is indicated for children with mild or moderate dehydration.
- Signs of mild dehydration are slightly dry mucous membranes and increased thirst. Signs of moderate dehydration are sunken eyes, sunken fontanelles, loss of skin turgor, and dry mucous membranes. Signs of severe dehydration include those previously mentioned plus one or more signs, such as rapid, thready pulse; cyanosis; rapid breathing; delayed capillary refill; lethargy; and coma.
- Children who live in warm environments with poor sanitation and refrigeration or in crowded, substandard environments are at risk for eating contaminated food.

Geriatric Considerations

- Age-related loss of elasticity in abdominal muscles and muscle tone in the perineal floor and anal sphincter can cause diarrhea in some older people.
- Refer to the Key Concepts of *Deficient Fluid Volume* related to dehydration.

Focus Assessment Criteria

Refer to *Constipation.*

Goal

NOC	Bowel Elimination, Electrolyte & Acid/Base Balance, Fluid Balance, Hydration, Symptom Control

The person will report less diarrhea.

Indicators
- Describe contributing factors when known.
- Explain rationale for interventions.
- Report less diarrhea.

General Interventions

NIC	Bowel Management, Diarrhea Management, Fluid/Electrolyte Management, Nutrition Management, Enteral Tube Feeding

Assess Causative Contributing Factors.

Tube feedings   Dietary indiscretions/contaminated foods
Dietetic foods   Food allergies
Foreign travel

Eliminate or Reduce Contributing Factors.
Side effects of tube feeding (Fuhrman, 1999)
Control infusion rate (depending on delivery set).

Administer smaller, more frequent feedings.

Change to continuous-drip tube feedings.

Administer more slowly if signs of gastrointestinal intolerance occur.

Control temperature.

If refrigerated, warm in hot water to room temperature.

Dilute strength of feeding temporarily.

Follow standard procedure for administration of tube feeding.

Follow tube feeding with specified amount of water to ensure hydration.

Be careful of contamination/spoilage (unused but opened formula should not be used after 24 h; keep unused portion refrigerated).

Contaminated foods (possible sources)

Raw seafood	Shellfish	Excess milk consumption
Raw milk	Restaurants	Improperly cooked/stored food

Dietetic foods: eliminate foods containing large amounts of the hexitol, sorbitol, and mannitol used as sugar substitutes in dietetic foods, candy, and chewing gum.

Reduce Diarrhea.

Discontinue solids.

Avoid milk (lactose) products, fat, whole grains, fried and spicy foods, and fresh fruits and vegetables.

Gradually add semisolids and solids (crackers, yogurt, rice, bananas, applesauce).

Avoid opiate-containing antidiarrheal drugs with acute infectious diarrhea (eg, Lomotil, Imodium).

For mild or moderate diarrhea, advise to use bismuth subsalicylate (Pepto-Bismol), 30 mL or 2 tablets every ½ to 1 h, up to 8 doses in 24 h. Avoid in individuals with salicylate contraindications.

Instruct to seek medical care if blood in stool and fever greater than 101°F.

Replace Fluids and Electrolytes.

Increase oral intake to maintain a normal urine specific gravity (light yellow in color).

Encourage liquids (tea, water, apple juice, flat ginger ale).

When diarrhea is severe, use an oral rehydration solution—over-the-counter or homemade (½ teaspoon salt, ½ teaspoon baking soda, 4 tablespoons sugar in 1 L of water; discard in 24 h).

Teach to monitor the color of urine to determine hydration needs. Increase fluids if urine color is amber or dark yellow.

Caution against use of very hot or cold liquids.

See *Deficient Fluid Volume* for additional interventions.

Conduct Health Teaching as Indicated.

Explain the interventions required to prevent future episodes.

Explain the effects of diarrhea on hydration.

Teach precautions to take when traveling to foreign lands.

    Avoid foods served cold, salads, milk, fresh cheese, cold cuts, and salsa.

    Drink carbonated or bottled beverages; avoid ice.

    Peel fresh fruits and vegetables.

    Avoid foods not stored at proper temperature.

Consult with primary health care provider for prophylactic use of bismuth subsalicylate (eg, Pepto-Bismol) 30 to 60 mL or 2 tablets qid during travel and 2 days after return; or antimicrobials, for prevention of traveler's diarrhea.

Explain how to prevent food-borne diseases at home.

    Refrigerate all perishable foods.

    Cook all food at high temperature (212°F) and boil for at least 15 min before serving.

    Avoid allowing food to stand at warm temperatures for several hours.

    Thoroughly clean kitchen equipment after contact with perishable foods (eg, meats, dairy, fish).

    Caution about foods at picnics in hot summer.

Explain that a diet primarily made up of dietetic foods containing sugar substitutes (hexitol, sorbitol, and mannitol) can cause diarrhea from slow absorption and rapid small bowel motility.

Teach to gently clean anal area after bowel movements lubricants (eg, petroleum jelly) can protect skin.

Rationales

- Most acute episodes of diarrhea are managed with symptomatic therapy with fluid and electrolyte replacement.

- Foods with complex carbohydrates (eg, rice, toast, cereal) facilitate fluid absorption into the intestinal mucosa (Bennett, 2000).
- Soft drinks (nondietetic or dietetic) and sport drinks are unsatisfactory for fluid replacement for moderate or severe fluid loss because of their sugar and salt content (Bennett, 2000).
- Opiate-containing antidiarrheals do not alter the natural cause of the disease and are harmful if invasive pathogens are the cause (Bennett, 2000).
- Bismuth subsalicylate (Pepto-Bismol) has been found safe in a variety of diarrheal illnesses and to have antibacterial activity as well. It is also effective in controlling symptoms of traveler's diarrhea (Bennett, 2000).
- Diarrheal stool can cause excoriation of the anal area because it is usually acidic and contains digestive enzymes.
- High-solute tube feedings may cause diarrhea if not followed by sufficient water.

Pediatric Interventions

Monitor Fluid and Electrolyte Losses.

Fluid volume lost

Skin color

Capillary refill time

Urine color and output

Mucous membranes

Consult with Primary Care Provider if:

Diarrhea persists.

Client has signs of moderate
  dehydration.

Client is vomiting.

Blood or mucus is in stools.

Stools suddenly increase.

Reduce Diarrhea.

Avoid milk (lactose) products, fat, whole grains, and fresh fruits and vegetables.

Avoid high-carbohydrate fluids (eg, soft drinks), gelatin, fruit juices, caffeinated drinks, chicken or
  beef broths.

Provide Oral Rehydration.

Use oral rehydration solutions (eg, Pedialyte, Lytren, Ricelyte, Resol; Larson, 2000).

Provide 60 to 80 mL/kg over 2-h period for mild to moderate diarrhea.

Reintroduce Food.

Begin with bananas, rice, cereal, and crackers in small quantities.

Gradually return to regular diet (except milk products) after 36 to 48 h; after 3 to 5 days, gradually
  add milk products (half-strength skim milk to skim milk to half-strength whole milk to whole milk).

Gradually introduce formula (half-strength formula to full-strength formula).

For Breast-Fed Infants:

Continue breast-feeding.

Use oral rehydration therapy if needed.

**Protect Skin from Irritation with Non–Water-Soluable Cream
(eg, Petroleum Jelly)**

Teach Parents Signs to Report (Refer to Key Concepts).

Rationales

- Children with signs of moderate or severe dehydration should be referred for possible parenteral therapy (Wong, 2003).
- Lactose-containing fluids or foods can worsen diarrhea in some children (Goepp & Santosham, 1994).
- Fluids high in carbohydrates can exacerbate diarrhea because of their high osmolality. They are also low in electrolytes (Wong, 2003).

- Early reintroduction of normal nutrients has nutritional advantages and may reduce number of stools, weight loss, and duration of disease, and enhance intestinal mucosal healing (Brown, 1991).
- Breast-feeding should be continued with fluid replacement therapy. Reduced severity and duration of the illness is attributed to breast milk's low osmolality and antimicrobial effects (Brown, 1991).
- Oral rehydration solution for acute diarrhea prevents subsequent unscheduled follow-up visits (Duggan et al., 1999).

DISUSE SYNDROME

DEFINITION

Disuse Syndrome: The state in which a person is experiencing or at risk for deterioration of body systems or altered functioning as the result of prescribed or unavoidable musculoskeletal inactivity

DEFINING CHARACTERISTICS

Presence of a cluster of actual or risk nursing diagnoses related to inactivity:

- *Risk for Impaired Skin Integrity*
- *Risk for Constipation*
- *Risk for Altered Respiratory Function*
- *Risk for Ineffective Peripheral Tissue Perfusion*
- *Risk for Infection*
- *Risk for Activity Intolerance*
- *Risk for Impaired Physical Mobility*
- *Risk for Injury*
- *Disturbed Sensory Perception*
- *Powerlessness*
- *Disturbed Body Image*

RELATED FACTORS
Pathophysiologic
Related to: (optional)

Decreased sensorium
Unconsciousness
Neuromuscular impairment

Multiple sclerosis	Muscular dystrophy	Parkinsonism
Partial/total paralysis	Guillain-Barré syndrome	Spinal cord injury

Musculoskeletal impairment

Fractures	Rheumatic diseases

End-stage disease

AIDS	Cardiac	Renal

Cancer
Psychiatric/mental health disorders

Major depression	Catatonic state	Severe phobias

Treatment-Related
Related to: (optional)

Surgery (amputation, skeletal)	Mechanical ventilation
Traction/casts/splints	Invasive vascular lines
Prescribed immobility	

Situational (Personal, Environmental)
Related to: (optional)

Depression   Debilitated state
Fatigue   Pain

Maturational
Related to: (optional)

Newborn / infant / child / adolescent

Down syndrome   Risser-Turnbuckle jacket   Legg-Calvé-Perthes disease
Juvenile arthritis   Osteogenesis imperfecta   Autism
Cerebral palsy   Mental/physical disability   Spina bifida
Older adult
Decreased motor agility   Muscle weakness   Presenile dementia

---

⦾ AUTHOR'S NOTE

Disuse Syndrome describes a person experiencing or at risk for the adverse effects of immobility. Syndrome nursing diagnoses should not be written as "Risk for," because risk and actual diagnoses are clustered under them. *Disuse Syndrome* identifies vulnerability to certain complications and also altered functioning in a health pattern. As a syndrome diagnosis, its etiology is within the diagnostic label (*Disuse*); a "related to" statement is not applicable. As discussed in Chapter 2, a syndrome diagnosis comprises a cluster of predicted actual or risk nursing diagnoses because of the situation. Eleven risk or actual nursing diagnoses are clustered under *Disuse Syndrome* (see Defining Characteristics).

The nurse no longer needs to use separate diagnoses, such as *Risk for Ineffective Respiratory Function* or *Risk for Impaired Skin Integrity,* because they are incorporated into the syndrome category. If an immobile person manifests signs or symptoms of impaired skin integrity or another diagnosis, however, the nurse should use the specific diagnosis. He or she should continue to use *Disuse Syndrome* so other body systems do not deteriorate.

⦾ ERRORS IN DIAGNOSTIC STATEMENTS

1. *Disuse Syndrome related to reddened sacral area (3 cm)*

A reddened sacral area is evidence of *Impaired Skin Integrity.* Thus, the nurse should use two diagnoses: *Impaired Skin Integrity related to effects of immobility, as evidenced by reddened sacral area (3 cm)* and *Disuse Syndrome.*

KEY CONCEPTS
Generic Considerations

- "Immobility is inconsistent with human life." Mobility provides control over the environment; without mobility, the person is at the mercy of the environment (Christian, 1982).
- Prolonged immobility decreases motivation to learn and ability to retain new material. Affective changes are anxiety, fear, hostility, rapid mood shifts, and disrupted sleep patterns (Porth, 2002).
- Immobility restricts the ability to seek out sensory stimulation. Conversely, immobile people may be unable to remove themselves from a stressful or noisy environment (Christian, 1982).
- Musculoskeletal inactivity or immobility adversely affects all body systems (Table II.7).
- A muscle loses about 3% of its original strength each day it is immobilized.
- Prolonged immobility adversely affects psychological health, learning, socialization, and ability to cope. Table II.8 illustrates these effects.
- Possible long-term complications in people with traumatic spinal cord injury are pneumonia, atelectasis, autonomic dysreflexia, deep vein thrombosis, pulmonary embolism, pressure ulcers, fractures, and renal calculi (McKinley et al., 1999).

TABLE II.7 Adverse Effects of Immobility on Body Systems

System	Effect
Cardiac	Decreased myocardial performance
	Decreased aerobic capacity
	Decreased heart rate and stroke volume
	Decreased oxygen uptake
Circulatory	Venous stasis
	Orthostatic intolerance
	Dependent edema
	Decreased resting heart rate
	Reduced venous return
	Increased intravascular pressure
Respiratory	Stasis of secretions
	Impaired cilia
	Drying of sections of mucous membranes
	Decreased chest expansion
	Slower, more shallow respirations
Musculoskeletal	Muscle atrophy
	Shortening of muscle fiber (contracture)
	Decreased strength/tone (eg, back)
	Decreased bone density
	Joint degeneration
	Fibrosis of collagen fibers (joints)
Metabolic/Hemopoietic	Decreased nitrogen excretion
	Decreased tissue heat conduction
	Decreased glucose tolerance
	Insulin resistance
	Decreased red blood cells
	Decreased phagocytosis
	Hypercalcemia
	Change in circadian release of hormones (eg, insulin, epinephrine)
	Anorexia
	Decreased metabolic rate
	Obesity
	Elevated creatine levels
Gastrointestinal	Constipation
Genitourinary	Urinary stasis
	Urinary calculi
	Urinary retention
	Inadequate gravitational force
Integumentary	Decreased capillary flow
	Tissue acidosis to necrosis
Neurosensory	Reduced innervation of nerves
	Decreased near vision
	Increased auditory sensitivity

Caswell, 1993; Porth, 2002; Tyler, 1984; Wong, 2003.

TABLE II.8 Psychosocial Effects of Immobility

Psychological	Increased tension
	Negative change in self-concept
	Fear, anger
	Rapid mood changes
	Depression
	Hostility
Learning	Decreased motivation
	Decreased ability to retain, transfer learning
	Decreased attention span
Socialization	Change in roles
	Social isolation
Growth and development	Dependency

Porth, 2002; Zubek & McNeil, 1967.

◆ Pediatric Considerations

- Mobility is essential for physical growth and development and mastery of developmental tasks (Wong, 2002). Restricted movement can thwart achievement of developmental tasks. Refer to Table II-12 in the diagnostic category *Delayed Growth and Development.*
- Physical activity serves as a means of communication and expression for children. Major psychological consequences of immobility include the following:
  - Sensory deprivation, leading to alterations in self-perception and environmental awareness
  - Isolation from peers
  - Feelings of helplessness, frustration, anxiety, and boredom (Wong, 2002; Wright, 1989)
- Children who are restrained by casts, splints, or straps during the first 3 years of life have more difficulty with language than children with unrestricted activities (Wong, 2002).
- Children's responses to immobility may range from active protest to withdrawal or regression (Wong, 2003; Wright, 1989).

● Geriatric Considerations

- Aging affects muscle function because of progressive loss of muscle mass, strength, and endurance.
- Age-related changes in joint and connective tissues include impaired flexion and extension movements, decreased flexibility, and reduced cushioning protection for joints (Whitbourne, 1985).
- After menopause, women experience an accelerated loss of trabecular and cortical bone of 9% to 10% per decade (Miller, 2004).
- Bed rest can cause an average vertical bone loss of 0.9% per week (Maher et al., 1998).

Focus Assessment Criteria

Subjective Data
Assess for Related Factors.

Neurologic	Cardiovascular
Musculoskeletal	Respiratory
Debilitating diseases	History of recent trauma or surgery
History of symptoms (complaints) of pain, muscle weakness, fatigue	

Objective Data
Assess for Defining Characteristics.

Dominant hand

Right	Left	Ambidextrous

Motor function

Right arm	Strong	Weak	Absent	Spastic
Left arm	Strong	Weak	Absent	Spastic
Right leg	Strong	Weak	Absent	Spastic
Left leg	Strong	Weak	Absent	Spastic

Mobility

Ability to turn self	Yes	No	Assistance needed (specify)
Ability to sit	Yes	No	Assistance needed (specify)
Ability to stand	Yes	No	Assistance needed (specify)
Ability to transfer	Yes	No	Assistance needed (specify)
Ability to ambulate	Yes	No	Assistance needed (specify)

Weight bearing (assess both right and left sides)
Full   Partial   As tolerated   Non–weight bearing

Gait
Stable   Unstable

Range of motion of shoulders, elbows, arms, hips, legs
Full   Limited (specify)   None

Assess for Related Factors.

Assistive devices

Crutches	Wheelchair	Cane
Prosthesis	Braces	Other
Walker		

Restrictive devices

Cast or splint	Foley	Traction
Intravenous line	Braces	Monitor
Ventilator	Dialysis	Drain

Motivation (as perceived by nurse, reported by person, or both)
Excellent   Satisfactory   Poor

For more information on Focus Assessment Criteria, visit http://connection.lww.com.

Goal

NOC Endurance, Immobility Consequences: Physiological, Immobility Consequences: Psycho-Cognitive, Mobility Level

The person will not experience complications of immobility.

Indicators

- Intact skin/tissue integrity
- Maximum pulmonary function
- Maximum peripheral blood flow
- Full range of motion
- Bowel, bladder, and renal functioning within normal limits
- Uses of social contacts and activities when possible
- Explain rationale for treatments
- Make decisions regarding care when possible
- Share feelings regarding immobile state

General Interventions

NIC Activity Therapy, Energy Management, Mutual Goal Settings, Exercise Therapy, Fall Prevention, Pressure Ulcer Prevention, Body Mechanics Correction, Skin Surveillance, Positioning, Coping Enhancement, Decision-Making, Support

Identify Causative and Contributing Factors.

Pain; refer also to *Impaired Comfort*.
Fatigue; refer also to *Fatigue*.
Decreased motivation; refer also to *Activity Intolerance*.
Depression; refer also to *Ineffective Coping*.

Promote Optimal Respiratory Function.

Vary the position of the bed, thus gradually changing the horizontal and vertical position of the thorax, unless contraindicated.
Assist client to reposition, turning frequently from side to side (hourly if possible).
Encourage deep breathing and controlled coughing exercises five times every hour.
Teach client to use blow bottle or incentive spirometer every hour when awake (with severe neuromuscular impairment, the person also may have to be awakened at night).
For child, use colored water in blow bottle; have him or her blow up balloons, soap bubbles, or cotton balls with straw.
Auscultate lung fields every 8 h; increase frequency if breath sounds are altered.
Encourage small, frequent feedings to prevent abdominal distention.

Maintain Usual Pattern of Bowel Elimination.

Refer to *Constipation* for specific interventions.

Prevent Pressure Ulcers (Maklebust & Sieggreen, 1996).

Use repositioning schedule that relieves vulnerable area most often (eg, if vulnerable area is the back, turning schedule would be left side to back, back to right side, right side to left side, and left side to back); post "turn clock" at bedside.

Turn client or instruct him or her to turn or shift weight every 30 min to 2 h, depending on other causative factors and the ability of the skin to recover from pressure.

Frequency of turning schedule should increase if any reddened areas that appear do not disappear within 1 h after turning.

Position person in normal or neutral position with body weight evenly distributed.

Keep bed as flat as possible to reduce shearing forces; limit Fowler's position to only 30 min at a time.

Use foam blocks or pillows to provide a bridging effect to support the body above and below the high-risk or ulcerated area so affected area does not touch bed surface; do not use foam donuts or inflatable rings because they increase the area of pressure.

Alternate or reduce the pressure on the skin surface with:

Foam mattresses	Air mattresses
Air-fluidized beds	Vascular boots to suspend heels

Use enough personnel to lift person up in bed or chair rather than pull or slide skin surfaces; use protectors to reduce friction on elbows and heels.

To reduce shearing forces, support feet with footboard to prevent sliding.

Promote optimum circulation when person is sitting.

Limit time spent sitting for person at high risk for ulcer development.

Instruct person to lift self using chair arms every 10 min if possible, or assist client to rise from the chair every 10 to 20 min, depending on risk factors.

Inspect areas at risk for ulcers with each position change.

Ears	Occiput
Heels	Sacrum
Scrotum	Elbows
Trochanter	Ischia
Scapula	

Observe for erythema and blanching and palpate for warmth and tissue sponginess with each position change.

Massage nonreddened, vulnerable areas gently with each position change.

Refer to *Impaired Skin Integrity* for additional interventions.

Promote Factors that Improve Venous Blood Flow.

Elevate extremity above the level of the heart (may be contraindicated in cases of severe cardiac or respiratory disease).

Ensure client avoids standing or sitting with legs dependent for long periods.

Consider the use of below-knee elastic stockings to prevent venous stasis.

Reduce or remove external venous compression, which impedes venous flow.

Avoid pillows behind the knees or suggest a bed that is elevated at the knees.

Tell client to avoid crossing the legs.

Remind client to change positions, move extremities, or wiggle fingers and toes every hour.

Ensure client avoids garters and tight elastic stockings above the knees.

Measure baseline circumference of calves and thighs daily if person is at risk for deep venous thrombosis, or if it is suspected.

Maintain Limb Mobility and Prevent Contractures (Maher et al., 1998).

Increase Limb Mobility.

Perform range-of-motion exercises (frequency to be determined by client's condition).

Support extremity with pillows to prevent or reduce swelling.

Encourage client to perform exercise regimens for specific joints as prescribed by physician or physical therapist.

Position Client in Alignment to Prevent Complications.

Avoid placing pillows under knee; support calf instead.

Point toes and knees toward ceiling when client is supine.

Use footboard to prevent footdrop.

Avoid prolonged periods of hip flexion (ie, sitting position).

To position hips, place rolled towel lateral to hip to prevent external rotation.

Keep arms abducted from the body with pillows.

Keep elbows in slight flexion.

Keep wrist neutral, with fingers slightly flexed and thumb abducted and slightly flexed.

Change position of shoulder joints during the day (eg, abduction, adduction, range of circular motion).

Prevent Urinary Stasis and Calculi Formation.

Provide a daily fluid intake of 2000 mL or more (unless contraindicated); see *Deficient Fluid Volume* for specific interventions.

Maintain urine pH below 6.0 (acidic) to reduce the formation of calcium calculi with acid ash foods (cereals, meats, poultry, fish, cranberry juice, apple juice).

Teach client to avoid foods high in calcium and oxalate (*very high):

> Milk, milk products, cheese
> Bran cereals
> *Spinach, cranberries, plums, raspberries, gooseberries
> Sardines, shrimp, oysters
> Legumes, whole-grain rice
> *Chocolate
> Asparagus, rhubarb, kale, Swiss chard, turnip greens, mustard greens, broccoli, beet greens
> Peanut butter, ripe olives

Reduce and Monitor Bone Demineralization.

Monitor for hypercalcemia.

> Serum levels
> Nausea/vomiting, polydipsia, polyuria, lethargy

Promote weight-bearing when possible (tilt-table).

Maintain vigorous hydration.

> Adults: 2000 mL/day
> Adolescents: 3000 to 4000 mL/day

Promote Sharing and a Sense of Well-Being.

Encourage client to share feelings and fears regarding restricted movement.

Encourage client to wear own clothes rather than pajamas, and unique adornments (eg, baseball caps, colorful socks) to express individuality.

Reduce the Monotony of Immobility.

Vary Daily Routine when Possible (eg, Give Bath in the Afternoon so the Person can Watch a Special Show or Talk with a Visitor During the Morning).

Include Client in Planning Daily Schedule.

Allow client to make as many decisions as possible.

Make daily routine as normal as possible (eg, have the person wear street clothes during the day, if feasible).

Encourage person to make a schedule for visitors so everyone does not come at once or at inconvenient times.

Spend quality time with the person (ie, not time that is task oriented; rather, sit down and talk).

Be Creative; Vary the Physical Environment and Daily Routine when Possible.

Update bulletin boards, change pictures on the walls, and move furniture within the room.

Maintain a pleasant, cheerful environment (eg, plenty of light, flowers).

Place the person near a window, if possible.

Provide reading material (print or audio), radio, and television.

Plan an activity daily to give person something to look forward to; always keep promises.

Discourage the use of television as the primary source of recreation unless it is highly desired.

Consider using a volunteer to spend time reading to the person or helping with an activity.

Encourage suggestions and new ideas (eg, "Can you think of things you might like to do?").

Provide Opportunities for Client to Control Decisions.

Allow person to manipulate surroundings, such as deciding what to keep where (shoes under bed, picture on window).

Keep needed items within reach (call bell, urinal, tissues).

Discuss daily plan of activities and allow person to make as many decisions as possible.

Increase decision-making opportunities as person progresses.

Respect and follow client's decision if you have given options.

Record specific choices on care plan to ensure that others on staff acknowledge preferences ("Dislikes orange juice," "Takes shower," "Plan dressing change at 7:30 before shower").

Keep promises.

Provide opportunities for person and family to participate in care.

Plan a care conference to allow staff to discuss methods of individualizing care; encourage each nurse to share at least one action that he or she discovered a particular client liked.

Shift emphasis from what one cannot do to what one can do.

Set goals that are short-term, practical, and realistic.

Rationales

* See Tables II-7 and II-8 for effects of immobility.
* Activity, mobility, and flexibility are integral to a person's lifestyle. Immobility seriously affects self-concept and lifestyle (Christian, 1982; Porth, 2002).
* The more portions of the body immobilized and the longer the immobilization, the greater the adverse effects.
* Joints without range of motion develop contractures in 3 to 7 days, because flexor muscles are stronger than extensor muscles.
* Increased serum calcium resulting from bone destruction caused by lack of motion and weight bearing increases blood coagulability. This, in addition to circulatory stasis, makes the person vulnerable to thrombosis formation.
* The peristaltic contractions of the ureters are insufficient when in a reclining position; thus, there is stasis of urine in the renal pelvis.
* Compression of nerves by casts, restraints, or improper positions can cause ischemia and nerve degeneration. Compression of the peroneal nerve results in footdrop; compression of the radial nerve results in wristdrop.
* Interventions to maintain hydration prevent hypercoagulability and clot formation and urine concentration of stone-forming elements (Porth, 2002).

Pediatric Interventions

Plan Appropriate Activities for Children.

Provide an environment with accessible toys that suit the child's developmental age; ensure they are well within reach.

Encourage family to bring in child's favorite toys, including items from nature that will keep the "real world" alive (eg, goldfish, leaves in fall).

Use Play Therapy to Encourage Child to Share Feelings (eg, Put Cast on Doll).

Transport Child Outside the Room as Much as Possible.

Engage Child to Participate in Self-Care.

Plan daily routine.

Select diet, snacks.

Select clothes (eg, baseball cap).

Allow Child to Wear Street Clothes as Soon as Possible.

Rationales

* Play therapy decreases the monotony of immobilization, tension, and frustration (Wong, 2003).
* Changes in the environment provide varied stimuli and increased social contact (Wong, 2003).
* Increasing self-care activities and decision making allows expressions of autonomy and individualization (Wong, 2003).

DEFICIENT DIVERSIONAL ACTIVITY

DEFINITION

Deficient Diversional Activity: The state in which a person or group experiences or is at risk of experiencing decreased stimulation from, or interest in, leisure activities

DEFINING CHARACTERISTICS
Major (Must Be Present)

Observed and/or statements of boredom/depression due to inactivity

Minor (May Be Present)

Constant expression of
  unpleasant thoughts/feelings
Flat facial expression
Restlessness/fidgeting

Hostility
Yawning or inattentiveness
Body language (shifts body away)
Weight loss or gain

RELATED FACTORS
Pathophysiologic

Related to difficulty accessing or participating in usual activities secondary to:
Communicable disease   Pain

Situational (Personal, Environmental)

Related to unsatisfactory social behaviors
Related to no peers or friends
Related to monotonous environment
Related to long-term hospitalization or confinement
Related to lack of motivation
Related to difficulty accessing or participating in usual activities secondary to:

Excessive stressful work
Career changes (eg, new job,
  retirement)
Immobility

Multiple role responsibilities
No time for leisure activities
Children leaving home ("empty nest")
Decreased sensory perception

Maturational
Infant/Child
Related to lack of appropriate stimulation toys/peers

Older Adult
Related to difficulty accessing or participating in usual activities secondary to:

Sensory/motor deficits
Lack of transportation
Fear of crime

Lack of peer group
Limited finances
Confusion

 AUTHOR'S NOTE

Only the client can express a deficit in diversional activities based on his or her determination that types and amounts of activity are problematic. Miller (2004) writes that activities associated with various roles affirm a person's self-concept.

    To validate *Deficient Diversional Activity,* explore the etiology of factors amenable to nursing interventions, keeping your main focus on improving the quality of leisure activities. For a person with personality problems that hinder relationships and decrease social activities, *Impaired Social Interactions* is more valid. In this case, focus on helping the person identify behavior that imposes barriers to socialization.

⊗ **ERRORS IN DIAGNOSTIC STATEMENTS**

1. *Deficient Diversional Activity related to boredom and reports of no leisure activities*
   This diagnosis does not reflect nursing interventions. Boredom and reports of no leisure activities are manifestations, not contributing factors, of the diagnosis. Thus, write the diagnosis as *Deficient Diversional Activity related to unknown etiology, as evidenced by reports of boredom and no leisure activities.*
2. *Deficient Diversional Activity related to inability to sustain meaningful relationships, as evidenced by "no one calls me to go out"*
   This diagnosis focuses nursing interventions on enhancing the person's diversional activities. In this situation, delay making a formal diagnosis and collect more data to explore more specifically the meaning of "no one calls me to go out." Other diagnoses may be more applicable, such as *Impaired Social Interactions, Disturbed Self-Concept,* and *Ineffective Coping.*

KEY CONCEPTS
Generic Considerations

- All human beings need stimulation. In adults, lack of stimulation leads to boredom and depression. In infants and children, it causes "failure to thrive" and may stunt growth severely.
- The relationship between informal activity and life satisfaction is significant. The quality or type of activity is more important than the quantity (Rantz, 1991).
- Boredom paralyzes a person's productivity and causes a feeling of stagnation. It is often a major contributing factor to addictive behaviors (eg, overeating, drug abuse, alcoholism, smoking).
- The bored person has introspective feelings of being oppressed and trapped, which give rise to conscious or unconscious anger or hostility.
- In recent years, pet therapy has been appreciated increasingly for ill and older clients.

♦ Pediatric Considerations

- Children at special risk for deficient diversional activity include the following:
  - Those who are bored
  - Those who are immobilized
  - Those who are hospitalized for long periods
  - Those who are isolated to protect themselves or others
  - Those who have diminished contact with family, friends, or both
- Age-appropriate activities should be provided to promote mental health and human development. Child life specialists—experts who are certified in early childhood, creative arts, or recreation therapies—provide psychosocial assessment and therapeutic activities in group contexts (they give advice on individual clients, playroom design, and activities). They are available in 98% of pediatric medical-surgical units, working with the multidisciplinary team to provide developmentally appropriate therapy and education to children and aiming to reduce the psychological trauma of illness (Rode, Capitulo, Fishman & Holden, 1998). You can visit a Child Life program Web site at http://www.mssm.edu/peds/childlif.html and http://www.childlif.org. Refer to Table II.12 in *Delayed Growth and Development.*
- Bored children may be at increased risk for injury. Refer to *Risk for Injury related to maturational age of the hospitalized child* for more information.
- See also Key Concepts, Pediatric Considerations for *Anxiety* and *Delayed Growth and Development.*

⊙ Geriatric Considerations

- Cultural background strongly influences the older client's use of diversional activities because of the value placed on work versus leisure. Older, less educated, rural people tend to place less value on leisure activities.

(continued)

Geriatric Considerations (continued)

- In Western society, retirement usually occurs between 62 and 70 years of age. About 80% of men and 90% of women older than 65 years are identified as retired. The lost work role can lead to depression, particularly if the client has engaged in no preretirement planning (Miller, 2004).
- Cultivating varied interests and activities throughout life enhances aging (Miller, 2004).
- A change in living arrangements or environment might subject the older adult to a diversional activity deficit. For example, an organic gardener with her own private yard moves to a senior high-rise apartment with no land for a garden. Or an older man who plays the drums moves in with his adult children who have neither the space for his drum set nor the inclination to listen to his drum solos.
- Social isolation resulting from death of a spouse, lack of transportation, hearing impairment, limited finances, fear of crime, or other physical or psychological disabilities places the older client at risk for diversional activity deficit (Rantz, 1991).
- Volunteer activities provide diversion for 21% of people 55 to 64 years of age and 14% of those 65 years and older. Those 65 years and older volunteered an average of 8 hours per week. Reasons cited for not volunteering included transportation difficulties, financial concerns, and age discrimination by some community organizations (Miller, 2004).

Focus Assessment Criteria

Subjective Data

Assess for Defining Characteristics.

Perception of person's current activity level: ask client to rate on a scale of 1 to 10 his or her satisfaction with current diversional activity level (1=not at all satisfied and 10=very satisfied).

Past activity patterns (type, frequency): work, leisure

Activities the person desires

Objective Data

Assess for related factors.

Motivation

Interested	Withdrawn
Uninterested	Hostile

Any barriers to recreational activities
Physical status

Immobility	Pain
Altered level of consciousness	Sensory deficits (visual, auditory)
Fatigue	Equipment (traction, intravenous [IV] lines)
Altered hand mobility	Communicable disease/isolation

Psychological/cognitive status

Depression	Lack of knowledge
Embarrassment	Fear

Socioeconomic status

Lack of support system	Financial limitations
Previous patterns of inactivity	Transportation difficulties
Language barrier	

For more information on Focus Assessment Criteria, visit http://connection.lww.com.

Goal

NOC Leisure Participation, Social Involvement

The person will rate that he or she is more satisfied with current activity level.

Indicators

- Relate methods of coping with anger or depression resulting from boredom.
- Report participation in one enjoyable activity each day.

General Interventions

 Recreation Therapy, Socialization Enhancement, Self-Esteem Enhancement

Assess Causative Factors.

Monotony
Diminished socialization (see *Social Isolation*)
Lack of motivation/depression
Inability to concentrate

Reduce or Eliminate Causative Factors.

Monotony

Refer to Interventions, "Reduce the monotony of immobility," under *Disuse Syndrome*.

Provide opportunities for reminiscence individually or in groups (eg, past trips, hobbies).

Provide music therapy with audio cassette players with lightweight headphones. For help with music therapy, call the American Music Therapy Association (AMTA) at 301-589-3300 or visit the Web site at www.namt.com. For group music therapy (Rantz, 1991):

1. Introduce a topic.
2. Play related music.
3. Develop the topic with discussion.
4. Discuss responses.

Consider using holistic and complementary therapies (eg, aromatherapy, pet therapy, therapeutic touch). For pet therapy (Rantz, 1991):

Animals must be well groomed, healthy, and clean.
Animals should be relaxed with strangers.
Animals should eliminate before entering the facility.
Sponsors always should ask the client if he or she likes the type of animal before approaching the person.

Lack of Motivation

Stimulate motivation by showing interest and encouraging sharing of feelings and experiences.
Explore fears and concerns about participating in activities.
Discuss likes and dislikes.
Encourage sharing of feelings of present and past experiences.
Spend time with the person purposefully talking about other topics (eg, "I just got back from the shore. Have you ever gone there?").
Point out the need to "get oneself going" and try something new.

Help the person work through feelings of anger and grief.
Allow him or her to express feelings.
Take the time to be a good listener.
See *Anxiety* for additional interventions.

Encourage client to join a group of possible interest or help (may have to participate by way of intercom or special arrangement).

Consider the use of music therapy or reminiscence therapy.

Inability to Concentrate

Plan a simple daily routine with concrete activities (eg, walking, drawing, folding linens).
If anxious, suggest solitary, noncompetitive activities (eg, puzzles, photography).

Identify Factors that Promote Activity and Socialization.

Encourage Socialization with Peers and All Age Groups (Frequently Very Young and Very Old Clients Mutually Benefit from Interactions).

Acquire Assistance to Increase the Person's Ability to Travel.

Arrange transportation to activities if necessary.
Acquire aids for safety (eg, wheelchair for shopping, walker for ambulating in hallways).

Increase Client's Feelings of Productivity and Self-Worth.

Encourage client to use strengths to help others and self (eg, assign him or her tasks to perform in a general project).
Acknowledge efforts (eg, "Thank you for helping Mr. Jones with his dinner").
Encourage open communication; value the person's opinion ("Mr. Jones, what do you think about . . . ?").
Encourage the person to challenge himself or herself to learn a new skill or pursue a new interest.

Refer to *Social Isolation* for Additional Interventions.

Rationales

- Informal activities promote well-being more than formally structured activities do. Solitary activities have few effects on life satisfaction (Longino & Kart, 1982).
- Being aware of boredom allows the person to redirect activities to increase stimulation.
- Music therapy can be valuable in relieving boredom, sparking interest, and assisting clients to cope with social problems (Rantz, 1991).
- Membership in a group or a support group can boost self-esteem and self-worth, provide a sense of belonging, and encourage activities that the person otherwise may have avoided. Support groups can often assist those with stressful, costly, or time-consuming problems.
- Reminiscing, or spending time focusing on significant memories, can be satisfying and stimulating for the bored, ill, confined, or elderly person (Rantz, 1991).
- Tasks that match the person's concentration and interest can increase contact with reality, promote socialization, and improve self-esteem (Varcarolis, 2002).

Pediatric Interventions

Provide an environment with accessible toys that suit the child's developmental age; ensure that they are well within reach.

Keep toys in all waiting areas.

Encourage family to bring in child's favorite toys, including items from nature that will help to keep the "real world" alive (eg, goldfish, leaves in fall).

Consult a child life specialist as indicated.

Consider using Starbright World, a private computer network in which children interact in a virtual community, articulating their experiences and escaping the day-to-day trials of hospitalization. Starbright World is one of many programs of the Starbright Foundation, a nonprofit organization whose mission is to improve quality of life for seriously ill children and their families by designing entertaining therapeutic interventions.

Rationales

- Play is essential to a child's emotional, developmental, and physical health (Kuntz et al., 1996).
- Play provides diversion and increases security (Wong, 2003).
- Play provides an expressive outlet for feelings.
- Play provides opportunities for choices and to be in control (Wong, 2003).

Geriatric Interventions

Explore Interests and the Feasibility of Trying a New Activity (eg, Mobility).

Arrange for Someone to Accompany or Orient Client During Initial Encounters.

Explore Possible Volunteer Opportunities (eg, Red Cross, Hospitals).

Initiate Referrals, if Indicated.

Suggest joining American Association of Retired Persons (AARP).

Write local health and welfare council or agencies.

Provide a list of associations with senior citizen activities:

YMCA	Sixty Plus Club	Churches
XYZ Group (Extra Years of Zest)	Golden Age Club	Young at Heart Club
SOS (Senior Outreach Services)	Encore Club	Leisure Hour Group
MORA (Men of Retirement Age)	Gray Panthers	

Rationales

- Cognitive impairment, musculoskeletal impairment, pain, metabolic abnormality, or sensory deficit may force an older adult to consider modifying long-time leisure activities or developing new activities. For example, a person who likes to cook but has poor eyesight might obtain large-print cookbooks, have a friend write favorite recipes in bold print, or tape-record recipes (Rantz, 1991).
- Change, although a welcome relief from boredom, increases anxiety initially.

DYSREFLEXIA

DEFINITION

Dysreflexia: The state in which a person with a spinal cord injury at T6 or above experiences or is at risk to experience a potential life-threatening uninhibited sympathetic response of the nervous system to a noxious stimulus

DEFINING CHARACTERISTICS
Major (Must Be Present)

Individual with spinal cord injury (T6 or above) with:

- Paroxysmal hypertension (sudden periodic elevated blood pressure in which systolic pressure is above 140 mm Hg and diastolic is above 90 mm Hg)
- Bradycardia or tachycardia (pulse rate less than 60 or more than 100 beats/min)
- Profuse diaphoresis (above the injury)
- Red splotches on skin (above the injury)
- Pallor (below the injury)
- Headache (a diffuse pain [dull to pounding] in different portions of the head and not confined to any nerve distribution area)
- Apprehension
- Dilated pupils

Minor (May Be Present)

Chilling
Conjunctival congestion
Horner's syndrome (pupillary contraction; partial ptosis of the eyelid; enophthalmos; sometimes, loss of sweating over the affected side of the face)
Paresthesia
Response pilomotor (gooseflesh)
Blurred vision
Chest pain
Metallic taste in mouth
Nasal congestion
Penile erection and semen emission

RELATED FACTORS
Pathophysiologic
Related to visceral stretching and irritation secondary to:

Gastrointestinal

Constipation	Fecal impaction	Acute abdominal condition
Gastric ulceration	Hemorrhoids	Anal fissure

Urologic

Distended bladder	Urinary calculi	Urinary tract infection

Cutaneous

Pressure ulcers	Burns	Sunburn
Insect bites	Ingrown toenails	Blister

Reproductive

Menstruation	Pregnancy or delivery	Vaginal infection
Epididymitis	Uterine contraction	Vaginal dilation

Related to fracture
Related to stimulation of skin (abdominal, thigh)
Related to spastic sphincter
Related to deep vein thrombosis

Treatment-Related
Related to visceral stretching secondary to:
Removal of fecal impaction
Clogged or nonpatent catheter
Visceral stretching and irritation secondary to surgical incision, enemas
Catheterization, enema

Situational (Personal, Environmental)
Related to lack of knowledge of prevention or treatment
Related to visceral stretching secondary to:
Boosting
Sexual activity
Menstruation
Pregnancy or delivery
Related to neural stimulation secondary to immersion in cold water

---

○○ **AUTHOR'S NOTE**

Dysreflexia represents a life-threatening situation that nurse-prescribed interventions can prevent or treat. Prevention involves teaching the client to reduce sympathetic nervous system stimulation and not using interventions that can cause such stimulation. Treatment focuses on reducing or eliminating noxious stimuli (eg, fecal impaction, urinary retention). If nursing actions do not resolve symptoms, initiation of medical intervention is critical. When a client requires medical treatment for all or most episodes of dysreflexia, the situation is labeled a collaborative problem: *PC: Dysreflexia.*

○○ **ERRORS IN DIAGNOSTIC STATEMENTS**

1. *Dysreflexia related to paroxysmal hypertension*
    Paroxysmal hypertension is a sign of dysreflexia, not a causative or contributing stimulus. The diagnosis should be restated: *Risk for Dysreflexia related to possible reflex stimulation by visceral or cutaneous irritation, as evidenced by (specify).*
    Clinically, *Risk for Dysreflexia* is more descriptive than *Dysreflexia*. The client usually is in a potential state, with associated nursing responsibilities of prevention, teaching, and early removal of stimulus.

KEY CONCEPTS
- The autonomic nervous system (sympathetic and parasympathetic) is located in the cerebrum, hypothalamus, medulla, brain stem, and spinal cord. With spinal cord injury, activity below the injury is deprived of the controlling effects from the higher centers. The result is poorly controlled responses (Travers, 1999).
- Stimulation of sensory receptors below a spinal lesion results in sympathetic discharge, mediated by the spinothalamic tract and posterior columns. This reflex stimulation of the sympathetic nervous system causes spasms of the pelvic viscera and arterioles. These spasms cause vasoconstriction below the level of injury. Baroreceptors in the aortic arch and carotid sinus respond to the

- hypertensive state with superficial vasodilatation, flushing, diaphoresis, and piloerection (goose-flesh) above the level of the spinal lesion (Bennett, 2003).
- Vagal stimulation slows the heart rate, but, because the cord is severed, vagal impulses to dilate vessels are prohibited (Teasell, Arnold & Delaney, 1996; Porth, 2002).
- Failure to reverse dysreflexia can result in status epilepticus, stroke, and death.
- Uncontrolled hypertension can cause systolic blood pressure to rise as high as 240 to 300 mm Hg (Porth, 2002).
- Three types of stimuli can initiate dysreflexia: visceral distention (eg, full bladder or rectum), stimulation of pain receptors (eg, diagnostic procedure, pressure), and visceral contractions (eg, ejaculation, bladder spasms, uterine contractions; Porth, 2002).
- Eighty-five percent of all clients with quadriplegia experience autonomic dysreflexia some time after spinal shock (Kavchak-Keyes, 2000).

Focus Assessment Criteria

Subjective Data
Assess for Defining Characteristics.

Initial Symptoms

Headache (severe, sudden)	Pallor
Sweating (where?)	Dyspnea
Chills	Cold extremities
Metallic taste in mouth	Pilomotor skin erections (goosebumps)
Nasal congestion	Blurred vision
Numbness	Other _____

Assess for Related Factors.

History of Dysreflexia, Triggered by

Bladder distention	Sexual activity
Bowel distention	Menstruation
Tactile stimulation	Diagnostic study
Skin lesion	Pressure
Knowledge of dysreflexia	
Cause	Medical treatment
Self-treatment	Prevention

For more information on Focus Assessment Criteria, visit http://connection.lww.com.

Goal

NOC Neurological Status, Neurological Status: Autonomic, Vital Signs Status

The individual/family will respond to early signs/symptoms.

Indicators
- State factors that cause dysreflexia.
- Describe the treatment for dysreflexia.
- Relate indications for emergency treatment.

General Interventions

NIC Dysreflexia Management, Vital Signs Monitoring, Emergency Care, Medication Administration

Assess for Causative or Contributing Factors.
See *Related Factors.*

Proceed as Follows if Signs of Dysreflexia Occur:
1. Stand or sit person up.
2. Lower client's legs.
3. Loosen all client's constrictive clothing or appliances.

Check for Distended Bladder.

If Client is Catheterized:
1. Check catheter for kinks or compression.
2. Irrigate catheter with only 30 mL of saline, very slowly.
3. Replace catheter if it will not drain.

If Client is Not Catheterized:
1. Insert catheter using dibucaine hydrochloride ointment (Nupercainal).
2. Remove 500 mL, then clamp for 15 min.
3. Repeat cycle until bladder is drained.

Check for Fecal Impaction.

First apply Nupercainal to the anus and into the rectum for 1 inch (2.54 cm).
Gently check rectum with a well-lubricated glove using index finger.
Insert rectal suppository or gently remove impaction.

Check for Skin Irritation.

Spray skin lesion that is triggering dysreflexia with a topical anesthetic agent.
Remove support hose.

Continue to Monitor Blood Pressure Every 3 to 5 min.

Immediately Consult Physician for Pharmacologic Treatment if Hypertension is Double Baseline or Noxious Stimuli are not Eliminated.

Initiate Health Teaching and Referrals as Indicated.

Teach signs, symptoms, and treatment of dysreflexia to client and family.
Teach indications that warrant immediate medical intervention.
Explain situations that trigger dysreflexia (menstrual cycle, sexual activity, elimination).
Teach to watch for early signs and to intervene immediately.
Teach to observe for early signs of bladder infections and skin lesions (pressure ulcers, ingrown toenails).
Advise consultation with physician for long-term pharmacologic management if client is very vulnerable.
Document frequency of episodes and precipitating factor(s).
Provide printed instructions to guide actions during crisis or to show to other health care personnel (eg, dentists, gynecologists; Kavchak-Keyes, 2000).
Advise athletes with high spinal cord injury about the danger of boosting (binding their legs, distending bladder to increase norepinephrine; McClain et al., 1999).

Rationales

- An upright position and removal of hose increase venous pooling, reduce venous return, and decrease blood pressure (Kavchak-Keyes, 2000; Porth, 2002).
- Failure to reverse severe hypertension can result in status epilepticus, retinal or intracerebral hemorrhage, and death (Black & DeSantis, 1999).
- Intravenous pharmacologic intervention may be warranted if noxious stimuli cannot be removed or hypertension is not reduced. Medications may include diazoxide (Hyperstat), hydralazine (Apresoline), sodium nitroprusside (Nipride), and ganglionic-blocking agents such as phenoxybenzamine (Dibenzyline) and guanethidine sulfate (Ismelin). Nifedipine capsule (10 mg) administered sublingually has been used to relieve hypertension in dysreflexia (Eisenhauer et al., 1997).
- Athletes can induce dysreflexia by boosting (McClain et al., 1999).
- Thorough teaching can help the client and family successfully prevent or treat dysreflexia at home.

RISK FOR DYSREFLEXIA

DEFINITION

Refer to *Dysreflexia*.

RISK FACTORS

Refer to *Dysreflexia—Related Factors*.

KEY CONCEPTS

Refer to *Dysreflexia*.

Focus Assessment Criteria

Refer to *Dysreflexia—Focus Assessment Criteria*.

Goal

Refer to *Dysreflexia*.

Interventions

Refer to *Dysreflexia*.

ENERGY FIELD DISTURBANCE

DEFINITION

Energy Field Disturbance: State in which a disruption of the flow of energy surrounding a person's being results in a disharmony of the body, mind, and/or spirit

DEFINING CHARACTERISTICS

Perception of changes in patterns of the energy flow, such as:

- *Temperature change:* warmth, coolness
- *Visual changes:* image, color
- *Disruption of the field:* vacant, hole, spike, bulge
- *Movement:* wave, spike, tingling, dense, flowing
- *Sounds:* tone, word

RELATED FACTORS
Pathophysiologic
Related to slowing or blocking of energy flows secondary to:

Illness (specify)	Pregnancy	Injury

Treatment-Related
Related to slowing or blocking of energy flows secondary to:

Immobility	Perioperative experience	Labor and delivery

Situational (Personal, Environmental)
Related to slowing or blocking of energy flows secondary to:

Pain	Fear	Anxiety
Grieving		

Maturational
Related to age-related developmental difficulties or crises (specify)

○○ **AUTHOR'S NOTE**

This diagnosis is unique for two reasons: it represents a specific theory (human energy field theory), and its interventions require specialized instruction and supervised practice. Meehan (1991) recommends the following preparation:

- At least 6 months of professional practice in an acute care setting
- Guided learning by a nurse with at least 2 years of experience
- Conformance with practice guidelines
- Thirty hours of instruction in the theory and practice
- Thirty hours of supervised practice with relatively healthy people
- Successful completion of written and practice evaluations

Some may consider this diagnosis unconventional. Perhaps nurses need to be reminded that there are many theories, philosophies, and frameworks of nursing practice, just as there are many definitions of clients and practice settings. Some nurses practice on street corners with homeless people, whereas others practice in offices attached to their homes. Nursing diagnosis should not represent only mainstream nursing (acute care, long-term care, home health). Rather than criticize a diagnosis as having little applicability, perhaps nurses should celebrate diversity. Fundamentally, nurses are all connected through the quest to improve the condition of individuals, families, groups, and communities.

KEY CONCEPTS
- Therapeutic touch is rooted in Eastern philosophy. The cultural orientation of Western medicine is to conduct research to explain a modality's effects. In the Eastern culture, if something works, research is unnecessary for proof.
- Therapeutic touch is derived from the basic premise that universal life energy sustains all living organisms. Health is defined as the state in which all a person's energies are in harmony or dynamic balance. Health is compromised when there is disequilibrium, blockage, or deficits in energy flow (Macrae, 1988).
- In nursing, the Rogerian conceptual system has provided the foundation for therapeutic touch. This model affirms that energy fields are fundamental units of human beings and their environment (Meehan, 1991).
- "Therapeutic touch is a knowledgeable and purposive patterning of the patient–environmental energy field process" (Meehan, 1991, p. 201). It requires specialized instruction and supervised practice. See the Author's Note for recommended preparation.
- Life-giving, healing energy flows within the universal flow of energy. Such energy, present in all living systems, is composed of intelligence, order, and compassion (Bradley, 1987).
- Rogers states that therapeutic touch is an example of how a nurse "seeks to strengthen the coherence and integrity of human and environmental fields and to knowingly participate in the

patterning of human and environmental fields for the realization of optimum well-being" (Meehan, 1991).

- In a pilot study, Quinn and Strelkauskas (1993) found that all the recipients of therapeutic touch experienced dramatic increases in all dimensions of positive affect (joy, vigor, contentment, and affection) and dramatic decreases in all dimensions of negative affect (anxiety, guilt, hostility, and depression). They also identified a shift in consciousness during therapeutic touch, which was measured by perception of time. The practitioner and the recipients reported the same time distortions, indicating a shift in consciousness.
- The use of healing touch with critically ill people resulted in no physiologic change before, during, or after therapy; however, recipients experienced significant improvements in relaxation and sleep (Umbreit, 2000).
- An intrinsic relationship may exist between therapeutic touch and the placebo effect. Therapeutic touch may enhance the placebo effect and reduce discomfort and distress (Meehan, 1998).
- Denison (2004) reported that persons with fibromyalgia syndrome reported a decrease in pain with therapeutic touch. Using thermography, there also was an increase in cutaneous skin temperature (Denison, 2004).

Focus Assessment Criteria

Because assessment of the energy field is quickly followed by the intervention and reassessment continues throughout, refer to Interventions for assessment.

Goal

NOC Spiritual Well-Being, Well-Being

The person will report relief of symptoms after therapeutic touch.

Indicators
- Report increased sense of relaxation.
- Report decreased pain, using a scale of 0 to 10 before and after therapies.
- Have slower, deeper respirations.

General Interventions

NIC Therapeutic Touch, Spiritual Support

Note: The following phases of therapeutic touch are learned separately but rendered concurrently. Presentation of these interventions is to describe the process for nurses who do not practice therapeutic touch. This discussion may help them to support colleagues who practice therapeutic touch and also to initiate referrals. As discussed before, preparation for therapeutic touch requires specialized instruction, which is beyond the scope of this book.

Prepare the Client and Environment for Therapeutic Touch.
Provide as much privacy as possible.
Explain therapeutic touch and obtain verbal permission to perform it.
Give person permission to stop the therapy at any time.
Allow person to assume a comfortable position (eg, lying on a bed, sitting on a couch).

Shift from a Direct Focus on the Environment to an Inner Focus, which is Perceived as the Center of Life within the Nurse (Centering).

Assess Client by Scanning His or Her Energy Field for Openness and Symmetry (Krieger, 1979).
Move palms of hands toward client, at a distance of 2 to 4 inches over his or her body, from head to feet in a smooth, light movement.
Use calm and rhyhmic hand movements.
Sense the cues to energy imbalance (eg, warmth, coolness, tightness, heaviness, tingling, emptiness).

Facilitate a Rhythmic Flow of Energy by Moving Hands Vigorously from Head to Toe (Unruffling/Clearing).

Focus Intent on the Specific Repatterning of Areas of Imbalance and Impeded Flow.

Using Your Hands as Focal Points, Move Them Gently, Sweeping from Head to Feet One Time.

Note energy flow over lower legs and feet.

If energy flow is not open in this area, continue to move hands or hold feet physically to facilitate energy flow.

Briefly shake hands to dispel congestion from field if needed.

When therapeutic touch is complete, place hands over the solar plexus area (just above the waist) and focus on facilitating the flow of healing energy to the person.

Provide the person with an opportunity to rest.

Encourage the Person to Provide Feedback.

Assess if the person exhibits a relaxation response. Signs include drops of several decibels in voice volume; slower, deeper respirations; audible sign of relaxation; and a peripheral flush perceived on face.

Document Both the Procedure and the Feedback.

Rationales

- Early beliefs regarding therapeutic touch attributed its effects to an energy transfer and exchange between practitioner and recipient (Quinn, 1989). Current beliefs are that the practitioner shifts "consciousness into a state that may be thought of as a 'healing meditation,' facilitates repatterning of the recipient's energy field through the process of resonance, rather than 'energy exchange or transfer' " (Quinn & Strelkauskas, 1993, p. 14).
- The practitioner of therapeutic touch facilitates the flow of healing energy (Umbreit, 2000).
- "At the core of the therapeutic touch process is the intent of the practitioner to help the recipient" (Quinn & Strelkauskas, 1993, p. 14). The practitioner focuses entirely on the recipient with unconditional love and compassion. The healer is intentionally motivated to help the recipient, who is willing to accept the change.

IMPAIRED ENVIRONMENTAL INTERPRETATION SYNDROME

DEFINITION

Impaired Environmental Interpretation Syndrome: Consistent lack of orientation to person, place, time, or circumstances over more than 3 to 6 months, necessitating a protective environment

DEFINING CHARACTERISTICS
Major

Consistent disorientation in known and unknown environments

Chronic confusional states

Minor

Loss of occupation or social functioning from memory decline

Inability to follow simple directions, instructions

Slow response to questions

Inability to reason

Inability to concentrate

RELATED FACTORS

Dementia (Alzheimer's disease, multiinfarct dementia, Pick's disease, acquired immunodeficiency syndrome [AIDS] dementia)

Parkinson's disease

Huntington's disease

Depression

Alcoholism

⊙⊙ AUTHOR'S NOTE

Impaired Environmental Interpretation Syndrome describes a person who needs a protective environment because of consistent lack of orientation to person, place, time, or circumstance. Interventions focus on maintaining maximum independence and preventing injury. This diagnosis is described already under *Chronic Confusion* and *Risk for Injury*. Until clinical research better differentiates it, use *Chronic Confusion, Risk for Injury,* or both depending on the data presented.

INTERRUPTED FAMILY PROCESSES

DEFINITION

Interrupted Family Processes: State in which a usually supportive family experiences, or is at risk to experience, a stressor that challenges its previously effective functioning

DEFINING CHARACTERISTICS
Major (Must Be Present)

Family system cannot or does not:
Adapt constructively to crisis
Communicate openly and effectively between family members

Minor (May Be Present)

Family system cannot or does not:
Meet physical needs of all its members
Meet emotional needs of all its members
Meet spiritual needs of all its members
Express or accept a wide range of feelings
Seek or accept help appropriately

RELATED FACTORS

Any factor can contribute to *Interrupted Family Processes.* Common factors are listed below.

Treatment-Related

Related to:
Disruption of family routines because of time-consuming treatments (eg, home dialysis)
Physical changes because of treatments of ill family member
Emotional changes in all family members because of treatments of ill family member
Financial burden of treatments for ill family member
Hospitalization of ill family member

Situational (Personal, Environmental)

Related to loss of family member

Death	Incarceration	Going away to school
Desertion	Separation	Hospitalization
Divorce		

Related to addition of new family member

Birth	Marriage	Adoption
Elderly relative		

Related to losses associated with:

Poverty	Economic crisis	Change in family roles
Birth of child with defect	Relocation	(eg, retirement)
Disaster		

Related to conflict (moral, goal, cultural)
Related to breach of trust between members
Related to social deviance by family member (eg, crime)

⦿ AUTHOR'S NOTE

Interrupted Family Processes describes a family that reports usual constructive function but is experiencing an alteration from a current stress-related challenge. The family is viewed as a system, with interdependence among members. Thus, life challenges for individual members also challenge the family system. Certain situations may negatively influence family functioning; examples include illness, an older relative moving in, relocation, separation, and divorce. *Risk for Interrupted Family Processes* can represent such a situation.

Interrupted Family Processes differs from *Caregiver Role Strain*. Certain situations require one or more family members to assume a caregiver role for a relative. Caregiver role responsibilities can vary from ensuring an older parent has three balanced meals daily to providing for all hygiene and self-care activities for an adult or child. *Caregiver Role Strain* describes the mental and physical burden that the caregiver role places on individuals, which influences all their concurrent relationships and role responsibilities. It focuses specifically on the individual or individuals with multiple direct caregiver responsibilities.

⦿ ERRORS IN DIAGNOSTIC STATEMENTS

1. *Interrupted Family Processes related to family not discussing the situation*
   A family's failure to discuss a situation does not represent a related factor, but a possible validation of the problem. If this situation is usual for the family, the nurse should examine *Disabled Family Coping*. If a failure to support one another represents a response to a stressor affecting the family system, *Interrupted Family Processes related to (specify stressor), as evidenced by report of family not discussing the situation* may be appropriate.

KEY CONCEPTS
Generic Considerations

- Each family has a personality to which each member contributes.
- The family unit may be viewed as a system with
  - Interdependence among members
  - Interactional patterns that provide structure and support for members
  - Boundaries between the family and the environment and between members, with varying degrees of permeability
- Families change with time. They must accomplish specific tasks that originate from the needs of their members. Table II.9 illustrates the tasks of the family.
- Each family responds to life challenges in ways that reflect past experiences and future goals.
- Within a family, members interact in various roles that result from individual and group needs: parent, spouse, child, sibling, friend, teacher, and so forth. Illness of one member may precipitate great changes, putting the family at high risk for maladaptation (Clemen-Stone et al., 2002).
- Each family member influences the entire family unit. Thus, the health of an individual influences the health of the family. Family equilibrium depends on a balance of roles in the family and reciprocation (Clemen-Stone et al., 2002; Duvall, 1977).
- *Stress* is defined as the body's response to any demand made on it. Stress has the potential to become a crisis when the person or family cannot cope constructively. A *crisis* is when a person's usual problem-solving methods are inadequate to resolve the situation.
- The family responding to crisis returns to precrisis functioning, develops improved functioning (adaptation), or develops destructive functioning (maladaptation).
  - Constructive or functional coping mechanisms of families facing a stress crisis are as follows (Clemen-Stone et al., 2002).
    - Greater reliance on one another
    - Maintenance of a sense of humor
    - Increased sharing of feeling and thoughts
    - Promotion of each member's individuality
    - Accurate appraisal of the meaning of the problem

TABLE II.9 Stage-Critical Family Developmental Tasks Through the Family Life Cycle

Stage of the Family Life Cycle	Positions in the Family	Stage-Critical Family Developmental Tasks
1. Married couple	Wife Husband	Establishing a mutually satisfying marriage Adjusting to pregnancy and the promise of parenthood Fitting into the kin network
2. Child-bearing	Wife–mother Husband–father Infant daughter or son or both	Having, adjusting to, and encouraging the development of infants Establishing a satisfying home for both parents and infant(s)
3. Preschool-aged	Wife–mother Husband–father Daughter–sister Son–brother	Adapting to the critical needs and interests of preschool children in stimulating, growth-promoting ways Coping with energy depletion and lack of privacy as parents
4. School-aged	Wife–mother Husband–father Daughter–sister Son–brother	Fitting into the community of school-aged families in constructive ways Encouraging children's educational achievement
5. Teenage	Wife–mother Husband–father Daughter–sister Son–brother	Balancing freedom with responsibility as teenagers mature and emancipate themselves Establishing postparental interests and careers as growing parents
6. Launching center	Wife–mother–grandmother Husband–father–grandfather Daughter–sister–aunt Son–brother–uncle	Releasing young adults into work, military service, college, marriage, etc. with appropriate rituals and assistance Maintaining a supportive home base
7. Middle-aged parents	Wife–mother–grandmother Husband–father–grandfather	Rebuilding the marriage relationship Maintaining kin ties with older and younger generations
8. Aging family members	Widow–widower Wife–mother–grandmother Husband–father–grandfather	Coping with bereavement and living alone Closing the family home or adapting it to aging Adjusting to retirement

Duvall, E. M. (1977). *Marriage and family development* (5th ed.). Philadelphia: J. B. Lippincott, reproduced with permission.

- Search for knowledge and resources about the problem
- Use of support systems
- Destructive or dysfunctional coping mechanisms of families facing a crisis are as follows (Smith-DiJulio, 1998):
  - Denial of the problem
  - Exploitation of one or more members (threats, violence, neglect, scapegoating)
  - Separation (hospitalization, institutionalization, divorce, abandonment)
  - Authoritarianism (no negotiation)
  - Preoccupation of family or members (who lack affection) with appearing close
- Parenthood is a crisis. Some common problems include the following:
  - Increased arguments in adults
  - Fatigue resulting from schedule
  - Disrupted social life
  - Disrupted sex life
  - Multiple losses—actual or perceived (eg, independence, career, appearance, attention)
- Characteristics of families prone to crisis include the following (Fife, 1985; Smith-DiJulio, 1998):
  - Apathy (resignation to state in life)
  - Poor self-concept
  - Low income
  - Inability to manage money
  - Unrealistic preferences (materialistic)
  - Lack of skills and education
  - Unstable work history
  - Frequent relocations
  - History of repeated inadequate problem solving
  - Lack of adequate role models
  - Lack of participation in religious or community activities
  - Environmental isolation (no telephone, inadequate public transportation)

- A time lag exists between identifying symptoms and help-seeking behavior, which may vary among families, depending on previous experience with the health care system, cultural interpretations of health and illness, and financial concerns.
- Successful outcomes of family efforts to achieve new adaptation after a crisis depend on the following (Nugent, Hughes, Ball & Davis, 1992):
  - Cohesiveness in response to past stressors
  - Interaction with others in support group
  - Belief that family can handle the crisis

❖ Pediatric Considerations

- Two of the most significant stresses a child and family may experience are illness and hospitalization. The stresses of separation from parents, loss of control in a strange environment, and fear of bodily injury and pain make children particularly vulnerable (Wong, 2003).
- Parents share many of the same stresses as hospitalized children. In addition, they may experience stress if hospital staff takes over their roles as primary caretakers. Parents are responsible as well for the care of siblings, who are affected by the crisis of illness and hospitalization (Craft & Craft, 1989; Wong, 2003). Parents of hospitalized children often are not aware of the number of changes that siblings experience (Wong, 2003).
- Keeping "family secrets" consumes a child's attention and energy.
- Family functioning has been found to deteriorate over 1 year after injury among children with severe traumatic head injuries (Burgess et al., 1999).
- "Chronic illnesses consume and deprive the parents of extra finances, time, energy, and privacy and can ultimately lead to emotional and social isolation" (Kurnat & Moore, 1999, p. 290).

🌐 Transcultural Considerations

- The dominant US culture values two goals for families: (1) encouragement and nurturance of each individual and (2) cultivation of healthy, autonomous children. Marital partners are expected to be supportive and share a sense of meaning. Each partner has the freedom for personality development. Children are encouraged to develop their own identity and life directions (Giger & Davidhizar, 2003).
- The family was found to be the principal source of support during illness in seven minority groups (Giger & Davidhizar, 2003).
- In Latin families, the needs of the family are more important than those of the individual. The father is provider, head of household, and decision maker (Andrews & Boyle, 2003).
- Arab-American families are supposed to be supportive. A family is often criticized as a failure if a member is sent to the hospital for psychiatric care. Arab-American families may appear overindulgent and interfering to compensate for criticism (Giger & Davidhizar, 2003).
- Japanese Americans identify themselves by the generation in which they are born. First- and second-generation Japanese Americans see the family as one of the most important factors in their lives. They manage problems within the family structure. The father and other male members are in the top position. Achievement or failure of one member reflects on the entire family. Caring for elderly parents, usually by the oldest son or unmarried child, is expected. Adult children freely provide their parents with goods, money, and assistance (Andrews & Boyle, 2003; Hashizume & Takano, 1983).
- The nuclear family and the greater Jewish community are the center of Jewish culture. Families are close knit and child oriented. The commandments dictate expected behavior toward parents and within the community (Giger & Davidhizar, 2003).
- For the Vietnamese, family has been the chief source of cohesion and continuity for hundreds of years. Immediate family includes parents, unmarried children, and sometimes the husband's parents and sons with their wives and children. Individual behavior reflects on the whole family. A member is expected to give up personal wishes or ambitions if they disrupt family harmony. Family loyalty is "filial piety," which commands children to obey and honor their parents even after death (Giger & Davidhizar, 2003).

Focus Assessment Criteria

Subjective/Objective

General

Family composition (who resides in home)
Family strengths
Rules/discipline
Financial status
Participation in community activities

How Does the Family

Integrate its roles, relationships?
Use information from outside the family?
Adapt to changes?
Make and implement decisions?
Respond to conflict or disagreements?
Preserve family integrity as well as family members' autonomy?

Assess for Defining Characteristics.

Communication patterns

Express feelings openly	Straight messages	No manipulation

Emotional/supportive pattern

Constructive

Appraise problem accurately	Rely on one another	Show optimism
Seek knowledge and resources	Share feelings, thoughts	Deal with problems
Use support systems		

Destructive

Deny problems	Use abandonment	Show authoritarianism
Exploit members (threats, violence, neglect, scapegoating)	Show apathy	

Socialization function

Family members develop in a healthy pattern.
Family members negotiate roles and responsibilities.

Parenting and marriage roles

Satisfying	Mutual agreement

Child behavior

Home	School

Assess for Related Factors.

Addition of new family member

Birth	Adoption	Marriage
Elderly relative		

Loss of family member

Relocation	Illness	Death

Change in family roles

Financial crisis
Disaster
Conflicts
Family member with a coping problem
Relocation history

For more information on Focus Assessment Criteria, visit http://connection.lww.com.

Goal

NOC Family Coping,
Family Environment: Internal,
Family Normalization, Parenting

The family will maintain functional system of mutual support for one another.

Indicators

- Frequently verbalize feelings to professional nurse and one another.
- Identify appropriate external resources available.

General Interventions

 NIC Family Involvement Promotion, Coping Enhancement, Family Integrity Promotion, Family Therapy, Counseling, Referral

Assess Causative and Contributing Factors.

Illness-related Factors

Sudden, unexpected nature of illness
Burdensome, chronic problems
Potentially disabling nature of illness
Symptoms creating disfiguring change in physical appearance
Social stigma associated with illness
Financial burden

Factors Related to Behavior of Ill Family Member

Refuses to cooperate with necessary interventions
Engages in socially deviant behavior associated with illness: suicide attempts, violence, substance abuse
Isolates self from family
Acts out or is verbally abusive to health professionals and family members

Factors Related to the Overall Family

Unresolved guilt, blame, hostility, jealousy
Inability to solve problems
Ineffective communication patterns among members
Changes in role expectations and resulting tension

Factors Related to Illness in Family (See also *Caregiver Role Strain*)

Lack of family members available for support
Inadequate finances
Lack of knowledge of caregiver
History of poor relationship between caregiver and ill member
Overburdened caregiver

Factors Related to Health Care Environment

Lack of expertise by intervening professionals in crisis intervention, counseling, or basic communication
Not enough health professionals to spend time with family
Lack of continuity of care
Lack of physical facilities in institution to ensure privacy or individualized care

Factors Related to the Community

Lack of support from spiritual resources (philosophical, religious, or both)
Lack of relevant health education resources
Lack of supportive friends
Lack of adequate community health care resources (eg, long-term follow up, hospice, respite)

Provide Ongoing Information.

Approach the family with warmth, respect, and support.
Avoid vague and confusing advice and clichés, such as, "Take it easy; everything will be OK."
Reflect family emotions to confirm these feelings ("This is very painful for you"; "You are very frightened").
Keep family members abreast of changes in ill member's condition when appropriate.
Avoid discussing what caused the problem or blaming.

Promote Cohesiveness.

Facilitate communication.
Encourage verbalization of guilt, anger, blame, and hostility and subsequent recognition of own feelings in family members.
Enlist help of other professionals (eg, social worker, clinical psychologist, nurse therapist, clinical specialist, psychiatrist, child care specialist, school nurse) when indicated.

Assist Family to Appraise the Situation.

What is at stake? Encourage family to have a realistic perspective by providing accurate information and answers to questions.

What are the choices? Assist family to reorganize roles at home and set priorities to maintain family integrity and reduce stress.

Initiate discussions regarding stressors of home care (physical, emotional, environmental, financial).

Initiate Health Teaching and Referrals, as Necessary.

Include family members in group education sessions.

Refer families to lay support and self-help groups

Al-Anon	Lupus Foundation of America
Syn-Anon	Arthritis Foundation
Alcoholics Anonymous	National Multiple Sclerosis Society
Sharing and Caring	American Cancer Society
(American Hospital	American Heart Association
Association)	American Diabetes Association
Ostomy Association	American Lung Association
Reach for Recovery	Alzheimer's Disease and Related Disorders Association

Facilitate family involvement with social supports.

Assist family members to identify reliable friends (eg, clergy, significant others); encourage seeking help (emotional, technical) when appropriate.

Rationales

- The goal of crisis management is to assist the family to return to precrisis functioning. If such functioning was destructive (eg, alcoholism), the goal is to develop improved functioning.
- Common sources of family stress are as follows (Smith-DiJulio, 1998):
  - External sources of stress (eg, job or school related) one member is experiencing
  - External sources of stress (eg, finances, relocation) influencing the family unit
  - Developmental stressors (eg, childbearing, new baby, childrearing, adolescence, arrival of older grandparent, marriage of single parents, loss of spouse)
  - Situational stressors (eg, illness, hospitalization, separation)

INTERRUPTED FAMILY PROCESSES

RELATED TO IMPACT (SPECIFY) OF ILL MEMBER ON FAMILY SYSTEM

Goals

See Goals for *Interrupted Family Processes.*

Interventions (see NIC for General Interventions)

Create a Supportive Environment.

Keep client's door closed if desired.

Provide family members with an alternative meeting place to the client's room.

Make sure family members are oriented to visiting hours, bathrooms, vending machines, cafeteria, and so forth.

If possible, provide pillows/blankets for family members spending the night.

Promote positive family visits (Harkulich & Calamita, 1986).

    Relate a positive experience you've observed representing a strength or individuality of the person.

    Encourage the person to be well dressed and groomed for visits.

    Encourage activities the person enjoys (eg, walking, crafts, card games).

    If appropriate, share the weekly schedule of activities.

    Elicit suggestions from family for unmet needs.

Facilitate Family Strengths.

Acknowledge these strengths to family when appropriate.

    "I can tell you are a very close family."

    "You know just how to get your mother to eat."

    "Your brother means a great deal to you."

Ask family members about care routine at home; determine how involved they want to be (Kurnat & Moore, 1999).

Involve family members in client care conferences, when appropriate.

Encourage family to find substitutes to care for the ill person, to provide the family with time away.

Promote self-esteem of individual members ("Your daughter may respond to your drawings if we place them in her crib"; see *Disturbed Self-Concept*).

If appropriate, help ill member identify how to give support to caregiver (eg, praise, listening).

Mobilize ill person to accept responsibility for some activities that contribute to family functioning (eg, create shopping list, phone inquiries, peel vegetables).

Facilitate Understanding, in Other Family Members, of How Ill Person Feels.

Discuss stresses of hospitalization.

Describe implications of "sick role" and how it will return to "well role."

Assist family members to have realistic expectations of the ill member.

Assist Family to Appraise the Situation.

Emphasize the importance of respites to prevent isolating behaviors that foster depression.

Discuss with nonprimary caregivers their responsibilities in caring for the primary caregiver.

Provide Anticipatory Guidance as Illness Continues.

Inform parents of effects of prolonged hospitalization on children (appropriate to developmental age).

Prepare family members for signs of depression, anxiety, and dependency, which are a natural part of the illness experience.

If the ill family member is an elderly parent undergoing surgery, inform children that the client may be confused or disoriented for a limited period after surgery.

Refer to *Caregiver Role Strain* if indicated.

Discuss the Implications of Caring for Ill Family Member.

Available resources (financial, environmental)

24-hour responsibility

Effects on other household members

Likelihood of progressive deterioration

Sharing of responsibilities (with other household members, siblings, neighbors)

Likelihood of exacerbation of long-standing conflicts

Effects on lifestyle

Alternative or assistive options (eg, community-based health care providers, life care centers, group living, nursing home)

Rationales

- Successful coping with illness requires the family to complete the following tasks: acknowledge the problem and seek help, accept the problem and its implications, and adjust as the member begins reconstruction (Kurnat & Moore, 1999).

- The family acknowledges the problem by identifying the symptoms as serious enough to warrant investigation, and gaining knowledge of accessible resources (Clark & Gwin, 2001).
- The family must face the diagnosis and its implications. This task is multidimensional:
  - Experiencing the initial shock
  - Engaging in open communication among members
  - Minimizing anxiety and its disabling consequences
  - Preventing prolonged despair, guilt, blame, hostility
  - Accepting a valid diagnosis
- Studies have shown that relatives of people with cancer "have perceived needs for information, communication skills, coping strategies and support services" (Clark & Gwin, 2001, p. 470).
- The family must adjust, as the member begins to recover, by:
  - Adapting to new ways of living and making appropriate changes as recovery ensues
  - Fostering independence of recovering member
  - Accepting residual disability and making any necessary accommodations
  - Recognizing depression and anxiety in relative during change from "sick role" to "well role"
- The family must return to normal by resuming previous activities as much as possible and incorporating the recovered member back into family activities and responsibilities.

DYSFUNCTIONAL FAMILY PROCESSES: ALCOHOLISM

DEFINITION

Dysfunctional Family Processes: Alcoholism: State in which the psychosocial, spiritual, economic, and physiologic functions of the family members and system are chronically disorganized because of the effects of alcohol abuse

DEFINING CHARACTERISTICS (LINDEMAN, HOKANSON & BARTEK, 1994)
Major (80% to 100%)

Behaviors

Inappropriate expression of anger	Inadequate understanding or knowledge of alcoholism	Manipulation
Dependency	Loss of control of drinking	Denial of problems
Impaired communication	Alcohol abuse	Refusal to get help
Enabling behaviors	Blaming	Rationalization
Inability to meet emotional needs	Broken promises	Ineffective problem solving
		Criticizing

Feelings

Decreased self-esteem	Hopelessness	Anger
Unhappiness	Hurt	Guilt
Powerlessness	Frustration	Tension
Emotional isolation	Worthlessness	Vulnerability
Suppressed rage	Repressed emotions	Anxiety
Shame	Mistrust	Loneliness
Responsible for alcoholic's behavior	Embarrassment	Rejection

Roles and Relationships

Deteriorated family relationships	Ineffective spouse communication	Intimacy dysfunction
Closed communication systems	Inconsistent parenting	Disturbed family dynamics
	Family denial	Marital problems
		Disruption of family roles

Minor (70% to 79%)

Behaviors
Cannot express or accept wide range of feelings
Inability to get or receive help appropriately
Orientation toward tension relief rather than goal achievement
Ineffective decision making
Contradictory, paradoxical communication
Family's special occasions are alcohol centered
Failure to deal with conflict
Harsh self-judgment
Escalating conflict
Isolation
Lying
Failure to send clear messages
Difficulty having fun
Immaturity
Disturbances in concentration
Chaos
Inability to adapt to change
Substance abuse other than alcohol
Difficulty with life cycle transitions
Power struggles
Verbal abuse of spouse or parent
Stress-related physical illnesses
Failure to accomplish current or past developmental tasks
Lack of reliability
Disturbances in academic performance in children

Feelings

Being different from other people	Lack of identity	Unresolved grief
Feelings misunderstood	Loss	Depression
Fear	Hostility	Abandonment
Moodiness	Confused love and pity	Emotional control by others
Dissatisfaction	Confusion	Failure
	Being unloved	Self-blaming

Roles and Relationships
Triangulating family relationship
Inability to meet spiritual needs of members
Reduced ability to relate to one another for mutual growth and maturation
Lack of skills necessary for relationships
Lack of cohesiveness
Disrupted family rituals or no family rituals
Inability to meet security needs of members
Does not demonstrate respect for individuality of its members
Decreased sexual communication and individuality of its members
Low perception of parental support
Pattern of rejection
Neglected obligations

RELATED FACTORS

Because the cause of this diagnosis is alcohol abuse by a family member, no related factors are needed.

◯◯ AUTHOR'S NOTE

Alcoholism is a family disease. This nursing diagnosis represents the consequences of the disturbed family dynamics related to alcohol abuse by a family member. The NANDA definition of *Interrupted Family Processes* is "the state in which a family that normally functions effectively experiences a dysfunction" (NANDA, 1992, p. 41). The alcoholic family does not have a history of effective functioning. *Disabled Family Coping* would be more descriptive of the alcoholic family. The diagnosis

(continued)

○○ **AUTHOR'S NOTE** (*Continued*)

could be stated as *Ineffective Family Coping: Alcoholism*. Further assessment will determine the physical, psychological, spiritual, financial, and developmental effects of alcoholism on the family unit. If clinical research validates that alcoholism affects all these dimensions in all or most families, the diagnosis *Alcoholic Family Syndrome* may prove very useful.

○○ **ERRORS IN DIAGNOSTIC CONSIDERATIONS**

Dysfunctional Family Processes: Alcoholism related to effects of alcohol on family
   The "related to" duplicates the diagnostic statement. The inclusion of *Alcoholism* in the diagnostic statement eliminates the need for related factors. Thus, the nurse should state the diagnosis as *Dysfunctional Family Processes: Alcoholism as evidenced by denial of severity of the problem, guilt, and repressed emotions.*

KEY CONCEPTS
Generic Considerations

- Alcoholism is a family disease. Approximately 10 million alcoholics are in the United States; at least 4 million others are affected intimately (Captain, 1989).
- Alcoholic family members "lack trust in each other, lack nurturing closeness and solve problems in a piecemeal fashion" (Smith-DiJulio, 1998, p. 784).
- Alcoholism and its denial dominate alcoholic families. When alcohol is the center of the family, developmental tasks are thwarted or ignored. "To keep the family unit intact, each member must change his or her cognitive perceptions to fit into the family's scheme of enabling the drinking to continue, while at the same time denying that it is a problem" (Starling & Martin, 1990, p. 16).
- Alcoholics initially use denial about alcohol to relieve stress. After dependence sets in, they use denial to conceal from self and others how important alcohol is to functioning (Smith-DiJulio, 1998).
- As destructive interactions continue, family members and the alcoholic move away from each other. The alcoholic turns to liquor, while the family finds other means of escape (Collins, Leonard & Searles, 1990).
- "Meaningful sobriety is characterized by more than just the abstinence of the alcoholic person. It necessitates an ongoing growth process for all family members to work together toward the goal of a well-functioning family" (Grisham & Estes, 1982, p. 257).
- Wegscheider (1981) described six roles typical in families affected by alcoholism:
  - Alcoholic
  - Chief enabler—often the spouse; super-responsible, takes on alcoholic's duties
  - Family hero—high achiever to provide family with some pride to cover up failures
  - Scapegoat—defiant, angry, diverts family focus from alcoholism
  - Lost child—helpless, powerless
  - Mascot—clowning, joking; a form of tension relief to mask underlying terror
- Wing (1991; 1994) describes a four-stage theory of alcoholism, recovery, and goal setting:
  - Stage I: Denial—alcoholics are coerced into treatment; their goals are to avoid punishment, with no sincere desire to stop drinking.
  - Stage II: Dependence—alcoholics admit that they have a drinking problem and seek treatment to maintain job or a relationship.
  - Stage III: Behavior change—alcoholics attempt to replace unhealthy behaviors with healthy behaviors.
  - Stage IV: Life planning—alcoholics integrate family, career, and educational goals with sobriety.
- Men entering treatment services perceive alcohol as the cause of their problems. Women reported that they drank because of their problems (Kellett et al., 2000).

◆ **Pediatric Considerations**

- Children learn definitions of love, intimacy, and trust in their families of origin. The environment in the alcoholic family is chaotic and unpredictable. Roles are unclear. Some-

(*continued*)

❖ Pediatric Considerations (continued)

times, children become the parents and the alcoholic member becomes an outsider in the family.
* Children report being more disturbed by parents arguing rather than one parent's drinking. Children can respond in varied ways (eg, peacemaker, aggression at school).
* Behavioral problems in children need to be assessed in the context of their purpose for the family.
* Children of alcoholics are accustomed to extra and inappropriate responsibilities (Smith-DiJulio, 1998).

🌐 Transcultural Considerations

* Alcoholism is the number one health problem in the black community, reducing longevity with high incidences of acute and chronic alcohol-related diseases. Unemployment has been identified as the primary factor. Treatment programs must be accessible within the community or by public transportation. Black churches serve a dual role as a site for therapy meetings and as a referral service (Giger & Davidhizar, 2003).
* Alcohol consumption is a way to celebrate life for Mexican Americans. Alcohol contributes to increased accidents and violence. Family pride protects the alcoholic male as long as he provides for the family (Giger & Davidhizar, 2003).
* Alcoholism is found among Native Americans in very high percentages. It is responsible for violence, suicides, and fetal alcohol syndrome. Studies have shown an increased sensitivity to alcohol in this group (Giger & Davidhizar, 2003).

Focus Assessment Criteria

This assessment focuses on individual family members and the family unit. For a specific assessment tool (eg, Michigan Alcoholism Screening Test [MAST], CAGE Screening Test), refer to *Ineffective Coping*. For general family assessment, refer to *Interrupted Family Processes*.

Subjective Data
General

Family roles (eg, breadwinner)	Family composition	Family strengths
Participation in community activities	Rules/discipline	Financial status
	Extended family	

Assess for Defining Characteristics.
Denial of problem
Responses of family members

Alcohol use influences decisions	Afraid	Worried
Overall feelings	Embarrassed	Effects on each member
	Behavior problems (children)	Guilt feelings

Characteristics of alcoholic person

Friends drink heavily	Justifies alcohol use	Promises to quit or reduce
Is verbally/physically abusive	Drives under influence	Fails to remember events
Avoids conversations about alcohol	Has periods of remorse	

Family/social functions

Unsatisfactory, tense	Always include alcohol	Financial, legal problems
Negative comments of others on drinking behavior		

Objective Data

Prepare a three-generation genogram.
Use symbols □ (male) and ○ (female).
Give name, age, birth date, death date, highest level of education, occupation, significant health problems, addictions, and date of diagnosis for parents, siblings, children of person, and spouse.

Link symbols with lines that indicate:

Marriage	Separation	Divorce
Living together		

Indicate death with × in symbol or miscarriage with △ or abortion with ×

For more information on Focus Assessment Criteria, visit http://connection.lww.com .

Goals

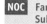 **NOC** Family Coping, Family Functioning, Substance Abuse Consequences

The family will acknowledge the alcoholism in the family.
The family will set short- and long-term goals.

Indicators

- Relate the effects of alcoholism on the family unit and individuals.
- Identify destructive response patterns.
- Describe resources available for individual and family therapy.

General Interventions

NIC Coping Enhancements, Referral, Family Process Maintenance, Substance Abuse Treatment, Family Integrity Promotion, Limit Setting, Support Group

Establish a Trusting Relationship.

Be consistent; keep promises.
Be accepting and noncritical.
Do not pass judgment on what is revealed.
Focus on family member responses.

Allow Family Members as Individuals and a Group to Share Pent-up Feelings.

Validate feelings as normal.
Correct inaccurate beliefs.

Emphasize that Family Members Are Not Responsible for the Person's Drinking (Starling & Martin, 1990; Smith & Julio, 1998).

Explain that emotional difficulties are relationship based rather than "psychiatric."
Instruct that their feelings and experiences are associated frequently with family alcoholism.

Explore the Family's Beliefs about Situation and Goals.

Discuss characteristics of alcoholism; review a screening test (eg, MAST, CAGE) that outlines characteristics of alcoholism.
Discuss causes and correct misinformation.
Assist to establish short- and long-term goals.

Discuss Ineffective Methods Families Use.

Hiding alcohol or car keys	Anger, silence, threats, crying
Making excuses for work, family, or friends	Bailing the person out of jail

Assist the Family to Gain Insight into Behavior.

Does not stop drinking
Increases family anger
Removes the responsibility for drinking from the person
Prevents the person from suffering the consequences of his or her drinking behavior

Emphasize that Helping the Alcoholic Means First Helping Themselves.

Focus on changing their response.
Allow the person to be responsible for his or her drinking behavior.
Describe activities that will improve their lives, as individuals and a family.
Initiate one stress management technique (eg, aerobic exercise, assertiveness course, meditation).
Plan time as a family together outside the home (eg, museum, zoos, picnic). If the alcoholic is included, he or she must contract not to drink during the activity and agree on a consequence if he or she does.

Discuss with Family that Recovery will Change Dramatically Usual Family Dynamics.

The alcoholic is removed from the center of attention.

All family roles will be challenged.

Family members will have to focus on themselves instead of the alcoholic person.

Family members will have to assume responsibility for their behavior, rather than blaming others.

Behavioral problems of children serve a purpose for the family.

Discuss Possibility of and Contributing Factors to Relapse (see Rationales).

If Additional Family or Individual Nursing Diagnoses Exist, Refer to Specific Diagnosis (eg, Child Abuse, Domestic Violence).

Initiate Health Teaching Regarding Community Resources and Referrals as Indicated.

Al-Anon	Alcoholics Anonymous	Family therapy
Individual therapy	Self-help groups	

Rationales

- Ending the drinking behavior threatens the family because equilibrium is centered around the alcoholism (Smith-DiJulio, 1998).
- Interventions focus on assisting the family to change their ineffective communication and response patterns (Smith-DiJulio, 1998).
- Family members use denial to avoid admitting the problem and dealing with their contribution to it, and in the hope that the problem will disappear if not disclosed (Collins et al., 1990).
- Alcoholism disturbs family communication. Sharing feelings is uncommon because of a history of disappointment. Diminished sharing and silence can maintain disturbed families for long periods. Communication focuses mainly on family members trying to control the other person's drinking behavior (Grisham & Estes, 1982).
- "The potential value of reaching the alcoholic person by first assisting family members should not be underestimated" (Grisham & Estes, 1982, p. 257). The family and health care professional must accept that no certain outcome can be promised for the alcoholic, even when the family gets help.
- Wing (1994) proposes that relapses occur for different reasons in each stage. In stage I, relapse accompanies removal of the threat of punishment. Relapse in stage II occurs when the object of dependence (eg, marriage, job) is secured or lost. Relapses in stages III and IV are less frequent and triggered by unexpected, stressful events. Nursing interactions for people in stages I and II focus on confronting denial and helping them become more internally focused. People in stages III and IV need assistance to learn how to cope with unexpected, stressful events (Wing, 1994).
- Common issues that families in therapy face are as follows (Vanicelli, 1987):
  - Coping with sudden disequilibrium
  - Feeling that they are strangers
  - Attributing all family problems to the alcohol problem
  - Losing the fantasy that everything will be fine when drinking ceases
  - Learning appropriate ways to express anger
- Self-help and support groups promote acceptance of the disease concept of alcoholism and can reduce burdens of guilt, shame, and hostility (Smith-DiJulio, 1998).
- The family is the unit of treatment when one member is an alcoholic. Referrals are needed for long-term therapy.

FATIGUE

DEFINITION

Fatigue: Self-recognized state in which a person experiences an overwhelming, sustained sense of exhaustion and decreased capacity for physical and mental work that is not relieved by rest

DEFINING CHARACTERISTICS
Major (80% to 100%)
Verbalization of an unremitting and overwhelming lack of energy
Inability to maintain usual routines
Verbalization of distress

Minor (50% to 79%)
Perceived need for additional energy to accomplish routine tasks
Impaired ability to concentrate

Lethargy or listlessness
Increased physical complaints
Emotional ability or irritability
Decreased performance
Sleep disturbances

RELATED FACTORS
Many factors can cause fatigue; combining related factors may be useful (eg, *Related to muscle weakness, accumulated waste products, inflammation, and infections secondary to hepatitis*).

Bio-Pathophysiologic
Related to hypermetabolic state secondary to:

Viruses (eg, Epstein-Barr)	Fever	Pregnancy

Related to inadequate tissue oxygenation secondary to:

Chronic obstructive lung disease	Congestive heart failure	Anemia
Peripheral vascular disease		

Related to biochemical changes secondary to:
Endocrine / metabolic disorders

Diabetes mellitus	Pituitary disorders	Acquired immunodeficiency syndrome (AIDS)
Hypothyroidism	Addison's disease	

Chronic diseases

Renal failure	Cirrhosis	Lyme disease

Related to muscular weakness/wasting secondary to:

Myasthenia gravis	Parkinson's disease	Multiple sclerosis
AIDS	Amyotrophic lateral sclerosis	

Related to hypermetabolic state, competition between body and tumor for nutrients, anemia, and stressors associated with cancer
Related to nutritional deficits or changes in nutrient metabolism secondary to:

Nausea	Side effects of medications	Vomiting
Gastric surgery	Diarrhea	Diabetes mellitus

Related to chronic inflammatory process secondary to:

AIDS	Cirrhosis	Arthritis
Inflammatory bowel disease	Lupus erythematosus	Renal failure
Hepatitis	Lyme disease	

Treatment-Related
Biochemical changes secondary to:
Chemotherapy
Radiation therapy
Side effects of (specify):
Related to surgical damage to tissue and anesthesia
Related to increased energy expenditure secondary to:

Amputation	Gait disorder	Use of walker, crutches

Situational (Personal, Environmental)
Related to prolonged decreased activity and deconditioning secondary to:

Anxiety	Social isolation	Fever
Nausea/vomiting	Diarrhea	Depression
Pain	Obesity	

Related to excessive role demands
Related to overwhelming emotional demands
Related to extreme stress
Related to sleep disturbance

Maturational
Child/Adolescent
Related to hypermetabolic state secondary to:
Mononucleosis   Fever

Related to chronic insufficient nutrients secondary to:
Obesity   Excessive dieting   Eating disorders
Related to effects of newborn care on sleep patterns and need for continuous attention
Related to hypermetabolic state during first trimester

⊗ AUTHOR'S NOTE

Fatigue as a nursing diagnosis differs from acute tiredness. Tiredness is a transient, temporary state (Rhoten, 1982) caused by lack of sleep, improper nutrition, increased stress, sedentary lifestyle, or temporarily increased work or social responsibilities. Fatigue is a pervasive, subjective, drained feeling that cannot be eliminated; however, the nurse can assist the person to adapt to it. Activity intolerance differs from fatigue in that the nurse will assist the person with activity intolerance to increase endurance and activity.

The focus for the person with fatigue is not on increasing endurance. If the cause resolves or abates (eg, acute infection, chemotherapy, radiation), *Fatigue* as a diagnosis is discontinued and *Activity Intolerance* can be initiated to focus on improving the deconditioned state.

⊗ ERRORS IN DIAGNOSTIC STATEMENTS

1. *Fatigue related to feelings of lack of energy for routine tasks*

When a person reports insufficient energy for routine tasks, the nurse performs a focus assessment and collects additional data to determine whether *Fatigue* is appropriate or actually a symptom of another diagnosis, such as *Activity Intolerance, Ineffective Coping, Interrupted Family Processes, Anxiety,* or *Ineffective Health Maintenance.* When acute or chronic conditions cause fatigue, the nurse must determine whether the person can increase endurance (which would call for *Activity Intolerance*) or needs energy conservation techniques to help accomplish desired activities. When fatigue results from ineffective stress management or poor health habits, *Fatigue* or *Activity Intolerance* is not indicated. During data collection to determine contributing factors, the nurse can record the diagnosis as *Possible Fatigue related to reports of lack of energy.* Using a "possible" diagnosis indicates the need for more data collection to rule out or confirm.

KEY CONCEPTS
Generic Considerations

- Fatigue is a subjective experience with physiologic, situational, and psychological components.
- Acute tiredness is an expected response to physical exertion, change in daily activities, additional stress, or inadequate sleep.
- US society values energy, productivity, and vitality. It views those without energy as sluggish or lazy. It views fatigue and tiredness negatively.
- Fatigue can be physical, mental, and motivational. Causes of fatigue are multifactorial. Careful assessment of the causes and interventions to reduce them are critical (Adinolfi, 2001).
- Fatigue can be manifested in areas of cortical inhibition (Jiricka, 2002; Rhoten, 1982):
  - Decreased attention
  - Slowed and impaired perception
  - Impaired thinking
  - Decreased motivation

TABLE II.10 Contributing Factors to Fatigue in Clients with Cancer

Pathophysiologic
Hypermetabolic state associated with active tumor growth
Competition between the body and the tumor for nutrients
Chronic pain
Organ dysfunction (eg, hepatic, respiratory, gastrointestinal)
Treatment-Related
Accumulation of toxic waste products secondary to radiation, chemotherapy
Inadequate nutritional intake secondary to nausea, vomiting
Anemia
Analgesics, antiemetics
Diagnostic tests
Surgery
Situational (Personal, Environmental)
Uncertainty about future
Fear of death, disfigurement
Social isolation
Losses (role responsibilities, occupational, body parts, function, appearance, economic)
Separation for treatments

- Decreased performance in physical and mental activities
- Loss of fine coordination
- Poor judgment
- Indifference to surroundings
- Hargreaves (1977) described a high incidence of "fatigue syndrome" in young married women moving to a new town. Contributing factors were increased physical work, changes in support systems, and other stresses in relocation.
- People with rheumatoid arthritis reported that their fatigue was related to joint pain. In addition, clients with flare were observed to awaken more often and take longer to walk and perform activities than nonflare clients and the control group (Crosby, 1991).
- Cancer-related fatigue has been reported in 35% to 100% of cases and is reported to be the most distressing side effect (Badger et al., 2001). Stressors contributing to fatigue in clients with cancer are illustrated in Table II.10.
- Women receiving localized radiation to the breast reported that fatigue decreased the second week but increased and reached a plateau after week 4 until 3 weeks after treatment ceased. Fatigue levels did not change significantly on weekends between treatments (Greenberg, Sawicka, Eisenthal & Ross, 1992).
- When fatigue is a side effect of treatment, it does not resolve when the treatment ends, but gradually lessens over months (Nail & Winningham, 1997).
- Depression slows thought processes and leads to decreased physical activities. Work output decreases, and endurance lessens. The effort to continue activity produces fatigue.
- Anxiety can interfere with thought processes, increase movements, and disturb gastrointestinal function, thus causing fatigue.

Pediatric Considerations

- Infants and small children cannot express fatigue. The nurse can elicit this information by interviewing the parents and carefully assessing key functional health patterns (eg, sleep–rest, activity–exercise [which may reveal respiratory difficulties or activity intolerance], and nutrition–metabolic [which may reveal feeding difficulties]).
- Children at risk for fatigue include those with acute or chronic illness, congenital heart disease, exposure to toxins, prolonged stress, or anemia.
- Children depend on parents/caregivers to modify the environment to mitigate effects of fatigue.

Maternal Considerations

Gardner reported that levels of fatigue in postpartum women increased at 2 weeks but decreased by 6 weeks. Factors associated with high postpartum fatigue were sleep alterations, additional children, child care problems, less household help, less education, low family income, and young age of mother (Gardner & Campbell, 1991).

Geriatric Considerations

- The normal effects of aging do not in themselves increase the risk of or cause fatigue. Fatigue in older adults has basically the same etiologies as in younger adults. The difference is that older adults tend to experience more chronic diseases than younger adults. Thus, fatigue in older adults is not the result of age-related factors, but related to such risk factors as chronic diseases and medications.
- Depression is the most common psychosocial impairment in older adults. Depression-related affective disturbances affect 27% of adults in a community-living setting (Miller, 2004).
- Chronic fatigue and diminished energy are functional consequences of late-life depression (Miller, 2004).
- According to Miller (2004), "the activity theory proposed that older adults would remain psychologically and socially fit if they remained active." Participation in activities affirms a person's self-concept.
- Chronic fatigue, reported by approximately 70% of older adults, can result in diminished motor activity and muscle tone. Note that anemia, very common in this population, is another possible contributor to complaints of chronic fatigue (Miller, 2004).

Focus Assessment Criteria

Subjective Data
Assess for Defining Characteristics.
Description of Fatigue
Onset
Pattern: morning, evening, transient, unfading
Precipitated by what?
Relieved by rest?

Effects of Fatigue on:

Activities of daily living	Libido	Concentration
Mood	Leisure activities	Motivation

Assess for Related Factors.
Medical Condition (Acute, Chronic; Refer to Key Concepts)

Nutritional Imbalances

Treatments

Chemotherapy	Medication side effects	Radiation therapy

Stressors

Excessive role demands	Financial	Depression
Career	Family	

For more information on Focus Assessment Criteria, visit http://connection.lww.com.

Goals

NOC Activity Tolerance, Endurance, Energy Conservation

The person will participate in activities
that stimulate and balance physical, cognitive, affective, and social domains.

Indicators

- Discuss the causes of fatigue.
- Share feelings regarding the effects of fatigue on life.
- Establish priorities for daily and weekly activities.

General Interventions

NIC Energy Management, Environmental Management, Mutual Goal Setting, Socialization Enhancement

Nursing interventions for this diagnosis are for people with fatigue of etiology that cannot be eliminated. The focus is to assist the individual and family to adapt to the fatigue state.

Assess Causative or Contributing Factors.

Lack of sleep; refer to *Disturbed Sleep Pattern*
Poor nutrition; refer to *Imbalanced Nutrition*
Sedentary lifestyle; refer to *Health-Seeking Behaviors*
Inadequate stress management; refer to *Health-Seeking Behaviors*
Physiologic impairment
Treatment (chemotherapy, radiation, medications)
Chronic excessive role or social demands

Quality or type of activity reportedly is more important than quantity. Informal activities promoted well-being the most, followed by formal structured activities, and last by solitary activities, which were found to have little or no effect on life satisfaction (Longino & Kart, 1982).

Explain the Causes of Fatigue (See Key Concepts).

Allow Expression of Feelings Regarding the Effects of Fatigue on Life.

Identify difficult activities.
Help client verbalize how fatigue interferes with role responsibilities.
Encourage client to convey how fatigue causes frustration.

Assist Client to Identify Strengths, Abilities, and Interests.

Identify values and interests.
Identify areas of success and usefulness; emphasize past accomplishments.
Use information to develop goals with the client.
Assist client to identify sources of hope (eg, relationships, faith, things to accomplish).
Assist client to develop realistic short- and long-term goals (progress from simple to more complex; use a "goals poster" to indicate type and time for achieving specific goals).

Assist Client to Identify Energy Patterns.

Instruct Client to Record Fatigue Levels Every Hour Over 24 h; Select a Usual Day.
Ask client to rate fatigue using the Rhoten fatigue scale (0 = not tired, peppy; 10 = total exhaustion).
Record the activities during each rating.

Analyze Together the 24-h Fatigue Levels.
Times of peak energy
Times of exhaustion
Activities associated with increasing fatigue

Explain Benefits of Exercise and Discuss What is Realistic.

Assist Client to Identify Tasks He or She Can Delegate.

Explore what activities the client views as important to maintain self-esteem.
Attempt to divide vital activities or tasks into components (eg, preparing menu, shopping, storing, cooking, serving, cleaning up); client can delegate some parts and retain others.
Plan important tasks during periods of high energy (eg, prepare all meals in the morning).

Explain the Purpose of Pacing and Prioritization.

Assist client to identify priorities and to eliminate nonessential activities.

Plan each day to avoid energy- and time-consuming, nonessential decision making.

Organize work with needed items within easy reach.

Distribute difficult tasks throughout the week.

Rest before difficult tasks and stop before fatigue ensues.

Teach Energy Conservation Techniques.

Modify the environment.

    Replace steps with ramps.

    Install grab rails.

    Elevate chairs 3 to 4 inches.

    Organize kitchen or work areas.

    Reduce trips up and down stairs (eg, put a commode on first floor).

Plan small, frequent meals to decrease energy required for digestion.

Use taxi instead of driving self.

Delegate housework (eg, employ a high school student for a few hours after school).

Promote Socialization with Family and Friends (Dzurec, 2000).

Encourage client to participate in one social activity, weekly.

Explain that feelings of connectedness decrease fatigue.

Explain Effects of Conflict and Stress on Energy Levels.

Teach the importance of mutuality in sharing concerns.

Explain the benefits of distraction from negative events.

Teach the value of confronting issues.

Teach and assist with relaxation techniques before anticipated stressful events. Encourage mental imagery to promote positive thought processes.

Allow client time to reminisce to gain insight into past experiences.

Teach to maximize aesthetic experiences (eg, smell of coffee, feeling warmth of the sun).

Teach to anticipate experiences the client takes delight in each day (eg, walking, reading favorite book, writing letter).

Provide Significant Others Opportunities to Discuss Feelings in Private Regarding:

Changes in person with fatigue

Caretaking responsibilities

Financial issues

Changes in lifestyle, role responsibilities, relationships

See *Caregiver Role Strain* for additional strategies for caregivers.

Initiate Health Teaching and Referrals, as Indicated.

Counseling

Community services (Meals-On-Wheels, housekeeper)

Financial assistance

Rationales

- In many chronic diseases, fatigue is the most common, disruptive, and distressing symptom because it interferes with self-care activities (Hart, Freel & Milde, 1990). Exploring the cause and effects of fatigue helps both nurse and client plan interventions (Adinolfi, 2001).
- Identifying times of peak energy and exhaustion can aid in planning activities to maximize energy conservation and productivity.
- Focusing the client on strengths and abilities may provide insight into positive events and lessen the tendency to overgeneralize the severity of disease, which can lead to depression (Beck, 1984).
- The client requires rest periods before or after some activities. Planning can provide for adequate rest and reduce unnecessary energy expenditure. Such strategies can enable continuation of activities, contributing to positive self-esteem.

- Many stressors are related to chronic illness (eg, pain; threats to independence, self-concept, future plans, role fulfillment). Clients who learn self-help responses face definable, manageable adversities by maintaining control of everyday problems (Braden, 1990).
- Reciprocity or returning support to one's support system is vital for balanced and healthy relationships (Tilden & Weinert, 1987). Clients with fatigue have difficulty with reciprocity.
- Winningham (1992) found the following in clients with cancer:
  Too much as well as too little rest contributes to feelings of fatigue.
  Too little as well as too much activity contributes to feelings of fatigue.
  A balance between activity and rest promotes restoration; an imbalance promotes fatigue and deterioration.
  Any symptom that contributes to decreased activity leads to increased fatigue and decreased functional status.
- Preparatory information clarifies expectations about chemotherapy or radiation therapy. Such information regarding fatigue, with suggestions about planning for rest, has positively affected clients' abilities to maintain usual activities (Nail, 1997; Nail & Winninghan, 1997).
- Dzurec (2000) found that relatedness was linked to fatigue. People with fatigue who became disconnected from interpersonal relationships became more fatigued.

Maternal Interventions

Explain reasons for fatigue in first and third trimesters:
- Increased basal metabolic rate
- Changes in hormonal levels
- Anemia
- Increased cardiac output (third trimester)

Emphasize the need for naps and 8 h of sleep each night.
Discuss the importance of exercise (eg, walking).
Advise client to avoid overexertion.
For postpartum women, discuss factors that increase fatigue:

Labor more than 30 h	Difficult labor or reports of high labor pain
Hemoglobin <10 g/dL or postpartum hemorrhage	Preexisting chronic disease Episiotomy, tear, or cesarean section
Sleeping difficulties	Ill newborn or a congenital anomaly
Nonsupportive partner	Dependent children at home
Child care problems	Unrealistic expectations

Rationale

Explaining the reasons for fatigue can allay fears.

Geriatric Interventions

Consider if chronic fatigue is the consequence of late-life depression.
Refer client with suspected depression for evaluation.

Rationale

Late-life depression causes chronic fatigue and diminishes energy (Miller, 2004).

FEAR

DEFINITION

Fear: State in which an individual or group experiences a feeling of physiologic or emotional disruption related to an identifiable source that is perceived as dangerous

DEFINING CHARACTERISTICS
Major (Must Be Present, One or More)

Feeling of dread, fright, apprehension and/or
Behaviors of
    Avoidance
    Narrowing of focus on danger
    Deficits in attention, performance, and control

Minor (May Be Present)

Verbal Reports of Panic, Obsessions

Behavioral Acts

Crying	Dysfunctional immobility	Increased questioning/
Compulsive mannerisms	Escape	verbalization
Hypervigilance	Aggression	

Visceral–Somatic Activity
Musculoskeletal

Shortness of breath	Muscle tightness	Fatigue/limb weakness

Respiratory

Increased rate	Trembling

Cardiovascular

Palpitations	Rapid pulse	Increased blood pressure

Skin

Flush/pallor	Sweating	Paresthesia

Gastrointestinal

Anorexia	Nausea/vomiting	Diarrhea/urge to defecate
Dry mouth/throat		

Central Nervous System (CNS)/Perceptual

Syncope	Irritability	Insomnia
Absentmindedness	Lack of concentration	Nightmares
Pupil dilation		

Genitourinary
Urinary frequency/urgency

RELATED FACTORS

Fear can be a response to various health problems, situations, or conflicts. Some common sources are indicated next.

Pathophysiologic

Related to perceived immediate and long-term effects of:

Terminal disease	Long-term disability	Loss of body function or part
Cognitive impairment	Disabling illness	Sensory impairment

Treatment-Related

Related to loss of control and unpredictable outcome secondary to:

| Hospitalization | Invasive procedures | Surgery and its outcome |
| Radiation | Anesthesia | |

Situational (Personal, Environmental)

Related to loss of control and unpredictable outcome secondary to:

Change or loss of significant	Pain	New environment
other	New people	Success
Divorce	Lack of knowledge	Failure

Related to potential loss of
  income

Maturational

Preschool
Related to:

Not being liked	Strangers	Age-related fears
Bodily harm	Being alone	(dark, strangers, ghosts)
Animals		

Separation from parents, peers

School-Age (6–12 years)
Related to:

| Being lost | Being in trouble | Thunder, lightening |
| Bad dreams | Weapons | |

Adolescent
Related to uncertainty of:

| Appearance | Scholastic success | Peer support |

Adult
Related to uncertainty of:

| Marriage | Job security | Pregnancy |
| Effects of aging | Parenthood | |

Older Adult
Related to anticipated dependence

| Prolonged suffering | Financial insecurity | Vulnerability to crime |
| Abandonment | | |

◎ AUTHOR'S NOTE

See *Anxiety*.

KEY CONCEPTS
Generic Considerations

- Psychological defense mechanisms are distinctly individual and can be adaptive or maladaptive.
- Fear differs from anxiety in that fear is aroused by an identified threat (specific object); anxiety is aroused by a threat that cannot be easily identified (nonspecific or unknown).
- Both fear and anxiety lead to disequilibrium.
- Anger may be a response to certain fears.
- A sense of adequacy in confronting danger reduces fear. Fear disguises itself. The expressed fear may substitute for other fears that are not socially acceptable. Awareness of factors that intensify fears enhances control and prevents heightened feelings. Confronting the safe reality of a situation reduces fear.
- Fear can become anxiety if it becomes internalized and serves to disorganize instead of becoming adaptive.
- Chronic physical reactions to stressors lead to susceptibility and chronic disease.

- Physiologic responses are manifested throughout the body primarily from the hypothalamus' stimulation of the autonomic and endocrine systems.
- People interpret the degree of danger from a threatening stimulus. The physiologic and psychological systems react with equal intensity (elevations in blood pressure and heart and respiratory rates).
- Fear is adaptive and a healthy response to danger.
- Fear differs from *phobia,* an irrational, persistent fear of a circumscribed stimulus (object or situation) other than having a panic attack (panic disorder) or of humiliation or embarrassment in certain social situations (social phobia) (American Psychiatric Association, 2000).

⬥ Pediatric Considerations

- "Fear is a part of normal development in children. Fear can be a positive adaptive force when it teaches children an awareness of potential danger" (Nicastro & Whetsell, 1999, p. 392).
- Infants and small children experience fear but cannot identify the threat verbally. Verbal (crying, protesting) and nonverbal (kicking, biting, holding back) responses are important indicators of children's fear (Broome, Bates, Lillis & McGahee, 1990; Wong, 2003).
- Fear behaviors are *consistent* and *immediate* on exposure to or mention of a specific stressor; if the response is erratic, the diagnosis more accurately might be anxiety. Refer to Table II.12 in *Delayed Growth and Development* or Key Concepts—Pediatric Considerations in *Anxiety.*
- Fears throughout childhood follow a developmental sequence and are influenced by culture, environment, and parental fears (Wong, 2003).
- Fears are most frequent in 8- to 10-year-old children (Nicastro & Whetsell, 1999).
- Main fears of different age groups are as follows (Nicastro & Whetsell, 1999; Wong, 2003):
  - *Infants and toddlers (birth to 2 years):* Fears evolve from physical stimuli (eg, loud noises, separation from parents/caregivers, strangers, sudden movements, animals, certain situations [doctor's office]).
  - *Preschoolers (3 to 5 years):* Fears evolve from real or imagined situations (eg, injury or mutilation, ghosts, devils, monsters, the dark, bathtub and toilet drains, being alone, dreams, robbers, wild animals, snakes).
  - *School-aged children (6 to 8 years):* Common fears are ghosts, monsters, dark, being alone, thunder, lightning, being lost, kidnapping, guns, and weapons.
  - *School-aged children (9 to 12 years):* Common fears are the dark, being lost or alone, bodily harm, strangers, bad dreams, punishment, grades and tests, and being in trouble.
  - *Adolescents:* Fears may be verbalized and include loss of self-control, disturbance to body image, death, separation from peers, inept social performance, sexuality gossip, acquired immunodeficiency syndrome (AIDS), being alone, and war.
- Fear is a momentary reaction to danger related to a low estimate of one's own power over the situation (Wong, 2003).

⬥ Maternal Considerations

The fears and concerns of pregnancy differ for each trimester:

First Trimester
- Uncertainty about timing of pregnancy
- Uncertainty about her or partner's adequacy as parent
- Concerns about material issues (eg, finances)

Second Trimester
- Fears diminish as fetus moves
- Decrease in physical symptoms

Third Trimester
- Fears for her own well-being and how she will tolerate labor
- Fears for the well-being of the fetus
- Obsessed with labor and delivery

Geriatric Considerations

Cesarone (1991) clustered the sources of fear in the elderly into five categories:

- Disease, suffering
- Dependence, abandonment
- Dying
- Illness or death of loved ones
- Miscellaneous reasons (crime, financial insecurity, diagnostic tests)

Focus Assessment Criteria

Subjective/Objective Data

Assess for Defining Characteristics.

Onset
Have the person tell you "story" about his or her fearfulness.

Thought process and content
Are thoughts clear, coherent, logical, confused, or forgetful?
Can client concentrate or is he or she preoccupied?

Perception and judgment
Does fear remain after stressor is eliminated?
Is the fear a response to a present stimulus or distorted by past influences?

Visceral–somatic activity
Musculoskeletal

Shortness of breath	Muscle tightness	Fatigue/limb weakness

Respiratory

Increased rate	Trembling

Cardiovascular

Palpitations	Rapid pulse	Increased blood pressure

Skin

Flush/pallor	Sweating	Paresthesia

Gastrointestinal

Anorexia	Nausea/vomiting	Diarrhea/urge to defecate

Dry mouth/throat

CNS/Perceptual

Syncope	Irritability	Insomnia
Absentmindedness	Lack of concentration	Nightmares

Pupil dilation

Genitourinary
Urinary frequency/urgency

For more information on Focus Assessment Criteria, visit http://connection.lww.com.

Goals

NOC Anxiety Control, Fear Control

The adult will relate increased psychological and physiologic comfort.

Indicators

- Show decreased visceral response (pulse, respirations).
- Differentiate real from imagined situations.
- Describe effective and ineffective coping patterns.
- Identify own coping responses.

The child will exhibit or relate increased psychological and physiologic comfort.

- Discuss fears.
- Exhibit less crying.

General Interventions

 NIC Anxiety Reduction, Coping Enhancement, Presence, Counseling, Relaxation Therapy

Nursing interventions for *Fear* represent interventions for any person with fear regardless of the etiologic or contributing factors.

Assess Possible Contributing Factors.

Perception of Threatening Stimulus (Realistic)
Unfamiliar environment (new home, hospital admission, new people)
Intrusion on personal space
Lifestyle change (promotion, marriage/divorce, retirement)
Biologic and physiologic change (dysfunction, disability, pain)
Threat to self-esteem (abandonment, rejection)
Distorted perceptions of dangerous stimulus

Reduce or Eliminate Contributing Factors.

Unfamiliar Environment
Orient client to environment using simple explanations.
Speak slowly and calmly.
Avoid surprises and painful stimuli.
Use soft lights and music.
Remove threatening stimulus.
Plan one-day-at-a-time, familiar routine.
Encourage gradual mastery of a situation.
Provide transitional object with symbolic safeness (security blanket, religious medals).

Intrusion on Personal Space
Allow personal space.
Move person away from stimulus.
Remain with person until fear subsides (listen, use silence).
Later, establish frequent and consistent contacts; use family members and significant others to stay with person.
Use touch as tolerated (sometimes holding person firmly helps him or her maintain control).

Threat to Self-esteem
Support preferred coping style when client uses adaptive mechanisms.
Initially, decrease the person's number of choices.
Use simple, direct statements (avoid detail).
Give direct suggestions to manage everyday events (some prefer details; others like general explanations).
Encourage expression of feelings (helplessness, anger).
Give feedback about expressed feelings (support realistic assessments).
Refocus interaction on areas of capability rather than dysfunction.
Encourage normal coping mechanisms.
Encourage sharing common problems with others.
Give feedback of effect person's behavior has on others.
Encourage person to face the fear.

Distorted Perceptions
Encourage responses that reflect reality.
Ask straightforward questions (eg, "Do you feel pain?" "Does asking you about your feelings make you uncomfortable?").
Provide information to reduce distortions (eg, "No, I will not harm you." "That was only a shadow and not a monster.").
Encourage specifics and discourage generalizations; have person give details, not vague general assumptions (eg, "Who are you referring to when you say 'they' are trying to kill you?").
Explore superficial interactions.
Examine the person's reason for avoiding feelings.
Allow client to know that it is okay to feel.
Share your reaction to the event (eg, "I can see why you're upset; if that happened to me, I would have felt like screaming.").
Provide an emotionally nonthreatening atmosphere.

Provide predictable situations.

Allow for consistency in personnel to enhance comfort and familiarity.

Announce changes in the environment.

When Intensity of Feelings has Decreased, Assist with Insight and Controlling Response.

Bring Behavioral Cues into Client's Awareness.

Teach signs that indicate increased fear (eg, "Your face flushes and you clench your fists when we discuss your discharge.").

Indicate adaptiveness of behavior.

Explain How Expressed Fear of One Thing May Hide Fear of Something Else.

Teach How to Solve Problems.

What is the problem?

Who or what is responsible?

What are the options?

What are advantages and disadvantages of each option?

Teach Ways to Enhance Control.

Include client in treatment process (eg, "Please raise your hand if the procedure causes pain.").

Share test results when appropriate.

Inform ahead of time about tests (time interval depends on ability to cope).

Identify activities that rechannel emotional energy to diffuse intensity.

Use night light or flashlight to diffuse fear (give child with fear of dark a flashlight to use as needed).

Before tests or surgery, prepare client as to what to expect, especially sensations; define this role and how to participate in it (eg, postoperative breathing exercises may distract from fears and dissipate physical reaction).

Initiate Health Teaching and Referrals as Indicated.

Recommend or Instruct Concerning Methods that Increase Comfort or Relaxation.

Progressive relaxation technique   Reading, music, breathing exercises

Desensitization, self-coaching   Thought stopping, guided fantasy

Yoga, hypnosis, assertiveness training

Participate in Community Functions to Teach Parents Age-related Fears and Constructive Interventions (Eg, Parent–school Organizations, Newsletters, Civic Groups).

Rationales

- Safety feelings increase when a person identifies with another person who has successfully dealt with a similar fearful situation.
- Open, honest dialogue may help initiate constructive problem solving and can instill hope.
- Support people and coping mechanisms are important tools in anxiety reduction.
- Minimizing environmental stimuli can help reduce escalation of fear (Varcarolis, 1998).
- Physical activity helps redirect and dissipate tension (Varcarolis, 1998).
- Severe fear or panic can interfere with concentrating and information processing (Varcarolis, 1998).
- A quiet, calm professional can communicate calm to the person (Varcarolis, 1998).

Pediatric Interventions

Provide child opportunities to talk and write about fears and to learn healthy outlets for anger or sadness, such as play therapy.

Acknowledge illness, death, and pain as real; refrain from protecting children from the reality of existence; encourage open, honest sharing.

Accept child's fear and provide an explanation, if possible, or some form of control; share with child that these fears are okay. Never make fun of the child.

> Fear of imaginary animals, intruders (eg, "I don't see a lion in your room, but I will leave the light on for you, and, if you need me again, please call.")
>
> Fear of parent being late (establish a contingency plan [eg, "If you come home from school and Mommy is not here, go to Mrs. S. next door."])
>
> Fear of vanishing down a toilet or bathtub drain
>
> > Wait until child is out of tub before releasing drain.
> >
> > Wait until child is off the toilet before flushing.
> >
> > Leave toys in bathtub and demonstrate how they do not go down the drain.
>
> Fear of dogs, cats
>
> > Allow child to watch a child and a dog playing from a distance.
> >
> > Do not force child to touch the animal.
>
> Fear of death (see Key Concepts for *Grieving*)
>
> Fear of pain (see *Pain* under Pediatric Interventions)
>
> Refusal to go to sleep (Wong, 1999)
>
> > Establish a realistic hour for retiring.
> >
> > Contract for a reward if child is successful.
> >
> > Do not sleep with child or take child to parent's room.

Discuss with parents the normality of fears in children; explain the necessity of acceptance and the negative outcomes of punishment, shaming, or of forcing the child to overcome the fear.

Provide child with opportunity to observe other children cope successfully with feared object.

Demonstrate strength and self-confidence.

> Take child's hand and gently guide into shallow water.
>
> Allow child to watch you pet a dog.

Rationales

- A familiar caregiver, comforts, and routines can reduce children's fears after a traumatic event (Nicastro & Whetsell, 1999).
- Desensitization by gradually facing a fearsome object or situation is effective with most children (Wong, 2003).
- Providing the child with some control (eg, flashlight) can help to reduce fear.
- The more successfully a child handles a fearful situation, the more confidence and less vulnerability the child feels (Nicastro & Whetsell, 1999).
- "Play-therapy facilitates the development of hardiness and resiliency, and the ability to master critical experiences" (Kuntz et al., 1996, p. 362).

Maternal Interventions

Provide opportunities to express fears during each trimester.
Provide opportunities for expectant father to share his concerns and fears.

Rationales

- Fears and concerns change with each trimester. Refer to Key Concepts—Maternal Considerations for specifics.
- Expectant fathers are concerned about changes in the relationship with their partner, their competence as a provider, and meeting the newly evolving expectations of the mother.

DEFICIENT FLUID VOLUME

DEFINITION

Deficient Fluid Volume: State in which a person who can take fluids (not NPO) experiences or is at risk of experiencing dehydration

DEFINING CHARACTERISTICS

Major (Must Be Present, One or More)

Insufficient oral fluid intake
Negative balance of intake
  and output

Dry skin/mucous membranes
Weight loss

Minor (May Be Present)

Increased serum sodium
Concentrated urine or
  urinary frequency

Thirst/nausea/anorexia
Decreased urine output or excessive urine output

RELATED FACTORS

Pathophysiologic

Related to excessive urinary output
Uncontrolled diabetes
Diabetes insipidus (inadequate antidiuretic hormone)

Related to increased capillary permeability and evaporative loss from burn wound (nonacute)
Related to losses secondary to:
Fever or increased metabolic rate   Peritonitis
Abnormal drainage   Diarrhea
  Wound
  Excessive menses

Situational (Personal, Environmental)

Related to vomiting/nausea
Related to decreased motivation to drink liquids secondary to:
Depression   Fatigue

Related to fad diets/fasting
Related to high-solute tube feedings
Related to difficulty swallowing or feeding self secondary to:
Oral or throat pain   Fatigue

Related to extreme heat/sun/dryness
Related to excessive loss through:
Indwelling catheters   Drains

Related to insufficient fluids for exercise effort or weather conditions
Related to excessive use of:
Laxatives or enemas   Diuretics, alcohol, or caffeine

Maturational

Infant/Child
Related to increased vulnerability secondary to:
Decreased fluid reserve and decreased ability to concentrate urine

Older Adult
Related to increased vulnerability secondary to:
Decreased fluid reserve and decreased sensation of thirst

◯◯ AUTHOR'S NOTE

Deficient Fluid Volume frequently is used incorrectly to describe people who are NPO, in hypovolemic shock, or experiencing bleeding, as well as those with insufficient oral fluid intake. The current NANDA-approved defining characteristics contribute to its clinical misuse in cases of hemoconcentration, change in serum sodium, or hypotension. Related factors are listed as active fluid volume loss and failure of regulatory mechanisms.

Should *Deficient Fluid Volume* be used to represent such clinical situations as shock, renal failure, or thermal injury? Most nurses would agree that these are collaborative problems to report to the physician.

◯◯ ERRORS IN DIAGNOSTIC STATEMENTS

1. *Risk for Deficient Fluid Volume related to increased capillary permeability, protein shifts, inflammatory process, and evaporation secondary to burn injuries*
   This diagnosis does not represent a situation for which nurses could prescribe interventions with achievable outcomes (eg, "Client will have stable vital signs and adequate urine output [0.5 to 1.0 mL/kg]"). Because both nurse- and physician-prescribed interventions are needed to accomplish this outcome, this situation is actually the collaborative problem *PC: Fluid/ Electrolyte Imbalance* with the nursing goal of "The nurse will monitor to detect fluid and electrolyte imbalances."
2. *Deficient Fluid Volume related to effects of NPO status*
   Managing fluid balance in an NPO client is a nursing responsibility involving both nurse- and physician-prescribed interventions. Thus, this situation is best described as *PC: Fluid/ Electrolyte Imbalance*. If the nurse wants to specify etiology, he or she can write *PC: Fluid/ Electrolyte Imbalance related to NPO state*. This usually is not necessary, however.
   When a person can drink but is not drinking sufficient amounts, *Deficient Fluid Volume related to decreased desire to drink fluids secondary to fatigue and pain* may apply.

KEY CONCEPTS
Generic Considerations

- Table II.11 shows average intake and output over 24 h for an adult. Ingested and excreted water and electrolytes (sodium, potassium, chloride) influence fluid balance.
- The two main causes of deficient fluid volume are inadequate fluid intake and increased fluid and electrolyte losses (eg, gastrointestinal, urinary, skin, third-space [edema]).
- Vomiting or gastric suctioning results in fluid, potassium, and hydrogen losses.
- The thirst sensation primarily regulates fluid intake. The kidneys' ability to concentrate urine primarily regulates fluid output.
- Urine specific gravity reflects the kidneys' ability to concentrate urine; the range of urine specific gravity varies with the state of hydration and the solids to be excreted. (Specific gravity is elevated with dehydration, signifying concentrated urine.) Normal values are 1.010 to 1.025. Diluted values are less than 1.010. Concentrated values are greater than 1.025.
- People at high risk for fluid imbalance include the following:
  - Those taking medication for fluid retention, high blood pressure, seizures, or "anxiety" (tranquilizers)

TABLE II.11 Average Intake and Output in an Adult for a 24-Hour Period

Intake		Output	
Oral liquids	1300 mL	Urine	1500 mL
Water in food	1000 mL	Stool	200 mL
Water produced by		Insensible	
metabolism	300 mL	Lungs	300 mL
TOTAL	2600 mL	Skin	600 mL
		TOTAL	2600 mL

Metheny N. (2000). *Fluid and electrolyte balance: Nursing considerations* (4th ed.). Philadelphia: Lippincott Williams & Wilkins.

- Those with diabetes, cardiac disease, excessive alcohol intake, malnourishment, obesity, or gastrointestinal distress
- Adults older than 60 years, and children younger than 6 years (decreased sensation of thirst)
- Those who are confused, depressed, comatose, or lethargic (no sensation of thirst)
- Athletes unaware of the need to replace electrolytes as well as fluids
- Excessive fluid and electrolyte loss can be expected during

Fever or increased meta-	Climate extremes
 bolic rate	 (heat/dryness)
Extreme exercise or	Excessive vomiting or diarrhea
 diaphoresis	Burns, tissue insult, fistulas

- Fluid balance maintenance is a major concern for all athletes competing in hot climates. The following is true for both men and women (Maughan, Leiper & Shirreffs, 1997):
  - Drinking large volumes of plain water will inhibit thirst and promote a diuretic response.
  - To maintain hydration during extreme exercise, high levels of sodium (as much as 50 to 60 mmol) and possibly some potassium to replace losses in sweat are needed.
  - Palatability of drinks is important to stimulate intake and ensure adequate volume replacement.
  - Because adequate hydration greatly affects athletic performance, the goal should be to be hydrated *at the beginning* of exercise, and to maintain hydration as well as possible thereafter, focusing on replacing salt loss as well as water.

Pediatric Considerations

- In determining the 24-h intake requirement for an infant or child, both caloric and fluid intake should be measured. The following calculations can be used:

Calorie Intake
For a child up to 10 kg of body weight: 100 cal/kg
For a child between 11 and 20 kg: 1000 cal plus 50 cal/kg for each kg above 10 kg

Fluid Intake for Maintenance
For daily fluid maintenance (Wong, 2003):
1–10 kg	100 mL/kg
11–20 kg	1000 mL plus 50 mL/kg for each kg >10 kg
>20 kg	1500 mL plus 20 mL/kg for each kg >20 kg
Abnormal fluid loss must be replaced in addition to the above.

- Infants are vulnerable to fluid loss because of the following:
  - They can lose more water rapidly because their bodies have a higher proportion of water.
  - More fluid is in the extracellular space, from where it is lost more easily.
  - They have a greater metabolic turnover of water.
  - Homeostatic regulation (ie, renal function) is immature.
  - They have a greater surface area relative to body mass (Wong, 2003).
- One gram wet diaper equals/mL of urine (Wong, 2003)

Geriatric Considerations

- A general decrease in thirst with aging puts older adults at risk for not drinking sufficient fluids to maintain adequate hydration.
- Older adults are more susceptible to fluid loss and dehydration because of (Sansevero, 1997):
  - Decreased percentage of total body water
  - Decreased renal blood flow and glomerular filtration
  - Impaired ability to regulate temperature
  - Decreased ability to concentrate urine
  - Increased physical disabilities (decrease access to fluids)
  - Self-limiting of fluids for fear of incontinence
  - Diminished thirst sensation
- About 75% of fluid intake in older adults occurs between 6 AM and 6 PM (Miller, 2004).
- Cognitive impairments can interfere with recognition of cues of thirst.
- Dehydration, defined as diminished total body water content, is the most common fluid and electrolyte disturbance among older adults (Sansevero, 1997). Because it is associated with morbidity and mortality rates, careful screening and prevention in primary care settings are essential.
- Older adults often have multiple physical and socioeconomic factors that predispose them to dehydration. Classic signs of dehydration may be present in a normally hydrated older population, requiring careful assessment (Sansevero, 1997).
- Dehydration in nursing home residents is a complex problem that requires a comprehensive approach, including facility-wide involvement and use of checklists to ensure adequate hydration (Zembruski, 1997).

Focus Assessment Criteria

Subjective Data

Assess for Defining Characteristics.

Fluid intake (amounts, type)   Skin (dry, turgor)
Thirst   Weight loss (How much? Since when?)
Urine output (decreased,
  increased)

Assess for Related Factors.

Refer to Related Factors.

Objective Data

Assess for Defining Characteristics.

Present weight/usual weight
Intake (last 2 to 48 h)
Output (last 24 to 48 h)
Skin
Mucosa (lips, gums) (dry)   Moisture (dry or diaphoretic)
Tongue (furrowed/dry)   Fontanelles of infants (depressed)
Turgor (decreased)   Eyeballs (sunken)
Color (pale or flushed)   Tachycardia

Urine output
Amount (varied; very large or minimal amount)
Color (amber; very dark or very light; clear?; cloudy?)
Specific gravity (increased or decreased)
Odor?

Assess for Related Factors.

Abnormal or excessive fluid loss
Liquid stools   Fever
Diuresis or polyuria   Vomiting or gastric suction (eg, fistulas, drains)

Abnormal or excessive	Diaphoresis
drainage	Loss of skin surfaces (eg, healing burns)

Decreased fluid intake related to

Fatigue	Decreased level of consciousness
Depression/disorientation	Nausea or anorexia
Physical limitations (eg, cannot hold glass)	

For more information on Focus Assessment Criteria, visit http://connection.lww.com.

Goal

NOC Electrolyte and Acid/Base Balance, Fluid Balance, Hydration

The person will maintain urine specific gravity within normal range.

Indicators

- Increase fluid intake to a specified amount according to age and metabolic needs.
- Identify risk factors for fluid deficit and relate need for increased fluid intake as indicated.
- Demonstrate no signs and symptoms of dehydration.

General Interventions

NIC Fluid/Electrolyte Management, Fluid Monitoring

Assess Causative Factors.

Inability to feed self
Dislike of available liquids
Sore throat/mouth
Extreme fatigue or weakness
Lack of knowledge (of the need for increased fluid and electrolyte intake)
Difficulty swallowing (see *Impaired Swallowing*)
Inadequate fluid intake before and during exercise (usually in athletes)

Reduce or Eliminate Causative Factors.

Inability to Feed Self (See *Deficient Self-Care*)

Dislike of Available Liquids

Assess likes and dislikes; provide favorite fluids within dietary restrictions.
Plan an intake goal for each shift (eg, 1000 mL during day; 800 mL during afternoon; 300 mL at night).
Set a schedule for supplementary liquids.

Sore Throat/Mouth

Offer warm or cold fluids; consider ices.
Consider warm saline gargle or anesthetic lozenges before fluids.

Extreme Fatigue or Weakness

Give small amounts of fluids frequently.
Provide for rest periods before meals.

Lack of Knowledge

Assess client's understanding of reasons to maintain adequate hydration and methods to reach fluid intake goal.
Include significant others.
Proceed with teaching.

See Key Concepts, *Health-Seeking Behaviors*.

Have Person Maintain a Record (Log).

Fluid intake
Urinary output
Daily weight

Prevent Dehydration in High-Risk Clients (see Key Concepts).

Monitor intake; ensure at least 2000 mL of oral fluids every 24 h.
Monitor output; ensure at least 1000 to 1500 mL every 24 h.

Monitor serum electrolyte studies as needed.

Offer fluids in large glasses, 120 or 240 mL.

Weigh daily in same clothes, at same time. A 2% to 4% weight loss indicates mild dehydration; 5% to 9% weight loss indicates moderate dehydration.

Monitor urine and serum electrolytes, blood urea nitrogen, osmolality, creatinine, hematocrit, and hemoglobin.

For people scheduled to fast before diagnostic studies, advise them to increase fluid intake 8 h before fasting.

Review client's medications. Do they contribute to dehydration (eg, diuretics)? Do they require increased fluid intake (eg, lithium)?

Teach that coffee, tea, and grapefruit juice are diuretics and can contribute to fluid loss.

Consider the additional fluid losses associated with vomiting, diarrhea, fever.

Initiate Health Teaching, as Indicated.

Give verbal and written directions for desired fluids and amounts.

Include the person/family in keeping a written record of fluid intake, output, daily weights.

Provide a list of alternative fluids (eg, ice cream, pudding).

Explain the need to increase fluids during exercise, fever, infection, and hot weather.

Teach how to observe for dehydration (especially in infants) and to intervene by increasing fluid intake (see Subjective and Objective Data for signs of dehydration).

Seek medical consultation for continued dehydration.

For Athletes, Stress the Need to Hydrate Before and During Exercise, Preferably with a High-Sodium-Content Beverage (Refer to Hyperthermia for Additional Interventions).

For Dehydration in the Terminally Ill (Parkash & Burge, 1997):

Help caregivers and families to discover client's wishes and attitudes concerning procedures for hydration (eg, intravenous [IV]).

Provide as accurate information as available about advantages and disadvantages of hydration.

Recognize and explore caregiver's concerns (eg, who will manage IV administration).

Rationales

- Output may exceed intake, which already may be inadequate to compensate for insensible losses.
- Dehydration may increase glomerular filtration rate, making output inadequate to clear wastes properly and leading to elevated BUN and electrolyte levels.
- Accurate daily weights can detect fluid loss.
- To monitor weight effectively, weights should be measured at the same time on the same scale with the same clothes.
- Large amounts of sugar, alcohol, and caffeine act as diuretics that increase urine production and may cause dehydration.
- People receiving tube feedings are at high risk for dehydration, because the high solute concentration of the tube feeding may cause diarrhea and diuresis. *Tube feedings must be supplemented with specific amounts of water to maintain adequate hydration.*
- Adequate protein intake is necessary to maintain normal osmotic pressures. Foods with high protein content are meats, fish, fowl, soybeans, eggs, legumes, and cheese.

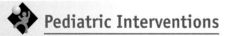 ## Pediatric Interventions

To increase fluid intake
Offer:
- Appealing fluids (popsicles, frozen juice bars, snow cones, water, milk, Jell-O); let child help make them
- Unusual containers (colorful cups, straws)
- A game or activity

Read a book to child and have him or her drink a sip when turning a page, or have a tea party.

Have child take a drink when it is his or her turn in a game.

Set a schedule for supplementary liquids to promote the habit of in-between-meal fluids (eg, juice or Kool-Aid at 10 AM and 2 PM each day).

Decorate straws.

Let child fill small cups with a syringe.

Make a progress poster; use stickers or stars to indicate fluid goals met.

For Fever in Children Younger than 5 Years:

Work to attain a temperature below 101°F (38.4°C) with medication* (acetaminophen or ibuprofen) only.

Use tepid water (85° to 90°F/29.4° to 37.7°C) to sponge or bathe the child.

Caution parents not to cover the child with blankets and to be aware of the increased risk of febrile seizures.

Give the child small amounts (15 mL) of *clear liquids only* frequently.

Teach parents how to protect the child should a seizure occur, and *instruct them to seek immediate medical consultation.*

For Fluid Replacement, Refer to Pediatric Interventions under *Diarrhea*.

Rationales

- Older children usually respond to the challenge of meeting a specific intake goal (Wong, 2003).
- Rewards and contracts are also effective (eg, sticker for drinking a certain amount).
- Young children usually respond to games that integrate drinking fluids.

DEFICIENT FLUID VOLUME

RELATED TO ABNORMAL FLUID LOSS

Abnormal fluid loss describes fluid loss by vomiting, diarrhea, excessive diaphoresis, or drains, not by hemorrhage or acute burns.

Goal

NOC Refer to General Interventions.

The person will maintain urine specific gravity within normal range.

Indicators

- Maintain adequate intake of fluid and electrolytes, as evidenced by (specify):
- Identify abnormal fluid loss, relate methods of decreasing (if possible), and replace fluids as needed.

---

*May require a primary care professional's order. Do not give aspirin or products containing aspirin to children **younger than** 18 years with flu symptoms because of risk of potentially fatal Reye's syndrome.

Interventions

 NIC Fluid/Electrolyte Management, Fluid Monitoring, Fever Treatment

Assess Causative Factors.

Vomiting	Diarrhea/loose stools
Fever	Impaired swallowing
Gastric suction	(see *Impaired Swallowing*)

Remove or Reduce Causative Factors.

Vomiting

Encourage small, frequent ice chips or clear liquids such as weak tea or apple juice (adults 30 mL, children 15 mL); see *Diarrhea* for replacement therapy.

Fever (See Also *Hyperthermia*)

Maintain temperature lower than 101°F (38.4°C) with medication (eg, ibuprofen or acetaminophen).*
  Eliminate excessive clothing and bed covers.
  Keep room temperature cool.
  Encourage cool, clear liquids when medication is at peak effectiveness and temperature is lowest.
  Substitute frozen ices or popsicles if necessary (be resourceful).
  If the temperature is extremely high (above 103°F [39.5°C]), sponge with tepid water.†

Gastric Suction (Nasogastric or Other)

Use only normal saline for irrigation of gastric tubes to minimize electrolyte imbalance.

Do not allow swallowing of water or ice chips; a "few small sips" can readily add up over time.

For the thirsty person with gastric suction, *unless contraindicated by surgery or renal failure,* consult with physician concerning ingestion of measured sips of Gatorade (1 oz/h).

Always subtract all fluid ingested (by either tube or mouth) from any total gastric drainage to attain net drainage.

Keep a careful, clear record of intake and output: amount, character, and color.

Offer frequent mouth care.

Diarrhea/Loose Stools

See *Diarrhea*.

Wound Drainage

Keep careful records of amount and type of drainage.

Weigh dressings, if necessary, to estimate fluid loss (weigh the wet dressing; weigh a dry dressing of the same type; compare the difference).

Weigh client daily if drainage is excessive and difficult to measure (eg, soaked sheets).

Replace fluid loss (may be contraindicated in cardiac failure, renal failure, or head trauma).

Initiate Health Teaching, as Indicated.

Assess client's understanding of the type of fluid loss he or she is experiencing (what electrolytes are lost) and the fluids that provide replacement (see Key Concepts).

Give verbal and written instructions for fluid replacement (eg, "Drink at least 3 quarts of liquid a day, including 1 quart of Gatorade.").

Teach client to:
  Avoid sudden exposure and overexposure to heat, sun, and exercise.
  Gradually increase exposure and activity in hot weather.
  Eat three balanced meals a day.
  Increase fluid intake during hot days.
  Decrease activity during extreme weather.

Rationales

- The focus of treatment is replacing both water and electrolytes lost (Porth, 2002).
- Fluids high in sugar (eg, soda, Jell-O) can cause osmotic diarrhea (Porth, 2002).
- Refer to Rationales in *Diarrhea*.
- For child, refer to Rationales under Pediatric Interventions in *Diarrhea*.

---

*May require a primary care professional's order. Do not give aspirin or products containing aspirin to children younger than 18 years with flu symptoms because of risk of potentially fatal Reye's syndrome.
† May require a primary care professional's order.

EXCESS FLUID VOLUME

DEFINITION

Excess Fluid Volume: State in which a person experiences or is at risk of experiencing intracellular or interstitial fluid overload

DEFINING CHARACTERISTICS
Major (Must Be Present, One or More)

Edema (peripheral, sacral)   Taut, shiny skin

Minor (May Be Present)

Intake greater than output   Shortness of breath   Weight gain

RELATED FACTORS
Pathophysiologic

Related to compromised regulatory mechanisms secondary to:
Renal failure (acute or chronic)   Systemic and metabolic abnormalities
Endocrine dysfunction   Lipedema

Related to portal hypertension, lower plasma colloidal osmotic pressure, and sodium retention secondary to:
Liver disease   Cirrhosis   Ascites
Cancer

Related to venous and arterial abnormalities secondary to:
Varicose veins   Phlebitis   Infection
Peripheral vascular disease   Immobility   Trauma
Thrombus   Lymphedema   Neoplasms

Treatment-Related

Related to sodium and water retention secondary to:
Corticosteroid therapy

Related to inadequate lymphatic drainage secondary to:
Mastectomy

Situational (Personal, Environmental)

Related to excessive sodium intake/fluid intake
Related to low protein intake
Fad diets   Malnutrition

Related to dependent venous pooling/venostasis secondary to:
Standing or sitting for   Immobility   Tight cast or bandage
  long periods

Related to venous compression from pregnant uterus

Maturational
Older Adult
Related to impaired venous return secondary to increased peripheral resistance and decreased efficiency of valves

⦿ ERRORS IN DIAGNOSTIC STATEMENTS

1. *Risk for Excess Fluid Volume related to left-sided mastectomy*

   For this diagnosis, the nurse would institute strategies to reduce edema and teach the client how to manage it. Thus, the nurse would write the diagnosis as *Risk for Excess Fluid Volume related to lack of knowledge of techniques to reduce edema secondary to compromised lymphatic function*. If edema were present, the nurse might use *Risk for Impaired Physical Mobility related to effects of lymphedema on motion*.

2. *Excess Fluid Volume related to portal hypertension and decreased colloid osmotic pressure secondary to cirrhosis*

   This diagnosis requires frequent monitoring, electrolyte replacement, diuretic therapy, dietary restrictions, and plasma expander therapy. These interventions call for three collaborative problems: (1) *PC: Ascites;* (2) *PC: Negative nitrogen balance;* (3) *PC: Hypokalemia*. Because edema predisposes skin to injury and breakdown, the nurse also could use *Risk for Impaired Skin Integrity related to vulnerability of skin secondary to edema*.

KEY CONCEPTS
Generic Considerations

- See *Deficient Fluid Volume*.
- Edema results from the accumulation of fluid in the interstitial compartment of the extravascular space. Without intervention, edema can progress to further tissue damage and permanent swelling.
  - Determining the underlying cause is essential to identifying specific interventions.
  - Peripheral edema should be classified as unilateral or bilateral. *Unilateral* usually results from venous and arterial abnormalities, lymphedema, infection, trauma, and neoplasms. *Bilateral* usually results from congestive heart failure, systemic and metabolic abnormalities, endocrine dysfunction, lipedema, and pregnancy (Terry, O'Brien & Kerstein, 1998).
- Distribution of peripheral edema is important to differentiating its etiology (Powell & Armstrong, 1997).
- People with cardiac pump failure are at high risk for excesses in both vascular and tissue fluids (ie, pulmonary and peripheral edema). Pulmonary edema is a medical emergency.
- The most frequent vascular cause of tissue edema is increased venous pressure, which leads to increased capillary blood pressure.

⦿ Maternal Consideration

Increased estrogen levels during pregnancy cause water retention of 6 to 8 L to supply tissue needs for water and electrolytes.

⦿ Geriatric Consideration

Older adults are prone to stasis edema of the feet and ankles as a result of increased vein tortuosity and dilatation and decreased valve efficiency (Miller, 2004).

Focus Assessment Criteria

Subjective Data
Assess for Defining Characteristics.

History of symptoms
Complaints of

Shortness of breath	Weakness/fatigue	Weight gain
Edema		

Onset/duration

Assess for Related Factors.
See Related Factors.

Objective Data
Assess for Defining Characteristics.

Signs of fluid overload
Pulse (bounding or dysrhythmic)
Respirations

Rate (tachypnea)	Lung sounds (rales or rhonchi)
Quality (labored or shallow)	

Blood pressure (elevated)
Edema
Press thumb for at least 5 s into the skin, and note any remaining indentations.
Rate edema according to the following scale:

    None = 0
    Trace = +1
    Moderate = +2
    Deep = +3
    Very deep = +4

Note degree and location (feet, ankles, legs, arms, sacral, generalized).
Weight gain (weigh daily on the same scale, at the same time)
Neck vein distention (distended neck veins at 45-degree elevation of head may indicate fluid overload or decreased cardiac output)

For more information on Focus Assessment Criteria, visit http://connection.lww.com.

Goals

NOC Electrolyte Balance, Fluid Balance, Hydration

The person will exhibit decreased edema (specify site).

Indicators
- Relate causative factors.
- Relate methods of preventing edema.

General Interventions

NIC Electrolyte Management, Fluid Management, Fluid Monitoring, Skin Surveillance

Identify Contributing and Causative Factors.

Improper diet (inadequate protein intake, excessive sodium intake)
Dependent venous pooling/venostasis
Venous pressure point (eg, tight cast or bandage)
Inadequate lymphatic drainage
Immobility/neurologic deficit
Lack of knowledge of or compliance with medical regimen

Reduce or Eliminate Causative and Contributing Factors.

Improper Diet
Assess dietary intake and habits that may contribute to fluid retention.
    Be specific; record daily and weekly intake of food and fluids.

Assess weekly diet for inadequate protein or excessive sodium intake.

Discuss likes and dislikes of foods that provide protein.

Teach client to plan weekly menu that provides protein at an affordable price.

Teach client to decrease salt intake.

Read labels for sodium content.

Avoid convenience, canned, and frozen foods.

Cook without salt; use spices (lemon, basil, tarragon, mint) to add flavor.

Use vinegar in place of salt to flavor soups, stews, etc. (eg, 2 to 3 teaspoons of vinegar to 4 to 6 quarts, according to taste).

Ascertain whether client may use salt substitute (caution that he or she must use the exact substitute prescribed).

Dependent Venous Pooling

Assess for evidence of dependent venous pooling or venostasis.

Encourage alternating periods of horizontal rest (legs elevated) with vertical activity (standing); this may be contraindicated in congestive heart failure.

Keep edematous extremity elevated above level of the heart whenever possible (unless contraindicated by heart failure).

Keep edematous arms elevated on two pillows or with intravenous (IV) pole sling.

Elevate legs whenever possible, using pillows under legs (avoid pressure points, especially behind knees).

Discourage leg and ankle crossing.

Reduce constriction of vessels.

Assess clothing for proper fit and constrictive areas.

Instruct client to avoid panty girdles/garters, knee-highs, and leg crossing and to practice elevating legs when possible.

Consider using antiembolism stockings or Ace bandages; measure legs carefully for stockings/support hose.*

Measure from back of heel to back of knee or top of thigh, depending on desired stocking length.

Measure circumference of calf and thigh.

Consider both measurements in choosing stockings, matching measurements with size requirement chart that accompanies the stockings.

Apply stockings while lying down (eg, in the morning before arising).

Check extremities frequently for adequate circulation and evidence of constrictive areas.

Venous Pressure Points

Assess for venous pressure points associated with casts, bandages, and tight stockings.

Observe circulation at edges of casts, bandages, and stockings.

For casts, insert soft material to cushion pressure points at edges.

Check circulation frequently.

Shift body weight in cast to redistribute weight within (unless contraindicated).

Encourage client to do this every 15 to 30 min while awake to prevent venostasis.

Encourage wiggling of fingers or toes and isometric exercise of unaffected muscles within the cast.

If the person cannot do this alone, assist him or her at least hourly to shift body weight.

See *Impaired Physical Mobility.*

Inadequate Lymphatic Drainage

Keep extremity elevated on pillows.

If edema is marked, the arm should be elevated, *but not in adduction* (this position may constrict the axilla).

The elbow should be higher than the shoulder.

The hand should be higher than the elbow.

Measure blood pressure in the unaffected arm.

Do not give injections or start IV fluids in affected arm.

Protect affected limb from injury.

Teach client to avoid using strong detergents, carrying heavy bags, holding cigarettes, injuring cuticles or hangnails, reaching into hot ovens, wearing jewelry or wristwatch, or using Ace bandages.

Advise client to apply lanolin or similar cream often daily to prevent dry, flaky skin.

Encourage client to wear a Medic-Alert tag engraved with *Caution: lymphedema arm—no tests—no needle injections.*

Caution client to visit a physician if arm becomes red, swollen, or unusually hard.

---

*May require a primary care professional's order.

After a mastectomy, encourage range-of-motion (ROM) exercises and use of affected arm to facilitate development of a collateral lymphatic drainage system (explain that lymphedema often decreases within 1 month, but that she should continue massaging, exercising, and elevating the arm for 3 to 4 months after surgery).

Immobility/Neurologic Deficit

Plan passive or active ROM exercises for all extremities every 4 h, including dorsiflexion of the foot to massage veins.

Change client's position at least every 2 h, using the four positions (left side, right side, back, abdomen), if not contraindicated (see *Impaired Skin Integrity*).

If client must remain in high Fowler's position, assess for edema of buttocks and sacral area; help client shift body weight every 2 h to prevent pressure on edematous tissue.

Lack of Knowledge

Assess client's knowledge of:

- Medical diagnosis (eg, congestive heart failure, renal failure)
- Diet
- Medications (eg, diuretics, cardiotonics)
- Activity
- Use of Ace bandages, antiembolism stockings

Proceed with health teaching, as indicated.

Protect Edematous Skin from Injury.

Inspect skin for redness and blanching.

Reduce pressure on skin areas; pad chairs, knee-high stockings, and footstools.

Prevent dry skin.

Use soap sparingly.

Rinse off soap completely.

Use a lotion to moisten skin.

See *Impaired Skin Integrity* for additional information on preventing injury.

Initiate Health Teaching and Referrals, as Indicated.

Give clear verbal and written instructions for all medications: what, when, how often, why, side effects; pay special attention to drugs that directly influence fluid balance (eg, diuretics, steroids).

Write down instructions for diet, activity, use of Ace bandages, stockings, and so forth.

Have client demonstrate the instructions.

Have client keep a written record of intake/output.

With severe fluctuations in edema, have client weigh himself or herself every morning and before bedtime daily; instruct client to keep a written record of weights. For less severe illness, the client may need to weigh himself or herself daily only and record.

Caution client to call physician for excessive edema/weight gain (>2 lb/day) or increased shortness of breath at night or on exertion. Explain that these signs may indicate early heart problems and may require medication to prevent them from worsening.

Consider home care or visiting nurses referral to follow at home.

Provide literature concerning low-salt diets; consult with dietitian if necessary.

Rationales

- Edema inhibits blood flow to the tissue, resulting in poor cellular nutrition and increased susceptibility to injury.
- High sodium intake leads to increased water retention. High-sodium foods include salted snacks, bacon, cheddar cheese, pickles, soy sauce, processed lunchmeats, monosodium glutamate (MSG), canned vegetables, ketchup, and mustard. Some over-the-counter drugs, such as antacids, also are high in sodium.
- Corticosteroids contain both glucocorticoid and mineralocorticoid elements. Mineralocorticoid promotes sodium resorption and potassium excretion from distal renal tubules. Resultant sodium retention expands extracellular fluid volume by preventing water excretion (Porth, 2002).
- Edema develops as increased extracellular fluid enters interstitial spaces and the blood, increasing interstitial fluid and blood volume.
- Contracting skeletal muscles propel lymph flow. Exercise increases muscle efficiency.
- In addition to the increased risk of injury to the skin from edema, loss of perivascular collagen in the small vessels of the skin makes them more susceptible to damage.

Maternal Interventions

Explain the cause of edema of ankles and fingers.

Advise client to limit salt intake moderately (eg, eliminate processed meats, chips) and to maintain water intake of 8 to 10 glasses daily unless contraindicated.

Instruct client to lie on left side for short periods several times a day and to take a warm tub bath daily.

Advise client to avoid reclining on back, sitting for prolonged periods without elevating feet, or standing for prolonged periods (Davis, 1996).

Instruct client how to apply support stockings.

Consult with an advanced practice nurse or physician if client has elevated blood pressure, proteinuria, facial puffiness, sacral or pitting edema, or weight gain of more than 2 lb in 1 week.

Rationales

- Limiting salt can decrease circulating volume to a point so low that kidney function decreases (Reeder et al., 1997).
- During pregnancy, possible causes of edema are peripheral arterial vasodilation, sodium and water retention, decreased thirst threshold, the enlarging uterus increasing capillary pressure in lower extremities, and changes in the renin–angiotensin–aldosterone system (Davis, 1996).
- Sodium is important to maintain adequate circulatory blood volume. A health care professional should supervise restrictions.
- Lying on the left side removes weight of gravid uterus from vessels, increases venous return to heart, and improves renal function.
- Research findings have suggested that rest periods in water (ie, baths) instead of bed rest may better reduce edema during pregnancy.

RISK FOR IMBALANCED FLUID VOLUME

DEFINITION

Risk for Imbalanced Fluid Volume: State in which a person is at risk to experience a decrease, increase, or rapid shift from one to the other of intravascular, interstitial, and/or intracellular fluid

RISK FACTORS

Major invasive procedures scheduled
Others need to be developed (NANDA, 2002)

✪ AUTHOR'S NOTE

This diagnosis can represent several clinical conditions, such as edema, hemorrhage, dehydration, and compartmental syndrome. If the nurse is monitoring a person for imbalanced fluid volume, labeling the specific imbalance as a collaborative problem, such as hypovolemia, compartmental syndrome, increased intracranial pressure, gastrointestinal bleeding, or postpartum hemorrhage, would be more useful clinically. For example, most intraoperative clients would be monitored for hypovolemia. If the procedure is neurosurgery, then cranial pressure also would be monitored. If the procedure is orthopedic, compartmental syndrome would be addressed. Refer to Section III for specific collaborative problems and interventions.

GRIEVING*

DEFINITION

Grieving: State in which an individual or family experiences a natural human response involving psychosocial and physiologic reactions to an actual or perceived loss (person, object, function, status, relationship)

DEFINING CHARACTERISTICS
Major (Must Be Present)

The person reports an actual or perceived loss (person, object, function, status, relationship)

Minor (May Be Present)

Denial	Suicidal thoughts	Guilt
Crying	Anger	Sorrow
Despair	Longing/searching behaviors	Inability to concentrate
Delusions	Phobias	Anergia
Hallucinations	Feelings of worthlessness	

RELATED FACTORS

Many situations can contribute to feelings of loss. Some common situations follow.

Pathophysiologic
Related to loss of function or independence secondary to:

Neurologic	Digestive	Cardiovascular
Respiratory	Sensory	Renal
Musculoskeletal	Trauma	

Treatment-Related
Related to losses associated with:

Long-term dialysis	Surgery (eg, mastectomy)

Situational (Personal, Environmental)
Related to the negative effects and losses secondary to:

Chronic pain	Death	Terminal illness

Related to losses in lifestyle associated with:

Childbirth	Child leaving home	Marriage
Divorce	Separation	

Related to loss of normalcy secondary to:

Handicap	Illness	Scars

---

*This diagnosis is not currently on the NANDA list but has been included for clarity or usefulness.

Maturational

Related to changes attributed to aging:

Friends   Function   Occupation
Home

Related to loss of hope, dreams

ⓧ AUTHOR'S NOTE

Grieving, Anticipatory Grieving, and *Dysfunctional Grieving* represent three types of responses of individuals or families experiencing a loss. *Grieving* describes normal grieving after a loss and participation in grief work. *Anticipatory Grieving* describes engaging in grief work before an expected loss. *Dysfunctional Grieving* represents a maladaptive process in which grief work is suppressed or absent or a person exhibits prolonged exaggerated responses. For all three diagnoses, the goal of nursing is to promote grief work. In addition, for *Dysfunctional Grieving,* the nurse directs interventions to reduce excessive, prolonged, problematic responses.

In many clinical situations, the nurse expects a grief response (eg, loss of body part, death of significant other). Other situations that evoke strong grief responses are sometimes ignored or minimized (eg, abortion, newborn death, death of one twin or triplet, death of illicit lover, suicide, loss of children to foster homes or adoption).

ⓧ ERRORS IN DIAGNOSTIC STATEMENTS

1. *Dysfunctional Grieving related to excessive emotional reactions (crying, anger) to recent death of son*

   Response to loss is highly individualized. Regardless of severity, no response to acute loss should be labeled "dysfunctional." *Dysfunctional Grieving* is characterized by a sustained or prolonged detrimental response; this diagnosis cannot be validated until several months to 1 year after the loss. The nurse should reword this diagnosis as *Grieving related to recent death of son, as evidenced by emotional responses of anger and profound sadness.*

2. *Anticipatory Grieving related to perceived effects of spinal cord injury on life goals*

   Using *Anticipatory Grieving* here focuses on anticipated, not actual losses. Because this person is grieving for both actual and anticipated losses, the nurse should rewrite this as *Grieving related to actual or anticipated losses associated with recent spinal cord injury.*

KEY CONCEPTS
Generic Considerations

- US culture is devoted to youth and life. Even though death surrounds each person, society views it as pertaining to someone else. Society today has been called "death defying," failing to recognize and confront the realities of death and grief.
- Caregivers must recognize that their attitudes and beliefs about death, dying, and grief significantly influence their care of people experiencing loss.
- Loss can occur without death; when a person experiences any loss (object, relationship), grief and mourning ensue.
- Grief is the emotional response to loss. *Grief work,* the adaptive process of mourning, involves the following: (Worden, 2002)
  - Accepting the reality of the loss
  - Experiencing the pain of grief
  - Adjusting to an environment from which the lost person or object is missing
  - Progressing with life.
- Many factors affect grief: personality, previous losses, intimacy of relationship, and resources.
- Zisook and Schochter's study (1992) of widows and widowers found that a depressive episode frequently occurs within 1 year after the death of a spouse. Those at highest risk for depressive episodes are young widows or widowers who have past histories of depression and believe themselves to be in poor health.

- Staging (of grieving process) can create problems if the nurse applies the stages universally, disregarding individual differences. Staging also may encourage the nurse to focus on the symptoms as opposed to the strength of the person/family. The following stages (Engle, 1964) are specific enough to assist the nurse to intervene and broad enough to prevent labeling:

  I.Shock and disbelief

Initial denial	Decreased activity
Numbed feelings	Sporadic periods of despair

  II.Developing awareness of loss

Sadness	Guilt
Anger	Crying

  III.Restitution (usually requires at least 1 year)

The work of mourning	Preoccupation with thoughts of loss
Painful void in life	

  IV.In the months to follow

  Putting the lost relationship in perspective (its positive and negative qualities)
- Research findings have refuted the notion that grief is neat, orderly, linear, and completed at an arbitrary point (Boyd, 2001).
- Terminal illness with its concurrent treatments and progression produces many losses:
  - Loss of function (all systems/roles)
  - Loss of financial independence
  - Change in appearance
  - Loss of friends
  - Loss of self-esteem
  - Loss of self
- Divorce poses many losses for the partners and their families: roles, relationships, homes, possessions, finances, control, routines, and patterns.
- When men lose their spouses, they respond as if they have lost a part of themselves, whereas women respond as if they been deserted or abandoned (Bateman, 1999).
- When social stigma is associated with a death or illness (eg, suicide, acquired immunodeficiency syndrome [AIDS]), the person may be alone to grieve (Bateman, 1999).
- Complex social issues of morality, sexuality, contagion, and shame associated with AIDS-related losses interfere with the healing process of bereavement (Mallinson, 1999).
- Gay men who have experienced multiple AIDS-related losses (eg, loss of friends and community, disintegrating family structures and social networks) may receive little understanding from heterosexuals (Mallinson, 1999).

❖ Pediatric Considerations

- Children respond to death depending on developmental stage and response of significant others:
  - *Younger than 3 years:* Cannot comprehend death, fear separation
  - *3 to 5 years of age:* View illness as punishment for real or imagined wrongdoing; have little concept of death as final because of immature concept of time; may view death as a kind of sleep; may believe they caused the event (magical thinking; eg, by bad thoughts about person)
  - *6 to 10 years of age:* Begin to fear death; attempt to give meaning to the event (eg, devil, ghost, God); associate death with mutilation and punishment; can feel responsibility for the event
  - *10 to 12 years of age:* Usually have an adult concept of death (inevitable, irreversible, universal); attitudes greatly influenced by reactions of parents and others; very interested in postdeath services and rituals
  - *Adolescence:* Have a mature understanding of death; may suffer from guilt and shame; least likely to accept death, particularly their own (Wong, 2003)
  - "The death of a child is emotionally, psychologically, and physically the most painful experience that one can encounter and is often philosophically unintelligible in today's society" (Vickers & Carlisle, 2000, p. 12).

Maternal Considerations

- The death of a fetus or infant presents multiple stresses for the family.
- Birth of a child with a congenital anomaly creates emotional difficulties for the parents, their relationship with the child, and family functioning.

Geriatric Considerations

- Grief in older adults often is related to losses within the self, such as changes in roles or body image or decreased body function. These losses sometimes are less easily accepted than is the loss of a significant other (Miller, 2004).
- Many cultures document the death of a mate as the most stressful life event. Increasing longevity brings increased potential for 50 years or more of marriage to the same spouse, with concomitantly greater effects of the loss of that spouse. The spouse may be the older person's only close family member and social contact.
- One study of people older than 50 years examined the following factors over 2 years after the loss of a spouse: emotional shock, helplessness/avoidance, psychological strength/coping, anger/guilt/confusion, and grief resolution behaviors. Statistically significant changes were seen in all areas except psychological strength/coping. There also was no significant change in life satisfaction scores (Caserta, Lund & Dimond, 1985).
- There seems to be some support for extending traditional bereavement periods to at least 24 months for older adults who have lost a spouse. Of greater influence than the loss of a significant other is the loss of a crucial relationship that provides meaning to the person's life. Even in young widows, the estimate of adjustment period has been extended, based on research showing movement at the 24-month mark from high distress to low distress (as measured on the Goldberg General Health Questionnaire; Caserta, Lund & Dimond, 1985).
- Bereavement is a risk factor for suicide. Older adults commit about 25% of all suicides. Suicide attempts are less frequent in older adults; however, the rate of attempted to successful suicide increases to 4:1 after 60 years of age, compared with 20:1 in those younger than 40 years. Men older than 65 years have the highest incidence of suicide; men 65 to 74 years of age have 30.4 suicides per 100,000; men 75 to 84 years of age have 42.3 suicides per 100,000; and men older than 85 years have 50.6 suicides per 100,000 (Miller, 2004).
- Death of a pet can be significant for an isolated older person and can result in a grieving process.
- Reminiscence therapy or life review can help integrate losses. Frequently, older adults use reminiscence to move through Erikson's eighth developmental stage, Ego Integrity versus Despair (Miller, 2004).
- Social supports, strong religious beliefs, and good prior mental health are resources that decrease psychosocial and physical dysfunction (Miller, 2004).

Transcultural Considerations

- Mourning, a behavioral response to death or loss, is culturally determined (Andrews & Hansen, 2004).
- "Even if bereavement is regarded as a universal stressor, the magnitude of the stress and its meaning to the individual varies significantly cross-culturally" (Andrews & Hansen, 2004, p. 96). The dominant US culture assumes that the death of a child is more stressful than that of an older relative.
- Puerto Ricans believe that a person's spirit is not free to enter the next life if he or she has left something unsaid before death. Heightened grieving may occur if closure has not been achieved, such as through sudden death (Andrews & Hansen, 2004).

(continued)

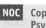 **Transcultural Considerations (continued)**

- Hispanics sometimes express grief with seizurelike behavior, hyperkinetic episodes, aggression, or stupor. This syndrome is called *elliptic* (Andrews & Hansen, 1998).
- The degree of mourning in the Chinese culture depends on the mourner's closeness to and the importance of the deceased person (Andrews & Hansen, 1998).
- Grief work for Haitians fequently includes taking on symptoms of the deceased person's last illness (Giger & Davidhizar, 2004).

Focus Assessment Criteria

Subjective Data

Assess for Defining Characteristics.

Present interactions between or among family members
Adults
Children

Maturational level	Understanding of crisis	Degree of participation

Knowledge of expected grief reactions
Relationship to ill or deceased person

Expressions of

Ambivalence	Anger	Denial
Depression	Fear	Guilt

Report of

Gastrointestinal disturbances	Insomnia	Preoccupation with sleep
Fatigue (decreased or) increased	Inability to carry out work, self-care, social responsibility	

Assess for Related Factors.

Family
Previous coping patterns for crisis
Quality of the relationship of the ill or deceased person with each family member
Position or role responsibilities of the ill or deceased person
Sociocultural expectations for bereavement
Religious expectations for bereavement

Individual family members
Previous experiences with loss or death (as child, adolescent, or adult)
Did family talk out their grief?
Did they practice any particular religious rituals associated with bereavement?

Objective Data

Assess for Defining Characteristics.

Normative

Shock	Disbelief, denial	Withdrawal
Anger	Preoccupation	Crying
Hopelessness	Sorrow	

Pathologic pattern (profound; progressively worsened responses) (subjective, objective)

Anger	Isolation	Hallucinations
Denial	Obsession	Suicidal thoughts
Despair	Delusions	Inability to go back to
Substance abuse	Regression	pre-bereavement funtioning

For more information on Focus Assessment Criteria, visit http://connection.lww.com.

Goals

NOC Coping, Family Coping, Grief Resolution, Psychosocial Adjustment: Life Change

The person will express his or her grief.

Indicators

- Describe the meaning of the death or loss to him or her.
- Share his or her grief with significant others.

General Interventions

 Family Support, Grief Work Facilitation, Coping Enhancement, Anticipatory Guidance, Emotional Support

Assess for Factors that may Delay Grief Work.

Unavailable or no support system

Uncertain loss (eg, missing child)

Failure to grieve for past loss

Nature of relationship

Dependency

Inability to grieve

Personality structure

Multiple losses

Previous emotional illness

Early object loss

Reduce or Eliminate Factors, if Possible.

Promote a Trust Relationship.

Promote feelings of self-worth through one-on-one or group sessions.

Allow for established time to meet and discuss feelings.

Communicate clearly, simply, and to the point.

Never try to lessen the loss (eg, "She didn't suffer long"; "You can have another baby").

Use feedback to assess what the person and family are learning.

Offer support and reassurance.

Create a therapeutic milieu ("convey that you care").

Establish a safe, secure, and private environment.

Demonstrate respect for the person's culture, religion, race, and values.

Provide privacy, but be careful not to isolate the person or family inadvertently.

Provide a presence of simply "being" with the bereaved.

Support Grief Reactions.

Explain grief reactions: shock and disbelief, developing awareness, and resolution.

Describe varied acceptable expressions.

    Elated or manic behavior as a defense against depression

    Elation and hyperactivity as a reaction of love and protection from depression

    Various states of depression

    Various somatic manifestations (weight loss or gain, indigestion, dizziness)

Assess for past experiences with loss (eg, losses in childhood and later life).

Determine Whether Family has Special Requests Regarding Viewing the Deceased (Vanezis & McGee, 1999).

Respect their requests.

Prepare them for any body changes.

Remove all equipment; change soiled linen.

Support their request (eg, holding, washing, touching, kissing).

Promote Family Cohesiveness.

Support the family at its level of functioning.

Encourage self-exploration of feelings with family members.

Explain the need to discuss behaviors that interfere with relationships.

Recognize and reinforce the strengths of each family member.

Encourage family members to evaluate their feelings and support one another.

Promote Grief Work with Each Response.

Denial

Recognize that response is useful and necessary.

Explain the use of denial by one family member to the other members.

Do not push client to move past denial without emotional readiness.

Isolation

Convey acceptance by allowing grief.

Create open, honest communications to promote sharing.

Reinforce the person's self-worth by allowing privacy.

Encourage client/family to increase social activities (eg, support groups, church groups) gradually.

Prepare client/family that they may experience avoidance from some friends and family who may not be comfortable with their situation of loss or their grief responses.

Encourage client/family to let significant others know their needs (eg, support, privacy, permission to share their experience).

Depression

Reinforce the person's self-esteem.

Identify the level of depression and develop the approach accordingly.

Use empathic sharing; acknowledge grief ("It must be very difficult").

Identify any indications of suicidal behavior (frequent statements of intent, revealed plan).

See *Risk for Self-Harm* for additional information.

Anger

Understand that this feeling usually replaces denial.

Explain to family that anger serves to try to control one's environment more closely because of inability to control loss.

Stress that the illness or death did not result from being bad or because the well child wished it.

Identify Clients at High Risk for Dysfunctional Grieving Reactions.

No emotion

Previous conflict with deceased person

History of ineffective coping patterns

Teach Client/Family Signs of Pathologic Grieving, Especially those at Risk.

Prolonged hallucinations

Continued searching for the deceased (frequent moves/relocations)

Delusions

Isolation

Egocentricity

Overt hostility (usually toward a family member)

Promote Physical Well-Being: Nutrition, Rest, Exercise.

For Survivors of Suicide:

Encourage them to see a primary care professional.

Elicit their interpretation of the event. Clarify distortions.

Discuss plans for funeral and notification of friends and relatives.

Discuss the hazards of secrecy.

Allow for expression of guilt, rage, and blame (eg, of professionals).

Follow up with telephone contacts to family.

Refer all survivors to counseling, especially those at high risk (surviving children; those with inadequate support; those who respond with blaming, scapegoating, or secrecy).

Provide Health Teaching and Referrals, as Indicated.

Teach Client and Family Signs of Resolution.

Grieving person no longer lives in the past but is future oriented and establishes new goals.

Grieving person redefines relationship with the lost object/person.

Grieving person begins to resocialize.

Identify Agencies that may be Helpful (eg, Community Agencies, Religious Groups).

Rationales

- Grief work cannot begin until the person acknowledges the loss. Nurses can encourage this acknowledgment by engaging in open, honest dialogue, providing the family an opportunity to view the dead person, and recognizing and validating the grief (Vanezis & McGee, 1999).
- *Life review* is a process by which a dying person reminisces about the past, especially unresolved conflicts, in an attempt to resolve them. It also provides an opportunity for the person to evaluate successes and failures.
- Anger is often perceived as negative; however, it can energize behavior, facilitate expression of negative feelings, and help defend against threats (Boyd, 2001).
- Sudden death or suicide is catastrophic. Interventions focus on helping survivors with valid perceptions of the event, and, in suicide, shame and embarrassment (Mohr, 2003).
- Interventions must begin immediately after a completed suicide, because those left behind experience guilt, rejection, and disillusionment.
- Interventions focus on projection of hope, facilitating a cathartic release, and experiencing a better ending (Cutcliffe, 2004).

- Death of a child can put extreme strain on a marriage (Pallikkathayil & Flood, 1991).
- Mourners who were very busy with the practical and necessary caregiving tasks of the dying person may not address the impending loss and, therefore, are at risk for delayed grieving response (Stuart & Sundeen, 2002).
- The purpose of mourning and related rituals is to acknowledge the loss, promoting a return of energy for reinvestment in daily life and for coping with the changes required.
- Silent presence and use of touch can covey acceptance of crying.
- Acknowledging that grief responses are expected and normal can support an anxious grieving person.
- Helping the person identify perceptions of dying and death can provide opportunities to examine their accuracy.
- Secrecy related to suicide impedes grief work because it thwarts open discussion (Boyd, 2001).

Pediatric Interventions

Explain What Caused the Death.
Clarify child's perceptions.
Openly clarify that the child did not cause the death.

Openly Discuss Possible Responses.
"Sometimes when someone dies we feel bad if we said or did something bad to them."
"Sometimes we feel glad we didn't die and then feel bad because _____ did."
"When someone dies, we can become afraid that we may die also."
"I remember when _____ said or did _____. What do you remember?"

Explain Rituals (eg, Read Children's Book on Death).

Assist Family with the Decision About the Child Attending the Funeral. Determine if the Following are Present (Boyd, 2001):
- Child has a basic understanding of death and good coping skills.
- Child is not afraid of adults' emotional responses.
- The ethnic group approaches death openly (eg, children commonly attend funerals).
- A familiar adult who is coping well with his or her own grief is available to monitor the child's needs.
- Child expresses a desire to attend and has a basic understanding of what will happen.

Explore the Child's Modified Involvement in Funeral Activities (eg, Visit Funeral Home Before Guests Come, Attend After-Service Gathering).

Allow Child to Grieve at Own Pace. Give Adolescents Permission to Grieve Openly.

Consider a Sibling Support Group, if Indicated.

Rationales

- Children need to be included in grief rituals based on their developmental level or "they may feel abandoned and left to face their fear alone" (Bateman, 1999, p. 144).
- Children can be encouraged to communicate symbolically through writing, telling stories, or drawing pictures.
- Children need to feel the joys and sorrows of life to begin to incorporate both in their lives appropriately (Boyd, 2001; Kübler-Ross, 1983).
- Children can feel rejected or unloved if parents or significant others fail to offer emotional support and nurturing because of their own grief (Bourne & Meier, 1988; Wong, 2003).
- Children of parents who commit suicide are at increased risk for future psychopathology and depression (Boyd, 2001).
- Siblings of deceased children may experience guilt, anger, jealousy, and fear (Wong, 2003).

Maternal Interventions

Assist Parents of a Deceased Infant, Newborn, or Fetus with Grief Work (Mina, 1985; Wong, 2003).

Promote Grieving.

Use baby's name when discussing the loss.

Allow parents to share the hopes and dreams they had for the child.

Provide parents with access to a hospital chaplain or religious leader of their choice.

Encourage parents to see and to hold their infant to validate the reality of the loss.

Design a method to communicate to auxiliary departments that the parents are in mourning (eg, rose sticker on door, chart).

Prepare a memory packet wrapped in a clean baby blanket (photograph [Polaroid], ID bracelet, footprints with birth certificate, lock of hair, crib card, fetal monitor strip, infant's blanket). Encourage them to take the memory packet home. If they prefer not to, keep the packet on file in case they change their minds later.

Encourage parents to share the experience with their other children at home (refer to pertinent literature for consumers).

Provide for follow-up support and referral services (eg, support group) after discharge.

Assist Others to Comfort Grieving Parents.

Stress the importance of openly acknowledging the death.

If the baby or fetus was named, use the name in discussions.

Never try to lessen the loss with discussions of future pregnancies or other healthy siblings.

Send sympathy cards.

Be sensitive to the gravity of the loss for both the mother and father.

Create a remembrance (eg, plant a tree).

Rationales

- Researchers have found 100% of parents who held their deceased babies reported positive experiences. Parents who did not hold their infants reported problems with resolution of the grief process (Ransohoff-Adler & Berger, 1989).
- In a study, 80% of the parents who did not hold their deceased infants reported it was the decision of a health care professional (Ransohoff-Adler & Berger, 1989).

ANTICIPATORY GRIEVING

DEFINITION

Anticipatory Grieving: State in which a person/group experiences reactions in response to an expected significant loss

DEFINING CHARACTERISTICS
Major (Must Be Present)

Expressed distress at potential loss

Minor (May Be Present)

Change in sleep patterns	Denial	Change in social patterns
Change in communication patterns	Guilt	Anger
	Sorrow	Change in eating habits
Decreased libido		

RELATED FACTORS

See *Grieving*.

KEY CONCEPTS

See *Grieving*.

Focus Assessment Criteria

See *Grieving*.

Goal

NOC Refer to *Grieving*

The person will express his or her grief.

Indicators

- Participate in decision making for the future.
- Share concerns with significant others.

General Interventions

NIC Refer to *Grieving*

Assess for Causative and Contributing Factors of Anticipated or Potential Loss.

Terminal illness	Body image changes	Self-esteem changes
Separation (divorce, hospitalization,marriage, relocation, job)	Aging	Socioeconomic status

Assess Individual Response.

Denial	Shock	Rejection
Anger	Bargaining	Depression
Isolation	Guilt	Helplessness/hopelessness
Fear		

Encourage Client to Share Concerns.

Use open-ended questions and reflection ("What are your thoughts today?" "How do you feel?").

Acknowledge value of the person and his or her grief by using touch, sitting with him or her, and verbalizing your concern ("This must be very difficult," "What is most important to you now?").

Recognize that some people may choose not to share their concerns, but convey that you are available if they desire to do so later ("What do you hope for?").

Assist Client and Family to Identify Strengths.

"What do you do well?"

"What are you willing to do to improve your life?"

"Is religion a source of strength for you?"

"Do you have close friends?"

"Whom do you turn to in times of need?"

"What does this person do for you?"

Promote Integrity of Client and Family by Acknowledging Strengths.

"Your brother looks forward to your visit."

"Your family is so concerned for you."

Support Client and Family with Grief Reactions.

Prepare them for grief reactions.

Explain grief reactions.

Focus on the current situation until the person or family indicates the desire to discuss the future.

Promote Family Cohesiveness.

Identify Availability of a Support System.

Meet consistently with family members.

Identify family member roles, strengths, and weaknesses.

Identify Communication Patterns within the Family Unit.

Assess positive and negative feedback, verbal and nonverbal communication, and body language.

Listen and clarify messages being sent.

Provide for the Concept of Hope.

Supply accurate information.

Resist the temptation to give false hope.

Discuss concerns willingly.

Promote Group Decision Making to Enhance Group Autonomy.

Establish consistent times to meet with person and family.

Encourage members to talk directly with and to listen to one another.

Initiate a Dialogue Regarding Options Available During Terminal Stage.

Home care

Institution

Hospice

Discuss Benefits of Home Care of Terminal Family Member (Vickers & Carlisle, 2000).

Family has unlimited access to person.

Family stays together.

Opportunities for support and assistance from extended family and friends are improved.

Dying person is less isolated.

Discuss the Problems of Home Care and Fears.

Family has 24-h responsibility.

Family is unprepared for experience.

Feelings of inadequacy are common.

Family cohesiveness may be disrupted.

Promote Grief Work with each Response.

Denial

Initially support and then strive to increase development of awareness (when person indicates readiness).

Isolation

Listen and spend designated time consistently with person and family.

Offer client and family opportunity to explore their emotions.

Reflect on past losses and acknowledge loss behavior (past and present).

Depression

Begin with simple problem solving and move toward acceptance.

Enhance self-worth through positive reinforcement.

Identify level of depression and indications of suicidal behavior or ideas.

Be consistent and establish times daily to speak with person and family.

Anger

Allow for crying to release this energy.

Listen to and communicate concern.

Encourage concerned support from significant others as well as professionals.

Guilt

Listen and communicate concern.

Promote more direct expression of feelings.

Allow for crying.

Explore methods to resolve guilt.

Fear

Help person and family recognize the feeling.

Explain that this will help them cope with life.

Explore attitudes about loss, death, and so forth.

Explore methods of coping.

Rejection

Allow for verbal expression of this feeling to diminish the emotional strain.

Recognize that expression of anger may cause rejection by significant others.

Provide for Expression of Grief.

Encourage Emotional Expressions of Grieving.

Caution Client About Use of Sedatives and Tranquilizers, which may Prevent or Delay Expressions.

Encourage Verbalization by Clients of all Age Groups and Families.

Support family cohesiveness.

Promote and verbalize strengths of the family group.

Encourage Person and Family to Engage in Life Review.

Focus and support the social network relationships.

Reevaluate past life experiences and integrate them into a new meaning.

Convey empathic understanding.

Explore unfinished business.

Identify Potential Dysfunctional Grieving Reactions.

Suicidal indications	Delusions	Hallucinations
Difficulty crying	Difficulty controlling crying	Phobias
Obsessions	Isolation	Conversion hysteria
Agitated depression	Restrictions of pleasure	Delay in grief work
Intense reaction (longer than 6 months with few signs of relief)	Loss of control of environment leading to hopelessness/ helplessness	

Provide Health Teaching and Referrals, as Indicated.

Refer Person with Potential for Dysfunctional Grieving Responses for Counseling (Psychiatrist, Nurse Therapist, Counselor, Psychologist).

Explain What to Expect.

Sadness	Rejection	Feelings of aloneness
Anger	Guilt	Labile emotions
Fear		

Teach Person and Family Signs of Resolution.

Grieving person no longer lives in past but is future oriented, establishing new goals.

Grieving person redefines relationship with the lost object/person.

Grieving person begins to resocialize.

Teach Signs of Dysfunctional Responses and Referrals Needed.

Defenses used in uncomplicated grief work that become exaggerated or maladaptive responses

Persistent absence of any emotion

Prolonged intense reactions of anxiety, anger, fear, guilt, helplessness

Identify Agencies that may Enhance Grief Work.

Self-help groups	Widow-to-widow groups	Parents of deceased children
Single-parent groups	Bereavement groups	

Rationales

- The knowledge that no further treatment is warranted and that death is imminent may give rise to feelings of powerlessness, anger, profound sadness, and other grief responses. Open, honest discussions can help the client and family members accept and cope with the situation and their response to it.
- Research validates that professional interventions and professionally supported voluntary and self-help services are capable of reducing the risk of psychiatric and psychoanalytic disorders resulting from bereavement (Boyd, 2001).
- Home care of a dying relative can provide the family with choice and control, reduce feelings of helplessness, and promote effective grieving after death (Vickers & Carlisle, 2000).

DYSFUNCTIONAL GRIEVING

DEFINITION

Dysfunctional Grieving: State in which a person or group experiences prolonged unresolved grief and engages in detrimental activities

DEFINING CHARACTERISTICS
Major (Must Be Present, One or More)

Unsuccessful adaptation
  to loss
Delayed emotional reaction

Prolonged denial, depression
Inability to assume normal patterns of living

Minor (May Be Present)

Social isolation or withdrawal
Failure to restructure life
  after loss

Failure to develop new relationships/interests

RELATED FACTORS

See *Grieving*.

KEY CONCEPTS
Generic Considerations

- Unresolved grief may be difficult to determine because the grief experience has no clearly defined end point, nor is there a "right way" to grieve (Varcarolis, 2002). Some people do experience factors that interfere with the natural progress of grief work and, therefore, its resolution. Rando (1984) outlines seven variations of unresolved grief:
  - *Absent grief:* as if the death never occurred
  - *Inhibited grief:* can mourn only certain aspects of the loss
  - *Delayed grief:* cannot experience grief at the time of loss (ie, mourner feels he or she cannot deal with grief at the time of loss: "I must be strong for my children now.")
  - *Conflicted grief:* often associated with a previous dependent or ambivalent relationship
  - *Chronic grief:* ongoing intense grief reaction, sometimes serves to keep the deceased "alive" through grief
  - *Unanticipated grief:* cannot grasp the full implications of loss; extreme bewilderment, anxiety, self-reproach, and depression
  - *Abbreviated grief:* often confused with unresolved grief, this shortened but normal form of grief might occur when significant grief work has been done before the loss
- Unresolved grief is a pathologic response of prolonged denial of the loss or a profound psychotic response. Examples include the following:
  - Refusal to remove possessions of deceased after reasonable time
  - Lasting loss of normal patterns of social behavior
  - Progressively deeper regression, depression
  - Progressively deeper isolation
  - Somatic manifestations (prolonged)
  - Obsessions, phobias
  - Delusions, hallucinations
  - Attempted suicide
- Predisposing factors attributed to *Dysfunctional Grieving* are as follows (Bateman, 1999; Worden, 1991):
  - A socially unspeakable or negated loss (eg, suicide, AIDS-related death)

- New feelings of dependency and neediness associated with the loss
- History of depressive illness or previous complicated grief reactions
- Sudden, uncertain, or overcomplicated circumstances surrounding the loss
- A highly ambivalent, narcissistic, or dependent relationship with the deceased
- Rando (1984) describes the social factors that can contribute to unresolved grief as social negation of the loss (eg, abortion, newborn, death of twin, death of frail elderly parent) and socially defined as inappropriate to discuss (eg, death of lover, suicide).

Focus Assessment Criteria

See *Grieving*.

Goal

NOC See *Grieving*

The person will verbalize intent to seek professional assistance.

Indicators

- Acknowledge the loss.
- Acknowledge an unresolved grief process.

General Interventions

NIC See also *Grieving*, Referral, Support Group

Assess for Causative and Contributing Factors.

Unavailable (or lack of) support system
History of dependency on deceased
History of a difficult relationship with the lost person or object
Multiple past losses
Ineffective coping strategies
Unexpected death
Expectations to "be strong"

Promote a Trust Relationship.

Implement the General Interventions under *Grieving*.

Support the Person and the Family's Grief Reactions.

Implement the General Interventions under *Grieving*.

Promote Family Cohesiveness.

Implement the General Interventions under *Grieving*.
Slowly and carefully identify the reality of the situation (eg, "After your husband died, who helped you most?").

Promote Grief Work with Each Response.

Denial
Explain the use of denial by one family member to the other members.
Do not force client to move past denial without emotional readiness.

Isolation
Convey a feeling of acceptance by allowing grief.
Create open, honest communications to promote sharing.
Reinforce the person's self-worth by allowing privacy.
Encourage client/family gradually to increase social activities (eg, support or church groups).

Depression
Implement the General Interventions under *Grieving*.

Anger
Understand that this feeling usually replaces denial.

Explain to family that anger serves to try to control one's environment more closely because of inability to control loss.

Encourage verbalization of the anger.

See *Anxiety* for additional information for anger.

Guilt/Ambivalence

Acknowledge client's expressed self-view.

Role play to allow client to "express" to dead person what he or she wants to say or how he or she feels.

Encourage client to identify positive contributions/aspects of the relationship.

Avoid arguing and participating in the person's system of shoulds and should nots.

Discuss the person's preoccupation with him and attempt to move verbally beyond the present.

Fear

Focus on the present and maintain a safe and secure environment.

Help the person to explore reasons for a meaning of the behavior.

Consider alternative ways of expressing his or her feelings.

Provide Health Teaching and Referrals, as Indicated.

Teach the Person and the Family Signs of Resolution.

Grieving person no longer lives in past but is future oriented and establishing new goals.

Grieving person redefines relationship with the lost object/person.

Grieving person begins to resocialize; seeks new relationships, experiences.

Teach Individual/Family to Recognize Signs of Pathologic Grieving, Especially for People who are at Risk, and to Seek Professional Counseling.

Continued searching for deceased	Prolonged depression	Denial
	Prolonged hallucinations	Delusions
Living in past	Egocentricity	Overhostility
Isolation		

Identify Agencies that May Be Helpful.

Support groups	Mental health agencies	Religious groups
Psychotherapists	Grief specialists	

Rationales

- Risk of death is greater in men than in women during the first 6 months of conjugal bereavement. Changes in health behavior patterns, such as nutrition, alcohol use, smoking, and decreased physical activity levels, may contribute to this increased mortality rate (Kaprio & Koskenvuo, 1987).
- The more dependent the person was on the deceased person, the more difficult the resolution (Varcarolis, 2002).
- Unresolved conflicts disrupt successful grief work (Varcarolis, 2002).
- People with few supportive relationships have more difficulty grieving (Varcarolis, 2002).

DELAYED GROWTH AND DEVELOPMENT

DEFINITION

Delayed Growth and Development: State in which a person has, or is at risk for, impaired ability to perform tasks of his or her age group or impaired growth

DEFINING CHARACTERISTICS
Major (Must Be Present, One or More)

Inability or difficulty performing skills or behaviors typical of his or her age group (eg, motor, personal/social, language/cognition; Table II.12)

and/or

Altered physical growth: weight lagging behind height by two standard deviations; pattern of height and weight percentiles indicate a drop in pattern

Minor (May Be Present)

Inability to perform self-care or self-control activities appropriate for age (see Table II.12)

Flat affect, listlessness, decreased responses, slow social responses, limited signs of satisfaction to caregiver, limited eye contact, difficulty feeding, decreased appetite, lethargy, irritability, negative mood, regression in self-toileting, regression in self-feeding (see Focus Assessment Criteria)

Infants: watchfulness, interrupted sleep pattern

RELATED FACTORS
Pathophysiologic

Related to compromised physical ability and dependence secondary to:

Congenital heart defects	Repeated acute or chronic illness	Acute illness
Cerebral damage	Congestive heart failure	Cerebral palsy
Malabsorption syndrome	Congenital neurologic defects	Cystic fibrosis
Congenital anomalies of extremities	Gastroesophageal reflux	Prolonged pain
	Muscular dystrophy	Inadequate nutritional intake

Treatment-Related

Related to separation from significant others or school, or inadequate sensory stimulation secondary to:

Confinement for ongoing treatment	Prolonged, painful treatment	Traction or casts
Repeat or prolonged hospitalizations	Prolonged bed rest	Isolation from disease

Situational (Personal and Environmental)

Related to parental stressor secondary to:

Insufficient knowledge

Change in usual environment

Separation from significant others (parents, primary caretaker)

School-related conflicts

Loss of significant other

Loss of control over environment (established rituals, activities, established hours of contact with family)

Related to Inadequate, inappropriate parental support (neglect, abuse)
Related to Inadequate sensory stimulation (neglect, isolation)

Maturational

Infant–Toddler (Birth to 3 Years)
Related to limited opportunities to meet social, play, or educational needs secondary to:

Separation from parents/   Restriction of activity secondary to (specify)
  significant others   Inability to trust significant other
Inadequate parental support   Multiple caregivers
Inability to communicate
  (eg, deafness)

Preschool Age (4 to 6 Years)
Related to limited opportunities to meet social, play, or educational needs secondary to:
Loss of ability to communicate   Lack of stimulation
Lack of significant other

Related to loss of significant other (death, divorce)
Related to loss of peer group
Related to removal from home environment

School Age (6 to 11 Years)
Related to loss of significant others
Peer group   Strange environment

Adolescent (12 to 18 Years)
Related to loss of independence and autonomy secondary to: (specify)
Related to disruption of peer relationships
Related to disruption of body image
Related to loss of significant others

◎◎ AUTHOR'S NOTE

Specific developmental tasks are associated with various age groups (eg, to gain autonomy and self-control [eg, toileting] from 1 to 3 years of age; to establish lasting relationships from 18 to 30 years of age). An adult's failure to accomplish a developmental task may cause or contribute to a change in functioning in a functional health pattern (eg, *Impaired Social Interactions, Powerlessness*). Because nursing interventions focus on altered functioning rather than achievement of past developmental tasks, the diagnosis *Delayed Growth and Development* has limited uses for adults. It is most useful for a child or adolescent experiencing difficulty achieving a developmental task.

◎◎ ERRORS IN DIAGNOSTIC STATEMENTS

1. *Delayed Growth and Development related to inability to perform toileting self-control appropriate for age (4 years)*
   Inability to perform toileting self-control is not a contributing factor but a diagnostic cue. The nurse should rewrite the diagnosis as *Delayed Growth and Development related to unknown etiology, as evidenced by inability to perform toileting self-control appropriate for age (4 years)*. The use of "unknown etiology" directs nurses to collect more data on reasons for the problem.
2. *Delayed Growth and Development related to mental retardation secondary to Down syndrome*
   When *Delayed Growth and Development* is used to describe a person with mental or physical impairment, what is the nursing focus? What client goals would nursing interventions achieve? If physical impairments represent barriers to achieving developmental tasks, the nurse can write the diagnosis as *Risk for Delayed Growth and Development related to impaired ability to achieve developmental tasks (specify—eg, socialization) secondary to disability*. For a child with mental impairment, the nurse should determine what functional health patterns are altered or at high risk for alteration and amenable to nursing interventions and address the specific problem (eg, *Toileting Self-Care Deficit*).

KEY CONCEPTS
Generic Considerations

- *Development* can be defined as the patterned, orderly, lifelong changes in structure, thought, or behavior that evolve from maturation of physical and mental capacity, experiences, and learning. It results in a new level of maturity and integration. *Growth* refers to an increase in body size, function, and complexity of body cell content (Wong, 2003). For *Delayed Growth and Development*, growth and development are synonymous, because any disruption that does not affect development most likely results in *Imbalanced Nutrition*.
- The following assumptions concerning development are relevant (Wong, 2003):
  - Growth and development is most rapid in the early stages of life.
  - Childhood is the foundation period that establishes the basis for successful or unsuccessful development throughout life.
  - Growth and development are continuous and occur in spurts, not straight and upward.
  - Development follows a definable, predictable, and sequential pattern.
  - Critical periods exist when development is rapid and the person's ability to respond to stressors is limited.
  - Growth proceeds in a cephalocaudal, proximodistal direction.
  - Development proceeds from simple to complex.
  - Development occurs in all components of a person (ie, motor, intellectual, personal, social, language).
  - Development results from biologic, maturational, and individual learning.
- Often development is defined in terms of stages or levels (eg, Erikson's and Piaget's theories). In addition, development may be defined in terms of tasks that must be accomplished. A *developmental task* is a growth responsibility at a particular point in life. Achievement of the task leads to success with later tasks. Various influences affect development, either by accelerating or slowing down the process. Physiologic disruptions, through either genetic malfunction or insult from illness, may potentially alter development, temporarily or permanently. Psychological and social influences also may alter development positively or negatively. Altered development in a child is particularly critical because it may establish a foundation that then remains faulty for life. Because of the rapid acceleration of development in childhood, several critical periods exist (Wong, 2003).

Focus Assessment Criteria

See Table II.12 for descriptions of appropriate developmental milestones/behaviors for each age group, as well as information for nursing interventions and parental guidance.

Subjective Data

Data should be verified with primary caregiver.

Assess for Defining Characteristics.

Developmental level: behaviors listed under developmental tasks (see Table II.12) may be assessed through direct observation or report of parent/primary caregiver. The Denver Developmental Screening Tool (DDST) may be used for children younger than 6 years.

Assess for Related Factors.

Current nutritional patterns

Diet recall for past 24 h (from parent or child, type of food, amounts)	Parental/child knowledge of nutrition
	Diet history
	Height/weight at birth
Intake pattern	Child's reaction to eating, feeding

Physiologic alterations

Any nausea, vomiting, diarrhea	Allergies
Food intolerances	Dysphagia
Fatigue	

TABLE II.12 Age-Related Developmental Tasks

Developmental Tasks/Needs	Parental Guidance	Implications for Nursing
Birth to 1 Year		

Personal/Social
Learns to trust and anticipate satisfaction
Sends cues to mother/caretaker
Begins understanding self as separate from others (body image)
 	
Motor
Responds to sound
Social smile
Reaches for objects
Begins to sit, creep, pull up, and stand with support
Attempting to walk
 	
Language/Cognition
Learns to signal wants/needs with sounds, crying
Begins to vocalize with meaning (two-syllable words: Dada, Mama)
Comprehends some verbal/nonverbal messages (no, yes, bye-bye)
Learns about words through senses
 	
Fears
Loud noises
Falling
	Encourage parent to respond to cry, meet infant's need *consistently*
	Teach parent not to be afraid of spoiling infant with too much attention
	Talk and sing to child; hold and cuddle often
	Provide variety of stimulation
	Allow infant to feed self (cereal, etc.)
	Do not prop bottle
	
	Toys
	Brightly colored crib toys, mobiles
	Stuffed toys of varied textures
	Music boxes
	
	Safety
	Be aware of rapidly changing locomotive ability (eg, child-proof kitchen, stairways; small objects within reach; tub safety)
		Encourage parent to participate in care:
		    Bathing
		    Feeding
		    Holding
		Teach parent guidance information
		Provide ongoing stimulation while confined through use of toys, mirrors, mobiles, music
		Hold, speak to infant, maintain eye contact
		Investigate crying
		Do not restrain

1 to 3½ Years		

Personal/Social
Establishes self-control, decision making, self-independence (autonomy)
Extremely curious, prefers to do things himself
Demonstrates independence through negativism
Very egocentric: believes he controls the world
Learns about words through senses
 	
Motor
Begins to walk and run well
Drinks from cup, feeds self
Develops fine motor control
Climbs
Begins self-toileting
 	
Language/Cognition
Has poor time sense
Increasingly verbal (4- to 5-word sentences by age 3½)
Talks to self/others
Misconceptions about cause/effect
 	
Fears
Loss/separation from parents
Darkness
Machines/equipment
Intrusive procedures
	Provide child with peer companionship
	Allow for brief periods of separation under familiar surroundings
	Practice safety measures that guard against child's increased motor ability and curiosity (poisoning, falls)
	Tell the truth
	Disciplining child for violation of safety rules:
	    Running in street
	    Touching electrical wires
	Allow child some control over fears:
	    Favorite toy
	    Night light
	Allow exploration within safe limits
	Explain as simply as possible why things happen
	Allow child to explain why he thinks things are happening
	Correct misconceptions
	Include child in domestic activities when possible:
	    Dusting
	    Cleaning spoons
	Discuss differences in opinions (between parents) in front of child
	Do not threaten child with what will happen if he does not behave
	Always follow through with punishment
		Allow child to take liquids from a cup (including medicines)
		Allow child to perform some self-care tasks:
		    Wash face and arms
		    Brush teeth
		Expect resistant behavior to treatments; reinforce treatments, not punishments
		Use firm, direct approach and provide child with choices only when possible
		Restrain child when needed
		Explain to parents methods for disciplining child:
		    Slap hand once (for dangerous touching, [eg, stove])
		    Sit in chair for 2 min (if child gets up, put him back and reset timer)
		Explain the need for consistency
		Allow expression of fear, pain, displeasure
		Assign consistent caregiver
		Let child play with simple equipment (stethoscope)
		Provide materials for play (favorite toy)
		Be honest about procedure
		Praise child for helping you:
		    Holding still
		    Holding the Band-Aid

(table continues on p. 354)

TABLE II.12 Age-Related Developmental Tasks (*Continued*)

Developmental Tasks/Needs	Parental Guidance	Implications for Nursing

	Toys
	Manipulative toys
	Puzzles
	Bright-colored, simple books
	Large-muscle devices (gym sets, etc.)
	Music (songs, records)
		Give child choices whenever possible
		Tell child he can cry or squeeze your hand, but you expect him to hold still
		Have parents present for procedures when at all possible
		Explore with child his fantasies of the situation:
		    Use play therapy
		    Explain the procedure immediately beforehand if short (eg, injection) and when appropriate if longer or intrusive (eg, x-ray, IV insertion)
		Follow home routines when possible

3½ to 5 Years

Developmental Tasks/Needs	Parental Guidance	Implications for Nursing

Personal/Social
Attempts to establish self as like his parents, but independent
Explores environment on his own initiative
Boasts, brags, has feelings of indestructibility
Family is primary group
Peers increasingly important
Assumes sex roles
Aggressive
 	
Motor
Locomotion skills increase, and coordinates easier
Rides tricycle/bicycle
Throws ball, but has difficulty catching
 	
Language/Cognition
Egocentric
Language skills flourish
Generates many questions: how, why, what?
Simple problem solving; uses fantasy to understand, problem solve
 	
Fears
Mutilation
Castration
Dark
Unknown
Inanimate, unfamiliar objects
	Teach parents to listen to child's fears, feelings
	Encourage hugs, touch as expressions of acceptance
	Provide simple explanations
	Limit stimulation from television to avoid intense material
	Focus on positive behaviors
	Allow child to help as much as possible
	Provide child with regular contact with other children (eg, nursery school)
	Explain that television, movies are make-believe
	Practice definite limit-setting behavior
	Offer child choices
	Allow child to express anger verbally but limit motor aggression ("You may slam a door but you may not throw a toy")
	Discipline (examples):
	    Sit in chair 5 minutes
	    Forbid a favorite pastime (no bicycle riding for 2 h)
	Be consistent and firm
	Teach safety precautions about strangers
	
	Toys and Games
	"Make-believe" play (play house, toy models, etc.)
	Simple games with others, books, puzzles, coloring
		Encourage expressing of fears
		Reinforce reality of body image
		Encourage self-care, decision making when possible
		Involve parents in teaching
		Provide peer stimulation
		Limit physical restraint
		Provide play opportunities for acting out fantasy, story-telling
		Explain to child how he can cooperate (eg, hold still), and expect that he will
		Use play therapy to allow child free expression
		Explain all procedures:
		    Use equipment if possible; allow therapeutic play
		    Encourage child to ask questions
		    Tell child the exact body parts that will be affected
		    Use models, pictures
		Explain when procedure will occur in relation to daily schedule (eg, after lunch, after bath)

5 to 11 Years

Developmental Tasks/Needs	Parental Guidance	Implications for Nursing
Personal/Social Learns to include values and skills of school, neighborhood, peers Peer relationships important Focuses more on reality, less on fantasy Family is main base of security and identity Sensitive to reactions of others Seeks approval, recognition	Teach appropriate foods needed each day; provide choices Encourage interaction outside home Include cooking and cleaning in home activities Teach safety (bicycle, street, playground equipment, fire, water, strangers) Maintain limit-setting and discipline	Promote family and peer interactions (eg, visiting, telephone) Explain all procedures and impact on body Encourage questioning, *active* participation in care Be direct about explanation of procedures (eg, body part involved, use anatomic names, pictures, etc.); explain step by step

(*table continues on p. 355*)

TABLE II.12 Age-Related Developmental Tasks (*Continued*)

Developmental Tasks/Needs	Parental Guidance	Implications for Nursing
Enthusiastic, noisy, imaginative, desires to explore Likes to complete a task Enjoys helping *Motor* Moves constantly Physical play prevalent (sports, swimming, skating, etc.) *Language/Cognition* Organized, stable thought Concepts more complicated Focuses on concrete understanding *Fears* Rejections, failures Immobility Mutilation Death	Prepare child for bodily changes of pubescence and provide with concrete sex education information (late childhood) Expect fluctuations between imma-ture and mature behavior Respect peer relationships but do not compromise your values (eg, "But, Mom, all the other girls are wearing makeup!") Promote responsibility, contribution to family (eg, duties for helping, etc.) Promote exploration and develop-ment of skills (eg, joining clubs, sports, hobbies, etc.) *Toys and Games* Group games, board games, art activities, crafts, video games, reading	Be honest Reassure child that he is liked Provide privacy Involve parents but make direction of care the child's decision Reason and explain Encourage continuance of school work, activities if condition permits (eg, homework, contact with class-mates) Encourage continuance of hobbies, interests

11 to 15 Years

Personal/Social
Family values continue to be signif-icant influence
Peer group values have increasing significance
Early adolescence: outgoing and enthusiastic
Emotions are extreme: mood swings, introspection
Sexual identity fully mature
Wants privacy/independence
Develops interests not shared with family
Concern with physical self
Explores adult roles
 	
Motor
Well developed
Rapid physical growth
Secondary sex characteristics
 	
Language/Cognition
Plans for future career
Able to abstract solutions and solve problems in future tense
 	
Fears
Mutilation
Disruption in body image
Rejection from peers
	Encourage independent problem solving, decision making within established values
	Be available
	Compliment child's achievements
	Listen to interests, likes, dislikes without passing judgment
	Respect privacy
	Allow independence while main-taining safety limits
	Provide concrete information about sexuality, function, bodily changes
	Teach about:
	  Auto safety
	  Drug abuse
	  Alcohol hazards
	  Tobacco hazards
	  Mechanical safety
	  Sexuality relations
	  Dating
	
	Games/Interests
	Intellectual games
	Reading
	Arts, crafts, hobbies
	Video games
	Problem-solving games
	Computers
		Respect privacy
		Accept expression of feelings
		Direct discussions of care and con-dition to child
		Ask for opinions, allow input into decisions
		Be flexible with routines; explain all procedures/treatments
		Encourage continuance of peer relationships
		Listen actively
		Identify impact of illness on body image, future functioning
		Correct misconceptions
		Encourage continuance of school work, hobbies, interests

Parental attitudes

What are the parents' expectations for the child?

What are the parents' feelings about being parents?

What is the parents' approach to care and discipline of the child?

How do the parents feel about the home situation?

How do the parents feel about child's illness, treatments/hospitalization?

Assess family functioning with an appropriate assessment tool.

Stressors in environment

Illness in family

History of illness or
  hospitalization of child

Child's peer/sibling relationships

Conflict in family

Child's behavior/success in school

Objective Data
Assess for Defining Characteristics.

General appearance

Cleanliness, grooming
Eye contact
Facial responses

Response to stimulation
Mood (eg, crying, elated)

Response/interaction with parent

Spontaneous, happy when
 comforted by parent

Response to procedures, strangers
Reaction when separated

Nutritional status

Height/weight (compare to norms)
Frontal/occipital circumference (also see Focus Assessment Criteria under *Imbalanced Nutrition: Less Than Body Requirements*)

Bowel and bladder control personal/social

Language/cognition
Motor activity: Assess for achievement of developmental skills in appropriate age group
 (see Table II.12)

Developmental level (see behaviors described under Developmental Tasks, Table II.12)

For more information on Focus Assessment Criteria, visit http://connection.lww.com.

Goal

NOC Child Development (specify age)

The child will demonstrate increased age-appropriate behaviors.

Indicators (Specify for Age)

- Socialization
- Language
- Motor skills
- Self-care
- Cognitive skills

General Interventions

 NIC Development Enhancement, Parenting Promotion, Infant/Child Care

Assess Causative or Contributing Factors.

Parental lack of knowledge
Inadequate stimulation

Acute or chronic illness
Parent–child conflict

Stress
Change in environment

Teach Parents Age-Related Developmental Tasks and Anticipatory Guidance Information (See Table II.12).

Carefully Assess Child's Level of Development in All Areas of Functioning by Using Specific Assessment Tools (eg, Brazelton Assessment Table, DDST).

Provide Opportunities for an Ill Child to Meet Age-Related Developmental Tasks (See Implications for Nursing in Table II.12 to Assist with Designing Interventions).

Birth to 1 Year

Increase stimulation by using various colored toys in crib (eg, mobiles, musical toys, stuffed toys of
 varied textures) and frequently holding and speaking to the infant.
Hold infant while feeding slowly and in a relaxed environment.
Provide rest periods before feeding.
Observe mother and child during interaction, especially feeding.
Investigate crying promptly and consistently.

Assign a consistent caregiver.

Encourage parental visits, calls, and, if possible, involvement in care.

Provide buccal experience (ie, thumb, pacifier) if infant desires.

Allow infant's hands and feet to be free, if possible.

1 to 3½ Years

Assign a consistent caregiver.

Encourage self-care activities (eg, self-feeding, self-dressing, bathing).

Reinforce word development by repeating words child uses, naming objects, and speaking to child often.

Provide frequent periods of play with peers and various toys (puzzles, books with pictures, manipulative toys, trucks, cars, blocks, bright colors).

Demonstrate all procedures on a doll before you do them to the child.

Provide a safe area where the child can move around.

Encourage parental visits, calls, and, if possible, involvement in care.

Provide comfort measures after painful procedures.

3½ to 5 Years

Encourage self-care: self-grooming, self-dressing, mouth care, hair care.

Provide frequent playtime with others and various toys (eg, models, musical toys, dolls, puppets, books, mini-slides, wagons, tricycles).

Read stories aloud. Ask for verbal responses and requests.

Say words for equipment, objects, and people; ask the child to repeat them.

Allow time for individual play and exploration of play environment.

Encourage parental visits, calls, and, if possible, involvement in care.

Monitor and use television as a means to help child understand time (eg, "After *Sesame Street,* your mother will come.").

5 to 11 Years

Talk with child about care provided.

Request input from child (eg, diet, clothes, routine).

Allow child to dress in clothes instead of pajamas.

Provide periods of interaction with other children.

Provide craft project that the child can complete each day or week.

Continue schoolwork at intervals each day.

Praise positive behaviors.

Read stories, and provide several independent games, puzzles, books, video games, and art projects.

Introduce child by name to people on unit.

Encourage visits with or telephone calls from parents, siblings, and peers.

11 to 15 Years

Speak frequently with child about feelings, ideas, and concerns over condition or care.

Provide opportunity for interaction with others of the same age.

Identify an interest or a hobby that the unit can support, and support it daily.

Allow health care facility routine to be altered to suit child's schedule.

Allow child to wear his or her own clothes if possible.

Involve child in decisions about his or her care.

Provide opportunity for involvement in several activities (eg, reading, video games, movies, board games, art, trips outside or to other areas).

Encourage visits or telephone calls from parents, siblings, and peers.

Initiate Health Teaching and Referrals, When Indicated.

Provide anticipatory guidance for parents regarding constructive handling of developmental problems and support of developmental process (see Table II.12 and *Impaired Parenting*).

Refer family to appropriate agency for counseling or follow-up treatment of abuse, parent–child conflict, chemical dependency, and so forth (see *Disabled Family Coping*).

Refer family to appropriate agency for structured, ongoing stimulation program (eg, schooling) when functioning is likely to be impaired permanently.

Refer to community programs specific to contributing factors (eg, Women, Infants, and Children Program [WIC], social services, family services, counseling).

Provide a list of parent support groups (eg, Down Syndrome Awareness, Muscular Dystrophy Association, National Epilepsy Association).

Rationales

- All dimensions of growth and development have a predictable, definite sequence. New behaviors or biologic parts evolve from those previously established. Each stage is affected by those before and influences those that follow (Wong, 2003).
- Of the range of physiologic, psychological, and social influences that may affect development, many exist within the context of illness and wellness care, and nurses often encounter them as they provide care to children. As a result, nursing interventions should be designed with particular developmental information and tasks as the basis. As part of such care, nurses also must consider the influence of the primary caregiver or parent figure on the child's development. Parents essentially control most psychological and social influences in the early years of childhood. By virtue of the child's dependence on parents, these influences can modify development (Wong, 2003).
- Illness, hospitalization, separation from family, conflict, or inadequate parental support, as well as specific pathophysiologic processes that interfere with growth, may ultimately affect a child's development. The nurse must support both family and child in ensuring continuance of the child's developmental processes throughout the illness if optimal recovery is to be achieved. In addition, the nurse must seek to stimulate as well as to maintain the child's unique developmental level to promote optimal recovery. Stimulation of the developmental process may occur through parental support or teaching, referral, or direct intervention (see also *Impaired Parenting*).

RISK FOR DELAYED DEVELOPMENT

DEFINITION

Risk for Delayed Development: State in which a person is at risk for an impaired ability to perform tasks (social or self-regulating behavior, cognitive, language, gross, or fine motor skills) of his or her age group

RISK FACTORS

Refer to *Delayed Growth and Development*—Related Factors.

Goal

NOC See *Delayed Growth and Development*

The child/adolescent will continue to demonstrate appropriate behavior.

Indicators (Specify for Age)

- Self-care
- Social skills
- Language
- Cognitive skills
- Motor skills

General Interventions

NIC See *Delayed Growth and Development*

Refer to *Delayed Growth and Development*.

RISK FOR DISPROPORTIONATE GROWTH

DEFINITION

Risk for Disproportionate Growth: State in which a person is at risk for impaired growth (above 97th percentile or below 3rd percentile for age)

RISK FACTORS

Refer to *Delayed Growth and Development—Related Factors*.

Goal

> **NOC** See *Delayed Growth and Development*

The child/adolescent will continue to demonstrate age-appropriate growth.

Indicators

- Height
- Weight
- Head circumference

General Interventions

> **NIC** Refer to *Delayed Growth and Development*

Refer to *Delayed Growth and Development*.

ADULT FAILURE TO THRIVE

DEFINITION

Adult Failure to Thrive: State in which a person experiences insidious and progressive physical and psychosocial deterioration characterized by limited coping and diminished resilience

DEFINING CHARACTERISTICS

Major (Must be Present, One or More)

Declining physical functioning	Social withdrawal	Declining cognitive function
Self-care deficit	Depression	Apathy
Weight loss	Anorexia	

RELATED FACTORS

The cause of failure to thrive in adults (usually older adults) is unknown. Researchers have identified some possible contributing factors, listed next.

Situational (Personal, Environmental)
Related to diminished coping abilities
Related to limited ability to adapt to effects of aging
Related to loss of social skills and resultant social isolation
Related to loss of social relatedness
Related to increasing dependency and feelings of helplessness

---

⊛ ERRORS IN DIAGNOSTIC STATEMENTS

1. *Adult Failure to Thrive related to dementia*
   Dementia does not cause *Adult Failure to Thrive,* but actually represents a response of the condition. Because the cause is uncertain, the nurse may find *Adult Failure to Thrive related to unknown etiology* clinically useful.

KEY CONCEPTS
Generic Considerations
- Optimal development across the life span depends on adaptation to personal and environmental changes (Bergland & Kirkevold, 2001; Newbern & Krowchuk, 1994).
- People predisposed to thrive (Felten, 2000; Haight et al., 2002; Wagnil & Young, 1990):
  - Have pride
  - Help others
  - Have family support
  - Are perseverant
  - Are self-reliant
  - Have experienced hardships
  - Have cultural, spiritual, and religious values
  - Regularly enhance their self-care activities
- Older adults who cannot cope with changes after a stressful life event will feel unprotected, empty, and lonely (Newbern & Krowchuk, 1994).
- "Interaction with the environment is as critical to thriving as a human being at the end of life as at the beginning" (Newbern & Krowchuk, 1994, p. 844).
- Older adults overwhelmed by a sense of helplessness and hopelessness give up.
- Failure to thrive implies that the older adult *should* thrive despite chronic illness and age-related changes. It is not a normal part of aging (Kimball & Williams-Burgess, 1995).
- Resilience is a combination of abilities and characteristics that allow an individual to bounce back and/or cope successfully in spite of significant stress or adverse events (Tusaie & Dyer, 2004).

Focus Assessment Criteria

Assessing and diagnosing *Adult Failure to Thrive* require evaluation for new pathology, or, if a condition is under treatment, a thorough functional assessment (physical, cognitive) and evaluation of the person's strengths and coping patterns (Kimball & Williams-Burgess, 1995). Focus assessment for these areas can be found under other nursing diagnoses in this book, such as:

- Self-Care Ability—refer to *Self-Care Deficit Syndrome*
- Cognition—refer to *Disturbed Thought Processes*
- Coping—refer to *Ineffective Coping*
- Socialization—refer to *Risk for Loneliness*
- Nutrition—refer to *Imbalanced Nutrition*

For more information on Focus Assessment Criteria, visit http://connection.lww.com.

Goal

NOC Physical Aging Status, Psychological Adjustment: Life Change, Will to Live

The person will participate to increase functioning.

Indicators

- Increase social relatedness.
- Maintain or increase present weight.

General Interventions

 NIC Coping Enhancement, Hope Instillment, Spiritual Support, Family Support, Referral

Consult with therapist to evaluate client
    for depression.
Promote socialization (refer to *Risk for Loneliness*).
Attemp to identify one activity that provides enjoyment.
Provide opportunities to increase social relatedness, such as music therapy, recreation therapy, and
    reminiscence therapy.
Maintain standards of empathic, respectful care.
Assist client to adapt to changes.
    Elicit unpleasant experiences and promote discussion of them.
    Encourage reminiscing about strengths and successes.
    Validate that adaptation to these changes is difficult.
Engage in useful and meaningful conversations about likes, dislikes, interests, hobbies, and work
    history.
Speak as one adult to another. Use average volume, appropriate eye contact, and slow rate of speech.
Provide respect and promote sharing.
    Pay attention to what the person is saying.
    Pick out meaningful comments and continue talking.
    Call person by name and introduce yourself each time you make contact; use touch if welcomed.
Encourage client to be as independent as possible.
For specific problems, refer to other nursing diagnoses, such as *Imbalanced Nutrition, Self-Care
    Deficits, Ineffective Coping, Disturbed Thought Processes,* and *Risk for Loneliness.*
Continually evaluate safety issues.
Institute health teaching and referrals, as indicated (eg, consult with home health agency for a home
    assessment).

Rationales

- Interventions that focus on strengths may help restore self-worth and reduce stress (Kimball &
  Williams-Burgess, 1995).
- Acknowledgment of feelings will increase the person's dignity.
- Interventions attempt to reverse feelings of uselessness.
- Loss of independence and reciprocity negatively affects self-esteem (Newbern & Krowchuk, 1994).

Ineffective Health Maintenance
Related to Insufficient Knowledge of Effects of Tobacco Use and Self-Help Resources Available
Related to Increased Food Consumption in Response to Stressors and Insufficient Energy
Expenditure for Intake

INEFFECTIVE HEALTH MAINTENANCE

DEFINITION

Ineffective Health Maintenance: State in which a person or group experiences or is at risk of experiencing a disruption in health because of an unhealthy lifestyle or lack of knowledge to manage a condition

DEFINING CHARACTERISTICS (IN THE ABSENCE OF DISEASE)
Major (Must Be Present, One or More)
Reports or demonstrates an unhealthy practice or lifestyle, such as:

Reckless driving	Excessive sun exposure	Inadequate dental care
High-fat diet	Substance abuse	Inadequate hygiene
Overeating	Sedenterry life style	Inadequate oral hygiene

Minor (May Be Present)
Reports or demonstrates:

Skin and nails

Malodorous	Skin lesions (pustules,
Unexplained scars	rashes, dry or scaly skin)
Sunburn	Unusual color, pallor

Respiratory system

Frequent infections	Dyspnea with exertion	Chronic cough

Oral cavity
Frequent sores (on tongue, buccal mucosa)
Loss of teeth at early age
Lesions associated with lack of oral care or substance abuse (leukoplakia, fistulas)

Gastrointestinal system and nutrition

Obesity	Chronic bowel irregularity	Chronic anemia
Chronic dyspepsia	Anorexia	Cachexia

Musculoskeletal system
Frequent muscle strain, backaches, neck pain
Diminished flexibility and muscle strength

Genitourinary system
Frequent sexually transmitted infections
Frequent use of potentially unhealthful over-the-counter products (eg, chemical douches, perfumed vaginal products, nasal sprays)

Constitutional

Chronic fatigue	Headaches	Apathy

Psychoemotional
Emotional fragility
Frequent feelings of being overwhelmed

RELATED FACTORS

Various factors can produce *Ineffective Health Maintenance*. Common causes are listed next.

Situational (Personal, Environmental)

Related to:

Information misinterpretation

Lack of motivation

Lack of education or readiness

Lack of access to adequate health care services

Inadequate health teaching

Impaired ability to understand secondary to: (specify)

Maturational

Table II.13 lists age-related conditions.

Related to lack of education of age-related risk factors. Examples include the following:

Child

Sexuality and sexual
  development

Inactivity

Substance abuse

Poor nutrition

Safety hazards

Adolescent

Same as children

Substance abuse

Vehicle safety practices

Adult

Parenthood

Safety practices

Sexual function

Older Adult

Effects of aging

Sensory deficits

⊚⊚ AUTHOR'S NOTE

The nursing diagnosis *Ineffective Health Maintenance* applies to both well and ill populations. Health is a dynamic, ever-changing state defined by the individual based on his or her perception of highest level of functioning (eg, a marathon runner's definition of health will differ from a paraplegic person's). Because clients are responsible for their own health, *Ineffective Health Maintenance* represents a diagnosis that the person is motivated to treat. An important associated nursing responsibility involves raising client consciousness that better health is possible.

This diagnosis is appropriate for a person expressing a desire to change an unhealthy lifestyle. Examples are excessive dissatisfaction with occupation; lack of exercise; failure to be refreshed after rest; diet high in fat, salt, simple carbohydrates; tobacco use; obesity; excessive alcohol use; and insufficient social support.

The nursing diagnosis *Risk for Ineffective Health Maintenance* is useful to describe a person who needs teaching or referrals before discharge from an acute care center to prevent problems with health maintenance after discharge or in community settings.

Health-Seeking Behaviors is used to describe a person or group desiring health teaching related to the promotion and maintenance of high-level wellness (eg, preventive behavior, age-related screening, optimal nutrition) or, according to NANDA, "seeking ways to alter personal health habits in order to move to a higher level of health." In most cases, this diagnosis describes an asymptomatic person. It also can be used in cases of chronic disease to help that person attain higher wellness in a particular area. Different from good health, high-level wellness is defined as an integrated method of functioning oriented toward maximizing potential (Dunn, 1959). For example, a woman with multiple sclerosis and many physical problems could learn breast self-examination or relaxation exercises using *Health-Seeking Behaviors: Breast self-examination.*

Health-Seeking Behaviors is best written as a one-part diagnostic statement with the sought-after health practice specified (eg, *Health-Seeking Behaviors: Breast self-examination*). Using "related to" is unnecessary; it is understood that all people with *Health-Seeking Behaviors* are motivated to achieve a higher level of health. Related factors could not represent causative or contributing factors, unless the nurse wants to repeat the same factors for each client (eg, *Health-Seeking Behaviors: Breast self-examination related to desire to maximize health*).

As focus shifts from an illness/treatment-oriented to a health-oriented health care system, *Ineffective Health Maintenance* and *Health-Seeking Behaviors* are becoming increasingly significant. The increasingly high acuity and shortened lengths of stay in hospitals require nurses to be creative in addressing health promotion (eg, by using printed materials, television instruction, and community-based programs).

(text continues on page 366)

TABLE II.13 Primary and Secondary Prevention for Age-Related Conditions

Developmental Level	Primary Prevention	Secondary Prevention

Infancy (0–1 year)	Parent education
	  Infant safety
	  Nutrition
	  Breast feeding
	Sensory stimulation
	  Infant massage and touch
	  Visual stimulation
	    Activity
	    Colors
	  Auditory stimulation
	    Verbal
	    Music
	Immunizations
	  DPT or DTaP
	  IPV, Hib
	  Hepatitis B
	  H. influenzae
	  Pneumococcal
	  Influenza
	Oral hygiene
	  Teething biscuits
	  Fluoride (if needed > 6 months)
	  Avoid sugared food and drink
		Complete physical examination every 2–3 months
		Screening at birth
		  Congenital hip dysplasia
		  PKU
		  G-6-PD deficiency in blacks, Mediterranean, and Far Eastern origin children
		  Sickle cell
		  Hemoglobin or hematocrit (for anemia)
		  Cystic fibrosis
		  Vision (startle reflex)
		  Hearing (response to and localization of sounds)
		  TB test at 12 months
		  Developmental assessments
		Screen and intervene for high risk
		  Low birth weight
		  Maternal substance abuse during pregnancy
		    Alcohol: fetal alcohol syndrome
		    Cigarettes: SIDS
		    Drugs: addicted neonate, AIDS
		  Maternal infections during pregnancy

Preschool (1–5 years)	Parent education
	  Teething
	  Discipline
	  Nutrition
	  Accident prevention
	  Normal growth and development
	Child education
	  Dental self-care
	  Dressing
	  Bathing with assistance
	  Feeding self-care
	Immunizations
	  DTaP
	  IPV
	  MMR
	  HIB
	  H. influenzae
	  Varicella
	  Hepatitis A (high risk)
	  Pneumococcal
	  Hepatitis B
	Dental/oral hygiene
	  Fluoride treatments
	  Fluoridated water
		Complete physical examination between 2 and 3 years and preschool (UA, CBC)
		TB test at 3 years
		Development assessments (annual)
		  Speech development
		  Hearing
		  Vision
		Screen and intervene
		  Lead poisoning
		  Developmental lag
		  Neglect or abuse
		  Strong family history of arteriosclerotic diseases (eg, MI, CVA, peripheral vascular disease), diabetes, hypertension, gout, or hyperlipidemia—fasting serum cholesterol at age 2 years, then every 3–5 years if normal
		  Strabismus
		  Hearing deficit
		  Vision deficit

School age (6–11 years)	Health education of child
	  "Basic 4" nutrition
	  Accident prevention
	  Outdoor safety
	  Substance abuse counsel
	  Anticipatory guidance for physical changes at puberty
	Immunizations
	  Tetanus age 11–12
	  MMR
	  DTaP } boosters between 4 and 6 years
	  TOPV
	  Pneumococcal (high risk)
	Varicella (at age 11–12 if no history of infection)
	Dental hygiene every 6–12 months
	  Continue fluoridation
	Complete physical examination
		Complete physical examination
		TB test every 3 years (at ages 6 and 9)
		Developmental assessments
		  Language
		  Vision: Snellen charts at school
		    6–8 years, use "E" chart
		    Over 8 years, use alphabet chart
		  Hearing: audiogram
		Cholesterol profile, if high risk, every 3–5 years
		Serum cholesterol one time (not high risk)

(table continues on p. 365)

TABLE II.13 Primary and Secondary Prevention for Age-Related Conditions (*Continued*)

Developmental Level	Primary Prevention	Secondary Prevention

Adolescence (12–19 years)	Health education
	  Proper nutrition and healthful diets
	  Sex education
	    Choices
	    Risks
	    Precautions
	  Sexually transmitted diseases
	Safe driving skills
	Adult challenges
	  Seeking employment and career choices
	  Dating and marriage
	  Confrontation with substance abuse
	Safety in athletics, water
	Skin care
	Dental hygiene every 6–12 months
	Immunizations
	  Hepatitis B series if needed
	  tOPV booster at 12–14 years
		Complete physical exam (prepuberty or age 13)
		  Blood pressure
		  Cholesterol profile
		  PPD test at 12 years and yearly if high risk
		  RPR, CBC, U/A
		  Female: breast self-exam (BSE)
		  Male: testicular self-exam (TSE)
		  Female, if sexually active: Pap and pelvic exam yearly (cervical gonorrhea and chlamydia culture and wet mount with pelvic)
		Screening and interventions if high risk
		  Depression
		  Suicide
		  Substance abuse
		  Pregnancy
		Family history of alcoholism or domestic violence
		Sexually Transmitted Infections

Young adult (20–39 years)	Health education
	  Weight management with good nutrition as BMR changes
	  Low-cholesterol diet
	Lifestyle counseling
	  Stress management skills
	  Safe driving
	  Family planning
	  Divorce
	  Sexual practices
	  Parenting skills
	  Regular exercise
	  Environmental health choices
	  Alcohol, drug use
	  Use of hearing protection devices
	Dental hygiene every 6–12 months
	Immunizations
	  Tetanus at 20 years and every 10 years
	  Female: rubella, if serum negative for antibodies
	  Hepatitis B for high-risk people
		Complete physical exam at about 20 years, then every 5–6 years
		Female: BSE monthly, Pap 1-2 years unless high risk
		Male: TSE monthly
		All females: baseline mammography between ages 35 and 40
		Parents-to-be: high-risk screening for Down syndrome, Tay-Sachs
		Female pregnant: RPR, rubella titer, Rh factor, amniocentesis for women 35 years or older (if desired)
		Screening and interventions if high risk
		  Female with previous breast cancer: annual mammography at 35 years and after
		  Female with mother or sister who has had breast cancer, same as above
		  Family history colorectal cancer or high risk: annual stool guaiac, digital rectal, and sigmoidoscopy
		  PPD if high risk
		  Glaucoma screening at 35 years and along with routine physical exams
		  Cholesterol profile every 5 years, if normal
		  Cholesterol profile every 1–2 years if borderline

Middle-aged adult (40–59 years)	Health education: continue with young adult
	Midlife changes, male and female counseling (see also Young adult)
	  "Empty nest syndrome"
	  Anticipatory guidance for retirement
	  Grandparenting
	Dental hygiene every 6–12 months
	Immunizations
	  Tetanus every 10 years
	  Influenza—annual if high risk (ie, major chronic disease [COPD, CAD])
	  Pneumococcal—every 5–6 years
		Complete physical exam every 5–6 years with complete laboratory evaluation (serum/urine tests, x-ray, ECG)
		Dexascan (screening for osteoporosis) once then as needed
		Female: BSE monthly
		Male: TSE monthly
		PSA yearly after age 40 for Blacks and Hispanics and after age 50 for others
		All females: mammogram every 1–2 years (40–49 years) then annual mammography 50 years and over
		Schiotz's tonometry (glaucoma) every 3–5 years
		Colonoscopy at 50 and 51, then every 4 years if negative
		Stool guaiac annually at 50 and yearly after

(*table continues on p. 366*)

TABLE II.13 Primary and Secondary Prevention for Age-Related Conditions (*Continued*)

Developmental Level	Primary Prevention	Secondary Prevention

Older adult (60–74 years)	Health education: continue with previous counseling
	  Home safety
	  Retirement
	  Loss of spouse, relatives, friends
	  Special health needs
	    Nutritional changes
	    Changes in hearing or vision
	  Dental/oral hygiene every 6–12 months
	Immunizations
	  Tetanus every 10 years
	  Influenza—annual if high risk
	  Pneumococcal—every 5–6 years
		Complete physical exam every 2 years with laboratory assessments
		Blood pressure annually
		Female: BSE monthly, Pap every 1–3 years annual mammogram
		Male: TSE monthly, PSA yearly
		Annual stool guaiac
		Colonoscopy every 4 years
		Complete eye exam yearly
		Dexascan once and as needed
		Screen for high risk
		  Depression
		  Suicide
		  Alcohol/drug abuse
		  "Elder abuse"

Old-age adult (75 years and over)	Health education: continue counseling
	Anticipatory guidance
	  Dying and death
	  Loss of spouse, relatives, friends
	  Increasing dependency on others
	Dental/oral hygiene every 6–12 months
	Immunizations
	  Tetanus every 10 years
	  Influenza—annual
	  Pneumococcal—if not already received
		Complete physical exam annually
		Female: annual mammogram, sigmoidoscopy every 4 years
		Schiotz's tonometry every 3–5 years
		Podiatrist PRN

ERRORS IN DIAGNOSTIC STATEMENTS

1. *Ineffective Health Maintenance related to refusal to quit smoking*

Refusal to quit smoking represents significant data that require further clarification. Is the person making an informed decision? Does the person know the effects of smoking on respiratory and cardiovascular functioning? Does the person know where to acquire assistance to stop smoking? If the answers are "yes," then *Ineffective Health Maintenance* is incorrect. On the other hand, if the person is not fully aware of the deleterious effects of smoking or the availability of self-help resources, *Ineffective Health Maintenance related to insufficient knowledge of effects of tobacco use and self-help resources available* may be appropriate.

Note: The nurse should be cautioned about timing attempts to encourage a person to quit smoking or control eating after an acute episode, such as myocardial infarction. In such a situation, denying the person his or her usual coping mechanism, no matter how unhealthy, may be more problematic to overall health. The nurse should emphasize teaching so the person can make informed choices, not merely prohibit certain choices.

2. *Health-Seeking Behaviors related to increased alcohol and tobacco use in response to marital break-up and heavy family demands*

This diagnosis is inappropriate for this person, who wants to alter personal habits but is not in good or excellent health. A more appropriate focus would be to promote constructive stress management without tobacco or alcohol through the nursing diagnosis *Ineffective Coping related to inability to constructively manage the stressors associated with marital break-up and family demands.*

KEY CONCEPTS
Generic Considerations

- Many people view health as the absence of disease. Rather, health can be viewed as a return (or recovery) to a previous state or to a heightened awareness of full potential and life meaning.
- Control of major health problems in the United States depends directly on modification of individual behavior and habits of living.

- In addition to addressing lifestyles to promote wellness, total health depends on (Edelman & Mandle, 2001):
  - Eradication of poverty and ignorance
  - Availability of jobs
  - Adequate housing, transportation, and recreation
  - Public safety
  - Aesthetically pleasing and beneficial environment
- The goals of prevention are as follows:
  - Avoidance of disease through healthy lifestyles
  - Decreased mortality from disease through early detection and intervention
  - Improved quality of life
- The three levels of prevention are primary, secondary, and tertiary.
- *Primary prevention* involves actions that prevent disease and accidents and promote well-being. Key concepts are as follows:

Concept	Examples
Wellness	Diet low in salt, sugar, and fat
A lifestyle that incorporates the principles of health promotion and is directed by self-responsibility	Regular exercise and stress management; elimination of smoking; minimal alcohol intake
Self-help	
Mutual sharing with others who have similar needs	LaLeche League; childbirth education; assertiveness training; specific written resources (books, pamphlets, magazines); public media
Safety	Adherence to speed limits; use of seat belts and car seats; proper storage of household poisons
Immunizations	*Children:* varicella *Nonpregnant women of childbearing age:* rubella if antibody titer is negative *Elderly:* influenza, pneumonia

- *Secondary prevention* concerns actions that promote early detection of disease and subsequent intervention: regular examination by a health professional and self-examination.
  - Tasks of screening are to
    - Identify major disabling conditions.
    - Investigate personal and social benefits of early detection and intervention for asymptomatic people with the condition (eg, facilitate family coping, minimize disability and cost, prevent premature death, improve productivity, decrease overall morbidity and mortality).
    - Identify those at high risk for specific conditions through *personal health history* (eg, concurrent disease such as diabetes mellitus means higher risk for hypertension), *family health history* (eg, breast cancer, diabetes, hypertension), and *social history* (eg, substance abuse—cancer, heart disease; sexual patterns—venereal disease; domestic violence—person abuse).
    - Identify tests and procedures that accurately detect the condition (Who will do them? How often are they done? Who bears the cost?).
    - Plan a strategy for disseminating screening information to health care professionals and the public.
    - Plan evaluation of screening effectiveness.
  - Types of screening include the following:
    - Physical findings (periodic examinations by health care professionals and self-examinations of breasts, testicles, and skin)
    - Survey of risk factors (smoking, alcohol abuse)
    - Laboratory tests (serum—eg, sickle cell in African-Americans, phenylketonuria in newborns; urine—eg, renal disease in older adults; x-ray—eg, dental caries, chest tuberculosis)
- *Tertiary prevention* involves actions that restore and rehabilitate and prevent complications in cases of illness. Examples for a person with coronary artery disease would be:
  - Restorative (surgery, such as coronary artery bypass, angioplasty, and medications)
  - Rehabilitative (stress management, exercise program, stop smoking)

- Potential barriers to prevention are found both in the health care system and in clients. The system may be
  - Disease oriented rather than health oriented
  - Composed of health care professionals who have learned to focus on fragmented systems of the human body rather than on a holistic approach
  - Functioning in a financial system that rewards treatment, not prevention, of illness
  - Difficult to reach or previously shown to be unsatisfactory
  - Clients may:
    - Believe that outside forces (fate, luck) determine health/illness (external locus of control)
    - Perceive the needed behavior as unacceptable or uncomfortable
    - Practice unhealthy sociocultural behaviors (eg, obesity considered desirable, salt prevalent in diet)
    - Experience psychological impediments to practicing healthy behaviors
    - Lack financial resources

Nutrition
See Key Concepts for *Imbalanced Nutrition.*

Exercise
- Regular exercise can increase

Cardiovascular–respiratory endurance	Delivery of nutrients to tissue
Muscle strength	Tolerance for psychological stress
Muscle endurance	Ability to reduce body fat content
Flexibility	

- Vigorous exercise sessions should include a warm-up phase (10 min at a slow pace), endurance exercises, and a cool-down phase (5 to 10 min of a slow pace and stretching).
- Current beliefs regarding optimal exercise are as follows:
  - Emphasize physical activity over "exercise."
  - Moderate physical activity is very beneficial.
  - Intermittent physical activity that accumulates to 30 or more minutes is beneficial.
- To enhance long-term exercise, the person should (Moore & Charvat, 2002):
  - Respond to relapses with a plan to prevent recurrences.
  - Set realistic goals.
  - Keep an exercise log.
  - Exercise with a friend.

Weight Reduction
- Overeating is a complex problem with physical, social, and psychological components.
- Eighty percent of children of two obese parents will become obese, as opposed to 40% with one obese parent and 7% with no obese parent (Buiten & Metzger, 2000).
- Body mass index (BMI) is a ratio of weight and height that estimates total body fat (Dudek, 2001). According to the third National Health and Nutrition Examination Survey (NHANES III), 54.9 million Americans 20 years and older are overweight (BMI 25 to 29.9) or obese (BMI >30; Dudek, 2001).
- An excess of 50 to 100 calories each day will cause a 5- to 10-lb gain in 1 year (Dudek, 2001).
- Excess weight contributes to hypertension, type 2 diabetes, heart disease, sleep apnea, osteoarthritis, gallstones, stress incontinence, and high LDL and low HDL levels (Dudek, 2001).
- To maintain ideal body weight, food consumed must equal physical activity daily (Roberts, 2000). Dieting without exercise decreases resting metabolic rate. Exercise, even without dieting, produces the best long-term effects (Roberts, 2000).
- Fluctuations in body weight are common, especially in women. Daily weights can be misleading and disheartening. Body measurements are a better gauge of losses.
- Regular exercise causes lean muscle mass to increase. Because muscle weighs more than fat, the scale may reflect a weight gain.
- Restrictive diets usually do not last and fail to establish healthy eating patterns. A better approach is modifying existing eating habits (Wierenga & Oldham, 2002).
- Weight loss of even 5% to 10% can lower blood pressure and improve glucose lipid profiles (Dennis, 2004).
- Dieting has and an end.
- Successful weight loss requires chaging once eating patterns for lifetime (Dennis, 2004).

Smoking

- Cigarette smoke causes more than 4000 chemicals to be absorbed in the blood and swallowed into the gastrointestinal (GI) tract to act directly in the oral cavity and respiratory system (Andrews, 1998).
- Smokers have a chronic cough, increased sputum production, dyspnea, and decreased lung capacity (Andrews, 1998).
- Tobacco use is the leading cause of preventable deaths n women (CDC, 2004).
- In the US, 25% of men and 21% of women smoke. In America Indian / Alaska Natives, the rate for women smokers is 42.5% (CDC, 2004).
- Smoking diring pregnancy is thought to be linked to 10% of all infant deaths in the US (CDC, 2004).
- Women who smoke have fertility problems and impaired uteroplacental function when pregnant. Tobacco use during pregnancy can adversely affect a child's physical growth and intellectual development. Women who smoke are at risk for early menopause, decreased bone density, and osteoporosis (Andrews, 1998).
- Smoking has immediate and long-term effects on the cardiovascular system. *Immediate effects* are vasoconstriction and decreased oxygenation of the blood, elevated blood pressure, increased heart rate and possible dysrhythmias, and increased work of the heart. *Long-term effects* are an increased risk for coronary artery disease, stroke, hyperlipidemia, and myocardial infarction. Smoking also contributes to hypertension, peripheral vascular disease (eg, leg ulcers), and chronically abnormal arterial blood gases (low oxygen, or Po_2, and high carbon dioxide, or Pco_2).
- Use of smokeless tobacco (snuff, chewing tobacco) is associated with oral leukoplakia (premalignant lesions), oral cancer, and nicotine addiction. At least 12 million Americans are at risk, mostly male teens and male adults.
- Tobacco use is a significant risk factor for cancers of the tongue and oral mucosa, larynx, lungs, bladder, and cervix. Combined with other carcinogens (eg, alcohol, asbestos, coal dust, radon), the health risk intensifies. The rate of cancer recurrence increases in clients who continue tobacco use during and after treatment.
- Nicotine is the primary addicting substance in tobacco smoke and juice. Clients with tobacco addiction need special assistance with short-term withdrawal and long-term maintenance of a tobacco-free life.
- *Passive smoking,* the inhalation of tobacco smoke by nonsmokers, has been shown to have negative health effects (Andrews, 1998; Pletsch, 2002):
  - People with angina experience more discomfort in a smoke-filled room.
  - Bronchospasm increases when a person with asthma is exposed to tobacco smoke.
  - Children living with smoking parents have more upper respiratory and ear infections than those living with nonsmokers.
  - Passive smoking causes lung cancer in nonsmokers.
  - Sudden infant death syndrome is two to four times more common in infants whose mothers smoked during pregnancy.
- In the last 25 years, most health professions have seen a significant decline in the smoking behavior of its members—*but not nursing.* Estimates show that 25% to 29% of nurses still smoke. Studies of nurses link occupational stress and social influences with tobacco use (Cinelli & Glover, 1988). A nurse who smokes sends the wrong signals to clients. According to Ash (1987), "a role model does not smoke, thus exemplifying behavior which is desired, and behaves in a way that provides guidance and that others will want to imitate."

Osteoporosis

- Age-related changes beginning around age 40 years decrease cortical bone by 3% per decade in men and women (Woodhead & Moss, 1998).
- Of all hip and vertebral fractures, 30% of hip fractures and 20% of vertebral fractures occur in men with osteoporosis (Eastell et al., 1998).
- Loss of trabecular bone begins in the fourth decade and progresses at 6% to 8% per decade. This rate accelerates in women after menopause (Woodhead & Moss, 1998).
- Osteoporosis is classified as primary (associated with age- and menopause-related changes) or secondary (caused by medications or diseases; Miller, 2004).
- Contributing factors to osteoporosis include loss of female hormones after menopause; hypogonadism; low calcium or vitamin D intake; insufficient exercise; small stature; fair skin; family history; cigarette smoking; excessive consumption of alcohol, caffeine, or protein; excessive use of aluminum-type antacids; long-term use of corticosteroids; therapy for chronic illness (bowel, kidney, liver); excessive thyroid replacement; excessive thyroid function (Woodhead & Moss, 1998).

Pediatric Considerations

- Anticipatory health promotion, or *anticipatory guidance,* is essential to comprehensive health care. It varies in content with a child's age and involves teaching families what is likely in upcoming weeks or months.
- Health maintenance begins with the prenatal visit and continues with comprehensive health supervision during the child's development (Wong, 2003).
- The child depends on a parent/adult caregiver to provide a safe environment and promote health (eg, immunizations, well check-ups, chronic disease management; Wong, 2003).
- Risk of ineffective health maintenance varies with a child's age and health status. For example, the toddler is at risk for accidental poisoning, whereas the adolescent is more likely to engage in high-risk behavior (Wong, 2003).
- Malnutrition, lack of immunizations, or an unsafe environment may be related to deficient parental knowledge, impaired parenting, or barriers to health care (Wong, 2003).
- Many factors can influence a child's nutritional needs, including periods of rapid growth, stress, illness, metabolic errors, medications, and socioeconomic factors (eg, inadequate income, poor housing, lack of food).
- By conservative estimates, more than one million youths run away from home each year. Alienated youth are frequently outside the health care system and tend to remain there unless efforts are made to identify and develop acceptable health services for them. The adoption of destructive lifestyles by many of these youths contributes heavily to physical and psychological morbidity and to alarmingly high mortality.
- Obesity rates are higher in Hispanic (56%) and African-American children (41%) than in white children (28%; Keller & Stevens, 1996).
- Good weight management for children and adolescents focuses on weight maintenance or slow loss, nutrient and energy needs, hunger prevention, preservation of lean body mass, and increased physical activity and growth.
- Obesity in children has increased astronomically. Contributing factors include decreased physical activity, increased television viewing and caloric intake, and parental obesity (Roberts, 2000).
- In a study of children who were clearly obese (> 90th percentile for weight and height), Myers and Vargas (2000) found that 35% of Hispanic parents did not perceive their child as obese. Eighteen percent of staff at the health center did not perceive the children as obese.
- About 3000 people younger than 18 years start smoking each day. About 75% of adolescents who smoke want to quit (DuRant & Smith, 1999).
- Approximately 80% of tobacco users start before 18 years of age (CDC, 2000).
- More than 33% of high school students (more than 3 million) smoke cigarettes; almost 10% (more than 1 million) use smokeless tobacco (DuRant & Smith, 1999).

Maternal Considerations

- Tobacco use in pregnancy is associated with intrauterine growth retardation, small size for gestational age, low birth weight, placental complications, premature rupture of membranes, prenatal mortality, spontaneous abortion, ectopic pregnancy, placental abruption, and sudden infant death syndrome (Mitchell et al., 1999).
- At least 14% (probably more) of pregnant women smoke (Mullen, 1999).

Geriatric Considerations

- According to Miller (2004), health is the ability of older adults to function at their highest capacity, despite age-related changes and risk factors. Of all age-related changes, osteoporosis is most likely to have serious negative functional consequences, even without additional risk factors.
- About 70% of people older than 65 years rate their health as excellent (Miller, 2004).
- Differentiating between age-related changes and risk factors that affect the functioning of older people is important. Such risk factors as inadequate nutrition, fluid intake, exercise,

(continued)

◉ Geriatric Considerations (continued)

and socialization can have more influence on functioning than can most age-related changes.

- The mortality rate from pneumonia and influenza for people older than 65 years is 9/100,000. For people who smoke or have kyphosis or chronic disease, the rate increases to 979/100,000. Older adults should be immunized yearly in the late fall against influenza (Miller, 2004).
- Oxygen consumption at anaerobic threshold varies inversely with age. Therefore, older adults have a lower anaerobic threshold, with earlier rise in accumulation of lactic acid and onset of muscle fatigue.
- Maximal aerobic capacity and maximal heart rate decline with age. For aerobic conditioning, an older person must exercise to reach target heart rate for at least 20 to 30 min three times a week. The following formula will obtain target heart rate: 220 – Person's Age × 60% to 70% = Target Training Heart Rate. Older adults must learn to monitor carotid pulse for rate and rhythm. Time threshold to return to baseline heart rate, blood pressure, and respiratory rate after exercise is greater for older people (Allison & Keller, 1997).
- Older adults have decreased thermoregulation and diminished ability to cool the body through perspiration, affecting tolerance of physical activity (Allison & Keller, 1997).
- There is an age-related increase in systolic blood pressure at rest and at submaximal workloads. Sensitivity of the cardiovascular system to the chronotropic, inotropic, and vasodilatory effects of catecholamines diminishes. Studies have shown that catecholamines or β-adrenergic stimulation, when administered during exercise, had greater effects on young people as opposed to those of advanced age (Miller, 2004).
- Regular exercise has been shown to correlate positively with increased self-esteem. Adult learning principles support encouraging exercise or regular activity that has meaning to the older person if compliance is expected. When exercising, the older adult should exercise to the point of mild intolerance and then cut back by 25% (Allison & Keller, 1997).

◉ Transcultural Considerations

- Health and illness are culturally prescribed. One culture may view an obese person as strong and healthy, whereas another culture views that same person as weak and unhealthy. Nurses must remember that treatment strategies consistent with a person's cultural beliefs may have a better chance of success (Andrews & Boyle, 2003).
- A future orientation to illness, disease, and health care is necessary for prevention. The dominant US culture is oriented to the future, whereas other cultures have a present-oriented perception (eg, African American, Hispanic, Southern Appalachian, traditional Chinese). Some members of these cultures, however, are future oriented.
- Some cultures believe that fate depends on God or other supernatural forces. Humans are at the mercy of these forces despite their behavior (Andrews & Boyle, 2003).
- Some Asian cultures believe in balance and harmony for health. They emphasize moderation and avoid excesses. In the *yin/yang theory,* the yin force in the universe represents female aspects of nature: cold and darkness. The yang force represents male aspects of nature: fullness, light, and warmth. An imbalance of yin and yang creates illness.
- In Hispanic and black cultures, health is maintained by the *hot/cold humoral theory.* This ancient Greek concept describes four body humors: yellow bile, black bile, phlegm, and blood. When these humors are balanced, health is present. Treatment of illness consists of restoring humoral balance by adding or deleting substances (eg, foods, beverages, herbs, drugs) that are either hot or cold. For example, an earache is classified as cold and thus needs hot substances for treatment (Andrews & Boyle, 2003).
- Because the family is usually the client's most important social unit, the nurse can promote their help to support lifestyle changes (Andrews & Boyle, 2003).
- Blacks, Hispanics, and Asians in the United States smoke more than whites and have higher death rates from cancer. More emphasis on creating culturally based cessation programs and materials is needed (Koepke, Flay & Johnson, 1990).
- Among Puerto Rican women, weight gain after marriage is considered positive, signifying that the husband is a good provider and that the wife is a good cook (Keller et al., 1996).

Focus Assessment Criteria

Subjective Data
Assess for Defining Characteristics.

Health status
Client's description of health
Immediate health concerns
Frequency of

Bowel irregularity	Respiratory infections	Influenza
Urinary tract infections	Headaches	Fatigue
Mouth lesions	Skin rashes	Feeling overwhelmed

Assess for Related Factors.

Influencing factors: health management and adherence behavior
What factors make it difficult to follow health advice?
What daily health management activities are practiced?
How much control does the person believe he or she has?

Risk factors
Family incidence of

Cardiovascular disease	Abuse or violence	Hypertension
Drug or alcohol abuse	Cancer	Genetic disorders
Diabetes mellitus	Depression	Other (specify)

Health habits
Smoking (how much)
Alcohol
Drug use (prescribed, over-the-counter)
Dietary consumption of fat/salt/sugar, carbohydrates, protein; frequency and amount of portions
Exercise program

Environmental risk factors
Do you use seat belts or child restraints?
Is home child-proofed? (If appropriate, determine measures taken.)
Could any factors in the home or at work cause falls or accidents?
Could any other factors potentially threaten your health or cause injury?

Preventive health screening activities
Self-examinations (breasts, testicles, blood pressure): indicate frequency and perceived problems
Last professional examination (dental, pelvic, rectal, vision, hearing, complete physical)
Last laboratory or other diagnostic testing (electrocardiogram, complete blood count, cholesterol, occult blood, Pap, chest x-ray, prostate-specific antigen [PSA])

Objective Data
Assess for Defining Characteristics.

General appearance	Weight	Height

For more information on Focus Assessment Criteria, visit http://connection.lww.com.

Goal

The person or caregiver will verbalize intent to engage in health maintenance behaviors.	**NOC** Health Promoting Behavior, Health Seeking Behaviors, Knowledge: Health Promotion, Knowledge: Health Resources, Participation: Health Care Decisions, Risk Detection, Treatment Behavior

Indicators
Identify barriers to health maintenance.

General Interventions

	NIC Health Education, Self-Responsibility Facilitation, Health Screening, Risk Identification, Family Involvement Promotion

Assess for Barriers to Health Maintenance.

Lack of knowledge	Lack of access or finances
Low priority	Family lifestyle patterns

Explain Primary and Secondary Prevention Measures for Age (see Table II.13).

Identify Strategies to Improve Access (eg, Community Centers, School-Based Clinics).

Assist Client or Family to Identify Health Behaviors Compatible With Their Lifestyle.

Rationales

- "Many of the most serious disorders can be prevented or postponed by immunizations, chemoprophylaxis and healthy lifestyles or detected early with screening and treated effectively" (USDHHS, 1994, p. xvii).
- Low-income families usually focus on meeting basic needs (food, shelter, and safety) and seeking help with curing illness, not preventing it (Hanson & Boyd, 1996).
- Lifestyle patterns are passed from one generation to the next. When one relative initiates a change (eg, diet, smoking cessation), it affects others (Hanson & Boyd, 1996).
- Providing information and resources can help foster a sense that change is possible.

INEFFECTIVE HEALTH MAINTENANCE

RELATED TO INSUFFICIENT KNOWLEDGE OF EFFECTS OF TOBACCO USE AND SELF-HELP RESOURCES AVAILABLE*

Goal

> NOC See *Ineffective Health Maintenance*

The person will decrease or eliminate tobacco use.

Indicators

- Identify short-term and long-term health effects of tobacco use.
- Identify benefits of abstinence from tobacco use.
- Verbalize commitment to personal health and desire to eliminate tobacco use.[†]
- Devise strategies to assist in smoking/chewing cessation.[†]

Interventions

> NIC See *Ineffective Health Maintenance*

Define Tobacco Use Behavior.

Type and Quantity
Cigarettes
Filter/nonfilter
Regular/reduced tar and nicotine
Pack-years

---

*This nursing diagnosis can be used in two different situations—for the person who does not know the hazards of tobacco use and for the person who desires to quit.
†These outcome criteria are established only *if* the client desires to quit tobacco use. For the client who does not wish to change tobacco use behaviors, provide information regarding health risks and benefits so he or she makes an *informed* choice. Avoid being judgmental. Always "keep the door open" should the client later change his or her mind.

Cigars
Inhaled/not inhaled
Number/day, number of years
Pipe
Inhaled/not inhaled
Number of bowls/day
Smokeless tobacco (chewing)
Number of minutes/day
Number of years

Associated Activities, Motivation, Previous Quitting Attempts (Leon, 1999)
- When do you smoke first cigarette of the day?
- What triggers you to want a cigarette?
- What happens if you can't smoke for a few hours?
- When you are sick, do you still smoke?
- When did you last try to stop smoking, and what motivated you?
- Have you had any successes, and for how long?
- What were your three toughest obstacles to quitting, and what could we do about them?
- What made you start again?
- What is your present motivation for quitting?
- What method(s) do you think would be best for you to try now?
- Who or what has helped you when you tried to stop in the past?

Take Opportunities to Discuss:
Risks of smoking
Relevance of smoking to present symptoms or illness
Rewards of cessation

Promote Understanding of Personal Tobacco Use Behavior.
Identify Negative Aspects of Tobacco Use with Client.
Physical: exercise intolerance, cough, sputum, frequent respiratory infections, dental disease, increased risk of diseases, premature facial wrinkling, bad breath
Environmental: burned clothing/furniture, discolored interiors of home/workplace, malodorous clothing/furniture, dirty ashtrays, house and occupational fires
Social: inability to smoke in public places; offensive nature of tobacco use behaviors to family members, friends, coworkers
Financial: calculate monetary cost of client's habit with client
Psychological: unpleasant withdrawal symptoms when tobacco is not available (eg, midnight "nicotine fits"), decreased self-esteem from dependency

Identify Positive Aspects of Tobacco Use with Client (Use Client's Own Words).

Have Person List all Reasons Why He or She Wants to Quit.

Provide Information.
Address Health Risks of Tobacco Use to Self.
Cancer (oral, lung, bladder)
Chronic obstructive pulmonary disease (COPD) and respiratory infections
Arteriosclerosis (coronary and peripheral)
Hypertension and cerebrovascular accident
Periodontal disease

Address Health Risks of Tobacco Use to Others (Refer to Key Concepts).

Unborn child	People with angina	Infants
People with allergies	Asthmatics	People sharing space

Discuss the Benefits of Quitting.

Decreased pulse and blood pressure	Improved taste/smell	Lower risk of cancer, stroke, COPD, myocardial infarction
Pulmonary mucosa regenerates	Decreased sputum production	Increased social acceptance
	Improved dental hygiene	Fewer respiratory infections
	Improved circulation	

Explore Strategies Available.
Individual methods: self-help books and tapes, "cold turkey"
Group methods: contact local chapters of American Cancer Society, American Lung Association, and state-funded hotlines
Hypnosis
Acupuncture
Over-the-counter products: filters, tablet regimens, nontobacco cigarettes, nicotine-containing chewing gum
Transdermal nicotine patch: stress the hazards of smoking with patch

Discuss Strategies to Minimize Weight Gain and to Increase Exercise.

Discuss Symptoms of Nicotine Withdrawal; Assist Client to Prepare for Them (McAndrew, 1998).

Craving for tobacco	Irritability	Anxiety
Difficulty concentrating	Restlessness	Headache
Drowsiness	GI upsets: diarrhea, cramps	

If client has experienced these symptoms before, suggest he or she choose a time to quit of relatively low stress.

Advise Client on Strategies to Help with Quitting.

Prepare to Stop.
List all reasons for wanting to quit.
Choose a quit date within next 1 to 2 weeks.
Enlist someone for support.
Reduce caffeine intake.
Throw away all tobacco, lighters, and ashtrays.
Clean car, clothes, and house of smell of smoke.
Have teeth cleaned.
Avoid tempting situations (eg, alcohol use).

Avoid Urges to Smoke.
Spend more time with nonsmokers.
Engage in activities that cannot include smoking (eg, exercising).
Keep low-calorie oral substitutes handy (eg, gum, fruit).
Use a relaxation technique such as deep breathing.

Engage in the Following if Relapse Occurs.
Stop smoking immediately.
Get rid of cigarettes.
Realize that relapse is common before successful quitting.
Learn from mistakes.
Set a new date.

Rationales

- Benefits of cessation extend to people of all ages. Quitting enhances life expectancy and quality, even in people older than 60 years. It is never too late to quit (Andrews, 1998).
- To assist a person to initiate a health behavior change, the nurse provides interventions to increase perceptions of the seriousness of the behavior and susceptibility to disease if behavior continues (Andrews, 1998).
- Information on the benefits of smoking cessation can be motivational (Andrews, 1998).
- Information that increases confidence in success may precipitate a decision to cease smoking (Andrews, 1998).

❖ Pediatric Interventions

Assess If Adolescent Knows Someone Who Smokes (Peers, Relatives).
Use an open-ended, nonjudgmental approach (eg, "What do you think about smoking?").

Relate Short-Term Rather Than Long-Term Consequences of Smoking (eg, Early Wrinkling of Skin, Yellow Stains on Teeth and Fingers, Tobacco Odor on Breath and Clothing, Gum Disease, Tooth Staining).

Emphasize Ostracization of Smokers (eg, Standing Outside Buildings in the Cold to Smoke).

Discuss Hazards of Smokeless Tobacco (Cancer of Mouth and Tongue, Tooth Erosion and Loss, Foul Breath, Gum Disease, Tooth Staining).

Assist Adolescent Not to Start Smoking (DuRant & Smith, 1999).
Counteract advertising images.
Practice assertive behavior.
Discuss smoking myths.
Address health consequences of tobacco use.

Rationales

- Helping teens to appreciate that most smokers would like to quit may deter them from starting (Wong, 2003).
- Programs that focus on negative long-term effects of smoking are not effective with teenagers.
- Teenagers are very preoccupied with appearance and peer acceptance (Wong, 2003).
- The incidence of use of smokeless tobacco has increased in school-aged children, many of whom see it as less of a health hazard than smoking cigarettes (Mitchell et al., 1999).

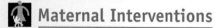 ## Maternal Interventions

Explain the Adverse Effects of Smoking (Mitchell et al., 1999).

During Pregnancy
- Crosses the placenta
- Reduces oxygen to the fetus
- Reduces transport of nutrients, calcium, glucose, hormones
- Causes low birth weight
- Causes stillbirths, congenital deformities

In Infants and Children
- Contributes to allergies, otitis media, bronchitis, asthma, and sudden infant death syndrome

If Desired, Establish a Plan to Decrease Number of Cigarettes Smoked per Day and, if Possible, Set a Date for Total Cessation.

Approach Relapses as Temporary Setbacks.

Identify Situations That Lead to Smoking.

Rationales

Adverse effects are proportional to daily cigarettes smoked; thus, any decrease is beneficial.

INEFFECTIVE HEALTH MAINTENANCE

RELATED TO INCREASED FOOD CONSUMPTION IN RESPONSE TO STRESSORS AND INSUFFICIENT ENERGY EXPENDITURE FOR INTAKE

Goal

NOC Refer to *Ineffective Health Maintenance*

The person will commit to a weight-loss program.

Indicators

- Identify patterns of eating associated with consumption/energy expenditure imbalance.
- Identify stressors and effective response patterns.
- Describe the relationship among metabolism, intake, and exercise.
- Commit to exercise program (specify type, amount).
- Commit to reduced caloric intake program (adults only).
- Commit to eating a balanced diet.

Interventions

NIC Refer also to *Ineffective Health Maintenance*, Weight Reduction Assistance, Counseling, Mutual Goal Setting, Referral, Support Group

Assess for Causative and Contributing Factors.

Lack of knowledge about
    Balanced nutritional intake
    Exercise requirements
Inappropriate response to external stressors
Lack of initiative, motivation
Imbalanced composition of foods (eg, excess fat or simple carbohydrate intake)
Cultural, familial, genetic factors
Poor eating habits (eg, eating out, eating on the run, skipping meals)
Sedentary lifestyle or occupation
Recent smoking cessation
Sabotage by family or significant others
Too much intake for energy expended

Increase Awareness of Components of Intake/Activity Balance.

Multiply female weight by 11 and male weight by 12 to determine calorie intake/day needed to maintain current weight. One pound of fat is roughly equivalent to 3500 cal. To lose 2 lb/week, a person must cut 7000 cal from weekly intake or increase exercise caloric expenditure.
Use exercise caloric expenditure charts to determine amount of calories burned per duration of activity.
Teach client that he or she may achieve weight-loss goals by combining reduction of caloric intake with energy expenditure (exercise).
Remind client that successful weight reduction/maintenance depends on a balance of reduced caloric intake and caloric expenditure through exercise.

Assist Client to Identify Realistic Weight-Loss Program.

Decide on amount of loss desired.
Establish time and duration of program.
Explore costs of various programs.
Evaluate nutritional soundness of program.
Discuss compatibility of program with client's lifestyle.

Assist Client to Anticipate Environmental Considerations.

What are the habits of friends, family, and coworkers? Will they be supportive?
What types of foods are found in the home, at parties, at work, and in the cafeteria?
In what types of leisure/recreational activities does the client engage? Is he or she sedentary?
What routes does the client take to work? Does he or she pass by fast-food establishments?
Who does the housework, gardening, yard work, and errands?
How much television does the client watch? Do commercials trigger eating?
Has the client responded to gimmick advertisements for rapid weight loss (eg, "sleep away," belts, garments, wraps, lotions)?

Advise Client to Keep a Food Intake and Exercise Diary for 1 week.

Food intake/exercise	Location/time of meals	Emotions around meal time
People with whom client eats	Skipped meals	Snacks

Familiarize Client with Cues that Often Trigger Eating.

Another activity (eg, watching TV)	Everyone else eating	Boredom or stress
	Standing up	

Teach Basics of Balanced Nutritional Intake.

Choose a plan that encourages high intake of complex carbohydrates and limited intake of fat.
Know what you are eating. The "basic four" label is misleading (eg, a chicken-fried steak is a protein converted to high fat content through its preparation [frying]).
Obtain more calories from fruits and vegetables than from meat and dairy products. Also, eat more chicken and fish, which contain less fat and fewer total calories than beef, removing the fat and skin.
Avoid salad dressings with mayonnaise (216 to 308 calories per 2-oz serving).
Avoid fast food (they have high fat and total caloric content).
Dine in or make special requests in restaurants for food selection/preparation (eg, salad dressing on side, no sauce on entree).
Plan meals in advance. If attending a party or restaurant, decide what to eat ahead of time and stick to it.
Adhere to grocery list.
Involve family in meal planning for better nutrition.
Buy the highest-quality beef (ground round = 10% fat; hamburger = 25% fat).
Choose a variety of foods.
Avoid serving family-style.
Drink eight to ten 8-oz glasses of water daily. Avoid sugary drinks (eg; juice, soda fruit drinks)
Measure foods and count calories; keep records.
Read labels on foods, noting amount and calories per serving.
Eat slowly.
Experiment with spices, substitutes, and low-calorie recipes.
Do not skip meals

Discuss Benefits of Exercise.

Reduces caloric absorption	Suppresses appetite	Improves self-esteem
Preserves lean muscle mass	Increases oxygen uptake	Increases restful sleep
Reduces depression, anxiety, stress	Increases caloric expenditure	Increases resistance to age-related degeneration
Improves body posture	Maintains weight loss	
Provides fun, recreation, diversion	Increases metabolic rate	

Assist Client to Identify Realistic Exercise Program.

Personality	Lifestyle	Time factor
Time of day	Season	Occupation
Safety	Costs	Age
Physical size	Physical condition	

Discuss Aspects of Starting the Exercise Program.

Start slow and easy. Obtain clearance from physician.
Choose an activity that uses many body parts and is vigorous enough to cause "healthful fatigue."
Read, consult experts, and talk with friends/coworkers who exercise.

Plan a daily walking program.

    Start at 5 to 10 blocks for 0.5 to 1 mile/day; increase 1 block or 0.1 mile/week.

    Gradually increase rate and length of walk; remember to progress slowly.

    Avoid straining or pushing too hard and becoming overly fatigued.

    Stop immediately if any of the following occur:

Lightness or pain in chest	Dizziness
Severe breathlessness	Loss of muscle control
Lightheadedness	Nausea

    If pulse is 120 beats/minute (bpm) at 5 min or 100 bpm at 10 min after stopping exercise, or if shortness of breath occurs 10 min after exercise, slow down either the rate or the distance of walking.

    If client cannot walk 5 blocks or 0.5 mile without signs of overexertion, decrease length of walking for 1 week to point before signs appear and then start to add 1 block/0.1 mile each week.

    Walk at same rate; time with stopwatch or second hand on watch; after reaching 10 blocks (1 mile), try to increase speed.

    Remember, increase only the rate or the distance of walking at one time.

    Establish a regular time for exercise, with the goal of three to five times/week for 15 to 45 min and a heart rate of 80% of stress test or gross calculation (170 bpm for 20 to 29 years of age; decrease 10 bpm for each additional decade [eg, 160 bpm for 30 to 39 years of age, 150 bpm for 40 to 49 years of age]).

Encourage significant others also to engage in walking program.

Add supplemental activity (eg, parking far from destination, gardening, using stairs, spending weekends at activities that require walking).

Work up to 1 h of exercise per day at least 4 days per week.

Avoid lapses of more than 2 days between exercise sessions.

Teach About the Risks of Obesity.

Vascular insufficiency	Arteriosclerosis	Heart disease
Hypertension	Left ventricular hypertrophy	Diabetes mellitus
Gallbladder disease	Complications of surgery	Respiratory disease
Joint degeneration	Cancer (eg, breast)	Risk of accident/injury
Increased LDL cholesterol	Decreased HDL cholesterol	

Assist Client to Increase Interest and Motivation.

Develop contract listing realistic short- and long-term goals.

Keep intake/activity records.

Hang an admired photograph on the refrigerator.

Get family involved in project.

Record body measurements; limit weighing to once per week.

Increase knowledge by reading and talking with health-conscious friends and coworkers.

Make new friends who are health conscious.

Get a friend to also follow program or be a source of support.

Avoid people who may sabotage attempts.

Reward self regularly.

Remind self that self-image and behavior are learned and can be unlearned.

Build a support system of people who value growth and you as an individual.

Be aware of rationalization (eg, a lack of time may be a lack of prioritization).

Keep a list of positive outcomes.

Reduce Inappropriate Responses to Stressors.

Distinguish between urge and hunger.

Use distraction, relaxation, and imagery.

Use alternative response training.

    Make a list of external cues/situations that lead to off-target behavior.

    List constructive behaviors (eg, take a walk) to replace off-target behaviors.

    Post the list of alternate constructive behaviors on the refrigerator.

    Reevaluate every 1 to 2 weeks whether plan is realistic and effective.

Assist Client to Plan for Life-Long Weight Maintenance.

Understand issues of dependency, control, and esteem.

Decide on *your* plan for *your* control.

Set realistic short- and long-term goals; revise as necessary.

Emphasize that dieting has a begining and an end.
Successful weight loss involves a change in habits for life.
Think positively; start slowly.
Give credit for each achievement; avoid perfectionism.
Build healthy support system.
Focus on quantity, not types of food.

Initiate Health Teaching and Referrals, as Indicated.

Refer client to support groups (eg, Weight Watchers, Overeaters Anonymous, TOPS).
Consult dietitian for meal planning.
Consult physician for morbid obesity and evaluation of other health problems.

Rationales

- Intake must be reduced to 500 cal/day less than requirement to obtain a 1 lb/week weight loss.
- Desirable weight loss rate is 1 to 2 lb/week.
- The US diet currently consists of 42% fat, 12% protein, 22% complex carbohydrates, and 24% simple carbohydrates. Recommended dietary goals are 30% fat, 12% protein, 48% complex carbohydrates, and 10% simple carbohydrates.
- Any increase in activity also increases energy output and caloric deficits.
- Weight loss without exercise decreases resting basal metabolism (Roberts, 2000).
- Often, inappropriate response to external cues, including stressors, facilitates or aggravates obesity. This response initiates an ineffective pattern in which the person eats in response to stress cues rather than physiologic hunger.
- The safest activities for the unconditioned obese person are walking, water aerobics, swimming, and cycling.
- A regular exercise program should
  - Be enjoyable
  - Use a minimum of 400 calories in each session
  - Sustain a heart rate of approximately 120 to 150 bpm
  - Involve rhythmic, alternating contracting and relaxing of muscles
  - Be integrated into the person's lifestyle 4 to 5 days/week for at least 30 to 60 min
- Before beginning an exercise program, the person must consider
  - Physical limitations (consult nurse or physician)
  - Personal preferences
  - Lifestyle
  - Community resources
  - Needed clothing and shoes
  - Clients must learn to monitor pulse before, during, and after exercise to assist them to achieve target heart rate and not to exceed maximum advisable heart rate for age.

Age	Maximum Heart Rate	Target Heart Rate
30	190	133 to 162
40	180	126 to 153
50	170	119 to 145
60	160	112 to 136

Pediatric Interventions

Assist child and family to realize the shared responsibility of weight control.
Discuss with family the hazards of overweight children.
- Childhood obesity leads to adult obesity.
- Excess weight elevates blood pressure, heart rate, and cardiac output in children (see Key Concepts, Pediatric Considerations for other health dangers).
- As weight increases, activity decreases.
Discuss the importance of balancing intake with activity. Explain that weight gain occurs with overeating, inadequate activity, or both.
Collaborate with family on a dietary plan (Keller & Stevens, 1996).
- Elicit the child's favorite foods; try to include reasonable amounts in the plan.
- Encourage child to try new foods (eg, yogurt).

- Teach child how to self-monitor intake, eating only when hungry.
- Encourage child to eat healthy snacks (eg, raw vegetables, no-fat popcorn).
- Advise that perfection is impossible.

Help child avoid prepared and sugared foods.
Advise parents to limit the high-calorie/high-fat foods in the house.
Ensure that the diet has ample fiber.
Advise parents to replace whole milk with skim milk after child is 2 years of age.
Advise parents not to force child to finish every bottle or meal.
Advise parents not to use sweets as reward for finishing meal.
Help child to avoid skipping meals.
Set realistic goals and rewards of 1 to 4 lb/month; collaborate with parents for reward for adherence.
Increase physical activity for entire family.
  Encourage them to decrease television watching (1 h/day); elicit favorite shows.
  Plan family activity regularly (adult walking, child riding or skating).
Initiate referrals as indicated.
  If desired, enlist the help of the school nurse (eg, weigh-ins, support).
  Consider summer camps for overweight teens.
  Make use of community resources (eg, adolescent support groups).

Rationales

- Sharply reduced calories can lead to loss of lean body mass and thus should be avoided.
- Replacing high-fat and high-calorie foods with healthy, low-fat, low-calorie choices while the child grows into his or her weight prevents an increase in body fat (Keller & Stevens, 1996).
- The most successful diets use ordinary foods in controlled portions rather than require the avoidance of any specific foods (Wong, 2003).
- Dietary fiber increases satiety and displaces fat in diet (Dudek, 2001).

HEALTH-SEEKING BEHAVIORS

DEFINITION

Health-Seeking Behaviors: State in which a person in stable health actively seeks ways to alter personal health habits and/or the environment to move toward a higher level of wellness*

DEFINING CHARACTERISTICS
Major (Must Be Present)

Expressed or observed desire to seek information for health promotion

Minor (May Be Present)

Expressed or observed desire for increased control of health
Expression of concern about current environmental conditions on health status
Stated or observed unfamiliarity with wellness community resources
Demonstrated or observed lack of knowledge of health-promotion behaviors

---

*Stable health status is defined as age-appropriate illness prevention measures are achieved, client reports good or excellent health, and signs and symptoms of disease, if present, are controlled.

RELATED FACTORS
Situational (Personal, Environmental)
Related to anticipated role changes (specify)

Marriage	"Empty-nest" syndrome
Parenthood	Retirement

Related to lack of knowledge of:

Preventive behavior (disease)	Regular exercise program
Screening practices for age and risk	Constructive stress management
	Supportive social networks
Optimal nutrition and weight control	

Maturational
See Table II.12 for age-related situations.

○○ **AUTHOR'S NOTE**

See *Ineffective Health Maintenance.*

KEY CONCEPTS
Generic Considerations

- A major focus of nursing care is to promote effective health-seeking behaviors in clients. Activities that do so include nurturing, encouraging, teaching, communicating, and providing.
- According to Nyamathi (1989), "The health goals of the client and desired goals of the nurse are mutually concerned with enhancing the individual's motivation to attain and maintain health and function, to avoid disease and disability, and to attain or retain the highest possible level of health, function or productivity."
- The third National Health and Nutrition Examination Survey found that of Americans 20 years and older, 32.6% are overweight (BMI 25 to 29.5) and 22.3% are obese (BMI >30; Dudek, 2001).
- Adequate dietary intake of complex carbohydrates, found in grains, fruits, legumes, and vegetables, improves human health in many ways (eg, decreases obesity, cardiovascular disease, cancer, malnutrition, diabetes, and dental caries). Current recommendations advise an increase in total dietary carbohydrates to 55% of daily calories, a decrease in total simple sugars (concentrated non-nutritive sweets) to only 10% of daily calories, and a decrease in fat to less than 30% of total calories (Dudek, 2001).
- Recent studies prove that decreasing serum cholesterol through diet and drugs (if necessary) can reduce the risk of heart disease (Woodhead, 1996). Recommended dietary changes to reduce serum cholesterol level include the following:
  - Decreased total fats, saturated fats, and cholesterol
  - In overweight people, reduced daily caloric intake to attain desired body weight
  - Increased intake of nutrients that may help decrease the risk of cardiovascular disease (eg, oat bran and other water-soluble fibers, fruit gums, vegetables, garlic, polyunsaturated fats, olive oil, legumes, fatty fish)
- Many people find it difficult to maintain health-seeking diets even when they have been successful. Examples of helpful approaches include designing behavioral contracts, engaging in positive self-talk, and strengthening family supports.
- Risk factors for cardiovascular disease include the following (Woodhead, 1996):
  - Male gender
  - Family history (parent or sibling) of myocardial infarction or sudden death younger than 55 years
  - Smoking
  - Hypertension
  - High-density lipoprotein level less than 35 mg/dL
  - History of definite occlusive vascular disease (peripheral or cerebral)
  - Obesity (more than 30% overweight)

- Guidelines for cholesterol screening are as follows (Woodhead, 1996):
  - Less than 200 mg/dL: Desirable
  - 200 to 239 mg/dL: Borderline high
  - 240 mg/dL and over: High
  - For all readings greater than 200 mg/dL, the test should be repeated within 8 weeks, along with lipoprotein analysis and follow-up with primary provider.
- Dietary recommendations for children older than 2 years are as follows (Wong, 2003):
  - Provide a variety of foods daily.
  - Maintain desirable body weight.
  - Limit total dietary fat to 30% of calories.
  - Limit total daily cholesterol to 100 mg/1000 calories and not more than 300 mg/day.
  - Limit daily protein intake to 15% of calories.
  - Limit daily carbohydrate intake to 55% of calories.
  - Limit sodium intake by reducing processed foods and keeping salt off the table.
- Research on both animals and human beings has suggested a link between nutrition and cancer (Dudek, 2001). To reduce the risk of diet-related cancers:
  - Eat five or more servings of fruits and vegetables daily.
  - Add grain products to every meal (eg, whole grains over refined).
  - Add soy-based foods to daily intake (eg, one glass of soy milk).
  - Substitute dried peas and beans for meat at some meals.
  - Limit intake of high-fat foods and animal fat.
  - Avoid high intake of alcohol (>14 drinks week/men, >7 drinks week/female).
  - Avoid excessive intake of nitrite-containing foods (eg, bacon, cured foods).
- The exact relationship between dietary sodium and essential hypertension has yet to be described unequivocally. Studies show, however, that blood pressure in many (not all) clients with hypertension decreases when they restrict dietary sodium. Thus, all people with hypertension should try a reduced sodium diet (2 g sodium/day).

Pediatric Considerations

- Children who are intrinsically motivated in their health behavior reinforce their sense of competency and self-determinism by choosing and accomplishing positive health behaviors.
- Children who are extrinsically motivated in their health behavior need interventions based on a program of external rewards for positive health behaviors.

Focus Assessment Criteria

Subjective Data
Assess for Defining Characteristics.
Does the person/family report good or excellent health?
Does the person/family desire to adopt a behavior to maximize health?

For more information on Focus Assessment Criteria, visit http://connection.lww.com.

Goal

NOC Adherence Behavior, Health Beliefs, Health Promoting Behaviors, Well-Being

The person will assume responsibility for own wellness (physical exercises, dental, safety, nutritional).

Indicators
- Describe screening appropriate for age and risk factors.
- Perform self-screening for cancer.
- Participate in a regular exercise program.
- State an intent to use positive coping mechanisms and constructive stress management.
- Eat a balanced, nutritious diet to maintain or achieve a BMI < 26.

General Interventions

NIC Health Education, Risk Identification, Values Classification, Behavior Modification, Coping Enhancement, Knowledge: Health Resources

Assess for Factors that Contribute to Health Promotion and Maintenance.

Knowledge of disease and preventive behavior
Appropriate screening practices for age and risk
Good nutrition and weight control
Regular exercise program
Constructive stress management
Supportive social networks

Promote Health Behaviors in Client and Family.

Determine Knowledge or Perception of

Specific diseases (eg, heart disease, cancer, respiratory disease, childhood diseases, infections, dental disease)
Susceptibility (eg, risk factors, family history)
Seriousness
Value of early detection

Determine Past Patterns of Health Care.

Expectations
Interactions with health care system or providers
Influences of family, cultural group, peer group, mass media

Provide Specific Information About Screening for Age-Related Conditions (see Table II.13).

Discuss the Role of Nutrition in Health Maintenance and Illness Prevention (see Key Concepts for *Imbalanced Nutrition* for Specific Explanations).

Basic food groups
Nutrient needs for age, level of physical activity, pregnancy, and lactation
Prudent use of

Salt (see *Excess Fluid Volume*)	Canned vegetables
Fried foods	Red meats
Fats (butter, margarines)	High-calorie desserts
Snack foods (potato chips, candy)	Refined sugar
Foods containing nitrosamines (smoked meats, preservatives)	Soda, fruit drinks, iced tea

Generous use of health-promoting foods
Cruciferous vegetables (broccoli, cabbage, cauliflower, Brussels sprouts)—protect against colorectal cancer
High-fiber foods—protect against colorectal cancer
Calcium-containing foods (eg, dairy, dark leafy vegetables)—protect against osteoporosis
Soy products—may reduce the risk of hormone-related cancers (eg, breast, prostate)
See *Ineffective Health Maintenance* for specific information concerning weight control.

Discuss the Benefits of a Regular Exercise Program.

See Key Concepts for *Ineffective Health Maintenance* for positive effects of regular exercise.
Determine optimal exercise for the client, considering physical limitations, preferences, and lifestyle.

Walking briskly	Aerobic dancing
Jogging	Swimming
Running	Bicycling
Skipping rope	

Stress the importance of beginning any physical activity slowly.

Discuss the Elements of Constructive Stress Management (Leon, 2002).

Maintain realistic expectations of self.
Set clear, realistic goals and subgoals.
Allow for interruptions.
Be aware of toxic thinking.
Acknowledge personal strengths.

Let go of unrealistic expectations of others.
Plan to manage time.

Discuss Strategies to Develop Positive Social Networks.

Relate the functions of a support system.

Provide love and affection.	Provide dependable assistance
Serve as buffers against life's	(emotional, economic, if appropriate).
stressors.	Share common social concerns.
Respect mutual pursuits of	Prevent isolation.
members.	Cooperate for a common purpose.

Suggest methods to strengthen this system:

Be supportive of others.
Practice active listening.
Don't interrupt the person.
Allow a few seconds to lapse between dialogue to provide time to gather thoughts and to reduce the "rush to speak."

Provide others with opportunities to share their concerns without judgment. Refrain from giving solutions; rather, discuss options (eg, "You have several options: You can quit your job, request a transfer, discuss the problem with your boss, or do nothing").

When confronted with a relationship problem, review the situation.

What is the problem?
Who/what is responsible?
What are the options?
What are the advantages and disadvantages of each option?

Show love and mutual respect to significant others.

Show unconditional love to own children.
Provide encouragement to significant others facing challenges.
Avoid criticism, punishment, excessive praise, or pampering.
Demonstrate genuine warmth and affection.

Practice mutual goal setting to direct common efforts; reevaluate them periodically.
Offer sincere assistance to others to promote trust.
Build relationships with people and families who share common interests and values.
Recognize when additional assistance is needed.

Marital counseling	Health professional
Self-help group	Religious affiliation

Allow self and each family member (children, spouse, parents) to enhance personal identity by pursuing individual interests (refer to *Delayed Growth and Development* for age-related needs of children).

Initiate Health Teaching and Referrals, as Indicated.

Review Client's Daily Health Practices.

Dental care
Food and fluid intake
Exercise regimen, leisure activities
Responsibilities in the family (eg, chores)
Use of

Tobacco	Alcohol
Salt, sugar, fat products	Drugs (over-the-counter, prescribed)

Knowledge of safety practices

Fire prevention	Water safety
Car (maintenance, seat belts,	Bicycle
car seats, air bags)	Poison control

Suggest Selective Disease-Preventing Behaviors When Appropriate.

Skin cancer
Avoid frequent sun exposure.
Avoid tanning salons.
Wear effective sunscreens and protective clothing.
Plan outdoor activities for before 10 AM and after 2 PM. During these hours, wear a hat and sunscreen.
Sexually transmitted diseases
Use barrier contraceptive methods.
Avoid casual sex.
Avoid high-risk partners (eg, history of multiple partners, no use of condoms).

Acquired Immunodeficiency Syndrome (AIDS) / Hepatitis B / Hepatitis C

Use condoms. Avoid use of contaminated needles.

Avoid high-risk sexual practices. Get hepatitis A and B vaccine.

Hearing loss

Use ear protection routinely (eg, mowing lawn, using machinery).

Avoid loud music (eg, headphones).

Avoid prolonged exposure to loud noises.

Treat infections promptly.

Congenital deformities

Avoid use of alcohol and drugs during pregnancy.

Oral cancers

Avoid tobacco chewing.

Avoid concurrent heavy use of alcohol and tobacco.

Lung cancers, chronic obstructive pulmonary disease (COPD)

Avoid tobacco smoking.

Avoid chronic exposure to known inhalable carcinogens (eg, asbestos).

Include carotene-rich foods in diet (eg, yellow vegetables and fruits).

Avoid smoke-filled rooms; discourage smoking in your living and work spaces.

Routinely test home for radon.

Coronary artery disease

Avoid obesity.

Avoid tobacco use.

Practice stress management.

Exercise regularly.

Avoid dietary cholesterol and saturated fats; reduce total dietary fats.

Maintain normal blood pressure.

Increase daily intake of water-soluble fibers in diet (eg, oat bran, fruit pectins, psyllium).

Stroke

Avoid tobacco use, especially if taking oral contraceptives.

Maintain normal blood pressure.

Avoid dietary cholesterol and saturated fats, and reduce total dietary fats.

Reye's syndrome

Avoid aspirin products in children with viral infections.

Osteoarthritis

Avoid obesity.

Avoid repeated trauma to joints.

Osteoporosis for high-risk women and men

Refer to *Ineffective Health Maintenance.*

Colorectal cancer

Avoid chronic constipation.

Avoid foods containing nitrites (cured and smoked meats); consume orange juice or other vitamin C-rich product with same meal when including nitrites in diet.

Include generous amounts of cruciferous vegetables and other sources of fiber in diet.

Breast cancer

Avoid high-fat diet.

Add soy products to daily intake.

Gastroenteritis from contaminated food

Avoid foods prepared with raw egg.

Avoid raw or incompletely cooked seafood, poultry, or meats.

Avoid shellfish from polluted waters.

Hematologic cancers

Avoid consumption of fish from dangerously polluted waters (mercury, polychlorinated biphenyl [PCBs]).

Lyme disease

Avoid tick-infested wooded or grassy areas during peak seasons (late spring, summer, early fall).

If entering hazardous areas, wear long sleeves, hat, long pants with socks pulled over cuffs of pants. Light colors make ticks more visible.

Use effective insect repellent (adults only).

Search clothes, body, and pets for ticks after hiking in hazardous areas.

Because deer ticks are the size of a dot, inspect all skin areas for reddened dots or rash. Have a physician or nurse evaluate bites or rashes.

Rationales

- Health-seeking and coping behaviors are closely intertwined; nurses assist clients to maximize their abilities to handle stress throughout life (Nyamathi, 1989).
- The process of seeking and attaining positive lifestyle change is known as "empowering potential" (Fleury, 1991). It occurs in three stages: appraising readiness, changing, and integrating change. As a person strives to improve health, he or she moves through a process of introspection; planning new, healthier activities; coping with barriers and setbacks; and ultimately absorbing these new behaviors into everyday life.
- The client is responsible for choosing a healthy pattern of living. The nurse is responsible for explaining the choices.
- Healthy eating can prevent disease and decrease complications. Regular exercise improves cardiovascular endurance, increases muscle strength and endurance, and lowers low-density lipoprotein cholesterol and triglyceride levels, blood pressure, and body fat.
- Social support helps maintain health and prevent disequilibrium (Clemen-Stone et al., 1997).
- Social support increases resiliency and positive coping (Tusaie & Dyer, 2004).

IMPAIRED HOME MAINTENANCE

DEFINITION

Impaired Home Maintenance: State in which a person or family experiences or is at risk to experience difficulty in maintaining a safe, hygienic, growth-producing home environment

DEFINING CHARACTERISTICS
Major (Must Be Present, One or More)

Expressions or observations of

Difficulty maintaining home hygiene	Difficulty maintaining a safe home	Inability to keep up home
		Lack of sufficient finances

Minor (May Be Present)

Repeated infections	Infestations	Accumulated wastes
Unwashed utensils	Offensive odors	Overcrowding

RELATED FACTORS
Pathophysiologic

Related to compromised functional ability secondary to chronic debilitating disease

Diabetes mellitus	Arthritis	Chronic obstructive pulmonary disease (COPD)
Multiple sclerosis	Congestive heart failure	
Cerebrovascular accident	Parkinson's disease	Muscular dystrophy
Cancer		

Situational (Personal, Environmental)

Related to change in functional ability of (specify family member) secondary to:

Injury (fractured limb, spinal cord injury)
Surgery (amputation, ostomy)
Impaired mental status (memory lapses, depression, anxiety–severe panic)
Substance abuse (alcohol, drugs)

Related to unavailable support system
Related to loss of family member
Related to lack of knowledge
Related to insufficient finances

Maturational

Infant
Related to multiple care requirements secondary to:
High-risk newborn

Older Adult
Related to multiple care requirements secondary to:
Family member with deficits (cognitive, motor, sensory)

⟲ AUTHOR'S NOTE

With rising life expectancy and declining mortality rates, the numbers of older adults are steadily increasing, with many living alone at home. Eighty percent of people 65 years or older report one or more chronic diseases. Of adults 65 to 74 years of age, 20% report activity limitations, and 15% cannot perform at least one activity of daily living (ADL) independently (Miller, 2004). The shift from health care primarily in hospitals to reduced lengths of stay has resulted in the discharge of many functionally compromised people to their homes. Often a false assumption is that someone will assume the management of household responsibilities until the client has recovered.

Impaired Home Maintenance describes situations in which a person or family needs teaching, supervision, or assistance to manage the household. Usually, a community health nurse is the best professional to complete an assessment of the home and the person's functioning there. Nurses in acute settings can make referrals for home visits for assessment.

A nurse who diagnoses a need for teaching to prevent household problems may use *Risk for Impaired Home Maintenance related to insufficient knowledge of (specify)*.

⟲ ERRORS IN DIAGNOSTIC STATEMENTS

Impaired Home Maintenance related to caregiver burnout

Caregiver burnout is not a sign of or related factor for *Impaired Home Maintenance*. It is associated with *Caregiver Role Strain*. *Impaired Home Maintenance* also may be present if multiple responsibilities overwhelm the caregiver. In this situation, both diagnoses are needed because the interventions for them differ.

KEY CONCEPTS
Generic Considerations

- Home care by professionals should be preventive, supportive, and therapeutic.
  - *Preventive* care includes health education, home safety, and stress management.
  - *Supportive* care can be legal, financial, nutritional, social, religious, and homemaking.
  - *Therapeutic* care involves nursing, therapy (occupational, speech), dentistry, and medicine.

✦ Pediatric Considerations

- Children depend on family members to manage home care.
- Trends in the treatment of children with chronic illness or disability include home care, early discharge, focus on developmental age, and assessment of strengths and uniqueness. Interventions are geared toward the entire family rather than just the ill child (Wong, 2003).
- High-risk graduates of neonatal intensive care units (NICUs) require technically complex home care. Discharge is planned as early as possible to contain cost and to help reduce adverse effects of hospitalization on the family system.

◉ Geriatric Considerations

- Older people have greater incidences of chronic disease, impaired function, and diminished economic resources, and a smaller social network than do younger people (Miller, 2004).
- After 75 years of age, most people living in the community live alone. Of older people living alone, 60% own their home (Miller, 2004).
- Functional ability includes ADLs and also instrumental activities of daily living (IADLs)—those skills needed to live independently (eg, procuring food, cooking, using the telephone, housekeeping, handling finances). IADLs are connected integrally to physical and cognitive abilities. The older adult who lives alone is at great risk of being institutionalized if he or she cannot perform IADLs. The possibility is great that no social network can meet these deficits (Miller, 2004).
- Approximately 9 of 10 older people have one or more chronic health problems with differing effects on function. Chronic conditions cause approximately 60% of people older than 75 years to limit their ADLs (Holzapfil, 1998).
- Along with diminished cognitive or physical ability, the older person frequently has diminished financial resources, sporadic kin, or few neighborhood social supports. He or she also may live in substandard housing or housing that does not allow simple adaptation to meet individual physical or cognitive deficits (Miller, 2004).
- In some cultures and family structures, older adults can seek assistance in some areas of home management and still retain a sense of independence. These people have determined that, by choosing selective resources to meet their needs, they will be able to maintain independent living for a longer time (Miller, 2004).

Focus Assessment Criteria

Subjective Data
Assess for Defining Characteristics.
Assessment of individual function
Housekeeping activities: ability to

Clean	Shop	Launder clothes
Prepare food		

Assess for Related Factors.
Assessment of individual function
Vision
Adequate
Corrected (date of last prescription)
Complaints of blurriness, difficulty focusing, loss of side vision, inability to adjust to darkness
Hearing

Adequate	Need to lip-read	Use of hearing aid

Thermal / tactile

Adequate	Sense of cold/hot

Mental status
Mobility
Ability to ambulate

Around room	Around house	Up and down stairs
Outside house		

Ability to travel

Drive car (last reevaluation)	Get in and out of vehicles	Use public transportation

Devices

Cane	Prosthesis	Wheelchair
Condition of devices	Walker	Competence in their use

Self-care activities: ability to

Dress and undress	Use the toilet	Groom self
Eat	Bathe	

Communication: ability to

Write	Reach emergency assistance	Use phone

Support system

Relatives, friends, neighbors	Club or religious contacts	Emergency help

Objective Data
Assess for Defining Characteristics.
Assessment of housing

Type (rent, own)

Apartment	Single-family house	Duplex

Appearance: presence of

Insects (flies, roaches)	Unwashed equipment	Rodents/vermin
Dirt, food, hygiene wastes	Offensive odors	

Physical facilities

Rooms (number)	Lighting	Toilet facilities (accessibility)
Water supply	Heating	Sewage disposal
Ventilation	Garbage disposal	Handrails (stairs)
Appliances: stove, refrigerator, sink	Screens	

Safety

Do any adaptations need to be made in the home for the person?

Refer to Focus Assessment Criteria for *Risk for Injury* for an assessment of hazards in the home.

Assessment of home environment of children

Provisions for play

Appropriate play materials	Safe play area (indoors, outdoors)
Special place for child's possessions	

Stimulating environment

Selected use of television (amount, type)

Activities for age-related development (see *Delayed Growth and Development*)

Family time (meal, joint activities)

Family outings

Affectionate environment

Touching, holding	Conversations convey positive feelings
Parent speaks with pride about child	

For more information on Focus Assessment Criteria, visit http://connection.lww.com.

Goal

 Family Functioning

The person or caretaker will express satisfaction with home situation.

Indicators
- Identify factors that restrict self-care and home management.
- Demonstrate ability to perform skills necessary for care of the home.

General Interventions

NIC Home Maintenance Assistance, Environmental Management: Safety, Environmental Management

The following interventions apply to many
with impaired home maintenance, regardless of etiology.

Assess for Causative or Contributing Factors.

Lack of knowledge

Insufficient funds

Lack of necessary equipment or aids

Inability (illness, sensory deficits, motor deficits) to perform household activities

Impaired cognitive functioning

Impaired emotional functioning

Reduce or Eliminate Causative or Contributing Factors, if Possible.
Lack of Knowledge

Determine with client and family the information they need to learn.

Monitoring skills (pulse, circulation, urine)

Medication administration (procedure, side effects, precautions)

Treatment/procedures
Equipment use/maintenance
Safety issues (eg, environmental)
Community resources
Follow-up care
Anticipatory guidance (eg, emotional and social needs, alternatives to home care)
Initiate teaching; give detailed written instruction.
Refer family to a community-nursing agency for follow-up.

Insufficient Funds

Consult with social service department for assistance.
Consult with service organizations (eg, American Heart Association, The Lung Association, American Cancer Society) for assistance.

Lack of Necessary Equipment or Aids

Determine type of equipment needed, considering availability, cost, and durability.
Seek assistance from agencies that rent or loan supplies.
Teach care and maintenance of supplies to increase length of use.
Consider adapting equipment to reduce cost.

Inability to Perform Household Activities

Determine type of assistance needed (eg, meals, housework, transportation); assist client to obtain it.
Meals
Discuss with relatives the possibility of freezing complete meals that require only heating (eg, small containers of soup, stews, casseroles).
Determine availability of meal services for ill people (eg, Meals on Wheels, church groups).
Teach people about nutritious foods that are easily prepared (eg, hard-boiled eggs, tuna fish, peanut butter).
Housework
Encourage client to contract with an adolescent for light housekeeping.
Refer client to community agency for assistance.
Transportation
Determine availability of transportation for shopping and health care.
Suggest client request rides with neighbors to places they drive routinely.

Impaired Cognitive Functioning

Assess client's ability to maintain a safe household.
Refer to *Risk for Injury* related to lack of awareness of hazards.
Initiate appropriate referrals.

Impaired Emotional Functioning

Assess severity of the dysfunction.
Refer to *Ineffective Coping* for additional assessment and interventions.

Initiate Health Teaching and Referrals, as Indicated.

Refer to support groups (eg, local Alzheimer's Association, American Cancer Society).
Refer to community-nursing agency.
Refer to community agencies (eg, visitors, meal programs, homemakers, adult day care).

Rationales

- Discharge planning begins at admission, with the nurse determining anticipated needs after discharge: client's self-care ability, availability of support, homemaker services, equipment needs, community nursing services, therapy (physical, speech, occupational; Green, 1998).
- The home environment must be assessed for safety before discharge: location of bathroom, access to water, cooking facilities, and environmental barriers (stairs, narrow doorways).
- In determining a person's ability to perform self-care at home, the nurse must assess his or her ability to function and protect self. The nurse considers motor and sensory deficits and mental status (Miller, 2004).

HOPELESSNESS

DEFINITION

Hopelessness: A sustained subjective emotional state in which a person sees no alternatives or personal choices available to solve problems or to achieve what is desired and cannot mobilize energy on own behalf to establish goals

DEFINING CHARACTERISTICS
Major (Must Be Present, One or More)

Expresses profound, overwhelming, sustained apathy in response to a situation perceived as impossible
Verbal cues of despondency

Physiologic

Slowed responses to stimuli   Lack of energy
Increased sleep

Emotional
Person feels:

Difficulty experiencing feelings   Incompetent or trapped
A lack of meaning or purpose in life   Unable to seek good fortune, luck, God's favor
Sense of loss and deprivation   Empty or drained
Helpless

Person exhibits:

Passivity and lack of involvement in care   Decreased verbalization
Decreased affect   Lack of ambition, initiative, and interest
"Giving up–given up complex"   Inability to accomplish anything
Lack of responsibility for decisions and life   Slowed thought processes
Isolating behaviors

Cognitive

Decreased problem solving and decision making
Focus on past and future, not here and now
Decreased flexibility in thought processes
Rigidity (eg, all-or-none thinking)
Lack of imagination and wishing capabilities
Inability to identify or accomplish desired objectives and goals
Inability to plan, organize, or make decisions
Inability to recognize sources of hope
Suicidal thoughts

Minor (May Be Present)
Physiologic

Anorexia   Weight loss

Emotional
Person feels:

A lump in the throat   Tense
Discouraged with self and others   Overwhelmed (just "can't . . .")
Loss of gratification from roles and relationships
At the end of his or her rope   Vulnerable

Person exhibits:

Poor eye contact (turns away, shrugs)
Sighing
Resignation

Decreased motivation
Regression
Depression

Cognitive

Decreased ability to integrate information received
Loss of time perception (past, present, and future)
Decreased ability to recall from the past
Confusion
Inability to communicate effectively
Distorted thought perceptions and associations
Unreasonable judgment

RELATED FACTORS
Pathophysiologic

Any chronic or terminal illness (eg, heart disease, kidney disease, cancer, acquired immunodeficiency syndrome [AIDS]) can cause or contribute to hopelessness.

Related to impaired ability to cope secondary to, eg:

Failing or deteriorating physiologic condition
New and unexpected signs or symptoms of previous disease process
Prolonged pain, discomfort, weakness
Impaired functional abilities (walking, elimination, eating)

Treatment-Related

Related to:

Prolonged treatments (eg, chemotherapy, radiation) that cause pain, nausea, discomfort
Treatments that alter body image (eg, surgery, chemotherapy)
Prolonged diagnostic studies
Prolonged dependence on equipment for life support (eg, dialysis, respirator)
Prolonged dependence on equipment for monitoring bodily functions (eg, telemetry)

Situational (Personal, Environmental)

Related to:

Prolonged activity restriction (eg, fractures, spinal cord injury)
Prolonged isolation (eg, infectious diseases, reverse isolation for suppressed immune system)
Abandonment by, separation from, or isolation from significant others (parents, spouse, children)
Inability to achieve valued goals in life (marriage, education, children)
Inability to participate in desired activities (walking, sports, work)
Loss of something or someone valued (spouse, children, friend, financial resources)
Prolonged caretaking responsibilities (spouse, child, parent)
Exposure to long-term physiologic or psychological stress
Loss of belief in transcendent values/God
Ongoing, repetitive losses in community related to AIDS

Maturational

Related to:

Child

Loss of caregiver
Rejection or abandonment by caregivers
Loss of bodily functions

Loss of trust in significant other
Loss of autonomy related to illness (eg, fracture)
Inability to achieve developmental tasks (trust, autonomy, initiative, industry)

Adolescent

Loss of significant other (peer, family)
Change in body image

Rejection by family
Loss of bodily functions
Inability to achieve developmental task (role identity)

Adult

Impaired bodily functions, loss of body part	Impaired relationships (separation, divorce)
Loss of job, career	Loss of significant others (death of spouse, child)
Inability to achieve developmental tasks (intimacy, commitment, productivity)	

Older Adult

Sensory deficits	Motor deficits
Cognitive deficits	Loss of independence
Loss of significant others, things	Inability to achieve developmental tasks (generativity)

◎ AUTHOR'S NOTE

Hopelessness describes a person who sees no possibility that his or her life will improve and maintains that no one can do anything to help. *Hopelessness* differs from *Powerlessness* in that a hopeless person sees no solution or no way to achieve what is desired, even if he or she feels in control. In contrast, a powerless person may see an alternative or answer, yet be unable to do anything about it because of lack of control or resources. Sustained feelings of powerlessness may lead to hopelessness. Hopelessness is commonly related to grief, depression, and suicide. For a person at risk for suicide, the nurse also should use the diagnosis *Risk for Suicide.*

◎ ERRORS IN DIAGNOSTIC STATEMENTS

1. *Hopelessness related to AIDS*

This diagnostic statement does not describe a situation the nurse can treat. The statement should include specific factors the person has identified as overwhelming, as in the following diagnostic statement: *Hopelessness related to recent diagnosis of AIDS and rejection by parents.*

KEY CONCEPTS
Generic Considerations

Hope

- Hope is an unconscious cognitive behavior that energizes and allows a person to act, achieve, and use crisis as an opportunity for growth. It activates motivation and defends against despair (Korner, 1970). It has been defined as any expectation greater than zero for achieving a given goal (Stotland, 1969). Hope is a "common human experience in that it is a way of propelling self towards envisioned possibilities in everyday encounters with the world" (Parse, 1990).
- Early childhood experiences influence a person's ability to hope. A trusting environment promotes hope.
- Hope is related to faith, because many people experience hope by recognizing their reliance on higher powers to restore meaning and purpose to their lives.
- Plummer (1988) found high indices of hope in people who have a relationship with a higher being, participate in religious services, and can control their immediate environment. Spiritual practices provide a source of hope.
- Watson (1979) has identified hope as both a curative and a "carative" factor in nursing. Hope, with faith and trust, provides psychic energy to draw on to aid the curative process.
- Researchers have observed that hope prolongs life in critical survival conditions, whereas loss of hope often results in death (Korner, 1970).
- A hoping person feels autonomous in making decisions.
- Kübler-Ross (1975) observed that those who expressed hope coped more effectively during their difficult dying periods. She also noted that death occurred soon after these people stopped expressing hope.

- A person's level of hope relates directly to his or her level of coping. Christman (1990) found uncertainty and less hope to be associated with adjustment problems during radiation therapy.
- According to Hickey (1986), hope enables the living to continue and the dying to die better.
- Notwotny (1989) identified six dimensions of hope: confidence in outcome, possibility of a future, relating to others, spiritual beliefs, emergence from within, and active involvement.
- Owen (1989) found hopeful clients with cancer able to set goals, be optimistic, redefine the future, find meaning in life, feel peaceful, and give out or use energy.
- Miller (1989) studied 60 critically ill clients to determine hope-inspiring strategies:
  - Thinking to buffer threatening perceptions
  - Using positive thinking
  - Feeling that life has meaning and growth results from crises
  - Engaging in beliefs and practices that enable transcendence of suffering
  - Receiving from caregivers a constructive view, expectations of client's ability to manage difficulty, and confidence in therapy
  - Sustaining relationships with loved ones
  - Perceiving that knowledge and actions can affect outcomes
  - Having desired activities and outcomes to attain
  - Other specific behaviors that thwart despair, including distraction and humor
- Researchers have found significant correlations between perceived level of control and hope and information seeking.
- Theorists have postulated that hope is a powerful resource that can promote wound healing through the electrochemical reaction that affects the autonomic, endocrine, and immune systems (Jackson, 1993).
- Hopeful people engage in health-promoting lifestyles and self-care.

Hopelessness

- Hopelessness is an emotional state in which a person feels that life is too much or impossible. A person without hope sees no possibility that life will improve and no solutions. He or she believes that no one can do anything to help. Hopelessness is related to despair, helplessness, doubt, grief, apathy, sadness, depression, and suicide. It is present and past oriented and a deenergizing state.
- Researchers have observed that hope reflected in clients' drawings is related directly to health improvement, whereas lack of hope is related to disease recurrence. Thus, nurses should help clients to find their resources of hope.
- Cancer has been predicted significantly in people based on identifying hopelessness in their lives before diagnosis. Therefore, terminal illness may lead to hopelessness, or a state of hopelessness may contribute to terminal illness.
- Hopelessness results in three basic categories of feeling:
  - Sense of the impossible: what a person feels compelled to do, he or she cannot; thus, he or she feels trapped
  - Overwhelmed: the person perceives tasks and others as too big and difficult to handle and self as small
  - Apathy: the person has no goals or sense of purpose
- Hopeless people lack internal resources and strengths (eg, autonomy, self-esteem, integrity). Regardless of age, they reach outside for help because their internal resources are depleted.
- Everyone's life has some degree of hopelessness. It occurs in various forms and is more common and usual than reported (eg, we all must die; hoping for anything else is hopeless).
- Hopelessness is observed most often in people who are rigid and inflexible in their thoughts, feelings, and actions.
- People may have ideals that are hopeless in reality (eg, not to die, trusting everyone, all people always act appropriately).
- Engel (1989) identified the "giving up–given up" complex as having five characteristics:
  - Experiencing the feeling of giving up as helplessness or hopelessness
  - Having a depreciated image of self
  - Experiencing a sense of loss of gratification from relationships or roles
  - Feeling disruption
  - Reactivating memories of earlier periods of giving up
  - Engel proposed that this state of coping activates neurally regulated biologic emergency patterns, which may decrease the capacity to fight off pathogenic processes. Therefore, the "giving up–given up" complex is a contributing factor to disease.

- Often, when internal and external resources are exhausted, a person relies on his or her relationship with God for hope. The person may feel more secure placing hope in God than in others or self. Hoping in God may not mean an abrupt end to the crisis, but it may give a sense of God's control of circumstances and ability to provide support during this time. Meaning and purpose for life and suffering may be found in a client's relationship with God and the knowledge of His control. Hope for a client's future may depend on his or her perception of a promise of eternal fellowship with God that continues after life on earth ends. With this eternal relationship comes the belief in God's promise to end all suffering and restore harmonious relationships—with God, self, and others (Jennings, 1997).
- Hope and hopelessness are not mutually exclusive. Hope is not the complete absence of hopelessness (LeGresley, 1991).
- Hopelessness can be found in the gay community in response to multiple AIDS-related losses, such as of friends and community and disintegrating family structures and social networks. These losses are unending and repetitive and receive little understanding from many heterosexuals (Mallinson, 1999).

Pediatric Considerations

- Consistent nurturing, trustworthiness, and achievement of hoped-for things and events nurture hope in children.
- Families of children with life-threatening diseases may feel hopeless and become dysfunctional. The nurse may need to identify dysfunctional family interactions, use strategies from family therapy, or make appropriate referrals.
- Hinds (1984) introduced a definition of hope for teens through the use of grounded theory methodology: the degree to which an adolescent believes that a personal tomorrow exists.
- To become an adult, the adolescent must first achieve hopefulness. Hinds and Martin (1988) found that adolescents with cancer progress through four sequential, self-sustaining phases to cope and achieve hopefulness:
  - Cognitive discomfort
  - Distraction
  - Cognitive comfort
  - Personal competence
- These phases have implications for nurses planning appropriate strategies to assist adolescents to achieve hopefulness.
- Hinds (1988) identified that adolescent hopefulness differs from adult hopefulness in that adolescents experience a wider range or greater intensity of hopefulness. In addition, they usually focus on hope for others and believe in the value of forced effort—that is, identifying an area of hope and fostering it.
- Nursing interventions that have been found to influence hopefulness in adolescents include truthful explanations, doing things with them, nursing knowledge of survivors, caring behaviors, focusing on future, competency, and conversing about less sensitive areas. In addition, humor has been identified as promoting cognitive distraction and facilitating hope. Nursing interventions that inhibit cognitive distraction, (eg, focusing on nursing tasks and on negative adolescent behaviors) promote hopelessness (Hinds, Martin & Vogel, 1987).

Geriatric Considerations

- Older adults are at risk for hopelessness because of the many psychosocial and physiologic changes that accompany normal aging, which often are perceived as losses. Older adults also have decreased energy, and energy is necessary for hopefulness.
- Healthy coping in older adults is related to acquiring developmental resources in later adulthood. Older adults must learn to give up less useful operations and acquire more effective resources to deal with age-related life changes (Reed, 1986).
- Stressors for older adults are unique and differ from those of other age groups. They include changes in personal care, longing for absent children or grandchildren, fear of being a victim of crime, and fear of being taken advantage of by the "system." The nurse may be able to assist older clients to identify stressors and locate resources to prevent hopelessness.

⊕ Transcultural Considerations

- Nurses who subscribe to the dominant US culture may misinterpret cultural differences related to values, expectations, and loci of control. A nurse who misdiagnoses a client as hopeless may not actively intervene—"Why even try?" (Leininger, 1978).
- Hopelessness focuses on an inability to achieve goals, which is future oriented. The concept of hopelessness may not be relevant to cultures that are not future oriented.
- Interventions for hopelessness vary among cultures (Miller & Wake, 1994).

Focus Assessment Criteria

Hopelessness is a subjective emotional state that the nurse must validate with the person. The nurse must assess emotional and cognitive areas carefully to infer that the person is experiencing hopelessness. Some of these same cues may be seen in people with diagnoses of *Social Isolation, Powerlessness, Disturbed Self-Concept, Spiritual Distress,* or *Ineffective Coping.* The nurse can use the Herth Hope Scale to determine the level of hope in adults of various ages and with different levels of illness (Herth, 1992).

Subjective Data
Assess for Defining Characteristics.

Activities of daily living

Exercise: amount, type

Hobbies: self-interest
 activities

Appetite: eating habits

Sleep: time, amount, quality

Self-care participation: grooming habits

Energy and motivation

Is the person exhausted, tired?

Does the person believe he or
 she can achieve goals?

Does he or she express an
 interest in any activities?

Does he or she have any goals or desires?

Does this person feel overwhelmed?

Meaning and purpose in life

What does this person value most in life? Why?

What does this person describe as his or her purpose or role in life?

Is this purpose or role fulfilled?

Are perceptions of his or her meaning and purpose realistic or achievable?

What kind of relationship does he or she have with God or a higher being?

Does this relationship give meaning or purpose to his or her life?

What does this illness mean to the person?

Choice or control in situations

What does the client perceive to be his or her most difficult problem? Why?

What does he or she believe is the solution? Is this solution realistic?

Is his or her perception of the problem distorted? If so, how?

Has the client considered or tried other alternatives?

Does this person believe he or she has any control in the situation?

How flexible or rigid are this person's thought processes?

Future options

What does the person believe the future will bring? Negative or positive things?

What does he or she see as worth living for?

How does the future look to this person?

How does this person perceive his or her present illness? Its effect on his or her life? Its effect on his or her relationships?

How does this person perceive current treatments for his or her illness? Promising, or stressful and useless?

Does this person recognize any sources of hope?

What does he or she want most in life?

Does this person have suicidal thoughts? If so, refer to *Risk for Suicide*.

Assess for Related Factors.

Presence of illness or treatment

Chronic, prolonged, deteriorating, exhausting

Significant relationships

Whom does this person perceive as the most significant other?

What is this person's current relationship with this significant other?

Has divorce or death of spouse, child, sibling, friend, or pet occurred recently?

Has this person moved away from or been rejected by significant others?

Objective Data

Assess for defining characteristics.

General appearance
- Grooming
- Posture

Eye contact

Speed of activities

Interaction with others

Involvement in self-care activities

For more information on Focus Assessment Criteria, visit http://connection.lww.com .

Goals

 NOC Decision Making, Depression Control, Hope, Quality of Life

The person will:

- Demonstrate increased energy, as evidenced by activities (eg, self-care, exercise, hobbies).
- Express positive expectations about the future, purpose, and meaning in life.
- Demonstrate initiative, self-direction, and autonomy in decision making and problem solving.
- Redefine the future and set realistic goals.
- Exhibit peace and comfort with situation.

Indicators

- Share suffering openly and constructively with others.
- Reminisce and review life positively.
- Consider values and the meaning of life.
- Express optimism about the present.
- Practice energy conservation.
- Develop, improve, and maintain positive relationships with others.
- Participate in a significant role.
- Express spiritual beliefs.

General Interventions

NIC Hope Instillation, Values Classification, Decision-Making Support, Spiritual Support, Support System Enhancement

Assist Client to Identify and Express Feelings.

Listen actively and treat the person as an individual.

Convey empathy to promote verbalization of doubts, fears, and concerns.

Validate and reflect impressions with the person. It is important to realize that clients with cancer often have their own reality, which may differ from the nurse's (Yates, 1993).

Accept the client's feelings (eg, trust will to live if it exists, accept anger).

Encourage client to verbalize why and how hope is significant in his or her life.

Encourage expressions of how hope is uncertain and areas in which hope has failed him or her.

Assist client to recognize that hopelessness is part of everyone's life and demands recognition. The client can use it as a source of energy, imagination, and freedom to consider alternatives. Hopelessness can lead to self-discovery.

Assist client to understand that he or she can deal with the hopeless aspects of life by separating them from the hopeful aspects. Help client to identify and to acknowledge areas of hopelessness. Help client to distinguish between the possible and impossible.

The nurse mobilizes a client's internal and external resources to promote hope. Assist clients to identify their personal reasons for living that provide meaning and purpose to their lives.

Assess and Mobilize Client's Internal Resources (Autonomy, Independence, Rationality, Cognitive Thinking, Flexibility, Spirituality).

Emphasize Strengths, Not Weaknesses.

Compliment Client on Appearance or Efforts as Appropriate.

Promote Motivation.

Identify reasons for living.

Identify areas of success and usefulness; emphasize past accomplishments. Use this information to develop goals with the client.

Assist client to identify things he or she has fun doing and perceives as humorous. Such activities can serve as distractions to discomfort and allow the client to progress to cognitive comfort (Hinds & Martin, 1988).

Assist client to identify sources of hope (eg, relationships, faith, things to accomplish).

Assist client to adjust and develop realistic short- and long-term goals (progress from simple to more complex; may use a "goals poster" to indicate type and time for achieving specific goals). Attainable expectations promote hope.

Teach client to monitor specific signs of progress to use as self-reinforcement.

Encourage "means–end" thinking in positive terms (ie, If I do this, then I'll be able to . . .).

Foster lightheartedness and the sharing of uplifting memories.

Assist Client with Problem Solving and Decision Making.

Respect client as a competent decision maker; treat his or her decisions and desires with respect.

Encourage verbalization to determine client's perception of choices.

Clarify client's values to determine what is important.

Correct misinformation.

Assist client to identify those problems he or she cannot resolve to advance to problems he or she can. In other words, assist client to move away from dwelling on the impossible and hopeless and to begin to deal with realistic and hopeful matters.

Assess client's perceptions of self and others in relation to size. (People with hopelessness often perceive others as large and difficult to deal with and themselves as small.) If perceptions are unrealistic, assist client to reassess them to restore proper scale.

Promote flexibility. Encourage client to try alternatives and take risks.

Assist Client to Learn Effective Coping Skills.

Assist with setting realistic, attainable short- and long-term goals.

Teach the importance of mutuality in sharing concerns.

Explain benefits of distraction from negative events.

Teach the value of confronting issues.

Teach and assist with relaxation techniques before anticipated stressful events.

Encourage mental imagery to promote positive thought processes.

Allow client time to reminisce to gain insight into past experiences.

Teach client to "hope to be" the best person possible today and to appreciate the fullness of each moment.

Teach client to maximize aesthetic experiences (eg, smell of coffee, back rub, feeling warmth of the sun or a breeze), which can inspire hope.

Teach client to anticipate experiences he or she delights in daily (eg, walking, reading favorite book, writing letter).

Assist client to express spiritual beliefs (Jennings, 1997).

Teach client ways to conserve and generate energy. Moderate physical exercise and rest can enhance hope (Owen, 1989).

Assess and Mobilize Person's External Resources (Significant Others, Health Care Team, Support Groups, God or Higher Powers).

Family or Significant Others

Involve them in plan of care.

Encourage client to spend increased time or thoughts with loved ones in healthy relationships.

Teach family members their role in sustaining hope through supportive, positive relationships (Johnson & Roberts, 1996).

Convey hope, information, and confidence to family, because they will convey their feelings to the client (Johnson & Roberts, 1996).

Discuss client's attainable goals with family (Johnson, Roberts & Cheffer, 1996).

Use touch and closeness with client to demonstrate to family its acceptability (provide privacy).

Herth (1993) found the following strategies to foster hope in caregivers of terminally ill people:

- *Cognitive reframing*—positive self-talk, praying/meditating, and envisioning hopeful images (this may involve letting go of expectations for things to be different)
- *Time refocusing*—focusing less on the future and more on living one day at a time
- *Belief in a power greater than self*—empowering the caregiver's hope
- *Balancing available energy*—listening to music or other favorite activities to empower the caregiver's hope through uplifting energy

Health Care Team

Develop positive, trusting nurse–client relationship by:

Answering questions	Touching
Respecting client's feelings	Providing comfort
Providing consistent care	Being honest
Following through on requests	Conveying positive attitude

Convey attitude of "We care too much about you to let you just give up," or "I can help you."

Hold conferences and share client's goals with staff.

Share advances in technology and research for treatment of diseases.

Have available a list of laughter resources (eg, books, films).

Support Groups

Encourage client to share concerns with others who have had similar problem or disease and positive experiences from coping effectively with it.

Provide information on self-help groups (eg, "Make today count"—40 chapters in United States and Canada; "I can cope"—series for clients with cancer; "We Can Weekend"—for families of clients with cancer).

God or Higher Powers

Assess belief support system (value, past experiences, religious activities, relationship with God, meaning and purpose of prayer; refer to *Spiritual Distress*).

Create environment in which client feels free to express spirituality (Dossey et al., 1994).

Allow client time and opportunities to reflect on the meaning of suffering, death, and dying.

Accept, respect, and support client's hope in God.

Identify Client at Risk for Self-Harm (Refer to *Risk for Suicide*).

Initiate Referrals, as Indicated.

Counseling (spiritual, family)   Crisis hotline

Rationales

- Hope is related to help from others, in that a person believes external resources may be supportive when his or her internal resources and strengths seem insufficient to cope (ie, a family or significant other is often a source of hope).
- Hope has been claimed capable of influencing physical, psychological, and spiritual health.
- Maintaining family role responsibilities is essential for hope and coping. In addition, hope is essential for families of the critically ill to facilitate coping and adjustment.
- Moderate physical exercise and adequate rest can enhance hope, because hope takes energy and gives energy (Owen, 1989).
- "Lightheartedness," humor, and uplifting memories were found to foster hope in terminally ill people.
- Hope maintained by family members has a contagious effect on clients (Miller, 1991).
- Isolation, concurrent losses, and poorly controlled symptom management hinder hope.
- A person experiencing hopelessness cannot imagine anything that can be done or is worth doing, nor can he or she imagine beyond what is current.
- If a person recognizes and deals with hopelessness imaginatively, movement, growth, and resourcefulness can result. Rigidity never overcomes hopelessness.
- People can cope with a part of life they view as hopeless if they realize that other factors in life are hopeful. For example, a person may realize he or she may never walk again, but will be able to go home, be with grandchildren, and move around. Therefore, hopelessness can lead to the discovery of alternatives that provide meaning and purpose in life. It is essential to keep hopelessness out of the way of hope.

- Motivation is essential to recovering from hopelessness. The client must determine a goal even if he or she has low expectations of achieving it. The nurse is the catalyst to encourage the client to take the first step to identify a goal. Then, the client must create another goal.
- The health care team must be hopeful if the client is to be hopeful; otherwise, the client views efforts of the team as a waste of time.

DISORGANIZED INFANT BEHAVIOR

DEFINITION
Disorganized Infant Behavior: The degree to which an infant has reached his or her organizational threshold and no longer is maintaining self, as reflected in his or her use of varying physiologic, postural, or state strategies, and as reflected across all subsystems of behavioral adaptation (ie, autonomic, motor, state, and attention–interaction systems)

DEFINING CHARACTERISTICS (VANDENBERG, 1990; WONG, 2003)
Autonomic System
Cardiac
Increased rate

Respiration
Pauses	Tachypnea	Gasping

Color Changes
Paling around nostrils	Perioral duskiness	Mottling
Cyanosis	Grayness	Flushing/ruddiness

Visceral
Hiccupping	Straining as if actually	Grunting
Spitting up	producing a bowel	
Gagging	movement	

Motor
Seizures	Sneezing	Tremoring/startling
Yawning	Twitching	Sighing
Coughing		

Motor System
Fluctuating Tone
Flaccidity of
Trunk	Face	Extremities

Hypertonicity
Extending legs	Arching	Saluting
Splaying fingers	Airplaning	Extending tongue
Sitting on air	Fisting	

Hyperflexions
Trunk	Fetal tuck	Extremities

Frantic Diffuse Activity
State System (Range)
difficulty maintaining state control
difficulty in transitions from one state to another

Sleep

Twitches	Whimpers	Makes sounds
Grimaces	Makes jerky movements	Fusses in sleep
Has irregular respirations		

Awake

Eyes floating	Panicky, worried, dull look	Glassy eyes
Weak cry	Strain, fussiness	Irritability
Staring	Abrupt state changes	Gaze aversion

Attention–Interaction System

Attempts at engaging behaviors elicit stress.
Impaired ability to orient, attend, engage in reciprocal social interactions
Difficulty consoling

RELATED FACTORS
Pathophysiologic

Related to immature or altered central nervous system (CNS) secondary to:

Prematurity	Infection	Prenatal exposure to drugs
Hyperbilirubinemia	Congenital anomalies	Decreased oxygen saturation
Hypoglycemia	Perinatal factors	

Related to nutritional deficits secondary to:

Reflux emesis	Swallowing problems	Colic
Feeding intolerance		

Related to excess stimulation secondary to:

Pain	Hunger	Oral hypersensitivity
Temperature variation		

Treatment-Related

Related to excess stimulation secondary to:

Invasive procedures	Restraints	Chest physical therapy
Movement	Noise (eg, prolonged alarm,	Feeding
Lights	voices, environment)	Tubes, tape
Medication administration		

Related to inability to see caregivers secondary to eye patches

Situational (Personal, Environmental)

Related to unpredictable interactions secondary to multiple caregivers
Related to imbalance of task touch and consoling touch
Related to decreased ability to self-regulate secondary to:

Sudden movement	Noise
Disrupted sleep–wake cycles	Fatigue

⊙⊙ **AUTHOR'S NOTE**

This diagnosis describes an infant who has difficulty regulating and adapting to external stimuli. This difficulty is from immature neurobehavioral development and increased environmental stimuli associated with neonatal units. When an infant is overstimulated or stressed, he or she uses energy to adapt, which depletes the supply of energy available for physiologic growth. The goal of nursing care is to assist the infant to conserve energy by reducing environmental stimuli, allowing the baby sufficient time to adapt to handling, and providing sensory input appropriate to the infant's physiologic and neurobehavioral status.

KEY CONCEPTS
Generic Considerations

- Als (1986) explained that an infant's primary route of communication of competency and efforts at self-regulation is through behavioral indices.

- Infant behavior is a continual interaction with the environment by means of fine subsystems (Blackburn, 1993; Merenstein & Gardner, 1998; Yecco, 1993):
  - *Autonomic/physiologic*—regulation of respiration, color, and visceral functions (eg, gastrointestinal, swallowing)
  - *Motor*—regulation of tone, posture, activity level, specific movement patterns of the extremities, head, trunk, and face
  - *State/organizational*—the range, transition between, and quality of states of consciousness (*eg,* sleep to arousal, awake to alert, crying)
  - *Attention–interactive*—ability to orient and to focus on sensory stimuli (eg, faces, sounds, objects) and to take in cognitive, social, and emotional information
  - *Self-regulatory*—maintenance of the integrity and balance of the other subsystems, smooth transitions between states, and relaxation among subsystems
- In full-term infants, these systems function smoothly and are synchronized and regulated with ease. Less mature or ill infants, however, can tolerate only one activity at a time. Loss of control results in instability or disorganization in one or more subsystems (Blackburn, 1993). The defining characteristics represent signs of the instability.
- Premature infants must adapt to the extrauterine environment with underdeveloped body systems, usually in a neonatal intensive care unit (NICU; Merenstein & Gardner, 1998).
- Although mortality and morbidity rates have been reduced greatly in high-risk infants, these babies experience various neurobehavioral problems. These problems have been labeled as *the new morbidities of low-birth-weight infants* and include hyperexcitability, language problems, attention-deficit disorders, higher-order cognitive problems, and schooling problems (Blackburn, 1993).
- The six stages of CNS development are dorsal induction, ventral induction, proliferation and neurogenesis, neuron migration, organization, and myelinization. The first three occur completely before the 4th month of gestation. The last three stages continue until development is complete. The *migration stage* involves the movement of millions of cells from their point of origin in the periventricular region to their terminal location within the cerebral cortex and cerebellum. The *organization stage* peaks from 6 months' gestation to 1 year after birth. The *myelinization stage* peaks from 8 months' gestation to 1 year after birth. Myelinization insulates individual nerve fibers to facilitate specificity of connections, increases the number of alternative pathways, and increases the speed of transmission (Blackburn, 1993).
- Neurologic dysfunctions resulting from neurologic underdevelopment include the following (Blackburn, 1993):

Sparse myelin	Long refractory period
Weak transmission	Decreased inhibitory potential
Decreased ability to use various systems	Slow nerve conduction
Slow synaptic conduction	Inability to sustain high firing rates
Incomplete cell differentiation	Decreased ability to process impulses for cell-to-cell communication

- These limitations result in the following behavior characteristics of immature infants (Blackburn, 1993; Merenstein & Gardner, 1998):

Irregular state of regulation	Increased and decreased tone
Deficits in primitive reflexes	Easy exhaustion
Irritability (difficult to soothe)	Inability to inhibit
Jerky movements	Low arousal
Difficulty sustaining alertness	Poor coordination
Altered autonomic regulation	Uncoordinated posture/movements

- For too long, researchers believed that newborns could not perceive, respond to, or remember pain. Findings have validated, however, that newborns do feel and express pain. Williamson and Williamson (1983) found that infants who received local anesthesia for circumcision cried less and had less variation in heart rate and higher oxygen saturation compared with infants who did not have a local anesthetic.
- Loudness of sound is measured in decibels (db). Adult speech is recorded at about 45 to 50 db. Sound levels in infant incubators have been reported to be 50 to 80 db. Hearing loss in adults has been associated with levels above 80 to 85 db (Blackburn, 1993).
- Incidence of sensorineural hearing impairment is 4% in low-birth-weight infants and 13% in very-low-birth-weight infants (Thomas, 1989).

Focus Assessment Criteria

Note: Experts recommend three assessment tools for neurobehavioral function: the Brazelton Neonatal Behavioral Assessment Scale (NBAS) for healthy, full-term newborns; Assessment of Preterm Infant Behavior (APIB) for preterm newborns; and NIDCAP (Newborn Individualized Developmental Care and Assessment Program). All tools require training in their use.

Objective Data

Assess for Defining Characteristics.

Autonomic system
Respirations (see Defining Characteristics)
Color changes (see Defining Characteristics)
Visceral (see Defining Characteristics)
Motor (see Defining Characteristics)

Motor system (fluctuating tone)
Flaccid trunk, extremities, face (see Defining Characteristics)
Hypertonic (see Defining Characteristics)
Hyperflexions (see Defining Characteristics)
Frantic, diffuse activity (see Defining Characteristics)

State system (range)
Sleep

Twitches	Jerky movements	Grimaces
Whimpers	Fussiness	

Awake

Lack of coordination	Glassy eyes	Unfocused eyes
Staring	Panicked look	Weak cry
Irritability		

Abrupt state changes

Attention–interaction system
Imbalance of withdrawal versus engaging behaviors
Impaired ability to orient, engage in reciprocal interactions, attend
Difficulty consoling

For more information on Focus Assessment Criteria, visit http://connection.lww.com.

Goal

> **NOC** Neurologic Status, Preterm Infant Organization, Sleep, Comfort Level

The infant will demonstrate increase signs of stability.

Indicators

- Exhibit smooth, stable respirations; pink, stable color; consistent tone; improve posture; calm, focused alertness-well-modulated sleep; responsive to authority, visual and social stimuli.
- Demonstrate self-regulatory skills as sucking, hand to mouth, hand holding, position changes.

The parent(s)/caregiver(s) will describe techniques to reduce environmental stress in agency, at home, or both.

- Describe situations that stress infant.
- Describe signs/symptoms of stress in infant.

General Interventions

> **NIC** Environmental Management, Neurologic Monitoring, Sleep Enhancement, Newborn Care, Parent Education: Newborn Positioning

Determine Causative/Contributing Factors.

Pain
Fatigue
Disorganized sleep–wake pattern
Feeding problems
Exessive stimulation (person, environment)

Reduce or Eliminate Contributing Factors, if Possible.

Pain

Observe infant before touching him or her.

Document infant's baseline behavioral manifestations.

Observe for responses different from baseline that have been associated with neonatal pain responses (Bozzette, 1993):

Facial responses (open mouth, brow bulge, grimace, chin quiver, nasolabial furrow, taut tongue)

Motor responses (flinch, muscle rigidity, clenched hands, withdrawal)

If unsure whether behavior indicates pain, but you suspect pain, consult with physician for an analgesic trial. Evaluate infant's response.

Aggressively manage obvious pain stimuli (eg, postsurgical, lack of feeding, painful procedures, hyperglycemia; Merenstein & Gardner, 1998).

Consult with physician for an analgesic.

Provide an analgesic before painful procedures.

Consider topical analgesia for frequent painful procedures (eg, heelstick, venipuncture).

When administering analgesics (Merenstein & Gardner, 1998):

Reduce initial dose and monitor respiratory response cautiously.

Determine optimal dose and interval.

Monitor when pain breaks through.

Determine if infant appears comfortable after the dose.

When indicated, wean infant slowly over a period of days from the drug. Assess response to withdrawal. Consult with physician to manage withdrawal symptoms if indicated.

Disrupted 24-h Diurnal Cycles

Evaluate the need for and frequency of each intervention.

Consider 24-h caregiving assignment and primary caregiving to provide consistent caregiving throughout the day and night for the infant from the onset of admission. This is important in terms of responding to increasingly more mature sleep cycles, feeding ability, and especially emotional development.

Consider supporting the infant's transition to and maintenance of sleep by avoiding peaks of frenzy and overexhaustion; continuously maintaining a calm, regular environment and schedule; and establishing a reliable, repeatable pattern of gradual transition into sleep in prone and side-lying positions in the isolette or crib.

Feeding Experience

Observe and record infant's readiness for participation with feeding.

Hunger cues

Transitioning to drowsy or alert state

Mouthing, rooting, or sucking

Bringing hands to mouth

Crying that is not relieved with pacifier or non-nutritive sucking alone

Physiologic stability

Look for regulated breathing patterns, stable color, and stable digestion.

Promote nurturing environment in support of coregulatory feeding experience.

Decrease environmental stimulation.

Provide comfortable seating (be especially sensitive to the needs of postpartum mothers: eg, soft cushions, small stool to elevate legs, supportive pillows for nursing).

Encourage softly swaddling the infant to facilitate flexion and balanced tone during feeding.

Explore feeding methods that meet the goals of both infant and family (eg, breast-feeding, bottle-feeding, gavage).

Support the Infant's Self-Regulatory Efforts.

When administering painful or stressful procedures, consider actions to enhance calmness.

Support the flexed position with another caregiver.

Provide opportunities to suck while shielding the infant from other stresses.

Consider the efficient execution of necessary manipulations while supporting the infant's behavioral organization.

Consider *unhurried* reorganization and stabilization of the infant's regulation (eg, position prone, give opportunities to hold onto caregiver's finger and suck, encase trunk and back of head in caregiver's hand, provide inhibition to soles of feet).

Consider removing extraneous stimulation (eg, stroking, talking, shifting position) to institute resta-
bilization. Consider spending 15 to 20 min after manipulation; over time, the infant's self-regulatory
abilities will improve, making the caregiver's intervention less important.

Consider supporting the infant's transition to and maintenance of sleep by avoiding peaks of frenzy
and overexhaustion; by continuously maintaining a calm, regular environment and schedule; and
by establishing a reliable, repeatable pattern of gradual transition into sleep in prone and side-
lying positions in the isolette or crib.

Consider initiating calming on the caregiver's body and then transferring the baby to the crib as necessary. For other infants, this may be too arousing, and transition is accomplished more easily in
the isolette with the provision of steady boundaries and encasing without any stimulation.

Critical review of use of the automatic swing may be indicated for irritable infants. For some
infants, it leads to momentary quieting, but not necessarily to increased internal regulatory
control over time.

Soothing, gentle instrumental music or the parent's voice is comforting for some infants during transition to sleep.

A nonstimulating sleep space with minimal exciting visual targets, social inputs, and so forth, may
need to be made available to facilitate relaxation before sleep. A regularly implemented sleep routine helps many infants.

Reduce Environmental Stimuli.

Noise (Merenstein & Gardner, 1998; Thomas, 1989)

Do not tap on incubator.

Place a folded blanket on top of the incubator if it is the only work surface available.

Slowly open and close porthole.

Pad incubator doors to reduce banging.

Use plastic instead of metal waste cans.

Remove water from ventilator tubing.

Speak softly at the bedside and only when necessary.

Slowly drop the head of the mattress.

Eliminate radios.

Close doors slowly.

Position the infant's bed away from sources of noise (eg, telephone, intercom, unit equipment).

Consider the following methods to reduce unnecessary noise in the NICU:

Perform rounds away from the bedsides.

Adapt large equipment to eliminate noise and clutter.

Alert staff when the decibel level in the unit exceeds 60 db (eg, by a light attached to a sound meter).
Institute quiet time for 10 min to lower noise.

Move more vulnerable infants out of unit traffic patterns.

Lights

Use full-spectrum instead of white light at bedside. Avoid fluorescent lights.

Cover cribs, incubators, and radiant warmers completely during sleep and partially during awake
periods.

Install dimmer switches, shades, and curtains. Avoid bright lights.

Shade infants' eyes with a blanket tent or cutout box.

Avoid visual stimuli on cribs.

Shield eyes from bright procedure lights. Avoid patches unless for phototherapy.

Position Baby in Postures that Permit Flexion and Minimize Flailing.

Consider gentle, *unhurried* reorganization and stabilization of infant's regulation by supporting
the infant in softly tucked prone position, giving opportunities to hold onto caregiver's finger and
suck, encasing trunk and back of head in caregiver's hand, and providing inhibition to soles
of feet.

Use the prone/side-lying position.

Avoid the supine position.

Swaddle baby, if possible, to maintain flexion.

Create a nest using soft bedding (eg, natural sheepskin, soft cotton, flannel).

Avoid oversized diapers to allow you to perceive normal hip alignment

Avoid tension on lines or tubing.

Reduce the Stress Associated with Handling.

When moving or lifting the infant, contain him or her with your hands by wrapping or placing rolled blankets around his or her body.

Maintain containment during procedures and caregiving activities.

Handle slowly and gently. Avoid stroking.

Initiate all interactions and treatments with one sense stimulus at a time (eg, touch), then slowly progress to visual, auditory, and movement.

Assess child for cues for readiness, impending disorganization, or stability; respond to cues.

Support minimal disruption of the infant's own evolving 24-h sleep–wake cycles.

Use PRN instead of routine suctioning or postural drainage.

Use minimal adhesive tape. Remove any carefully.

Reduce Disorganized Behavior During Active Interventions and Transport.

Have a plan for transport, with assigned roles for each team member.

Establish behavior cues of stress on this infant with the primary nurse before transport.

Minimize sensory input.

> Use calm, quiet voices.
>
> Shade the infant's eyes from light.
>
> Protect infant from unnecessary touch.

Support the infant's softly tucked postures with your hands and offer something to grasp (your finger or corner of a soft blanket or cloth).

Swaddle the infant or place him or her in a nest made of blankets.

Ensure that the transport equipment (eg, ventilator) is ready. Warm mattress or use sheepskin.

Carefully and smoothly move the infant. Avoid talking, if possible.

Consider conducting caregiving routines while parent(s) or designated caregiver hold infant, whenever possible.

Reposition in 2 to 3 hours or sooner if infant behavior suggests discomfort.

Engage Parents in Planning Care.

Encourage them to share their feelings, fears, and expectations.

Consider involving parents in creating the family's developmental plan (Cole & Frappier, 1985)

> My strengths are: These things stress me:
>
> Time-out signals: How you can help me:

Teach caregivers to continually observe the changing capabilities to determine the appropriate positioning and bedding options, eg, infant may fight containment (Wong, 2003).

Initiate Health Teaching and Referrals as Indicated.

Review the Following Information Relating to Growth and Development of the Infant and Family in Anticipatory Guidance for Home.

Health concerns

Feeding	Hygiene	Illness
Infection	Safety	Temperature
Growth and development		

State modulation

Appropriate stimulation	Sleep–wake patterns

Parent–infant interaction

Behavior cues	Signs of stress

Infant's environment

Animate, inanimate stimulation	Playing with infant	Role of father and siblings

Parental coping and support

Support network	Challenges	Problem solving

Discuss Transition to Community Supports (Nursing Respite, Social and Civic Groups, Religious Affiliations).

Refer for Follow-Up Home Visits.

Rationales

- When a premature newborn is ill, the combination of immature CNS, exposure to inappropriate and unexpected patterned sensory input, and multiple caregivers leads to disorganization and imbalance of the behavioral indices to regulation.
- Preterm infants may have difficulty or demonstrate disorganization in the progression of their feeding behaviors (eg, readiness, availability of hunger cues) and gastrointestinal motility (eg, esophageal motility, intestinal motility, gastric emptying time).
- "If care providers are unsure whether a behavior indicates pain, and if there is a reason to suspect pain, an analgesic trial can be diagnostic as well as therapeutic" (Acute Pain Management Guideline Panel, 1992a, p. 12).
- Pharmacologic treatments may not be the first line of intervention with all infants. Nonpharmacologic methods (eg, rocking) may be appropriate.
- Noise levels in NICUs are hazardous because of potential damage to the cochlea with subsequent hearing loss, and because of arousal effects on infants who cannot inhibit their responses. Noise interferes with sleep, increases heart rate, and leads to vasoconstriction (Blackburn, 1993). The infant expends energy he or she needs to grow and to supply the brain with glucose and oxygen (Thomas, 1989).
- Thomas (1989) found that NICUs have a loud, continuous pattern of background noise. In addition, peak noises over the continuous noise level can raise the decibel level 10-fold. Examples of peak noises are monitor alarms (67 db), NICU radios (62 db), openings of plastic sleeves (67 db), tappings of hoods (70 db), and sinks (66 db).
- Stroking preterm infants who are unstable results in decreased levels of oxygen saturation (Harrison et al., 1996).
- "Vision is the least mature of newborn's senses" (Wong, 2003 p. 365). The preterm infant cannot adjust visually and will be stressed (Wong, 2003).
- Fluorescent lighting and lights over 150 ftc should be avoided.

RISK FOR DISORGANIZED INFANT BEHAVIOR

DEFINITION
Risk for Disorganized Infant Behavior: State in which the neonate is at risk for an alteration in integration and modulation of the physiologic and behavioral systems of adaptation (autonomic, motor, state, organizational, self-regulatory, and attentional–interactional)

RISK FACTORS
Refer to Related Factors.

RELATED FACTORS
Refer to *Disorganized Infant Behavior*.

Focus Assessment Criteria

Refer to *Disorganized Infant Behavior*.

General Interventions

Refer to *Disorganized Infant Behavior*.

READINESS FOR ENHANCED ORGANIZED INFANT BEHAVIOR

DEFINITION

Readiness for Enhanced Organized Infant Behavior: A pattern of modulation of the physiologic and behavioral systems of functioning of an infant (ie, autonomic, motor, state, organizational, self-regulatory, and attentional–interactional) that is satisfactory but that can be improved, resulting in higher levels of integration in response to environmental stimuli

DEFINING CHARACTERISTICS (BLACKBURN & VANDENBERG, 1993)
Autonomic System

Regulated color and respiration	Reduced tremors, twitches
Reduced visceral signals (eg, smooth)	Digestive functioning, feeding tolerance

Motor System

Smooth, well-modulated posture and tone
Synchronous smooth movements with:

Hand/foot clasping	Suck/suck searching
Grasping	Hand holding
Hand-to-mouth activity	Tucking

State System

Well-differentiated range of states	Clear, robust sleep states
Active self-quieting/consoling	Focused, shiny-eyed alertness with intent or animated facial expressions
"Ooh" face	Attentional smiling
Cooing	

RELATED FACTORS

Because this is a diagnosis of effective functioning, the use of related factors is not warranted.

⊕ AUTHOR'S NOTE

This diagnosis describes an infant who is responding to the environment with stable and predictable autonomic, motor, and state cues. The focus of interventions is to promote continued stable development and to reduce excess environmental stimuli that may stress the infant. Because this is a wellness diagnosis, use of related factors is not needed. The nurse can write the diagnostic statement as *Readiness for Enhanced Organized Infant Behavior as evidenced by ability to regulate autonomic, motor, and state systems to environmental stimuli.*

KEY CONCEPTS
Generic Considerations

See *Disorganized Infant Behavior.*

Focus Assessment Criteria

Objective Data
Assess for Defining Characteristics.

Ability to regulate

Respiratory rate	Color	Cardiac rate

Autonomic/visceral stability

Smooth digestive functioning	Reduced twitches, tremors

Posture/tone

Smooth	Well modulated	Balanced flexion/extension
Midline oriented		

Synchronous, smooth movements

Hand/foot clasping	Grasping	Hand-to-mouth activity
Suck/suck searching	Hand holding	Tucking
Symmetric movements		

Sleep–wake states

Well-differentiated range	Organized alertness	Clear states from deep sleep
Robust cry		

Self-regulatory ability

Balance of engaging and withdrawal
Ability to orient and arouse to visual or auditory stimuli

Reciprocal interactions

Eye contact	Exploratory behavior	Mutual gazing
Easy consolation	Reaching toward	Attending to social stimuli

Goals

> **NOC** Child Development: Specify Age, Sleep, Comfort Level

The infant will continue age-appropriate growth and development and not experience excessive environmental stimuli.
The parent(s) will demonstrate handling that promotes stability.

Indicators
- Describe developmental needs of infant.
- Describe signs of stress or exhaustion.
- Demonstrate:
  - Gentle, soothing touch
  - Melodic tone of voice, coos
  - Mutual gazing
  - Rhythmic movements
  - Acknowledgment of all baby's vocalizations
  - Recognition of soothing qualities of actions

General Interventions

> **NIC** Developmental Care, Infant Care, Sleep Enhancement, Environmental Management: Comfort, Parent Education: Infant, Attachment Promotion, Caregiver Support, Calming Technique

Explain to Parents the Effects of Excess Environmental Stress on the Infant.

Provide a list of signs of stress for their infant.
Teach them to terminate stimulation if infant shows signs of stress.
Instruct parents to, when providing developmental intervention(s):
  Offer only when the infant is alert (if possible, show parents examples of alert and not alert).
  Begin with one stimulus at a time (touch, voice).
  Provide intervention for a short time.
  Increase interventions according to infant's cues.
  Provide frequent, short interventions instead of infrequent, long-term ones.

Explain to Parents the Developmental Needs of Infants.
Stimulation (visual, auditory, vestibular, tactile, olfactory, gustatory)
Periods of alertness
Sleep requirements

Explain, Role-Model, and Observe Parents Engaging in Developmental Interventions.

Visual
Eye-to-eye contact
Face-to-face experiences
High-contrast colors, geometric shapes (eg, black and white shapes on paper mobile); up to 4 weeks, simple mobiles of four dessert-size paper plates with stripes, four-square checkerboards, a black dot, and a simple bull's eye, hung 10 to 13 inches from baby's eyes.

Auditory
Use high-pitched vocalizations.
Play classical music softly.
Use a variety of voice inflections.
Avoid loud talking.
Call infant by name.
Avoid monotone speech patterns.

Vestibular (Movement)
Rock baby in chair.
Place infant in sling and rock.
Close infant's fist around a soft toy.
Slowly change position during handling.
Provide head support.

Tactile
Use firm, gentle touch as initial approach.
Use skin-to-skin contact in a warm room.
Provide alternative textures (eg, sheepskin, velvet, satin).
Avoid stroking if responses are disorganized.

Olfactory
Wear a light perfume.

Gustatory
Allow non-nutritive sucking (eg, pacifier, hand in mouth).

Promote Adjustment and Stability to Caregiving Activities (Blackburn & Vandenberg, 1993; Merenstein & Gardner, 1998).

Waking
Enter room slowly.
Turn on light and open curtains slowly.
Avoid waking baby if he or she is asleep.

Changing
Keep room warm.
Gently change position: contain limbs during movement.
Stop changing if infant is irritable.

Feeding
Time feedings with alert states.
Eliminate unnecessary noise.
Hold infant close and, if needed, swaddle in blanket.

Bathing
Ventral openness may be stressful. Cover body parts not being bathed.
Proceed slowly; allow for rest.
Offer a pacifier or hand to suck.
Eliminate unnecessary noise.
Use a soft, soothing voice.

Explain Need to Reduce Environmental Stimuli When Taking Infant Outside.

Shelter eyes from light.
Swaddle the infant so his or her hands can reach the mouth.
Protect from loud noises.

Praise Parent(s) on Interaction Patterns; Point Out Infant's Engaging Responses.

Initiate Health Teaching and Referrals if Needed.

Explain that developmental interventions will change with maturity. Refer to *Delayed Growth and Development* for specific age-related developmental needs.
Provide parent(s) with resources for assistance at home (eg, community resources).

Rationales

Refer to Rationales under *Disorganized Infant Behavior.*

RISK FOR INFECTION

DEFINITION

Risk for Infection: State in which a person is at risk to be invaded by an opportunistic or pathogenic agent (virus, fungus, bacteria, protozoa, or other parasite) from endogenous or exogenous sources

RISK FACTORS

See Related Factors.

RELATED FACTORS

Various health problems and situations can create favorable conditions that would encourage the development of infections.* Some common factors follow.

Pathophysiologic

Related to compromised host defenses secondary to:

Cancer	*Altered or insufficient leukocytes*	Arthritis
Respiratory disorders	*Periodontal disease*	Renal failure
Hematologic disorders	Hepatic disorders	Diabetes mellitus
Acquired immunodeficiency syndrome (AIDS)		
Alcoholism		
Immunosuppression		
Immunodeficiency secondary to: specify		

Related to compromised circulation secondary to:

Lymphedema	Obesity	Peripheral vascular disease

Treatment-Related

Related to a site for organism invasion secondary to:

Surgery	Invasive lines	Dialysis
Intubation	Total parenteral nutrition	Enteral feedings

*See Key Concepts.

Related to compromised host defenses secondary to:
Radiation therapy
Organ transplant
Medication therapy (specify; eg, chemotherapy, immunosuppressants)

Situational (Personal, Environmental)
Related to compromised host defenses secondary to:

History of infections	Malnutrition	Prolonged immobility
Stress	Increased hospital stay	Smoking

Related to a site for organism invasion secondary to:
Trauma (accidental, intentional)
Postpartum period
Bites (animal, insect, human)
Thermal injuries
Warm, moist, dark environment (skin folds, casts)

Related to contact with contagious agents (nosocomial or community acquired)

Maturational
Newborns
Related to increased vulnerability of infant secondary to:
Lack of maternal antibodies (dependent on maternal exposures)
Lack of normal flora
Open wounds (umbilical, circumcision)
Immature immune system

Infant/Child/Adolescent
Related to increased vulnerability secondary to:

Lack of immunization	Multiple sex partners

Older Adult
Related to increased vulnerability secondary to:

Diminished immune response	Debilitated condition	Chronic diseases

---

◯◯ AUTHOR'S NOTE

All people are at risk for infection. Secretion control, environmental control, and handwashing before and after client care reduce the risk of transmission of organisms. Included in the population at risk for infection is a smaller group at high risk for infection. *Risk for Infection* describes a person whose host defenses are compromised, thus increasing susceptibility to environmental pathogens or his or her own endogenous flora (eg, a person with chronic liver dysfunction or with an invasive line). Nursing interventions for such a person focus on minimizing introduction of organisms and increasing resistance to infection (eg, improving nutritional status). For a person with an infection, the situation is best described by the collaborative problem *PC: Sepsis.*

Risk for Infection Transmission describes a person at high risk for transferring an infectious agent to others. Some people are at high risk both for acquiring opportunistic agents and for transmitting infecting organisms, warranting the use of both *Risk for Infection* and *Risk for Infection Transmission.*

◯◯ ERRORS IN DIAGNOSTIC STATEMENTS

1. *Risk for Infection related to progression of sepsis secondary to failure to treat infection*
   Sepsis is a collaborative problem, not a nursing diagnosis. This person is not at risk for infection; rather, he or she requires medical and nursing interventions to treat the sepsis and prevent septic shock.
2. *Risk for Infection related to direct access to bladder mucosa secondary to Foley catheter and lack of staff knowledge of aseptic technique*

⊙⊙ ERRORS IN DIAGNOSTIC STATEMENTS (*Continued*)

If the staff's lack of knowledge of aseptic technique is valid, the nurse should proceed with reporting the situation to nursing management in an incident report. Adding this to a nursing diagnosis statement would be legally and professionally inadvisable. Nurses never should use nursing diagnostic statements to criticize a client, group, or member of the health team or to expose unsafe or unprofessional practices or behavior. Nurses must use other organizational channels of communication for these purposes.

KEY CONCEPTS
Generic Considerations

- Resistance to infection depends on the host's immune response (*susceptibility*), dose of the infecting agent, and virulence of the organism. Factors influencing the host's immune response include the following:
  - Anatomic barriers—each system has specific lines of defenses.
  - Therapies—pose a threat to normal lines of defense by either invasiveness or alteration of body function.
  - Developmental and heritable factors—factors that negatively affect the person's immune system function (eg, newborn status; agammaglobulinemia).
  - Hormonal factors—males are more vulnerable to infection than are females; pregnancy increases the female's vulnerability; steroid therapy increases vulnerability in both sexes.
  - Age—includes both extremes (immaturity or degeneration of immune system).
  - Nutrition—influences protein synthesis and phagocytosis, decreasing the body's vulnerability to infection.
  - Fever—hyperthermia may inhibit the growth of organisms; hypothermia may decrease the effects of the fever.
  - Secretions such as mucus, saliva, and skin secretions—contain substances that are bactericidal, decreasing the risk of infection and colonization.
  - Endotoxins, a product of some gram-negative bacteria—have a limited ability to kill other bacteria or increase a person's resistance to some infections.
  - Interference—the interaction between two distinct organisms that are parasitizing the host leads to interference, in which one remains dominant and the other is suppressed.
- The inflammatory response consists of (1) activation of leukocytes, (2) plasma proteins, which localize and phagocytize the infectious process, and (3) increased blood and lymph flow, which dilutes and flushes out toxic materials; this process causes a local increase in temperature.
- Phagocytosis is the process by which parasites are removed by engulfment and digestion.

Host Defenses
Specific host defenses of each system that influence the immune response include the following:

Central nervous system (CNS)
Because the most common route for both bacterial and viral infections of the CNS is the hematogenous route, blood host defenses play an important primary role.
Cutaneous
- Skin provides a first line of defense against organisms, both anatomically and chemically.
- Sweat glands and sebaceous glands do not allow overgrowth of bacteria.
- The acid pH of the skin does not allow pathogenic organisms to grow or survive on the skin for any length of time.
- The flushing and lysozyme actions of tears control eye infections. The lacrimal duct flushes out organisms and deposits them in the nasopharynx.

Blood
- Circulating blood is the major vehicle for transporting internal defense mechanisms.
- The febrile response is associated with the circulation of pyrogens to the hypothalamus.

Genitourinary tract
- Anatomic structure eliminates easy ascent of perineal microorganisms into the bladder.
- Mucous layer allows entrapment of organisms and engulfment by bladder cells.
- The pH and osmolality of urine prevent bacterial multiplication.
- The ability to empty the bladder completely eliminates stasis of invading organisms and allows continual flushing.

Respiratory tract
- The nares entrap most foreign matter on the mucous membranes as a result of turbulence caused by the turbinates and hairs.
- The mucociliary transport system consists of cilia and mucus, which remove additional matter passing to the upper and lower bronchi.
- Lysozymes and immunoglobulin A (IgA), a secretion of phagocytes, are found in nasal secretions and assist in the prevention of colonization.
- Particles reaching as far as the alveoli can be removed through the expulsive action of sneezing and coughing, and the gag reflex.
- Phagocytosis occurs in the alveoli, with the macrophages used as a major defense mechanism.

Gastrointestinal tract
- A mucous layer traps ingested microbes in the epithelium of the gastrointestinal (GI) tract.
- Gastric acids kill most organisms.
- Peristalsis aids in the removal of organisms.
- Intestinal secretions contain antibody (IgA), bile salts, lysozyme, glycolipids, and glycoproteins that prevent proliferation and adherence.
- Normal gut flora interact to restrict overproliferation.

Wounds
- Skin provides a first line of defense; the opening of the skin, either surgically or traumatically, potentiates infection.
- A wound essentially closes within 24 h, eliminating the risk of direct inoculations of organisms.
- Wound infections rely on the capabilities of other host defenses to assist in healing.
- Risk factors associated with wound infections depend on (1) endogenous factors such as the presence of confounding factors, skin preparation, and the use of prophylactic antibiotics; and (2) exogenous factors such as the preoperative scrub, barrier techniques, airborne contamination, environmental disinfection, wound care, and the condition of the wound at the time of closure.
- Wounds are at risk for infection owing to the following factors:
  - Sutures and staples, unlike tape, create their own wounds, act like drains, and cause their own inflammatory response.
  - Drains provide a site for microorganism entry.
  - The incidence of infection in clients who are not shaved or clipped is 0.9%. It increases to 1.4% with electric shaving, 1.7% with clipping, and 2.5% with razor shaving (Kovach, 1990).

Pediatric Considerations

- Congenital infections, those acquired in utero, usually result from exposure to such viruses as cytomegalovirus, rubella, hepatitis B, herpes simplex, herpes zoster, varicella, and Epstein-Barr. Nonviral agents also may cause some infections, such as toxoplasmosis, syphilis, tuberculosis, trypanosomiasis, and malaria.
- Congenital bacterial infections may arise from bacterial organisms that travel to the fetus through the placenta. The fetus also may become infected by organisms that reach the amniotic cavity through the mother's cervix (Reeder et al., 1997).
- Fetal skin and mucous membranes, intervillous placenta spaces, the umbilical cord, and respiratory airways (through aspiration) provide other avenues of infection.
- Approximately 80% of all childhood illnesses are infections, with respiratory infections occurring two to three times as often as other illnesses combined (Wong, 2003).
- In general, acute illness is less frequent in children younger than 6 months, increases from then until 3 or 4 years of age, and then gradually decreases throughout childhood (Wong, 1999).
- According to Kliegman (1990), newborns are at increased risk for infections. By the time a child is a toddler, production of antibodies is well established. Phagocytosis is much more efficient in toddlers than in infants (Wong, 2003).
- Children who attend day care centers are at increased risk for infections caused by *Shigella*, rotavirus, *Haemophilus influenzae* type b, and hepatitis A (Wong, 2003).
- Good hygiene, optimal nutrition, immunizations, and strict sanitary practices can reduce the incidence of infectious disease during childhood.
- Perinatal transmission of HIV occurs in utero, intrapartum, or after delivery through breastfeeding. Rate of transmission can range from 15% to 30% (Wong, 2003).

Pediatric Considerations (continued)

- Perinatal HIV transmission can be reduced with antiviral treatment of the pregnant woman and her newborn (Wong, 2003).
- Perinatally inflicted children have a more rapid progression of the disease because of the immaturity of their immune system (Wong, 2003).
- They develop symptoms by 18 to 24 months of age. Malabsorption of carbohydrates, portions, and fats is seen in both symptomatic and asymptomatic HIV-infected children (Wong, 2003).
- The high prevalence of risky sexual behavior among teenagers contributes to the high rates of sexually-transmitted infections and pregnancy (CDC, 2000).
- Each year 1 in 6 teenagers acquires an STD (CDC, 2000).

Geriatric Considerations

- A slower rate of epidermal proliferation causes injured skin to take twice as long to heal in older adults.
- Older adults also have compromised dermal immunologic responses because of a reduced number of Langerhans cells and reduced microcirculation (Miller, 2004).
- In older adults, the lung's alveolar surface and elastic recoil are slightly decreased, and gas exchange in lower lung regions is decreased (Miller, 2004).
- Age-related changes in respiratory function do not significantly increase risk for infection. Rather, non–age-related risk factors, such as smoking and exposure to occupational toxins, increase risk.
- Studies have shown 5% to 20% of residents in long-term care facilities to have infections. The most frequent are those of the urinary tract, respiratory system, and skin and soft tissues (usually pressure ulcers; Miller, 2004).
- The increased susceptibility of older adults to infections is multifactorial (either host factors or environmental). Host factors include underlying diseases, invasive treatment modalities, indiscriminate use of antibiotics, malnutrition, dehydration, impaired mobility, and incontinence. Environmental factors in institutions include limited surveillance for infection, crowded areas, cross-contamination, and delay in early detection.
- Skin and urinary tract colonization is a greater problem in older than in younger clients. Changes in immune competence with aging increase susceptibility to fungal, viral, and mycobacterial pathogens (Miller, 2004).
- Older adults do not exhibit the usual signs of infection (fever, chills, tachypnea, tachycardia, leukocytosis) but, instead, present with anorexia, weakness, change in mental status, normothermia, or hypothermia (Miller, 2004).

Transcultural Considerations

- The incidence of tuberculosis in American Indians is 7 to 15 times that of non-Indians. African-Americans have an incidence 3 times that of white Americans. Urban American Jews are the most resistant to tuberculosis.
- Susceptibility to disease may also be environmental or a combination of genetic, psychosocial, and environmental factors (Giger & Davidhizar, 2004).
- Among Americans with AIDS, 1 of every 4 persons is African-American, while 1 in 7 infected with AIDS is Hispanic (CDC, 2001).
- African-American women are the fastest-growing segment of the population to be infected by HIV (CDC, 2001).
- American Indians and Alaskan natives have twice the reported rate of gonorrhea and syphilis than other Americans (Giger & Davidhizar, 2004).
- Patient education regarding safe sex in many religions is difficult because according to the Torah, the Bible, and other "holy books," homosexuality is an abomination and premarital sexual activity is not permitted (Giger & Davidhizar, 2004).

Focus Assessment Criteria

Subjective Data
Assess for Related Factors.

Does the person complain of:
Previous infections
Pain or swelling (generalized, localized)
Hemoptysis
Productive, prolonged cough
Chest pain associated with other criteria
Systemic symptoms

Fever, continuous or intermittent	Easy fatigability	Chills
	Night sweats	Weight loss
Loss of appetite		

History of recent travel
Within United States
Outside United States

History of exposure to infectious diseases
Airborne (most childhood infections result from communicable diseases [eg, chickenpox, tuberculosis])
Vector-borne and other vector-associated infections (malaria, plague)
Vehicle-borne and other food- and water-borne infections (hepatitis A, salmonellas)
Contact spread (most common type of exposure)
    Direct (person to person)
    Indirect (eg, by instruments, clothing, and so forth)
Contact droplet (eg, pneumonias, colds)

History of risk factors associated with infections (see Related Factors)

Objective Data
Assess for Related Factors.
Presence of wounds
    Surgical
    Burns
    Invasive devices (tracheostomy, intravenous (IV), drains)
    Self-induced
Temperature, abnormal
Nutritional deficiency

For more information on Focus Assessment Criteria, visit http://connection.lww.com.

Goal

NOC Infection Status, Wound Healing: Primary Intention, Immune Status

The person will report risk factors associated with infection and precautions needed.

Indicators
- Demonstrate meticulous handwashing technique by the time of discharge.
- Describe methods of transmission of infection.
- Describe the influence of nutrition on prevention of infection.

General Interventions

NIC Infection Control, Wound Care, Incision Site Care, Health Education

Identify Clients at High Risk for Nosocomial Infections (Owen & Grier, 1987).
Assess for Predictors that Increase the Risk of Infection.
Remote site of infection
Abdominal or thoracic surgery

Surgical procedure longer than 2 h
Genitourinary procedure
Instrumentation (ventilator, suction, catheters, nebulizers, tracheostomy, invasive monitoring)
Anesthesia

Assess for Confounding Factors.
Age younger than 1 year or older than 65 years
Obesity
Underlying disease conditions (chronic obstructive pulmonary disease [COPD], diabetes, cardio-
  vascular, blood dyscrasias)
Substance abuse
Medications (steroids, chemotherapy, antibiotic therapy) that modify immune response
Nutritional status (intake less than minimum daily requirements)
Smoking

Consider a Person with One or More Predictors and One or More Confounding Factors to be at Risk for Infection.

Consider Those with the Following Factors at Risk for Delayed Wound Healing:

Malnourishment	Tobacco Use	Obesity
Anemia	Diabetes	Cancer
Corticosteroid therapy	Renal insufficiency	Hypovolemia
Hypoxia	Surgery >3 h	Night or emergency surgery
Zinc, copper, magnesium deficiency	Immune system compromise	

Reduce Entry of Organisms into Clients (Owen & Grier, 1987).

Surgical Wound
Before surgery, assess client for risk of remote site of infection.
If surgery is abdominal, teach client (preoperatively) the importance of and correct technique for
  coughing, turning, and deep breathing.
If surgery is longer than 2 h, assess client every shift for signs and symptoms of infection at the
  surgical site.
Monitor temperature every 4 h; notify physician if temperature is greater than 100.8°F.
Assess nutritional status to provide adequate protein and caloric intake for healing.
Assess wound site every 24 h and during dressing changes; document any abnormal findings.
Evaluate all abnormal laboratory findings, especially culture/sensitivities and complete blood
  count (CBC).
Notify epidemiologist of any abnormal findings related to the development of infection.
Administer all prophylactic antibiotics within 15 min of scheduled administration to ensure ade-
  quate therapeutic levels at surgery.
Instruct client and family on appropriate aseptic practice.
Use aseptic technique during dressing changes.
Use universal precautions with all body fluids from client.

Urinary Tract
Evaluate all abnormal laboratory findings, especially cultures/sensitivities and CBC.
Assess for abnormal signs and symptoms after any urologic procedure, including frequency, urgency,
  burning, abnormal color, and odor.
Monitor client's temperature at least every 24 h for elevation; notify physician if temperature is
  greater than 100.8°F.
Encourage fluids when appropriate.
Notify epidemiologist of any abnormal findings related to the development of infection.
Assess other wounds and systems to evaluate client's increased risk for development of infections at
  other sites.
Instruct client and family as to risk for development of urinary tract infections.
Use universal precautions with all fluids from client.
Use aseptic technique when emptying any urinary drainage device; keep bag off the floor, but below
  bladder or clamped during transport.
Administer all antibiotics within 15 min of scheduled administration to maintain adequate thera-
  peutic levels.
Reassess need for indwelling urinary catheter daily.

Circulatory

Assess all invasive lines every 24 h for redness, inflammation, drainage, and tenderness.

Monitor client's temperature at least every 24 h; notify physician if greater than 100.8°F.

Maintain aseptic technique for all invasive devices, changing sites, dressings, tubing, and solutions per policy schedule.

Evaluate all abnormal laboratory findings, especially cultures/sensitivities and CBC.

Notify epidemiologist of any abnormal findings related to the development of infection.

Administer all antibiotics within 15 min of scheduled administration.

Instruct client and family on appropriate aseptic practices to prevent infection.

Use universal precautions with all body fluids from client.

Assess client's nutritional status to provide adequate protein and caloric intake for healing.

Evaluate client for secondary sites of infection, either to bloodstream from another site or from bloodstream to other risk sites.

Respiratory Tract

Evaluate risk for infection after any instrumentation of the respiratory tract for at least 48 h after procedure.

Notify epidemiologist of any abnormal findings related to the development of infection.

Monitor temperature at least every 8 h and notify physician if greater than 100.8°F.

Evaluate sputum characteristics for frequency, purulence, blood, odor.

Evaluate sputum and blood cultures, if done, for significant findings.

Evaluate CBC for significant shift in white blood cell counts.

Assess lung sounds every 8 h or PRN.

If client has abdominal/thoracic surgery, instruct before surgery on importance of coughing, turning, and deep breathing.

If client has had anesthesia, monitor for appropriate clearing of secretions in lung fields.

Administer cardiopulmonary treatments as ordered, with assessment of response to treatment documented.

Evaluate need for suctioning if client cannot clear secretions adequately.

Use universal precautions with all body fluids from client.

Use aseptic technique with all invasive procedures of the respiratory tract.

Assess for risk of aspiration, keeping head of bed elevated 30 degrees unless otherwise contraindicated.

Assess client's nutritional status to provide adequate protein and caloric intake for healing.

If oral feedings are not tolerated without aspiration, contact physician for further action.

Instruct on principles of cough and deep breathing and prevention of infection.

Protect the Client with Immune Deficiency from Infection.

Place client in private room.

Instruct client to ask all visitors and personnel to wash their hands before approaching.

Limit visitors when appropriate.

Screen all visitors for known infections or exposure to infections.

Limit invasive devices to those that are necessary.

Teach client and family members signs and symptoms of infection.

Evaluate client's personal hygiene habits.

Provide immune globulin to those exposed to specific diseases that might be life-threatening (eg, chickenpox, hepatitis, measles).

Reduce Client's Susceptibility to Infection.

Encourage and maintain caloric and protein intake in diet (see *Imbalanced Nutrition*).

Assess client for adequate immunizations against childhood diseases, bacterial infections (eg, pneumonia, *Haemophilus influenzae*), and other viral infections (eg, influenza).

Monitor use or overuse of antimicrobial therapy.

Administer prescribed antimicrobial therapy within 15 min of schedule.

Observe for clinical manifestations of infection in clients at high risk.

Minimize length of stay in hospital to prevent colonization with nosocomial organisms.

Observe for superinfection in clients receiving antimicrobial therapy.

Initiate Health Teaching and Referrals, as Indicated.

Instruct client and family regarding the causes, risks, and communicability of the infection.

Report communicable diseases as appropriate to public health department.

Collaborate with nurse epidemiologist on needs of client and family.

Rationales

- Intervention can be implemented to control or influence the degree of risk associated with predictors and confounding factors (Owen & Grier, 1987).
- Nurses must use precautions with blood and body fluids from all clients to protect themselves from exposure to all potentially infectious organisms (CDC, 2000).
  - Wash hands before and after all client or specimen contact.
  - Handle the blood of all clients as potentially infectious.
  - Wear gloves for potential contact with blood and body fluids.
  - Place used syringes immediately in nearby impermeable container; avoid recapping or manipulating needle! Recapping or needle removal must be accomplished through the use of a mechanical device or a one-handed technique.
  - Wear protective eyewear and mask if splatter with blood or body fluids is possible (eg, bronchoscopy, oral surgery).
  - Wear gowns when splash with blood or body fluids is anticipated.
  - Handle all linen soiled with blood or body secretions as potentially infectious.
  - Process all laboratory specimens as potentially infectious.
  - Wear mask for tuberculosis and other respiratory organisms (human immunodeficiency virus [HIV] is not airborne).
  - Place resuscitation equipment where respiratory arrest is predictable.
  - Wear shoe covers or surgical caps or hoods when gross contamination can reasonably be anticipated (eg, autopsy, orthopedic surgery, obstetrics).
- Antibiotics administered at proper intervals ensure maintenance of therapeutic levels.
- Handwashing reduces the risk of cross-contamination.
- Subtle changes in vital signs may be early signs of sepsis, particularly fever.
- Wound healing by primary intention requires a dressing to protect it from contamination until the edges seal (usually 24 h). Wound healing by secondary intention requires a dressing to maintain adequate hydration; the dressing is not needed after wound edges seal.
- To repair tissue, the body needs increased protein and carbohydrate intake and adequate hydration for vascular transport of oxygen and wastes.

Risk for Infection Transmission
Related to Lack of Knowledge of Reducing the Risk of Transmitting the AIDS Virus

---

RISK FOR INFECTION TRANSMISSION*

DEFINITION
Risk for Infection Transmission: The state in which an individual is at risk for transferring an opportunistic or pathogenic agent to others

RISK FACTORS
Presence of risk factors (see Related Factors)

RELATED FACTORS
Pathophysiologic
Related to:
Colonization with highly antibiotic-resistant organism
Airborne transmission exposure
Contact transmission exposure (direct, indirect, contact droplet)
Vehicle transmission exposure
Vector-borne transmission exposure

Treatment-Related
Related to contaminated wound
Related to devices with contaminated drainage:
Urinary, chest, endotracheal tubes
Suction equipment

Situational (Personal, Environmental)
Related to:
Unsanitary living conditions (sewage, personal hygiene)
Areas considered high risk for vector-borne diseases (malaria, rabies, bubonic plague)
Areas considered high risk for vehicle-borne disease (hepatitis A, *Shigella, Salmonella*)
Lack of knowledge of sources or prevention of infection
Intravenous drug use
Multiple sex partners
Natural disaster (*e.g.,* flood, hurricane)
Disaster with hazardous infectious material

Maturational
Newborn
Related to birth outside hospital setting in uncontrolled environment
Related to exposure during prenatal or perinatal period to communicable disease through mother

---

*This diagnosis is not currently on the NANDA list but has been included for clarity or usefulness.

KEY CONCEPTS
Generic Considerations

- To spread an infection, three elements are required (Figure II.2):
  - A source of infecting organism
  - A susceptible host
  - A means of transmission for the organism
- Sources of infecting organisms include the following:
  - Clients, personnel, and visitors with acute disease, incubating infection, or colonized organisms without apparent disease
  - Person's own endogenous flora (autogenous infection)
  - Inanimate environment, including equipment and medications
- Susceptibility of the host varies according to
  - Immune status
  - Ability to develop a commensal relationship with the infecting organism and become an asymptomatic carrier
  - Preexisting diseases
- Means of transmission for the organism include one or more of the following:
  - Contact transmission, the most frequent method of transferring organisms, can be divided into three subgroups:

    Direct contact—involves direct physical transfer between a susceptible host and an infected or colonized person

    Indirect contact—involves the exchange of organisms between a host and contaminated objects, usually inanimate

    Droplet contact—involves an infected person transferring organisms into the conjunctivae, nose, or mouth of a susceptible host by coughing, sneezing, or talking. Droplets travel no more than 3 feet.

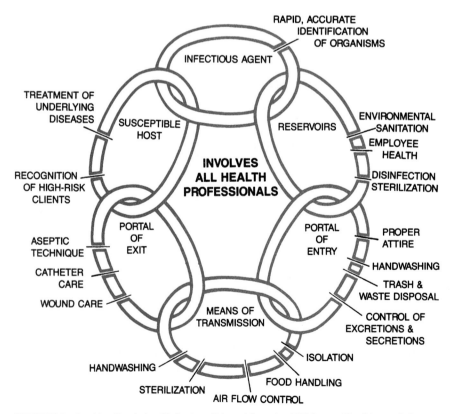

FIGURE II.2 Breaking the chain of infection. (Adapted from the APIC Starter Kit with permission from the Association for Professionals in Infection Control and Epidemiology. Washington, DC, copyright APIC, 1978.)

- Vehicle route transmission infections are spread through means such as:
  Food (eg, hepatitis A, *Salmonella*)
  Water (eg, *Legionella*)
  Drugs (eg, IV-contaminated products)
  Blood (eg, hepatitis B, hepatitis C, HIV)
  - Airborne infections are disseminated by droplet nuclei (residue of evaporated droplets that may remain suspended in the air for long periods) or dust particles in the air containing the infectious agent.
  - Vector-borne infections are spread through vectors such as animals or insects.
- Universal body substance precautions require precautions with all blood and body fluids. Those clients with a suspected or confirmed medical diagnosis indicative of an infectious disease process, however, need documentation with a comprehensive plan of care for that infection or potential infection. The nursing diagnosis *Risk for Infection Transmission* can be used to document specific universal precaution practices.

Human Immunodeficiency Virus (HIV)

- The cause of AIDS is a retrovirus labeled human immunodeficiency virus (HIV). Transmission is by exposure to contaminated semen, vaginal fluids, or blood.
- HIV infection has a latency or incubation period of 18 months to 5 years. During this period, the person transmits disease through sexual activity or contaminated blood.
- HIV destroys the body's T and B lymphocytes, thus making the host susceptible to a select group of diseases (Table II.14).

TABLE II.14 Most Frequent Infections and Neoplasms in Acquired Immunodeficiency Syndrome (AIDS)

Problem	Site
AIDS-Related Complex	
Candida albicans	Mouth (thrush), throat
Herpes simplex	Mucocutaneous; may be severe
Herpes zoster	Disseminated; may be severe
Lymphadenopathy	Generalized (always more than one lymph node)
Fevers	Usually greater than 100°F; persistent over months
Diarrhea	No organisms recovered, or conventional organisms recovered
Weight loss	Progressive and sustained
Night sweats	Characteristically severe and drenching; persistent and sustained over months
Thrombocytopenia	Often accompanied by petechia; may be severe and life threatening
Human immunodeficiency virus (HIV) encephalopathy	Clinical findings of disabling cognitive or motor dysfunction in absence of concurrent illness or condition other than HIV infection
HIV wasting syndrome	Profound, in the absence of concurrent illness or condition other than HIV infection
Infections	
Candida albicans	Mouth (thrush); throat
Cryptococcus neoformans	Central nervous system (CNS); pulmonary; disseminated
Pneumocystis carinii	Pneumonia
Toxoplasma gondii	CNS
Histoplasma gondii	CNS
Cryptosporidium	Intestine; diarrhea
Cytomegalovirus	Retinas; intestine; pulmonary; disseminated
Herpes simplex	Mucocutaneous; severe
Herpes zoster	Disseminated; severe
HIV dementia	CNS, disseminated
Progressive multifocal leukoencephalopathy	CNS
Mycobacterium avium-intracellulare	Disseminated
Mycobacterium tuberculosis	Pulmonary (TB)
Neoplasms	
Kaposi's sarcoma	Skin; disseminated
Burkitt's lymphoma	Lymphatic system
Non-Hodgkin's lymphoma	Lymphatic system
Mycosis fungoides	Skin (dermal lymphoma)

◆ Pediatric Considerations

- Infections in newborns can be acquired transplacentally or transcervically. They can occur before, during, or after birth.
- Children are at greater risk for transmission of disease because of the following factors:
  - Close contact with other children
  - Frequency of infectious disease in children
  - Lack of hygienic habits (eg, not washing hands after toileting or before eating)
  - Frequent hand-to-mouth activity, increasing risk for infection and reinfection (eg, pinworms) (Wong, 2003)

Focus Assessment Criteria

Refer to *Risk for Infection*.

Goal

NOC Infection Status, Risk Control, Risk Detection

The person will describe the mode of transmission of disease by the time of discharge.

Indicators

- Relate the need to be isolated until noninfectious.
- Demonstrate meticulous handwashing during hospitalization.

General Interventions

NIC Teaching: Disease Process, Infection Protection

Identify People Who are Susceptible Hosts Based on Focus Assessment for Risk for Infection and History of Exposure.

Identify the Mode of Transmission Based on Infecting Agent.
Airborne
Contact
   Direct
   Indirect
   Contact droplet
Vehicle-borne
Vector-borne

Reduce the Transfer of Pathogens.
Isolate clients with airborne communicable infections (Table II.15).
Secure appropriate room assignment depending on the type of infection and hygienic practices of the infected person.
Use universal precautions to prevent transmission to self or other susceptible host.

Discuss the Mode of Transmission of Infection with Client, Family and Significant Others.

Evaluate Client for Secondary Sites of Infection.

Initiate Health Education and Referrals as Indicated.

Rationales

- Nurses must use precautions with blood and body fluids from all clients to protect themselves from exposure to HIV and hepatitis B and C.
- To prevent transmission of infection, the mode of transmission (ie, airborne, contact, vehicle-borne, or vector-borne) must be known.

TABLE II.15 Air-borne Communicable Diseases

Disease	Apply Air-borne Precautions for How Long	Comments
Anthrax, inhalation	Duration of illness	Promptly report to infection control office.
Chickenpox (varicella)	Until all lesions are crusted	Immune person does not need to wear a mask. Exposed susceptible clients should be placed in a private special air-flow room on STOP SIGN alert status beginning 10 days after initial exposure until 21 days after last exposure. Report to epidemiology.
Diphtheria, pharyngeal	Until two cultures from both nose and throat taken at least 24 h after cessation of antimicrobial therapy are negative for *Corynebacterium diphtheriae*	Promptly report to epidemiology.
Epiglottis, due to *Haemophilus influenzae*	For 24 h after cessation of anti-microbial therapy	Report to epidemiology.
Erythema infectiosum	For 7 days after onset	Report to epidemiology.
Hemorrhagic fevers	Duration of illness	Call epidemiology office immediately. Physician may call the State Health Department and Centers for Disease Control and Prevention for advice about management of a suspected case.
Herpes zoster (varicella zoster), disseminated	Duration of illness	Localized; does not require STOP SIGN.
Lassa fever Marburg virus disease	Duration of illness	Call epidemiology office immediately. Physician may call the State Health Department and Centers for Disease Control and Prevention for advice about management of a suspected case.
Measles (rubeola)	For 4 days after start of rash, except in immunocompromised patients, for whom precautions should be maintained for duration of illness	Immune people do not need to wear a mask. Exposed susceptible clients should be placed in a private special air flow room on STOP SIGN alert status beginning the 5th day after exposure until 21 days after last exposure. Call epidemiology to report.
Meningitis *Haemophilus influenzae* known or suspected	For 24 h after start of effective antibiotic therapy	
Neisseria meningitidis (meningococci) known or suspected	For 24 h after start of effective antibiotic therapy	Promptly report to epidemiology.
Meningococcal pneumonia	For 24 h after start of effective antibiotic therapy	Promptly report to epidemiology.
Meningococcemia	For 24 h after start of effective antibiotic therapy	Consult with epidemiology.
Multiply resistant organisms	Until culture negative or as determined by epidemiology	Consult with epidemiology.
Mumps (infectious parotitis)	For 9 days after onset of swelling	People with history do not need to wear a mask. Call epidemiology office to report.
Pertussis (whooping cough)	For 7 days after start of effective therapy	Call epidemiology to report.
Plague, pneumonic	For 3 days after start of effective therapy	Promptly report to epidemiology.
Pneumonia, *Haemophilus* in infants and children any age	For 24 h after start of effective therapy	Call epidemiology.
Pneumonia, meningococcal	For 24 h after start of effective antibiotic therapy	Promptly report to epidemiology.
Rubella (German measles)	For 7 days after onset of rash	Immune people do not need to wear a mask. Promptly report to epidemiology.
Tuberculosis, bronchial, laryngeal, pulmonary, confirmed or suspect	Clients are not considered infectious if they meet all these criteria: Adequate therapy received for 2–3 weeks Favorable clinical response to therapy Three consecutive negative sputum smear results from sputum collected on different days	Call epidemiology to report; prompt use of effective antituberculosis drugs is the most effective means of limiting transmission.
Varicella (chickenpox)	Until all lesions crusted over	See chickenpox

Centers for Disease Control and Prevention. www.cdc.gov.

RISK FOR INFECTION TRANSMISSION

RELATED TO LACK OF KNOWLEDGE OF REDUCING THE RISK OF TRANSMITTING THE AIDS VIRUS

Goal

NOC Refer to *Risk for Infection*

The person will relate practices that reduce the transmission of HIV.

Indicators

- Describe the causes of AIDS and factors contributing to its transmission.
- Describe how to disinfect equipment.

Interventions

NIC Refer also to *Risk for Infection* Sexual Counseling, Behavior Management: Sexual Behavior

Identify Susceptible Host Individual.

Homosexual practices	Bisexual practices	Intravenous drug users
Blood transfusions before 1985	People with HIV	Multiple sexual partners
High-risk behaviors	Sexually transmitted diseases	

Counsel Susceptible Individuals to be Tested for AIDS.

Discuss the Mode of Transmission of the Virus.

Vaginal, anal, or oral sex with infected hosts
Unprotected sex with infected person
Sharing intravenous needles and syringes
Contact of infected fluids with broken skin or mucous membrane
Breast feeding, perinatal transmission

Prevent the Transfer of Virus and Infection.

Teach client the following:
    Abstain from sexual activity.
    Engage in sexual activity with one, mutually faithful, uninfected partner.
    Avoid IV (street) drug use.
Use appropriate universal body substance precautions for all body fluids.
    Wash hands before and after all contact with client or specimen.
    Handle the blood of all clients as potentially infectious.
    Wear gloves for potential contact with blood and body fluids.
    Place used syringes immediately in nearby impermeable container; do not recap or manipulate needle in any way! Use retractable needle syringes when possible.
    Wear protective eyewear and mask if splatter with blood or body fluids is possible (eg, bronchoscopy, oral surgery).
    Wear gowns when splash with blood or body fluids is anticipated.
    Handle all linen soiled with blood or body secretions as potentially infectious.
    Process all laboratory specimens as potentially infectious.
    Wear mask for tuberculosis and other respiratory organisms (HIV is not airborne).
    Place resuscitation equipment where respiratory arrest is predictable.
Administer all antibiotics within 15 minutes of scheduled administration to ensure adequate maintenance of therapeutic levels.

Monitor temperature at least every 4 hours during infectious process.

Evaluate all abnormal laboratory findings and report to physician, including culture with sensitivities to antibiotic administration.

Evaluate client for secondary sites of infection related to spread of infection from primary site.

Reduce the Risk of Transmission of HIV.

Explain low-risk sexual behaviors.
   Mutual masturbation
   Massage
   Vaginal intercourse with condom

Explain the risk of ejaculate contact with broken skin or mucous membranes (oral, anal).

Teach client to use condoms of latex rubber, not "natural membrane"; teach appropriate storage to preserve latex. Avoid spermicides with nonoxynol-9.

Explain the need for water-based lubricants to reduce prophylactic breaks. Avoid petroleum-based lubricants, which dissolve latex.

Explain that a condom with a spermicide may provide additional protection by decreasing the number of viable HIV particles.

Teach Client How to Disinfect Equipment at Home (Needles, Syringes, Sex Aids).

Wash under running water.

Fill or wash with household bleach.

Rinse well with water.

Provide Facts to Dispel Myths Regarding HIV Transmission.

The AIDS virus is not transmitted by mosquitoes, swimming pools, clothes, eating utensils, telephones, toilet seats, or close contact (eg, at work, school).

Saliva, sweat, tears, urine, and feces do not transmit the AIDS virus.

AIDS cannot be contracted during blood donations.

Blood for transfusions is tested to reduce substantially the risk of contracting the AIDS virus.

Initiate Health Teaching and Referrals as Indicated.

Provide client with AIDS hotline (1-800-342-AIDS) for more information.

Emphasize the need to be careful about sex partners (past sexual partners, experimentation with drugs).

Provide the community and schools with facts regarding AIDS transmission, and dispel myths.

In case of acute exposure to HIV (eg, sexual assault, needlestick, break in barrier with HIV-infected person), immediately refer to health care facility for immediate initiation of post-exposure prophylaxis of antiviral therapy (Sharbaugh, 1999).

Educate clients about the chain of infection and responsibilities both in the hospital and at home.

Rationales

- Handwashing is one of the most important means to prevent the spread of infection.
- Masks prevent transmission by aerosolization of infectious agents if oral mucosal lesions are present; gowns prevent soiling of clothes if contact with secretions/excretions is likely.
- Gloves provide a barrier from contact with infectious secretions and excretions.
- Eye coverings protect the eyes from accidental exposure to infectious secretions.
- It is advisable that family members and others caring for or coming into contact with the client take simple precautions.
- Testing can predict onset of infection, enabling the person to receive medications prophylactically to slow disease progression.
- HIV is transmitted by sexual contact, by contact with infected blood and blood products, and perinatally (from mother to fetus).
- These measures aim to prevent contact of body fluids with mucous membranes.
- Exposure to disinfecting agents rapidly inactivates HIV. Household bleach solution (dilute 1:10 with water) is an inexpensive choice.
- Dispelling myths and correcting misinformation can reduce anxiety and allow others to interact more normally with the client.
- Nonoxynol-9 spermicides may increase the risk of HIV transmission (Hollander, 2000).

Risk for Injury
    Related to Lack of Awareness of Environmental Hazards
    Related to Lack of Awareness of Environmental Hazards Secondary to Maturational Age
    Related to Vertigo Secondary to Orthostatic Hypotension
Risk for Aspiration
Risk for Falls
Risk for Poisoning
Risk for Suffocation
Risk for Trauma
Risk for Perioperative Positioning Injury

RISK FOR INJURY

DEFINITION
Risk for Injury: State in which a person is at risk for harm because of a perceptual or physiologic deficit, a lack of awareness of hazards, or maturational age

RISK FACTORS
Presence of risk factor (see Related Factors)

RELATED FACTORS
Pathophysiologic
Related to altered cerebral function secondary to:

Tissue hypoxia	Syncope	Vertigo

Related to altered mobility secondary to:

Unsteady gait	Loss of limb	Amputation
Cerebrovascular accident	Arthritis	Parkinsonism

Related to impaired sensory function (specify)

Vision	Thermal/touch	Hearing
Smell		

Related to fatigue
Related to orthostatic hypotension
Related to vestibular disorders
Related to lack of awareness of environmental hazards secondary to:

Confusion	Depression	Hypoglycemia
Electrolyte imbalance		

Related to tonic–clonic movements secondary to:
Seizures

Treatment-Related
Related to effects of (specify) on mobility or sensorium:
Medications

Sedatives	Diuretics	Vasodilators
Phenothiazine	Antihypertensives	Psychotropics
Hypoglycemics		

Related to casts/crutches, canes, walkers

Situational (Personal, Environmental)
Related to decrease in or loss of short-term memory
Related to faulty judgment secondary to:

Stress	Alcohol, drugs	Dehydration

Related to prolonged bed rest
Related to household hazards (specify)

Unsafe walkways	Stairs	Unsafe toys
Slippery floors	Inadequate lighting	Faulty electric wires
Bathrooms (tubs, toilets)	Improperly stored poisons	

Related to automotive hazards
Lack of use of seat belts or child seats
Mechanically unsafe vehicle

Related to fire hazards
Related to unfamiliar setting (hospital, nursing home)
Related to improper footwear
Related to inattentive caretaker
Related to improper use of aids (crutches, canes, walkers, wheelchairs)
Related to history of accidents

Maturational
Infant/Child
Related to lack of awareness of hazards

Older Adult
Related to faulty judgments secondary to motor and sensory deficits, medication, cognitive deficits

---

⊕ AUTHOR'S NOTE

This diagnosis has four subcategories: *Risk for Aspiration, Poisoning, Suffocation,* and *Trauma.* Interventions to prevent poisoning, suffocation, and trauma are included under the general category *Risk for Injury.* Should the nurse choose to isolate interventions only for prevention of poisoning, suffocation, or trauma, then the diagnosis *Risk for Poisoning, Risk for Suffocation,* or *Risk for Trauma* would be useful.

Nursing interventions related to *Risk for Injury* focus on protecting a person from injury and teaching precautions to reduce the risk of injury. When the nurse is teaching a client or family safety measures to prevent injury, but is not providing on-site protection (as in the community or outpatient department, or for discharge planning), the diagnosis *Risk for Injury related to insufficient knowledge of safety precautions* may be more appropriate.

⊕ ERRORS IN DIAGNOSTIC STATEMENTS

1. *Risk for Injury: Hemorrhage related to abnormal blood profile secondary to cirrhosis*
This diagnosis does not represent a situation that a nurse can prevent, but one that he or she monitors and comanages as the collaborative problem *PC: Hemorrhage related to altered clotting factors.*

KEY CONCEPTS
Generic Considerations

- Injury is the fourth leading cause of death in the general population (40.1 deaths per 100,000) and the leading cause of death in children and young adults (US Public Health Services [USPHS], 1998).

TABLE II.16 Poisonous Substances Around the House

Drugs

Aspirin	Cough medicines	Laxatives
Tranquilizers	Vitamins	Oral contraceptives
Barbiturates	Acetaminophen	

Petroleum Products

Cleaning Agents

Soaps and polishes	Disinfectants	Drain cleaners

Poisonous Plants

Amaryllis	Iris	Philodendron
Azalea	Jack-in-the-pulpit	Poinsettia
Baneberry	Jerusalem cherry	Poison hemlock
Belladonna	Jimsonweed	Poison ivy
Bittersweet	Lily of the valley	Pokeweed
Bloodroot	Marijuana	Potato leaves
Castor-bean plant	Mistletoe	Rhododendron
Climbing nightshade	Morning glory	Rhubarb leaves
Daffodil	Mountain laurel	Schefflera
Devil's ivy	Mushrooms	Tomato leaves
Dieffenbachia	Oleander	Wisteria
Foxglove	Peacelily	Yew
Holly		

Miscellaneous

Baby powder	Cosmetics	Lead paint

- Health education activities that focus on fire safety, home safety, water safety, seat belt use, motor vehicle safety, cardiopulmonary resuscitation (CPR) training, poison control, and first aid can reduce the rate of accidents (Clemen-Stone, Eigasti & McGuire, 2001).
- Table II.16 lists common sources of poisoning in the home.

Orthostatic Hypotension
- Postural hypotension refers to a sudden drop in blood pressure of 20 mm Hg or more for at least 1 min when standing.
- Studies have shown that postprandial hypotension occurs in about one third of healthy adults 1 h after eating breakfast and lunch (Lipsitz & Fullerton, 1986).
- Postural hypotension can affect quality of life if it contributes to falls or fear of falling. It also can precipitate stroke and myocardial infarction (Porth, 2002).

Pediatric Considerations

- Injury is the leading cause of death in people 1 to 19 years of age (Wong, 2003). Six leading types are traffic accidents, drownings, burns and fires, chokings, poisonings, and falls (Wong, 2003).
- Each year, car crashes injure and kill more children than does any disease. Used properly, safety seats and belts protect children in crashes and help save lives (National Safety Council, 2000).
- Injury accounts for 72% of total fatalities among late adolescents (15 to 19 years of age), the pediatric age group at highest risk for injury mortality (National Safety Council, 2000).
- Between 70% and 80% of infants will use a walker, usually between 5 and 12 months of age. Of them, 30% to 40% will have an accident (American Medical Association [AMA] Board of Trustees, 1991). Most walker accidents are minor; however, serious trauma from head

(continued)

✤ Pediatric Considerations (continued)

injuries, lacerations, and burns occurs occasionally. Nurses should counsel parents on the risk of injury from use of infant walkers (AMA Board of Trustees, 1991).

- Every day, more than 1000 children are injured, and one dies, in bicycle accidents. School-aged children are at greatest risk. One third of children treated in emergency rooms for bicycle accidents have head injuries. Use of bicycle helmets could reduce incidence of these injuries.
- Drowning is the second leading cause of death from injury during childhood. Children younger than 4 years of age are at especially high risk (National Safety Council, 2000).
- Children should be taught early (2 years of age) and reminded constantly about rules for streets, playground equipment, fires, water (pools, bathtubs), animals, and strangers.
- Many near-drownings take place while a parent is supervising the child but has a momentary lapse of attention (Wong, 2003).
- Effective swimming depends on intellectual as well as physical maturity. Organized swimming lessons may give parents a false sense of security that their child "can swim."
- Swimming programs that use total submersion put infants at risk for water intoxication, hypothermia, and bacterial infections. In addition, infants may learn to fear the water.
- Children 1 to 3 years of age are at greatest risk for scalds. More than one third of children 3 to 8 years of age are burned while playing with matches. When a fire strikes, young children need help to escape (Wong, 2003).
- For children younger than 3 years, choking is the fourth leading cause of accidental death.
- Toddlers are at highest risk for poisoning. Children are poisoned by medications as well as by common household items (eg, plants, makeup, cleaning products).
- For children 1 to 4 years of age, the leading cause of accidental death and serious injury is falls in the home (Wong, 2003).

Ⓒ Geriatric Considerations

- Falls are more frequent in older adults, and the mortality, dysfunction, disability, and need for medical services that result are greater than in younger age groups. Unintentional injury, a category including falls, motor vehicle collisions, and burns, is the seventh leading cause of death in older adults, and the incidence of falls represents more than 60% of that category.
- Approximately 25% of hospital admissions for older adults are directly related to falling; 47% of these people are admitted to long-term care facilities (Miller, 2004).
- "Fallaphobia" refers to fears related to a person's loss of confidence to perform activities without falling. These fears actually increase the risk for falling, and the person eventually becomes housebound (Miller, 2004).
- A fall-free existence is not always possible for some people. Increased independence and mobility may be an important and valuable trade-off for increased risk of falling. Collaboration among client, family, and team members helps arrive at the decision of a less restricted environment.
- With age comes some loss of the postural control system. To not fall, a person must be able to keep his or her center of gravity over an adequate base, as well as to rapidly process and respond to sensory information (Baumann, 1999).
- Older adults frequently lack muscle strength in lower extremities and have insufficient torque in their ankles (Baumann, 1999).
- Regular walking, as little as 60 min twice a week, can improve sensory function, balance, stability, hip flexion strength, hip extension, and dorsiflexion, all of which can reduce falls (Schoenfelder, 2000).
- The following factors increase the risk for falls in older adults (Miller, 2004; Moss, 1992):
  - History of falls
  - Sensory–motor deficits (eg, vision, hearing, hemianopia [loss of half of visual field], paresis, aphasia)
  - Gait instability

(continued)

⊙ **Geriatric Considerations (continued)**

- Improper footwear or foot problems (corns, bunions, calluses)
- Postural hypotension, especially with complaints of dizziness
- Confusion (persistent or acute)
- Incontinence, urinary urgency
- Cardiovascular disease affecting cerebral perfusion and oxygenation: dysrhythmias, syncopal episodes, congestive heart failure, fibrillation
- Neurologic disease affecting movement or judgment: cerebrovascular accident with impulsivity; parkinsonism; moderate Alzheimer's disease; seizure disorder, vertigo
- Orthopedic disorders or devices affecting movement or balance: casts, splints, slings, prostheses, recent surgery, severe arthritis
- Medications affecting blood pressure or level of consciousness: psychotropics, sedatives, analgesics, diuretics, antihypertensives, medication change, more than five drugs
- Agitation, increased anxiety, emotional lability
- Willfulness, uncooperativeness
- Situational factors: new admission, room change, roommate change

Focus Assessment Criteria

This entire assessment is indicated only when the client is at high risk for injury because of personal deficits, alterations (eg, mobility problems), or maturational age. In households without such a family member, the functional assessment of the individual can be deleted with the focus on the environment.

Subjective Data

These consist of the person's physical capabilities (as reported by person or caretaker).

Assess for Related or Risk Factors.

Vision
Corrected (date of last prescription)
Complaints of
   Blurriness   Difficulty focusing   Loss of side vision
   Inability to adjust to darkness

Hearing
   Need to read lips   Use of hearing aid
   Inadequate   (condition, batteries)

Thermal/tactile
   Altered sense of hot/cold

Mental status
   Drowsy
   Confused
   Oriented to time, place, events
   Complaints of
      Vertigo   Orthostatic hypotension
   Altered sense of balance
   Cognitive stage (immature reasoning/judgment)

Mobility
Reports of
Feeling lightheaded, dizzy   Losing balance   Difficulty standing, sitting
Wandering   Falling or almost falling
Ability to ambulate
Around room   Around house   Up and down stairs
Outside house
Ability to travel
Drive car (date of last   Use public transportation
  reevaluation)

Devices

Cane	Walker	Condition of devices
Wheelchair	Prosthesis	Competence in their use

Shoes / slippers

Condition	Nonskid soles	Fit

Abilities related to developmental milestones

Turning over	Climbing	Sitting
Crawling	Standing	Walking

Miscellaneous

Drug therapy

Type	Dosage	Storage
Labeling	Ability to self-medicate safely	

Communication

Write	Use phone	Make needs known

Contact emergency assistance

Support system / primary caregiver

Help available from relatives, friends, neighbors, club and church contacts

History of "blackouts"

Urinary frequency or incontinence

Objective Data

Assess for Related Factors.

Blood pressure (left, right, sitting/lying more than 5 min, 1 min after standing)
Gait

Steady	Requires aids	Unsteady

Strength

Can stand on one leg	Can sit-stand-sit

Cognitive processes

Can communicate needs	Can interact	History of wandering (witnessed and reported by others)
Can understand cause and effect		

Presence of

Anger	Withdrawal	Depression
Faulty judgment		

Ability for self-care activities

Dress and undress	Bathe	Groom self
Feed self	Reach toilet	

Assess for Related Factors in the Home.

Safety

Toilet facilities	Water supply	Heating
Sewage	Ventilation	Garbage disposal

Safety of walkways (inside and outside)

Sidewalks (uneven, broken)

Stairs (inside and outside)

Broken steps	Lighting	No hand rails
Protection for children		

Halls

Cluttered	Poor lighting

Electrical hazards

No outlet covers

Cords frayed and unanchored

Outlets overloaded; accessible to children; near water

Switches too far from bedside

Inadequate lighting

At night	Outdoors	To bathroom at night

Unsafe floors

Even or uneven	Highly polished	Rugs not anchored

Kitchen hazards
Pot handles not turned inward
Stove (grease or flammable objects on stove)
Refrigerator (improperly stored food; inadequate temperatures)

Toxic substances
Stored in food containers; not properly labeled; accessible to children
Medications kept beyond date of expiration
Poisonous household plants

Fire hazards
Matches/lighters accessible to children
No fire extinguishers
Improper storage of corrosives, combustibles
Lack of furnace maintenance
No fire escape plan, no fire extinguishers
Emergency telephone numbers not accessible (fire, police)

Hazards for children in nursery
Cribs near drapery cords
Cribs with wide slat openings
Plastic bags
Pillows in crib
Unattended without crib rails up
Space between mattress and crib rails
Unattended on changing table
Pacifier hung around infant's neck
Propped bottle placed in infant's crib
Toys with pointed edges, removable parts

Hazards for children in household
Accessible medications, lighters, matches, cleaning products
Objects with lead paint
Poisonous plants (see Table II.16)
Open windows with loose or no screens
Plastic bags
Furniture with glass or sharp corners
Open doorways, stairways

Outdoor hazards for children

Porches without rails	Play area without fence	Backyard pools
Domestic/wild animals	Poisonous plants	

For more information on Focus Assessment Criteria, visit http://connection.lww.com.

Goal

NOC	Risk Control, Safety Status: Falls Occurrence, Safety Behavior: Home Physical Environment, Safety Behavior: Personal

The person will relate fewer falls and less fear of falling.

Indicators

- Identify factors that increase risk for injury.
- Relate intent to use safety measures to prevent injury (eg, remove or anchor throw rugs).
- Relate intent to practice selected prevention measures (eg, wear sunglasses to reduce glare).
- Increase daily activity, if feasible.

General Interventions

NIC Fall Prevention, Environmental Management: Safety, Health Education, Surveillance: Safety, Risk Identification

Assess for Causative or Contributing Factors.

Unfamiliar surroundings
Impaired vision
   Altered spatial judgment
   Diplopia
   Cataracts
   Hemianopia
   Decreased ability to tell
     object from background

   Blurred vision
   Blind spots
   Altered peripheral vision
   Increased susceptibility to visual glare

Decreased hearing acuity
Decreased tactile sensitivity (touch)
Orthostatic hypotension
Decreased strength/flexibility
Unstable gait
Pain
Fatigue
Improper shoes or slippers
Improper use of crutches, canes, walkers
Joint immobility
Side effects of medication (eg, tranquilizers, diuretics)
Hazardous environmental factors

Reduce or Eliminate Causative or Contributing Factors, if Possible.

Unfamiliar Surroundings

Orient each client to surroundings on admission; explain the call system, and assess client's ability to use it.
Closely supervise client during the first few nights to assess safety.
Use night-light.
Encourage person to request assistance during the night.
Teach about side effects of certain drugs (eg, dizziness, fatigue).
Keep bed at lowest level during the night.
Consider use of a movement detection monitor, if needed.

Impaired Vision

Provide safe illumination and teach client to
   Ensure adequate lighting in all rooms, with soft light at night.
   Have light switch easily accessible, next to bed.
   Provide background light that is soft.
Teach client how to reduce glare.
   Avoid glossy surfaces (eg, glass, highly polished floors).
   Use diffuse rather than direct light; use shades that darken the room.
   Turn head away when switching on a bright light.
   Wear sunglasses or hats with brims, or carry umbrellas, to reduce glare outside.
   Avoid looking directly at bright lights (eg, headlights).
Teach person or family to provide sufficient color contrast for visual discrimination and to avoid green and blue.
   Color-code edges of steps (eg, with colored tape).
   Avoid white walls, dishes, and counters.
   Avoid clear glasses (ie, use smoked glass).
   Choose objects colored black on white (eg, black phone).
   Avoid colors that merge (eg, beige switches on beige walls).
   Paint doorknobs bright colors.

Decreased Tactile Sensitivity

Teach preventive measures.
   Assess temperature of bath water and heating pads before use.
   Use bath thermometers.

Assess extremities daily for undetected injuries.

Keep feet warm and dry and skin softened with emollient lotion (lanolin, mineral oil).

See *Ineffective Peripheral Tissue Perfusion* for additional interventions.

Decreased Hearing Acuity

Determine if client has had hearing evaluated professionally.

Assist him or her to make a decision concerning the use or type of hearing aid if indicated.

Teach, when driving, to leave car window partially open to allow warning signals (eg, sirens) to be heard and to set air conditioner, heater, or radio low so outside noises are audible.

Orthostatic Hypotension

See *Risk for Injury Related to Vertigo Secondary to Orthostatic Hypotension* for additional interventions.

Decreased Strength/Flexibility

Perform ankle-strengthening exercises daily (Schoenfelder, 2000).

Stand behind a straight chair, with feet slightly apart.

Slowly raise both heels until body weight is on balls of feet, hold for count of 3 (eg, 1 Mississippi, 2 Mississippi, 3 Mississippi).

Do 5 to 10 repetitions; increase repetitions as strength increases.

Walk at least two or three times a week.

Use ankle exercises as a warm-up before walking.

Begin walking with someone at side, if needed, for 10 min.

Increase time and speed according to capabilities.

Use of Assistive Devices

Crutches

Teach exercises to strengthen arm and shoulder muscles to facilitate use of crutches; use weights and parallel bars.

Measure and fit crutches to each person (2 to 3 inches between top of crutch and armpit); improper length of crutches may cause nerve damage or falls.

Instruct person to wear shoes that fit properly and have nonskid soles.

Assess ability to walk and climb up and down stairs.

Consult with physical therapist for proper gait training.

Canes

Teach person to hold cane in hand opposite affected leg and move cane and impaired limb together.

Cane should be proper length to allow person to extend elbow and bear weight on hand.

Cane should be fitted with rubber tip.

Consult with physical therapist for proper gait training.

Walkers

Teach person exercises to strengthen triceps muscles used in proper crutch walking.

See that floors are clean, dry, and free of obstacles and that rugs are anchored.

Instruct person to wear properly fitted shoes with nonslip soles.

Consult with physical therapist for proper gait training.

Prosthesis

Teach person to bathe and inspect stump daily.

Instruct him or her to put on prosthesis soon after rising to minimize stump swelling.

Prepare person for crutch walking with triceps exercises using weights and parallel bars.

Consult with physical therapist for proper gait training.

Side Effects of Medications

Assess for any side effects of drugs that may cause vertigo.

Hypotension	Vasodilation	Sedation
Vasoconstriction	Hypokalemia	

Hazardous Environmental Factors

Teach client to:

Eliminate throw rugs, litter, and highly polished floors.

Ensure nonslip surfaces in bathtub or shower by applying commercially available traction tapes.

Install handgrips in bathroom.

Install railings in hallways and on stairs.

Remove protruding objects (eg, coat hooks, shelves, light fixtures) from stairway walls.

Instruct staff to:

Keep siderails on bed in place and bed at the lowest position when person is left unattended.

Keep bed at lowest position with wheels locked when stationary.

Teach person in wheelchair to lock and unlock wheels.
Ensure that person's shoes or slippers have nonskid soles.

Describe and Document Falls, Injuries, Previous Falls, Medications, and Measures Taken.

Rationales

- An unfamiliar environment and problems with vision, orientation, mobility, and fatigue can increase risk of falling.
- Identifying the types of visual disturbances and options available allows the client to take the necessary precautions.
- A client with mobility problems needs safety devices installed and hazards eliminated to aid in activities of daily living (ADLs).
- Goals to prevent and manage falls focus on reducing their likelihood by minimizing environmental hazards, strengthening individual competence to resist falls and fall-related injury, and providing postfall injury care.
- Visual difficulty because of glare is often responsible for falls in older adults, who have increased susceptibility to glare. Incandescent (nonfluorescent) lighting produces less glare and therefore provides better illumination for older clients.
- An unfamiliar environment coupled with vision and mobility difficulties can increase a client's risk of injury (eg, falls, burns).
- Ankle strengthening and a walking program can improve balance, increase ankle strength, improve walking speed, decrease falls and fear of falling, and increase confidence in performing ADLs (Schoenfelder, 2000).

RISK FOR INJURY

RELATED TO LACK OF AWARENESS OF ENVIRONMENTAL HAZARDS

Goal

NOC Safety Behavior: Home Physical Environment, Risk Control, Parent Education

The person or family will identify and reduce environmental hazards.

Indicators

- Teach children safety habits.
- Safely store hazardous items.
- Repair hazards as needed.
- Remove environmental hazards when possible.
- Install safety measures (eg, locks, rails).

Interventions

NIC Area Restriction, Surveillance: Safety, Environmental Management: Safety, Home Maintenance Assistance, Risk Identification, Teaching: Safety

Identify Situations that Contribute to Accidents.

Unfamiliar setting (homes of others, hotels)
Peak activity periods (meal preparation, holidays)

New equipment (bicycle, chain saw, lawn mower, snow blower)
Lack of awareness of or disregard for environmental hazards

Reduce or Eliminate Hazardous Situations.

Teach About New Equipment.
Teach client to read directions completely before using a new appliance or piece of equipment.
Determine the limitations of the equipment.
Unplug and turn off any appliance that is not functioning before examining it (eg, lawn mower, snow blower, electric mixer).

Review Unsafe Practices.
Automobiles
Driving a mechanically unsafe vehicle
Not using or misusing seat restraints
Driving after partaking of alcohol or drugs
Driving with unrestrained babies and children in the car
Driving at excessive speeds
Driving without necessary visual aids
Driving with unsafe road or road crossing conditions
Not using or misusing necessary headgear for motorcyclist
Allowing children to ride in front seat of car
Backing up without checking location of small children
Warming a car in a closed garage
Flammables
Igniting gas leaks
Delayed lighting of gas burner or oven
Experimenting with chemicals or gasoline
Using unscreened fires, fireplaces, heaters
Inadequately storing combustibles, matches, or oily rags
Smoking in bed or near oxygen
Buying highly flammable children's toys or clothing
Playing with fireworks or gunpowder
Playing with matches, candles, cigarettes, lighters
Wearing plastic aprons or flowing clothing around open flame
Kitchen
Allowing grease waste to collect on stoves
Wearing plastic aprons or flowing clothing around open flame
Using cracked glasses or dishware
Using improper canning, freezing, or preserving methods
Storing knives uncovered
Keeping pot handles facing front of stove
Using thin or worn potholders or oven mitts
Placing stove controls on front
Using dishes that have lead in them
Bathroom
Keeping medicine cabinet unlocked
Not having grab rails in bathtub
Not having nonskid mats or emery strips in bathtub
Maintaining poor lighting in bathroom and hallways
Improperly placing electrical outlets
Chemicals and irritants
Improperly labeling medication containers
Keeping medications in containers other than original ones
Maintaining poor illumination at the medicine cabinet
Improperly labeling containers of poisons and corrosive substances
Keeping expired medications that dangerously decompose
Storing toxic substances in accessible areas (eg, under sink)
Storing corrosives (eg, lye) inadequately
Having contact with intense cold
Being overexposed to sun, sunlamps, heating pads

Lighting and electrical
Using uncovered outlets
Using unanchored electrical wires
Overloading electrical outlets
Overloading fuse boxes
Using faulty electrical plugs, frayed wires, or defective electrical appliances
Maintaining inadequate lighting over landings and stairs
Maintaining inaccessible light switches (eg, bedside)
Using machinery or appliances without prior instruction

Initiate Health Teaching and Referral, as Indicated.

Teach Measures to Prevent Car Accidents.
Frequently reevaluate ability to drive.
Wear good-quality sunglasses (gray or green) to reduce glare.
Keep windshields clean and wipers in good condition.
Place mirrors on both sides of car.
Stop periodically to stretch and to rest eyes.
Know the effects of medications on driving ability.
Do not smoke while driving or drive after drinking.
Do not use cellular phone while driving.

Teach Measures to Prevent Pedestrian Accidents.
Allow enough time to cross streets.
Wear garments that reflect light (beige, white) at night.
Wait to cross on the sidewalk, not the street.
Look both ways.
Do not rely solely on green traffic lights to provide safe crossing (right turn on red light may be legal, or driver may disobey traffic regulations).

Teach Measures to Prevent Burns.
Equip home with smoke alarm system and check its function each month.
Have a hand-held fire extinguisher.
Set thermostats for water heater to provide warm, but not scalding, water.
Use baking soda or a lid cover to smother a kitchen grease fire.
Do not wear loose-fitting clothing (eg, robes, nightgowns) when cooking.
Do not smoke when sleepy.
Ensure that portable heaters are safely used.
See *Risk for Injury Related to Lack of Awareness of Environmental Hazards* for additional safety measures.

Refer Clients With Motor or Sensory Deficits for Assistance in Identifying Environmental Hazards.
Local fire company
Community nursing agency
Accident-prevention information (see References/Bibliography)

Assist Person and Family to Evaluate Environmental Hazards and Effects of Restrictions on Quality of Life.

Refer Client to Public Health or Visiting Nurse for Home Visit.

Refer Client to Physical Therapist for Evaluation of Gait.

Rationales

- The distinction between accident and injury is useful for nurses to understand. *Accident* implies lack of control of external forces. Nursing focuses on identifying controllable variables (host, agent, environment) to prevent injuries (Green, 1989).
- The nurse can reduce host variables that increase risk for injury, such as lack of knowledge; agent variables, such as shear forces in bed; and environmental variables, such as spills and other hazards.
- Accidents occur more frequently
  - During the initial period of hospitalization and between 6 and 9 pm
  - During peak activity periods (meals, playtime)
  - In unfamiliar surroundings
  - With inadequate lighting

- At holidays
- On vacations
- During home repairs
- Color contrast between object and background increases visualization (eg, white on black).

❖ Pediatric Interventions

Teach Parents Basic Safety Measures and Assessments.

Instruct parents to expect frequent changes in infants' and children's abilities and to take precautions (eg, infant who suddenly rolls over for the first time might be on a changing table unattended).

Discuss the necessity of constantly monitoring small children.

Provide information to assist parents in selecting a babysitter.

    Determine previous experiences and knowledge of emergency measures.

    Observe interaction of sitter with child (eg, pick up sitter 30 min before you are ready to leave).

Teach parents to expect children to mimic them and to teach what children can do with or without supervision.

    Tell child to ask you before attempting a new task.

    Do not take pills in front of children.

Explain and expect compliance with certain rules (depending on age) concerning

Streets	Fire	Playground equipment
Animals	Water (pools, bathtubs)	Strangers
Bicycles		

Role-play with children to assess understanding of the problem.

    "You're walking home. A strange man pulls up in a car near you. What do you do?"

    "While walking past a barbecue, your dress catches on fire. What do you do?"

Identify Situations that Contribute to Accidents.

Bicycles, Wagons, Skateboards, and Skates

No reflectors or lights	Not in single file
Riding a too-large bicycle	Lack of knowledge of rules of the road
Use of skateboards or skates in heavily traveled areas	Lack of helmet, protective pads

Water and Pools

Discourage use of flotation or swim aids (water wings, tubs) with children who cannot swim.

Teach safe water behavior:

No running, pushing	No jumping on others
No swimming alone	No playful screaming for help
No diving in water less than 8 feet deep	No swimming after meals
No swimming during electrical storms	No excessive alcohol use

Enclose pool:

    Use a 5- to 5½-foot fence.

    Use a fence that children cannot climb.

    Use self-locking gates.

Remove pool cover completely.

Avoid free-floating pool covers.

Teach safe diving and sliding techniques.

    Allow diving only from diving boards.

    Discourage running dives.

    Teach to steer upward with hands and head.

    Descend pool slide sitting with feet first.

Have lifesaving equipment at poolside (life preserver, rope, or hook).

Learn CPR and how to respond to accidental submersion.

    Remove from water.

    If spinal injury is suspected, immobilize on a board and apply a cervical collar.

    Clear airway of debris.

If person is unresponsive, place on side if vomiting occurs.
Remove wet clothes, dry, and cover with blankets (including head)
Begin CPR and continue until help arrives.

Miscellaneous
Unsupervised contact with animals and poisons in environment (plants, pool chemicals, pills)
Obstructed passageways
Unsafe window protection in home with young children
Guns or ammunition stored in unlocked fashion
Large icicles hanging from roof
Icy walkways
Glass sliding doors that look open when closed
Low-strung clothesline
Discarded or unused refrigerators or freezers without removed doors

Infants and Toddlers
Household
Pillows in crib
Staircases without stair gates
Crib mattresses that do not fit snugly
Cribs with slat opening to allow child's body to fall through, catching the head
Glass or sharp-edged tables
Porches and decks without railings
Poisonous plants (see Table II.16)
Furniture painted with lead paint
Unsupervised bathing
Open windows
Propped bottle in crib
Toys

Sharp edges	Balloons	Easily breakable parts
Lollipops	Removable small pieces	Pacifier around neck

Miscellaneous
Unattended in shopping cart
Unattended in car
Cribs, walkers, high chairs with movable parts that trap child (eg, springs)
Put in car safety seat in back seat only

Assist Parents to Analyze an Accident.

What happened?
How did it happen?
Where, when?
Why did the accident happen?

Teach How to Prevent Poisoning.

Instruct how to "childproof" the home.
Instruct to keep poisons and corrosive substances in tightly closed, carefully marked containers in locked closets.
Parents should discard unused supplies of medications and keep needed medications in locked, inaccessible medicine closet.
Parents should be taught how to administer antidotes for specific toxic substances, if advised by Poison Control Center.
Parents should also have the phone number of the Poison Control Center in a convenient place.
Refer individuals to local poison control center for "Mr. Yuk" poison warning stickers and advice on emergency procedures; teach the child what a Mr. Yuk sticker means.
Instruct parents on the use of ipecac and its availability.

Initiate Health Teaching and Referrals, as Indicated.

Assist family to evaluate environmental hazards in home and when visiting others.
Install specially designed locks to prevent children from opening closets where combustible, corrosive, or flammable materials or medications are stored.
Instruct to use socket covers to prevent accidental electrical shocks to children.

Teach about hazards of lead paint ingestion and how to identify "pica" in a child.
Refer parents to public health department if lead paint screening is necessary.
Encourage use of childproof caps.
Advise to avoid storing dangerous substances in containers ordinarily used for foods.

Rationales

• The nurse should assess each child's unique risk of potential for injury. This includes the child with sensory or motor deficits and developmental delay. Environmental changes, such as hospitalization, visiting relatives' homes, and celebrating holidays, pose special hazards for children.
• All environmental hazards cannot be removed. Strategies that include supervision and education of parents can reduce accidents (Clemen-Stone et al., 1997).
• Analysis of an accident may prevent recurrence.
• Injury prevention requires anticipation and recognition of where safety measures are applicable. Passive strategies provide automatic protection without choice (eg, air bags, product design). Active strategies require persuasion through teaching or legislation to practice safety measures (Wong, 2003).
• Prevention strategies to decrease serious injuries resulting from skateboarding include warnings against skateboard use by children younger than 5 years of age, prohibition of skateboards on streets and highways, and the promotion of use of helmets and other protective gear (Wong, 2003).

RISK FOR INJURY

○○ RELATED TO LACK OF AWARENESS OF ENVIRONMENTAL HAZARDS SECONDARY TO MATURATIONAL AGE

Goals

NOC Refer to *Risk for Injury*

• The child/adolescent will be free from injury from potentially hazardous factors identified in the hospital environment.
• The family will reinforce and demonstrate safe practices in the hospital.

Interventions

NIC Refer also to *Risk for Injury, Related to Lack of Awareness of Environmental Hazard,* Teaching: Toddler Safety

Protect the Infant/Child from
Injury in the Hospital by Controlling Age-Related Hazards.

Infant (1 to 12 Months)
Ensure that infant can be identified by an identification band and a tag on his or her crib.
Do not shake powder directly on infant; rather, place powder in hand and then on infant's skin.
Keep powder out of infant's reach.
Keep unsafe toys out of reach (eg, buttons, beads, balloons, broken toys, sharp-edged toys, other small toys).
Use mitts to prevent infant from removing catheters, eye patches, intravenous (IV) infusions, dressings, and feeding tubes, as needed.

Keep siderails up in locked position when child is in crib.

Pad siderails if infant can move out of bed or is at risk for seizures.

Use a cool-mist vaporizer.

Do not use an infant walker.

Ascertain identity of all visitors.

Use a firm mattress that fits crib snugly.

Do not feed honey to infants younger than 12 months because of the danger of botulism.

Fasten safety straps on infant seats, swings, highchairs, and strollers.

Do not allow bottles to be propped. The infant should be held with his or her head upright.

Do not place pillows in crib.

Place one hand over the child while weighing, changing diapers, and so forth, to keep him or her safe.

Do not allow infant to wear pacifier on a string around the neck.

Check bath water to make sure the temperature is appropriate. Never leave infant alone while bathing! Support the small infant's head out of the water.

Check the temperature of formula, especially if you have heated it in the microwave.

Position crib away from bedside stand, infusion pumps, and so forth, to prevent child from reaching unsafe objects (eg, suction machine, electrical outlets, flowers, dials on infusion pump).

Do not allow parents to smoke or drink hot beverages in infant's room.

Do not offer the child foods that must be chewed or are small enough to occlude the airway (eg, nuts, popcorn, hard candy, whole hot dogs). Forks and knives are not appropriate utensils for infants.

Discard syringes, needles, med packets, and plastic bags safely.

Protect the feet of the infant who can walk with shoes or slippers.

Transport the infant safely to other areas of the hospital (eg, x-ray, laboratory).

Remind parents to have approved car seat in their automobile to transport the child home.

Assess each unique situation for risk for injury to the infant. Inform parents of the infant's risk for injury.

Early Childhood (13 Months to 5 Years)

Ensure that the young child is identifiable by name band and name tag on crib.

Keep siderails up in locked position when child is in crib—top and bottom compartments; use siderails on youth beds.

Monitor child at all times when eating, bathing, playing, and toileting.

Keep cleaning agents, sharp items, and plastic bags out of reach.

Secure thermometer while taking temperature (use rectal or axillary method with toddler, oral method when child is old enough not to bite down on thermometer) or use infrared instant thermometer in the ear canal.

Assess for loose teeth, and document on records.

Check the temperature of bath water before immersing child.

Use electric beds with extreme caution. For example, children may get their fingers caught or get under the bed and be at risk for a crushing injury.

Position crib/bed away from bedside stand, infusion pumps, flowers, and so forth, to prevent child from reaching unsafe objects.

Keep child safe when mobile:

  Protect child's feet with shoes or slippers when ambulating.

  Keep bathroom and closet doors firmly shut.

  Check any tubing attached to child to prevent kinking or dislodgment.

  Apply safety straps when child is in highchair or stroller or on a cart.

  Transport safely to other areas of the hospital (eg, x-ray).

  Use mitts to prevent child from removing catheters, eye patches, IV infusion, dressings, and feeding tubes, as needed.

  Place one hand over child when weighing, changing diapers, and so forth, to prevent falls.

Do not call medications "candy."

Do not permit the child to chew gum or eat hard candy, nuts, whole hot dogs, or fish with bones.

Set limits. Enforce and repeat what the child can do in the hospital and areas he or she can go.

Provide age-appropriate, safe toys (see manufacturer's guidelines).

Do not allow parents to smoke or drink hot beverages in the child's room.

Feed the child in a quiet environment; ensure that he or she sits while eating, to prevent choking.

Remind parents to have an approved car seat in automobile to transport child home.

Ascertain identity of all visitors.

Assess each unique situation for risk for injury to the young child. Inform parents of the young child's risk for injury.

School-Aged/Adolescent (6 to 12 Years/13 to 18 Years)

Ensure that the child or adolescent can be identified by a name band and a tag on his or her bed. School-aged children may claim to be someone else as a joke, not realizing the danger of this.

Assess for loose teeth; document findings on records.

Assess for self-care deficits and activity intolerance, because the school-aged child or adolescent may not ask for help when ambulating, bathing, toileting, and so forth.

Apply safety straps when transporting by cart or wheelchair.

Set limits. Enforce and repeat what the child can do and areas he or she can go in the hospital.

Provide age-appropriate activities. Supervise therapeutic play closely. Do not allow child to use syringes as squirt guns.

Do not allow parents to smoke or drink hot beverages in the child's room.

Encourage child or adolescent to wear Medic-Alert necklace or bracelet, if appropriate. Encourage him or her to carry identification in a wallet or purse.

Remind child to wear his or her seat belt in the car when discharged.

Discourage smoking and use of illicit drugs, including alcohol.

Assess each unique situation for risk for injury to the school-age child or adolescent. Inform parents of their child's risk for injury.

Rationale

To protect children from injury, caretakers must be aware of the age-related behavioral characteristics that increase the child's vulnerability to injury (Wong, 2003).

Anatomically, children are more susceptible to head injuries because of their large head, to liver and spleen trauma because these organs are larger, and to being thrown more easily (in a car) because of their small, light bodies (Wong, 2003).

Infants explore the environment through taste and touch.

Children have a natural curiosity, seek attractive objects, and frequently challenge rules.

Children cannot comprehend danger to self or others.

RISK FOR INJURY

⊕ RELATED TO VERTIGO SECONDARY TO ORTHOSTATIC HYPOTENSION

Goal

NOC Refer to *Risk for Injury*

The person will relate fewer episodes of dizziness or vertigo.

Indicators

- Identify situations that cause vertigo.
- Relate methods of preventing sudden decreases in cerebral blood flow from orthostatism.
- Demonstrate maneuvers to change position and avoid sudden drop in cerebral pressure.

Interventions

NIC Refer to *Risk for Injury*

Identify Contributing Factors.

Cardiovascular disorders (hypertension, cerebral infarct, anemia, dysrhythmias)
Fluid or electrolyte imbalances
Peripheral neuropathy, Parkinson's disease
Diabetes
Certain medications (antihypertensives, anticholinergics, barbiturates, vasodilators, tricyclic anti-
  depressants, levodopa, nitrates, monoamine oxidase inhibitors, phenothiazine)
Alcohol use
Age 75 years or older
Prolonged bed rest
Surgical sympathectomy
Valsalva maneuver during voiding (Miller, 2004)
Arthritis (spurs on cervical vertebrae)

Assess for Orthostatic Hypotension.

Take bilateral brachial pressures with the person supine.
If the brachial pressures are different, use the arm with the higher reading and take the blood pres-
  sure immediately after the client stands up quickly. Report differences to the physician.
Ask the client to describe sensations (eg, lightheaded, dizzy).
Assess skin and vital signs.

Discuss Physiology of Orthostatic Hypotension with Client.

Age-related changes in vessel
Sympathetic nervous system
  response
Postprandial effects
Volume of blood in lower extremities
Effects of prolonged bed rest
Vasomotor paralysis in clients with
  spinal cord injury

Teach Client Techniques to Reduce Orthostatic Hypotension.

Change positions slowly.
Move from lying to an upright position in stages.
  1. Sit up in bed.
  2. Dangle first one leg, then the other over the side of the bed.
  3. Allow a few minutes before going on to each step.
  4. Gradually pull oneself from a sitting to a standing position.
  5. Place a chair, walker, cane, or other assistive device nearby to use to steady oneself when
     getting out of bed.
Sleep with head of bed elevated up to 30 degrees.
During day, rest in a recliner rather than in bed.
Avoid prolonged standing.
Avoid stooping to pick something up from the floor; use an assistive device available from an
  orthotics department or a self-help store.
Evaluate the possible effectiveness of waist-high stockings.
    Wrap legs from below toes to top of thigh with elastic compression bandages. Check compression
      effectiveness before purchase.
    Put stockings on in morning before getting out of bed if compression is advised.
    Avoid sitting for long periods.
    Remove stockings when supine.

Encourage Person to Increase Daily Activity, if Permissible.

Discuss the value of daily exercise (increases circulation and energy levels, decreases stress and the
  process of osteoporosis, and contributes to overall well-being).
Establish an exercise program.

Teach Client to Avoid Dehydration and Vasodilation.

Replace fluids during periods of excess fluid loss (eg, hot weather).
Minimize diuretic fluids (eg, coffee, tea, cola).
Minimize alcohol consumption.
Avoid sources of intense heat (eg, direct sun, hot showers, baths, electric blankets).
Avoid taking nitroglycerin while standing.

Teach Client to Reduce Postprandial Hypotension (Miller, 2004).

Take antihypertensive medications after meals rather than before.

Eat small, frequent meals.

Remain seated or lie down after meals.

Institute Environmental Safety Measures (Refer to *Risk for Injury Related to Lack of Awareness of Environmental Hazards*).

Rationales

- Older adults cannot compensate for hypertensive or hypotensive stimuli as efficiently as younger adults and are thus more sensitive to these states (see also Orthostatic Hypotension under Key Concepts).
- The client's understanding of orthostatic hypotension may help him or her modify behavior to reduce the frequency and severity of episodes.
- Use of the arm with the higher pressure gives a more accurate assessment of the mean blood pressure.
- Prolonged bed rest increases venous pooling. Gradual position change allows the body to compensate for venous pooling (Porth, 2002).
- Adequate hydration is necessary to prevent decreased circulating volume.
- Certain medications (eg, vasodilators, antihistamines) can precipitate orthostatic hypotension.
- Studies have shown that in healthy older adults blood pressure is reduced by 20 mm Hg within 1 h of eating the morning or afternoon meal. This is thought to result from an impaired baroreflex compensatory response to splanchnic blood pooling during digestion (Miller, 2004).
- External heat may dilate the superficial vessels sufficiently to shunt blood from the brain, causing neurologic symptoms.
- Extensive isomotor paralysis results in decreased vascular tone (lower blood pressure; Hickey, 2002).

RISK FOR ASPIRATION

DEFINITION

Risk for Aspiration: State in which a person is at risk for entry of secretions, solids, or fluids into the tracheobronchial passages.

Risk Factors

Presence of favorable conditions for aspiration (see Related Factors)

RELATED FACTORS
Pathophysiologic

Related to reduced level of consciousness secondary to:

Presenile dementia	Parkinson's disease	Seizures
Head injury	Alcohol-/drug-induced	Anesthesia
Cerebrovascular accident	Coma	

Related to depressed cough/gag reflexes
Related to increased intragastric pressure secondary to:

Lithotomy position	Obesity	Enlarged uterus
Ascites		

Related to impaired swallowing or decreased laryngeal and glottic reflexes secondary to:

Achalasia	Muscular dystrophy	Scleroderma
Cerebrovascular accident	Esophageal strictures	Parkinson's disease
Myasthenia gravis	Debilitating conditions	Guillain-Barré syndrome
Catatonia	Multiple sclerosis	

Related to tracheoesophageal fistula
Related to impaired protective reflexes secondary to:

Facial/oral/neck surgery or trauma	Paraplegia or hemiplegia

Treatment-Related

Related to depressed laryngeal and glottic reflexes secondary to:

Tracheostomy/endotracheal tube	Sedation	Tube feedings

Related to impaired ability to cough secondary to:

Wired jaw	Imposed prone position

Situational (Personal, Environmental)

Related to inability/impaired ability to elevate upper body
Related to eating when intoxicated

Maturational

Premature
Related to impaired sucking/swallowing reflexes

Neonate
Related to decreased muscle tone of inferior esophageal sphincter

Older Adult
Related to poor dentition

◯◯ AUTHOR'S NOTE

Risk for Aspiration is a clinically useful diagnosis for people at high risk for aspiration because of reduced level of consciousness, structural deficits, mechanical devices, and neurologic and gastrointestinal disorders. People with swallowing difficulties often are at risk for aspiration; the nursing diagnosis *Impaired Swallowing* should be used to describe a client with difficulty swallowing who also is at risk for aspiration. *Risk for Aspiration* should be used to describe people who require nursing interventions to prevent aspiration, but do not have a swallowing problem.

◯◯ ERRORS IN DIAGNOSTIC STATEMENTS

1. *Risk for Aspiration related to bronchopneumonia*
   This diagnostic statement does not direct the nurse to the risk factors that could be reduced. If the nurse were monitoring and comanaging bronchopneumonia, the correct statement would be the collaborative problem *PC: Bronchopneumonia*.
2. *Risk for Aspiration related to difficulty swallowing*
   Difficulty swallowing is validation for *Impaired Swallowing*; thus, *Impaired Swallowing* would be correct. Nursing measures also would include prevention of aspiration.

KEY CONCEPTS
Generic Considerations

- Swallowing is a complicated mechanism with three stages:
  - The *voluntary stage* is the moving of the food from the palate to the pharynx.
  - The *pharyngeal stage* is automatic:
    - The soft palate is pulled up to close the posterior nares.
    - Palatopharyngeal folds on the sides of the pharynx constrict to permit passage of properly masticated food.
    - The epiglottis swings backward over the larynx opening to prevent aspiration into the trachea.
    - Relaxation of hypopharyngeal sphincter stretches the opening of the esophagus.
    - Rapid peristaltic wave forces food into the upper esophagus.
  - The *esophageal stage* moves the food from the pharynx to the stomach by peristaltic movements controlled by vagal reflexes.
- Central nervous system (CNS) depression interferes with the protective mechanism of the sphincters.
- Nasogastric and endotracheal tubes cause incomplete closure of the esophageal sphincters and depress the gag and cough reflexes.
- Clients with debilitating conditions who aspirate are at high risk for aspiration pneumonia.
- The volume and characteristics of the aspirated contents influence morbidity and mortality. Food particles can cause mechanical blockage. Gastric juice erodes alveoli and capillaries and causes chemical pneumonitis.

Pediatric Considerations

- A proportionately oversized airway diameter in infants and small children increases the risk of aspiration of foreign objects (Wong, 2003).
- Common household objects and food items that are aspirated include balloons (toy rubber balloons are the leading cause of choking deaths from children's products), baby powder, hot dogs, candy, nuts, grapes, and small batteries.
- Children with certain congenital anomalies (eg, tracheoesophageal fistula, cleft palate, gastroesophageal reflux) are at greater risk for aspiration.

Focus Assessment Criteria

Subjective Data
Assess for Related Factors.

History of a problem with swallowing or aspiration
Presence or history of: (see Pathophysiologic Related Factors)

Objective Data
Assess for Related Factors.

Ability to swallow, chew, feed self
Neuromuscular impairment
    Decreased/absent gag reflex
    Decreased strength on excursion of muscles involved in mastication
    Perceptual impairment
    Facial paralysis
Mechanical obstruction
    Edema
    Tracheostomy tube
    Tumor
Perceptual patterns/awareness
Level of consciousness
Condition of oropharyngeal cavity
Nasal regurgitation
Hoarseness

Aspiration
Coughing 1 or 2 s after swallowing
Dehydration
Apraxia

For more information on Focus Assessment Criteria, visit http://connection.lww.com.

Goal

| NOC | Aspiration Control |

The person will not experience aspiration.

Indicators

- Relate measures to prevent aspiration.
- Name foods or fluids that are high risk for causing aspiration.

General Interventions

| NIC | Aspiration Precautions, Airway Management, Positioning, Airway Suctioning |

Assess Causative or Contributing Factors.

Susceptible Individual

| Reduced level of consciousness | Autonomic disorders | Debilitated |
| Newborn | | |

Tracheostomy/Endotracheal Tubes

Gastrointestinal Tubes/Feedings

Reduce the Risk of Aspiration in:

Clients with Decreased Strength, Decreased Sensorium, or Autonomic Disorders

Maintain a side-lying position if not contraindicated by injury.

If the person cannot be positioned on the side, open oropharyngeal airway by lifting the mandible up and forward, tilting the head backward (for a small infant, hyperextension of the neck may not be effective).

Assess for position of the tongue, ensuring it has not dropped backward, occluding the airway.

Keep the head of the bed elevated, if not contraindicated by hypertension or injury.

Maintain good oral hygiene. Clean teeth and use mouthwash on cotton swab; apply petroleum jelly to lips, removing encrustations gently.

Clear secretions from mouth and throat with a tissue or gentle suction.

Reassess frequently for obstructive material in mouth and throat.

Reevaluate frequently for good anatomic positioning.

Maintain side-lying position after feedings.

Tracheostomy or Endotracheal Tubes

Inflate cuff:
  During continuous mechanical ventilation
  During and after eating
  During and 1 h after tube feedings
  During intermittent positive-pressure breathing treatments
Suction every 1 to 2 h and PRN.

Gastrointestinal Tubes and Feedings

Confirm that tube placement has been verified by radiography or aspiration of greenish fluid.

Confirm that tube position has not changed since it was inserted and verified.

Elevate head of bed 30 to 45 min during feeding periods and 1 h after to prevent reflux by use of reverse gravity.

Aspirate for residual contents before each feeding for tubes positioned gastrically.

Administer feeding if residual contents are less than 150 mL (intermittent), or administer feeding if residual is no greater than 150 mL at 10% to 20% of hourly rate (continuous).

Regulate gastric feedings using an intermittent schedule, allowing periods for stomach emptying between feeding intervals.

For an Older Adult with Difficulties Chewing and Swallowing, see *Impaired Swallowing*.

Initiate Health Teaching and Referrals, as Indicated.

Instruct person and family on causes and prevention of aspiration.

Have family demonstrate tube-feeding technique.

Refer family to community nursing agency for assistance at home.

Teach client about the danger of eating when under the influence of alcohol.

Teach the Heimlich or abdominal thrust maneuver to remove aspirated foreign bodies.

Rationales

- Regurgitation is often silent in people with decreased sensorium or depressed mental states.
- Increased intragastric pressure can contribute to regurgitation and aspiration. Causes include bolus tube feedings, obstructions, obesity, pregnancy, and autonomic dysfunction.
- Verifying correct placement of feeding tubes is done most reliably by radiography. Aspiration of green-colored fluid or gastric aspirant with a pH of 6.5 or lower is also reliable. Verifying placement by instilling air and simultaneously auscultating or by aspirating nongreen fluid has proved inaccurate.
- After radiographic verification of correct feeding tube placement and knowledge that the position of the tube has not changed, routine testing of placement before feeding is not needed.
- Tracheostomy tubes interfere with the synchrony of the glottic closure. Inadequate cuff inflation provides a path for aspirate.
- Such regulation is necessary to prevent overfeeding and increased risk of reflux and aspiration. Gastric feedings should be administered intermittently when the potential for aspiration is high. Continuous feedings increase the risk of aspiration because the stomach contains a constant supply of formula.

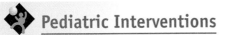 **Pediatric Interventions**

For Newborns with Cleft Lip, Palate, or Both:

Position infant's head upright.

Use a special feeding device for infants with cleft lip / cleft palate such as a cleft lip / cleft palate nurser, the Haberman Feeder, or a gravity flow nipple.

Position the nipple so it is compressed by the infant's tongue and existing palate.

Observe for signs to stop feeding momentarily, such as elevated eyebrows, wrinkled forehead (Wong, 2003).

Do not position the nipple through the cleft.

Apply gentle counter pressure on the base of the bottle to assist the infant with tongue and palate control of the milk flow.

Burp frequently because of excessive air swallowing.

If nipple feeding is unsuccessful, use a rubber-tipped syringe to deposit the formula on the back of the tongue.

Rationales

- All newborns have poor muscle tone of the cardiac sphincter of the esophagus, thus causing regurgitation easily (Wong, 2003).
- These infants cannot apply enough suction to use normal nipples.
- Sucking is important for muscle development for later speech development (Wong, 2003).
- Excessive air swallowing necessitates frequent burping.
- Gentle pressure at the base of bottle assists the infant with tongue and palate control.

RISK FOR FALLS

DEFINITION

Risk for Falls: State in which a person has increased susceptibility to falling

RISK FACTORS

Presence of risk factors (see Related Factors for *Risk for Injury*)

⊚ AUTHOR'S NOTE

This new nursing diagnosis can be used to specify a person at risk for falls. If the person is at risk for various types of injuries (eg, a cognitively impaired person), the broader diagnosis *Risk for Injury* is more useful.

⊚ ERRORS IN DIAGNOSTIC STATEMENTS

Risk for Falls related to inadequate supervision

    This diagnosis represents a legally inappropriate statement. Even if it is true, the diagnosis should be rewritten as *Risk for Falls related to inability to identify environmental hazards as a result of dementia*.

KEY CONCEPTS

Refer to *Risk for Injury*.

Focus Assessment Criteria

Refer to *Risk for Injury*.

Goals

Refer to *Risk for Injury*.

General Interventions

Refer to *Risk for Injury*.

RISK FOR POISONING

DEFINITION
Risk for Poisoning: State in which a person is at risk of accidental exposure to or ingestion of drugs or dangerous substances

RISK FACTORS
Presence of risk factors (see Related Factors for *Risk for Injury*)

RISK FOR SUFFOCATION

DEFINITION
Risk for Suffocation: State in which a person is at risk for smothering and asphyxiation.

RISK FACTORS
Presence of risk factors (see Related Factors for *Risk for Injury*)

RISK FOR TRAUMA

DEFINITION
Risk for Trauma: State in which a person is at risk of accidental tissue injury (eg, wound, burns, fracture)

RISK FACTORS
Presence of risk factors (see Related Factors for *Risk for Injury*)

RISK FOR PERIOPERATIVE POSITIONING INJURY

DEFINITION

Risk for Perioperative Positioning Injury: State in which a person is at risk for harm as a result of positioning requirements for surgery and loss of usual protective responses secondary to anesthesia

RISK FACTORS

Presence of risk factors (see Related Factors)

RELATED FACTORS
Pathophysiologic

Related to increased vulnerability secondary to:

Chronic disease	Radiation therapy	Renal, hepatic dysfunction
Cancer	Osteoporosis	Infection
Thin body frame	Compromised immune system	

Related to compromised tissue perfusion secondary to:

Diabetes mellitus	Cardiovascular disease	Peripheral vascular disease
Anemia	Hypothermia	History of thrombosis
Ascites	Dehydration	Edema

Related to vulnerability of stoma during positioning
Related to pre-existing contractures or physical impairments secondary to:

Rheumatoid arthritis	Polio

Treatment-Related

Related to position requirements and loss of usual sensory protective responses secondary to anesthesia*
Related to surgical procedures of 2 hours or longer
Related to vulnerability of implants or prostheses (eg, pacemakers) during positioning

Situational (Personal, Environmental)

Related to compromised circulation secondary to:

Obesity	Pregnancy	Cool operating suite
Tobacco use		

Maturational

Related to increased vulnerability to tissue injury secondary to:

Infant status	Elder status

⊕⊕ AUTHOR'S NOTE

This diagnosis focuses on identifying the vulnerability for tissue, nerve, and joint injury resulting from required positions for surgery. The addition of *perioperative positioning* to *Risk for Injury* adds etiology to the label.

If a client has no pre-existing risk factors that make him or her more vulnerable to injury, this diagnosis could be used with no related factors because they are evident. If related factors are

(continued)

---

*This risk factor is always present and may be deleted from the diagnostic statement.

⊙ **AUTHOR'S NOTE** (*Continued*)

desired, the statement could read *Risk for Perioperative Positioning Injury related to position requirements for surgery and loss of usual sensory protective measures secondary to anesthesia.*

When a client has pre-existing risk factors, the statement should include these—for example, *Risk for Perioperative Positioning Injuries related to compromised tissue perfusion secondary to peripheral arterial disease.*

⊙ **ERRORS IN DIAGNOSTIC STATEMENTS**

Risk for Perioperative Positioning Injury related to inadequate protective measures

These related factors are legally problematic. Even if inadequate protective measures are a problem, they must not be included in the diagnostic statement. Instead, this problem should be referred to nursing management.

KEY CONCEPTS
Generic Considerations

- The physiologic effects of positioning for surgical procedures vary with the specific position. Overall, positioning affects the cardiovascular, respiratory, neurologic, and integumentary systems.
- Prolonged immobility diminishes the pulmonary capillary blood flow volume. Positional pressure on the ribs or the diaphragm's ability to force abdominal contents downward limits lung expansion.
- Anesthesia causes peripheral blood vessels to dilate, resulting in hypotension, and decreases blood return to heart and lungs. Prolonged immobility causes pooling in vascular beds.
- People with obesity are at increased risk for injury from surgical positions as a result of the following (Fuller, 1994):
  - Lifting them into position is difficult.
  - Massive tissue and pressure areas need extra padding.
  - The mechanics of manipulating adipose tissue may prolong length of surgery.
  - Recovery period may be prolonged because adipose tissue retains fat-soluble agents and slows elimination of agents.
  - Venous stasis decreases circulation, and adipose tissue has a poor blood supply.

⊙ Geriatric Considerations

Osteoarthritis, loss of subcutaneous fat, decreased peripheral circulation, and wasted flaccid muscles can contribute to injury or trauma to bones, joints, nerves, and skin when on the operating table (Stanley & Beare, 1995).

Focus Assessment Criteria

Subjective Data
Assess for Pre-existing Risk Factors.

Refer to Related Factors.

Objective Data
Assess for Presurgical Risk Factors.

Skin

Temperature (cool, warm)

Color (pale, dependent rubor, flushed, cyanotic, brown discolorations)

Ulcerations (size, location, description of surrounding tissue)

Bilateral pulses (radial, posterior tibial, dorsalis pedis)
Rate, rhythm
Volume
+0 = Absent, nonpalpable
+1 = Thready, weak, fades in and out
+2 = Present but diminished
+3 = Normal, easily palpable
+4 = Aneurysmal

Paresthesia (numbness, tingling, burning)
Edema (location, pitting)
Capillary refill (normal less than 3 s)
Range of motion (normal, compromised)

For more information on Focus Assessment Criteria, visit http://connection.lww.com.

Goal

> **NOC** Circulation Status, Neurologic Status, Tissue Perfusion: Peripheral

The person will have no neuromuscular damage or injury related to the surgical position.

Indicators

- Padding is used as indicated for procedure.
- Limbs are secured when at risk.
- Limbs are flexed when indicated.

General Interventions

> **NIC** Positioning: Intraoperative, Surveillance, Pressure Management

Determine Whether Client has Pre-existing Risk Factors (Refer to Risk Factors); Communicate Findings to Surgical Team.

Before Positioning, Assess and Document:

Range-of-motion ability
External/internal prostheses
  or implants

Circulatory status
Physical abnormalities
Neurovascular status

Move the Person From the Transport Stretcher to the Operating Room (OR) Bed.
Have a minimum of two people with their hands free (eg, not holding an IV bag).
Explain the transfer to the client. Lock all wheels on the stretcher and bed.
Ask person to move slowly to the OR bed. Assist during the move. Do not pull or drag person.
When client is on the OR bed, attach a safety belt a few inches above the knees with a space of three fingerbreadths.
Check that legs are not crossed and that feet are slightly separated and not over the edge.
Ensure that the person is not touching any metal of table or equipment.
Do not leave the person unattended.

Discuss with the Surgeon the Surgical Position Desired.

Advise if Any Pre-existing Factors Exist. Determine if the Position will be Arranged Before or After Anesthesia.

Always Ask the Anesthesiologist or Nurse Anesthetist for Permission Before Moving or Repositioning an Anesthetized Person.

Reduce Vulnerability to Injury (Soft Tissue, Joint, Nerves, Blood Vessels).
Align the neck and spine at all times.
Gently manipulate joints. Do not abduct more than 90 degrees.
Do not let limbs extend off the OR bed. Reposition slowly and gently.

Use a draw-sheet above the elbows to tuck in arms at side or abduct arm on an arm board with padding.

Protect Eyes and Ears From Injury.

Use padding or a special headrest to protect ears, superficial nerves, and blood vessels of face if the head is on its side.

Ensure that the ear is not bent when positioned.

If needed, protect eyes from abrasions with an eye patch or shield.

Depending on the Surgical Position Used, Protect Vulnerable Areas; Document Position and Protection Measures Used.

Supine

Pad the calcaneus, sacrum, coccyx, olecranon process, scapula, ischial tuberosity, and occiput.

Keep arms at side, palms down or abducted on arm board.

Protect the head and ears if the head is turned to the side.

Trendelenburg

Use a well-padded shoulder brace over the acromion process, not soft tissue, and away from neck.

Reverse Trendelenburg

Use a padded foot board.

Jack-Knife (Modified Prone)

Use padded arm boards at correct heights to allow elbows to bend comfortably.

Place a soft pillow under the down ear.

Cushion hips and thighs with large pillows.

Cushion breasts.

Cushion male genitalia in natural position.

Use a large pillow under the lower legs and ankles to raise the toes off the bed.

Use additional padding on the shoulder girdle, olecranon, anterosuperior iliac spine, patella, and dorsum of the foot.

Apply a safety strap across the thighs.

Prone

Position two large body rolls longitudinally from the acromioclavicular joint to the iliac crest.

Refer to jack-knife for additional information.

Laminectomy

After induction of anesthesia, at least six people help roll the person from the stretcher to the OR bed onto laminectomy brace.

Keep body aligned.

Protect limbs from torsion.

Place rolled towels in axillary regions.

Follow precautions for jack-knife.

Lithotomy

Prepare stirrups with padding.

Have two people simultaneously and slowly raise legs with slight rotation of the hips. Gently position the knees slightly flexed.

Position buttocks about 1 inch over the end of the table.

Use a small lumbar pad and extra padding in sacral area.

Cover legs with cotton boots.

Position arms on arm boards or loosely over abdomen, supported with a sheet.

Fowler

Position the neck in straight alignment.

Use a padded foot board.

Support the knees with a pillow.

Cross arms loosely over the abdomen and tape on pillow.

Sims (Lateral)

Position on the side with arms extended on double arm boards.

Flex the lower leg.

Use a small pillow under the head.

Use a rolled towel in the axillary area of the downside arm.

Elevate and pad the flank.

Flex the lower leg and place a long pillow the length of the leg to the groin.

Use a 4-inch strip of adhesive tape attached to one side of the table, over iliac crest and to other side.

Protect ankles and feet from pressure.

Protect male genitalia, female breasts, and ear as for jack-knife position.

If Feasible, Ask Client if He or She Feels Pain, Burning, Pressure, or Any Discomfort After Positioning.

Continually Assess that Team Members are Not Leaning on the Client, Especially Limbs.

Ensure That the Head is Lifted Slightly Every 30 Min.

When Repositioning or Returning Person to Supine Position After Certain Surgical Positions (eg, Trendelenburg, Lithotomy, Reverse Trendelenburg, Jack-Knife, Lateral), Slowly Change Position to Prevent Severe Hypotension.

Assess Skin Condition When Surgery is Over. Document Findings. Inform Postanesthesia Nurses of Any Pre-existing Risk Factors That Increase Postoperative Vulnerability.

Continue to Assess and to Relieve Pressure to Vulnerable Areas Postoperatively.

Rationales

- Prolonged positioning can cause mechanical pressure on peripheral and superficial nerves. Hyper-extension (>90-degree angle) of a limb of an anesthetized person can cause nerve injuries (Fairchild, 1993; Rothrock, 1996).
  - Hyperextension of the arm on an arm board can injure the brachial plexus (in the arm). Improper positioning of the brace also can injure the brachial plexus.
  - Ulnar nerve injuries occur when an elbow slips off the mattress and is compressed between the table and the medial epicondyle.
  - Radial nerve injuries occur when the nerve is compressed between the client and the table surface or from striking the table.
  - Saphenous and peroneal nerve damage occurs with the use of stirrups with lithotomy— compression of the peroneal nerve against the stirrups or of the saphenous nerve between the metal popliteal knee support stirrup and the medial tibial condyle.
- Tissue and skin can be injured by excessive pressure or bruised by hitting a hard surface. People more vulnerable to pressure injuries are the very young, older adults, dehydrated, very thin or obese, and those undergoing more than 2 h of immobility.
- Anesthetic agents interfere with normal vasodilation and constriction, thus reducing perfusion to bony prominences or compressed or dependent limbs.
- Excessive pressure of position, equipment, or surgery can cause injury to the face and eyes. Excessive pressure to the eyes can cause thrombosis of the central renal artery. Eyes should be kept closed and lubricated to prevent drying and scratching.
- If repositioning is necessary after induction, lifting, rather than rolling or pulling, the person prevents shearing forces and friction. Shearing occurs when the dermal layers stay fixed because of the friction between linen and skin, and tissues attached to bony structures move with the weight of the torso (Fairchild, 1993). Tissue layers slide on each other, resulting in the kinking or stretching of subcutaneous blood vessels, thus obstructing blood flow to and from areas (Porth, 2002).
- Prolonged immobilization of and pressure on the head can cause alopecia. Postoperatively, it first appears as edema and painful seroma leading to ulceration and localized hair loss (transient or permanent).
- Most surgical positions, except supine and prone, cause massive circulatory pooling. If the surgical position is reversed too quickly, severe hypotension can occur. Gradual and slow changes in position allow the person's cardiovascular system to adjust to the change (Rothrock, 1996).

DEFICIENT KNOWLEDGE

DEFINITION

Deficient Knowledge: State in which a person or group experiences a deficiency in cognitive knowledge or psychomotor skills concerning the condition or treatment plan

DEFINING CHARACTERISTICS
Major (Must Be Present, One or More)

Verbalizes a deficiency in knowledge or skill/request for information
Expresses "inaccurate" perception of health status
Does not correctly perform a desired or prescribed health behavior

Minor (May Be Present)

Lack of integration of treatment plan into daily activities
Exhibits or expresses psychological alteration (eg, anxiety, depression) resulting from misinformation or lack of information

---

⦾ AUTHOR'S NOTE

Deficient knowledge does not represent a human response, alteration, or pattern of dysfunction, but a related factor.* All people have knowledge deficits. It is when this lack of knowledge causes or could cause a problem that requires nursing interventions. Lack of knowledge can contribute to various responses (eg, anxiety, self-care deficits, noncompliance). All nursing diagnoses have related client/family teaching as part of nursing interventions (eg, *Impaired Verbal Communication*). When teaching directly relates to a specific nursing diagnosis, the nurse incorporates it in the plan. When lack of or insufficient knowledge is the primary cause of a diagnosis or a risk factor for a potential diagnosis, the nurse lists lack of knowledge as a "Related to." For example, when specific teaching is indicated before a procedure, the nurse can use *Anxiety related to unfamiliar environment and procedures.* When information giving is directed to assist a person or family with a decision, *Decisional Conflict* may be indicated. Conley (1998) proposed that a nursing diagnosis of *Information-Seeking Behaviors* serve as an alternative to *Deficient Knowledge.*† Other examples of diagnostic statements with lack of knowledge as the "Related to" are *Risk for Ineffective Therapeutic Regimen Management related to lack of knowledge of diabetes mellitus, management, and signs/symptoms of complications; Risk for Impaired Home Maintenance related to lack of knowledge of home care and community resources;* and *Risk for Injury related to lack of knowledge of bicycle safety.*

---

*Jenny, J. (1987). Knowledge deficit: Not a nursing diagnosis. *Image, 19*(4), 184–185.
†Conley, V. (1998) Beyond *Knowledge Deficit* to a proposal for *Information-Seeking Behaviors. Nursing Diagnosis, 9*(4), 129–135.

LATEX ALLERGY RESPONSE

DEFINITION

Latex Allergy Response: State in which a person experiences an immunoglobin E (IgE)–mediated response to latex

DEFINING CHARACTERISTICS
Major (Must be Present)

Positive skin test to natural rubber latex (NRL) extract

Minor

Allergic conjunctivitis   Urticaria   Rhinitis
Asthma

RELATED FACTORS
Biopathophysiologic

Related to hypersensitivity
Response to the protein component of natural rubber latex

KEY CONCEPTS
Generic Considerations

- NRL has been used widely in many products for more than 100 years. The first case of immediate hypersensitivity to latex was reported in 1979 (Reddy, 1998).
- Use of latex gloves and condoms has increased dramatically since 1985. The increase in total exposure to latex has led to more people with latex sensitivity (Reddy, 1998).
- Risk groups for *Latex Allergy* are health care workers; rubber industry workers; people with spina bifida, history of barium enema, history of indwelling catheter, repeated catheterizations, urogenital abnormalities, or history of repeated or prolonged surgeries or mucous membrane exposure to latex; and people with atopic history or history of food allergy (banana, avocado, mango, kiwi, passion fruit, chestnut, melon, tomato, celery).
- Some reactions to latex products are delayed immunologic responses caused by chemical irritants used in the manufacture of latex gloves. This is a type IV allergic reaction, which is not a true latex allergy (Kleinbeck et al., 1998). A true latex allergy (type I reaction) occurs shortly after exposure to the proteins in NRL (Kleinbeck et al., 1998).

Focus Assessment Criteria

Subjective Data
Assess for Defining Characteristics.

History of swelling, itching, sneezing, itchy throat, watery eyes, or redness of skin or mucous membranes upon exposure to any of the following:

Dental work   Condom use   Blowing up a balloon
Adhesive tape   Rubber cement   Elastic underwear

Rubber gloves	Shoes	Tennis racket
Golf grip	Garden hose	

Personal history of any of the following:

Asthma	Urticaria	Contact dermatitis
Conjunctivitis	Eczema	Rhinitis
Anaphylactic reaction		

Allergies to any of the following:

Avocado	Passion fruit	Peach
Chestnut	Tomato	Banana
Mango	Raw potato	Kiwi
Papaya		

History of adverse reaction or complication to surgery
Positive diagnostic testing (eg, antilatex IgE)

Assess for Risk Factors.

Occupation with frequent contact with latex (present? past?)
History of surgeries, urinary catheterizations, barium enema (before 1992)
Congenital abnormalities; spina bifida

For more information on Focus Assessment Criteria, visit http://connection.lww.com.

Goal

 NOC Immune Hypersensitivity Control

The person will report no exposure to latex.

Indicators

- Describe products of NRL.
- Describe strategies to avoid exposure.

General Interventions

NIC Allergy Management, Latex Precautions, Environmental Risk Protection

Assess for Causative and Contributing Factors (Refer to Focus Assessment).

Eliminate Exposure to Latex Products.

Use Nonlatex Alternative Supplies.
Clear disposable amber bags
Silicone baby nipples
2×2 gauze pads with silk tape in place of adhesive bandages
Clear plastic or Silastic catheters
Vinyl or neoprene gloves
Kling-like gauze

Protect from Exposure to Latex.
Cover skin with cloth before applying blood pressure cuff.
Do not allow rubber stethoscope tubing to touch person.
Do not inject through rubber parts (eg, heparin locks); use syringe and stopcock.
Change needles after each puncture of rubber stopper.
Cover rubber parts with tape.

Teach Which Products Are Commonly Made of Latex.
Health care equipment
Natural latex rubber gloves, powdered or unpowdered, including those labeled "hypoallergenic"

Blood pressure cuffs	Stethoscopes	Tourniquets
Electrode pads	Airways, endotracheal tubes	Syringe plunges, bulb syringes
Masks for anesthesia	Rubber aprons	Catheters, wound drains
Injection ports	Tops of multidose vials	Adhesive tape
Ostomy pouches	Wheelchair cushions	Briefs with elastic
Pads for crutches		

Office / household products

Erasers	Rubber bands	Dishwashing gloves
Balloons	Condoms, diaphragms	Baby bottle nipples, pacifiers
Rubber balls and toys	Racquet handles	Cycle grips
Tires	Hot water bottles	Carpeting
Shoe soles	Elastic in underwear	Rubber cement

Initiate Health Teaching as Indicated.

Explain the importance of completely avoiding direct contact with all NRL products.

Advise that a person with a history of a mild skin reaction to latex is at risk for anaphylaxis.

Instruct client to wear a Medic-Alert bracelet stating "Latex Allergy" and to carry autoinjectable epinephrine.

Instruct client to warn all health care providers (eg, dental, medical, surgical) of allergy.

Rationales

- Any exposure (tactile, inhaled, ingested) can precipitate an anaphylactic reaction.
- Products containing latex are very common in health care environments and the home.

RISK FOR LATEX ALLERGY RESPONSE

DEFINITION

Latex Allergy Response, Risk for: State in which a person is at risk for experiencing an immunoglobin E (IgE)-mediated allergic response to latex.

RISK FACTORS
Biopathophysiologic

Related to history of atopic eczema
Related to history of allergic rhinitis
Related to history of asthma

Treatment-Related

Related to frequent urinary catheterizations
Related to frequent rectal impaction removal
Related to frequent surgical procedures
Related to barium enema (before 1992)

Situational (Personal, Environmental)
Related to

History of food allergy to banana, kiwi, avocado, tomato, raw potato, peach, chestnuts, mango, papaya, passion fruit

History of allergy to gloves, condoms, and so forth

Frequent occupational exposure to Natural Rubber Latex (NRL), such as:

Workers making NRL products	Food handlers	Greenhouse workers
	Health care workers	Housekeepers

KEY CONCEPTS
Generic Considerations
Refer to *Latex Allergy Response.*

Focus Assessment Criteria

Refer to *Latex Allergy Response.*

Goals

Refer to *Latex Allergy Response.*

General Interventions

Refer to *Latex Allergy Response.*

SEDENTARY LIFESTYLE

DEFINITION
Sedentary Lifestyle: The state in which an individual or group reports a habit of life that is characterized by a low physical activity level

DEFINING CHARACTERISTICS
Major (Must Be Present, One or More)
Chooses a daily routine lacking physical exercise
Demonstrates physical deconditioning
Verbalized preference for activities low in physical activity

RELATED FACTORS
Pathophysiologic-related decreased endurance secondary to obesity.

Situational (Personal, Environment)
Related to inadequate knowledge of health benefits of physical activity
Related to inadequate knowledge of exercise routines
Related to insufficient resources (money, facilities)
Related to perceived lack of time
Related to lack of motivation
Related to lack of interest
Related to lack of injury

> ◎ AUTHOR'S NOTE
>
> This is the first nursing diagnosis submitted by a nurse from another country and accepted by NANDA. Congratulations to J. Adolf Guirao-Goris of Valencia, Spain.

KEY CONCEPTS
Generic Considerations

- Regular exercise can increase

Cardiovascular-respiratory endurance	Delivery of nutrients to tissue
Muscle strength	Tolerance for psychological stress
Muscle endurance	Ability to reduce body fat content
Flexibility	

- Vigorous exercise sessions should include a warm-up phase (10 minutes at a slow pace), endurance exercise, and a cool-down phase (5 to 10 minutes of a slow pace and stretching).
- Current beliefs regarding optimal exercise are as follows (Allison & Keller, 1997):
  Emphasize physical activity over "exercise."
  Moderate physical activity that accumulates to 30 or more minutes is beneficial.
  To enhance long-term exercise, the person should (Moore & Charvat, 2002):
  Respond to relapse with a plan to prevent recurrences.
  Set realistic goals.
  Keep an exercise log.
  Exercise with a friend.
- A regular pattern of moderate intensity physical activity of 30 minutes or more, which can be accumulated throughout the day, 4 to 5 times a week, can be beneficial. Previously, vigorous exercise was recommended for a continuous 30 minutes or more (Belza & Warms, 2004).
- Forty percent of adults are completely sedentary in their leisure time (Nies & Chruscial, 2002).
- At least 1 hour of walking per week can lower the risk of coronary heart disease in women (Lee et al., 2001).

Geriatric Considerations

- Physical activity, healthful eating, social connections, meaningful involvement and access to health care can increase healthy aging (Young & Cochrane, 2004).
- Physical activity contributes to well-being, flexibility, strength, function, and chronic disease management (Taggart, 2002).
- Only 24% of older women exercise (Rogers et al., 2002).
- Tai Chi improved balance, functional mobility and fear of falling among older women (Taggart, 2002).
- Falls in older women are a major health concerns (Young & Cochrane, 2004).

Focus Assessment Criteria

Subjective Data
Assess for Defining Characteristic.
Regular exercise pattern (none, daily weekly).
Reports fatigue, shortness of breath with increased activity.

Goal

 Knowledge: Health Behaviors, Physical Fitness

The person will verbalize intent to or engage in increased physical activity.

Indicators
- Set a goal for weekly exercise.
- Identify a desired activity or exercise.

General Intervention

NIC Exercise Promotion, Exercise Therapy

Discuss Benefits of Exercise

Reduces caloric absorption	Suppresses appetite	Improves self-esteem
Preserves lean muscle mass	Increases oxygen uptake	Increases restful sleep

Reduces depression, anxiety stress	Increases caloric expenditure	Increases resistance to age-related degeneration
Improves body posture	Maintains weight loss	
Provides fun, recreation, diversion	Increases metabolic rate	

Assist Client to Identify Realistic Exercise Program. Consider:

Physical limitations (consult nurse or physician)
Personal preferences
Lifestyle
Community resources
Needed clothing and shoes
Clients must learn to monitor pulse before, during, and after exercise to assist them to achieve target heart rate and not to exceed maximum advisable heart rate for age.

Age	Maximum Heart Rate	Target Heart Rate
30	190	133 to 162
40	180	126 to 153
50	170	119 to 145
60	160	112 to 136

Discuss Aspects of Starting the Exercise Program.

Start slow and easy; obtain clearance from physician.
Read, consult experts, and talk with friends/coworkers who exercise.
Plan a daily walking program.
   Start at 5 to 10 blocks for 0.5 to 1 mile/day; increase 1 block or 0.1 mile/week.
   Gradually increase rate and length of walk; remember to progress slowly.
   Avoid straining or pushing too hard and becoming overly fatigued.
   Stop immediately if any of the following occur:

Lightness or pain chest	Dizziness
Severe breathlessness	Loss of muscle control
Lightheadedness	Nausea

If pulse is 120 beats/minute (bpm) at 4 minutes or 100 bpm at 10 minutes after stopping exercise, or if shortness of breath occurs 10 minutes after exercise, slow down either the rate or the distance of walking for 1 week to point before signs appear and then start to add 1 block/0.1 mile each week.
Walk at same rate; time with stopwatch or second hand on watch; after reaching 10 blocks (1 mile), try to increase speed.
Remember, increase only the rate or the distance of walking at one time.
Establish a regular time for exercise, with the goal of three to five times/week for 15 to 45 minutes and a heart rate of 80% of stress test or gross calculation (170 bpm for 20 to 29 years of age.) Decrease 10 bpm for each additional decade (eg, 160 bpm for 30 to 39 years of age, 150 bpm for 40 to 49 years of age).
Encourage significant others also to engage in walking program.
Add supplemental activity (eg, parking far from destination, gardening, using stairs, spending weekends at activities that require walking).
Work up to 1 hour of exercise per day at least 4 days per week.
Avoid lapses of more than 2 days between exercise sessions.

Assist Client to Increase Interest and Motivation.

Develop contact listing realistic short- and long-term goals.
Keep intake/activity records.
Increase knowledge by reading and talking with health-conscious friends and coworkers.
Make new friends who are health conscious.
Get a friend to also follow the program or be a source of support.
Be aware of rationalization (eg, a lack of time may be a lack of prioritization).
Keep a list of positive outcomes.

Rationales

- The process of seeking and attaining positive lifestyle change is known as "empowering potential" (Fleury, 1991). It occurs in three stages: appraising readiness, changing, and integrating change.

As a person strives to improve health, he or she moves through a process of introspection; planning new, healthier activities; coping with barriers and setbacks; and ultimately absorbing these new behaviors into everyday life.

- The client is responsible for choosing a healthy pattern of living. The nurse is responsible for explaining the choices.
- Intake must be reduced to 500 cal/day less than requirement to obtain a 1-lb/week weight loss.
- Prescribed weight loss rate is 1 to 2 lb/week.
- Any increase in activity also increases energy output and caloric deficits.
- Often, inappropriate response to external cues, including stressors, facilitates or aggravates obesity. This response initiates an ineffective pattern in which the person eats in response to stress cues rather than physiologic hunger.
- The safest activities for the unconditioned obese person are walking, water aerobics, and swimming.
- A regular exercise program should be:
  Enjoyable
  Use a minimum of 400 calories in each session
  Sustain a heart rate of approximately 120 to 150 bpm
  Involve rhythmic, alternating contracting and relaxing of muscles
  Be integrated into the person's lifestyle 4 to 5 days/week for at least 30 to 60 minutes.

RISK FOR LONELINESS

DEFINITION
Risk for Loneliness: State in which a person is at risk for experiencing discomfort associated with a desire or need for contact with others

RISK FACTORS
See Related Factors.

RELATED FACTORS
Pathophysiologic
Related to fear of rejection secondary to:
Obesity
Cancer (disfiguring surgery of head or neck, superstition from others)
Physical handicaps (paraplegia, amputation, arthritis, hemiplegia)
Emotional handicaps (extreme anxiety, depression, paranoia, phobias)
Incontinence (embarrassment, odor)
Communicable diseases (acquired immunodeficiency syndrome [AIDS], hepatitis)
Psychiatric illness (schizophrenia, bipolar affective disorder, personality disorders)

Related to difficulty accessing social events secondary to:
Debilitating diseases   Physical disabilities

Treatment-Related
Related to therapeutic isolation

Situational (Personal, Environmental)
Related to insufficient planning for retirement
Related to death of a significant other
Related to divorce
Related to disfiguring appearance

Related to fear of rejection secondary to:

Obesity
Extreme poverty

Hospitalization or terminal illness (dying process)
Unemployment

Related to moving to another culture (eg, unfamiliar language)
Related to history of unsatisfactory social experiences secondary to:

Drug abuse
Delusional thinking

Unacceptable social behavior
Immature behavior

Alcohol abuse

Related to loss of usual means of transportation
Related to change in usual residence secondary to:

Long-term care

Relocation

Maturational

Child
Related to protective isolation or a communicable disease

Older Adult
Related to loss of usual social contacts secondary to:

Retirement
Loss of driving ability

Death of (specify)

Relocation

AUTHOR'S NOTE

Risk for Loneliness was added to the NANDA list in 1994. Currently, *Social Isolation* is also on the NANDA list. *Social Isolation* is a conceptually incorrect diagnosis, because it does not represent a response but a cause. *Loneliness* and *Risk for Loneliness* better describe the negative state of aloneness.

Loneliness is a subjective state that exists whenever a person says it does and perceives it as imposed by others. Social isolation is *not* the voluntary solitude necessary for personal renewal, nor is it the creative aloneness of the artist or the aloneness—and possible suffering—a person may experience from seeking individualism and independence (eg, moving to a new city, going away to college).

ERRORS IN DIAGNOSTIC STATEMENTS

1. *Loneliness related to inability to engage in satisfying personal relationships since death of wife 1 year ago*
   When a person fails to resume activities or to renew or to initiate social relationships after the death of a spouse, the nurse should suspect *Dysfunctional Grieving*. Prolonged social isolation after a death is a cue for unresolved grief. The nurse should conduct a focus assessment to identify other cues, such as prolonged denial, depression, or other evidence of unsuccessful adaptation to the loss. Until additional data are confirmed, the diagnosis *Possible Dysfunctional Grieving related to failure to resume or initiate relationships after wife's death 1 year ago* would be appropriate.
2. *Loneliness related to multiple sclerosis*
   Using multiple sclerosis as a related factor clusters all people with this condition as socially isolated and for the same reasons. This not only violates the uniqueness of each person but also does not specify how a nurse can intervene. If mobility and incontinence problems are present but no data support social isolation, the nurse can record the diagnosis as *Risk for Loneliness related to mobility and incontinence problems secondary to multiple sclerosis*.

KEY CONCEPTS
Generic Considerations

- Loneliness is an affective statement involving an awareness of being apart from others with an accompanying vague need for them (Leiderman, 1969).

- Loneliness differs from aloneness, solitude, and grief. *Aloneness* refers to being without company (not necessarily a negative state). *Solitude* involves being alone with a positive affective state. *Grief* is a response to traumatic loss (Hillestad, 1984).
- Social isolation can result in intense feelings of loneliness and suffering. Suffering associated with social isolation is not always visible. To diagnose this state, nurses must first be able to identify those at risk.
- The lonely or isolated person often aggravates his or her condition by suffering alone. Lonely people tend to shun one another. They may resign themselves to their situation and never seek companionship or help. They may deny their feelings. Illness, whether physical or psychiatric, may be the only legitimate way a socially isolated person can get attention.
- Lonely people are preoccupied with self, are hypervigilant to threats, and tend to interpret social cues as hostile.
- Loneliness may become part of a person's self-image. Although ego dystonic, he or she may find the state familiar, so that fear of the social risks may outweigh the discomfort level to overcome loneliness.
- The lonely often see the rest of the world (including health care providers) as a socially interactive milieu. They usually are not exposed to others who suffer from loneliness and so believe that their pain is unique. As a result, they tend to resent nurses, who seem to enjoy what lonely people see as unobtainable.
- A person cannot focus on meeting social needs until he or she has met more basic ones (shelter, food, safety; Maslow, 1968).
- Human immunodeficiency virus (HIV)-negative gay men may experience multiple ongoing loss of friends that causes them to suffer alone because of associated stigma (Mallinson, 1999).

◆ Pediatric Considerations

- Children at high risk for social isolation include the chronically ill or disabled, terminally ill, and disfigured, and their siblings.
- A child in protective isolation or with a communicable disease may not understand the rationale for separation from others.
- Gay or lesbian teenagers often suffer emotional isolation and lack access to information specific to their needs (eg, they are at increased medical risk for sexually transmitted diseases, substance use, and violence; Bidwell & Deisher, 1991).

◉ Geriatric Considerations

- "Resources valued by this society include knowledge, skills, power, and position, and the elderly may be ignored because they no longer have these in their control. This lack of control is noted in at least two contrasting views of the elderly. Some view the elderly as free to relax and enjoy freedom from worries and responsibilities. Others see the elderly as being slow and worthless, having nothing to contribute to society. In neither of these views is the older person seen as a contributing member of society" (Elsen & Blegen, 1991, p. 519).
- Older adults are at high risk for loneliness because they often have fewer natural opportunities to be among others. Retirement from work, difficulty securing transportation, health problems that restrict visiting, sensory deficits that make communication laborious or frustrating, or isolation from the mainstream in institutions (hospitals or nursing homes) can significantly limit natural interpersonal encounters.
- Family roles become altered and stressed when parents become dependent on their children and children begin to assume traditional parental tasks or decision making. To help older adults meet affiliative needs and increase satisfaction with social encounters, it is suggested that small groups (rather than large, noisy crowds) be formed to promote interaction and that one or two meaningful relationships (confidantes) be encouraged.
- Factors increasing social isolation in older adults include hearing impairment, limited mobility, fatigue, caregiving responsibilities, inability to drive, mental or psychosocial

(continued)

⊙ Geriatric Considerations (continued)

impairments, and separation from spouse, friends, and/or relatives by death, illness, or physical distance (Miller, 2004).
- Impaired ability to drive from impaired vision, financial hardship, musculoskeletal functioning, or central nervous system functioning can increase an older adult's social isolation and dependency on others (Miller, 2004).
- Sensory deficits rate highest on the list of problems in the older adult with the potential to cause social isolation (Miller, 2004).

Focus Assessment Criteria

Subjective Data
Assess for Related Factors.

Social resources (support)
"Who lives with you?"

"About how many times did you talk to someone—friends, relatives, or others—on the telephone in the past week (either you called them or they called you)?" If subject has no phone, ask "How many times during the past week did you spend some time with someone who does not live with you; that is, you went to see them, or they came to visit you, or you went out to do things together?"

To whom does the person turn in time of need?

Does the client rely on friends or neighbors for such things as meals and transportation?

"Do you see your relatives and friends as often as you want to, or are you somewhat unhappy about how little you see them?"

If institutionalized: "In the past year, about how often did you leave here to visit your family or friends for weekends or holidays or to go on shopping trips or outings, or are most of your friends here in the institution with you?"

Desire for more human contact
What kind of relationships would he or she like? (Same sex or opposite sex? Same age? Someone with same situational or maturational problem?)

Can the person make the effort to meet new people and go to new places?

What kind of group activities does he or she most enjoy? (Travel? Religious service or activity?)

Has divorce or death (of spouse, child, sibling, friend, pet) occurred recently?

Barriers to social contacts
Does the person lack knowledge of resources available, where to meet others, how to initiate conversation with strangers?

Is client housebound? (Illness or incapacity—lack of mobility on steps or curbs—and weather hazards can physically isolate older adults, as can loss of usual transportation, living in dangerous area, and lack of access to public transportation.)

Are there changes in the person's sensory ability (tactile sense, hearing, visual acuity, ability to write letters)?

Change in living arrangement
Has the person moved recently (to nursing home, child's home, apartment, strange location)?

Objective Data
Assess for Related Factors.

Aesthetic problems
Mutilating surgery	Extreme obesity	Odor (eg, ulcerating tumor)
Incontinence		

Personality problems
Does this person lack certain social skills or have personality features (eg, aggression, egocentricity, racism, sexism, complaining, critical, problem drinker) that may discourage others from befriending him or her?

For more information on Focus Assessment Criteria, visit http://connection.lww.com.

Goal

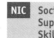 Loneliness, Social Involvement

The person will report decreased feelings of loneliness.

Indicators

- Identify the reasons for his or her feelings of isolation.
- Discuss ways to increase meaningful relationships.

General Interventions

NIC Socialization Enhancement, Spiritual Support, Behavior Modification: Social Skills, Presence, Anticipatory Guidance

The nursing interventions for various contributing factors that might be associated with *Risk for Loneliness* are very similar.

Identify Causative and Contributing Factors (see Focus Assessment Criteria).

Reduce or Eliminate Causative and Contributing Factors.

Promote social interaction.

Support the person who has experienced a loss as he or she works through grief (see *Grieving*).

Validate the normality of grieving.

Encourage person to talk about feelings of loneliness and their causes.

Encourage development of a support system or mobilize person's existing family, friends, and neighbors to form one.

Discuss the importance of high-quality, rather than high-quantity, socialization.

Refer to social skills teaching (see *Impaired Social Interaction*).

Offer feedback on how the person presents himself or herself to others (see *Impaired Social Interaction*).

Decrease Barriers to Social Contact.

Help identify transportation options.

Determine available transportation in the community (public, church-related, volunteer).

Determine if person must learn how to use alternative transportation. Help desensitize client to fear/stigma of using public transportation.

Assist with the development of alternative means of communication for people with compromised sensory ability (eg, amplifier on phone, taped instead of written letters; see *Impaired Communication*).

Assist with management of aesthetic problems (eg, consult enterostomal therapist if ostomy odor is a problem; teach client with cancer to control odor of tumors by packing area with yogurt or pouring in buttermilk, then rinsing well with saline solution).

Help locate stores that sell clothing specially made for those who have had disfiguring surgery (eg, mastectomy).

Refer to *Impaired Urinary Elimination* for specific interventions to control incontinence.

Identify Strategies to Expand the World of the Isolated.

Senior centers and church groups

Foster grandparent programs

Adult day care centers

Retirement communities

House sharing, group homes, community kitchens

Adult education classes, special interest courses

Pets

Regular contact to diminish the need to obtain attention through a crisis (eg, suicidal gesture)

Psychiatric day hospital or activity program

Implement the Following for People With Poor or Offensive Social Skills:

Engage in one-to-one social dialogue. Explain the difference between casual and meaningful conversation.

Discuss characteristics of meaningful conversation:

Initiating interactions	Using appropriate tone
Being alert	and nonverbal behavior
Giving and receiving	Being spontaneous
compliments	Showing interest

Requesting help when needed	Showing interest in others, in activities
	Using increased eye contact

Allow the person opportunities to observe others engaged in meaningful conversation.

Observe the person socializing, and discuss the interactions afterward. Offer praise. Gently discuss alternative approaches. Role-play skills.

Discuss the Anticipatory Effects of Retirement; Assist with Planning.

Plan to ensure adequate income.

Decrease time at work the last 2 to 3 years (eg, shorter days, longer vacations).

Cultivate friends outside work.

Develop routines at home to replace work structure.

Rely on others rather than spouse for leisure activities.

Cultivate realistic leisure activities (energy, cost).

Prepare for ambivalent feelings and short-term negative effects on self-esteem.

Initiate Referrals, as Indicated.

Community-based groups that contact the socially isolated

Self-help groups for clients isolated because of specific medical problems (eg, Reach to Recovery, United Ostomy Association)

Wheelchair groups

Psychiatric consumer rights associations

Rationales

- A socially isolated person usually cannot independently initiate or coordinate various isolation-reduction activities.
- Functional ability of the senses strongly influences a person's perception of the world, behavior, and treatment from others. A person with visible deficits may be shunned.
- Chronic illness can contribute to social isolation because of lack of energy, decreased mobility, discomforts, fear of exposure to pathogens, and distancing by previous friends who are uncomfortable with the ill person's disabilities or the stigma associated with psychiatric problems (Miller, 2004).
- "Retirement is a significant life event that requires preplanning and realistic expectations of life changes" (Stanley & Beare, 1994, p. 365).
- Longino and Karl (1982) reported that type and quality of social interactions are more important than quantity. Informal activities promote well-being more than do formal, structured activities.

EFFECTIVE THERAPEUTIC REGIMEN MANAGEMENT: INDIVIDUAL

DEFINITION

Effective Therapeutic Regimen Management: Individual: Pattern in which a person integrates into daily living a program for treatment of illness and its sequelae that is satisfactory for meeting health goals

DEFINING CHARACTERISTICS

Appropriate choices of daily activities to meet the goals of a treatment or prevention program

Illness symptoms within a normal range of expectation

Verbalized desire to manage the treatment of illness and prevention of sequelae

Verbalized intent to reduce risk factors for progression of illness and sequelae

RELATED FACTORS

Refer to Author's Note for an explanation.

⊘ AUTHOR'S NOTE

Effective Therapeutic Regimen Management describes a person who is managing an illness or a condition successfully. The concept of "enhanced" is appropriate: the nurse can assist the person to enhance his or her management. The focus is anticipatory guidance (eg, teaching what events could negatively affect the person's management and how to reduce them).

⊘ ERRORS IN DIAGNOSTIC STATEMENTS

Effective Therapeutic Regimen Management related to internal locus of control
This diagnosis does not need related factors, which would serve only to repeat characteristics of people who manage their conditions well (eg, motivated, knowledgeable).

KEY CONCEPTS

See *Ineffective Therapeutic Regimen Management.*

Focus Assessment Criteria

Subjective and Objective Data

Assess for Defining Characteristics.

Is knowledgeable about
  Illness/condition (severity, susceptibility to complications, prognosis, ability to cure it or control its progression)
  Treatment/diagnostic studies
  Preventive measures
Has a pattern of adherence to recommended health behaviors or regimen
Expresses a desire to increase ability to manage condition (progression, sequelae)
Reports that symptoms of condition are stable or diminished

For more information on Focus Assessment Criteria, visit http://connection.lww.com.

Goal

NOC Compliance Behaviors, Knowledge: Treatment Regimen, Participation: Health Care Decisions, Risk Control

The person will describe strategies to
address progression or complications of condition should they arise.

Indicators

• Discuss situations that can challenge continued successful management.
• Describe or demonstrate self-care techniques needed.

General Interventions

NIC Behavior Modification, Mutual Goal Setting, Teaching: Individual, Decision-Making Support, Health System Guidance, Anticipatory Guidance

Discuss Possible Changes in Client's Condition that may Affect Illness and Usual Management.

Exacerbation   Complications   Side effects of medication

Advise Early Contact With Care Provider to Discuss Possible Changes in Management Regimen.

Discuss How Increased Stress Can Negatively Affect Previous Successful Management and Possibly Decrease Resistance to Colds or Influenza.

Explore With Client His or Her Usual Level of Stress.

Usual level of stress   Signs of overload

Emphasize That Stress Accompanies Favorable and Unfavorable Life Events (eg, Marriage, Divorce, Birth, Death, Vacations, Work).

Teach Client That, When Facing Upcoming Additional Stresses, He or She Should Plan to:

Reduce stress in other aspects of life, if possible.
Increase adherence to healthy habits.
    Sleep 7 to 8 h.
    Eat breakfast.
    Exercise daily (at least a 30-min brisk walk).
    Eliminate or minimize alcohol intake.
    Increase complex carbohydrates intake.
    Decrease fat intake.
    Decrease caffeine intake.
Increase spiritually related activities.
    Meditate.
    Listen to relaxing music.
    Go on nature walks (eg, woods, near water, mountains).
    Read poetry.

Initiate Health Teaching and Referrals Regarding Stress Reduction Techniques.

Rationales

- The dynamic nature of chronic conditions necessitates knowledge of how to balance one's life to keep symptoms under control as much as possible (Lubin, 1995).
- "Disease" refers to the state of unhealth related to biologic dysfunction. "Illness" is a personal perspective of the effects or experiences related to the disease (Lubin, 1995). Health care professionals can assist the person to reduce the illness experiences.
- Assisting the person to evaluate the effects of stress realistically can promote stress reduction activities (Edelman & Mandle, 2001).

INEFFECTIVE THERAPEUTIC REGIMEN MANAGEMENT

DEFINITION

Ineffective Therapeutic Regimen Management: Pattern in which a person experiences or is at risk to experience difficulty integrating into daily living a program for treatment of illness and the sequelae of illness that meets specific health goals

DEFINING CHARACTERISTICS
Major (Must Be Present, One or More)

Verbalized desire to manage the treatment of illness and prevention of sequelae
Verbalized difficulty with regulation/integration of one or more prescribed regimens for treatment of illness and its effects or prevention of complications

Minor (May Be Present)

Acceleration (expected or unexpected) of illness symptoms
Verbalized to include treatment regimens in daily routines
Verbalized to reduce risk factors for progression of illness and sequelae

RELATED FACTORS
Treatment-Related

Related to:

Complexity of therapeutic regimen	Complexity of health care system	Financial cost of regimen
		Side effects of therapy

Situational (Personal, Environmental)

Related to:

Previous unsuccessful experiences	Mistrust of health care personnel	Health belief conflicts
Questions seriousness of problem	Insufficient knowledge	Questions susceptibility
	Family conflicts	Mistrust of regimen
Questions benefits of regimen	Insufficient social support	Insufficient confidence
		Decisional conflicts

Related to barriers to comprehension secondary to:

Cognitive deficits	Fatigue	Hearing impairments
Motivation	Anxiety	Memory problems

Maturational

Child/Adolescent
Related to fear of being different

⊗ AUTHOR'S NOTE

Ineffective Therapeutic Regimen Management is a very useful diagnosis for nurses in most settings. Individuals and families experiencing various health problems, acute or chronic, usually face treatment programs that require changes in previous functioning or lifestyle. These changes or adaptations can be instrumental in influencing positive outcomes.

This diagnosis describes individuals or families experiencing difficulty achieving positive outcomes. The nurse is the primary professional who, with the client, determines available choices and how to achieve success. The primary nursing interventions are exploring the options available and teaching the client how to implement the selected option.

When a person faces a complex regimen or has compromised functioning that impedes successful management, the diagnosis *Risk for Ineffective Therapeutic Regimen Management* would be appropriate. In addition to teaching how to manage the regimen, the nurse also must assist the client to identify the adjustments needed because of a functional deficit.

⊗ ERRORS IN DIAGNOSTIC STATEMENTS

Ineffective Therapeutic Regimen Management related to a decision not to follow low-salt diet

When client makes a decision not to adhere to a therapeutic regimen, the nurse must explore with the client the circumstances surrounding this decision. The diagnosis *Ineffective Therapeutic Regimen Management related to unknown etiology as evident by not adhering to low-salt diet* is useful. The nurse must collect more data to determine if the client wants to adhere to the diet, or if the client understands the rationale for it. Did the client desire to adhere to the diet but encounter difficulty? Did the client adhere to the diet but experience no positive effects? Nursing intervention strategies would differ with each contributing factor. The following nursing diagnosis is an example of a client who desires to comply but is having difficulty: *Ineffective Therapeutic Regimen Management related to unplanned meals associated with frequent air travel schedule.*

KEY CONCEPTS
Generic Considerations

- The Stages of Change Model (Transtheoretical Model of Change) can provide interventions to assist people with lifestyle modifications for disease prevention and management. The five stages are *precontemplation, contemplation, action, maintenance,* and *relapse* (Prochasaska et al., 1992). People in the precontemplation stage are not considering change because of denial or past failures. People in the contemplation stage are ambivalent about change. Once they decide to make a specific change, they reach the preparation, action, and maintenance stages. The relapse stage is expected (Zimmerman et al., 2000).
- Self-efficacy is a theory that describes a person's evaluation of his or her capacity to manage or to change behaviors to manage stressful situations. Successful management depends on the person believing that the behavior change will improve the situation (outcome expectancy) and that he or she can make the behavior change (self-efficacy expectancy; Bandura, 1982).
- Health education is the teaching–learning process of influencing client and family behavior through changes in knowledge, attitudes, and beliefs and by acquiring psychomotor skills. The goal of client teaching is to help the client assume responsibility for self-care.
- Physical factors that affect learning or the learner include the following (Redman & Thomas, 1992):
  - Acute illness
  - Fluid and electrolyte imbalance
  - Nutritional status
  - Illness or treatments that interfere with mental alertness (pain, medications)
  - Illness or treatments that interfere with motor abilities (fatigue, equipment)
  - Activity tolerance (endurance)
- Personal factors that affect learning or the learner include the following:

Age	Past experiences or knowledge
Intelligence	Locus of control
Reading ability	Perceived seriousness of condition

Level of motivation	Level of anxiety
Denial of disease process	Perceived susceptibility to complications
Prognosis	Depression
Stage of adaptation to illness	Ability to control progression or to cure condition

- Socioeconomic factors that affect learning include the following:

Language	Cultural background
Lifestyle	Transportation
Support system	Health care facility
Financial status	Drugstore
Past health care experiences	

- Factors resulting in ineffective teaching include the following (Redman & Thomas, 1996):
  - Inadequate or no assessment before teaching
  - Assessment data not communicated or not considered when teaching (the most influential assessment factors are psychological status, physical stability, educational level, cultural background, socioeconomic status)
  - Teaching not individualized
  - Information not presented at a level consistent with the client's ability
  - Tendency to talk down to client
  - Use of misunderstood terms
  - Fragmented presentation of information
  - Too much information given, with important information hidden or lost among irrelevant information
  - No repetition of information
  - No feedback given in relation to process (or client is punished for not learning)
  - No evaluation made of client learning

Geriatric Considerations

- The ability to manage one's therapeutic regimen profoundly influences self-esteem and independence. Using education to increase the self-care capacity of older adults can be an effective way to meet their self-esteem needs (Rakel, 1991).
- It is a myth that older adults cannot learn new concepts and skills. Some changes during aging may deter learning, such as decreased visual acuity, decreased hearing, slowing of information processing, decreased attention span, difficulty in unlearning habits, fear of uncertainty or failure, decreased problem solving, and the need for a longer time and more repetition to retain learning (Rakel, 1991).

Transcultural Considerations

- Because the dominant US culture is future oriented, it values a lifestyle that promotes health and prevents disease. This value is challenged when a client or family of another culture is oriented to the present (Andrews & Boyle, 2003).
- Clients with an external locus of control believe that outside factors or forces determine health. This belief challenges the entire concept of health promotion (Andrews & Boyle, 2003).
- Folk remedies are treatments or practices that cultural groups use to stay healthy or to treat illnesses. Spector (1985) questioned students of various cultures to determine health and illness behaviors. Table II.17 illustrates some of her findings.
- Folk remedies are used to treat many illnesses, such as headaches, colds, rashes, coughs, sore throats, constipation, fever, warts, and menstrual cramps. Examples of folk remedies for headaches include lying down and resting in complete darkness (Canadian); boiling a beef bone, breaking up toast in the broth, and drinking (German); applying a cold or hot face cloth to the forehead and resting (Irish); putting a kerchief with ice around the head (Italian); and taking aspirin and hot liquids (Spector, 1985).
- Some folk remedies may be misdiagnosed as abuse. Three folk practices of Southeast Asians leave marks on the body that providers may interpret as signs of violence or abuse. *Cao gio*

(continued)

TABLE II.17 Folk Remedies to Maintain Health

Wine: It
Eat wholesome, balanced foods: It, P, S, A, BA, EB, FC, G, I, IC
Dress right for weather: BA, NA, EB, FC, FCC, G, IC
Cleanliness: BA, CC, EC, G, I, IC, N
Daily walks: EB, EC, S
Pray daily: BA, CC
Read: EB
Take baths: EC
Open bedroom windows at night: EC
Enough sleep: FCC, IC
Cod liver oil daily: FC, N, P, S
Exercise: FCC, IC, It
Take aspirin: G
Wear holy medals: IC
Brush teeth: I
Early to bed: It
Hard bread: It
Routine medical examination: S
Medical care when sick: EE, P
Rest: EC, FC, IC, N, P

Spector, R. E. (1985). *Cultural diversity in health and illness* (2nd ed.). Norwalk, CT: Appleton-Century-Crofts.

Code: A, Asian; BA, black African; CC, Canadian Catholic; EE, Eastern Europe, Jewish; EB, English Baptist; EC, English Catholic; FC, French Catholic; FCC, French Canadian Catholics; G, German Catholics; I, Iran Islam; IC, Irish Catholic; It, Italian; N, Norwegian; P, Polish; S, Swedish; NA, Native American.

🌐 Transcultural Considerations (continued)

is rubbing the skin with a coin to produce dark blood or ecchymotic strips; it is done to treat colds and flulike symptoms. *Bat gio* is skin pinching on the temples to treat headaches or on the neck for sore throat; if petechiae or ecchymoses appear, the treatment is a success. *Poua* is burning the skin with the tip of a dried, weedlike grass; it is believed the burning will cause the noxious element that causes the pain to exude (Andrews & Boyle, 2003).

Focus Assessment Criteria

Subjective Data

Assess for Defining Characteristics.

Determine present knowledge of

Illness
  Severity   Susceptibility to complications   Prognosis
  Ability to cure it or control
    progression
Treatment/diagnostic studies
Preventive measures

What is the pattern of adhering to prescribed health behaviors?
Complete   Modified

Does anything interfere with adherence to the prescribed health behavior?
Learning needs (perceived by client, family)

Assess for Related Factors.

History of disease
Onset
Effects on lifestyle (relationships, work, leisure, finances)
Symptoms

Stage of adaptation to disease
Disbelief   Anger   Denial
Awareness   Depression   Acceptance

Learning ability (client, family)

Level of education	Language spoken	Ability to read
Language understood		

Cultural factors

Health care beliefs and	Values	Lifestyle
practices	Traditions	

Objective Data
Assess for Related Factors.

Ability to perform prescribed procedures

Competency	Accuracy

Level of cognitive and psychomotor development

Age	Ability to read and write

Presence of sensory deficits

Vision	Taste (altered or lost)	Hearing
Touch	Smell (altered or lost)	

For more information on Focus Assessment Criteria, visit http://connection.lww.com.

Goal

NOC	Compliance Behavior, Knowledge: Treatment Regimen, Participation: Health Care Decisions, Treatment Behavior: Illness or Injury

The person/family will relate the intent to
practice health behaviors needed or desired for recovery from illness and prevention of recurrence or complications.

Indicators

- Relate less anxiety related to fear of the unknown, fear of loss of control, or misconceptions.
- Describe disease process, causes of and factors contributing to symptoms, and regimen for disease or symptom control.

General Interventions

Identify Causative or Contributing Factors That Impede Effective Management.

Lack of trust
Insufficient confidence (self-efficacy)
Insufficient knowledge
Insufficient resources

Build Trust and Strength (Zerwich, 1992).

Gain Entrance to Family System.
Behave as a guest.
Do not take over.
Gently ease in.

Avoid Impression of Pressuring.
Give space.
Cease discussion when client shows indicators of closure or uneasiness.

Listen to Discover Concerns, Not to Impose Expectations.

Attempt to Discover a Match Between Expressed Needs and Services Nurses Can Provide.
Start where they are.
Give a good "excuse" to continue relationship.

Discover and Affirm Strengths.

Accept People Where They Are.
Avoid judging.
Avoid setting expectations for others.

Demonstrate Persistence.
Proceed slowly.
Plan short, frequent visits.

Demonstrate Honesty, Consistency, and Stability.
Follow through on promises.
Maintain pre-established contacts in person or by phone.

Identify and Emphasize Strengths.

Survival skills	Parent–child relationship	Family caregiving abilities

Consider Cultural Preferences or Practices.
What does family do to maintain health?
What does family do to prevent illness?
What home remedies do you or your family use?

Promote Confidence and Positive Self-Efficacy (Bandura, 1982).

Explore past successful management of problems.
Emphasize past successful coping.
Tell stories of other "successes."
If appropriate, encourage opportunities to witness others successfully coping in a similar situation.
Encourage participation in self-help groups.

Reduce or Eliminate Barriers to Learning.

Assist in Meeting Basic Physiologic Needs, if Necessary.

Support Progression Through Stages of Psychosocial Adaptation to Illness.
Stage of disbelief (denial)
Orient person to hospital setting, routines.
Teach with a focus on the present.
Provide simple explanations of procedures as you perform them.
Help person feel safe and secure.
Concentrate on one-to-one rather than group teaching.
Teach family about denial that the person is having.
State of developing awareness (guilt, anger)
Listen carefully to person.
Continue teaching with a present-tense focus.
Allow client to express hostility safely.
Avoid arguing.

Delay Teaching Until Person is Ready.

Adapt Teaching to Person's Physical and Psychological Status.
Comfort levels
Fatigue levels
Not concurrent with peaks of medications that alter perception or cognition

Allow Person to Work Through and Express Intense Emotions Before Beginning to Teach.

Examine Person's Health Beliefs and Past Experiences Related to Illness; Assess Their Effects on Desire to Learn.

Reduce Anxiety.

Encourage verbalization.
Listen attentively.
Meet person's expressed needs before giving other information.
Develop trust with frequent, consistent interactions.
Give correct, relevant information.
Give nonthreatening information before delivering more anxiety-producing information.
Explain reason for and intended effect of treatment; emphasize the positive.
Explore with person the effects of a new diagnosis, treatment, or surgery on significant others.
Do not overwhelm person with too much information if anxiety is high or physical condition is unstable.
Allow person to maintain some control over self and routines by involving him or her in care.
Prepare person and family for what to expect concerning environment, routines, personnel giving care, sensations experienced, and so forth.
Provide interventions dependent on stages of change (Prochasaska et al., 1992; Zimmerman et al., 2000.)

Precontemplation stage
Focus on building a relationship of trust.
Educate in small bits.
Elicit the advantages of changing behaviors.
Associate symptoms with risk behaviors (eg, bronchitis with smoking).
Contemplation stage
Elicit reasons for wanting to change.
Acknowledge ambivalence.
Discuss barriers.
Elicit possible solutions to barriers.
Preparation stage
Elicit what strategies the person has decided to try.
Set date for beginning.
Acknowledge that relapses are expected.
Action stage
Reinforce the decision.
Acknowledge any success (eg, reduced number of cigarettes, lost 1 lb).
Maintenance stage
Continue reinforcement.
Elicit what strategies have been helpful.
Relapse stage
Emphasize that this is not a failure.
Re-engage in the change process.

Promote Personal/Family Learning.

Individualize the teaching approach after a thorough assessment.
Plan and share need for learning outcomes.
Follow the principles of teaching–learning (refer to Key Concepts).
Explain and discuss:
    Disease process
    Treatment regimen (medications, diet, procedures, exercises, equipment)
    Rationale for regimen
    Expectations (client, family) of regimen
    Side effects of regimen
    Lifestyle changes needed
    Methods to monitor condition
    Follow-up care needed
    Signs/symptoms of complications
    Resources, support available
    Home environment alterations needed
Evaluate personal/family behaviors as evidence that learning outcomes have been achieved.

Proceed with Referrals, as Indicated.

Community nursing services

Rationales

- A major determinant of self-efficacy is past successful coping in a similar situation (Bandura, 1982). In contrast, past unsuccessful management of a similar situation is a deterrent.
- In addition to past successful coping experiences, Bandura (1982) identified three other factors that promote positive self-efficacy:
  - Witnessing others successfully coping
  - Belief by others that they can successfully cope or manage
  - Not experiencing high autonomic arousal in response to the situation
- Zerwich (1992) has identified family caregiving competencies that provide the essential groundwork to promote family self-help as building trust and strength.
- Vulnerable families have poor self-esteem and are "starved for validation" that they have capabilities (Zerwich, 1992).
- Research has shown that, when family members are involved in care, client cooperation and positive adjustment to the experience increase (Leske, 1993).

- Teaching should be incorporated routinely as an integral part of nursing care whenever a new diagnosis or change in regimen is made, or when the client faces an unfamiliar situation.
- An assessment before beginning teaching facilitates the meaningfulness, efficacy, and overall success of the teaching–learning process by defining *what* content should be present, *how* the content should be given, *when* the client is ready to learn, and *who* should be included.
- Learning depends on physical and emotional readiness. The client needs to be relatively free of pain and extreme anxiety. High anxiety decreases learning, whereas slight anxiety may increase learning.
- Client motivation is one of the most important variables affecting how much learning takes place.

INEFFECTIVE THERAPEUTIC REGIMEN MANAGEMENT: FAMILY

DEFINITION

Ineffective Therapeutic Regimen Management, Family: Pattern in which the family experiences or is at risk to experience difficulty integrating into daily living a program for treatment of illness and the sequelae of illness that meets specific health goals

DEFINING CHARACTERISTICS

Major (Must Be Present)

Inappropriate family activities for meeting the goals of a treatment or prevention program

Minor

Acceleration (expected or unexpected) of illness symptoms of a family member
Lack of attention to illness and its sequelae
Verbalized desire to manage the treatment of illness and prevention of sequelae
Verbalized difficulty with regulation/integration of one or more prescribed regimens for treatment of illness and its effects or prevention of complications
Verbalized that family did not take action to reduce risk factors for progression of illness and sequelae

RELATED FACTORS

Refer to *Ineffective Therapeutic Regimen Management.*

AUTHOR'S NOTE

Refer to *Ineffective Therapeutic Regimen Management.*

ERRORS IN DIAGNOSTIC STATEMENTS

Refer to *Ineffective Therapeutic Regimen Management.*

KEY CONCEPTS

Refer to *Ineffective Therapeutic Regimen Management.*

Focus Assessment Criteria

Refer to *Ineffective Therapeutic Regimen Management.*

GENERAL INTERVENTIONS

Refer to *Ineffective Therapeutic Regimen Management.*

INEFFECTIVE THERAPEUTIC REGIMEN MANAGEMENT: COMMUNITY

DEFINITION

Ineffective Therapeutic Regimen Management: Community: Pattern in which the community experiences or is at risk to experience difficulty integrating a program for treatment of illness and the sequelae of illness and reduction of risk situations (eg, safety, pollution)

DEFINING CHARACTERISTICS
Major (Must Be Present, One or More)

Verbalized difficulty in meeting health needs in communities
Acceleration (expected or unexpected) of illness(es)
Morbidity, mortality rates above norm

RELATED FACTORS
Situational (Environmental)

Related to availability of community programs for (specify):

Prevention of diseases	Screening for diseases	Immunizations
Dental care	Accident prevention	Fire safety
Smoking cessation	Substance abuse	Alcohol abuse
Child abuse		

Related to problem accessing program secondary to:

Inadequate communication	Limited hours	Lack of transportation
Insufficient funds		

Related to complexity of population's needs
Related to lack of awareness of availability
Related to environmental or occupational health hazards
Related to multiple needs of vulnerable groups (specify):

Homeless	Pregnant teenagers	Below poverty level
Home-bound individuals		

Related to unavailable or insufficient health care agencies

⊗ AUTHOR'S NOTE

This diagnosis describes a community with evidence that a population is underserved because of lack of availability of, access to, or knowledge of health care resources. Community nurses, using the results of community assessments, can identify at-risk groups and overall community needs. In addition, they assess health systems, transportation, social services, and access.

KEY CONCEPTS
Generic Considerations
Refer to Key Concepts under *Readiness for Enhanced Community Coping* and *Ineffective Community Coping*.

Focus Assessment Criteria (Community Health Assessment [Allender & Spradley, 2001; Helvie, 1991; Kriegler & Harton, 1992])

Subjective and Objective Data
Population
Percentage in each age group (years)

0–5	45–54
5–14	55–64
15–24	65–75
25–34	75+
35–44	

Gender and race distribution
Vital statistics
Births (mother's age, unwed parents)
Death rate (newborns, infants, maternal, suicides, general)

Health Perception–Health Maintenance Pattern
Vital statistics

Communicable disease incidence
Ten leading causes of death

Immunization percentages by age
Rate of chronic diseases

Health care services (adequate, inadequate)
Hospital services (general, maternity, psychiatric, pediatric, rehabilitation)
Nursing home services
Ambulatory services
Occupational services
School health services
Health department services
Community services
Health centers (types, frequency)
Home services (types, number of agencies)

Protective services
Police
Fire
Disaster response plan
Ambulance service
Environment protection services (air, water, industrial, wastes, food services, housing)

Nutritional–Metabolic Pattern
Food sources (stores, markets, restaurants)
Nutritional assistance programs (WIC, Meals on Wheels)
Nutrition educational programs

Elimination Pattern
Sanitation (water supply, sewage disposal, trash and garbage disposal, rodent and vermin control)
Ecologic concerns (recycling, hazardous wastes)

Activity–Exercise Pattern
Transportation options
Recreation and fitness facilities (types for various age groups)

Sleep–Rest Pattern
Noise (traffic, airline, trains, industry)

Cognitive–Perceptual Pattern

Process of community decisions (government, schools)
Educational facilities (public, private, adult education, higher education, health education programs)
Communication (publications, radio and TV stations, informal network)

Self-Perception–Self-Concept Pattern

Population characteristics (ethnic origins, race)
Socioeconomic (primary occupations, average income level, percentage below poverty level, unemployment rate, percentage of homeowners vs renters)

Role–Relationship Pattern (Intergenerational, Interracial, Interethnic)

Community-sponsored events

Sexuality–Reproductive Pattern

Average size of family
Reproduction (birth rate, teen pregnancies, prenatal care, abortion facilities)
Birth control resources
Educational programs (sex education, childbirth education classes, parenting classes)

Coping–Stress Tolerance Pattern

Assistance programs (federal, state)
Community-based programs (self-help, telephone help-lines, crisis centers)

Value–Belief Pattern

Religious distribution
Religious outreach
Social programs

Fundraising	Service organizations	Senior citizen programs
Handicap services	Shelters	

Cultural–ethnic programs (services, social)

For more information on Focus Assessment Criteria, visit http://connection.lww.com.

Goals

NOC Participation: Health Care Decisions, Risk Control, Risk Detection

The community will:

- Identify needed community resources.
- Promote the use of community resources for health problems.

General Interventions

NIC Decision-Making Support, Health System Guidance, Risk Identification, Community Health Development, Risk Identification

Create a Survey to Determine:

Health problem identification
Awareness of health services
Use of health services
Interest in health promotion programs
Recommendation for funding sources

Survey Samples of the Target Population.

Mail survey
One-to-one survey at community center, sports field, supermarket
Group survey (eg, church groups, clubs)
Key community leaders

Design Survey for Easy Reading and Answering (eg, Circle the Number That Best Describes Your Answer: 1—No Concern; 2—Medium; 3—High)

How concerned are you about _____ (eg, hypertension, stress, alcohol misuse)?

Organize Response Data.

Rank-order entire sample
Group responses of selected groups (eg, age, gender, income level, disabled)

Analyze the Findings.
What Overall Health Problems are Reported?

What are the Health Concerns of:

Older population	Households with children up to 20 years of age
Single-parent households	Respondents younger than 45 years
People below poverty level	

Evaluate Community Resources.

What resources are available for the health problems identified?
Are there utilization or access problems with the services?
How does the population learn about services?
Identify problems that do not have community services available.

If Services Are Available But Are Underutilized, Evaluate:

Hours of operation (convenient?)	Location of services (access, aesthetics)
Efficiency and atmosphere	Advertising strategies

If Services Are Unavailable, Pursue Program Development.
Examine and Evaluate Similar Programs in Other Communities.

Basic information	Purpose, goals	Services available
Funding	Cost to participants	Accessibility of services
Satisfaction (citizen, employees)		

Meet With Appropriate People to Discuss Findings (Survey, On-Site Visits). Address the Following:
Presence of community support
Available expertise and technology in community
Financial support

Identify Appropriate Community Sources of Assistance.

Hospital departments	Health departments	Industry
Chamber of Commerce	Health care professionals	Schools of nursing
Private foundations	Public assistance agencies	Professional societies

Plan the Program (Refer to *Effective Community Coping* for Interventions for Community Planning).

Evaluate Vulnerable Population's Access to Health Care and Knowledge of Risk Factors.

Rural families, elderly	Migrant workers	New immigrants
Homeless	Those below poverty level	

Make a Priority of Ensuring that Basic Needs for Food, Shelter, Clothing, and Safety Are Met Before Attempting to Address Higher Health Needs.

Provide Information Regarding Illness Prevention, Health Promotion, and Health Services to Vulnerable Populations.

Be sure reading material is appropriate for targeted group (eg, reading level, language, pictures).
Use posters, flyers.
Select locations that the targeted population uses regularly:

Grocery, convenience stores	Day care centers	School activities
Religious services, meetings	Laundromat	Community fairs
	Sporting events	

Rationales

- In community base planning, it is necessary to conduct a needs assessment, set priorities, and establish objectives (Clemen-Stone et al., 2002).
- Community involvement is necessary to validate which problems warrant attention and to ensure successful outcomes (Clemen-Stone et al., 2002).
- Incentives to mobilize the community to change are integrated into the planning.
- Evaluation of resources available is needed to match activities planned (Edelman & Mandle, 2001).
- Liaisons with community leaders and other sources of support are integral to successful program outcomes (Edelman & Mandle, 2001).

IMPAIRED PHYSICAL MOBILITY

DEFINITION
Impaired Physical Mobility: State in which a person experiences or is at risk of experiencing limitation of physical movement but is not immobile

DEFINING CHARACTERISTICS (LEVIN, KRAINOVITCH, BAHRENBURG & MITCHELL, 1989)
Major (80% to 100%)
Compromised ability to move purposefully within the environment (eg, bed mobility, transfers, ambulation)
Range-of-motion (ROM) limitations

Minor (50% to 80%)
Imposed restriction of movement
Reluctance to move

RELATED FACTORS
Pathophysiologic
Related to decreased strength and endurance secondary to:
(Neuromuscular impairment)
    Autoimmune alterations (eg, multiple sclerosis, arthritis)
    Nervous system diseases (eg, Parkinson's disease, myasthenia gravis)
    Muscular dystrophy
    Partial paralysis (spinal cord injury, stroke)
    Central nervous system (CNS) tumor
    Increased intracranial pressure
    Sensory deficits
    Musculoskeletal impairment
    Fractures
    Connective tissue disease (systemic lupus erythematosus)

Related to edema

Treatment-Related
Related to external devices (casts or splints, braces, intravenous (IV) tubing)
Related to insufficient strength and endurance for ambulation with (specify)
Prosthesis   Crutches   Walker

Situational (Personal, Environmental)
Related to:
Fatigue   Motivation   Pain

Maturational

Children

Related to abnormal gait secondary to:

Congenital skeletal
  deficiencies

Legg-Calvé-Perthes disease
Congenital hip dysplasia

Osteomyelitis

Older Adult

Related to decreased motor agility
Related to muscle weakness

⊚⊚ AUTHOR'S NOTE

Impaired Physical Mobility describes a person with limited use of arm(s) or leg(s) or limited muscle strength. Nurses should not use this diagnosis to describe complete immobility; in this case, *Disuse Syndrome* is more applicable. Limitation of physical movement also can be the etiology of other nursing diagnoses, such as *Self-Care Deficit* and *Risk for Injury*. Nursing interventions for *Impaired Physical Mobility* focus on strengthening and restoring function and preventing deterioration.

⊚⊚ ERRORS IN DIAGNOSTIC STATEMENTS

1. *Impaired Physical Mobility related to traumatic amputation of left arm*

    Listing traumatic amputation of the left arm as a related factor does not describe the problem. Rather, the diagnostic statement should reflect how the loss has affected functioning. A more appropriate diagnosis might be *Self-Care Deficit: Feeding related to insufficient knowledge of adaptations needed secondary to loss of left arm.*

2. *Impaired Physical Mobility related to limited muscle strength secondary to cerebrovascular accident (CVA)*

    Limited muscle strength is a sign of *Impaired Physical Mobility,* not a related factor.

Related factors should represent direction for nursing intervention, as reflected in the diagnosis *Impaired Physical Mobility related to insufficient knowledge of techniques needed to increase motor function secondary to upper motor neuron damage.*

KEY CONCEPTS
Generic Considerations

- According to Miller (2004), mobility is one of the most significant aspects of physiologic functioning, because it greatly influences the maintenance of independence.
- Activity, mobility, and flexibility are integral to a person's lifestyle. Compromised mobility seriously affects self-concept and lifestyle.
- The four ROM categories are passive, active assistive, active, and active resistive (Addams & Clough, 1998).
    - *Passive ROM* is movement of the client's muscles by another person with the client's help.
    - *Active assistive ROM* is active contraction of a muscle with assistance by an external force such as a therapist, mechanical appliance, or the uninvolved extremity.
    - *Active ROM* is active contraction of a muscle against the force of gravity, such as straight leg lifts.
    - *Active resistive ROM* is active contraction of a muscle against resistance, such as weights.
- Isometric exercises are when muscles contract or tense without joint movement. They are contraindicated for people with cardiac conditions because they increase left ventricular function. When done, muscles should be tensed for 5 to 15 s (Pellino et al., 1998).
- *Ambulation* is a complex, three-dimensional activity involving the legs, pelvis, trunk, and upper extremities. *Gait* is a complex movement involving the musculoskeletal, neurologic, and cardiovascular systems. Cognitive factors such as mentation and orientation are critical for safe ambulation (Addams & Clough, 1998).

> ### ❖ Pediatric Considerations
>
> See *Disuse Syndrome.*

> ### ⊙ Geriatric Considerations
>
> - About 10% of noninstitutionalized older adults report some limitation in mobility; of institutionalized older adults, more than 90% are dependent in at least one activity of daily living (Miller, 2004). Mobility problems are often the reason for nursing home admission or extensive in-home care. Assessment of mobility determines the extent of functional impairment as a result of disease or disability.
> - Effects of immobility are particularly dangerous in older adults. Muscle weakness, atrophy, and decreased endurance occur quickly, and biochemical and physiologic effects such as nitrogen loss and hypercalciuria are important to consider (Porth, 2002). Permanent functional loss is more likely with prolonged immobility, and older adults also are vulnerable to new morbidity such as pneumonia, pressure sores, falls and fracture, osteoporosis, incontinence, confusion, and depression. Every effort toward prevention and mobilization should be made (Miller, 2004).
> - Age-related changes in joint and connective tissue impair flexion and extension movements, decrease flexibility, and reduce cushioning protection for joints (Miller, 2004).

Focus Assessment Criteria

Subjective Data

Assess for Defining Characteristics.

History of symptoms (complaints of)

Pain
Muscle weakness
Fatigue

Attributed to?	Amount of time out of bed
Induced by?	Amount of time sleeping or resting

Assess for Related Factors.

History of systemic disorders

Neurologic

Head trauma	Birth defect	Multiple sclerosis
Increased intracranial pressure	CVA	Guillain-Barré syndrome
	Polio	Tumor
Myasthenia gravis	Spinal cord injury	

Cardiovascular

Myocardial infarction	Congenital heart anomaly	Congestive heart failure

Musculoskeletal

Osteoporosis	Arthritis	Fractures

Respiratory

Chronic obstructive pulmonary disease (COPD)	Pneumonia	Dyspnea on exertion
	Orthopnea	

Debilitating diseases

Cancer	Renal disease	Endocrine disease

History of symptoms that interfere with mobility

Onset	Frequency	Duration
Precipitated by what?	Location	Relieved by what?
Description	Aggravated by what?	

History of recent trauma or surgery
Current drug therapy

Objective Data
Assess for Defining Characteristics.

Dominant hand
Motor function

Right arm	Strong	Weak	Absent	Spastic
Left arm	Strong	Weak	Absent	Spastic
Right leg	Strong	Weak	Absent	Spastic
Left leg	Strong	Weak	Absent	Spastic

Mobility

Ability to turn self	Yes	No	Assistance needed (specify)
Ability to sit	Yes	No	Assistance needed (specify)
Ability to stand	Yes	No	Assistance needed (specify)
Ability to get up	Yes	No	Assistance needed (specify)
Ability to transfer	Yes	No	Assistance needed (specify)
Ability to ambulate	Yes	No	Assistance needed (specify)

Weight-bearing (assess both right and left sides)

    Full   As tolerated   Partial   Non–weight-bearing

Gait

    Stable   Unstable

Assistive devices

Crutches	Wheelchair	Cane	Prosthesis
Braces	Walker	Other	

Restrictive devices

Cast or splint	Foley	Traction	IV
Braces	Monitor	Ventilator	Dialysis
Drain			

Range of motion (neck, shoulders, elbows, arms, spine, hips, legs)

    Full   Limited (specify)   None

Assess for Related Factors.

Endurance (see *Activity Intolerance* for additional information)

Assess

Resting pulse, blood pressure, respirations

Blood pressure, respirations, and pulse immediately after activity

Pulse every 2 min until pulse returns to within 10 beats of resting pulse

After activity, assess for indicators of hypoxia (showing intensity, frequency, or duration of activity must be decreased or discontinued) as follows:

Blood pressure

Failure of systolic rate to increase	Increase in diastolic of 155 mm Hg

Respirations

Excessive rate increases	Decrease in rate	Dyspnea
Irregular rhythm		

Cerebral and other changes

Confusion	Pallor	Weakness
Change in equilibrium	Uncoordination	Cyanosis

Peripheral circulation

Capillary refill time (normal, less than 3 s)

Skin color, temperature, and turgor

Peripheral pulses (rate, quality)

Brachial	Posterior tibial	Radial
Popliteal	Femoral	Pedal

Motivation (as perceived by nurse and/or stated by person)

Excellent	Satisfactory	Poor

For more information on Focus Assessment Criteria, visit http://connection.lww.com.

Goal

NOC Ambulation: Walking, Joint Movement: Active, Mobility Level

The person will report increased strength and endurance of limbs.

Indicators

- Demonstrate the use of adaptive devices to increase mobility.
- Use safety measures to minimize potential for injury.
- Describe rationale for interventions.
- Demonstrate measures to increase mobility.

General Interventions

 NIC Exercise Therapy: Joint Mobility, Exercise Promotion: Strength Training, Exercise Therapy: Ambulation, Positioning, Teaching: Prescribed Activity: Exercise, Teaching: Assistive Device, Teaching: Safety

Assess Causative Factors.

Trauma (eg, cartilage tears, fractures, amputations)

Surgical procedure (eg, joint replacement, reduction of fractures, vascular surgery)

Debilitating disease (eg, diabetes, cancer, rheumatoid arthritis, multiple sclerosis, stroke)

Promote Optimal Mobility and Movement.

Promote Motivation and Adherence (Addams & Clough, 1998).

Explain the problem and the objective of each exercise.

Ensure that initial exercises are easy and require minimal strength and coordination.

Progress only if the client is successful at the present exercise.

Provide written instructions for prescribed exercises after demonstrating and observing return demonstration.

Document and discuss improvement specifically (eg, can lift leg 2 inches higher).

Increase Limb Mobility. Determine Type of ROM Appropriate for Person (Passive, Active Assistive, Active, Active Resistive).

Perform passive or active assistive ROM exercises (frequency determined by client's condition):

Teach client to perform active ROM exercises on unaffected limbs at least four times a day, if possible.

Perform passive ROM on affected limbs. Do the exercises slowly to allow the muscles time to relax, and support the extremity above and below the joint to prevent strain on joints and tissues.

During ROM, the client's legs and arms should move gently to within his or her pain tolerance; perform ROM slowly to allow the muscles time to relax.

For passive ROM, the supine position is most effective. The client who performs ROM himself or herself can use a supine or sitting position.

Do ROM daily with bed bath, three or four times daily if there are specific problem areas. Try to incorporate into activities of daily living.

Support extremity with pillows to prevent or reduce swelling.

Medicate for pain as needed, especially before activity* (see *Impaired Comfort*).

Apply heat or cold to reduce pain, inflammation, and hematoma (after 48 h).*

Apply cold to reduce swelling after injury (usually first 48 h).*

Encourage client to perform exercise regimens for specific joints as prescribed by physician or physical therapist (eg, isometric, resistive).

Position in Alignment to Prevent Complications.

Use a foot board.

Avoid prolonged sitting or lying in the same position.

Change position of the shoulder joints every 2 to 4 h.

Use a small pillow or no pillow when in Fowler's position.

Support the hand and wrist in natural alignment.

If the client is supine or prone, place a rolled towel or small pillow under the lumbar curvature or under the end of the rib cage.

Place a trochanter roll or sandbags alongside the hips and upper thighs.

If the client is in the lateral position, place pillow(s) to support the leg from groin to foot, and a pillow to flex the shoulder and elbow slightly; if needed, support the lower foot in dorsal flexion with a sandbag.

For upper extremities:

Arms abducted from the body with pillows

Elbows in slight flexion

Wrist in a neutral position, with fingers slightly flexed, and thumb abducted and slightly flexed

Position of shoulder joints changed during the day (eg, adduction, abduction, range of circular motion)

---

*May require a primary care professional's order.

Maintain Good Body Alignment when Mechanical Devices are Used.

Traction devices

Assess for correct position of traction and alignment of bones.

Observe for correct amount and position of weights.

Allow weights to hang freely, with no blankets or sheets on ropes.

Assess for changes in circulation; check pulse quality, skin temperature, color of extremities, and capillary refill (should be less than 3 s).

Assess for changes in circulation (numbness, tingling, pain).

Assess for changes in mobility (ability to flex/extend unaffected joints).

Assess for signs of skin irritation (redness, ulceration, blanching).

Assess skeletal traction pin sites for loosening, inflammation, ulceration, and drainage; clean pin insertion sites (procedure may vary with type of pin and physician's order).

Encourage isometrics* and prescribed exercise program.

Casts

Assess for proper fit of cast (should not be too loose or too tight).

Assess circulation to the encased area every 2 h (color and temperature of skin, pulse quality, capillary refill less than 2 s).

Assess for changes in sensation of extremities every 2 h (numbness, tingling, pain).

Assess motion of uninvolved joints (ability to flex and extend).

Assess for skin irritation (redness, ulceration, or complaints of pain under the cast).

Keep cast clean and dry; do not allow sharp objects to be inserted under cast; petal rough edges with adhesive tape; place soft cotton under edges that seem to be causing pressure points.

Allow cast to air dry while resting on pillows to prevent dents.

Observe cast for areas of softening or indentation.

Exercise joints above and below cast if allowed (eg, wiggle fingers and toes every 2 h).

Assist with prescribed exercise regimens and isometrics of muscles enclosed in casts.*

Keep extremities elevated after cast application to reduce swelling.

Braces

Assess for correct positioning of braces.

Observe for signs of skin irritation (redness, ulceration, blanching, itching, pain).

Assist with exercises as prescribed for specific joints.

Have the client demonstrate correct application of the brace.

Prosthetic devices

Observe for signs of skin irritation of the stump before applying prosthetic device (stump should be clean and dry; Ace bandage should be rewrapped and securely in place).

Have the client demonstrate correct application of the prosthesis.

Assess for gait alterations or improper walking technique.

Proceed with health teaching, if indicated.

Ace bandages

Assess for correct position of Ace bandage.

Apply Ace bandage with even pressure, wrapping from distal to proximal portions, and making sure that the bandage is not too tight or too loose.

Observe for bunching of the bandage.

Observe for signs of irritation of skin (redness, ulceration, excessive tightness).

Rewrap Ace bandage twice daily or as needed, unless contraindicated (eg, if the bandage is a postoperative compression dressing, it should be left in place).

When wrapping lower extremity, leave the heel exposed, using figure-8 technique.

Slings

Assess for correct application; sling should be loose around neck and should support elbow and wrist above level of the heart.

Remove slings for ROM.*

Note: Some mechanical devices may be removed for exercises, depending on nature of injury or type and purpose of device. Consult with the physician to ascertain when the person may remove the device.

Provide Progressive Mobilization.

Assist slowly to sitting position.

Allow client to dangle legs over the side of the bed for a few minutes before standing.

---

*May require a primary care professional's order.

Limit time to 15 min, three times a day, the first few times out of bed.

Increase time out of bed, as tolerated, by 15-min increments.

Progress to ambulation with or without assistive devices.

If client cannot walk, assist him or her out of bed to a wheelchair or chair.

Encourage ambulation for short, frequent walks (at least three times daily), with assistance if unsteady.

Increase lengths of walks progressively each day.

Encourage Use of Affected Arm When Possible.

Encourage the person to use affected arm for self-care activities (eg, feeding self, dressing, brushing hair).

For post-CVA neglect of upper limb, see *Unilateral Neglect.*

Instruct client to use unaffected arm to exercise the affected arm.

Use appropriate adaptive equipment to enhance the use of arms.

> Universal cuff for feeding in clients with poor control in both arms, hands
>
> Large-handled or padded silverware to assist clients with poor fine motor skills
>
> Dishware with high edges to prevent food from slipping
>
> Suction-cup aids to prevent sliding of plate

Use a warm bath to alleviate early-morning stiffness and improve mobility.

Encourage client to practice handwriting skills, if able.

Allow time to practice using affected limb.

Provide Health Teaching, as Indicated.

Teach Methods of Transfer from Bed to Chair or Commode and to Standing Position.

Before transferring anyone, assess the number of personnel needed for assistance.

The person should transfer toward unaffected side.

Position the client on the side of the bed. His or her feet should be touching the floor, and he or she should be wearing stable shoes or slippers with nonskid soles.

For getting in and out of bed, encourage weight-bearing on the uninvolved or stronger side.

Lock wheelchair before transfer. If using a regular chair, be sure it will not move.

Instruct client to use the arm of the chair closer to him or her for support while standing.

Place arm around client's rib cage and keep back straight, with knees slightly bent.

Tell client to place his or her arms around the nurse's waist or rib cage, *not the neck.*

Support client's legs by bracing his with yours. (While facing the person, lock his or her knees with your knees.)

Instruct clients with hemiplegia to pivot on the uninvolved foot.

For clients with lower limb weakness or paralysis, a sliding board transfer may be used.

> The person should wear pajamas so he or she will not stick to the board.
>
> The person needs good upper extremity strength to be able to slide the buttocks from the bed to the chair or wheelchair. (Wheelchairs should have removable arms.)

When the person's arms are strong enough, he or she should progress to a sitting transfer without the board, if he or she can lift buttocks enough to clear bed and chair seat.

If the person's legs give out, guide him or her gently to the floor and *seek additional assistance.*

Teach Client How to Ambulate with Adaptive Equipment (eg, Crutches, Walkers, Canes).

Instruct client in weight-bearing status.

Observe and teach the use of:

Crutches

Do not exert pressure on axilla; use hand strength.

Type of gait varies with client's diagnosis.

Measure crutches 2 to 3 inches below axilla and tips 6 inches away from feet.

Walkers

Use arm strength to support weakness in lower limbs.

Gait varies with client's problems.

Wheelchairs

Practice transfers.

Practice maneuvering around barriers.

Prostheses (teach about the following)

Stump wrapping before application of the prosthesis

Application of the prosthesis

Principles of stump care

Importance of cleaning the stump, keeping it dry, and applying the prosthesis only when the stump is dry

Teach client safety precautions.

Protect areas of decreased sensation from extremes of heat and cold.

Practice falling and how to recover from falls while transferring or ambulating.

For decreased perception of lower extremity (post-CVA "neglect"), instruct the person to check where limb is placed when changing positions or going through doorways; and check to make sure both shoes are tied, that affected leg is dressed with trousers, and that pants are not dragging.

Instruct people who are confined to wheelchair to shift position and lift up buttocks every 15 min to relieve pressure; maneuver curbs, ramps, inclines, and around obstacles; and lock wheelchairs before transferring.

Practice proper positioning, ROM (active or passive), and prescribed exercises.

Practice climbing stairs if person's condition permits.

Rationales

- A regular exercise program including ROM, isometrics, and selected aerobic activities can help maintain the integrity of joint function (Addams & Clough, 1998).
- A warm-up period of local heat or gentle stretching before strengthening and endurance exercises allows muscles to become ready gradually for more intense work.
- Exercises are needed to improve circulation and strengthen muscle groups needed for ambulation.
- Ambulatory aids must be used correctly and safely to ensure effectiveness and prevent injury.
- Promoting the client's feelings of control and self-determination may improve compliance with the exercise program.
- Exercise enhances independence. Incorporating ROM exercises into a person's daily routine encourages regular performance.
- Active ROM increases muscle mass, tone, and strength and improves cardiac and respiratory functioning. Passive ROM improves joint mobility and circulation.
- Prolonged immobility and impaired neurosensory function can cause permanent contractures.
- Prolonged bed rest or decreased blood volume can cause a sudden drop in blood pressure (orthostatic hypotension) as blood returns to peripheral circulation. Gradual progression to increased activity reduces fatigue and increases endurance (Kasper, 1993; Porth 2002).
- Effective management of pain and depression is sometimes necessary. Inadequate pain relief may be a primary factor leading to depression in some people, but depression should not be discounted as a secondary feature of pain. Depression may require aggressive management, including drugs and other therapies.

IMPAIRED BED MOBILITY

DEFINITION

Impaired Bed Mobility: State in which a person experiences, or is at risk of experiencing, limitation of movement in bed

DEFINING CHARACTERISTICS

Impaired ability to turn side to side

Impaired ability to move from supine to sitting to supine

Impaired ability to "scoot" or reposition self in bed

Impaired ability to move from supine to prone or prone to supine

Impaired ability to move from supine to long sitting or long sitting to supine

> ⊚ AUTHOR'S NOTE
>
> *Impaired Bed Mobility* may be a clinically useful diagnosis when a person is a candidate for rehabilitation to improve strength, range of motion, and movement. The nurse can consult with a physical therapist for a specific plan. This diagnosis is inappropriate for an unconscious or terminally ill person.

RELATED FACTORS
Refer to *Impaired Physical Mobility*.

KEY CONCEPTS
Refer to *Impaired Physical Mobility*.

Focus Assessment Criteria

Refer to *Impaired Physical Mobility*.

Goals

Refer to *Impaired Physical Mobility*.

General Interventions

Refer to *Impaired Physical Mobility*.

IMPAIRED WALKING

DEFINITION
Impaired Walking: State in which a person experiences, or is at risk of experiencing, limitation in walking

DEFINING CHARACTERISTICS
Impaired ability to climb stairs
Impaired ability to walk required distances
Impaired ability to walk on an incline
Impaired ability to walk on uneven surfaces
Impaired ability to navigate curbs

RELATED FACTORS
Refer to *Impaired Physical Mobility*.

KEY CONCEPTS
Refer to *Impaired Physical Mobility*.

Focus Assessment Criteria

Refer to *Impaired Physical Mobility*.

Goal

 **NOC** Refer to *Impaired Physical Mobility*

The person will increase walking distances (specify distance goal).

Indicators
- Demonstrate safe mobility.
- Use mobility aids correctly.

General Interventions

NIC Refer to *Impaired Physical Mobility*

Explain that safe ambulation is a complete movement involving the musculoskeletal, neurologic, and cardiovascular systems and cognitive factors such as mentation and orientation.

A person who is deconditioned needs a progressive exercise program. Consult with a physical therapist for evaluation and planning.

Ascertain that client is using ambulatory aids (eg, cane, walker, crutches) correctly and safely.
    Wears well-fitting shoes
    Can ambulate on inclines, uneven surfaces, and up and down stairs
    Is aware of hazards (eg, wet floors, throw rugs)
    Refer to *Impaired Physical Mobility*.

Provide progressive mobilization if indicated.
    Assist slowly to a sitting position.
    Allow person to dangle legs over the side of the bed for a few minutes before standing.
    Limit the time to 15 min, three times a day, the first few times out of bed.
    Increase time out of bed, as tolerated, by 15-min increments.
    Progress to ambulation, with or without assistive devices.

If client cannot walk, assist him or her out of bed to a wheelchair or chair.

Encourage ambulation for short frequent walks (at least three times daily), with assistance if unsteady.

Increase lengths of walks progressively each day.

Evaluate response to ambulation.

Refer to *Activity Intolerance* if needed.

Refer to *Activity Intolerance* and *Risk for Falls*.

Rationale

See *Impaired Physical Mobility*.

IMPAIRED WHEELCHAIR MOBILITY

DEFINITION

Impaired Wheelchair Mobility: State in which a person experiences or is at risk for experiencing difficulty with wheelchair mobility and safety

DEFINING CHARACTERISTICS

Impaired ability to operate manual or power wheelchair on an even or uneven surface
Impaired ability to operate manual or powered wheelchair on an incline
Impaired ability to operate wheelchair on curbs

RELATED FACTORS

Refer to *Impaired Physical Mobility.*

KEY CONCEPTS
Refer to *Impaired Physical Mobility.*

Focus Assessment Criteria

Refer to *Impaired Physical Mobility*

Goal

The person will report satisfactory, safe wheelchair mobility.

Indicators

- Demonstrate safe use of wheelchair.
- Demonstrate safe transfer to wheelchair.

General Interventions

Determine factors interfering with proper wheelchair use (ie, knowledge, strength, mentation).
Consult with physical therapist if strengthening exercises are indicated.
Teach transfer techniques (weight-bearing and non–weight-bearing).
Have person demonstrate technique; evaluate effectiveness and safety.

Rationale

See *Impaired Physical Mobility.*

IMPAIRED WHEELCHAIR TRANSFER ABILITY

DEFINITION

Impaired Wheelchair Transfer Ability: State in which a person experiences or is at risk for experiencing difficulty with transfer to and from the wheelchair

DEFINING CHARACTERISTICS

Impaired ability to transfer from bed to chair and chair to bed
Impaired ability to transfer on or off a toilet or commode
Impaired ability to transfer in and out of tub or shower
Impaired ability to transfer between uneven levels
Impaired ability to transfer from chair to car or car to chair
Impaired ability to transfer from chair to floor or floor to chair
Impaired ability to transfer standing to floor or floor to standing

RELATED FACTORS

Refer to *Impaired Physical Mobility.*

Focus Assessment Criteria

Refer to *Impaired Physical Mobility*.

Goal

NOC Transfer Performance

The person will demonstrate transfer to and from the wheelchair.

Indicators

* Identify when assistance is needed.
* Demonstrate ability to transfer in varied situations (eg, toilet, bed, car, chair, uneven levels).

General Interventions

NIC See also *Impaired Physical Mobility*, Positioning: Wheelchair

Explain that safe ambulation is a complete movement involving the musculoskeletal, neurologic, and cardiovascular systems and cognitive factors such as mentation and orientation.
A person who is deconditioned needs a progressive exercise program; consult with a physical therapist for evaluation and planning.
Explain that one always should transfer toward the unaffected side.
Determine whether client needs an assistive device (eg, walking belt with handles, mechanical lift, transfer sheets).
Consult with a physical therapist to determine how much assistance the client needs.
    None
    Verbal cuing
    Support by clinician's hand
    Physical assistance
    Mechanical device (eg, lifts)
Refer to *Impaired Physical Mobility*.
Advise that ability may fluctuate; encourage client to request assistance to prevent injury.

Rationale

See *Impaired Physical Mobility*.

NONCOMPLIANCE

DEFINITION

Noncompliance: State in which an individual or group desires to comply but factors are present that deter adherence to health-related advice given by health professionals

DEFINING CHARACTERISTICS
Major (Must Be Present, One or More)

Verbalization of noncompliance or nonparticipation or confusion about therapy
and/or
Direct observation of behavior indicating noncompliance

Minor (May Be Present)

Missed appointments

Partially used or unused medications

Persistence of symptoms

Progression of disease process

Undesired outcomes (postoperative morbidity, pregnancy, obesity, addiction, regression during rehabilitation)

RELATED FACTORS
Pathophysiologic

Related to impaired ability to perform tasks because of disability secondary to:

Poor memory   Motor and sensory deficits

Related to increasing disease-related symptoms despite adherence to advised regimen

Treatment-Related

Related to:

Side effects of therapy	Past unsuccessful experiences with advised regimen
Impersonal aspects of referrals	Nontherapeutic environment
Financial cost of therapy	Complex, unsupervised, prolonged therapy

Situational (Personal, Environmental)

Related to barriers to access secondary to:

Mobility problems	Transportation problems	Financial issues
Inclement weather	Lack of child care	

Related to concurrent illness of family member

Nonsupportive family, peers, community

Related to barriers to care secondary to homelessness
Related to change in employment status
Related to change in health insurance coverage
Related to barriers to comprehension secondary to:

Cognitive deficits	Anxiety	Visual deficits
Fatigue	Hearing deficits	Decreased attention span
Poor memory	Motivation	

⊛ AUTHOR'S NOTE

Compliance depends on various factors, including motivation, perception of vulnerability, and beliefs about controlling or preventing illness; environment; quality of health instruction; and ability to access resources (cost, accessibility). The diagnosis *Noncompliance* describes a person desiring to comply but prevented from doing so by certain factors (eg, lack of understanding, inadequate finances, overly complex instructions). The nurse must attempt to reduce or eliminate these factors to ensure successful interventions.

The process of *informed consent* protects a person's right to self-determination. Informed consent has three conditions: the person must be capable of giving consent, understand the advantages and disadvantages of consent, and not be coerced (Cassells & Redman, 1989). When a person refuses to comply with advice or instructions, it is important for the nurse to assess for and validate the presence of all required elements for informed consent. The nurse is cautioned against using *Noncompliance* to describe a person who has made an informed autonomous decision not to comply. As Cassells and Redman (1989) state, "human dignity is respected by granting individuals the freedom to make choices in accordance with their own values." When a person must change habits or lifestyle or perform certain activities to manage a health problem, *Risk for Ineffective Therapeutic Regimen Management* is very useful.

⊚ ERRORS IN DIAGNOSTIC STATEMENTS

Noncompliance related to reports of not following low-salt diet and resulting increased edema

The above factors would not have caused or contributed to noncompliance. Rather, they represent evidence. If the reason for noncompliance is unknown, *Noncompliance related to unknown etiology, as evidenced by reports of (specify)* would be appropriate.

When the reasons are identified, the nurse must determine whether these factors can be reduced or eliminated. If the person has made an informed decision not to follow the prescribed diet, *Noncompliance* may not be the correct nursing diagnosis. Perhaps the nurse and client could examine the prescribed diet. Is it realistic? What is the probability that compliant behavior will improve quality of life?

KEY CONCEPTS
Generic Considerations

- Compliance is a positive behavior that clients exhibit when moving toward mutually defined therapeutic goals.
- Compliance should be viewed on a continuum rather than as separate states of compliance or noncompliance.
- Partnerships between health care provider and client involve choices and compromises. Some clients desire a passive role, whereas others want complete autonomy.
- Compliance involves a behavioral change, which the following can influence positively:
  - Initial and continuing trust in the health care professional
  - Reinforcement from significant others
  - Perception of own susceptibility to the disease
  - Perception that the disease is serious
  - Evidence that compliance helps control symptoms or the disease
  - Tolerable side effects
  - Less interference with daily activities of client or significant others
  - More benefit than harm provided by therapy
  - Positive sense of self
- The following factors hinder compliance (Blevins & Lubkin, 1999; Hussey & Gilliland, 1989):
  - Inadequate explanation
  - Disagreement between client and provider
  - Long duration of therapy
  - High complexity or expense of regimen
  - Great number and severity of side effects
- Motivation, "the pre- and post-decisional processes which guide the initiation and maintenance of health behaviors," is important for nurses to act on (Fleury, 1992, p. 229). Aspects of motivation to consider include the following:
  - What does the prescribed health behavior change mean to the client?
  - What environmental factors may interfere with the new behavior?
  - What future events may challenge the client's motivation?
  - How will personal values affect the client's ability to remain motivated?
- *Self-efficacy,* the client's beliefs about his or her ability to adopt, perform, and maintain a healthy behavior change, also has been shown to contribute to long-term compliance (Kavanagh & Gooley, 1993; Redland & Stuifbergen, 1993). The nurse can evaluate a client's self-efficacy with questions such as:
  - How many days per week do you think you can take a walk?
  - At what interval do you feel comfortable enough to breast-feed your baby?
  - How often do you think you can check your sugar?
- Noncompliance that follows a period of compliant behavior is termed *relapse.* It usually happens when nonsupportive environmental influences overcome the person's desire to perform the newly adopted behavior (Redland & Stuifbergen, 1993). Causes of relapse can be any of the related factors already listed.
- When evaluating noncompliance related to medication, the nurse must consider the following factors that may affect drug absorption, metabolism, effectiveness, side effects, and excretion: body

weight, age, time of administration, route of administration, genetic factors, basal metabolic rate, interactions with other drugs and foods, presence of organ disease (eg, liver, kidneys), altered body chemistry (eg, hypokalemia), and infection. For example, serum theophylline levels are diminished in a person who smokes cigarettes.

Pediatric Considerations

- Transfer of responsibility for self-care of a child with chronic illness is difficult when noncompliance increases risks to the child, anxiety to the parents, and costs to the family. The child should progress gradually to self-care to increase self-confidence and reduce overdependence (Wong, 2003).
- Compliance is lower during adolescence, when following a regimen competes with self-consciousness and concerns over peer reactions (Whatley, 1991).
- Following a particular treatment regimen can be difficult and trying for an ill child and family. For example, certain drugs may affect behavior, alertness, or school performance (Scipien, Chard, Howe & Barnard, 1990).

Geriatric Considerations

Factors influencing noncompliance in older adults are functional deficits, complicated regimens, costs, inconvenience, and side effects that decrease functional status (eg, strength, alertness).

Transcultural Considerations

Refer to Transcultural Considerations under *Impaired Communication* and *Ineffective Health Maintenance*.

Focus Assessment Criteria

Subjective Data

Assess for Defining Characteristics.

Unacceptable side effects of therapy

Unpleasant taste	Pain	Difficulty swallowing
Too expensive	Time-consuming	Inconvenient

Does family member report any of the above problems?
What does the client want from the nurse or physician?

Assess for Related Factors.

What is the person's general health motivation?
Does client seek help as needed?
Does client intend to make advised lifestyle alterations?
Does client accept diagnosis?

What is the client's perception of his or her present state of health?
Does client consider self to be generally well?
Does he or she fear a specific illness?
Does client believe his or her illness is severe?

How does client view the advised treatment regimen? (eg, does it make personal sense?)
Situations that interfere with prescribed behavior

Family demands	Travel (hotels, restaurants)	Stress
Lack of transportation	Occupations	Denial

Objective Data
Assess for Defining Characteristics.

Evidence of noncompliance
Persistence of symptoms
Problems with medications (pill count, serum drug levels)
Progression of disease
Missed appointments

Assess for Related Factors.

Obstacles to self-care

Inability to read	Musculoskeletal deficits	Immaturity
Cognitive deficits	Memory lags	Pain

Evidence of obstacles in caregiving environment
Long waiting period   Hurried atmosphere

Goal

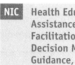

NOC Adherence Behavior, Compliance Behavior, Symptom Control, Treatment Behavior: Illness/Injury

The person will report a desire to change or initiate change.

Indicators

- Describe reasons for suggested regimen.
- Identify barriers to adhering to regimen.

General Interventions

NIC Health Education, Self-Modification Assistance, Self-Responsibility Facilitation, Coping Enhancement, Decision Making Support, Health System Guidance, Mutual Goal Setting, Teaching: Disease Process

Determine Person's Understanding of:
Presence of or risk for health problem (prognosis, disability)
 Vulnerability to problem
 Prevention or treatment measures available
 Effectiveness of preventive measures
 Effectiveness of treatment measures

Explore Client's Feelings Regarding:
Past attempts at compliance
Present concerns regarding prevention or treatment modalities
Which recommendations are feasible
Level of guidance desired from professional
Support from significant others

Refer to *Ineffective Therapeutic Regimen Management* for additional interventions.

Address the benefits of antiviral medications and the risks of nonadherence with HIV medications.
Emphasize that HIV/AIDS can be a chronic disease.
Describe the actions of the medications on the virus.
Explain and track CD4 and viral load counts.
Explain how resistance to medications occurs (eg, missed doses).
Design a system and schedule with the person that will decrease missed doses.
Advise, if he or she is regularly missing doses, to stop all HIV medications and to call the nurse.

Encourage Positive Thinking About New Health-Related Behaviors.

Collaborate with Client to Set Goals.
Short-term goals are most useful.
Be flexible.
Be realistic, considering each person's uniqueness.
Avoid imposing your goals for client.

Consider Using a *Contract,* a Written Statement of Expected Behaviors.
Initially, use short-term contracts with family member, coworker, friend, or nurse.
For the longer term, self-contracts work well; the client finds his or her own rewards and reinforces his or her own positive behavior changes.

Self-Monitoring is Useful to Determine Positive and Negative Influences on Compliance.
Daily records
Charts
Diary of progress or symptoms, clinical values (eg, blood pressure), or dietary intake

Review Present Medication Therapy (Prescribed and Over-the-Counter).

Discuss present therapy (names, dosages, time taken, side effects). Don't ask, "Are you taking your medications?" Ask:
    "What medications did you take today? Yesterday?"
    "What time of day is it difficult for you to take your medications?"
    "Are there times when you decide not to take one of the doses?"
Determine person's understanding of the need for medication.
    Emphasize life-long therapy when indicated (eg, hypertension, diabetes mellitus).
    Explain the complications of unmanaged disease.
Identify possible adverse interactions among drugs (consult pharmacist).
Commit to work with person to reduce or eliminate side effects (eg, change agents or dose).
Help the person identify a reminder to take the medication (eg, brushing teeth at night, daily favorite TV show, watch timer).
Ask person to call primary provider with problems rather than stopping the medication.
Emphasize that unavoidable side effects are still better than the consequences of no therapy (eg, stroke, blindness, renal failure).

Help to Reduce Side Effects.

For gastric irritation, administer drug with milk or food; yogurt may be advisable (unless contraindicated).
For drowsiness, administer medication at bedtime or late in afternoon; consult primary provider for dose reduction.
For leg cramps (hypokalemia), increase foods high in potassium (eg, oranges, raisins, tomatoes, bananas).
For other side effects, consult pertinent references.
Use long-acting intramuscular preparations whenever possible; this includes some antibiotics and antipsychotic medications.
Suggest use of combination pills if available (eg, Maxzide [hydrochlorothiazide and triamterene] and Triavil [perphenazine and amitriptyline]).
When appropriate, be sure client is taking the fewest pills possible (check dosages to provide the largest dose available in the fewest pills).
To decrease frequency of oral medications, suggest longer-acting drug preparations, including the transdermal patch (eg, nitroglycerin).
Encourage prescription of generic drugs for people with financial concerns. Determine if client needs assistance (eg, pharmaceutical patient assistance program such as Merck, Bristol-Myers).
When treatments require more than one set of hands, evaluate home help situation.
When expensive equipment is involved for treatments at home, make appropriate referrals to social workers and local agencies.

If Indicated, Focus on Emotional Responses that Interfere With Compliance (eg, Situational Anxiety, Depression, Denial, Relationship Problems).

Initiate Health Teaching and Referrals, as Indicated.

Teach importance of adhering to prescribed regimen.
Provide written drug information tailored to client's needs. Include drug names, dosages, number of tablets to take and when, purpose of drugs, potential side effects and adverse reactions, and directions for relief of side effects.
Offer praise for honesty about compliance and for sharing reasons. For example:
    "I'm glad you told me that you stopped taking Motrin because it made your stomach hurt. Now I understand why your hands still ache. Let's talk about ways we can get you some comfort."
    "It's good that you told me about your stopping the blood pressure pills. That explains your headaches and higher pressure today. Let's discuss how those pills made you feel."
At discharge from hospital or outpatient setting, provide written name and phone number of professional to call with questions or concerns about prescribed drug regimen.

Rationales

- Evidence exists that "compliance at initiation of the medication regimen is predictive of future compliance" (DeGreest et al., 1998, p. 474).
- Perceived success as a result of one's own efforts enhances self-confidence, which helps to increase adherence.
- Lack of understanding of the health problem, complications, and the client's own vulnerability contribute to noncompliance.
- Involving the client in decision making places some responsibility on him or her to make sure the plan works, promoting compliance with treatment.
- Increasing the person's beliefs that the health behavior change is possible contributes to long-term compliance.
- Lack of understanding regarding reasons for drug therapy and options available contributes to noncompliance.
- Open discussions about side effects can encourage the person to report problems before discontinuing treatment.
- Coping problems take priority and prevent the person from incorporating health behavior changes.
- Establishing a consensual regimen and goals validates that the client is the decision maker and the health care professional is the advisor.
- Contracting involves a commitment to make changes and to be accountable for choices (Blevins & Lubkin, 1999).
- Missing one or two doses of HIV medications a week can cause resistance to the medications.

❖ Pediatric Interventions

Talk with the child to help him or her understand the need for the treatment and likely problems if it is not followed.

Keep information short, simple, and concrete; attempt minimal disruption in lifestyle.

Emphasize visible benefits of compliance. Attempt to minimize side effects and/or teach how to manage side effects.

Design a reminder system with child and family (checklist); write down simple instructions in steps.

Avoid being punitive; instead, problem solve with the family to improve compliance.

Discuss how the child can participate in self-care according to developmental level (Wysocki & Wayne, 1992).

   Put stars on chart when exercises are completed.
   Draw up insulin.
   Select food choices.
   Establish accountability for child or family members.

Discuss conflicts (see *Impaired Parenting*).

Elicit problems in compliance and possible solution or compromises (Wong, 2003).

Use age-related behavioral strategies (Wong, 2003).

   Earning tokens or stickers
   Contracting with positive reinforcers
   Disciplinary techniques (eg, time-out for young children, withholding privileges for older children)

Rationales

- Compliance increases when expectations, responsibilities, and consequences are discussed (Wong, 2003).
- Attempts to engage the child in some aspect of self-care can increase independence, initiative, and self-confidence (Wysocki & Wayne, 1992).
- Contracting is an effective method with older children when they are involved in defining the rules of the agreement (Wong, 2003).
- Strategies to improve compliance must include the child and caregivers in the home (Wong, 2003).

Imbalanced Nutrition: Less Than Body Requirements
    Related to Anorexia Secondary to (Specify)
    Related to Difficulty or Inability to Procure Food
Altered Dentition
Impaired Swallowing
Ineffective Infant Feeding Pattern
Imbalanced Nutrition: More Than Body Requirements
Imbalanced Nutrition: Potential for More Than Body Requirements

IMBALANCED NUTRITION: LESS THAN BODY REQUIREMENTS

DEFINITION

Imbalanced Nutrition: Less Than Body Requirements: State in which a person who is not NPO experiences or is at risk of experiencing reduced weight related to inadequate intake or metabolism of nutrients for metabolic needs

DEFINING CHARACTERISTICS
Major (Must Be Present, One or More)

Person who is not NPO reports or has food intake less than recommended daily allowance (RDA)
    with or without weight loss
and/or
Actual or potential metabolic needs in excess of intake with weight loss

Minor (May Be Present)

Weight 10% to 20%+ below ideal for height and frame
Triceps skinfold, mid-arm circumference, and mid-arm muscle circumference less than 60% standard
    measurement
Muscle weakness and tenderness
Mental irritability or confusion
Decreased serum albumin
Decreased serum transferrin or iron-binding capacity

RELATED FACTORS
Pathophysiologic
Related to increased caloric requirements and difficulty in ingesting sufficient calories secondary to:

Burns (postacute phase)	Cancer	Infection
Trauma	Chemical dependence	AIDS

Related to dysphagia secondary to:

Cerebrovascular accident (CVA)	Muscular dystrophy	Amyotrophic lateral sclerosis
Parkinson's disease	Cerebral palsy	Neuromuscular disorders

Related to decreased absorption of nutrients secondary to:

Crohn's disease	Lactose intolerance	Cystic fibrosis

Related to decreased desire to eat secondary to altered level of consciousness
Related to self-induced vomiting, physical exercise in excess of caloric intake, or refusal to eat secondary to anorexia nervosa

Related to reluctance to eat for fear of poisoning secondary to paranoid behavior
Related to anorexia, excessive physical agitation secondary to bipolar disorder
Related to anorexia and diarrhea secondary to protozoal infection
Related to vomiting, anorexia, and impaired digestion secondary to pancreatitis
Related to anorexia, impaired protein and fat metabolism, and impaired storage of vitamins secondary to cirrhosis

Treatment-Related

Related to protein and vitamin requirements for wound healing and decreased intake secondary to:

Surgery	Surgical reconstruction
Radiation therapy	of mouth
Wired jaw	Medications (chemotherapy)

Related to inadequate absorption as a medication side effect of (specify)

Colchicine	Neomycin	Pyrimethamine
Para-aminosalicylic acid	Antacid	

Related to decreased oral intake, mouth discomfort, nausea, and vomiting secondary to:

Radiation therapy	Tonsillectomy	Chemotherapy

Situational (Personal, Environmental)

Related to decreased desire to eat secondary to:

Anorexia	Social isolation	Depression
Nausea and vomiting	Stress	Allergies

Related to inability to procure food (physical limitations, financial or transportation problems)
Related to inability to chew (damaged or missing teeth, ill-fitting dentures)
Related to diarrhea secondary to (specify)

Maturational

Infant/Child

Related to inadequate intake secondary to:
Lack of emotional/sensory stimulation
Lack of knowledge of caregiver

Related to malabsorption, dietary restrictions, and anorexia secondary to:

Celiac disease	Lactose intolerance	Cystic fibrosis

Related to sucking difficulties (infant) and dysphagia secondary to:

Cerebral palsy	Cleft lip and palate

Related to inadequate sucking, fatigue, and dyspnea secondary to:

Congenital heart disease	Viral syndrome	Prematurity

⊗ AUTHOR'S NOTE

Nurses usually are the primary diagnosticians and prescribers for improving nutritional status. Although *Imbalanced Nutrition* is not a difficult diagnosis to validate, interventions for it can challenge the nurse.

Many factors influence food habits and nutritional status: personal, family, cultural, financial, functional ability, nutritional knowledge, disease and injury, and treatment regimens. *Imbalanced Nutrition: Less Than Body Requirements* describes people who can ingest food but eat an inadequate or imbalanced quality or quantity. For instance, the diet may have insufficient protein or excessive fat. Quantity may be insufficient because of increased metabolic requirements (eg, cancer, pregnancy) or interference with nutrient use (eg, impaired storage of vitamins in cirrhosis).

The nursing focus for *Imbalanced Nutrition* is assisting the person or family to improve nutritional intake. Nurses should not use this diagnosis to describe people who are NPO or cannot ingest food. They should use the collaborative problems *PC: Electrolyte Imbalance* or *PC: Negative Nitrogen Balance* to describe those situations.

ERRORS IN DIAGNOSTIC STATEMENTS

1. *Imbalanced Nutrition: Less Than Body Requirements related to insulin deficiency, altered consciousness, and hypermetabolic state*

   This diagnosis represents a client with diabetes experiencing diabetic ketoacidosis. In such a situation, nursing responsibility focuses on two major problems: managing the ketoacidosis with the physician and teaching client and family how to prevent future episodes. The first is described by the collaborative problem *PC: Ketoacidosis,* for which the nurse would be responsible to monitor for physiologic instability, initiate timely interventions, and evaluate the client's response. The nurse would investigate the second problem, described by the nursing diagnosis *Possible Ineffective Management of Therapeutic Regimen related to adherence to diabetic diet and insufficient knowledge of adaptation needed when sick,* after the client was stable.

2. *Imbalanced Nutrition: Less Than Body Requirements related to parenteral therapy and NPO status*

   This diagnosis represents a situation with which nurses are intricately involved (parenteral therapy). From a nutritional perspective, however, what interventions do nurses prescribe to improve the nutritional status of an NPO client? Parenteral nutrition in a client who is NPO influences several actual or potential responses that nurses treat, representing both nursing diagnoses, such as *Risk for Infection* and *Impaired Comfort,* and the collaborative problems *PC: Hypo/hyperglycemia* and *PC: Negative Nitrogen Balance.*

KEY CONCEPTS
Generic Considerations

- For proper metabolic functioning, the body requires adequate carbohydrates, protein, fat, vitamins, minerals, electrolytes, and trace elements. Figure II.3 depicts the Food Pyramid developed by the United States Department of Agriculture. It recommends daily servings of five food groups. The sixth group—fats, oils, and sweets—should be eaten sparingly and should not exceed 30% of total calorie intake.
- Overall, 54.9% of adult Americans are overweight (15% over ideal weight for height); 18% to 25% of adolescents are overweight. The rate for children is 25% to 30% (Dudek, 2001).
- Obesity is a risk factor for hypertension; type 2 diabetes mellitus; coronary artery disease; cancer of the breast, endometrium, cervix, ovary, colon, rectum, prostate, gallbladder, and biliary tract; and joint and foot disorders (Dudek, 2001).
- Studies report that US women consume insufficient iron, calcium, and vitamins A and C (Lo, 1995).
- Americans eat half of the fiber requirement and 20% more fat than needed (Dudek, 2001).
- The National Research Council (1989) compiled the dietary recommendations outlined in Table II.18.
- Factors influencing nutrient requirements include age, activity, gender, health status (presence of disease, injuries), and nutrient metabolism (storage, absorption, use, excretion).
- Factors influencing nutrient intake include personal (appetite, chewing and swallowing ability, functional ability, psychological status, culture) and structural (socialization, finances, ability to obtain and prepare food, kitchen facilities, transportation; Miller, 2004).
- Drugs can reduce nutrient intake by altering the following (White & Ashworth, 2000):
  - Appetite (eg, metformin, digoxin, paroxetine)
  - Absorption (eg, neomycin, cimetidine)
  - Metabolism (eg, metformin, isoniazid, phenytoin)
- The body requires a minimum level of nutrients for health and growth. During the life span, nutritional needs vary, as indicated in Table II.19 (Wong, 2003; Dudek, 2001).
- Table 11.20 shows the basal metabolic index (BMI) for height.
- The person with cancer experiences disease- and treatment-related nutritional problems:

Disease-Related

| Malabsorption | Diarrhea | Constipation |
| Anemia | Protein deficits | Fatigue |

Treatment-Related

| Stomatitis | Diarrhea | Nausea and vomiting |
| Anorexia | Fatigue | |

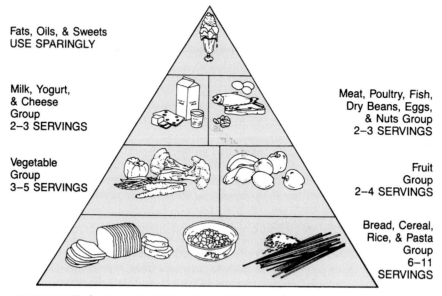

Fats, Oils, & Sweets
USE SPARINGLY

Milk, Yogurt,
& Cheese
Group
2–3 SERVINGS

Meat, Poultry, Fish,
Dry Beans, Eggs,
& Nuts Group
2–3 SERVINGS

Vegetable
Group
3–5 SERVINGS

Fruit
Group
2–4 SERVINGS

Bread, Cereal,
Rice, & Pasta
Group
6–11
SERVINGS

FIGURE II.3   The food pyramid. (U.S. Department of Agriculture.)

Pediatric Considerations

- Changes in nutritional needs characterize each growth period (see Table II.18).
- Nonadolescent children should not be put on diets. The goal for growing children is to maintain, not lose, weight. Healthy food choices of fruit, vegetables, and low-fat snacks (eg, pretzels) can replace foods high in salt, fats, and sugar (Wilson, 1994). Refer to *Ineffective Health Maintenance* for specific interventions for weight loss.

(continued)

TABLE II.18 Dietary Recommendations of the National Research Council Report

Reduce total fat intake to 30% or less of calories; saturated fatty acid intake to less than 10% of kilocalories, and cholesterol to less than 300 mg daily.*
Drink 8–10 glasses of water or noncaffeinated beverages.
Increase intake of starches and other complex carbohydrates.
Maintain protein intake at moderate levels.[†] Increase dry beans, fish.
Increase fiber intake to 25–35 g daily.
Eat 2–4 servings of fruit daily.
Eat 3–5 servings of vegetables daily.
Limit total daily intake of salt (sodium chloride) to 6 g or less.[‡]
Maintain adequate calcium and iron intake.
Avoid taking dietary supplements in excess of the recommended daily allowance (RDA) in any one day.
Balance food intake and physical activity to maintain appropriate body weight.
For those who drink alcoholic beverages, limit consumption to the equivalent of less than 1 oz of pure alcohol in a single day.[§]

*The intake of fat and cholesterol can be reduced by substituting fish, poultry without skin, lean meats, and low-fat or nonfat dairy products for fatty meats and whole-milk dairy products; by choosing more vegetables, fruits, cereals, and legumes; and by limiting oils, fats, egg yolks, and fried and other fatty foods.

[†]Meet at least the RDA for protein, do not exceed twice the RDA.

[‡]Limit the use of salt in cooking, and avoid adding it to food at the table. Salty, highly processed salty, salt-preserved, and salt-pickled foods should be consumed sparingly.

[§]The Committee does not recommend alcohol consumption. One ounce of pure alcohol is the equivalent of two cans of beer, two small glasses of wine, or two average cocktails.

National Research Council, Committee on Diet and Health of Food and Nutrition Board. (1989). Diet and health: Implications for reducing chronic disease risk. *Nutrition Reviews, 47,* 142–149; *Food guide pyramid: A guide to daily food choices.* Leaflet No. 572. Washington, DC: US Department of Agriculture; Dudek, S.G. (2001). *Nutrition essentials for nursing practice.* (4th ed.) Philadelphia: Lippincott Williams and Wilkins.

TABLE II.19 Age-Related Daily Nutritional Requirements

Age	Daily Nutritional Requirements
Infants	
Newborn	12–18 oz milk
2–3 months	20–30 oz milk
4–5 months	25–35 oz milk; strained vegetables and fruits; egg yolks
6–7 months	28–40 oz milk; above solids, plus meat, finger foods
8–11 months	24 oz milk; three regular meals, chopped table food
1–2 years	24 oz milk; 100 cal/kg same as 8–11 months
Children	
Preschool (3–5 years)	90 cal/kg; 1.2g/kg protein Basic food groups Calcium 800 mg

School (6–12 years)	80 cal/kg; 1.2 g/kg protein
	Basic food groups (as preschool)
	  1.5–2 g calcium
	  400 units vitamin D
	  1.5–3 L water

Adolescent (13–17 years)	2,200–2,400 cal for girls
	3,000 cal for boys
	Basic food groups (as preschool)
	  50–60 g protein
	  1,200–1,500 mg calcium (to age 25)
	  400 units vitamin D

Adults	
	1,600–3,000 calorie range (based on physical activity, emotional state, body size, age, and individual metabolism) Basic food groups Refer to Figure II.4 Men need increased protein, ascorbic acid, riboflavin, and vitamins E and B_6 Women need the above and also increased iron, calcium, and vitamins A and B_{12}

Pregnant women (2nd and 3rd trimesters)	Daily calorie requirement
	  11–15 years, 2,500
	  16–22 years, 2,400
	  23–50 years, 2,300
	Increase protein 10 g or 1 serving meat
	1.2–3.5 g calcium
	Increase vitamins A, B, and C
	30–60 mg iron

Lactating women	2,500–3,000 cal (500 over regular diet)
	Basic food groups
	  4 servings protein
	  5 servings dairy
	  4+ servings grain
	  5+ servings vegetables
	    2+ servings vitamin C-rich
	    1+ green leafy
	    2+ others
	Fluids 2–3 qt (1 qt milk)
	Increase in vitamin A, C, niacin

Over 65 years	Basic food groups (same as adult) Caloric requirements decrease with age (1,600–1,800 for women, 2,000–2,400 for men), but dependent on activity, climate, and metabolic needs Ensure intake of essential amino acids, fatty acids, vitamins, elements, fiber, and water 60 mg ascorbic acid 40–60 mg protein 1,200 mg calcium (1,500 mg for women not taking estrogen) 10 mg iron

TABLE II.20 Weight for Height and Body Frame

		Men					Women		
Height (Feet)	(Inches)	Small Frame	Medium Frame	Large Frame	Height (Feet)	(Inches)	Small Frame	Medium Frame	Large Frame
5	2	128–134	131–141	138–150	4	10	102–111	109–121	118–131
5	3	130–136	133–143	140–153	4	11	103–113	111–123	120–134
5	4	132–138	135–145	142–156	5	0	104–115	113–126	122–137
5	5	134–140	137–148	144–160	5	1	106–118	115–129	125–140
5	6	136–142	139–151	146–164	5	2	108–121	118–132	128–143
5	7	138–145	142–154	149–168	5	3	111–124	121–135	131–147
5	8	140–148	145–147	152–172	5	4	114–127	124–138	134–151
5	9	142–151	148–160	155–176	5	5	117–130	127–141	137–155
5	10	144–154	151–163	158–180	5	6	120–133	130–144	140–159
5	11	146–157	154–166	161–184	5	7	123–136	133–147	143–163
6	0	149–160	157–170	164–188	5	8	126–139	136–150	146–167
6	1	152–164	160–174	168–192	5	9	129–142	139–153	149–170
6	2	155–168	164–178	172–197	5	10	132–145	142–156	152–173
6	3	158–172	167–182	176–202	5	11	135–148	145–159	155–176
6	4	162–176	171–187	181–207	6	0	138–151	148–162	158–179

Pediatric Considerations (continued)

- Children at special risk for inadequate nutritional intake include those with
  - Congenital anomalies (eg, tracheoesophageal fistula, cardiac or neurologic anomalies)
  - Prematurity, intrauterine growth retardation
  - Inborn errors of metabolism (eg, phenylketonuria)
  - Malabsorption disorders
  - Developmental disorders (eg, cerebral palsy)
  - Chronic illness (eg, cystic fibrosis, chronic infections, diabetes)
  - Accelerated growth rates (eg, prematurity, infancy, adolescence)
  - Parents who have inadequate attachment
- Parents must follow sound feeding practices to prevent nutritional deficits in their infants (Anderson, 1989; Wong, 2003):
  - Feeding the infant breast milk or iron-fortified formula for the first year
  - Adding solid foods by 5 to 6 months of age
  - Assessing the infant's cues for burping or satiety
  - Holding the infant during feeding versus propping the bottle
  - Selecting foods appropriate to the infant's physiologic and motor development
  - Preparing formula correctly
- The frequent eating of fast food (high in salt, sugar, fat) and the increasing rate of obesity in children has created a problem that needs specific interventions (Wong, 2003).

Maternal Considerations

- Nutritional needs change during pregnancy (refer to Table II.19).
- Recommendations for total weight gain during pregnancy vary. Women underweight before pregnancy should gain 28 to 40 lb; women at a desirable weight, 25 to 35 lb; women who are moderately overweight, 15 to 25 lb; women who are very overweight (BMI >29), 15 lb (Pilliteri, 2003).
- Dieting during pregnancy may result in insufficient maternal intake to provide the fetus with the necessary energy for growth. The fetus depends on the mother's dietary intake for growth and development, taking only iron and folate from maternal stores.

⊙ Geriatric Considerations

- In general, older adults need the same kind of balanced diet as any other group, but fewer calories. Diets of older clients, however, tend to be insufficient in iron, calcium, and vitamins. The combination of long-established eating patterns, income, transportation, housing, social interaction, and the effects of chronic or acute disease influence nutritional intake and health (Miller, 2004).
- The decreased energy needs of many older adults require a change in nutrient intake:

	25 to 50 years of age	50 years or older
Carbohydrates	60%	55%
Protein	10%	20%
Fat	30%	25%
Kcal/day		
Women	2,200	1,900
Men	2,900	2,300

- People taking diuretics must be observed closely for adequate hydration (intake and output) and electrolyte balance, especially sodium and potassium. Potassium-rich foods should be included regularly in the diet.
- Iron-deficiency anemia usually occurs over time and may be related to chronic diseases and insufficient dietary iron. Increasing the intake of foods rich in vitamin C, folic acid, and dietary iron can improve the conditions necessary for optimal absorption of iron. Iron supplementation is often necessary.

⊙ Transcultural Considerations

- Many cultures have used diet for centuries to treat specific diseases, promote health during pregnancy, foster growth and development in children, and prolong life (Andrews & Boyle, 2003).
- Some cultures view health as a state of balance among the body humors (blood, phlegm, black bile, and yellow bile). In this framework, a humoral imbalance that causes excessive dryness, cold, hot, or wetness leads to illness. For example, an upset stomach is believed to result from eating too many foods identified as cold. Foods, herbs, and medicines are classified as hot or cold or wet or dry. They are used to restore the body to its natural balance. For example, bananas are classified as a cold food, whereas corn meal is a hot food (Andrews & Boyle, 2003).
- Adult lactose intolerance has been reported among most populations, affecting 94% of Asians, 90% of African blacks, 79% of American Indians, 75% of American blacks, 50% of Mexican Americans, and 17% of American whites (Overfield, 1985).
- Nutritional practices can be categorized as beneficial, neutral, or harmful. Beneficial and neutral practices should be encouraged. Harmful practices should be approached with sensitivity and their detrimental effects explained (Andrews & Boyle, 2003).
- Group dining, which is encouraged in some settings (eg, rehabilitation, long-term, mental health), may be in conflict with certain cultures (eg, women eating with men; Andrews & Boyle, 2003).
- Maintaining a kosher diet for a Jewish client is possible even if the agency does not have a kosher kitchen. Fish with fins or scales will meet dietary requirements. Dairy products are also possible. Paper plates with disposable utensils should be used so that meat and milk dishes are not mixed (Giger & Davidhizar, 2004).

Focus Assessment Criteria

Subjective Data
Assess for Defining Characteristics.

Usual intake
Diet recall for 24 h
Is this the usual intake pattern?

Is intake of basic five food groups sufficient?
Is fluid intake sufficient?

Assess for Related Factors.

Appetite (usual, changes)
Dietary patterns
Food/fluid dislikes, preferences, taboos
Religious dietary practices
Frequency of fast food consumption

Activity level
Occupation, exercise (type, frequency)

Food procurement/preparation (who)

Functional ability	Kitchen facilities	Transportation
Income adequate for food needs		

Knowledge of nutrition
Basic five food groups
Recommended intake of carbohydrates, fats, salt
Relationship of activity and metabolism

Physiologic risk factors (Evans-Stoner, 1997)
Neurologic impairment
Chronic illness (renal failure, chronic obstructive pulmonary disease [COPD], human immuno-
  deficiency virus [HIV], liver disease)
Malabsorption
Inflammatory bowel disease

Psychosocial conditions (Evans-Stoner, 1997)

Alcohol abuse	Drug use	Household status
Isolation	Depression	Institutionalization

Medications (prescribed, over-the-counter)
Reports of

Allergies	Dysphagia	Nausea
Indigestion	Vomiting	Chewing problems
Anorexia	Constipation	Fatigue
Diarrhea	Sore mouth	Pain

Objective Data
Assess for Defining Characteristics.

General

Appearance	Muscle mass	Fat distribution
Hair	Skin	Nails
Height	Weight	Body mass index
Mouth	Teeth	Edema

Anthropometric measurements

Mid-arm circumference	Triceps skinfold	Mid-arm muscle circumference

Laboratory studies

Decreased serum prealbumin	Decreased serum transferrin

Assess for Related Factors.
Ability to chew, swallow, feed self
For more information on Focus Assessment Criteria, visit http://connection.lww.com.

Goal

NOC Nutritional Status, Teaching: Nutrition

The client will ingest daily nutritional requirements in accordance with activity level and metabolic
needs.

Indicators

- Relate importance of good nutrition.
- Identify deficiencies in daily intake.
- Relate methods to increase appetite.

General Interventions

| NIC | Nutrition Management, Nutrition Monitoring |

Explain the Need for Adequate Consumption of Carbohydrates, Fats, Protein, Vitamins, Minerals, and Fluids.

Consult With a Nutritionist to Establish Appropriate Daily Caloric and Food Type Requirements for the Client.

Discuss With the Client Possible Causes of Decreased Appetite.

Encourage the Client to Rest Before Meals.

Offer Frequent, Small Meals Instead of a Few Large Ones; Offer Foods Served Cold.

With Decreased Appetite, Restrict Liquids With Meals and Avoid Fluids 1 h Before and After Meals.

Encourage and Help the Client to Maintain Good Oral Hygiene.

Arrange to Have High-Calorie and High-Protein Foods Served at the Times that the Client Usually Feels Most Like Eating.

Take Steps to Promote Appetite.

Determine client's food preferences and arrange to have them provided, as appropriate.
Eliminate any offensive odors and sights from the eating area.
Control any pain and nausea before meals.
Encourage the client's support people to bring permitted foods from home, if possible.
Provide a relaxed atmosphere and some socialization during meals.

Give Client Printed Materials Outlining a Nutritious Diet That Includes the Following:

High intake of complex carbohydrates and fiber
Decreased intake of sugar, salt, cholesterol, total fat, and saturated fats
Alcohol use only in moderation
Proper caloric intake to maintain ideal weight

Rationales

- Nutrients provide energy sources, build tissue, and regulate metabolic processes.
- Consultation can help ensure a diet that provides optimal caloric and nutrient intake.
- Factors such as pain, fatigue, analgesic use, and immobility can contribute to anorexia. Identifying a possible cause enables interventions to eliminate or minimize it.
- Fatigue further reduces an anorectic client's desire and ability to eat.
- Even distribution of total daily caloric intake helps prevent gastric distention, possibly increasing appetite.
- Restricting fluids with meals helps prevent gastric distention.
- Poor oral hygiene leads to bad odor and taste, which can diminish appetite.
- Presenting high-calorie and high-protein food when the client is most likely to eat increases the likelihood that he or she will consume adequate calories and protein.
- Diet planning focuses on avoiding nutritional excesses. Reducing fats, salt, and sugar can reduce the risk of heart disease, diabetes, certain cancers, and hypertension.

Pediatric Interventions

Teach parents the age-related nutritional needs of their children (consult an appropriate textbook on pediatrics or nutrition for specific recommendations).

Discuss the importance of limiting snacks high in salt, sugar, or fat (eg, soda, candy, chips) to limit risks for cardiac disorders, obesity, and diabetes mellitus. Advise families to substitute healthy snacks (eg, fresh fruits, plain popcorn, frozen fruit juice bars, fresh vegetables).

Assist families to evaluate their nutritional patterns.

Discuss strategies to make meals a social event and to avoid struggles (Dudek, 2001; Wong, 2003).

   Allow child to select one type of food he or she doesn't have to eat.

   Provide small servings (eg, one tablespoon of each food for every year of age).

   Make snacks as nutritiously important as meals (eg, hard-boiled eggs, raw vegetable sticks, peanut butter/crackers, fruit juices, cheese, fresh fruit).

   Offer a variety of foods.

   Encourage all members to share their day.

Involve child in monitoring healthy eating (eg, create a chart where child marks off intake of healthy foods daily).

Replace passive television watching with a group activity (eg, Frisbee, biking, walking).

Address strategies to improve nutrition when eating fast foods:

   Drink skim milk.

   Avoid fries.

   Choose grilled foods.

   Eat salads and vegetables.

   Substitute quick, nutritious fast meals (eg, frozen dinners).

Rationales

- Nutritional requirements vary greatly for each age group. Periods of accelerated physical growth (eg, infancy, puberty) may necessitate doubling iron, calcium, zinc, and protein intake (Wong, 2003).
- During periods of slow growth (eg, preschool, elementary school), appetite is diminished (Dudek, 2001).
- Increasing healthy snacks reduces the pressure for the child to eat a certain amount at mealtime (Wong, 2003).
- Family nutritional patterns are the primary influence on the development of food habits (eg, unhealthy snacks, excessive television watching; Dudek, 2001).

Maternal Interventions

Explain physiologic changes and nutritional needs during pregnancy (see Table II.19).

Discuss the effects of alcohol, caffeine, and artificial sweeteners on the developing fetus.

Explain the different nutritional requirements for pregnant girls 11 to 18 years of age, pregnant young women 19 to 24 years of age, and women older than 25 years.

Determine if a woman needs more calories because of daily activity.

Rationales

- Explanations about metabolic changes can increase awareness of nutritional requirements.
- Studies have shown that alcohol consumption (two to four drinks/day) can cause low birth weight. Larger amounts cause fetal alcohol syndrome.
- Studies have shown caffeine to have few effects on pregnancy outcome, but moderation is recommended (Dudek, 2001).
- Consumption of artificial sweeteners during pregnancy has not been found to be contraindicated, but moderation is suggested (Dudek, 2001).

- Adolescent girls need increased nutritional intake because of their own accelerated growth, and pregnancy increases the requirements even more (Dudek, 2001).
- Resting caloric needs for pregnant women differ according to age (Pilliteri, 2003):
  - 28.5 kcal/kg for 11 to 14 years
  - 24.9 kcal/kg for 15 to 18 years
  - 23.3 kcal/kg for 19 to 24 years
  - 21.9 kcal/kg for 25 to 50 years
- More calories are needed depending on activity level (Pilliteri, 2003): multiply resting caloric needs by
  - 1.5 for light activity
  - 1.6 for moderate activity
  - 1.9 for heavy activity

Geriatric Interventions

Determine Person's Understanding of Nutritional Needs with:

Aging   Medication use   Illness
Activity

Assess if Any Factors Interfere With Procuring or Ingesting Foods (Miller, 2004).

Anorexia from medications, grief, depression, illness
Impaired mental status leading to inattention to hunger or selecting insufficient kinds/amounts of food
Impaired mobility or manual dexterity (paresis, tremors, weakness, joint pain, or deformity)
Voluntary fluid restriction for fear of urinary incontinence
Small frame or history of undernutrition
Inadequate income to purchase food
Lack of transportation to buy food or facility to cook
New dentures or poor dentition
Dislike of cooking and eating alone
Regularly eats alone
Has more than 2 alcoholic drinks daily

Explain Decline in Sensitivity to Sweet and Salty Tastes.

If Indicated, Consult With Home Health Nurse to Evaluate Home Environment (eg, Cooking Facilities, Food Supply, Cleanliness).

Access Community Agencies as Indicated (eg, Nutritional Programs, Community Centers, Home-Delivered Grocery Services).

Rationales

- With age, nutritional requirements do not diminish, but overall caloric needs do. High-quality, nutritious foods are very important (Miller, 2004).
- Multiple factors can interfere with access or ingestion of food. Strategies to improve nutrition should address specific factors (Dudek, 2001).
- Older adults can consume excessive salt and sugar to compensate for loss of sensitivity to these tastes (Miller, 2004).
- A home assessment may provide valid data in cases of suspected nutritional problems (Miller, 2004).
- Certain medications or illnesses may require an adjustment in diet (eg, potassium, sodium, fiber).

IMBALANCED NUTRITION: LESS THAN BODY REQUIREMENTS

RELATED TO ANOREXIA SECONDARY TO (SPECIFY)

Goal

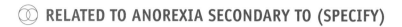

NOC Nutritional Status, Teaching: Nutrition, Symptom Control

The person will increase oral intake as evidenced by (specify).

Indicators

- Describe causative factors when known.
- Describe rationale and procedure for treatments.

Interventions

NIC Nutrition Management, Weight Gain Assistance, Nutritional Counseling

Assess Causative Factors.

Diminished sense of taste or smell
Social isolation
Radiation therapy or chemotherapy
Altered body image or self-concept
Early satiety
Noxious stimuli (pain or painful or unpleasant procedures, fatigue, odors, nausea and vomiting)

Reduce or Eliminate Contributing Factors, if Possible.

Diminished Sense of Taste or Smell

Explain to client the importance of consuming adequate nutrients.

Teach client to use spices (eg, lemon juice, mint, cloves, basil, thyme, cinnamon, rosemary, bacon bits) to help improve the taste and aroma of food.

Teach protein sources that the client may find more acceptable than red meat:
  Eggs and dairy products
  Chicken and turkey
  Fish (if not strong-smelling)
  Marinated meat (in wine, vinegar)
  Soy products (tofu)

Chopped or ground meats/protein sources may be more acceptable.

Mixing protein and vegetables may be more acceptable.

Refer to meals as "snacks" to make them sound smaller.

Social Isolation

Encourage client to eat with others (meals served in dining room or group area at local meeting place such as community center, by church groups).

Provide daily contact through phone calls by support system.

See *Risk for Loneliness* for additional interventions.

Noxious Stimuli (Pain, Fatigue, Odors, Nausea, and Vomiting)

Pain

Plan care so unpleasant or painful procedures do not take place before meals.

Schedule pain relief medications so optimal relief without drowsiness is achieved at meal time.

Provide pleasant, relaxed atmosphere for eating (no bedpans in sight; don't rush); try a "surprise" (eg, flowers with meal).

Arrange plan of care to decrease or eliminate nauseating odors or procedures near mealtimes.

Fatigue

Teach or assist client to rest before meals.

Teach client to expend minimal energy in food preparation (cook large quantities and freeze several meals at a time; request assistance from others).

Odor of food

Teach client to avoid cooking odors—frying foods, brewing coffee—if possible (take a walk; select foods that can be eaten cold).

Suggest using foods that require little cooking during periods of anorexia.

Nausea and vomiting

See *Impaired Swallowing* for Additional Interventions.

Promote Foods That Stimulate Eating and Increase Protein Consumption (Foltz, 1997).

Maintain good oral hygiene (brush teeth, rinse mouth) before and after eating.

Offer frequent small feedings (six per day plus snacks) to reduce the feeling of a distended stomach.

Allow client to choose food items as close to actual eating time as possible.

Arrange to serve the highest protein/calorie nutrients served when the client feels most like eating (eg, if chemotherapy is in early morning, serve food in late afternoon).

Encourage significant others to bring in favorite home foods.

Instruct client to:

    Eat dry foods (toast, crackers) on arising.

    Eat salty foods, if permissible.

    Avoid overly sweet, rich, greasy, or fried foods.

    Try clear, cool beverages.

    Sip slowly through straw.

    Take whatever he or she feels can be tolerated.

    Eat small portions low in fat. Eat more frequently.

Try commercial supplements available in many forms (liquids, powder, pudding); keep switching brands until some are found that are acceptable to the client in taste and consistency.

Teach techniques for home food preparation to client and family.

    Add powdered milk or egg to milkshakes, gravies, sauces, puddings, cereals, meatballs, or milk to increase protein and calorie content.

    Add blenderized or baby foods to meat juices or soups.

    Use fortified milk (ie, 1 cup instant nonfat milk to 1 qt fresh milk).

    Use milk or half-and-half instead of water when making soups and sauces; soy formulas also can be used.

    Add cheese or diced meat.

    Add cream cheese or peanut butter to toast, crackers, or celery sticks.

    Add extra butter or margarine to soups, sauces, or vegetables.

    Spread butter on toast while hot.

    Use mayonnaise (100 cal/T) instead of salad dressing.

    Add sour cream or yogurt to vegetables or as dip.

    Use whipped cream (60 cal/T).

    Add raisins, dates, nuts, and brown sugar to hot or cold cereals.

    Have extra food (snacks) easily available.

Review high-calorie versus low-calorie foods. Avoid empty-calorie foods (eg, soda).

For clients with lactose intolerance, explore alternative dairy source to drinking milk (eg, cheese, yogurt, acidophilus milk).

Initiate Health Teaching and Referrals, as Indicated.

Dietitian for meal planning	Psychiatric therapy when indicated
Community meal centers	Support groups for clients with anorexia

Rationales

- For most people, meals are social events. Loneliness at meals can reduce the incentive to prepare nutritious meals.
- The client should have as much control as possible over his or her diet—for example, have the client make a list of food and fluid preferences and dislikes and try to incorporate these into the prescribed diet.

- Maintaining good oral hygiene before and after meals decreases microorganisms that can cause foul taste and odor, inhibiting appetite.
- Fluid restrictions at meals can help prevent gastric overdistention and can enhance appetite.
- Nausea can be reduced by controlling environmental conditions and promoting positions that minimize abdominal pressure.
- Certain measures can increase the nutritional content of foods even when intake is limited.

IMBALANCED NUTRITION: LESS THAN BODY REQUIREMENTS

⊙⊙ RELATED TO DIFFICULTY OR INABILITY TO PROCURE FOOD

Altered ability to procure food is the inability to acquire food because of physical, economic, or sociocultural barriers.

Goal

NOC Nutritional Status

The person will identify a method to acquire food on a regular schedule.

Indicators

- Describe causative factors when known.
- Relate importance of good nutrition.

Interventions

NIC Nutritional Counseling, Nutrition Management, Teaching: Individual, Family, Referral, Environmental Management

Assess Causative Factors.

Inadequate economic resources to obtain adequate nutrition
Sociocultural barriers
Physical inability to procure food related to health problem such as COPD, CVA, or quadriplegia

Eliminate or Reduce Contributing Factors, If Possible.

Inadequate Economic Resources

Assess client's eligibility for food stamps or other government-funded programs for low-income groups; consult with social services.
Suggest cooperatives or local farmers' markets for shopping.
Buy foods and meats on sale and freeze; use cheaper cuts and tenderize.
Suggest foods that are low in cost and high in nutrients; decrease use of prepackaged or prepared items.
    Beans and legumes as protein source
    Powdered milk (alone or mixed half-and-half with whole milk)
    Seasonal foods when plentiful
Encourage growing a small garden or participating in a community plot.
Freeze or can fruits and vegetables in season (refer to county agricultural agent for information on canning and freezing).

Sociocultural Barriers

Introduce client to locally available foodstuffs; instruct in their preparation.
Suggest substitutions of locally available foodstuffs for those to which client is accustomed.
Refer client to adult education home economics classes for food preparation.

Assist client to recognize and use additional outlets and sources of food (grocery stores, meat and fruit markets).

Encourage peer group meetings among people of similar backgrounds to allow learning and exchange of ideas.

Acquaint client with ethnic food store locations, if available.

Physical Deficits

Promote alternative methods of food procurement and preparation.

Support systems of people willing to purchase or prepare food for client or take him or her to store

Supermarkets that deliver

Meals on Wheels or similar service

Homemaker

Group housing

Door-to-store bus service

Teach client or others to cook enough for six meals at once and freeze; make own complete "frozen dinners."

Aid client to plan daily activities that allow enough energy for shopping and cooking.

Rest periods before and after activity

Rest periods during activity, if needed

Teach Techniques for Meal Planning and Preparation for One.

Buy small cans of food (they may seem more expensive, but spoiled food is costly).

When buying fruit, select three stages of ripeness (ripe, medium ripe, green).

Family-sized packages of meat or fresh vegetables can be broken down and frozen.

When buying in large quantity, make soups and stews with the extra.

Use powdered instead of fresh milk in recipes.

Buy fresh milk in pints or quarts.

Store large-quantity items (rice, flour, corn meal, dry milk, cereal) in glass jars. Place tightly sealed jars in the freezer for one night to kill any organisms and their eggs.

Experiment with stir-frying vegetables (eg, Chinese cabbage, celery) in a little chicken broth.

If freezer space is available, prepare four to six times as much as you need and freeze in individual portions, dating the packages.

Store half a loaf of bread well wrapped in freezer. (It will become stale in the refrigerator.)

Buy large bags of frozen vegetables, use small amounts, and close with twist ties.

Finely chop and freeze fresh herbs (parsley, dill, basil) in small freezer bags. Flatten so small portions can be broken off after freezing.

Buy large quantities of meat and freeze in foil wrap (not freezer paper).

Initiate Health Teaching and Referrals, as Indicated.

Refer to social worker, occupational therapist, or visiting nurse, as needed.

Refer to local extension office for information on vegetable gardening, community gardens, and techniques of freezing and canning foods.

Refer to dietitian for meal planning.

Rationales

- People who are impaired either physically or cognitively should receive the necessary support and supervision in selecting foods and self-feeding.
- Activities needed to procure food depend on skills of cognition, balance, mobility, manual dexterity, and all five senses (Miller, 2004).
- Nurses must be familiar with available local resources so they can initiate referrals (Miller, 2004).
- People with difficulty preparing meals can be assisted to reduce daily preparation time through specific planning (Mahan & Arlin, 1996).

ALTERED DENTITION

DEFINITION

Altered Dentition: State in which a person experiences a disruption in tooth development/eruption patterns or structural integrity of individual teeth

DEFINING CHARACTERISTICS

Excessive plaque

Halitosis

Toothache

Excessive calculus

Malocclusion or tooth
  misalignment

Premature loss of primary teeth

Missing teeth or complete
  absence

Asymmetric facial expression

Crown or root caries

Tooth enamel discoloration

Loose teeth

Incomplete eruption for age (may be
  primary or permanent teeth)

Tooth fracture(s)

Erosion of enamel

 AUTHOR'S NOTE

Altered Dentition describes a multitude of problems with teeth. It is unclear how nurses or any health care professional would use this diagnosis. If the client had caries, abscesses, misaligned teeth, or malformed teeth, the nurse would refer the client to a dental professional. If the tooth problem is affecting comfort or nutrition, *Impaired Comfort* or *Imbalanced Nutrition* would be the appropriate nursing diagnosis, not *Altered Dentition*.

IMPAIRED SWALLOWING

DEFINITION

Impaired Swallowing: State in which a person has decreased ability voluntarily to pass fluids and/or solid foods from the mouth to the stomach

DEFINING CHARACTERISTICS (JENG ET AL., 2001)
Major (Must Be Present, One or More)

Observed evidence of difficulty in swallowing

and/or

Stasis of food in oral cavity   Coughing after food or fluid intake   Choking

Minor (May Be Present)

Nasal-sounding voice   Drooling
Slurred speech

RELATED FACTORS
Pathophysiologic

Related to decreased/absent gag reflex, mastication difficulties, or decreased sensations secondary to:

Cerebral palsy   Muscular dystrophy
Poliomyelitis   Parkinson's disease
Guillain-Barré syndrome   Myasthenia gravis
Amyotrophic lateral sclerosis   CVA
Neoplastic disease affecting brain Right or left hemispheric brain damage
Cranial nerve damage (V, VII, IX, X, XI)

Related to tracheoesophageal tumors, edema
Related to irritated oropharyngeal cavity
Related to decreased saliva

Treatment-Related

Related to surgical reconstruction of the mouth, throat, jaw, or nose
Related to decreased consciousness secondary to anesthesia
Related to mechanical obstruction secondary to tracheostomy tube
Related to esophagitis secondary to radiotherapy

Situational (Personal, Environmental)

Related to fatigue
Related to limited awareness, distractibility

Maturational

Infants/Children
Related to decreased sensations or difficulty with mastication

Older Adult
Related to reduction in saliva, taste

⊗ **AUTHOR'S NOTE**

See *Imbalanced Nutrition: Less Than Body Requirements.*

⊗ **ERRORS IN DIAGNOSTIC STATEMENTS**

See *Imbalanced Nutrition: Less Than Body Requirements.*

KEY CONCEPTS
Generic Considerations

- Swallowing has an intellectual as well as a physical component.
- The swallowing process occurs in three stages with select cranial nerve involvement (Porth, 2002).
  - *Stage 1*—Oral: Food is placed in oral cavity, the lips close, and swallowing is initiated as a reflex. The tongue maneuvers the food, and the soft palate and uvula close off the nasopharynx.
  - *Stage 2*—Pharyngeal: The food passes the anterior fossa arches and triggers the swallow reflex. The tongue prevents the food from returning to the oral cavity by elevation and contraction of the soft palate. Pharyngeal peristalsis begins, causing the food to move downward.

- *Stage 3*—Esophageal: Pharyngeal peristalsis pushes the food downward. The larynx elevates and the cricopharyngeal muscles relax, allowing the food to move from the pharynx into the esophagus. The larynx wave pushes the food down the esophagus to the stomach.
- Cranial nerves V, VII, IX, X, and XI are involved in swallowing.
- Impairment of cranial nerve function can cause the following swallowing problems:
  - Trigeminal (V)—loss of sensation and ability to move mandible
  - Facial (VII)—Increased salivation; inability to pucker lips, pouching of foods
  - Glossopharyngeal (IX)—diminished taste sensation, salivation, and gag reflex
  - Vagus (X)—decreased peristalsis, decreased gag reflex
  - Hypoglossal (XI)—poor tongue control, poor movement of food to the throat
- A cough reflex is essential for rehabilitation, but a gag reflex is not.
- Do not confuse the ability to chew with the ability to swallow. See also *Imbalanced Nutrition: Less Than Body Requirements*.

Focus Assessment Criteria

Subjective Data
Assess for Defining Characteristics.

History of problem with swallowing
   Onset
   History of nasal regurgitation, hoarseness, choking, or coughing
Problem foods or liquids
Nonproblem foods or liquids

Assess for Related Factors.

CVA	Parkinson's disease	Multiple sclerosis
Brain lesions	Head trauma	Tracheoesophageal tumors
Oral surgery		

Objective Data
Assess for Defining Characteristics.

Decreased or absent swallowing, cough, or gag reflex
Poor coordination of tongue
Observed choking or coughing with food or fluid

Assess for Related Factors.

Facial muscle weakness	Impaired use of tongue	Chewing difficulties
Decreased saliva production	Thick secretions	Impaired cognition

For more information on Focus Assessment Criteria, visit http://connection.lww.com.

Goal

NOC Aspiration Control, Swallowing Status

The person will report improved ability to swallow.

Indicators
The person and/or family will

- Describe causative factors when known.
- Describe rationale and procedures for treatment.

NIC Aspiration Precautions, Swallowing Therapy, Surveillance, Referral, Positioning

General Interventions

Assess for Causative or Contributing Factors.

Mechanical Impairment of Oropharyngeal Structures

Congenital anomalies	Decreased/absent gag reflex	Fatigue
Surgical reconstruction of mouth	Cleft lip/palate	Cranial nerve damage

Red, irritated oropharyngeal cavity	CVA	Altered level of consciousness

Muscle Paralysis or Paresis

Post-CVA	Cranial nerve damage	Decreased/no gag reflex

Impaired Cognition or Awareness

Cortical damage	Apraxia	Aphasia

Reduce or Eliminate Causative/Contributing Factors in People With:

Mechanical Impairment of Mouth

Assist client with moving the bolus of food from the anterior to the posterior part of mouth. Place food in the posterior mouth where swallowing can be ensured, using:

A syringe with a short piece of tubing attached

A glossectomy spoon

Soft, moist food of a consistency that can be manipulated by the tongue against the pharynx, such as gelatin, custard, or mashed potatoes

Prevent/decrease thick secretions.

Artificial saliva

Papain tablets dissolved in mouth 10 min before eating

Meat tenderizer made from papaya enzyme applied to oral cavity 10 min before eating

Frequent mouth care

Increase fluid intake to 8 glasses of liquid (unless contraindicated)

Check medications for potential side effects of dry mouth/decreased salivation

Muscle Paralysis or Paresis

Establish a visual method to communicate at bedside to staff that client is dysphagic.

Plan meals when client is well rested; ensure that reliable suction equipment is on hand during meals. Discontinue feeding if client is tired.

If indicated, use modified supraglottic swallow technique (Emick-Herring & Wood, 1990).

1. Position the head of the bed in semi- or high Fowler's position, with the neck flexed forward slightly and chin tilted down.
2. Use cutout cup (remove and round out one third of side of foam cup).
3. Take bolus of food and hold in strongest side of mouth for 1 to 2 s. Then immediately flex the neck with chin tucked against chest.
4. Without breathing, swallow as many times as needed.
5. When mouth is emptied, raise chin and clear throat.

Offer highly viscous foods (eg, mashed bananas, potatoes, gelatin, gravy) first.

Offer thick liquids (eg, milkshakes, slushes, nectars, cream soups).

Establish a goal for fluid intake.

If drooling is present, use a quick-stretch stimulation just before and toward the end of each meal (Emick-Herring & Wood, 1990).

Digitally apply short, rapid, downward strokes to edge of bottom lip, mostly on affected side.

Use a cold washcloth over finger for added stimulation.

If a bolus of food is pocketed in the affected side, teach client how to use tongue to transfer food or apply external digital pressure to cheek to help remove the trapped bolus (Emick-Herring & Wood, 1990).

Impaired Cognition or Awareness

General

Remove feeding tube during training if increased gag reflex is present.

Concentrate on solids rather than liquids, because liquids usually are less well tolerated.

Minimize extraneous stimuli while eating (eg, no television or radio, no verbal stimuli unless directed at task).

Have person concentrate on task of swallowing.

Have person sit up in chair with neck slightly flexed.

Instruct person to hold breath while swallowing.

Observe for swallowing and check mouth for emptying.

Avoid overloading mouth, because this decreases swallowing effectiveness.

Give solids and liquids separately.

Progress slowly. Limit conversation.

Provide several small meals to accommodate a short attention span.

Person with aphasia, or left hemispheric damage
Demonstrate expected behavior.
Reinforce behaviors with simple, one-word commands.
Person with apraxia, or right hemispheric damage
Divide task into smallest units possible.
Assist through each task with verbal commands.
Allow to complete one unit fully before giving next command.
Continue verbal assistance at each eating session until no longer needed.
Incorporate written checklist as a reminder to person.

Note: Person may have both left and right hemispheric damage and require a combination of the above techniques.

Reduce the Possibility of Aspiration.

Before beginning feeding, assess that the client is adequately alert and responsive, can control the mouth, has cough/gag reflex, and can swallow own saliva.
Have suction equipment available and functioning properly.
Position client correctly.
> Sit client upright (60 to 90 degrees) in chair or dangle his or her feet at side of bed if possible (prop pillows if necessary).
> Client should assume this position 10 to 15 min before eating and maintain it for 10 to 15 min after finishing eating.
> Flex client's head forward on the midline about 45 degrees to keep esophagus patent.

Keep client focused on task by giving directions until he or she has finished swallowing each mouthful.
> "Take a breath."
> "Move food to middle of tongue."
> "Raise tongue to roof of mouth."
> "Think about swallowing."
> "Swallow."
> "Cough to clear airway."
> Reinforce voluntary action.

Keep client's mouth fresh and clean. Mix 1 teaspoon baking soda in 1 qt water. Client should rinse and gargle every 2 h.
Avoid very hot fluids.
Start with small amounts and progress slowly as person learns to handle each step.
> Ice chips
> Eyedropper partly filled with water
> Whole eyedropper filled with water
> Juice in place of water
> ¼ teaspoon semisolid food
> ½ teaspoon semisolid food
> 1 teaspoon semisolid food
> Pureed or commercial baby foods
> One half cracker
> Soft diet
> Regular diet; chew food well

For client who has had a CVA, place food at back of tongue and on side of face he or she can control.
> Feed slowly, making certain client has swallowed the previous bite.
> Some clients do better with foods that hold together (eg, soft-boiled eggs, ground meat and gravy).

If the above strategies are unsuccessful, consultation with a physician may be necessary for alternative feeding techniques such as tube feedings or parenteral nutrition.

Initiate Health Teaching and Referrals, as Indicated.

Teach Exercises to Strengthen (Grober, 1984):

Lips and facial muscles
Alternate a tight frown with a broad smile with lips closed.
Puff out cheeks with air and hold.
Blow out of pursed lips.
Practice pronouncing *u, m, b, p, w.*
Suck hard on a popsicle.

Tongue
Lick a popsicle or lollipop.
Push tip of tongue against roof of mouth and floor.
Count teeth with tongue.
Pronounce *la, la, la; ta, ta, ta; d; n; z; s.*
Consult with speech pathologist.
Consult with dietitian for meal planning.
Explain to client and significant others rationale for treatment and how to proceed with it.

See *Impaired Oral Mucous Membranes.*
See *Imbalanced Nutrition: Less Than Body Requirements.*

Rationales

- Interventions vary depending on the causative or contributing factors.
- A speech pathologist has the expertise needed to perform the dysphagia evaluation.
- Alerting all staff can reduce the risk of aspiration.
- Impaired reflexes and fatigue increase the risk of aspiration.
- Upright position uses the force of gravity to aid downward motion of food and decreases the risk of aspiration.
- Straws and thin fluids hasten transit time and increase the risk of aspiration.
- Thicker fluids have a slower transit time and allow more time to trigger the swallow reflex.
- Poor tongue control with impaired oral sensation allows food into affected side.
- A confused client needs repetitive, simple instructions.
- Exercise can strengthen muscles to improve chewing and tongue movement of bolus to back of mouth to stimulate swallowing reflex (Porth, 2002).
- Avoid foods that do not form a bolus (eg, sticky foods, pureed foods, applesauce, dry foods) or do not stimulate the swallowing reflex (eg, thin liquids).

INEFFECTIVE INFANT FEEDING PATTERN

DEFINITION

Ineffective Infant Feeding Pattern: State in which an infant (birth to 9 months) demonstrates an impaired ability to suck or coordinate the suck/swallow response, resulting in inadequate oral nutrition for metabolic needs

DEFINING CHARACTERISTICS
Major (Must Be Present, One or More)

Inability to initiate or sustain an effective suck; inability to coordinate sucking, swallowing, and breathing
Actual metabolic needs in excess of oral intake with weight loss or need for enteral feeding supplement

Minor (May Be Present)

Inconsistent oral intake (volume, time interval, duration)
Oral motor developmental delay
Tachypnea with increased respiratory effort
Regurgitation or vomiting after feeding

RELATED FACTORS
Pathophysiologic
Related to increased caloric need secondary to:

Body temperature instability Growth needs

Tachypnea with increased Wound healing
  respiratory effort Major organ system disease or failure

Infection

Related to muscle weakness/hypotonia secondary to:

Malnutrition Congenital defects

Prematurity Major organ system disease or failure

Acute/chronic illness Neurologic impairment/delay

Lethargy

Treatment-Related
Related to hypermetabolic state and increased caloric needs secondary to:

Surgery Painful procedures

Related to muscle weakness and lethargy secondary to:

Medications

Muscle relaxants (antiseizure medications, paralyzing agents in past, sedatives, narcotics)

Sleep deprivation

Related to oral hypersensitivity
Related to previous prolonged NPO state

Situational (Personal, Environmental)
Related to inconsistent caretakers (feeders)
Related to lack of knowledge or commitment of caretaker (feeder) to special feeding needs or regimen
Related to presence of noxious facial#stimuli or absence of oral stimuli

---

(◯◯) **AUTHOR'S NOTE**

Ineffective Infant Feeding Pattern describes an infant with sucking or swallowing difficulties. This infant experiences inadequate oral nutrition for growth and development, which is exacerbated when caloric need increases, as with infection, illness, or stress. Nursing interventions assist infants and their caregivers with techniques to achieve nutritional intake needed for weight gain. In addition, the goal is for the intake eventually to be exclusively oral.

Infants with sucking or swallowing problems who have not lost weight need nursing interventions to prevent weight loss. *Ineffective Infant Feeding Pattern* is clinically useful for this situation.

(◯◯) **ERRORS IN DIAGNOSTIC STATEMENTS**

1. *Risk for Ineffective Infant Feeding Pattern related to inconsistent oral intake with or without weight loss*

   Inconsistent oral intake is a defining characteristic for *Ineffective Infant Feeding Pattern*, not *Risk for Ineffective Infant Feeding Pattern*. *Ineffective Infant Feeding Pattern* may not be useful as a risk nursing diagnosis because this actual diagnosis exists whenever an infant has sucking or suck/swallow response difficulties, whether mild or severe. The diagnosis would be appropriate as *Ineffective Infant Feeding Pattern related to (specify contributing factors, eg, lethargy) as evidenced by inconsistent oral intake.*

KEY CONCEPTS
Generic Considerations

- There are two goals for the infant with an ineffective feeding pattern:
  - The infant will receive adequate and appropriate calories (carbohydrate, protein, fat) for age with weight gain at a rate consistent with an individualized plan based on age and needs.
  - The infant will take all feedings orally.
- For an infant with an ineffective feeding pattern (with or without a demonstrable oral motor impairment), conversion from a catabolic state to an anabolic state with consistent weight gain from appropriate calories is a prerequisite for goal attainment.
- Identification of contributing physiologic factors assists in evaluating and adapting the feeding plan. For example, fever increases caloric needs; mechanical ventilation can decrease caloric needs; infants with impaired renal function or fluid retention can experience weight gain without meeting nutritional metabolic needs; dysfunction in major organ systems or infection affects feeding patterns adversely and increases caloric needs.
- Some infants with oral motor impairment or weakness feed adequately by mouth when their metabolic need for calories is normal. But in cases of increased caloric need (eg, congestive heart failure, infection, major organ system dysfunction, wound healing, malnutrition), they cannot take in adequate calories by increasing their volume intake sufficiently because of their ineffective feeding skills. Intervention with these infants is based on providing adequate calories, promoting oral feeding skills, and decreasing (if possible) caloric needs.
- Knowledge of normal infant feeding patterns is necessary to promote effective feeding patterns. For example, a quiet, awake state is ideal for feeding; non-nutritive sucking preceding nutritive sucking can enhance feeding behaviors; and there is a relation between sucking–swallowing– gastric emptying–bowel emptying during feeding. Over time, each infant develops an effective unique feeding pattern.
- For newborns, a lactation specialist should explore with mothers options to promote breast-feeding (either by using previously pumped breast milk or feeding directly from the breast). Many infants who initially have oral motor delays or lack of coordination of suck and swallow can successfully breast-feed with appropriate early intervention.
- High-calorie formulas (up to 32 cal/oz) or calorie-enhanced breast milk can be administered safely to most infants, provided the preparation is consistent with the child's age and needs. For example, concentrating formula to increase calories can increase the protein load disproportionately; therefore, additives (carbohydrate or fat) are often used to increase calories safely. The appropriate use of high-calorie formulas can reduce the target volume/day goal for an infant, making it easier to attain the goal of total oral feedings. Serum protein, albumin, and renal function need to be assessed periodically when high-calorie formulas are used.
- Enteral feedings often are required initially to ensure adequate caloric intake, weight gain, and anabolic state. Identifying a total plan for feeding from the beginning that includes both enteral and oral feeding (or oral stimulation if feeding is not possible) is instrumental in promoting the goal of total oral feeding. Infants who are exclusively enterally fed in the first months of life, with no effort to develop oral feeding skills, can become behaviorally disinterested in oral feeding and may remain enterally fed indefinitely.

Focus Assessment Criteria

Subjective and Objective Data
Assess for Defining Characteristics.

General
Current weight and height
Weight gain daily/weekly goal
Calorie/kg daily goal

Feeding history
Previous oral feeding pattern (volume, time interval, duration)
Previous enteral feeding pattern (continuous or bolus, volume, time interval, duration)
Gastrointestinal tolerance of feedings (oral, enteral, emesis, stool pattern)

Assess for Related Factors.

Presence/absence of noxious stimuli to face and mouth (including NG/NJ feedings, endotracheal intubation, oral or NP suction, nasal cannula oxygen)

Physiologic factors

Hyperthermia or hypothermia

Oral motor developmental delay

Infection

Gastroesophageal reflux

Congestive heart failure

Colic

Prematurity

Prolonged NPO state with or without enteral feedings

Neurologic dysfunction

Elevated body temperature

Increased respiratory rate and effort

Strength and coordination of non-nutritive sucking

Strength and coordination of nutritive sucking

Impaired sleep patterns

Irritability

Lethargy

For more information on Focus Assessment Criteria, visit http://connection.lww.com.

Goal

NOC Muscle Function, Nutritional Status, Swallowing Status

The infant will receive adequate nutrition for growth appropriate to age and need.

Indicators

- Parent demonstrates increasing skill.
- Parent identifies techniques that increase effective feeding.

General Interventions

 NIC Nonnutritive Swallowing, Swallowing Therapy, Aspiration Precautions, Bottle Feeding, Parent Education: Infant

Assess the Infant's Feeding Pattern and Nutritional Needs.

Assess volume, duration, and effort during feeding; respiratory rate and effort; signs of fatigue.

Assess past caloric intake, weight gain, trends in intake and output, renal function, fluid retention.

Identify physiologic risk factors.

Identify physiologic ability to feed:

Can infant stop breathing when sucking and swallowing?

What happens to oxygen level, heart rate, and respiratory rate when sucking/swallowing?

Does the infant need rest periods? How long? Are there problems in initiating sucking/swallowing again?

Assess nipple-feeding skills:

Does the infant actively suck with a bottle?

Does the infant initiate a swallow in coordination with suck?

Does the infant coordinate sucking, swallowing, and breathing?

Is the feeding completed in a reasonable time?

Collaborate with clinical dietitian to set calorie, volume, and weight gain goals.

Collaborate with occupational therapist to identify oral motor skills and planned intervention, if needed.

Collaborate with parent(s) about effective techniques used with this infant or other children, temperament, and responses to environmental stimuli.

Promote Adequate Caloric Intake and Anabolic State With Consistent Weight Gain Per Goals (Wong, 2003).

High-risk neonate: 120 to 150 cal/kg

Normal neonate: 100 to 120 cal/kg

Provide Specific Interventions to Promote Effective Oral Feeding (Wong, 2003).

Encourage non-nutritive sucking not in response to noxious stimuli.

Ensure nutritive sucking for an identified period (to prevent overtiring and unnecessary caloric expenditure).

Choose nipple according to individual needs and successes; assess effects of changes in formula/breast milk temperature and thickness.

Consider timing of feedings and competition in the environment.

Specific interventions for facilitating feeding are as follows:

   Position infant semi-upright, with trunk approximately 45 to 60 degrees (do not use a "head-back" position because it makes swallowing and sucking coordination more difficult).

   Stroke infant's lips, cheeks, and tongue before feeding.

   Use non-nutritive sucking before feeding to promote an awake and alert state.

   Use fingers to provide inward and forward support for infant's cheeks during feeding.

   Provide support for the base of the tongue (by placing fingers halfway between the chin and the throat, the nurse can provide a slight upward lift under the base of the tongue); *do not* provide strong upward pressure; steady support is most helpful; avoid moving fingers because it may interfere with the infant's own tongue movements.

Implement specific interventions for oral motor delays (position, equipment, jaw/mouth manipulation).

Control adverse environmental stimuli and noxious stimuli to face and mouth.

The following actions hinder, not help, feeding:

   Twisting or turning the nipple

   Moving the nipple up, down, around in the mouth

   Putting the nipple in and out of the mouth

   Putting pressure on the jaw or moving the infant's jaw up and down

   Placing the infant in a head-back position

Promote sleep and reduce unnecessary energy expenditure.

If needed, the plan for enteral feeding should include guidelines for increasing oral feeding and decreasing enteral feeding as the infant eats more effectively by mouth.

Promote consistency in approach to feeding.

As infant ages, revise and change feeding plan (including calorie and weight goals) to encourage normal feeding patterns for age when possible. For example, change type of formula, add solid foods, and so forth, when age appropriate.

Refer to *Risk for Aspiration* for interventions for feeding an infant with cleft lip and/or palate.

Establish Partnership with Parent(s) in All Stages of Plan.

Clearly identify and negotiate mutual goals for intervention.

Create a supportive environment for the parents to have the primary role in providing feeding-related intervention, when they are present. Whenever possible, nurses use the parents' approach when a parent is not present. In addition, when parents are not present, nurses can support the parents' role by imitating their approach to the infant, and communicate the infant's responses to the parents at a later time.

Negotiate and Identify Plans for Discharge With Parents and Incorporate Into the Overall Feeding Plan; Provide Ongoing Information About Special Needs and Assist Parents to Establish Needed Resources (Equipment, Nursing Care, Other Caretakers) When Needed.

Rationales

- Establishing parents as essential participants in the feeding plan gives them a role, place, and reason to be present so they can develop a closer relationship with the child.
- An infant who receives adequate calories will be more able physically to eat orally; if parents support and value the way calories are delivered and recognize milestones toward the goal, the child will be more likely to receive adequate calories after discharge. In addition, interactions will be more rewarding for both infant and parent during the intervention period.
- Calm, quiet, dim environments offer less distraction; attempt to decrease the negative effects of painful or very stimulating experiences shortly before or after feedings by timing them.

- Fever, infection, wound healing, malnutrition, and congestive heart failure increase caloric need beyond the goals listed for normal or high-risk newborns.
- For infants with demonstrable oral motor impairment, early intervention with an identified consistent approach to promoting oral feeding (equipment, body position, jaw and mouth manipulation, volume, time interval, duration) is essential for goal attainment.
- Identification of ineffective feeding patterns should be based on systematic assessment of the infant, in collaboration with other professionals. Behaviors that are cues to feeding dysfunction include ineffective coordination of suck/swallow/breathing, low energy or stamina, poor ability or inability to initiate sucking, disorganized rhythm in suck/swallow pattern, inadequate neurobehavioral control, and difficulty shifting back and forth from non-nutritive sucking and nutritive sucking.
- Close collaboration with a clinical dietitian to assess, plan, set, and evaluate calorie goals, weight gain goals, calorie distribution, and formula preparation is necessary for infants at risk.
- Close collaboration with a professional skilled in the assessment of infant oral motor skills (eg, occupational therapist, speech therapist) is necessary to assess, plan, intervene, and evaluate progress toward appropriate oral motor skills in infants with oral motor impairment.
- Close collaboration with parents from the beginning about identified needs, negotiation of priorities, and development of interventions is crucial to establishing effective feeding patterns in the infant and strengthening the infant–parent relationship.
- Environmental factors, including light, noise, inconsistent caretakers (feeders), and noxious stimuli, contribute significantly to ineffective feeding patterns.
- Efforts to promote sleep and reduce energy expenditure (primarily by controlling environmental stimuli) can substantially improve the infant's strength and stamina during feeding.
- Non-nutritive sucking (pacifier) should not be used exclusively to comfort infants during or after painful procedures or exposure to noxious stimuli. In addition, care and attention to reducing noxious stimuli to the face and mouth (type, frequency, intensity) should be initiated long before attempts to feed orally begin (Wong, 2003).

IMBALANCED NUTRITION: MORE THAN BODY REQUIREMENTS

DEFINITION

Imbalanced Nutrition: More Than Body Requirements: State in which a person experiences or is at risk of experiencing weight gain related to an intake in excess of metabolic requirements

DEFINING CHARACTERISTICS
Major (Must Be Present, One or More)

Overweight (weight 10% over ideal for height and frame), or
Obese (weight 20% or more over ideal for height and frame)
Triceps skinfold greater than 15 mm in men and 25 mm in women

Minor (May Be Present)

Reported undesirable eating patterns
Intake in excess of metabolic requirements
Sedentary activity patterns

RELATED FACTORS
Pathophysiologic

Related to altered satiety patterns secondary to (specify)
Related to decreased sense of taste and smell

Treatment-Related
Related to altered satiety secondary to:
Medications (corticosteroids, antihistamines, estrogens)
Radiation (decreased sense of taste and smell)

Situational (Personal, Environmental)
Related to risk to gain more than 25 to 30 lb when pregnant
Related to lack of basic nutrition knowledge

Maturational
Adult/Older Adult
Related to decreased activity patterns, decreased metabolic needs

---

⟲⟲ AUTHOR'S NOTE

Using this diagnosis to describe people who are overweight or obese places the focus of interventions on nutrition. Obesity is a complex condition with sociocultural, psychological, and metabolic implications. When the focus is primarily on limiting food intake, as with many weight-loss programs, the chance of permanent weight loss is slim. To be successful, a weight-loss program must focus on behavior modification and lifestyle changes.

The nursing diagnosis *Imbalanced Nutrition: More Than Body Requirements* does not describe this focus. Rather, *Ineffective Health Maintenance related to intake in excess of metabolic requirements* better reflects the need to increase metabolic requirements through exercise and decreased intake. For some people who desire weight loss, *Ineffective Coping related to increased eating in response to stressors* could be useful in addition to *Ineffective Health Maintenance*.

The nurse should be cautioned against applying a nursing diagnosis for an overweight or obese person who does not want to participate in a weight-loss program. Motivation for weight loss must come from within. Nurses can gently and expertly teach the hazards of obesity but must respect a person's right to choose, the right of self-determination.

Imbalanced Nutrition: More Than Body Requirements does have clinical usefulness in people at risk for or who have experienced weight gain because of pregnancy, taste or smell changes, or medications (eg, corticosteroids).

⟲⟲ ERRORS IN DIAGNOSTIC STATEMENTS

1. *Imbalanced Nutrition: More Than Body Requirements related to excessive calorie intake and sedentary lifestyle*

   As discussed in the Author's Note, *Imbalanced Nutrition* does not describe the complex nature of obesity or overweight conditions. Obesity is not a nutritional problem but a problem with coping and lifestyle choices. *Ineffective Health Maintenance* and *Ineffective Coping* are more useful diagnoses for the focus of nursing interventions.

2. *Imbalanced Nutrition: More Than Body Requirements related to reports of gaining 50 lb with first pregnancy*

   A report of gaining 50 lb during first pregnancy should prompt the nurse to initiate a focus assessment to explore other variables. For example, the nurse could ask, "What do you think contributed to your weight gain during your first pregnancy?" "What was the pattern of weight gain during each trimester?" The nurse also should discuss the difference between dieting during pregnancy versus a diet not excessive in simple carbohydrates or fat. After additional data collection, the following diagnosis possibly could prove valid: *Risk for Imbalanced Nutrition: More Than Body Requirements related to lack of knowledge of nutrition and exercise needed during pregnancy and history of 50-lb weight gain during previous pregnancy.*

KEY CONCEPTS
Generic Considerations
- Certain medications (eg, steroids, antihistamines, androgens, antipsychotics, hyperglycemics antidepressants) can cause weight gain (Abrams, 1997).
- Medications that can affect taste include amphetamines, clofibrate, lithium, griseofulvin, methicillin, phenindione, phenytoin, and probucol (Dudek, 2001).

Focus Assessment Criteria

See *Imbalanced Nutrition: Less Than Body Requirements.*

Goal

NOC Nutritional Status, Weight Control

The person will describe why he or she is at risk for weight gain.

Indicators
- Describe reasons for increased intake with taste or olfactory deficits.
- Discuss the nutritional needs during pregnancy.
- Discuss the effects of exercise on weight control.

General Interventions

NIC Nutritional Management, Weight Management, Teaching: Individual, Behavioral Modification, Exercise Promotion

Assess for Causative or Contributing Factors.
Decreased sense of smell or taste
Effects of medications
History of weight gain more than 30 lb during pregnancy

Explain the Effects of Decreased Sense of Taste and Smell on Perception of Satiety After Eating. Encourage Client to:
Evaluate intake by calorie counting, not feelings of satiety.
If not contraindicated, season foods heavily to satisfy decreased sense of taste. Experiment with seasonings (eg, dill, basil).
When taste is diminished, concentrate on food smells.

Explain the Rationale for Increased Appetite Owing to Use of Certain Medications (eg, Steroids, Androgens).

Discuss Nutritional Intake and Weight Gain During Pregnancy.
See Key Concepts under *Imbalanced Nutrition: Less Than Body Requirements.*

Assist Client to Decrease Unnecessary Calorie Intake and to Increase Metabolic Activity.

Increase Client's Awareness of Actions That Contribute to Excessive Food Intake.
Request that client write down all the food he or she ate in the past 24 h.
Instruct client to keep a diet diary for 1 week that specifies the following:
  What, when, where, and why eaten
  Whether he or she was doing anything else (eg, watching television, cooking) while eating
  Emotions before eating
  Others present (eg, snacking with spouse, children)
Review the diet diary to point out patterns (eg, time, place, emotions, foods, persons) that affect food intake.
Review high- and low-calorie food items.

Teach Behavior Modification Techniques to Decrease Caloric Intake.
Eat only at a specific spot at home (eg, the kitchen table).
Do not eat while performing other activities.
Drink an 8-oz glass of water immediately before a meal.

Decrease second helpings, fatty foods, sweets, and alcohol.
Prepare small portions, just enough for one meal, and discard leftovers.
Use small plates to make portions look bigger.
Never eat from another person's plate.
Eat slowly and chew food thoroughly.
Put down utensils and wait 15 s between bites.
Eat low-calorie snacks that must be chewed to satisfy oral needs (eg, carrots, celery, apples).

Instruct Client to Increase Activity Level to Burn Calories.
Use the stairs instead of elevators.
Park at the farthest point in parking lots and walk to buildings.
Plan a daily walking program with a progressive increase in distance and pace.

Note: Urge client to consult with a primary provider before beginning any exercise program.

Initiate Referral to a Community Weight Loss Program (eg, Weight Watchers), if Indicated.

Rationales

- The ability to lose weight while undergoing corticosteroid therapy likely depends on limiting sodium intake and maintaining reasonable caloric intake.
- Increased activity promotes weight loss.
- People with altered smell or taste may consume more food in an attempt to satisfy their taste (Dudek, 2001).

IMBALANCED NUTRITION: POTENTIAL FOR MORE THAN BODY REQUIREMENTS

DEFINITION
Imbalanced Nutrition: Potential for More Than Body Requirements: State in which a person is at risk of experiencing an intake of nutrients that exceeds metabolic needs

DEFINING CHARACTERISTICS
Reported or observed obesity in one or both parents
Rapid transition across growth percentiles in infants or children
Reported use of solid food as major food source before 5 months of age
Observed use of food as reward or comfort measure
Reported or observed higher baseline weight at beginning of each pregnancy
Dysfunctional eating patterns

> ⊗ **AUTHOR'S NOTE**
>
> This nursing diagnosis is similar to *Risk for Imbalanced Nutrition: More Than Body Requirements*. It describes a person who has a family history of obesity, is demonstrating a pattern of higher weight, or has had a history of excessive weight gain (eg, previous pregnancy). Until clinical research differentiates this diagnosis from other currently accepted diagnoses, use *Ineffective Health Maintenance (Actual or Risk for)* or *Risk for Imbalanced Nutrition: More Than Body Requirements* to direct teaching to assist clients and families to identify unhealthy dietary patterns.

IMPAIRED PARENTING

DEFINITION
Impaired Parenting: State in which one or more caregivers demonstrate a real or potential inability to provide a constructive environment that nurtures the growth and development of his/her/their child (children)

DEFINING CHARACTERISTICS
Major (Must Be Present, One or More)
Inappropriate and/or non-nurturing parenting behaviors
Lack of parental attachment behavior

Minor (May Be Present)
Frequent verbalization of dissatisfaction or disappointment with infant/child
Verbalization of frustration with role
Verbalization of perceived or actual inadequacy
Diminished or inappropriate visual, tactile, or auditory stimulation of infant
Evidence of abuse or neglect of child
Growth and development lag in infant/child

RELATED FACTORS
Individuals or families who may be at risk for developing or experiencing parenting difficulties

Parent(s)

Single	Addicted to drugs	Adolescent
Terminally ill	Abusive	Acutely disabled
Psychiatric disorder	Accident victim	Alcoholic

Child

Of unwanted pregnancy	With undesired	Terminally ill
With hyperactive	characteristics	Of undesired gender
characteristics	Mentally handicapped	Physically handicapped

Situational (Personal, Environmental)
Related to interruption of bonding process secondary to:

Illness (child, parent)	Relocation	Incarceration

Related to separation from nuclear family
Related to lack of knowledge
Related to inconsistent caregivers or techniques
Related to relationship problems (specify):

Marital discord	Stepparents	Divorce
Live-in partner	Separation	Relocation

Related to little external support and/or socially isolated family
Related to lack of available role model

Related to ineffective adaptation to stressors associated with

Illness

Substance abuse

Economic problems

Elder care

New baby

Maturational

Adolescent

Related to the conflict of meeting own needs over child's

Related to history of ineffective relationships with own parents

Related to parental history of abusive relationship with parents

Related to unrealistic expectations of child by parent

Related to unrealistic expectations of self by parent

Related to unrealistic expectations of parent by child

Related to unmet psychosocial needs of child by parent

⊕ AUTHOR'S NOTE

The family environment should provide the basic needs for a child's physical growth and development: stimulation of the child's emotional, social, and cognitive potential; consistent, stable reinforcement to learn impulse control; reality testing; freedom to share emotions; and moral stability (Pfeffer, 1981). This environment nurtures a child to develop, as Pfeffer (1981) states, "the ability to disengage from the family constellation as part of a process of lifelong individualization." It is the role of parents to provide such an environment. Most parenting difficulties stem from lack of knowledge or inability to manage stressors constructively. The ability to parent effectively is at high risk when the child or parent has a condition that increases stress on the family unit (eg, illness, financial problems).

Impaired Parenting describes a parent experiencing difficulty creating or continuing a nurturing environment for a child. *Parental Role Conflict* describes a parent or parents whose previously effective functioning is challenged by external factors. In certain situations, such as illness, divorce, or remarriage, role confusion and conflict are expected. If parents do not receive assistance in adapting their role to external factors, *Parental Role Conflict* can lead to *Impaired Parenting*.

⊕ ERRORS IN DIAGNOSTIC STATEMENTS

Impaired Parenting related to child abuse

Child abuse is a sign of family dysfunction. Usually, each situation involves an abusing adult and a knowing nonabusing adult; the treatment plan must include both. Thus, the diagnosis *Disabled Family Coping* would be more descriptive. *Impaired Parenting* is most appropriate when an external factor challenges the parents. External factors do not cause child abuse; rather, emotional disturbances and ineffective coping do.

KEY CONCEPTS
Generic Considerations

- In the past, because of living in extended families, young children observed and assisted frequently in the birth and care of infants. Today in the United States, because of social mobility and the more isolated nuclear family lifestyle, young men and women often approach parenthood with only a vague recollection of their own childhood, little knowledge of the birthing process, and limited, if any, experience in infant and child care.
- Parenting is a learned behavior; generally, people parent as they were parented.
- Successful adaptation to the stress of the new role of parenthood involves internal resources of adaptability and integration and positive external resources of social support, effective sources of advice and information, and a future orientation (Wong, 2003).
- Integration is an attempt by the couple to engage in some activities they enjoyed before parenthood and to continue to nurture the husband–wife relationship.

- Strong families appreciate and encourage all members. There is a commitment toward each member and the family unit. There is a clear set of family rules, values, and beliefs.
- Families acquire children through birth, adoption, and remarriage. Sometimes grandparents assume the parenting role for grandchildren because of the loss of parents, substance abuse, or a history of ineffective parenting (Clemen-Stone et al., 2002).
- Although many parents anticipate the birth of their child with pleasure, most are unprepared for the accompanying changes. After a child is born, parental self-concepts develop. For a woman, her role as parent often overshadows her role as wife and individual. For a man, parenthood strengthens his role as husband and worker. Parenting often becomes a dominant role for women and a secondary role for men (Clemen-Stone et al., 2002).
- Situations that contribute to abuse are often related to ineffective individual or family coping. (See *Disabled Family Coping,* as evidenced by child abuse.)
- Perceptions of a child's vulnerability affect parental behaviors. Early life-threatening events (eg, illness, accident, prematurity) may lead to disturbed parent–child relationships, which may result in problematic psychosocial development. This phenomenon, termed the "vulnerable child syndrome," has important implications for nurses working with parents during recovery from illness (Merenstein & Gardner, 1998).

Focus Assessment Criteria

Subjective and Objective Data

Assess for Defining Characteristics.

Parent does not:

Prenatal

Verbalize anticipation	Seek prenatal care	Select a name
Decide about feeding (breast, bottle)	Follow the regimen	Plan layette

Intrapartum

Participate in decisions and birthing process
Verbalize positive feelings
Attempt to see infant as soon as delivered
Respond positively (happy) or negatively (sad, apathetic, disappointed, angry, ambivalent)
Hold and talk to infant
Use baby's name
Talk to baby's father or mother

Postpartum

Verbalize positive feelings
Seek proximity by holding infant closely; touch and hug
Smile and gaze at infant; seek eye-to-eye contact
Seek family resemblance (eg, "has my eyes," "sleeps like his father")
Refer to infant by name and sex
Express interest in learning infant care
Perform nurturing behavior (ie, feeding, changing)

Parent–child relationship

Subjective

Parental level of satisfaction with child
Amount of play activities between mother and child, father and child
Amount of caretaking activities between mother and child, father and child
Provisions for child development (toys, verbal stimulation)
Reasons for discipline
Methods of discipline or punishment
Assess for at-risk factors in parent and child (see Related Factors).

Objective

Child's affect (animated, warm, apathetic, cold, withdrawn)
Touching/holding behavior
Injuries
    Explanation by child and parent
    Correlation of explanation to injury
    History of injuries (type, causes)

Observe

Parent–child interactions

Parental participation in caretaking activities

Parental comforting of child

Parental gathering and assimilation of information related to child and self

Family communication patterns

Visiting patterns and any changes

Assess for Related Factors.

Family structure/roles

Characteristics of family: age and sex of members, cultural and religious backgrounds, occupations of parents

Roles of parents within and outside family structure; identify potential for role conflicts

Demands of daily living (employment, financial)

Social support systems of parent(s)

> Location of most relatives
>
> Frequency of visits with relatives
>
> Length of time at present residence
>
> Patterns of parental socialization with friends and relatives
>
> Interrelationship between parents

Parenting knowledge/experience

Parents' recall of their relationship with their parents or caretakers and types of discipline and punishment used

Experiences with previous pregnancies

Knowledge of developmental needs and demands

Parental expectations of child

What effects has a child had on

Personal freedom	Marital relations	Leisure time
Career		

For more information on Focus Assessment Criteria, visit http://connection.lww.com.

Goal

NOC	Child Development (Specify), Family Coping, Family Environment: Internal, Family Functioning, Parent-Infant Attachment

The parent/primary caregiver will acknowledge a problem with parenting skills.

Indicators

- Provide a safe environment for child.
- Describe resource available for assistance with improvement of parenting skills.

General Interventions

NIC	Parenting Promotion, Developmental Enhancement, Anticipatory Guidance, Parent Education, Behavior Management

Encourage Parents to Express Frustrations Regarding Role Responsibilities, Parenting, or Both.

Convey empathy.

Reserve judgment.

Explore Parent's Expectations of Self, Partner, and Child.

Help foster realistic expectations.

Encourage discussion of feelings regarding unmet expectations.

Discuss strategies that might increase the likelihood of expectations being met (eg, discussing with partner, child; setting personal goals).

Educate Parents on Normal Growth and Development and Age-Related Expected Behaviors (Refer to *Delayed Growth and Development*).

Explore with Parents the Child's Problem Behavior.

Frequency, duration

Context (when, where, triggers)

Consequences (parental attention, discipline, inconsistencies in response)
Behavior desired by parents

Discuss Positive Parenting Techniques.

Convey to child that he or she is loved.
Catch child being good; use good eye contact.
Set aside "special time" when parent guarantees a time with child without interruptions.
Ignore minor transgressions by having no physical contact, eye contact, or discussion of the behavior.
Practice active listening. Describe what child is saying, reflect back the child's feelings, and do not judge.
Use "I" statements when disapproving of behavior. Focus on the act, not the child, as undesirable.

Explain the Discipline Technique of "Time Out," Which is a Method to Stop Misconduct, Convey Disapproval, and Provide Both Parent and Child Time to Regroup (Christophersen, 1992; Herman-Staab, 1994).

Outline the Procedure.

Place or bring the child to a chair in a quiet place with few distractions (not the child's room or an isolated place).
Instruct child to stay in the chair. Set timer for 1 min of quiet time for each year of age.
Start the timer when the child is quiet.
If the child misbehaves, cries, or gets off the chair, reset the timer.
When the timer goes off, tell the child it is okay to get up.

Explain to the Child.

This is not a game.
Practice it once when the child is behaving.
Explain rules and then ask the child questions to ensure understanding (if older than 3 years).

Remember:

Do not warn child before sending for time out. If time out is appropriate, use it; do not threaten.
If child laughs during time out, ignore it.
Be sure no television is on or can be seen.
Do not look at or talk to or about child during time out.
Do not act angry; remain calm.
Keep yourself busy; let the child see you and what he or she is missing.
Do not give up or give in.

If Additional Sources of Conflict Arise, Refer to the Specific Nursing Diagnosis (eg, *Caregiver Role Strain, Fatigue, Ineffective Sexuality Patterns*).

Take Opportunities to Role-Model Effective Parenting Skills; If Relevant, Share Some Frustrations You've Experienced with Your Child to Help Normalize the Frustrations.

Clarify the Strengths of the Parents or Family.

Role-Play Asking for Help or Disciplining a Child.

Provide General Parenting Guidelines.

Practice open, honest dialogues. Never threaten (eg, "If you are bad, I won't take you to the movies").
Do not lecture. Tell the child he or she was wrong and let it go. Spend time talking about pleasant experiences.
Compliment children on their achievements. Make each child feel important and special. Especially tell a child when he or she has been good; try not to focus on negative behavior.
Do not be afraid to hold and hug (boys as well as girls).
Set limits and keep them. Expect cooperation. Encourage the child to participate in activities that conform to your values. Do not be trapped by, "But everybody else can."
Let the child help you as much as possible.
Discipline the child by restricting activity. Sit a younger child in a chair for 3 to 5 min. If the child gets up, reprimand once and put him or her back. Continue until the child sits for the prescribed time. For an older child, restrict bicycle riding or movie going (pick an activity that is important to him or her).
Make sure the discipline corresponds to the unacceptable behavior. Allow children opportunities to make mistakes and to express anger verbally.

Stay in control. Try not to discipline when you are irritated.

When long explanations are needed, give them after the discipline.

Remember to examine what you are doing when you are not disciplining your child (eg, enjoying each other, loving each other).

Never reprimand a child in front of another person (child or adult). Take the child aside and talk.

Never decide you cannot control a child's destructive behavior. Examine your present response. Are you threatening? Do you follow through with the punishment or do you give in? Has the child learned you do not mean what you say?

Be a good model (the child learns from you whether you intend it or not). Never lie to a child even when you think it is better; the child must learn that you will not lie, no matter what.

Give each child a responsibility suited to his or her age, such as picking up toys, making beds, or drying dishes. Expect the child to complete the task.

Share your feelings with children (happiness, sadness, anger). Respect and be considerate of the child's feelings and of his or her right to be human.

Initiate Health Teaching and Referrals as Indicated.

Community resources—counseling, social service, parenting classes

Support groups—self-help, church

Rationales

- Parents need confidence, as well as skill, to be comfortable in their new role. The nurse is in the enviable position of being able to assist families by providing information on parenting.
- Observations of parent–child interactions should be guided by attention to the reciprocal aspect. Interactive "mismatch" may hamper parenting behaviors, evidenced when an infant is demanding and a parent lacks resilience or when the child's behavior is normal and the parents' expectations are unrealistic.
- Certain levels of stress interfere with the parent's ability to show patience and understanding (Wong, 2003).
- Parents who are encouraged to discuss their parenting expectations and who agree to support each other's decisions have less family tension (Wong, 2003).
- Behavioral modification techniques can be implemented effectively only when parents are consistent (Wong, 2003).
- Discipline should be implemented at the time of an undesired behavior to increase effectiveness (Wong, 2003).
- Reasoning is not appropriate with young children, who cannot "see the other side" (Wong, 2003).
- Ignoring problem behavior can minimize or eliminate it (Wong, 2003).
- The "time out" approach avoids many problems of other disciplinary approaches (eg, arguing, physical punishment, loss of control; Wong, 2003).
- Children learn to be responsible adults by having responsibilities as children.

RISK FOR IMPAIRED PARENT–INFANT ATTACHMENT

DEFINITION

Risk for Impaired Parent–Infant Attachment: State in which there is a risk for a disruption of a nurturing, protective, interactive process between a parent/primary caregiver and infant

RISK FACTORS

Refer to Related Factors.

RELATED FACTORS
Pathophysiologic
Related to interruption of attachment process secondary to:

Parental illness   Infant illness

Treatment-Related
Related to barriers to attachment secondary to:

Lack of privacy	Intensive care monitoring	Structured "visitation"
Equipment	Restricted visitors	

Situational (Personal, Environmental)
Related to unrealistic expectations (eg, of child, of self)
Related to unplanned pregnancy
Related to disappointment with infant (eg, gender, appearance)
Related to life event stressors associated with new baby and other responsibilities secondary to:

Health issues	Substance abuse	Mental illness
Relationship difficulties	Economic difficulties	

Related to lack of knowledge and/or available role model for parental role
Related to physical disabilities of parent (eg, blindness, paralysis, deafness)
Related to being emotionally unprepared due to premature delivery of infant

Maturational
Adolescent
Related to difficulty delaying own gratification for the gratification of the infant

---

(X) **AUTHOR'S NOTE**

This new diagnosis describes a parent or caregiver at risk for attachment difficulties with his or her infant. Barriers to attachment can be the environment, knowledge, anxiety, and health of parent or infant. This diagnosis is appropriate as a risk or high-risk diagnosis. If the nurse diagnoses a problem in infant–parent attachment, the diagnosis *Risk for Impaired Parenting related to difficulties in parent–child attachment* would be more useful so that the nurse could focus on improving attachment and preventing destructive parenting patterns.

(X) **ERRORS IN DIAGNOSTIC STATEMENTS**

Risk for Impaired Parent–Infant Attachment related to husband not being the biologic father
    The related factor is certainly a risk factor associated with attachment problems; however, this information is confidential and requires caution to protect its disclosure. If a family shares this information during an assessment or interaction, the nurse should record it exactly in quotes in the progress notes. The nurse can write the nursing diagnosis as *Risk for Impaired Parent–Infant Attachment related to possible rejection of infant by father.*

KEY CONCEPTS
Generic Considerations
- Attachment cannot be determined "by particular behaviors but from patterns of behavior" (Goulet et al., 1998, p. 1072). Parent–infant attachment is interactional. Attachment requires proximity, reciprocity, and commitment (Goulet et al., 1998).
- "Children who are cared for in a relatively consistent and predictable way develop confidence in their ability to have a positive influence on their environment and are more likely to express their need for love and security" (Goulet et al., 1998, p. 1078).
- The mother–child relationship begins before conception: planning, confirming, and accepting the pregnancy; feeling fetal movement, accepting the fetus as an individual; giving birth; hearing and seeing the baby; touching and holding the baby; and caring for the baby.

- Participation of the father in caregiving activities has increased in the United States. Fathers who choose a traditional role (allowing the mother to be totally responsible for caretaking activities) must be assessed in their sociocultural context.
- The attachment process is impeded when the parent(s) and child are separated because of the condition of the infant or a parent (Klaus & Kennell, 1976). Neonatal intensive care units (NICUs) should be structured to support the process of the parent–infant relationship (Brown, Pearl & Carrasco, 1991). Thurman (1991) describes a family-centered NICU as a setting adhering to the following parameters:
  - It provides services based on family-identified and family-perceived needs.
  - Fit between the family system and the service delivery system is adaptive.
  - It fosters family empowerment while providing a stable ongoing support system.
  - It recognizes the dynamism and complexity of the family system.
- Mercer and Ferketich (1990) studied parental attachment of 121 high-risk women, 61 partners of high-risk women, 182 low-risk women, and 117 partners of low-risk women. They found that the major predictor of parental attachment for all four groups was parental competence.
- Parents of a premature infant or an infant with malformations may feel a sense of failure, leading to low self-esteem and subsequent difficulties with attachment (Klaus & Kennell, 1976).
- Disorders of attachment may lead to nonorganic failure to thrive—failure of a child to grow without an organic cause.
- In multiple births, attachment takes longer because a mother can attach optimally only to one infant at a time. Mothers may feel differently about each infant of a multiple birth based on characteristics, such as health status or birth weight (Reeder et al., 1997).

Focus Assessment Criteria

Refer to *Impaired Parenting* for assessment of attachment behaviors.

Goal

NOC Refer to *Impared Parenting*

The parent will demonstrate increased attachment behaviors, such as holding infant close, smiling and talking to infant, and seeking eye contact with infant.

Indicators
- Be supported in his or her need to be involved in infant's care.
- Begin to verbalize positive feelings regarding infant.

General Interventions

NIC Refer to *Impared Parenting*

Assess Causative or Contributing Factors.

Maternal
Unwanted pregnancy
Prolonged or difficult labor and delivery
Postpartum pain or fatigue
Lack of positive support system (mother, spouse, friends)
Lack of positive role model (mother, relative, neighbor)
Inability to prepare emotionally for an unexpected delivery

Inadequate Coping Patterns (One or Both Parents)
Alcoholic
Drug addict
Marital difficulties (separation, divorce, violence)
Change in lifestyle related to new role
Adolescent parent
Career change (eg, working woman to mother)
Illness in family

Infant
Premature, defective, ill
Multiple birth

Eliminate or Reduce Contributing Factors, if Possible.

Illness, Pain, Fatigue

Establish with mother what infant care activities are feasible.

Provide mother with uninterrupted sleep periods of at least 2 h during the day and 4 h at night.

Provide relief for discomforts.

Episiotomy

Evaluate degree of pain.

Assess for hematomas and abscesses.

Provide with comfort measures (ice, warm compresses, analgesics*).

Hemorrhoids

Prevent and treat constipation.

Provide comfort measures (compresses with witch hazel, suppositories,* analgesics*).

Breast engorgement of nursing mother

Encourage woman to nurse as frequently as possible.

Apply warm compresses (shower) before nursing.

Apply cold compresses after nursing.

Try hand massage, hand expressing, or breast pump between nursing.

Offer mild analgesics.

See *Ineffective Breast-feeding*.

Breast engorgement of non-nursing mother

Offer analgesics as ordered.

Apply ice packs.

Encourage use of a good supporting brassiere that covers the entire breast.

Lack of Experience or Positive Mothering Role Model

Explore with mother her feelings and attitudes concerning her own mother.

Assist her to identify someone who is a positive mother; encourage her to seek that person's aid.

Outline the teaching program available during hospitalization.

Determine who will assist her at home initially.

Identify community programs and reference material that can increase her learning about child care after discharge (see References/Bibliography).

Lack of Positive Support System

Identify parent's support system; assess its strengths and weaknesses.

Assess the need for counseling.

Encourage parents to express feelings about the experience and about the future.

Be an active listener to the parents.

Observe the parents interacting with the infant.

Assess for resources (financial, emotional) already available to the family.

Be aware of resources available both within the hospital and in the community.

Counsel the parents on assessed needs.

Refer to hospital or community services.

Barriers to Practicing Cultural Beliefs That May Affect the Family Unit During Hospitalization

Support mother—infant—family beliefs.

Integrate culture and traditions into routine care.

Identify community resources.

Elimination of Institutional Barriers That Inhibit Individualizing of Care

Sensitize staff to practicing family-centered care.

Use families to review practice and policies.

Encourage cultural sensitization of staff.

Provide Opportunities for the Process of Mutual Interaction.

Promote Bonding in the Immediate Postdelivery Phase.

Encourage mother to hold infant after birth (may need a short recovery period).

Provide skin-to-skin contact if desired; keep room warm (72°F to 76°F) or use a heat panel over the infant.

Provide mother with an opportunity to breast-feed immediately after delivery, if desired.

---

*May require a primary care professional's order.

Delay administration of silver nitrate to allow for eye contact.

Give family as much time as they need together with minimum interruption from staff (the "sensitive period" lasts from 30 to 90 min).

Encourage father to hold infant.

Facilitate the Attachment Process During the Postpartum Phase.

Check mother regularly for signs of fatigue, especially if she had anesthesia.

Offer flexible rooming-in to the mother; establish with her the care she will assume initially and support her requests for assistance.

Discuss future involvement of the father in the infant's care (if desired, plan opportunities for father to participate in his child's care during visits).

Provide Support to the Parents.

Listen to the mother's replay of her labor and delivery experience.

Allow for verbalization of feelings.

Indicate acceptance of feelings.

Point out the infant's strengths and individual characteristics to the parents.

Demonstrate the infant's responses to the parents.

Have a system of follow-up after discharge, especially for families considered at risk (eg, phone call or a home visit by the community health nurse).

Be aware of resources and support groups available within the hospital and community; refer the family as needed.

Assess the Need to Support the Parents' Emerging Confidence in Child Care.

Observe the parents interacting with the infant.

Support each parent's strengths.

Assist each parent in those areas in which he or she is uncomfortable (role modeling).

Have handouts and audiovisual aids available for parents to view at odd hours.

Assess for level of knowledge in growth and development; provide information as needed.

Help parents understand infant's cues and temperament.

See References/Bibliography for recommended printed material on parenting and child care.

When Immediate Separation of the Child from the Parents is Necessary Because of Prematurity or Illness, Provide for Bonding/Attachment Experiences, as Possible.

Invite parents to see and touch infant as soon as possible.

Encourage parents to spend prolonged time with infant.

Support activities such as skin-to-skin holding, containment of infant with parental hands in the isolette, and basic caregiving activities.

If infant is transported to another facility and separated from mother:

  Have staff make frequent calls to mother.

  Encourage family to spend time in NICU; bring back verbal reports and pictures of infant.

  Explore family and community resources to provide means of rejoining mother and infant as soon as possible.

For Adoptive Parents:

Counsel adoptive parents that many emotions are normal on first interaction with their children.

Counsel adoptive parents about the possibility of postadoption depression.

Encourage adoptive parents to seek parenting classes before receiving their infant.

Initiate Referrals, as Needed.

Consult with community agencies for follow-up visits if indicated.

Refer parents to pertinent organizations (see References/Bibliography).

Rationales

- Research indicates that there is a "sensitive period" during the newborn's first minutes and hours of life during which the child is beautifully equipped to meet and interact with the parents. Close contact at this time and in the days to follow is most beneficial to the bonding process (Klaus & Kennell, 1976).
- The period from birth to 3 days is important for the father–child relationship.
- Seeing, touching, and caring for the infant promotes attachment (Klaus & Kennell, 1976).

- When caring for families of high-risk newborns, nurses can foster attachment and reduce anxiety by letting parents know through frequent communication that they are welcome partners in their child's care.
- In a longitudinal study of the interaction between 49 premature infants and their mothers, Zahr (1991) found that maternal rating of the infant's temperament and availability of support system were the most significant variables that correlated with a positive mother–infant interaction at 4 and 8 months postpartum.
- Parents are reluctant to form attachments to a sick infant because of their fear of loss. This reluctance creates tremendous guilt.
- Parents must be given the opportunity for grief work in the case of an ill or impaired infant before attachment can begin.
- The use of birthing rooms enhances the bonding process because of the decrease in interruptions.
- In a research study of 24 first-time adoptive mothers, Koepke, Anglin, Austin, and Delesalle (1991) found that adoptive mothers began developing affectional ties to their babies at much the same time and in as individual a way as birth mothers. Adoptive mothers may be as susceptible as birth mothers to periods of sadness and maternal depression.

PARENTAL ROLE CONFLICT

DEFINITION

Parental Role Conflict: State in which a parent or primary caregiver experiences or perceives a change in role in response to external factors (eg, illness, hospitalization, divorce, separation), pitch of child with special needs

DEFINING CHARACTERISTICS
Major (Must Be Present, One or More)

Parent(s) express(es) concerns about changes in parental role
Demonstrated disruption in care and/or caretaking routines

Minor (May Be Present)

Parent(s) express(es) concerns/feelings of inadequacy to provide for child's physical and emotional needs during hospitalization or in the home
Parent(s) express(es) concerns about effect of child's illness on other children
Parent(s) express(es) concerns about care of siblings at home
Parent(s) express(es) concern about perceived loss of control over decisions relating to the child

RELATED FACTORS
Situational (Personal, Environmental)

Related to separation from child secondary to:
Birth of a child with a congenital defect and/or chronic illness
Hospitalization of a child with an acute or chronic illness
Change in acuity, prognosis, or environment of care (eg, transfer to or from ICU)

Related to fear of involvement secondary to invasive or restrictive treatment modalities (eg, isolation, intubation)
Related to interruption of family life secondary to:
Home care of a child with special needs (eg, apnea monitoring, postural drainage, hyperalimentation)
Frequent visits to hospital
Addition of new family member (aging relative, newborn)

Related to change in ability to parent secondary to:

Illness of parent	Remarriage	Travel requirements
Dating	Work responsibilities	Death
Divorce		

⊚ AUTHOR'S NOTE

See *Impaired Parenting.*

KEY CONCEPTS
Generic Considerations

- Parental tasks for successful adaptation to children with special needs are:
  - Realistically perceive infant's condition and caregiver's needs
  - Adapt to hospital environment
  - Assume primary caregiver role
  - Progress to total responsibility for care at discharge
- Parenting behaviors are learned through role modeling, role rehearsal, and reference group interaction. External factors, both developmental (birth of a child) and situational (illness and/or hospitalization of a child), require the acquisition of new behaviors or the modification of existing behaviors. Difficulty in mastering the behaviors required for the role transition leads to role strain. Uncertainty about what behaviors the new role requires leads to lack of role clarity. Incompatibility between the new role expectations and already existing expectations leads to role conflict (Reeder et al., 1997).
- Parents experiencing their child's illness in an acute or a chronic situation face the challenge of role transition to continue effective parenting on either a temporary or permanent basis. The parent must give up the role of parenting a well child and acquire the role of parenting a sick child.
- Role conflicts can develop easily when a child receives home care from a parent or a combination of parents and health care professionals. Role diffusion caused by the intrusion of treatments, providers, or both into the home is a source of stress for the entire family and requires careful role negotiation (Hochstadt & Yost, 1989; Melnyk et al., 2001).
- Unhealthy outcomes resulting from maladaptation to family crisis are as follows:
  - Disturbed parent–child relationship
  - Failure to thrive
  - Vulnerable child syndrome
  - Disturbed marital and family equilibrium
  - Child abuse or neglect
- Clements, Copeland, and Loftus (1990) report in a study of 30 families with chronically ill children that parenting is more difficult at certain critical times: initial diagnosis; increase in physical symptoms; relocation of the child, such as rehospitalization; developmental changes for the child, such as entrance into school; and the physical or emotional absence of one parent (eg, illness, pregnancy).
- Caring for a child with special needs places high demands on parents' energy, time, and financial resources (Wong, 2003).
- Fathers of children with special needs are challenged with a situation that they could not protect their family from or control. They have more difficulty adjusting to a son with special needs because of the loss of future joint recreation.
- In a study of 45 mothers of acutely ill hospitalized children, Schepp (1991) found that predictability of events and anxiety influenced the mothers' coping effort. Mothers who knew what to expect were less anxious.
- Using the Family Adaptation Model, Gallo (1991) postulates the following strategies for preventive intervention useful to nurses working with families adapting to childhood chronic illness:
  - Focus on the family crisis.
  - Assist family to gain a conscious grasp of the crisis to enhance problem solving.
  - Offer medical information and education about the problem.
  - Help parents master physical care.
  - Help parents overcome doubts of adequacy.

- Assist family members with interpersonal communication.
- Assist family to develop social support and bridge access to community referral.
- Many parents of children with chronic illness experience stress as they watch their children struggle to achieve developmentally appropriate tasks (Melnyk, 2001).

Focus Assessment Criteria

Subjective Data
Assess Family System.

Family structures/roles
Characteristics of the family unit (as defined by the family): members, relationships, ages, sex, cultural and religious backgrounds
Living accommodations, distance from hospital, transportation
Roles and responses of each member
Employment, means of support
Change (relocation, addition, deletion, economic)
Family social support systems
Presence of extended family
Support from neighbors, church group, parent support group

Assess for Related Factors.

Recent changes, events

Change in household members	Occupation	Marital status

Child illness or hospitalization
History of illness

Acute or chronic	Resulting from an accident	Congenital or acquired

When diagnosis first made
Parent's knowledge / experiences
Experience with own hospitalizations
Experiences with previous hospitalizations of this child or other children
Involvement with medical/nursing care in the home
Communication style and level
Knowledge of child development and understanding of effect of hospitalization on child
Understanding of need for this hospitalization
Desired outcomes from current hospitalization
Involvement in case management for child, if any

Assess for Defining Characteristics.

Plans for dealing with this hospitalization
Visiting plans and travel arrangements
Desired involvement in care
Plans for acquiring information about child
Plans for self-care
Plans for payment of medical and hospital bills
Plans for meeting other roles while child is hospitalized (eg, working, care of home and other children)
Other emergent family situations that will affect time and energy needed for parenting the ill child
Concerns and fears

Objective Data
Assess for Defining Characteristics.

Parent–child interaction (observe each parent / caretaker)
Involvement in caretaking
Comforting of child
Discipline of child
Interpreting hospitalization/illness-related events to child
Support of child's development

For more information on Focus Assessment Criteria, visit http://connection.lww.com.

Goal

The parent and child will demonstrate control over decision making.

| NOC | Caregiver Adaptation to Child's Hospitalization, Caregiver Home Care Readiness, Coping, Family Environment: Internal Family Functioning, Parenting |

Indicators

- Express feelings regarding the situation.
- Identify sources of support.

General Interventions

| NIC | Caregiver Support, Role Enhancement, Anticipatory Guidance, Family Involvement Promotion, Counseling Referrals |

Assess the Present Situation.

Parents' and children's perceptions of and responses to situation

Parental understanding of the effects of the situation on children and their typical responses

Changes in parenting practices and daily routines (employment or change in child care arrangements)

Other related stressors (financial, job-related)

Level of conflict between parents

Social support for both parents

Encourage the Involvement of Fathers in Care.

Foster his strengths.

Provide an appropriate place for grieving.

Encourage the sharing of grief.

Include the father in care.

Help Parents With Limit Setting With the Child.

Explain the boundaries of acceptable behavior.

Expect the child to perform age-appropriate self-care activities when able.

Assign age-appropriate chores.

Expect the child to participate in his or her care.

Encourage Parents to Address Siblings' Responses.

Help parents talk to siblings about the child's condition.

Encourage parents to spend special time with siblings, acknowledge that negative feelings are normal, and allow some participation in the child's care.

Allow siblings a life outside of caregiving.

Assist Family to Increase Decision-Making Abilities (Dunst, Trivette & Deal, 1988a; Smith, 1999).

Emphasize parental responsibility for meeting needs and solving problems.

Emphasize building on parental strengths.

Provide active and reflective listening.

Offer normative help that is congruent with parental appraisal of need.

Promote acquisition of competencies.

Use parent–professional collaboration as the mechanism for meeting needs.

Allow locus of control to reside with the parent.

Accept and support parental decisions.

Support Siblings (Wong, 2003).

Listen to the siblings' feelings. Accept reasonable anger. Praise when they have been patient or very helpful.

Explain their sibling's condition and limit their responsibilities of care taking.

Encourage Expression of Feelings (Wong, 2003).

Describe behavior, eg, "You seem angry most of the time."

Provide understanding, eg, "Being angry is only natural."

Help focus on feelings: "Do you wonder why this has happened to your child (or siblings)?"

Facilitate Parent–Nurse Partnerships.

Attempt primary nursing (Wong, 2003) with consistent staff.

Acknowledge the parents' overall competence and their unique expertise.

Explain everything related to care.

Engage parents in team meetings.

Negotiate differences, be flexible, and offer respite.

Initiate Teaching and Referrals as Needed.

Ensure that the school nurse is aware of the situation.

Initiate referrals as needed, eg, in home care, day care, respite care.

Identify local and national disease—oriented organizations, eg, National Information Center for children and youth with disabilities (800-695-0285, www.Nichcy.org).

Refer to *Caregiver Role Strain* for additional interventions.

Rationales

- Nursing strategies based on an empowerment model are the most effective in helping parents resolve role conflict and move through role transition.
- These strategies can help parents acquire parenting behaviors that will be effective in caring for their ill child in the hospital or the home on a temporary or long-term basis.
- Respecting parents as the experts in caring for their child promotes more confidence and collaboration with caregivers (Baker, 1994).
- Adjustment to the condition may be accompanied by feelings of quilt, self-accusation, anger, and bitterness (Wong, 2003).
- Siblings need age—appropriate explanations of the situation. They need to be prepared for the physical changes and possible role changes (Wong, 2003).
- Siblings will experience being pushed to the background and a disruption in special events, eg, holidays, vacations. Their parents may be emotionally and physically unavailable for them (Wong, 2003).
- Siblings experience loneliness, increased responsibilities, fear, jealousy, guilt and resentment (Wong, 2003).

PARENTAL ROLE CONFLICT

○○ RELATED TO EFFECTS OF ILLNESS AND/OR HOSPITALIZATION OF A CHILD

Goals

NOC See *Parental Role Conflict*

The parent will demonstrate control over decision making concerning the child and collaborate with health professionals to make decisions about the care of the child.

Indicators

- Relate information about the child's health status and treatment plan.
- Participate in caring for the child in the home/hospital setting to the degree desired.

- Verbalize feelings about the child's illness and the hospitalization.
- Identify and use available support systems that allow parent time and energy to cope with ill child's needs.

General Interventions

NIC See *Parental Role Conflict*

Help Adapt Parenting Role During Illness (Newton, 2000).

Use role-supplementation strategies and role cues to help parents adapt parenting role to meet the child's needs.

Role model parenting behaviors appropriate to child's developmental stage and medical condition.

Instruct parents to continue limit-setting strategies and demonstrations of caring behaviors (eg, touching, hugging despite hospitalization and equipment).

Provide information to empower parents to adapt parenting role to the situation of hospitalization and/or chronic illness.

Provide information about hospital routines and policies, such as visiting hours, mealtimes, division routines, medical and nursing routines, rooming-in, and so forth.

Introduce self and other health care workers involved in the child's care; explain the role of each team member.

Explain procedures and tests to parents; help them interpret these activities to the child; discuss child's age-appropriate range of responses.

Assess usual parenting role or interpretation of real or perceived parental role.

Assess parental knowledge about child's normal growth and development, safety issues, and so forth; offer supplemental information as appropriate (see *Delayed Growth and Development*).

Teach parents special skills needed to provide for the physical and health care needs of the child.

Facilitate Communication About Condition and Treatment Plan.

Foster open communication between self and parents, allowing time for questions, frequent repetition of information; provide direct and honest answers.

Facilitate open communication between parents and other members of the health care team.

Approach parents with new information; do not make them assume the responsibility for seeking the information.

When parents cannot be with their child, facilitate communication through telephone calls; allow parents to call primary nurse or nurse caring for child.

Facilitate interdisciplinary communication so all members of the health care team have congruent and consistent information to share with the family.

Minimize waiting time for parents whenever possible.

Assess parental understanding of the child's illness.

Explain and interpret medical terminology to parents to foster their understanding of the child's condition.

> What is the reason for the child's hospitalization?
> What is going to be done to the child during hospitalization?
> Will the child be awake for the procedures?
> Will the child feel pain or discomfort?
> Where will it hurt?
> What will be done for the discomfort?
> Will the procedure change the child in any way? Is the change temporary or permanent?
> Who may visit the child? When?
> What may be brought to the hospital from home?
> How long will the child be in the hospital?
> Will there be any restrictions for the child at home?

Role-model interpreting events to child; help parents interpret to child and other family members.

Respect confidentiality of information; share information about child with parents only; instruct other family members to obtain information from parents.

Support Continued Decision Making.

Allow parents to help formulate plan of care for their child.

Use parents as a source of information about the child, his or her usual behaviors, reactions, and preferences.

Recognize parents as experts about their child.

Allow parents to be present during treatments and procedures if they desire.

Involve parents in decisions about the child's care, giving them choices whenever possible.

Allow Parents to Participate in Care of Their Child to the Degree They Desire.

Provide for 24-h rooming-in for at least one parent and extended visiting for other family members.

Collaborate and negotiate about parental tasks they wish to continue to do, tasks they wish others to assume, tasks they wish to share, and tasks they want to learn.

Assess parental ability to comfort the child; use comfort strategies that parents have indicated for the child.

Allow parents to have uninterrupted time with the child.

Provide consistent caregivers for the family through primary nursing; explain the primary nurse's role, responsibilities, and commitment to the parent and child.

Explore with parents their personal responsibilities (ie, work schedule, sibling care, household responsibilities, responsibilities to extended family); assist them to establish a schedule that allows sufficient caregiving time for the child or visiting time with the hospitalized child without frustration in meeting other role responsibilities (eg, if visiting is not possible until evening hours, delay child's bath time and allow parent to bathe child then).

Support Parental Ability to Normalize the Hospital/Home Environment.

Orient parents and child to hospital setting before admission, if possible, through prehospitalization or pretransfer tour.

Orient parents to the hospital environment: kitchen, playroom, tub room, treatment room, parents' lounge.

Instruct parents how to obtain needed supplies for self and child.

Orient parents to other hospital areas: cafeteria, chapel, gift shop, library, Ronald McDonald House.

Encourage parents to bring clothing and toys from home.

Allow parents to prepare home-cooked food or bring food from home if desired.

Encourage families to eat meals together.

Provide for sibling visitation. Help parents prepare siblings for the visit.

Construct daily routine around home routine as indicated by parent(s).

Provide privacy for parent–child interactions (eg, privacy for breast-feeding, family time for teens and parents).

Provide parents with comfortable visiting and sleeping accommodations at the bedside, if possible, for easy access to the child.

Attempt to minimize stressors of the unit/division (eg, noise level, overaccess by hospital personnel, unplanned patient care) that disrupt quiet/rest periods.

Provide age-appropriate developmental (school) and diversional activities for the child to provide for parenting opportunities.

Encourage parents to take the child on leaves from the hospital, including visits home, as possible.

Use an interdisciplinary approach to care planning to minimize the length of hospitalization.

Help Verbalize Feelings About the Child's Illness or Hospitalization.

Encourage parents to express feelings and concerns about the child's illness or hospitalization and about the perceived need for parental role change.

Provide opportunities for parents to be alone, not in the presence of the child, so they may feel free to express feelings, frustrations, and fears.

Indicate acceptance of parental feelings.

Identify staff members who have established a therapeutic relationship with the parents.

Provide opportunities for parents to talk about themselves, events related to hospitalization/illness, and real/perceived conflicts and changes in their role, whether temporary or permanent.

Provide for Physical and Emotional Needs of Parents.

Assess and facilitate parental ability to meet self-care needs (eg, rest, nutrition, activity, privacy).

Allow parents to determine the caregiving schedule to correspond with a schedule to meet their own needs.

Assess support systems: parent to parent, family, friends, minister, and so forth.

Assess, acknowledge, and facilitate family strengths.

Facilitate and reinforce effective coping strategies used by parents.

Continue to listen to parental concerns regarding the child and parental role.

Continue to assess additional stressors in the family setting.

Initiate Referrals, if Indicated.

Chaplain, social service, community agencies (respite care), parent self-help groups
Provide information to parents for self-referral.

Rationales

- Parents may be hampered in their acquisition of new effective parenting behaviors by feelings of anxiety, guilt, powerlessness, and diminished competence, and by lack of information or unfamiliarity with hospital surroundings, personnel, and systems.
- Nurses are in an exceptional position to assist parents to acquire effective parenting skills for their ill child by providing role cues and role supplementation strategies such as role rehearsal and role modeling.
- Support and enhancement of role transition for parents of an ill child can best be achieved in a setting that is guided by principles of family-centered care and by a nursing process that also is guided by this family-focused philosophy.
- Based on the promotion of self-determination, decision-making capabilities, and self-efficacy, the family-centered empowerment model requires three beliefs: (1) parents are competent in or have the capacity to become competent in the care of their child; (2) parents must be given opportunities to display competencies in the care of their children; and (3) parents need the necessary information to make informed decisions and to obtain resources to meet needs, and thus acquire control over their child's care (Dunst, Trivette, Davis & Wheeldreyer, 1988).
- Nursing interventions should be oriented to preparing the parent for potential stressors in an effort to decrease anxiety, thus enabling parents to spend more energy on normalizing the environment for their hospitalized children.
- Parental stress may be mediated by
  - Helping parents feel they are part of the team caring for their child and that they have all the information that is known about their child's condition
  - Allowing parents to comfort their child
  - Comforting the parent
  - Treating the child as an individual, such as using the child's name, approaching the child in an age-appropriate manner, and talking to the child even if the child is comatose
- Alexander and coworkers (1988) found significantly higher anxiety levels in non–rooming-in parents of hospitalized children, especially as the duration of hospitalization increased.
- Knafl and Dixon (1984) found that 24% of the fathers in their study reported role expansion as a result of the hospitalization of their child. Expansion included the responsibility for monitoring the child's care.
- Pass and Pass (1987) suggest providing parents with a list of questions they should be asking about their child's hospitalization.
- Alexander and coworkers (1988) found a significant level of high anxiety in non–rooming-in fathers with greater numbers of children at home, suggesting a shift in home responsibilities.

RISK FOR PERIPHERAL NEUROVASCULAR DYSFUNCTION

DEFINITION

Risk for Peripheral Neurovascular Dysfunction: State in which a person is at risk of experiencing a disruption in circulation, sensation, or motion of an extremity

RISK FACTORS

Presence of risk factor (see Related Factors)

RELATED FACTORS
Pathophysiologic
Related to increased volume of (specify extremity) secondary to:

Bleeding (eg, trauma, fractures)	Arterial obstruction	Coagulation disorder
	Venous obstruction/pooling	

Related to increased capillary filtration secondary to:

Allergic response (eg, insect bites)	Frostbite	Hypothermia
	Trauma	Nephrotic syndrome
Severe burns (thermal, electrical)	Venomous bites (eg, snake)	

Related to restrictive envelope secondary to:

Circumferential burns of extremities	Excessive pressure

Treatment-Related
Related to increased volume secondary to:

Infiltration of intravenous infusion	Excessive movement
	Dislocated prosthesis (knee, hip)
Nonpatent wound drainage system	

Related to increased capillary filtration secondary to:

Total knee replacement	Total hip replacement

Related to restrictive envelope secondary to:

Tourniquet	Antishock trousers	Blood pressure cuff
Circumferential dressings	Ace wraps	Excessive traction
Cast	Brace	Air splints
Premature or tight closure of fascial defects	Restraints	

⊗ **AUTHOR'S NOTE**

This diagnosis represents a situation that nurses can prevent by identifying who is at risk and implementing measures to reduce or eliminate causative or contributing factors. *Risk for Peripheral Neurovascular Dysfunction* can change to compartmental syndrome. *PC: Compartmental Syndrome* is inadequate tissue perfusion in a muscle, usually an arm or leg, caused by edema, which obstructs venous and arterial flow and compresses nerves. The nursing focus for compartmental syndrome is diagnosing its presence and notifying the physician. The medical interventions required to abate the problem are surgical, such as evacuation of hematoma, repair of damaged vessels, or fasciotomy. Refer to *PC: Compartmental Syndrome,* if indicated.

⊗ **ERRORS IN DIAGNOSTIC STATEMENTS**

1. *Risk for Peripheral Neurovascular Dysfunction related to thrombus in left leg*
   This situation does not represent a high-risk situation that a nurse can prevent; rather, it is a situation that requires nurse- and physician-prescribed interventions. The collaborative problem *PC: Thrombus Left Leg* would accurately describe this situation.
2. *Risk for Peripheral Neurovascular Dysfunction related to cast*
   Although the cast is an influencing factor, this diagnosis implies that the cast is the problem. The problem is edema formation. The cast aggravates the condition because, as edema increases, the cast provides external compression. The diagnosis should contain both risk factors as *High Risk for Peripheral Neurovascular Dysfunction related to the effects of edema formation secondary to fractured tibia and compression effect of cast.*

KEY CONCEPTS
Generic Considerations

- The most frequent cause of medical litigation in North America is failure to diagnose neurovascular compromise, which advances to compartmental syndrome (Bourne & Rorabeck, 1989).
- After trauma or surgery or with certain therapeutic measures, obstruction of blood flow can result from:
  Edema
  Embolus (air, fat, blood)
  Clot formation
  Blood vessel trauma
  Pressure on the vessels (cast, tourniquet, restraints, constrictive nature of burned tissue)
- Neurovascular compromise occurs when tissue pressure increases in a space-limiting envelope or site (Pellino et al., 1998).
- Factors that can limit a space are anatomic, such as skin or muscle fascia; pathophysiologic, such as circumferential burns of extremities; or treatment-related, such as casts (Fahey & Milzarek, 1999).
- Factors that can increase tissue pressure or envelope content are bleeding, edema formation, or anything that decreases arterial pressure or increases venous pressure (Pellino et al., 1998).
- Vascular insufficiency and nerve compression from edema can reduce blood supply to an extremity and result in peripheral nerve damage. Permanent damage can result within 4 to 12 h (Fahey & Milzarek, 1999).
- Compartments are areas of muscle, nerve, and blood vessels encased in inelastic boundaries of skin, muscle, fascia, and bone. The body has 46 compartments, with 38 found in the arms or legs (Kracun & Wooten, 1998).
- The effects of venous compression and the resulting signs and symptoms are outlined in Figure II.4.
- Lower leg pain that is worse after running may indicate chronic compartmental syndrome. The achy, pounding leg pain occurs after muscles warm up (usually 5 to 10 min) and can persist for several minutes to hours.

Focus Assessment Criteria

Subjective Data
Assess for Risk Factors.

History of
  Compromised peripheral   Peripheral thrombosis
    circulation
Tobacco use

Objective Data
Assess for Risk Factors.

Edema; postoperative
Pressure on vessels
  Cast   Restraints
Bleeding within compartment   Trauma
Venipuncture

For more information on Focus Assessment Criteria, visit http://connection.lww.com.

Goal

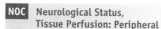
NOC Neurological Status,
Tissue Perfusion: Peripheral

The person will report changes in peripheral sensation or movement.

Indicators

- Palpable peripheral pulses
- Warm extremities
- Capillary refill less than 3 s

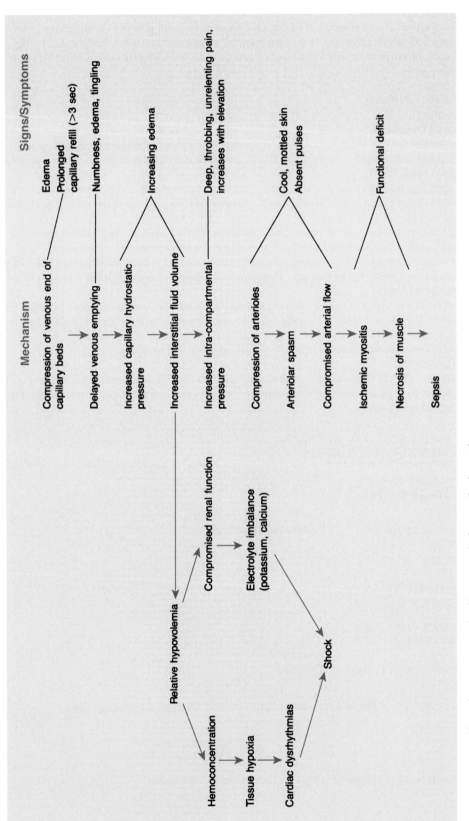

FIGURE II.4   The effects of venous compression (Ross, 1991; Peck, 1991; Porth, 2002).

General Interventions

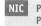 **NIC** Peripheral Sensation Management, Positioning, Embolus Precautions

Assess and Evaluate Neurovascular Status at Least Every Hour for First 24 h; Compare to Unaffected Limb, if Possible.

Skin

Temperature (cool, warm)

Color (pale, dependent, rubor, flushed, cyanotic)

Bilateral Pulses (Radial, Posterior Tibial, Dorsalis Pedis)

Rate, rhythm

Volume

0 = Absent, nonpalpable	Present but diminished
Thready, weak, fades in and out	Normal, easily palpable
	Aneurysmal

Edema (Location, Pitting); Measure Circumference at Widest Diameter of Leg or Arm

Capillary Refill (Normal Less than 3 s)

For Injured Arms (Pellino et al., 1998; Ross, 1991):

Assess for Movement Ability.

Hyperextension of thumbs, wrist, and four fingers

Abduction (fanning out) of all fingers

Touch thumb to small finger

Assess Sensation with Pressure from a Sharp Point.

Web space between thumb and index finger

Distal fat pad of small finger

Distal surface of the index finger

For Injured Legs (Pellino et al., 1998; Ross, 1991):

Assess for Movement Ability.

Dorsiflex (upward movement) ankle and extend toes at metatarsal-phalangeal joints.

Plantarflex (downward movement) ankle and toes.

Assess Sensation with Pressure from a Sharp Point.

Web space between great toe and second toe

Medial and lateral surfaces of the sole (upper third)

Instruct Client to Report Unusual, New, or Different Sensations, Such as Tingling, Numbness, Decreased Ability to Move Toes or Fingers.

Reduce Edema or Its Effects on Function.

Remove jewelry from affected limb.

Elevate limbs unless contraindicated.

Advise client to move fingers or toes of affected limb two to four times per hour.

Monitor drainage (characteristics, amount) from wounds or incision.

Maintain patency of the wound drainage system.

Apply ice bags around injured site if not contraindicated. Place cloth between ice bag and skin.

Notify the Physician if the Following Occur:

Change in sensation

Change in movement ability

Pale, mottled, or cyanotic skin

Capillary refill slower than 3 s

Diminished or absent pulse

Increasing pain or pain not controlled by medication

Pain with passive stretching of muscle

Pain increased with elevation

If Above Signs or Symptoms Occur, Discontinue Elevation and Ice Application.

Promote circulation in affected limb.

Ensure optimal hydration to maximize circulation.

Monitor traction apparatus and splints for pressure on vessels or nerves.

If using wrist or ankle restraints, monitor for pressure on vessels or nerves. Remove at least every hour and perform range of motion.

Encourage active range of motion of unaffected body parts and ambulation, if permissible.

After Hip or Knee Joint Replacement:

Maintain Correct Positioning to Prevent Prosthetic Dislocation.

Hip: keep in abduction at 45 degrees or less.

Knee: slightly elevate from hip; do not flex or hyperextend.

Keep the Affected Joint in Neutral Position with Rolls, Pillows, or Specified Devices.

Initiate Health Teaching, as Indicated.

Teach Client and Family to Watch for and Report the Following Symptoms:

Severe pain

Numbness or tingling

Swelling

Skin discoloration

Paralysis or reduced movement

Cool, white toes or fingertips

Foul odor, warm spots, soft areas, or cracks in the cast

Emphasize the Importance of Follow-Up Evaluations.

Rationales

- Swelling that cannot be controlled causes increased tissue pressure and occlusion of the blood supply to nerve and muscle tissue, resulting in anoxia. This complication is compartmental syndrome.
- Dehydration or hypovolemia decreases circulating volume and tissue perfusion, thus increasing neurovascular compromise.
- Neurovascular compromise often begins as minor sensations; early detection can enable prompt intervention to prevent serious complications (Pellino et al., 1998).
- A sudden change in temperature, drop in pressure, or no pulse indicates graft thrombosis. Changes in sensation or motor function can indicate compartmental syndrome (Kracun & Wooten, 1998).
- After a period of ischemia comes a period of increased capillary wall permeability. Restoration of arterial flow causes plasma and extracellular fluid to flow into the tissues, producing massive swelling in calf muscles. Pain and muscle tension result as the fascia prevent tissues from extending outward, and inward pressure obliterates the circulation. The nerves become anoxic, causing paresthesias and motor deficits (Kracun & Wooten, 1998).
- Edema at the fracture site can compromise muscular vascular perfusion. Stretching of the damaged muscle causes pain. Sensory deficit is an early sign of nerve ischemia; the specific area of change indicates the affected compartment (Pellino et al., 1998).
- Damaged tissue and muscles may not provide adequate support of the hip joint, resulting in displacement.
- Edema impairs circulation; however, if the extremity is elevated above heart level, this may decrease arterial blood flow. In a partial-thickness burn, edema may diminish blood flow.
- Postoperative edema is expected in the newly vascularized limb. Careful assessment alerts the nurse to edema severe enough to cause compartmental syndrome. Treatment must be initiated within 8 h to preserve function of the extremity.

POST-TRAUMA SYNDROME

DEFINITION

Post-Trauma Syndrome: State in which a person experiences a sustained painful response to one or more overwhelming traumatic events that have not been assimilated

DEFINING CHARACTERISTICS
Major (Must Be Present, One or More)

Reexperience of the traumatic event, which may be identified in cognitive, affective, and/or sensory motor activities for more than 1 month such as:

Flashbacks, intrusive thoughts
Repetitive dreams/nightmares
Excessive verbalization of the traumatic event(s)
Survival guilt or guilt about behavior required for survival
Painful emotion, self-blame, shame, or sadness
Vulnerability or helplessness, anxiety, or panic
Fear of repetition, death, or loss of bodily control
Angry outbursts/rage, startle reaction
Hyperalertness or hypervigilance
Persistent avoidance of stimuli

Minor (May Be Present)

Psychic/Emotional Numbness

Impaired interpretation of reality, impaired memory
Confusion, dissociation, or amnesia
Vagueness about the traumatic event(s)
Narrowed attention or inattention/daze
Feeling of numbness, constricted affect
Feeling detached/alienated
Reduced interest in significant activities

Altered Lifestyle

Submissiveness, passiveness, or dependency
Self-destructiveness (eg, alcohol/drug abuse, suicide attempts, reckless driving, illegal activities)
Thrill-seeking activities
Difficulty with interpersonal relationships
Development of phobia regarding trauma
Avoidance of situations or activities that arouse recollection of the trauma
Social isolation/withdrawal, negative self-concept
Sleep disturbances, emotional disturbances
Irritability, poor impulse control, or explosiveness
Loss of faith in people or the world, feeling of meaninglessness in life
Chronic anxiety or chronic depression
Somatic preoccupation/multiple physiologic symptoms

RELATED FACTORS
Situational (Personal, Environmental)
Related to traumatic events of natural origin, including

Floods	Earthquakes	Volcanic eruptions
Storms	Avalanches	Epidemics
Other natural disasters		

Related to traumatic events of human origin, such as

Concentration camp confinement	Wars	Airplane crashes
Torture	Serious car accidents	Assault
Large fires	Rape	Bombing
	Witnessing violence	

Related to industrial disasters (nuclear, chemical, or other life-threatening accidents)

◉◉ AUTHOR'S NOTE

Post-Trauma Syndrome represents a group of emotional responses to a traumatic event of either natural origin (eg, floods, volcanic eruptions, earthquakes) or human origin (eg, war, rape, torture). The emotional responses (eg, guilt, shame, fear, anger) interfere with interpersonal relationships and can precipitate self-destructive behavior (eg, substance abuse, suicide). The nurse may find it necessary to use additional diagnoses when specific interventions are indicated (eg, *Compromised Family Coping, Risk for Self-Harm*).

The diagnosis *Rape Trauma Syndrome* was described in 1975 as encompassing an acute phase of disorganization and a long-term phase of reorganization. Based on the most recent definition of syndrome nursing diagnoses as a cluster of associated nursing diagnoses, this diagnosis does not represent a syndrome and would be more accurately labeled *Rape Trauma Response*. The inclusion of causative or contributing factors with this category is unnecessary, because the etiology is always rape. Thus, the nurse omits the second part of the diagnostic statement; however, he or she can add the client's report of the rape to the statement. For example, *Rape Trauma Syndrome as evidenced by the report of a sexual assault and sodomy on June 22 and multiple facial bruises* (refer to ER record for description).

◉◉ ERRORS IN DIAGNOSTIC STATEMENTS

Post-Trauma Response related to expressions of survival guilt and recurring nightmares of auto accident

Survival guilt and nightmares of a traumatic event represent possible manifestations of post-trauma response, not related factors. The nurse should restate the diagnosis as *Post-Trauma Response related to auto accident, as evidenced by recurring nightmares and expressions of survival guilt.*

KEY CONCEPTS
Generic Considerations

- Trauma is defined in terms of the subjective experience of an event that cannot be dealt with or assimilated in the usual way. Traumatic situations differ from ordinary experiences in that they involve realistic danger of physiologic or psychological destruction, which could mobilize fear of death. A traumatic event may affect only one person or many people at once. It may be of human origin (eg, rape, wars) or natural origin (eg, avalanches, volcanoes).
- In general, traumatic events of natural origin are less severe or long-lasting than are those of human origin. Those of human origin are often perceived as resulting from indifference, negligence, or malice.

- Horowitz (1986a, 1986b) conceptualized these phenomena and postulated a phasic tendency in human responses to traumatic events.
  - The initial response to trauma is to survive and to function in the immediate life-threatening situation by using all resources.
  - The powerful coping method of "numbing" reduces psychological and emotional effects.
  - In an attempt to master the traumatic experience, intrusive recollection or reenactment of the trauma erupts into conscious awareness.
  - There is a pattern of oscillation between "numbing" and intrusive reactions peculiar to each person.
  - Gradually, the person works through the trauma by using a broader perception and rationale for the event and the aftermath.
  - Finally, the person assimilates such an experience into a meaningful whole congruent with basic beliefs and values.
- Severity of trauma is associated with intensity, duration, and frequency. It involves a complex interaction of environmental conditions and the person's subjective experiences, such as degree of warning, threat to life, exposure to the grotesque, bereavement, displacement, and moral conflict about the role of the survivor.
- Individual characteristics, such as early childhood experience, developmental phase, and character strength, may affect the outcome of responses to trauma.
  - The current trauma may reactivate unresolved childhood conflicts.
  - Age can be a crucial factor, because trauma can interrupt a stage of human development.
  - Individual coping resources are important when a person confronts a traumatic situation, and they influence the effectiveness of adaptation.

Pediatric Considerations

- A child's response to trauma depends on the nature and the extent of the trauma, developmental age, and response of significant others (Wong, 2003).
- Children can experience post-traumatic stress symptoms after a friend or acquaintance is killed (Pfefferbaum et al., 2000).

Focus Assessment Criteria

Subjective and Objective Data

Assess for Defining Characteristics.

History of the trauma*
Exposure to a very stressful, disturbing situation (see *Related Factors*)
List all traumas, including dates and duration.

The person's responses to the traumatic event(s)
Thoughts, feelings, or actions that he or she believes have been different since the traumatic experience, to assess signs and symptoms of reexperiencing or numbing responses
Changes in general lifestyle or pattern since the traumatic event(s), to assess any readjustment difficulties

Observe or consult with family members or other appropriate people, as possible.
Excessive verbalization of the traumatic events
Preoccupation with trauma reminders, such as sorting through pictures or other trauma-related objects
Use of denial, distortion, minimization, exaggeration, disavowal, fantasy, or avoidance
Evidence of indifference or dissociation to stimuli (questions, noise, activities around him or her)
Sudden or significant behavioral/personality changes since the traumatic event

---

*The purpose of securing a history is to substantiate evidence of trauma and not to explore details of trauma. This should be done in an appropriate therapy session.

Goals

The person will assimilate the experience into a meaningful whole and go on to pursue his or her life, as evidenced by goal setting.

Indicators

- Report a lessening of reexperiencing the trauma or numbing symptoms.
- Acknowledge the traumatic event and begin to work with the trauma by talking about the experience and expressing feelings such as fear, anger, and guilt.
- Identify and make connection with support persons/resources.

General Interventions

Determine if the Person has Experienced a Traumatic Event.

During the interview, secure a quiet room where there will be no interruptions but easy access to other staff in case of management problems.

Be aware that talking about a traumatic experience may cause significant discomfort to the person.

If the person becomes too anxious, discontinue the assessment and help the person to regain control of the distress or provide other appropriate interventions.

Evaluate the Severity of the Responses and Effects on Current Functioning.

Assist Client to Decrease Extremes of Reexperiencing or Numbing Symptoms.

Provide a safe, therapeutic environment where the person can regain control.

Reassure the person that others who have experienced such traumatic events often experienced these feelings/symptoms.

Stay with the person and offer support during an episode of high anxiety (see *Anxiety* for additional information).

Assist client to control impulsive acting-out behavior by setting limits, promoting ventilation, and redirecting excess energy into physical exercise or activity (eg, walking, jogging). (See *Risk for Self-Harm* and *Risk for Violence* for additional information.)

Recognize that psychic/emotional numbness provides a cushion.

Provide techniques to reduce anxiety, eg, progressive relaxation, deep breathing.

Assist Client to Acknowledge and Begin to Work Through the Trauma by Discussing the Experience and Expressing Feelings Such as Fear, Anger, and Guilt.

Provide a safe, structured setting.

Explain that talking about the traumatic event may intensify the symptoms (eg, nightmares, flashbacks, painful emotions, numbness).

Assist person to proceed at an individual pace.

Listen attentively with empathy and an unhurried manner.

Assist client to talk about trauma, to understand what has occurred, and to validate the reality of personal involvement.

Help client to express feelings associated with the traumatic event and to become aware of the link between the experience and anger, depression, or anxiety.

Assist client to differentiate reality from fantasy and to look back and talk about the areas of his or her life that have changed.

Recognize and support cultural and religious values in dealing with the traumatic event.

Assist Client to Identify and Make Connections with Support People and Resources.

Help client to identify his or her strength and resources.

Explore available support system.

Assist client to make connections with support and resources according to his or her needs.

Assist client to resume old activities and begin some new ones.

Assist Family/Significant Others.

Assist them to understand what is happening to the victim.

Encourage expression of their feelings.

Provide counseling sessions or link them with appropriate community resources, as necessary.

Provide Nursing Care Appropriate to Each Person's Traumatic Experience and Needs (see *Rape Trauma Syndrome* for Additional Information, if Relevant).

Provide or Arrange Follow-Up Treatment in Which Person can Continue to Work Through the Trauma and to Integrate the Experience into a New Self-Concept.

Rationales

- Short-term crisis intervention should begin as soon as victims are identified.
- Careful recording of psychological responses assists in documenting progress in therapy, planning treatment, or identifying those at greatest risk. Behavior can differ among individuals. Feelings can be fast and furious or slow, trancelike, mixed, or clear (Charron, 1998).
- Attempts to decrease extreme symptoms can help person regain some control (Charron, 1998).
- Interventions that focus on helping the person cope can reduce powerlessness (Charron, 1998).
- Assisting the person to recall and clarify the event puts that event in perspective and helps prevent repression.
- Lack of support or additional stresses may interrupt the process of working through the trauma.
- Victims need to work through trauma at their own pace.
- Unhurried, confident actions and eye contact help calm the victim and provide reassurance that he or she is alive and safe.
- Providing immediate and ongoing empathy and support prepares victims for referral to more in-depth psychological counseling. Main issues in the acute stage are being in control, fear of being left alone, and having someone to listen.
- Follow-up counseling and long-term support therapy in the community should be arranged.
- Anxiety management offers one way to maintain some control over their bodies (Boyd, 2005).

Pediatric Interventions

Assist children to understand and to integrate the experience in accordance with their developmental stage.

Assist them to describe the experience and to express feelings (eg, fear, guilt, rage) in safe, supportive places, such as play therapy sessions.

Provide accurate information and explanations in terms child can understand.

Evaluate risk for suicide, especially in male adolescents (see *Risk for Suicide*).

Provide family counseling to promote understanding of the child's needs.

Rationales

- Nursing assessment should include the child's symbolic or nonverbal language communication (Wong, 2003).
- Play therapy, such as writing, drawing, telling stories, or playing with dolls, should be offered so children can act out, express feelings, and communicate their experience safely.

RISK FOR POST-TRAUMA SYNDROME

DEFINITION

Risk for Post-Trauma Syndrome: State in which a person experiences a sustained painful response to one or more overwhelming traumatic events that have not been assimilated

RISK FACTORS

Refer to Related Factors in *Post-Trauma Syndrome.*

Goal

The person will continue to function appropriately after the traumatic event.

Indicators

- Identify signs or symptoms that necessitate professional consultation.
- Express feelings regarding traumatic event.

General Interventions

Refer to *Post-Trauma Syndrome.*

RAPE TRAUMA SYNDROME

DEFINITION

Rape Trauma Syndrome: State in which a person experiences a forced, violent sexual assault (vaginal or anal penetration) against his or her will and without his or her consent. The trauma syndrome that develops from this attack or attempted attack includes an acute phase of disorganization of the victim and family's lifestyle and a long-term process of reorganization of lifestyle (Holmstrom & Burgess, 1975).

DEFINING CHARACTERISTICS
Major (Must Be Present)

Reports or evidence of sexual assault

Minor (May Be Present)

If the victim is a child, parents may experience similar responses.

Acute Phase
Somatic responses
Gastrointestinal irritability (nausea, vomiting, anorexia)

Genitourinary discomfort (pain, pruritus)
Skeletal muscle tension (spasms, pain)
Psychological responses
Denial
Emotional shock
Anger
Fear—of being alone or that the rapist will return (a child victim fears punishment, repercussions,
   abandonment, rejection)
Guilt
Panic on seeing assailant or scene of the attack
Sexual responses
Mistrust of men (if victim is a woman)
Change in sexual behavior

Long-Term Phase
Any response of the acute phase may continue if resolution does not occur.

Psychological responses

| Nightmares or sleep disturbances | Depression | Suicidal ideation |
| | Phobias | Anxiety |

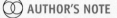 **AUTHOR'S NOTE**

See *Post-Trauma Syndrome.*

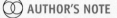 **ERRORS IN DIAGNOSTIC STATEMENTS**

See *Post-Trauma Syndrome.*

KEY CONCEPTS
Generic Considerations
- Estimates are that more than 100,000 cases of rape are reported in the United States yearly
  (Statistical Abstract of the United States, 1996). One of every six women will be raped during her
  lifetime (Petter & Whitehill, 1998).
- Rape is a crime using sexual means to humiliate or degrade the victim. Someone commits sexual
  acts against a nonconsenting person. Rape violates the victim's right of privacy, sense of security,
  safety, and well-being.
- Rape is a crime that health care providers must report. Estimates are that only 4 of 10 rapes are
  reported (Smith-DiJulio, 1998; Symes, 2000).
- Our past culture (and some cultures today) supported that (Heinrich, 1987)
  - A woman's rightful place in society is to fulfill man's destiny.
  - Women are property of men and responsible for retaining value (therefore, women who allow
    themselves to get raped are bad).
  - Women are important to men, as symbols of their power and status and as prizes of prowess.
- "Fraternity members have more rape-supportive attitudes and are more coercive than other men"
  (Foubert, 2000, p. 158). Men who report a higher likelihood of raping also have higher levels of
  anger, aggression, and a desire to hurt women (Foubert, 2000).
- Some myths about rape include the following (Heinrich, 1987):
  - The rapist is a sexually unsatisfied man who cannot control his urges.
  - Rape is a one-time incident, representing a momentary lapse in judgment.
  - Rapists are strangers.
  - The victim provokes rape.
  - Only promiscuous women get raped.

- Rapes happen to women out alone at night. If a woman stays home, she will be safe.
- Women cannot be raped against their will—they can avoid rape by resistance.
- Most rapes involve black men and white women.
- Women respect men for overpowering them; they may even enjoy the rape.
- Rapists are mentally ill or retarded and, therefore, not responsible for their acts.
- Victims, families, society, and caregivers who subscribe to these myths may not view themselves as victims or recognize the criminality of rape, may not seek help, or may be denied supportive interventions (Heinrich, 1987).
- Rapists can be divided into three broad categories (Whitehill, 1998):
  - Power rapists (55% of sexual assaults). They attack persons near their age and use intimidation and minimal violence to control. The attack is premeditated.
  - Anger rapists (40% of sexual assaults). They target the very young or elderly. They use extreme force and restraints, resulting in physical injury.
  - Sadistic rapists (5% of sexual assaults). The attack is premeditated. They derive erotic satisfaction from torturing.
- Burgess (1995) categorized three main types of rape:
  - *Rape:* Sex without consent in which the assailant uses confidence, coercion, or violence.
  - *Accessory to sex:* Survivors collaborate in a secondary manner with the sexual activity, and consent or lack of consent is from cognitive or personality development. (Mentally retarded people and children are susceptible.)
  - *Sex-stress situation:* Sex is agreed on initially, but then one party decides not to go through with it, usually because of exploitation, but this change of heart is not heeded.
- Rape occurs in all age groups, races, and educational and economic groups (Smith-DiJulio, 1998).
- Male rape victims (including homosexuals) are unlikely to report the rape but are most likely to experience symptoms of rape trauma syndrome (Anderson, 1981–82; Kaufman, 1980; Smith-DiJulio, 1998).
- "Many child and adult survivors of sexual assaults never report the crime or seek help" (Symes, 2000, p. 30).
- Survivors of sexual assault are more likely to attempt suicide, experience an eating disorder, be sexually assaulted again, and have substance abuse, depressive episodes, and anxiety disorders (Symes, 2000).

 ## Pediatric Considerations

- The female adolescent is particularly at risk for sexual assault; estimates are that more than 50% of rape victims are between 10 and 19 years of age (Wong, 2003).
- The assailant of a child is most likely someone the child knows, and the assaults usually have occurred for some time within the child's own home or neighborhood (Pownall, 1985).
- Adolescents, particularly boys, are more prone to attempt suicide in the aftermath of rape (Holmes, 1999).
- Acquaintance rape is very prevalent among college-age women and is believed to be underrecognized and underreported (Ellis, 1994).
- Greater emotional distress and long-term effects have been reported when a child knew and trusted the abuser (Holmes, 1999).
- Adolescent girls frequently underreport acquaintance rape because they believe they may have contributed to the act in some way (eg, alcohol use; Wong, 2003).
- Drug—facilitated sexual assaults are caused by slipping a drug in a drink. "Date rape" drugs are Rohypnol, GHB, and Ketamine. They cause disinhibition, passivity, relaxation of muscles, and amnesia (Smith, 1999).

Maternal Considerations

Refer to *Disabled Family Coping—Domestic Violence.*

> ### ⊙ Geriatric Considerations
>
> - Incidences of rape frequently are unreported among older adults (US Department of Justice, 1989).
> - Older adults experience reactions to rape similar to those of other adult victims but may have increased dependency, powerlessness, and depression (Fielo, 1987).
> - Residents of nursing homes are the most vulnerable to abuse. The failure to address the problem of sexual abuse may be the result of the incomprehensibility of sexual assault of nursing home residents and generalized negative attitudes or hostility toward older and cognitively impaired persons (Burgess et al., 2000).
> - Burgess found that, of 20 nursing home victims of sexual assault, 11 died within 1 year of the assault. These victims are not equipped physically, constitutionally, or psychologically to defend themselves or to cope with the aftermath (Burgess et al., 2000).

Focus Assessment Criteria

Subjective Data (Must Be Recorded)

Assess for Defining Characteristics.

History of the Undesired Sexual Activity (Child, Adolescent, Adult)*

Time and place of event
Identity or description of assailant
Sexual contact (type, amount, coercion, weapon)
Witnesses, if any
Activities that may alter evidence (changing clothes, bathing, urinating, douching)
Sexual history

Date of last menses	Contraceptive use	Menstrual history
Date of last sexual contact	History of venereal disease	

Response to the assault during acute phase

Assess person and family for

Somatic symptoms	Psychological symptoms	Sexual reactions

Assess child for

Understanding of the event
Knowledge of the identity of the molester
Possibility of previous assaults

Assess parents, spouse, others for

Understanding of the event	Ability to help victim cope	Ability to cope

Response to the assault during long-term phase

Assess person and family for reactions.

Objective Data

Assess for Injury (Ecchymoses, Lacerations, Abrasions).

Gastrointestinal system (mouth, anus, abdomen)
Skeletal muscle system
Genitourinary system

Assess the Emotional Responses.

Crying	Detachment	Hysteria
Composure	Withdrawal	

Assess for Change in Behavior in Cognitively Impaired (Burgess et al., 2000).

Avoidance behavior with males	Staying near nurses' station Fear of men	Lying in fetal position Withdrawal behavior

For more information on Focus Assessment Criteria, visit http://connection.lww.com.

---

*The purpose of securing a history is to substantiate evidence of trauma and not to explore details of trauma. This should be done in an appropriate therapy session.

Goals

NOC Abuse Protection, Abuse Recovery, Coping

The person will return to precrisis level of
  functioning.
The child will express feelings concerning the assault and the treatment.
The parents, spouse, or significant other will return to precrisis level of functioning.

Indicators

Short-term goals

- Share feelings.
- Describe rationale and treatment procedures.
- Identify members of support system and use them appropriately.

Long-term goals

- Report sleeping well.
- Report return to former eating pattern.
- Report no or occasional somatic reactions.
- Demonstrate calmness and relaxation.

NIC Abuse Protection Support, Coping Enhancement, Rape-Trauma Treatment, Support Group, Anxiety Reduction, Presence, Emotional Support, Calming Technique, Active Listening, Family Support, Grief Work Facilitation

General Interventions

Psychological Responses
Explore for Psychological Responses.

General

Phobias, nightmares	Enuresis	Denial, emotional shock
Anger, fear, anxiety	Depression, guilt	

Subjective

Expressions of numbness, shame, self-blame	Suicidal ideation

Objective
Crying
Silence
Trembling hands
Excessive bathing (particularly child or adolescent)
Avoiding interaction with others (staff, family)
Wearing excessive clothing (two or three pairs of pants or panties)

Assist Client to Identify Major Concerns (Psychological, Medical, Legal) and Perception of Help Needed.

Explain the Care and Examination.
Conduct examinations in an unhurried manner.
Explain every detail before acting.
If this is the person's first pelvic examination, explain the position and the instruments.
Discuss the possibility of pregnancy and sexually transmitted disease, and treatments available.

Explain the Legal Issues and Police Investigation (Heinrich, 1987).
Explain the need to collect specimens for future possible court use.
Explain that the choice to report the rape is the victim's.
If the police interview is permitted
  Negotiate with victim and police for an advantageous time.
  Explain to victim what kind of questions will be asked.
  Remain with the victim during the interview; do not ask questions or offer answers.
  If the officer is insensitive, intimidating, or offensive or asks improper questions, discuss this with
    the officer in private. If the behavior continues, use proper channels and make a complaint.

Eliminate or Reduce Psychological Responses, When Possible.

Promote a Trusting Relationship.
Stay with person during acute stage or arrange for other support.
Brief person on police and hospital procedures during acute stage.

Assist during medical examination; explain all procedures in advance.

Help person to meet personal needs (bathing *after* examination and evidence has been acquired).

Listen attentively to person's requests.

Maintain unhurried attitude toward person and family.

Avoid rescue feelings toward person.

Maintain nonjudgmental attitude.

Support person's beliefs and value system and avoid labeling.

Initiate play therapy with a child to explain treatments and allow child to express feelings.

Whenever Possible, Provide Crisis Counseling Within 1 h of Rape.

Ask permission to contact the rape crisis counselor.

Be flexible and individualize approach according to person's needs.

Observe person's behavior carefully and record objective data.

Encourage victim to verbalize thoughts, feelings, or perceptions of the event.

Discuss treatment as victim; express empathy.

Assess person's verbal style (expressive, controlled).

Discuss with person previous coping mechanism.

Explore available support system; involve significant others if appropriate.

Assess stress tolerance.

Reassure person about manner in which she or he reacted.

Explore with person her or his strengths and resources.

Convey confidence in person's ability to return to prior level of functioning.

Assist person in decision making and problem solving; involve person in own treatment plan.

Help restore person's dignity by calmly exploring together basis for feelings.

Reassure person that rape trauma victims often experience these feelings/symptoms: fear of rapist or death, guilt, loss of control, shame, short attention span, anger, anxiety, phobias, depression, flashbacks, embarrassment, and eating/sleeping pattern disturbances.

Respect victim's rights; honor wishes to restrict unwanted visitors; offer privacy when appropriate.

Explain to person that this experience will disrupt her or his life, and that feelings that occurred during acute phase may recur; encourage person to proceed at her or his own pace.

Explain any papers that need to be signed.

Briefly counsel family and friends at their level.

    Share the immediate needs of the victim for love and support.

    Encourage them to express their feelings and ask questions.

Support Person's Efforts to Overcome Feelings.

Change residence, telephone number, or both.

Use objects that symbolize safety (nightlight).

Take a trip.

Turn to support system.

Plan a day at a time.

Avoid highly stressful situations.

Engage in diversional activities.

Identify previous coping mechanisms that proved effective.

Fulfill Medical–Legal Responsibilities by Documentation (Peter & Whitehill, 1998).

Document

History of rape (date, time, place)

Nature of injuries, use of force, weapons used, threats of violence or retribution, restraints used

Nature of assault (fondling, oral, anal, vaginal penetration, ejaculation, use of condom)

Postassault activities (douching, bathing/showering, gargling, urinating, defecating, changing clothes, eating, or drinking)

Present state (use of drugs, alcohol)

Medical history, tetanus immunization status, gynecologic history (last menstrual period), last voluntary intercourse

Emotional state, mental status

Examination findings, smears/cultures taken, blood tests, evidence collected, and photographs (if appropriate)

Document to whom, when, and what evidence is delivered

Ascertain that the Following Are Addressed:

Sexually transmitted diseases (specimens, blood tests, prophylaxis)

Gonorrhea	Human immunodeficiency	Trichomoniasis
Syphilis	virus (HIV)	Hepatitis B
Chlamydia		

Pregnancy (test, emergency contraception)

Follow-up

Tests	Vaccines

Proceed with Follow-Up Until Victim is in Control of Reactions and Feelings (Andrews, 1992).

Before person leaves hospital, provide card with information about follow-up appointments and names and telephone numbers of local crisis and counseling centers.

Plan home visit or telephone call.

Arrange for legal or pastoral counseling, if appropriate.

Recommend and make referrals to psychotherapist, mental health clinic, citizen action and community group advocacy-related services.

Sexual Responses

Assess Responses.

General

Fear of intercourse

Family's fear that assault will affect person's future sexual health

Subjective

Mistrust of men

Objective

Change in sexual behavior

Lack of sexual desire (especially if victim never had intercourse before)

Promote Helping Relationship.

Encourage client to express feelings openly.

Provide accepting atmosphere.

Reassure person that rape trauma victims frequently experience her or his symptoms.

Offer feedback on feelings verbalized.

Encourage client to recognize positive responses or support from sexual partner or members of opposite sex.

Discuss possible fear of rejection by significant others.

Discuss potential anxiety about resuming sexual relations with partner.

Explore sexual concerns with person.

Do not tell victim what to do.

Proceed with Referrals.

Recommend couples therapy.

Recommend sexual counseling.

Somatic Responses

Assess for Somatic Responses.

Gastrointestinal irritability

Genitourinary discomfort

Rectal discomfort

Skeletal muscle tension

Vaginal discharge

Bruising and edema

Reports of:

Headaches	Fatigue	Itching
Anorexia	Nausea	Pain
Burning on urination		

Eliminate or Reduce Somatic Symptomatology.

Gastrointestinal Irritability

Anorexia

Offer small, frequent feedings.

Provide appealing foods.

Record intake.
Refer to *Imbalanced Nutrition* if anorexia is prolonged.
Nausea
Avoid gas-forming foods.
Restrict carbonated beverages.
Observe for abdominal distention.
Offer antiemetic per physician's order.

Genitourinary Discomfort
Pain
Assess for quality and duration.
Monitor intake and output.
Inspect urine and external genitalia for bleeding.
Listen attentively to person's description of pain.
Give pain medication per physician's order (see *Impaired Comfort*).
Discharge
Assess amount, color, and odor of discharge.
Allow person time to wash and change garments after initial examination has been completed.
Itching
Encourage bathing in cool water.
Avoid use of detergent soaps.
Avoid touching area causing discomfort.

Skeletal Muscle Tension
Headaches
Avoid any sudden change of person's position.
Approach person calmly.
Slightly elevate bed (unless contraindicated).
Discuss pain-reducing measures that have been effective in the past.
Fatigue
Assess present sleeping patterns if altered (see *Disturbed Sleep Pattern*).
Discuss precipitating factors for sleep disturbance; try to eliminate them, if possible.
Provide frequent rest periods throughout the day.
Avoid interruptions during sleep.
Avoid stress-producing situations.
Emotional responses
Provide emotionally secure environment.
Discuss person's daily routines and adhere to them as much as possible.
Avoid any sudden movements, and approach in calm manner.
Provide frequent quiet periods throughout the day.

Generalized Bruising and Edema
Avoid constrictive garments.
Handle affected body parts gently.
Elevate affected body part if edema is present.
Apply cool, moist compress to edematous area the first 24 h, then warm compress after 24 h.
Encourage person to verbalize discomfort.
Record any bruises, lacerations, edema, or abrasions.

Proceed with Health Teaching to Person and Family.

Gastrointestinal irritability: Explain side effects of diethylstilbestrol (DES): nausea and vomiting.
Genitourinary discomfort: Advise against scratching the area causing discomfort.
Skeletal muscle tension
    Explain potential causes of discomfort.
    Explain measures that may help release tension.
    Teach relaxation methods.
    Explain that rape trauma victims often experience these symptoms.

Rationales

- The sooner intervention begins with a rape victim, the less psychological damage she or he will incur. Many victims try to suppress the memory of the assault, so postponing counseling even

1 day may weaken their pursuit of follow-up care. Immediate contact with a counselor may overcome this reluctance.

- Because the victim's right to deny or consent to sexual activity has been violently violated, it is important to seek permission for subsequent care (Heinrich, 1987). It is important to tell the client as much as is practical or possible about what is happening, and why. Even in life-threatening situations, any sense of control given to the victim is helpful.
- Careful recording of psychological responses assists in recording progress in therapy, planning treatment, or identifying those at greatest risk. Behavior can differ among individuals. Feelings can be fast and furious or slow, trancelike, mixed, or clear.
- The interventions for rape trauma syndrome are listed for usefulness under the three types of responses: psychological, sexual, and somatic. The nurse must assess and intervene with each response for each victim and minimize any further trauma.
- Rape crisis centers provide rape victims and significant others with information concerning the medical examination, police interrogation, and court procedures; with escort service to hospital, police department, and courts; and with counseling.
- The medical–legal examination serves to assess the condition of the victim and to gather documentary evidence. It consists of a general examination; oral, pelvic, and rectal examinations; a culture for sperm and sexually transmitted diseases; serum pregnancy test; blood typing; and a drug and alcohol screen. Obvious debris is placed in separate envelopes. Dried sperm is collected. The victim's pubic hair and head hair are combed, and samples are placed in separate envelopes. Fingernail scrapings are placed in separate envelopes for each hand (Heinrich, 1987).
- Rape crisis centers work in the community to educate the public on rape and rape prevention, improve the response of hospitals and the police to rape victims, and improve rape-related legislation.
- Short-term rape crisis intervention should begin during the acute phase.
- Follow-up intervention is usually counselor-initiated.
- Nurses in community settings can teach primary prevention concepts by reviewing with clients measures to take to reduce the possibility of rape.
- Some destruction can be prevented if the victim's family and friends recognize symptoms as normal (Adams & Fay, 1989). Responses of others can help or hinder recovery greatly. Significant others also face a crisis and the need for recovery (Adams & Fay, 1989).
- After rape, people have profound feelings of loss of control and victimization. Interventions focus on restoring a sense of control and safety (Smith-DiJulio, 1998).
- Emotional support and presence validate the person's worth and prevent escalation of anxiety (Smith-DiJulio, 1998).
- Crisis counseling can provide accurate information and ongoing assessment of emotional state (Smith-DiJulio, 1998).
- Detailed follow-up instructions are given because the person cannot assimilate the information at this time (Andrews, 1992).
- Follow-up counseling provides support over time and may lessen the intrapsychic effects of the rape (Smith-DiJulio, 1998).
- Providing accurate information about the medical–legal procedures and their relevance can reduce feelings of physical intrusion and loss of control.
- Therapeutic alliances help the person express feelings and fears.
- Helping the person identify methods to increase his or her sense of safety can reduce panic levels of anxiety.
- When working with young rape victims, nurses should be cognizant of individual developmental levels, because the effects of the event vary according to developmental stage (Wong, 2003).
- The child's reaction depends on age, degree of physical trauma, relation to assailant, and parental (caretaker) reaction (Wong, 2003).
- Play therapy should be an integral part of the treatment regimen for children. The child can act out the assault with dolls of appropriate sex. Puppets are also beneficial for play therapy (Wong, 2003).

POWERLESSNESS

DEFINITION
Powerlessness: State in which an individual or group perceives a lack of personal control over certain events or situations that affects outlook, goals, and lifestyle

DEFINING CHARACTERISTICS
Major (Must Be Present)
Overt or covert (anger, apathy) expressions of dissatisfaction over inability to control a situation (eg, work, illness, prognosis, care, recovery rate) that is negatively affecting outlook, goals, and lifestyle

Minor (May Be Present)
Lack of information-seeking behaviors

Unsatisfactory dependence on others	Passivity	Resignation
	Apathy	Anxiety
Acting-out behavior	Anger	Depression
Violent behavior		

RELATED FACTORS
Pathophysiologic
Any disease process, acute or chronic, can cause or contribute to powerlessness. Some common sources are as follows.

Related to inability to communicate secondary to eg cerebrovascular accident (CVA), Guillain-Barré syndrome, intubation

Related to inability to perform activities of daily living secondary to eg CVA, cervical trauma, myocardial infarction, pain

Related to inability to perform role responsibilities secondary to surgery, trauma, arthritis

Related to progressive debilitating disease secondary to eg multiple sclerosis, terminal cancer, AIDS

Related to substance abuse

Related to cognitive distortions secondary to depression

Situational (Personal, Environmental)
Related to change from curative status to palliative status

Related to feeling of loss of control and lifestyle restrictions secondary to (specify)

Related to overeating patterns

Related to personal characteristics that highly value control (eg, internal locus of control)

Related to effects of hospital or institutional limitations

Related to lifestyle of helplessness

Related to fear of disapproval

Related to unmet dependency needs

Related to consistent negative feedback

Related to long-term abusive relationship

Maturational
Adolescent

Related to childrearing problems

Older Adult

Related to multiple losses secondary to aging (eg, retirement, sensory deficits, motor deficits, money, significant others)

⟲⟲ AUTHOR'S NOTE

Powerlessness is a feeling that all people experience to varying degrees in various situations. Stephenson (1979) described two types of powerlessness. *Situational powerlessness* occurs in a specific event and is probably short-lived. *Trait powerlessness* is more pervasive, affecting general outlook, goals, lifestyle, and relationships. The nursing diagnosis *Powerlessness* may be more useful clinically when describing a person experiencing trait rather than situational powerlessness.

Hopelessness differs from powerlessness in that a hopeless person sees no solution to problems or no way to achieve what is desired, even if he or she feels in control. A powerless person may see an alternative or answer, yet is unable to do anything about it because of perception of lack of control and resources. Prolonged powerlessness may lead to hopelessness.

⟲⟲ ERRORS IN DIAGNOSTIC STATEMENTS

Powerlessness related to hospitalization

Hospitalization evokes varied responses in people and families, including anxiety, fear, and powerlessness. If the hospitalization is expected to be short, the diagnosis of *Anxiety related to unfamiliar environment, loss of usual routines, and invasion of privacy* may be useful to describe situational powerlessness. If the hospitalization is a readmission for a continuing problem, *Powerlessness* may be more appropriate to describe trait powerlessness. The nurse should restate the diagnosis as *Powerlessness related to readmission for pulmonary infection and effects of illness on career and marriage.*

KEY CONCEPTS
Generic Considerations

- A person's response to loss of control depends on the meaning of the loss, individual coping patterns, personal characteristics (psychological, sociologic, cultural, spiritual), and response of others.
- Each person, whether well or ill, has a desire for control. Feelings of powerlessness are sometimes appropriate.
  - Stressors in the here-and-now precipitate powerlessness; however, the conflicts that emerge are often reminiscent of childhood issues (Boyd, 2005).
- When a person does not expect to be able to control outcomes, attention to and retention of information are poor.
- Powerlessness is very closely related to, but not synonymous with, the concept of external versus internal locus of control. Locus of control is a rather stable personality trait, whereas powerlessness is situationally determined.
- People with an internal locus of control believe they can affect outcomes by actively manipulating themselves or the environment. Examples of internal behavior are participating in regular exercise, acquiring printed literature about a new diagnosis, or learning assertiveness skills.
- People with external locus of control believe that outcomes are outside their control and attribute what happens to them to others or to fate. Examples of external behavior are losing weight because of fear of professional's response and blaming others for his present position (eg, depression, anger).
- Internally controlled people motivate themselves, whereas externally controlled people usually need others to motivate them. Young children are usually internally controlled but can learn to be externally controlled. For example, a child can learn to keep a record of the nutrients needed daily and his intake of them to help him understand the concept of good nutrition and to encourage him to take responsibility for his eating patterns.
- People with an internal locus of control may experience the loss of decision-making ability more profoundly than those with an external locus of control. Clients with external locus of control seem to be more prone to develop powerlessness.

- Powerlessness is part of a continuum with hopelessness and helplessness.
- Simmons and West (1984–1985) reported that older adults with high self-efficacy and occupational status had more difficulty with uncontrollable situations than their counterparts with lower self-efficacy. Younger adults were found to cope more effectively with uncontrollable situations if high efficacy, high income, and high occupational status were present.
- Miller (1985) postulates that if powerlessness is not contained, a cycle of lowered self-esteem and depression occurs, followed by hopelessness. Unrelieved states of powerlessness may lead to hopelessness and eventually may affect survival (Seligman, 1975).

Pediatric Considerations

- Hospitalized children commonly experience powerlessness.
- Differentiating *Powerlessness* from *Anxiety* and *Fear* may be difficult, especially in children. Refer to Key Concepts, Pediatric Considerations under *Anxiety* and *Fear*.

Geriatric Considerations

- Older adults are at high risk for powerlessness because multiple losses (previous roles, family, health, and functioning) may accompany the aging process. The added stressors of illness and institutionalization only compound feelings of powerlessness (O'Heath, 1991). Miller describes seven sources of power: physical strength and reserve, psychological stamina and support network, positive self-concept, energy, knowledge, motivation, and belief system (Miller, 1983).
- Internal locus of control and desired amount of control correlate with health status and high morale and life satisfaction (Chang, 1978; Fuller, 1978).
- Personality traits, various effects of diseases, and environmental conditions affect powerlessness. For older adults, disease states might restrict mobility. Changes in environment (eg, relocating to an extended care facility) can remove opportunities for decision making and autonomy. Institutional policy may require physical or chemical restraints for certain agitated behaviors (Miller, 2004).
- Late life changes in role, resources, and responsibility can contribute to feelings of loss of control.
- Extensive interactions with caregivers, rather than peers, can lead to a sense of powerlessness. This has implications for the older person, who, with an increased chance of multiple chronic illnesses, might be in the sick role for an extended period (Lambert & Lambert, 1981; Miller, 2004).

Transcultural Considerations

- The diagnosis of *Powerlessness* can be problematic with clients from various cultures. In Latin cultures, the concept of fatalism (eg, what will be will be) may be a challenge to a nurse who is trying to initiate a lifestyle change for better health (Andrews & Boyle, 2003; Giger & Davidhizar, 2004).
- The powerlessness associated with fatalism is accepted, and this usually does not constitute a problem for the person.
- Nurses must distinguish their goals for the client from those of the client. Nurses should address those areas that are of greatest concern to clients and family members (Andrews & Boyle, 2003).

Focus Assessment Criteria

Because powerlessness is subjective, the nurse must validate with the client all inferences concerning the client's feelings of powerlessness. The nurse assesses each client to determine his or her usual level of control and decision making and the effects that losing elements of control has had.

Subjective Data
Assess for Defining Characteristics.
Decision-making patterns
"How would you describe your usual method of making decisions (career, financial, health care)?"
  Make them alone
  Consult with others for advice (who?)
  Allow others to make them for me (spouse? children? others?)

Individual and role responsibilities
"What responsibilities did you have
  . . . as a school child and adolescent?"
  . . . at home?"
  . . . at work?"
  . . . in community and religious organizations?"

Assess for Related Factors.
Perception of control
"How would you describe your ability—high, moderate, fair, or poor—to control or cure your present health problem (eg, diabetes mellitus, aphasia, activity intolerance, obesity)?"
"To what do you attribute your (high, moderate, fair, poor) ability to control?"

Preventive measures		
Good nutrition	Stress management	Weight control
Exercise program		
Others		
Physician	Significant others	Nurse
Peer group		
No control		
Fate	Luck	

Objective Data
Assess for Defining Characteristics.
Participation in grooming and hygiene care (when indicated)

Actively seeks involvement	Requires encouragement
Reluctant to participate	Refuses to participate

Information-seeking behaviors
Actively seeks information and literature from others concerning condition
Refuses to receive information
Requires encouragement to ask questions
Expresses lack of interest

Response to limits placed on decision-making and self-control behaviors

Acceptance	Increases attempts to exercise control
Apathy	Depression
Attempts to circumvent limits	Anger
Ignores limits	Withdrawal

Nonverbal language

Posture	Tone of voice	Eye contact
Gestures		

For more information on Focus Assessment Criteria, visit http://connection.lww.com.

Goal

NOC	Depression Control, Health Beliefs, Health Beliefs: Perceived Control, Participation: Health Care Decisions

The person will verbalize ability to control or influence situations and outcomes.

Indicators

- Identify factors that the client can control.
- Make decisions regarding his or her care, treatment, and future when possible.

General Interventions

| NIC | Mood Management, Teaching: Individual, Decision-Making Support, Self-Responsibility Facilitation, Health System Guidance, Spiritual Support |

Assess for Causative and Contributing Factors.

Lack of knowledge

Previous inadequate coping patterns (eg, depression; for discussion, see *Ineffective Coping related to depression*)

Insufficient decision-making opportunities

Eliminate or Reduce Contributing Factors, If Possible.

Lack of Knowledge

Increase effective communication between person and health care provider.

Explain all procedures, rules, and options to person; avoid medical jargon. Help client anticipate sensations that will occur during treatments (provides reality-oriented cognitive images that bolster a sense of control and coping strategies).

Allow time to answer questions; ask client to write questions down so he or she does not forget them.

Provide a specific time (10 to 15 min) each shift that person knows can be used to ask questions or discuss subjects as desired.

Anticipate questions/interest and offer information. Help to anticipate events and outcomes.

While being realistic, point out positive changes in person's condition, such as serum enzymes decreasing after myocardial infarction or surgical incision healing well.

Be an active listener by allowing person to verbalize concerns and feelings; assess for areas of concern.

Provide consistent staffing.

Single out one nurse to be responsible for 24-h plan of care, and provide opportunities for person and family to identify with this nurse.

Contact self-help support groups if available (eg, mastectomy, ostomy clubs, paraplegics).

If contributing factors are pain or anxiety, provide information on how to use behavioral control techniques (eg, relaxation, imagery, deep breathing).

Provide Opportunities for Person to Control Decisions and to Identify Personal Goals of Care.

Allow person to manipulate surroundings, such as deciding what is to be kept where (shoes under bed, picture on window).

If person desires, and as hospital policy permits, encourage person to bring personal effects from home (eg, pillows, pictures).

Keep needed items within reach (call bell, urinal, tissues).

Do not offer options if there are none (eg, a deep intramuscular [IM] Z-track injection must be rotated). Offer options that are personally relevant.

Discuss daily plan of activities and allow person to make as many decisions as possible about it.

Increase decision-making opportunities as person progresses.

Respect and follow person's decision if you have given him options.

Record person's specific choices on care plan to ensure that others on staff acknowledge preferences ("dislikes orange juice," "takes showers," "plan dressing change at 7:30 before shower").

Keep promises.

Provide opportunity for person and family to express feelings.

Provide opportunities for person and family to participate in care.

Be alert for signs of paternalism/maternalism in health care providers (eg, making decisions for clients).

Plan a care conference to allow staff to discuss methods of individualizing care; encourage each nurse to share at least one action that she discovered a particular person liked.

Shift emphasis from what one cannot do to what one can do.

Set goals that are short-term, behavioral, practical, and realistic (walk 5 more feet every day; then, in 1 week, client can walk to television room).

Provide daily recognition of progress.

Praise gains/achievements.

Assist in identifying factors that are controllable and those that are not. Assist in accepting what cannot be changed and altering what can.

Emphasize positive aspects when the person becomes focused on fears of the worst (reduces fear by shifting perspective and allowing person to regain control).

Allow person to experience outcomes that result from his own actions.

Assess the Person's Usual Response to Problems (see Focus Assessment Criteria).

Internal control (seeks to change own behaviors or environment to control problems)

External control (expects others or other factors—fate, luck—to control problems)

Provide Person with Internal Locus of Control the Needed Information to Alter Behavior or Environment.

Explain the problem as explicitly as the person requests.

Explain the relationship of prescribed behavior and outcome (eg, need for salt restriction, physiologic effects of exercise, effects of bed rest on impaired cardiac function).

Monitor a Person with External Locus of Control to Encourage Participation.

Have him keep a record (eg, food intake for 1 week; weight loss chart; exercise program—type and frequency; medications taken).

Use telephone contact to monitor if feasible.

Provide explicit written directions (eg, meal plans; exercise regimen—type, frequency, duration; speech practice lessons—for aphasia).

Teach significant others methods to manipulate behaviors, if appropriate.

Provide reward for each goal reached.

Assist Client in Deriving Power from Other Sources.

Give permission to use other power sources to both client and significant others (eg, prayer, stress reduction techniques).

Self-help groups

Support groups

Offer referral to religious leader.

Provide privacy and support for other measures client may request (eg, meditation, imagery, special rituals).

Initiate Health Teaching and Referrals as Indicated (Social Worker, Psychiatric Nurse/Physician, Visiting Nurse, Religious Leader, Self-Help Groups).

Evaluate the Situation with the Client.

Once the outcome criteria have been accomplished or feelings of powerlessness are diminishing, discuss the process used to relieve powerlessness. Explain how factors contributed to the powerlessness, review why certain strategies were effective, and discuss how person will manage feelings of powerlessness in the future.

Advocate within the system to eliminate policies and routines that contribute to powerlessness.

Rationales

- To plan effective interventions, the nurse must determine whether the client usually seeks to change his own behaviors to control problems, or whether he expects others or external factors to control problems.
- Self-image changes negatively because of a restricted lifestyle, social isolation, unmet expectations, and dependence on others.
- People with chronic illness need to be assisted not to see themselves as helpless victims. People with a sense of hope, self-control, direction, purpose, and identity are better able to meet the challenges of their disease.
- Self-concept can be enhanced when clients actively engage in decisions regarding health and lifestyle.
- Setting realistic goals can increase motivation and hope.
- Loss of or decrease in power in one area may be counterbalanced by the introduction of a new source of power or by an increase in power in an existing area.
- Averill (1973) describes three types of control: behavioral, cognitive, and decisional. Interventions that allow people to participate in their care are enhancing their behavioral control. Interventions that provide the person with knowledge, solicit their input into situations, and provide feedback

are examples of increasing a person's cognitive control. Interventions that allow the person to make choices are providing decisional control.

- Research has shown that 75% of clients with chronic obstructive pulmonary disease do not think about the cause of their illness. People who do not engage in causal thinking may be in denial. This denial may produce a feeling of control, enabling them to be more functional. Contemplating causes may produce feelings of powerlessness, depression, and decreased functional status (Weaver & Narsavage, 1992).

Pediatric Interventions

Provide opportunities for child to make decisions (eg, set time for bath, hold still for injection). Engage child in play therapy before and after a traumatic situation (refer to *Delayed Growth and Development* for specific interventions for age-related development needs).

Rationales

- The goals of nursing interventions to treat powerlessness include modifying the environment to resemble the child's home and providing opportunities for acceptable control (Wong, 2003).
- Children can gain mastery over stressful situations by participating in play activities while ill or hospitalized (Wong, 2003).

Ineffective Protection
Impaired Tissue Integrity*
Impaired Skin Integrity
  Related to the Effects of Pressure, Friction, Shear, Maceration
Impaired Oral Mucous Membrane
Risk for Impaired Oral Mucous Membrane
  Related to Inadequate Oral Hygiene or Inability to Perform Oral Hygiene

INEFFECTIVE PROTECTION

DEFINITION

Ineffective Protection: State in which a person experiences a decrease in the ability to guard against internal or external threats, such as illness or injury

DEFINING CHARACTERISTICS

Major (Must Be Present, One or More)

Deficient immunity
Maladaptive stress response
Impaired healing
Neurosensory alterations
Altered clotting

Minor (May Be Present)

Chills
Fatigue
Cough
Immobility
Pressure sores
Insomnia
Dyspnea
Weakness
Restlessness
Perspiration
Anorexia
Itching
Disorientation

AUTHOR'S NOTE

This broad diagnosis describes a person with compromised ability to defend against microorganisms, bleeding, or both because of immunosuppression, myelosuppression, abnormal clotting factors, or all these. Use of this diagnosis entails several potential problems.

The nurse is cautioned against substituting *Ineffective Protection* for an immune system compromise, acquired immunodeficiency syndrome (AIDS), disseminated intravascular coagulation, diabetes mellitus, or other disorders. Rather, the nurse should focus on diagnoses describing the person's functional abilities that are or may be compromised by altered protection, such as *Fatigue, Risk for Infection,* and *Risk for Social Isolation.* The nurse also should address the physiologic complications of altered protection that require nursing and medical interventions for management, identifying appropriate collaborative problems.

For example, the nurse could use *Ineffective Protection* in each of these three cases: Mr. A, who has leukemia, leukopenia, and no evidence of infection; Mr. B, who is experiencing sickle cell crisis; and Mr. C, who has AIDS. The problem is that this diagnosis does not describe the specific focus of nursing, but describes situations in which more specific responses can be diagnosed. For Mr. A, the nursing diagnosis of *Risk for Infection related to compromised immune system* would apply. For

(continued)

*This diagnosis was developed and submitted to NANDA by the Clinical Nurse Specialist Group, Harper Hospital, in the Detroit Medical Center.

IMPAIRED TISSUE INTEGRITY

DEFINITION

Impaired Tissue Integrity: State in which a person experiences or is at risk for damage to the integumentary, corneal, or mucous membranous tissues of the body

DEFINING CHARACTERISTICS
Major (Must Be Present)

Disruptions of corneal, integumentary, or mucous membranous tissue or invasion of body structure (incision, dermal ulcer, corneal ulcer, oral lesion)

Minor (May Be Present)

Lesions (primary, secondary)	Dry mucous membrane	Edema
Leukoplakia	Erythema	Coated tongue

RELATED FACTORS
Pathophysiologic

Related to inflammation of dermal–epidermal junctions secondary to:

Autoimmune alterations

Lupus erythematosus	Scleroderma	

Metabolic and endocrine alterations

Diabetes mellitus	Jaundice	Hepatitis
Cancer	Cirrhosis	Thyroid dysfunction
Renal failure		

Bacterial

Impetigo	Folliculitis	Cellulitis

Viral

Herpes zoster [shingles]	Herpes simplex	Gingivitis
AIDS		

Fungal

Ringworm [dermatophytosis]	Athlete's foot	Vaginitis

Related to decreased blood and nutrients to tissues secondary to:

Diabetes mellitus

Peripheral vascular alterations	Anemia	Cardiopulmonary disorders
	Venous stasis	Arteriosclerosis

Nutritional alterations

Obesity	Emaciation	Dehydration
Malnutrition	Edema	

Treatment-Related

Related to decreased blood and nutrients to tissues secondary to:

Therapeutic extremes in body temperature	NPO status	Surgery

Related to imposed immobility secondary to sedation
Related to mechanical trauma
Therapeutic fixation devices

Wired jaw	Casts	Traction
Orthopedic devices/braces		

Related to effects of radiation on epithelial and basal cells
Related to effects of mechanical irritants or pressure secondary to:

Inflatable or foam donuts	Tourniquets	Footboards
Restraints	Dressings, tape, solutions	External urinary catheters
Nasogastric (NG) tubes	Endotracheal tubes	Oral prostheses/braces
Contact lenses		

Situational (Personal, Environmental)

Related to chemical trauma secondary to:

Excretions	Secretions	Noxious agents/substances

Related to environmental irritants secondary to:

Radiation–sunburn	Humidity	Bites (insect, animal)
Poisonous plants	Temperature	Parasites
Inhalants		

Related to the effects of pressure of immobility secondary to:

Pain	Fatigue	Motivation
Cognitive, sensory, or motor deficits		

Related to inadequate personal habits (hygiene/dental/dietary/sleep)
Related to impaired mobility secondary to (specify)
Related to thin body frame

Maturational

Related to dry, thin skin and decreased dermal vascularity secondary to aging

---

ⓧ AUTHOR'S NOTE

Impaired Tissue Integrity is the broad diagnosis under which the more specific diagnoses of *Impaired Skin Integrity* and *Impaired Oral Mucous Membranes* fall. Because tissue is composed of epithelium, connective tissue, muscle, and nervous tissue, *Impaired Tissue Integrity* correctly describes some pressure ulcers that are deeper than the dermis. *Impaired Skin Integrity* should be used to describe disruptions of epidermal and dermal tissue only. (Refer to page 590 for definitions of stages.)

When a pressure ulcer is stage IV, necrotic, or infected, it may be more appropriate to label the diagnosis a collaborative problem, such as *PC: Stage IV Pressure Ulcer*. This would represent a situation that a nurse manages with physician- and nurse-prescribed interventions. When a stage II or III pressure ulcer needs a dressing that requires a physician's order in an acute care setting, the nurse should continue to label the situation a nursing diagnosis, because it would be appropriate and legal for a nurse to treat the ulcer independently in other settings (eg, in the community).

If a client is immobile and multiple systems are threatened (respiratory, circulatory, musculoskeletal as well as integumentary), the nurse can use *Disuse Syndrome* to describe the entire situation. If a client is at risk for damage to corneal tissue, the nurse can use a diagnosis such as *Risk for Impaired Corneal Tissue Integrity related to corneal drying and lower lacrimal production secondary to unconscious state.*

ⓧ ERRORS IN DIAGNOSTIC STATEMENTS

1. *Impaired Skin Integrity related to surgical removal of skin/tissues*
   Impaired Skin Integrity should not be used as a new label for surgical incisions, tracheostomies, or burns. Surgical incisions disrupt the skin's protective mechanism, increasing vulnerability to microorganism invasion; a more clinically useful diagnosis would be *Risk for Infection related to surgical incision.*

(continued)

> ⊗ **ERRORS IN DIAGNOSTIC STATEMENTS** (*Continued*)
>
> 2. *Impaired Skin Integrity related to fecal diversion*
>   The nurse should not rename fecal diversions such as colostomy or ileostomy with the nursing diagnosis *Impaired Skin Integrity*. Instead, the nurse should assess the person's actual or potential responses to the surgical procedure that the nurse can treat. For example, the skin around an ostomy is at risk for erosion from effluent, calling for *Risk for Impaired Skin Integrity related to chemical irritation of effluent on adjacent skin.* If the adjacent skin exhibits lesions from irritants (chemical or mechanical), *Impaired Skin Integrity related to exposure to ostomy effluent, as evidenced by 2-cm ulcer left midline of stoma* would be appropriate.

KEY CONCEPTS
Generic Considerations

- At any given time, more than 1 million Americans are estimated to have pressure ulcers. Pressure ulcer incidence ranges from 2.7% to 29.5% in acute care settings, as high as 41% in critical care populations, and from 2.4% to 23% in skilled nursing facilities and nursing homes (Maklebust & Sieggreen, 2000).
- Tissues are groupings of specialized cells that unite to perform specific functions. The human body is composed of four basic types of tissue: epithelial, connective (including skeletal tissue and blood), muscle, and nervous.
- The external covering of the body is composed of epithelial tissue, called the integument. Wherever the body exposes large openings to the outside (eg, the mouth), its outer covering changes from integument to an inner lining called the mucous membrane. Each layer of the integument has its counterpart in a complete mucous membrane. The integument includes both the skin and the subcutaneous tissue.
- The skin is a complex organ consisting of two layers: the outer epidermis and the deeper dermis. The epidermis is approximately 0.04 mm thick, and the dermis is about 0.5 cm thick (Porth, 2002).
- The epidermis functions as a barrier to protect inner tissues (from injury, chemicals, organisms); as a receptor for a range of sensations (touch, pain, heat, cold); as a regulator of body temperature through radiation (giving off heat), conduction (transfer of heat), and convection (movement of warm air molecules away from the body); as a regulator of water balance by preventing water and electrolyte loss; and as a receptor for vitamin D from the sun (Maklebust & Sieggreen, 2000).
- A water-soluble mitotic inhibitor called *chalone* depresses epidermal regeneration. Chalone levels are high during daytime stress and activity and lower during sleep. Therefore, healing is promoted during rest and sleep (Maklebust & Sieggreen, 2000).
- Beneath the avascular epidermis lies the highly vascularized dermis. The dermis contains epithelial tissue, connective tissue, muscle, and nervous tissue. The dermis is rich in collagen, which imparts toughness to the skin. Hair follicles extend into the dermis and serve as islands of cells for rapid reepithelialization of minor wounds. Sweat glands in the dermis contribute to control of body water and temperature. Small muscles within the dermis serve to produce goose pimples. Specialized dermal nerve endings for pain, touch, heat, and cold cannot be replaced once destroyed (Maklebust & Sieggreen, 2000).
- The subcutaneous tissue, which lies beneath the dermis, stores fat for temperature regulation and contains the remainder of the sweat glands and hair follicles (Porth, 2002).
- The skin's responses to antigens are capillary dilation (erythema), arteriole dilation (flare), and increased capillary permeability (wheal), which all contribute to localized edema, spasms, and pruritus.
- Causes of tissue destruction can be mechanical, immunologic, bacterial, chemical, or thermal. Mechanical destruction includes physical trauma and surgical incision. Immunologic destruction occurs as an allergic response. Bacterial destruction results from an overgrowth of organisms. Chemical destruction results when a caustic substance contacts unprotected tissue. Thermal destruction occurs when tissue is exposed to temperature extremes that are incompatible with cell life (Maklebust & Sieggreen, 2000).

Wound Healing
- Wound healing is a complex sequence of events initiated by injury to the tissues. The components are coagulation of bleeding, inflammation, epithelialization, fibroplasia and collagen metabolism, collagen maturation, scar remodeling, and wound contraction (Wysocki, 1999).

- A wound must be considered in relation to the entire person. Major factors that affect wound healing are nutrition, vitamins, minerals, anemia, blood volume and tissue oxygenation, steroids and anti-inflammatory drugs, diabetes mellitus, chemotherapy, and radiation.
- Wound healing requires the following intrinsic factors (Dudek, 2006):
  - Increased protein–carbohydrate intake sufficient to prevent negative nitrogen balance, hypoalbuminemia, and weight loss
  - Increased daily intake of vitamins and minerals
    - Vitamin A, 10,000 to 50,000 IU
    - Vitamin B_1, 0.5 to 1.0 mg/1,000 diet calories
    - Vitamin B_2, 0.25 mg/1,000 diet calories
    - Vitamin B_6, 2 mg
    - Niacin, 15 to 20 mg
    - Vitamin B_{12}, 400 mg
    - Vitamin C, 75 to 300 mg
    - Vitamin D, 400 mg
    - Vitamin E, 10 to 15 IU
    - Traces of zinc, magnesium, calcium, copper, manganese
  - Adequate oxygen supply and the blood volume and ability to transport it

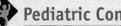

Pediatric Considerations

- A newborn commonly exhibits normal skin variations, such as mongolian spots, milia, and stork bites, which can be upsetting to parents but are clinically insignificant.
- Several common skin conditions affect children in specific age groups. These include atopic, seborrheic, and diaper dermatitis in infancy and acne in adolescence.
- Infants and young children have a thin epidermis and require special protection from the sun.

Geriatric Considerations

- Elastin, which gives the skin flexibility, elasticity, and tensile strength, decreases with age. It is found in tissues associated with body movement, such as the walls of major blood vessels, heart, lungs, and skin (Boynton et al., 1999).
- Collagen, found in all connective tissue, such as blood, lymph, and bone, binds together and supports other tissues. The extracellular matrix of connecting tissue is composed primarily of collagen and elastin, and approximately 80% of the dermis consists of collagen. With aging, skin strength decreases owing to age-related loss of collagen from the dermis and the degeneration of the elastic properties of the remaining collagen.
- Some older adults exhibit shiny, loose, thin, transparent skin, primarily on the backs of the hands and the forearms. Subcutaneous fat decreases with aging, reducing the cushioning of bony prominences and putting older adults at increased risk for pressure ulcers.
- Aging causes diminished immunocompetence and decreased angiogenesis, which delays wound healing (Boynton et al., 1999).
- Age-related decreases in sebum secretion and the number of sebaceous glands cause drier, coarser skin that is more prone to fissures and cracks.
- In older adults, cells are larger and proliferate more slowly, fibroblasts decrease in number, and dermal vascularity decreases. All these factors contribute to slower wound healing.
- With aging, the thermal threshold for sweating increases and the sweat output decreases.
- Aging nails become dull, brittle, and thickened owing to decreased blood supply to the nailbed. Splitting of the nails can occur, increasing the risk of infection. Thickening of the toenails causes the distal portion of the nail to lift from the nailbed; debris collection creates a risk of fungal infection.

🌐 Transcultural Considerations

- The darker the person's skin, the more difficult it is to assess for changes in color. A baseline must be established in daylight or with at least a 60-watt bulb. Baseline skin color should be assessed in areas with the least amount of pigmentation (eg, palms of hands, soles of feet, underside of forearms, abdomen, and buttocks; Weber & Kelley, 2003).
- All skin colors have an underlying red tone. Pallor in black-skinned people is seen as an ashen or gray tone. Pallor in brown-skinned people appears as a yellowish-brown color. Pallor can be assessed in mucous membranes, lips, nailbeds, and conjunctiva of the lower eyelids (Andrews & Boyle, 2003).
- Assessment of capillary refill time can be done on the second or third finger, lips, or earlobes (Andrews & Boyle, 2003).
- To assess for rashes and skin inflammations in dark-skinned people, the nurse should rely on palpation for warmth and induration, not observation (Giger & Davidhizar, 2004).
- Mongolian spots are dark-blue or black areas of pigmentation seen on the skin of black, Asian, Native American, or Mexican American newborns. They are often mistaken for bruises. By adulthood, they are lighter but still visible (Giger & Davidhizar, 2004).
- Some folk remedies may be misdiagnosed as injuries. Three folk practices of Southeast Asians leave marks on the body that can be taken for signs of violence or abuse. *Cao gio* is rubbing of the skin with a coin to produce dark blood or ecchymotic strips; it is done to treat colds and flulike symptoms. *Bat gio* is skin pinching on the temples to treat headaches or on the neck for a sore throat; if petechiae or ecchymoses appear, the treatment is a success. *Poua* is the burning of the skin with the tip of a dried weedlike grass; it is believed the burning will cause the noxious element that causes the pain to exude (Andrews & Boyle, 2003).

Focus Assessment Criteria

Subjective Data

Assess for Related Factors.

History of symptoms
Onset
Precipitated by what?
Relieved by what?
Frequency

History of exposure (if allergy is suspected)
Carrier of contagious disease
Chemicals, paints, cleaning agents, plants, animals
Heat or cold

Medical, surgical, and dental history; use of tobacco, alcohol
Current drug therapy
What drugs? How often? When was last dose taken?
Effects on symptoms

Factors contributing to the development or extension of tissue destruction (assess for)

Skin deficits

Dryness	Thinness	Edema
Excessive perspiration	Obesity	Aging skin

Mucous membrane deficits

Mouth pain	Oral lesions or ulcers	Bleeding gums
Oral plaque	Coated tongue	Dryness

Corneal deficits

Absence of blink reflex	Excessive tearing	Ptosis
Contact lens wear	Diminished tearing	Sensory deficits

Impaired oxygen transport
Edema
Anemia
Peripheral vascular disorders

Arteriosclerosis	Venous stasis	Cardiopulmonary disorders

Chemical / mechanical irritants

Radiation	Contact lenses	Casts, splints, braces
Oral prostheses	Incontinence (feces, urine)	

Nutritional deficiencies

Protein	Vitamin	Mineral and trace elements
Dehydration		

Systemic disorders
Refer to Related Factors (Pathophysiologic).

Sensory deficits

Decreased level of	Neuropathy	Visual or taste alterations
consciousness	Brain or cord injury	Confusion

Immobility

Objective Data
Assess for Defining Characteristics.

Skin

Color	Texture	Turgor
Vascularity	Moisture	Temperature
Lesions		
Type	Shape	Location
Size	Distribution	Drainage
Color		

Circulation
 Do capillaries refill within 3 s after blanching?
 Does erythema subside within 30 min after pressure is removed?
Edema
 Note degree and location.
 Palpate over bony prominences for sponginess (indicates edema).

Oral Mucous Membrane
Refer to Focus Assessment Criteria for *Impaired Oral Mucous Membrane.*

For more information on Focus Assessment Criteria, visit http://connection.lww.com.

Goal
[NOC] Tissue Integrity

The person will demonstrate progressive healing of tissue.

Indicators
- Participate in risk assessment.
- Express willingness to participate in prevention of pressure ulcers.
- Describe etiology and prevention measures.
- Explain rationale for interventions.

General Interventions
[NIC] Teaching: Individual, Surveillance

Identify Causative/Contributing Factors.
Removal of adhesives
Pressure dressings
NG tubes
Endotracheal tubes
Skeletal prominences with little overlying soft tissue
Hard, supporting sleep or sitting surfaces
Prolonged sitting or lying in same position
Dragging across bed linens
Sitting in Fowler's position
Bladder and bowel incontinence (see *Incontinence*)
Profuse diaphoresis
Cognitive, sensory, motor deficits

Fixation devices
    Skeletal traction
    Oral prostheses
Contact lens wear

Reduce Contributing Factors to Mechanical Irritants to Skin.

Encourage highest degree of mobility to avoid prolonged periods of pressure.
For neuromuscular impairment:
    Teach client/significant other appropriate measures to prevent pressure, shear, friction, maceration.
    Teach client to recognize early signs of tissue damage.
    Change position at least every 2 h around the clock.
    Use 30-degree lateral side-lying position.
    Frequently supplement full-body turns with minor shifts in body weight.
Keep client clean and dry.
Reduce environmental sources of pressure (drains, tubes, dressings).
Avoid stripping of epidermis when removing adhesives.
Use pressure-dispersing devices as appropriate.
Limit semi-Fowler's position in high-risk clients (limit elevation of head of bed to less than
  30 degrees.
Avoid use of knee gatch on bed.
Use lift sheet to reposition client.
Install overhead trapeze to allow clients increased mobility.
Use cornstarch to reduce friction.

Reduce Causative Factors if Possible.

For casts
    Monitor common pressure sites in relationship to cast application.
    Apply padding over bony prominence.
    Keep cast edges smooth and away from skin surfaces.
    Inspect for loose plaster and shifting of padding.

Protect Skin Around Feeding Tubes or Endotracheal Tubes with a Protective Barrier.

Change skin barrier when loose or leaking.
Instruct to report discomforts.

Teach How to Reduce Mechanical Irritation with Contact Lens Use.

Have person review care of lens.
If irritation occurs
    Remove lens.
    Clean with proper solution.
    Check for tears or chips.
    Reinsert lens after rewetting.

Rationales

- Contributing factors to tissue destruction can be intrinsic (eg, vulnerable skin, systemic disorders) or extrinsic (eg, mechanical, chemical). The more factors present, the more vulnerable is the client.
- Principles of pressure ulcer prevention include reducing or rotating pressure on soft tissue. If pressure on soft tissue exceeds intracapillary pressure (approximately 32 mm Hg), capillary occlusion and resulting hypoxia can cause tissue damage.
- Exercise and mobility increase blood flow to all areas.
- Keeping the bed as flat as possible (lower than 30 degrees) and supporting feet with a foot board help prevent shear, the pressure created when two adjacent tissue layers move in opposition. If a bony prominence slides across the subcutaneous tissue, the subepidermal capillaries may become bent and pinched, resulting in decreased tissue perfusion.
- Prolonged pressure of the cast on neurovascular structures and other body parts can cause necrosis, pressure sores, and nerve palsies.

- Padding over bony prominences is essential to prevent pressure ulcers.
- Rough or improperly bent plaster edges may cause damage to surrounding skin by friction. When an extremity is not elevated properly, cast edges press into the skin and cause pain.
- Loose plaster or wrinkled padding can irritate skin under casts.
- An NG tube can irritate skin and mucosa. Gastric juices can cause severe skin breakdown.
- Because contact lenses are foreign bodies, teaching should focus on prevention of infection and irritation.
- If irritation continues, remove lens and contact eye specialist.
- Urge client not to use tap water or saliva to lubricate lens.
- Emphasize need to follow disinfection procedures strictly, to rinse case daily and air dry, and to replace case every 3 to 6 months.

IMPAIRED SKIN INTEGRITY

DEFINITION

Impaired Skin Integrity: State in which a person experiences or is at risk for damage to the epidermal and dermal tissue

DEFINING CHARACTERISTICS
Major (Must Be Present)

Disruptions of epidermal and dermal tissue

Minor (May Be Present)

Denuded skin	Erythema	Pruritus
Lesions (primary, secondary)		

RELATED FACTORS

See *Impaired Tissue Integrity.*

○○ **AUTHOR'S NOTE**

See *Impaired Tissue Integrity.*

○○ **ERRORS IN DIAGNOSTIC STATEMENTS**

See *Impaired Tissue Integrity.*

KEY CONCEPTS

See *Impaired Tissue Integrity.*

Focus Assessment Criteria

See *Impaired Tissue Integrity.*

Goal

NOC Tissue Integrity: Skin and Mucous Membrane

The person will demonstrate skin integrity free of pressure ulcers (if able).

Indicators

- Participate in risk assessment.
- Express willingness to participate in prevention of pressure ulcers.
- Describe etiology and prevention measures.
- Explain rationale for interventions.

General Interventions

NIC Pressure Management, Pressure Ulcer Care, Skin Surveillance, Positioning

Use a Formal Risk Assessment Scale to Identify Individual Risk Factors in Addition to Activity and Mobility Deficits (eg, The Braden Scale, Worton Score [AHCPR, 1992]); Refer to Focus Assessment.

Assess for Skin Deficits.

Dryness	Edema	Obesity
Thinness	Excessive perspiration	

Assess for Impaired Oxygen Transport.

Edema	Anemia	Peripheral vascular disorders
Arteriosclerosis	Cardiopulmonary disorders	

Assess for Chemical/Mechanical/Thermal Irritants.

Radiation	Incontinence (feces, urine)	Casts, splints, braces
Spasms		

Assess for Nutritional Deficits.

Protein	Vitamin	Mineral and trace element
Dehydration		

Assess for Systemic Disorders.

Infection	Diabetes mellitus	Cancer
Hepatic or renal disorders		

Assess for Sensory Deficits.

Neuropathy	Confusion	Head injury
Cord injury		

Assess for Immobility.

Attempt to Modify Contributing Factors to Lessen the Possibility of a Pressure Ulcer Developing.

Incontinence of Urine or Feces

Determine etiology of incontinence.

Maintain sufficient fluid intake for adequate hydration (approximately 2,500 mL daily, unless contraindicated); check oral mucous membranes for moisture and check urine specific gravity.

Establish a schedule for emptying bladder (begin with every 2 h).

If person is confused, determine what his or her incontinence pattern is and intervene before incontinence occurs.

Explain problem to client; secure his or her cooperation for the plan.

When incontinent, wash perineum with a liquid soap that does not alter skin pH.

Apply a protective barrier to the perineal region (incontinence film barrier spray or wipes).

Check person frequently for incontinence when indicated.

For additional interventions, refer to *Impaired Urinary Elimination*.

Immobility

Encourage range-of-motion exercises and weight-bearing mobility, when possible, to increase blood flow to all areas.

Promote optimal circulation when in bed.

  Use repositioning schedule that relieves vulnerable area most often (eg, if vulnerable area is the back, turning schedule would be left side to back, back to right side, right side to left side, and left side to back); post "turn clock" at bedside.

Turn or instruct client to turn or shift weight every 30 min to 2 h, depending on other causative factors and the ability of the skin to recover from pressure.

Increase frequency of the turning schedule if any reddened areas that appear do not disappear within 1 h after turning.

Place person in normal or neutral position with body weight evenly distributed. Use 30-degree laterally inclined position when possible.

Keep bed as flat as possible to reduce shearing forces; limit semi-Fowler's position to only 30 min at a time.

Use foam blocks or pillows to provide a bridging effect to support the body above and below the high-risk or ulcerated area so affected area does not touch bed surface. Do not use foam donuts or inflatable rings because these increase the area of pressure.

Alternate or reduce the pressure on the skin with an appropriate support surface.

Suspend heels off bed surface.

Use enough personnel to lift person up in bed or chair rather than pull or slide skin surfaces.

Have person wear long-sleeved top and socks to reduce friction on elbows and heels.

To reduce shearing forces, support feet with footboard to prevent sliding.

Promote optimal circulation when person is sitting.

Limit sitting time for person at high risk for ulcer development.

Instruct person to lift self using chair arms every 10 min, if possible, or assist person in rising up off the chair at least every hour, depending on risk factors present.

Do not elevate legs unless calves are supported, to reduce the pressure over the ischial tuberosities.

Pad chair with pressure-relieving cushion.

Inspect areas at risk of developing ulcers with each position change.

Ears	Elbows	Occiput
Trochanter*	Heels*	Ischia
Sacrum	Scapula	Scrotum

Observe for erythema and blanching and palpate for warmth and tissue sponginess with each position change.

Do not rub reddened areas. To avoid damaging the capillaries, do not perform massage.

Malnourished State

Consult a dietitian.

Increase protein and carbohydrate intake to maintain a positive nitrogen balance; weigh the person daily and determine serum albumin level weekly to monitor status.

Ascertain that daily intake of vitamins and minerals is maintained through diet or supplements (see Key Concepts for recommended amounts).

See *Imbalanced Nutrition: Less Than Body Requirements* for additional interventions.

Sensory Deficit

Inspect person's skin daily, because he will not experience discomfort.

Teach person or family to inspect skin with mirror.

Initiate Health Teaching, as Indicated.

Instruct person and family in specific techniques to use at home to prevent pressure ulcers.

Consider the use of long-term pressure-relieving devices for permanent disabilities.

Rationales

- Pressure is a compressing downward force on a given area. If pressure against soft tissue is greater than intracapillary blood pressure (approximately 32 mm Hg), the capillaries can be occluded, and the tissue can be damaged as a result of hypoxia.
- Shear is a parallel force in which one layer of tissue moves in one direction and another layer moves in the opposite direction. If the skin sticks to the bed linen and the weight of the sitting body makes the skeleton slide down inside the skin, the subepidermal capillaries may become angulated and pinched, resulting in decreased perfusion of the tissue.
- Friction is the physiologic wearing away of tissue. If the skin is rubbed against the bed linens, the epidermis can be denuded by abrasion.
- Maceration is a mechanism by which the tissue is softened by prolonged wetting or soaking. If the skin becomes waterlogged, the cells are weakened and the epidermis is easily eroded.

---

*Areas with little soft tissue over a body prominence are at greatest risk.

- Pressure reduction is the one consistent intervention that must be included in all pressure ulcer treatment plans.
- A pressure-reducing surface must not be able to be fully compressed by the body. To be effective, a support surface must be capable of first being deformed and then redistributing the weight of the body across the surface. Comfort is not a valid criterion for determining adequate pressure reduction. A hand check should be performed to determine if the product is effectively reducing pressure. The palm is placed under the pressure-reducing mattress; if the client can feel the hand or the caregiver can feel the client, the pressure is not adequate (AHCPR, 1992; Bergstrom et al., 1994).
- Adequate nutrition (protein, vitamins, minerals) is vital for healing wounds, preventing infection, preserving immune function, and minimizing loss of strength (Maklebust & Sieggreen, 2000).

IMPAIRED SKIN INTEGRITY

RELATED TO THE EFFECTS OF PRESSURE, FRICTION, SHEAR, MACERATION

Goal

NOC See *Impaired Skin Integrity*

The person will demonstrate progressive healing of dermal ulcer.

Indicators

- Identify causative factors for pressure ulcers.
- Identify rationale for prevention and treatment.
- Participate in the prescribed treatment plan to promote wound healing.

General Interventions

NIC See *Impaired Skin Integrity*

Identify the Stage of Pressure Ulcer Development (AHCPR, 1992).
Stage I: Nonblanchable erythema of intact skin
Stage II: Ulceration of epidermis and/or dermis
Stage III: Ulceration involving subcutaneous fat
Stage IV: Extensive ulceration penetrating muscle, bone, or supporting structure

Reduce or Eliminate Factors that Contribute to the Extension of Pressure Ulcers; Refer to *Risk for Impaired Skin Integrity Related to Immobility.*

Prevent Deterioration of the Ulcer.
Wash reddened area gently with mild soap, rinse area thoroughly to remove soap, and pat dry.
Avoid massage of bony prominence to stimulate circulation.
Protect the healthy skin surface with one or a combination of the following:
    Apply a thin coat of liquid copolymer skin sealant.
    Cover area with moisture-permeable film dressing.
    Cover area with a hydrocolloid wafer barrier and secure with strips of 1-inch tape; leave in place for 2 to 3 days.
Increase dietary intake to promote wound healing.
    Initiate calorie count. Consult dietitian.

Increase protein and carbohydrate intake to maintain a positive nitrogen balance. Weigh daily and determine serum albumin level weekly to monitor status.

Ascertain that client maintains daily intake of vitamins and minerals through diet or supplements (see Key Concepts for recommended amounts).

See *Imbalanced Nutrition: Less Than Body Requirements* for additional interventions.

Devise Plan for Pressure Ulcer Management Using Principles of Moist Wound Healing (Maklebust & Sieggreen, 2000).

Assess status of pressure ulcer. (Bates-Jensen, 1990).*

Assess size—measure longest and widest wound surface.

Assess depth:

- No break in skin
- Abrasion or shallow crater
- Deep crater
- Necrosis
- Involved tendon, joint capsule

Assess edges.

- Attached
- Not attached
- Fibrotic

Assess undermining:

- <2 cm
- 2 to 4 cm
- >4 cm
- Tunneling

Assess necrotic tissue type (color, consistency, adherence) and amount.

Assess exudate type and amount.

Assess surrounding skin color.

Check for any peripheral edema and induration.

Assess for granulation tissue.

Assess for epithelialization.

Débride necrotic tissue (collaborate with physician).

Flush ulcer base with sterile saline solution. Avoid use of harsh antiseptic solutions.

Protect granulating wound bed from trauma and bacteria. Insulate wound surface.

Cover pressure ulcer with a sterile dressing that maintains a moist environment over the ulcer base (eg, film dressing, hydrocolloid wafer dressing, moist gauze dressing). Do not occlude ulcers on immunocompromised patients.

Avoid the use of drying agents (heat lamps, Maalox, Milk of Magnesia).

Monitor for clinical signs of wound infection.

Measure pressure ulcer weekly to determine progress of wound healing.

Consult with Nurse Specialist or Physician for Treatment of Necrotic, Infected, or Deep Pressure Ulcers.

Initiate Health Teaching and Referrals, as Indicated.

Instruct person and family on care of ulcers.

Teach the importance of good skin hygiene and optimal nutrition.

Refer to community nursing agency if additional assistance at home is needed.

Rationales

- See Rationale for *Impaired Skin Integrity*.
- Wound healing occurs most efficiently with the following extrinsic factors (Maklebust & Sieggreen, 2000):
  - Humidity affects the rate of epithelialization and the amount of scar formation. A moist environment provides optimal conditions for rapid healing.
  - When wounds are left uncovered, epidermal cells must migrate under the scab and over the fibrous tissue below. When wounds are semioccluded and the surface of the wound remains moist, epidermal cells migrate more rapidly over the surface.

*Refer to citation for the complete Pressure Sore Status tool and directions for scoring.

- Appropriate use of dressings may promote moist wound. Use of semiocclusive film dressings or hydrocolloid barrier wafers mechanically protect and properly humidify wounds that are epidermal or dermal. These dressings bathe the wound in serous exudate and do not adhere to the wound surface when they are removed. A physician's order may be required.
- Rationales for topical treatment (Maklebust & Sieggreen, 2000) are as follows:
  - Remove necrotic tissue, which delays wound healing by prolonging the inflammatory phase.
  - Cleanse wound bed to decrease bacterial count. Bacterial counts above 10^5 may produce infection by overwhelming the host.
  - Obliterate dead space in wound, which prevents premature closure and abscess formation.
  - Absorb excess exudate, which macerates surrounding skin and increases risk of infection in wound bed.
  - Maintain a moist wound surface, which promotes cellular migration. Dry wound surfaces delay epithelialization secondary to difficult cellular migration.
  - Insulate the wound surface; this enhances blood flow and increases epidermal migration.
  - Protect the healing wound from trauma and bacterial invasion. Open wounds are vulnerable to abrasion, contamination, drying, and shear mechanisms.

IMPAIRED ORAL MUCOUS MEMBRANE

DEFINITION

Impaired Oral Mucous Membrane: State in which a person experiences or is at risk for disruptions in the oral cavity

DEFINING CHARACTERISTICS
Major (Must Be Present)

Disrupted oral mucous membranes

Minor (May Be Present)

Coated tongue	Leukoplakia	Xerostomia (dry mouth)
Edema	Stomatitis	Hemorrhagic gingivitis
Taste changes	Purulent drainage	

RELATED FACTORS
Pathophysiologic

Related to inflammation secondary to:

Diabetes mellitus	Periodontal disease	Oral cancer
Infection		

Treatment-Related

Related to drying effects of:

NPO more than 24 h
Radiation to head or neck
Prolonged use of steroids or other immunosuppressives
Use of antineoplastic drugs

Related to mechanical irritation secondary to:

Endotracheal tube	NG tube

Situational (Personal, Environmental)

Related to chemical irritants secondary to:

Acidic foods
Alcohol

Drugs
Tobacco

Noxious agents

Related to mechanical trauma secondary to:

Broken or jagged teeth

Ill-fitting dentures

Braces

Related to malnutrition
Related to dehydration
Related to mouth breathing
Related to inadequate oral hygiene
Related to lack of knowledge of oral hygiene
Related to decreased salivation

○○ **AUTHOR'S NOTE**

See *Impaired Tissue Integrity.*

○○ **ERRORS IN DIAGNOSTIC STATEMENTS**

See *Impaired Tissue Integrity.*

KEY CONCEPTS
Generic Considerations

- Oral health directly influences many activities of daily living (eating, fluid intake, breathing) and interpersonal relations (appearance, self-concept, communication).
- Many oral diseases begin quietly and are painless until significant involvement has taken place.
- Common causes of decreased salivation are dehydration, anemia, radiation treatment to head and neck, vitamin deficiencies, removal of salivary glands, allergies, and side effects of drugs (eg, antihistamines, anticholinergics, phenothiazine, narcotics, chemotherapy).
- Excessive use of hydrogen peroxide for mouth care may predispose client to an oral yeast infection. Rinse afterward with normal saline (Kemp & Brackett, 2001).
- Lemon and glycerin swabs should be used only on clean, healthy mouths as a source of refreshment for an NPO client.
- Alcohol and tobacco are chronic irritants to oral mucosa and may lead to oral carcinoma.
- Stomatitis and mucositis denote inflammation and ulceration of the oral cavity. Stomatitis is associated with chemotherapy; mucositis is associated with radiation therapy. Mucositis refers to any oral mucosal inflammation, regardless of cause. It may progress from dry, red, inflamed, cracked areas to open sores of the mucosa and bleeding ulcers anywhere in the mouth, esophagus, vagina, or rectum. Mucous membranes are highly susceptible to toxicity because of their rapidly proliferating cells. Persons exposed to multiple therapies or who have predisposing risk factors such as poor oral hygiene, dental caries, and tobacco or alcohol use are more likely to develop mucositis. Stomatitis usually begins 2 to 5 days after chemotherapy; mucositis usually occurs 1 to 2 weeks after radiation therapy.
- Chemotherapy or direct radiation also can cause xerostomia, which is a decrease in the quality and quantity of saliva (Beck, 2001).

Pediatric Considerations

- Oral candidiasis (thrush) is common in newborns. It can be acquired by person-to-person transmission, from a maternal vaginal infection during delivery, or from use of contaminated nipples or other articles (Wong, 2003).
- Teething may cause discomfort and make gums appear red and swollen.

⊙ Geriatric Considerations

- Age-related changes in oral mucosa include loss of elasticity, atrophy of epithelial cells, and diminished blood supply to connective tissue (Miller, 2004).
- Dry mouth and vitamin deficiencies in older adults increase vulnerability to oral ulcerations and infection (Miller, 2004).
- Older adults commonly exhibit increased saliva viscosity and diminished saliva quantity (Miller, 2004).

Focus Assessment Criteria

Subjective Data

Assess for Defining Characteristics.

Complaints of

Mouth pain, irritation, burning, or dryness

Bad taste or odor in mouth

Change in tolerance to temperature of food (cold, hot)

Change in tolerance to acidic or highly seasoned food

Inability to eat, drink, or swallow own saliva

Xerostomia (dry mouth)

Chewing difficulties

Change in taste

Poorly fitting dentures

Assess for Related Factors.

History

Medical/surgical

Medication use (prescribed, over-the-counter)

Use of tobacco

Type (cigarettes, pipe, cigars, snuff)

Frequency (packs per day, how many years)

Use of alcohol

Type

Amount (daily, weekly)

Oral hygiene

Frequency of dental checkups

Personal hygiene

"Describe your oral care procedure."

Type of equipment (brush, floss)

Frequency

Possible barriers to performing oral care

Cannot hold standard brush

Cannot close hand

Limited arm movement

Semicomatose

Lack of knowledge

Nutritional status (Refer to *Imbalanced Nutrition* for specific assessment criteria.)

Daily intake of basic five food groups

Daily fluid intake

Difficulty in chewing or swallowing

Are certain foods avoided? Why?

Objective Data

Assess for Defining Characteristics.

Lips

Color	Cracks	Blisters
Fissures	Ulcers/lesions	

Tongue

Color	Masses	Cracks, dryness

Lesions	Exudates	Hairy extensions
Blisters		

Oral mucosa (gums, floor of mouth, inner cheeks, palate)

Color	Moisture	Bleeding
Plaques	Swelling (along gum line)	Lesions (red, white patches)

Saliva

Watery	Absent	Thick
Color		

Assess for Related Factors.

Teeth

Sharp edges	Looseness	Chips
Missing teeth	Cracks	

Dentures/prosthetics

Condition	Fit	Sharp edges
Cracks	Loose parts	Chips

For more information on Focus Assessment Criteria, visit http://connection.lww.com .

Goal

 NOC Oral Tissue Integrity, Oral Health

The person will be free of oral mucosa irritation or exhibit signs of healing with decreased inflammation.

Indicators

- Describe factors that cause oral injury.
- Demonstrate knowledge of optimal oral hygiene.

General Interventions

NIC Oral Health Restoration, Chemotherapeutic Management, Oral Health Maintenance

Assess for Causative or Contributing Factors.

Poor oral hygiene, pre-existing dental problems
Malnourishment
History of heavy alcohol intake and tobacco use
Chemotherapeutic drugs with mucous membrane toxicity
Radiation to head or neck
Immunosuppression
Dehydration
Steroid therapy
Antibiotics

Teach Preventive Oral Hygiene to Clients at Risk for Development of Stomatitis.

Refer to *Impaired Oral Mucous Membrane Related to Inadequate Oral Hygiene* for Specific Instructions on Brushing and Flossing.

Instruct client to:

Perform the regimen after meals and before sleep (if exudate is excessive, perform regimen before breakfast also).
Avoid mouthwashes with high alcohol content, lemon/glycerin swabs, or prolonged use of hydrogen peroxide.
Rinse mouth with flavored saline solution.
Apply lubricant to lips every 2 h and PRN (eg, lanolin, A&D ointment, petroleum jelly).
Inspect mouth daily for lesions and inflammation and report alterations.

Teach Person Who Cannot Tolerate Brushing or Swabbing to Irrigate Mouth (Every 2 h and PRN).

With normal saline, use an enema bag (labeled for oral use only) with a soft irrigation catheter tip.

Place catheter tip in mouth and slowly increase flow while standing over a basin or having a basin held under chin.

Remove dentures before irrigation and do not replace in person with severe stomatitis.

Consult with Physician for Possible Need of Prophylactic Antifungal or Antibacterial Agent for Clients at Risk for Radiation-Induced Stomatitis (Beck, 2001).

Instruct client to see a dentist 2 to 3 weeks before therapy begins for diagnosis and treatment of infections and to ensure adequate time for healing.

Consult with dentist for a regimen of daily fluoride treatments and oral hygiene.

Instruct client to see a dentist during treatment as needed and 2 months after treatment.

Promote Healing and Reduce Progression of Stomatitis.

Inspect oral cavity three times daily with tongue blade and light; if stomatitis is severe, inspect mouth every 4 h.

Ensure that oral hygiene regimen is done every 2 h while awake and every 6 h (every 4 h if severe) during the night.

Use normal saline solution as a mouthwash.

Floss teeth only once in 24 h.

Omit flossing if bleeding is excessive; use extreme caution with people with platelet counts less than 50,000.

Reduce Oral Pain and Maintain Adequate Food and Fluid Intake.

Assess person's ability to chew and swallow.

Administer mild analgesic every 3 to 4 h as ordered by physician.

Instruct client to:

    Avoid commercial mouthwashes, citrus fruit juices, spicy foods, extremes in food temperature (hot, cold), crusty or rough foods, alcohol, mouthwashes with alcohol.

    Eat bland, cool foods (sherbets).

    Drink cool liquids every 2 h and PRN.

Consult with dietitian for specific interventions.

Refer to *Impaired Nutrition: Less Than Body Requirements related to anorexia* for additional interventions.

Consult with physician for an oral pain relief solution.

    Xylocaine Viscous 2% oral, swish and expectorate every 2 h and before meals (if throat is sore, the solution can be swallowed; if swallowed, Xylocaine produces local anesthesia and may affect the gag reflex).

    Mix equal parts of Xylocaine Viscous, 0.5 aqueous Benadryl solution, and Maalox, swish and swallow 1 oz of mixture every 2 to 4 h PRN.

    Mix equal parts of 0.5 aqueous Benadryl solution and Kaopectate; swish and swallow every 2 to 4 h PRN.

Initiate Health Teaching and Referrals, as Indicated.

Teach person and family the factors that contribute to stomatitis and its progression.

Teach diet modifications to reduce oral pain and to maintain optimal nutrition.

Have client describe or demonstrate home care regimen.

Rationales

- The frequency of oral health maintenance varies according to a person's health status and self-care ability. All clients should have their teeth and mouths cleaned at least once after meals and at bedtime. High-risk clients (eg, NG tubes, cancer, poorly nourished) should have oral assessments daily. Clients in chronic care settings should have oral assessment at least once a week.
- Decreased salivary flow and increased viscosity of saliva reduce the removal of debris (food, bacteria) from the mouth (Kemp & Brackett, 1997).
- Factors that contribute to stomatitis are poor oral hygiene, pre-existing oral disease, irritants (spicy foods, citrus fruits, coarse foods [hard bread, pizza], ill-fitting dental prostheses, too-cold or too-hot foods, tobacco or alcohol), dehydration, malnutrition, and drug therapy (antibiotics, steroids; Beck, 1996).
- Proper hydration must be maintained to liquefy secretions and prevent drying of oral mucosa.
- Dry oral mucosa causes discomfort and increases the risk of breakdown and infection.
- Sodium bicarbonate neutralizes acidity and decreases redness (Kemp & Brackett, 1997).

RISK FOR IMPAIRED ORAL MUCOUS MEMBRANE

RELATED TO INADEQUATE ORAL HYGIENE OR INABILITY TO PERFORM ORAL HYGIENE

Goal

NOC Refer to *Impaired Oral Mucous Membrane*

The person will demonstrate integrity of the oral cavity.

Indicators
- Be free of harmful plaque to prevent secondary infection.
- Be free of oral discomfort during food and fluid intake.
- Demonstrate optimal oral hygiene.

General Interventions

NIC Refer to *Impaired Oral Mucous Membrane*

Assess for Causative or Contributing Factors.
Lack of knowledge
Lack of motivation
Impaired ability to use hands
Fatigue
Altered consciousness

Discuss the Importance of Daily Oral Hygiene and Periodic Dental Examinations.
Explain the relationship of plaque to dental and gum disease.
Evaluate person's ability to perform oral hygiene.
Allow person to perform as much oral care as possible.

Teach Correct Oral Care.

Have Person Sit or Stand Upright Over Sink (If He or She Cannot Get to a Sink, Place an Emesis Pan Under the Chin).

Remove and Clean Dentures and Bridges Daily.
Fill wash bowl half full of water (place washcloth on bottom to keep denture from breaking if dropped).
Brush dentures with a denture brush or stiff, hard toothbrush inside and outside; rinse in cool water before replacing.
Remove stains and odors from dentures by soaking them overnight in 8 oz of water and 1 tsp of laundry bleach (avoid bleach on any appliance with metal).
Remove hard deposits by soaking dentures in white (not brown) vinegar overnight.
Commercial liquid denture cleaners still require brushing.

Floss Teeth (Every 24 h).
With a piece of dental floss approximately 25 inches long, floss each tooth by wrapping the floss around the second and third fingers of each hand.
Begin with the back teeth; insert the floss between each tooth gently to avoid injuring the gum.
Wrap floss around tooth, making a C, and gently pull floss up and down over the back of each tooth.
Repeat this in reverse to floss the front of the tooth.
Remove the floss either by pulling straight up or by releasing one end and pulling the floss through (minor bleeding may occur).
Rinse.
Floss holders can make flossing easier (back teeth cannot be reached with a floss holder).

Brush Teeth (After Meals and Before Sleep).

Use a soft toothbrush (avoid hard brushes) with a nonabrasive toothpaste or sodium bicarbonate (1 tsp in 8 oz of water; may be contraindicated in people with sodium restrictions).

Brush back and forth or in a small circle, starting at the back of the mouth and brushing one or two teeth at a time.

Gently brush tongue and inner sides of cheeks.

Rinse with water.

Inspect Mouth for Lesions, Sores, or Excessive Bleeding.

Perform Oral Hygiene on Person Who Is Unconscious or at Risk for Aspiration as Often as Needed.

Preparation

Tell person what you are going to do.

Turn person on the side, supporting the back with a pillow (protect bed with an absorbent pad).

Place a tongue blade or bite block to keep mouth open.

Wear gloves to protect self.

Brushing Procedure

For people with their own teeth, brush following the procedure outlined above. Instead of toothpaste, use hydrogen peroxide and water (1 : 4), sodium bicarbonate (1 tsp : 8 oz water), or normal saline solution (may be contraindicated in people with sodium restrictions).

For people with dentures, remove dentures and clean as above. Leave dentures out for people who are semicomatose and store in water (in denture cup).

If gums are inflamed, use moist cotton-tipped applicators or soft foam Toothettes.

Use a bulb syringe to rinse mouth; aspirate rinse with suction or use an aspirating toothbrush.

Move tongue blade or bite block for access to other areas; do not put fingers on tops or edges of teeth.

Brush tongue and inner cheek tissue gently.

Pat mouth dry and apply lip lubricant.

Lightly wipe gums and teeth four to six times a day to prevent drying (eg, swab with mineral oil or saline, but use sparingly to prevent aspiration).

Initiate Health Teaching and Referrals, as Indicated.

Identify Clients Who Need Toothbrush Adaptations to Perform Own Mouth Care.

For clients with difficulty closing hands tightly (Danielson, 1988), tape a wide elastic band to toothbrush tightly enough so client can hold brush snugly in hand.

For clients with limited hand mobility, enlarge toothbrush handle with a sponge hair roller, wrinkled aluminum foil, or a bicycle handlebar grip attached with a small amount of plaster of Paris.

For clients with limited arm movement, extend handle of standard toothbrush by attaching handle of an old toothbrush (after cutting off bristle end) to a new toothbrush with strong cord or plastic cement, or by attaching toothbrush to a plastic rod (the toothbrush can be curved by gently heating and then bending it).

Refer Clients with Tooth and Gum Disorders to a Dentist.

Rationales

- Refer also to *Impaired Oral Mucous Membrane.*
- Factors that contribute to oral disease are excessive use of alcohol and tobacco, microorganisms, inadequate nutrition (quantity, quality), inadequate hygiene, and trauma (NG tubes, ill-fitting dentures, sharp-edged teeth, sharp-edged prostheses, improper use of cleaning devices).
- Plaque, microbial flora found in the mouth, is the primary cause of dental cavities and periodontal disease. Daily removal of plaque through brushing and flossing can help prevent dental decay and disease.

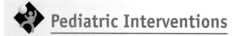 **Pediatric Interventions**

Teach Parents to:

Provide their child with fluoride supplements if not present in concentrations over 0.7 parts per million (ppm) in drinking water.

Avoid taking tetracycline drugs during pregnancy or giving them to children younger than 8 years.

Refrain from putting an infant to bed with a bottle of juice or milk.
Provide child with safe objects for chewing during teething.
Replace toothbrushes frequently (every 3 months).
Schedule dental checkups every 6 months after 2 years of age.
Supervise and assist preschool child with brushing and flossing in front of mirror.
   Talk to child when brushing.
   "Ask child to 'tweet like a bird' to brush front teeth and 'roar like a lion' to brush back teeth"
      (Wong, 2003).
   Incorporate brushing and flossing teeth into bedtime rituals.

Teach Child:

Why tooth care is important
To avoid highly sugared liquids, foods, and chewing gum
To drink water and extra fluid
To brush teeth using fluoride toothpaste

Rationales

- The objective of oral hygiene is to remove plaque, which causes decay and periodontal disease (Wong, 2003).
- Flossing removes plaque from gum line.
- Fluoride makes enamel more resistant to caries by decreasing the effects of acid on surface (Wong, 2003).

Maternal Interventions

Stress the importance of good oral hygiene and continued dental examinations. Advise woman to
   increase intake of vitamin C.
Remind client to advise dentist of her pregnancy.
Explain that gum hypertrophy and tenderness are normal during pregnancy.

Rationales

Gum hypertrophy, tenderness, and bleeding during normal pregnancy may be the result of vascular swelling called *epulis of pregnancy* (Pillitteri, 2003).

Geriatric Interventions

Explain High-Risk Age-Related Factors (Miller, 2004).

Degenerative bone disease	Diminished oral blood supply
Dry mouth	Vitamin deficiencies

Explain That Some Medications Cause Dry Mouth.

Laxatives	Antibiotics	Antidepressants
Anticholinergics	Analgesics	Iron sulfate
Cardiovascular medications		

Determine any Barriers to Dental Care.

Financial	Mobility	Dexterity
Lack of knowledge		

Rationales

Age-related changes and nutritional deficiencies increase vulnerability to oral ulcerations and infection (Miller, 2004).

RELOCATION STRESS [SYNDROME]

DEFINITION

Relocation Stress [Syndrome]: State in which a person experiences physiologic and/or psychological disturbances as a result of transfer from one environment to another.

Other terms found in the literature that describe relocation stress include admission stress, post-relocation crisis, relocation crisis, relocation shock, relocation trauma, transfer stress, transfer trauma, translocation syndrome, and transplantation shock.

DEFINING CHARACTERISTICS*
Major (80% to 100%)

Responds to transfer or relocation with

Loneliness	Depression	Anger
Apprehension	Anxiety	

Increased confusion (older adult population)

Minor (50% to 79%)

Change in former eating habits	Decrease in self-care activities
Change in former sleep patterns	Decrease in leisure activities
	Gastrointestinal disturbances
Demonstration of dependency	Increased verbalization of needs
Demonstration of insecurity	Need for excessive reassurance
Demonstration of lack of trust	Restlessness
Vigilance	Withdrawal
Weight change	Allergic symptoms
Sad affect	

Unfavorable comparison of post-transfer to pretransfer staff
Verbalization of being concerned/upset about transfer
Verbalization of insecurity in new living situation

RELATED FACTORS
Pathophysiologic

Related to compromised ability to adapt to changes secondary to:
Decreased physical health status
  Physical difficulties
Decreased psychosocial health status
  Increased/perceived stress before relocation
  Depression
  Decreased self-esteem

---

*Harkulich, J., & Brugler, C. (1988). *Nursing diagnosis—translocation syndrome: Expert validation study.* Partial funding granted by the Peg Schlitz Fund, Delta Xi Chapter, Sigma Theta Tau International; Barnhouse, A. (1987). *Development of the nursing diagnosis of translocation syndrome with critical care patients.* Unpublished master's thesis, Kent State University, Kent, OH.

Situational (Personal, Environmental)
Related to moderate to high degree of environmental change in new environment secondary to:
Loss of privacy
Decreased control of individual care
Decrease and/or change in available caregivers
Decrease/increase in client-monitoring equipment
Increased noise/activities in post-transfer environment
Decreased privacy as a result of changes in lifestyle

Related to concurrent, recent, and past interpersonal losses secondary to:
Negative experiences dealing with earlier separation(s) (for adults as well as children)
Loss of social and familial ties
Abandonment
Perceived/actual rejection by caregivers
Anticipation of lengthy and/or permanent stay in new environment
Threat to financial security
Change in relationship with family members

Related to little or no preparation for the impending move
Lack of predictability in new environment
Little or no time between when the person is notified of an impending move and the actual move
Unrealistic expectations of individual/family members regarding facility and staff
Lack of decision making and control on behalf of the person who is moving

Maturational
School-Aged Children and Adolescents
Related to losses associated with moving secondary to:
Fear of rejection, loss of peer group or school-related problems
Decreased security in new adolescent peer group and school

ⓓ AUTHOR'S NOTE

NANDA has accepted *Relocation Stress* as a syndrome diagnosis. It does not fit the criterion for a syndrome diagnosis, which is a cluster of actual or risk nursing diagnoses as defining characteristics. The defining characteristics associated with *Relocation Stress* are observable or reportable cues consistent with *Relocation Stress,* not *Relocation Stress Syndrome.* The author recommends deleting "Syndrome" from the label.

Relocation represents a disruption for all parties involved. It can accompany a transfer from one unit to another, or from one facility to another. It can involve a permanent move to a long-term care facility or new home. The relocation disturbs all age groups involved. When physiologic and psychological disturbances compromise functioning, the nursing diagnosis *Relocation Stress [Syndrome]* is appropriate.

The optimal nursing approach to relocation stress is to initiate preventive measures using *Risk for Relocation Stress* as the diagnosis.

ⓓ ERRORS IN DIAGNOSTIC STATEMENTS

Relocation Stress related to apprehension and sadness associated with impending family move
Apprehension and sadness are appropriate responses for children involved in a family move. Adolescents specifically are very disrupted because of peer relationships. Apprehension and sadness are not related factors but manifestations. The nurse should write the diagnosis as *Relocation Stress related to effects of family move on peer relationships, as evidenced by statements of apprehension and sadness.*

KEY CONCEPTS
Generic Considerations

- The process of relocation represents a transition for all involved parties (Miller, 1995; Puskar, 1986).
- Annually, 20% of all people in the United States either choose or are forced to relocate (Puskar & Rohay, 1999).
- Relocation stress can accompany any type of move. Types include previous home to new home (house, apartment); home to institution (hospital, long-term care nursing facility); institution to home (especially after an extended illness); moves within an institution (from one bed to another in the same room; from one room to another on the same unit/floor; from one room to another on different units/floors); and moves between institutions (hospital to long-term care facility, one long-term nursing care facility to another).
- Relocation stress typically occurs shortly before and after the move. Not all relocated people experience relocation stress, because the related factors are not present to the same degree in all those experiencing relocation.
- When a move results from a husband's change of employment, a relocated husband often finds satisfaction with his new job. The relocated wife seeks new neighbors, friends, home, and community activities as a primary source of satisfaction. If previously employed, she often feels isolated over the unavailability of jobs in the new environment (Puskar, 1990). Relocated wives who coped well demonstrated active behaviors (problem solving, support seeking from family and friends, volunteer activities); wives who coped poorly showed passive behaviors (eating, sleeping, crying, watching television, becoming angry at self and others; Puskar, 1990).
- Relocation stress has been compared to separation anxiety as a result of separation from monitors and nurse and physician surveillance, which results in an inability to cope.
- Houser (1974) reported the following in a study of 12 clients transferred from a coronary care unit: 6 of 12 people required readmission for cardiovascular complications, and 5 of the 6 had a high anxiety rating when transferred. Those who did not discuss their feelings were most likely to experience complications after transfer. After instituting a program aimed at reducing transfer stress, clients had fewer complications, and observed complications were less dangerous than those that the control group experienced.
- The incidence of psychophysiologic responses to relocation stress was higher for clients transferred during the afternoon and evening than for those transferred in the morning (Lethbridge et al., 1976).
- In their study of 177 clients with myocardial infarction in six hospitals, Minckley et al. (1979) found that:
  - The duration for which the client had been notified of the transfer was related inversely to the need for reassurance.
  - Clients with abnormal blood pressure readings on admission to the coronary care unit were at higher risk for negative effects of transfer.
  - Women had more physiologic indicators of stress with relocation than did men.
- Clients as well as families were found to be very anxious about transfer from an intensive care unit (ICU).
- During interviews of 15 parents of premature infants transferred between Level 1, 2, and 3 nurseries and home, McDonald Gibbins, and Chapman (1996) documented the following parental responses:
  - Sources of parental stress included lack of information about their infants' condition and events of the transfer between units and discharge home, insecurity about their own comfort in a new unit, inconsistencies in care within the different nurseries, and dependency on particular caregivers within the neonatal intensive care unit (NICU).
  - Parents had ambivalent feelings about transfer from a NICU (Level 3 nursery) to an intermediate care unit (Level 2 nursery). Parents also became more judgmental about the NICU care near the time of transfer to the Level 2 nursery and rationalized the transfer from the NICU.
- Forty-one mothers of infants transferred from a tertiary-care NICU to a community hospital nursery reported mild to moderate stress with the transfer and perceived the transfer as fairly positive. The higher the mothers viewed the quality of the transfer, the less stress they reported with this transfer (Flanagan et al., 1996).
- Clients who are more dependent are more likely to experience negative effects with relocation than clients who are less dependent (Adshead et al., 1991).
- Physically frail clients are more accident-prone in a new environment than are more physically adept clients (Adshead et al., 1991).
- For many clients with severe and chronic mental illness, involuntary transfers "exacerbate their feelings of defeat and their sense that there was nothing helpful about the transfer" (Osborne et al., 1990, p. 226).

◆ Pediatric Considerations

- When families need to relocate, their social attachment systems may be disrupted, thus producing slight changes in health status, daily functioning, and loneliness (Puskar, 1986).
- Because of age and maturation, children of different ages experience relocation in different ways.
- A relocated child's stress and frustration may lead to aggression, withdrawal, and deterioration in schoolwork, which may lead to future adjustment problems if the child is not well socialized in the new environment.
- Relocated children and adults may experience pains of past separations, which may arouse feelings of insecurity (Puskar & Dvorsak, 1991).
- When relocated, toddlers and preschoolers often demonstrate changes in eating and sleeping patterns along with minor disabilities (Puskar & Dvorsak, 1991).
- Relocated adolescent boys may experience more difficulties with peers (diminished contact, rejection, teasing, meanness) in the new environment (Vernberg, 1990). Relocated adolescent girls, however, may verbalize more stress and loneliness (Raviv et al., 1990).
- The adolescent has a developmental task of becoming independent, which impedes relocation (Puskar & Rohay, 1999).

◉ Geriatric Considerations

- Reactions to relocation are related to the person's psychological resources before the move and the move's context. Findings from older women relocating to an independent location, but not their own private home, were as follows:
  - Women with a greater ability to manage the world to meet their needs, as well as with more pressure to relocate and more prerelocation autonomy, were less sad and aggravated after the move than was expected.
  - Women with less autonomy or personal growth before the move were less sad after the move than was expected if they also experienced many unexpected gains, such as ease in making friends and opportunities for involvement in activities (Smider et al., 1996).
- Relocating rural older adults frequently identified perceived choice, environmental predictability, and social support from family, residential neighbors, and friends as factors associated with positive adjustment (Armer, 1996).
- Relocation of older adults to long-term care facilities was not associated with increased mortality rates.
- Transition to nursing home life is a process that occurs over time and varies.
- Positive appraisal of relocation to a nursing home is associated with positive morale; a negative appraisal is associated with negative morale.
- Highly educated nursing home residents have been found to view relocation more negatively than less educated residents (Gass et al., 1992).
- Nursing home residents' view of relocation and later adaptation are reported to be related to psychological and physical health, prior and new support systems, morale, and functional independence (Beirne et al., 1995; Gass et al., 1992).
- Older adults may use a variety of coping strategies, ranging from aggressive anger to passive resignation, when relocated to a nursing home.
- Uncontrollable events in nursing home relocation generally stimulate emotion and cognitive-focused responses. Events that are at least somewhat controllable usually stimulate problem solving and positive coping strategies.
- Any nursing interventions related to relocation stress should reflect the resident's effective coping strategies.
- Clients may refuse nursing interventions to minimize relocation stress.
- Living in a nursing home has been shown to be a cause of suicide in older adults. The person at risk for suicide when relocating to a nursing home is depressed and hopeless, with decreased life satisfaction and psychological well-being, as well as anger at the loss of control over his or her own life.

(continued)

ⓒ Geriatric Considerations (continued)

- Lack of a confidante in a nursing home has been correlated with suicidal ideation. High self-esteem, arthritis, and a mean age of 85 years also have been found to be significant indicators of suicide risk in older adults in nursing homes (Haight, 1995).
- The greatest incidence of relocation stress typically occurs shortly before and up to 3 months after the move (Beirne et al., 1995; Reinardy, 1995).
- In a study conducted by Rodgers (1997), the process of nursing home placement began with families recognizing and ultimately accepting the need to admit their loved ones to a nursing home. Concerns over safety provided a means to justify, rather than an initial incentive to seek, the placement.
- Relocated long-term care residents with a diagnosis of cognitive impairment demonstrated decreased self-care and withdrawal 3 months after relocation.
- Long-term care residents very familiar with their environments (median length of stay of 36 months) were more prone to falls after a secondary relocation than those residents with a shorter length of stay (24 months; Lander et al., 1997).
- Some minimal familiarity with a nursing home before relocation (eg, having driven by it over the years; Reed et al., 1998) or viewing a video about the facility (Kaisik & Ceslowitz, 1996) made the move less threatening for older people. Also, proximity of a nursing home to the resident's previous home assisted residents in feeling continuity with their previous lifestyle and in developing new relationships with other residents from the same geographic area (Reed et al., 1998).
- An older couple experiences complex changes in their roles, relationships, life structure (routine, activities, and so forth), time management, support systems, and self-esteem when one spouse is admitted to a nursing home (Rosenkoetter, 1996).
- In a study of nursing home rehabilitation after acute rehabilitation, clients had favorable outcomes under the care of the same shared group of therapists between the two settings (Kosasih et al., 1998).
- Advance planning and preparation are critical for decreasing the stress of both the involved older adults and their families.
- Residents whose admission to a long-term care facility was unplanned experienced a longer phase of being overwhelmed (focus on self, emotional response, crying, and loneliness) than residents with a planned admission.

🌐 Transcultural Considerations

- Relocation stress is a transcultural phenomenon that occurs in all age groups. Of 33 nurses practicing in China, 100% reported that relocation stress exists; 23 nurses from 12 different countries also reported that relocation stress exists (Harkulich & Brugler, 1991).
- Israeli adolescents were found to experience relocation stress after moving (Raviv et al., 1990).
- Children from Sweden experiencing a 1-year international relocation significantly reduced their leisure activities, experienced a loss of identity, and developed a more negative attitude toward international assignments after the move. They also demonstrated significant increases in atopic sensitization and subjective symptoms of allergies, including dry skin, eczema, and prickling sensations after 1 year in the foreign country (Anderzén et al., 1997).
- Relocation did not pose adverse psychological effects when children from Armenia were relocated after a major earthquake. They were found to have similar levels of post-traumatic stress disorder and depression as children who remained in the disaster area (Najarian et al., 1996).
- In her Soviet Jewish resettlement experience, Hulewat (1996) identified three control concepts to address when families relocate internationally: stages of resettlement (splitting, actual migration, arrival in new home, decompensation, and transgenerational stage); cultural styles and psychological dynamics of the population being resettled; and individual family dynamics based on the ability to tolerate cultural dissonance and to manage the tasks necessary to proceed through the resettlement stages.

(continued)

> 🌐 **Transcultural Considerations (continued)**
>
> • Cultural beliefs regarding family obligations influence a person's relocation to a long-term care facility. For example, Lee (1997) reported that Chinese older adults view caregiving as part of family duty. Therefore, many of them equate admission to a residential care home with family rejection, powerlessness, and a devalued sense of self.

Focus Assessment Criteria

Subjective Data

Assess for Defining Characteristics.

The relocated person complains of:

Dissatisfaction with new environment	Increased family conflicts
	Loneliness
Problems adjusting	Loss of control
Feelings of insecurity	Anger at loss of control over own life
Anger toward people responsible for placement	

Changes in

Sleep patterns	Nutritional intake
Socialization	Cognition
Orientation	

Assess for Related Factors.

History of:

One or more changes in environment in last 3 months
Multiple moves in last 5 years
Traumatic experiences after previous moves
Being in the same environment for more than 40 years

Risk factors

Moderate to severe confusion/disorientation
Perceived poor health
Lack of support/family/friends/staff
Low self-esteem
Functional deterioration
Involuntary move
Communication difficulties
Lack of continuity of care
Expression of dissatisfaction with life
Lack of preparation for move(s)
Lack of choices or input on the part of the relocating person
Multiple chronic illnesses
Lack of familiarity with nursing home before relocation
Nursing home location far from previous residence

Objective Data

Assess for Defining Characteristics.

Change in weight	Sleep problems	Change in eating patterns
Increased medical visits	Change in cognition	Decline in self-care activities

For more information on Focus Assessment Criteria, visit http://connection.lww.com.

Goals

> **NOC** Anxiety Control, Coping, Loneliness, Psychosocial Adjustment: Life Change, Quality of Life

The person/family will:

• Report adjustment to the new environment without physiologic and/or psychological disturbances.

Indicators

- Share in decision-making activities regarding the new environment.
- Express concerns regarding the move to a new environment.
- Verbalize one positive aspect of the relocation.
- Establish new bonds in the new environment.
- Become involved in activities in the new environment.

General Interventions

 NIC Anxiety Reduction, Coping Enhancement, Counseling, Family Involvement Promotion, Support System Enhancement, Anticipatory Guidance, Family Integrity Promotion

Encourage Each Family Member to Share Feelings About the Move.

Provide privacy for each individual.

Encourage family members to share feelings with one another.

Discuss the possible and different effects of the move on each family member.

Inform parents regarding potential changes in children's conduct with relocation, such as regression, withdrawal, acting-out, and changes with eating (breast/bottle-feeding).

Instruct parents to obtain all pertinent documents regarding children's medical/dental history (eg, immunizations, communicable diseases, dental work).

Allow for some ritual(s) when leaving the old environment. Encourage reminiscing, which will bring closure for many family members.

Teach Parents Techniques to Assist Their Children with the Move.

Remain positive about the move before, during, and after, accepting that the child may not be optimistic.

Explore various options with children on how to communicate with friends/families in previous environment. Children's relationships with friends in the previous community are very important, especially for "peer reassurance" after relocation.

Keep regular routines in the new environment; establish them as soon as possible.

Acknowledge the difficulty of peer losses with the adolescent.

Join the organizations to which the child previously belonged (eg, Girl Scouts, sports).

Assist children to focus on similarities between old and new environments (eg, clubs, Scouts, church groups).

Plan a trip to school during a class and lunch period to reduce fear of unknown.

Allow children some choices regarding room arrangements, decorating, and the like.

Ask teacher or counselor at new school to introduce adolescent to a student who recently relocated to that school.

Allow children to mourn their losses as a result of the move.

Assess the Following Areas When Counseling a Relocated Adolescent: Perceptions About the Move; Concurrent Stressors; Usual and Present Coping Skills; and Family, Peers, and Community Support Groups.

Initiate Health Teaching and Referrals, as Indicated.

Alert family to the possible need for counseling before, during, or after the move.

Furnish a written directory of relevant community organizations such as area churches, children's groups, Parents Without Partners, senior citizens' groups, and Welcome Wagon or other local new-neighbor groups.

Instruct the family about appropriate community services.

Consult school nurse regarding school programs for new students.

Rationales

- Many researchers report that relocation stress is preventable (Lander et al., 1997). Therefore, eliminating and/or minimizing the causative, contributing, and risk factors can decrease the occurrence of relocation stress.
- Assessing individuals before relocation is important to identify those most at risk.
- Early relocation planning is paramount in ensuring a smooth transfer for all involved individuals.
- Children need early notification, predictability, and decision-making opportunities when an upcoming relocation is planned.
- Peer networks are important during adolescence because the relocated adolescent needs additional parental and peer reassurance.

RELOCATION STRESS

RELATED TO CHANGES ASSOCIATED WITH HEALTH CARE FACILITY TRANSFERS OR ADMISSION TO LONG-TERM CARE FACILITY

Goals

> **NOC** See also *Relocation Stress, Adaptation to New Environment*

The person will:

- Make positive statements about acceptance of the new environment and reasons for leaving the previous environment.
- Adjust to the new environment without physiologic and/or psychological disturbance.
- Establish new bonds in the new environment.
- Become involved in activities in the new environment.

Indicators

- Participate in decision-making activities regarding the new environment.
- Voice concerns regarding the move to a new environment.
- Describe realistic expectations of the new environment.

General Interventions

> **NIC** See also *Relocation Stress*

Prevention is Key. Strategize How Best to Prevent Stress for Each Person Before Relocation.

All staff members must be aware of and alert to the complex process of relocation for both the person and family before proactively decreasing stress factors (Maun, 1996; Morgan, 1996).

Assess for Factors that May Contribute to Relocation Stress (See Related Factors and Focus Assessment Criteria).

Reduce or Eliminate Causative and Contributing Factors.

Environmental Differences Between Old and New Settings/Minimal Continuity of Care in New Environment

Design a program to prepare relocated residents and staff for the move, orienting them to the physical layout many times until they feel familiar with the new environment.

Provide visual presentations (through bulletin boards, posters, letters, and so forth) and first-hand accounts of new environment for those who cannot view the area before relocation.

Seek input from former staff regarding client and plan of care.

Initially maintain client on same activity level and diet through pretransfer and post-transfer units.

Transfer person to similar, proximal area when possible.

Wean any monitoring equipment gradually before transfer.

Transfer all personal items with the person, such as mobility aids, eyeglasses, hearing aids, dentures, prostheses, and belongings.

Transfer person during daytime hours.

Maintain similar heights of furnishings/beds.

Clearly mark steps and other potential environmental hazards.

Maintain people in familiar groups at mealtimes and in living arrangements.

Promote a welcoming, warm, and clean receiving environment.

Allow time for discussions regarding living spaces in old and new environments.

Gradually decrease nursing attention before ICU transfer, when possible.

Involuntary Relocation/Lack of Control in Decision Making

Offer decision-making opportunities throughout relocation experience.

Promote person's input regarding new environment when possible, such as use of decorations and arrangement of furniture.

Present transfer from a critical care unit as an indicator of improvement.

Inform hospitalized person of signs of daily progress.

Transfer client in an unhurried manner.

Establish mutual goals before relocation to nursing home.

Provide opportunities for questions/answers with relocation preparation.

Hold regular staff/resident meetings after relocation, encouraging new members to be involved with the facility's rules and regulations (Wilson, 1997).

Include parents in the care of their hospitalized premature infant as much as possible.

Promote use of support systems both inside and outside the hospital for parents of hospitalized infants.

Recent or Concurrent Interpersonal Loss

Discuss adaptation to the relocation with family members.

Assess responses of all family members to the relocation.

Identify family members who may need additional help with adjustment.

Encourage family members to share their perceptions of relocation with one another.

Offer the person help in maintaining contact with significant others by telephone calls, letters, and visits with previous roommates when applicable.

Introduce person to nurse from post-transfer unit before transfer.

Accompany client to post-transfer unit.

Provide follow-up visit of nurse from pretransfer unit to person on post-transfer unit.

Encourage family members to visit person during and after relocation.

Minimize number of transfers in the health care facility.

Visit resident daily.

Promote formation of friendships in new environment.

Encourage family involvement in resident's care.

Visit person in own home before nursing home placement.

Support the client's efforts to adjust to the new environment.

Assist client to remember past relocations that were positive (Johnson & Hlava, 1994).

Provide gatherings for clients and staff experiencing closure of their facility (Craig, 1997).

Decreased Physical and/or Psychosocial State

Promote discussion of feelings regarding relocation.

Encourage use of problem-solving skills.

Offer potential solutions to problems when person cannot do so.

Promote sleep with use of previous bedtime routines, back rubs, white noise, music, warm milk, and minimization of noise in surrounding areas.

Encourage positive eating habits with use of favorite foods, a pleasant eating environment, and any appropriate supplements.

Orient the client fully to the new environment.

When possible, retain highly anxious person in pretransfer unit until anxiety decreases.

Provide for spiritual needs (eg, visit from clergy, hanging religious symbols in new location, transporting client to a religious ceremony).

Use cues such as signs and arrows for the relocated.

Assist person in learning to view the relocation more positively.

Teach/mobilize coping strategies.

Reassess relocation perceptions periodically.

Residents diagnosed with pneumonia have more effective outcomes when treated at the nursing home compared with those who were hospitalized (Fried et al., 1997).

Reduce the Physiologic Effects of Relocation (Refer to Key Concepts).

Assess Before Relocation:

Blood pressure, temperature	Respiratory function	Orientation
Signs of infection	Level of discomfort	

Identify Person at High Risk for Selected Physiologic Responses.

Musculoskeletal/neurologic deficits

Advanced age

Cardiovascular disorders

Changes in orientation

Cardiovascular complications (eg, ischemia, dysrhythmias)

Prevent or Reduce Confusion and Activity Intolerance.

Promote Integration After Transfer into a Long-Term Care Nursing Facility.

Allow as many choices as possible regarding physical surroundings and daily routines.

Encourage person or family to bring familiar objects from person's home.

Orient to physical layout of environment.

Introduce relocated individuals to new staff and fellow residents.

Encourage interaction with other people in new facility.

Assist client to maintain previous interpersonal relationships.

Clearly state smoking rules and orient client to areas where smoking is permitted.

Promote the development or maintenance of a relationship with a confidante.

Reestablish normal routines, while initially increasing staffing and lighting, when a large number of long-term care residents are involved in a secondary relocation.

Assist nursing home residents to meet people from their previous geographic area.

Arrange frequent contacts by a volunteer or staff member with each newly admitted resident.

  Also, match a successfully relocated resident with the new resident to begin the networking process.

Initiate Health Teaching and Referrals, as Indicated.

Prepare person for relocation.

  Notify him or her as early as possible to increase predictability regarding eventual relocation.

  Provide ongoing and structured teaching regarding:

    Characteristics of new environment

    Staff capabilities

    Mechanisms for continuity of care

    Rationale for relocation and less constant professional attention when applicable

    Expectations of person in new environment

    Any increasing stages of activity/independence

Include family in teaching.

Offer information about positive health habits and resources during illness.

Make appropriate professional referrals as needed, as well as suggesting a phone monitoring system such as "Lifeline."

Refer relocated families to community agencies related to newcomers and to mental health agencies when at risk for relocation stress syndrome.

Assess the perceptions of parents of hospitalized infants regarding an upcoming transfer and their interest in related information.

Maintain at least daily communication with parents about their hospitalized infant (eg, condition, timing of transfer, mechanisms for continuity of care between the pre- and post-transfer nurseries) and their concerns.

Suggest that parents of hospitalized infants visit the nursery where their child will be transferred before the event.

Develop and use a mechanism for a thorough exchange of information between pre- and post-transfer nurseries.

Rationales

- Open communication with older adults both before and after a move is necessary, assessing their experiences with change and adjustment, coping history and style, and decisional control.

- With the influx of people who have chronic mental illness into the community, it is important that their needs and problems be assessed accurately so interventions and services that ensure successful relocation and adjustment can be planned and implemented.
- Before nursing home placement of a loved one, family members should be assessed regarding their perceptions of this decision. Areas of conflict and vulnerability can serve as the foci for family-centered nursing interventions.
- Minor changes between intrainstitutional settings may be challenging for relocating people within the context of decreased behavioral competence and few remaining opportunities to exercise autonomy—the loss of any opportunity could be critical.
- Wilson (1997) and Meacham and Brandriet (1997) found older adults made an effort to protect their significant others by hiding their feelings about relocation and attempting to maintain a sense of normalcy. Therefore, it is critical for new residents to develop trusting relationships with others to discuss the stressors of relocation.
- Case management by way of telephone calls to residents or family members and prompt attention to resident problems after nursing home admission can help to prevent adjustment problems.
- Parents of hospitalized infants frequently reported lack of information and communication with staff as sources of overall and relocation stress.
- The stress of a negative transfer from an NICU to a community hospital can affect parent–infant bonding adversely or increase stress regarding parental roles (Flanagan et al., 1996).
- Parents of preterm infants want to protect their child during hospitalization in addition to wanting to receive information about each new environment where their child will be transferred (McDonald Gibbins & Chapman, 1996).
- Gatherings for reminiscence and closure between clients and staff can assist them to move forward emotionally during a psychiatric hospital closure and relocation (Craig, 1997).
- Residents who were allowed choices regarding room location and favorite objects had an increased sense of control and less stress (Mitchell, 1999).
- Parents of children facing transfer from the ICU to a general unit who were given a verbal explanation 1 to 2 h before the transfer had significantly less anxiety than parents who were informed immediately before the transfer (Miles, 1999).

Risk for Ineffective Respiratory Function*
  Related to Allergic Response
Dysfunctional Ventilatory Weaning Response
Risk for Dysfunctional Ventilatory Weaning Response
Ineffective Airway Clearance
Ineffective Breathing Patterns
Impaired Gas Exchange
Impaired Spontaneous Ventilation

RISK FOR INEFFECTIVE RESPIRATORY FUNCTION

DEFINITION

Risk for Ineffective Respiratory Function (ARF): State in which a person is at risk of experiencing a threat to the passage of air through the respiratory tract and/or to the exchange of gases (O_2–CO_2) between the lungs and the vascular system

RISK FACTORS

Presence of risk factors that can change respiratory function (see Related Factors)

RELATED FACTORS
Pathophysiologic

Related to excessive or thick secretions secondary to:

Infection	Inflammation	Allergy
Cardiac or pulmonary disease	Smoking	

Related to immobility, stasis of secretions, and ineffective cough secondary to:

Diseases of the nervous system (eg, Guillain-Barré syndrome, multiple sclerosis, myasthenia gravis)
Central nervous system (CNS) depression/head trauma
Cerebrovascular accident (stroke)
Quadriplegia

Treatment-Related

Related to immobility secondary to:
Sedating effects of medications (specify)
Anesthesia, general or spinal

Related to suppressed cough reflex secondary to (specify)
Related to effects of tracheostomy (altered secretions)

Situational (Personal, Environmental)

Related to immobility secondary to:

Surgery or trauma	Fatigue	Pain
Perception/cognitive impairment	Fear	Anxiety

Related to extremely high or low humidity
For infants, related to placement on stomach for sleep
Exposure to cold, laughing, crying, allergens, smoke

---

*This diagnosis is not currently on the NANDA list but has been included for clarity or usefulness.

⟨⟨⟩⟩ **AUTHOR'S NOTE**

Nursing's many responsibilities associated with problems of respiratory function include identifying and reducing or eliminating risk (contributing) factors, anticipating potential complications, monitoring respiratory status, and managing acute respiratory dysfunction.

The author has added *Risk for Ineffective Respiratory Function* to describe a state that may affect the entire respiratory system, not just isolated areas, such as airway clearance or gas exchange. Allergy and immobility are examples of factors that affect the entire system; thus, it is incorrect to say *Impaired Gas Exchange related to immobility,* because immobility also affects airway clearance and breathing patterns. The nurse can use the diagnoses *Ineffective Airway Clearance* and *Ineffective Breathing Patterns* when nurses can definitely alleviate the contributing factors influencing respiratory function (eg, ineffective cough, stress).

The nurse is cautioned not to use this diagnosis to describe acute respiratory disorders, which are the primary responsibility of medicine and nursing together (ie, collaborative problems). Such problems can be labeled *PC: Acute hypoxia* or *PC: Pulmonary edema.* When a person's immobility is prolonged and threatens multiple systems—for example, integumentary, musculoskeletal, vascular, as well as respiratory—the nurse should use *Disuse Syndrome* to describe the entire situation.

⟨⟨⟩⟩ **ERRORS IN DIAGNOSTIC STATEMENTS**

1. *Ineffective Breathing Patterns related to respiratory compensation for metabolic acidosis*
   This diagnosis represents the respiratory pattern associated with diabetic ketoacidosis. Related nursing responsibilities would include monitoring, early detection of changes, and rapid initiation of nursing and medical interventions. This does not represent a situation for which nurses diagnose and are accountable to prescribe treatment. Rather, the collaborative problem *PC: Ketoacidosis* would represent the nursing accountability for the situation.
2. *Ineffective Airway Clearance related to mucosal edema and loss of ciliary action secondary to thermal injury*
   After sustaining burns of the upper airway, a person is at risk for pulmonary edema and respiratory distress. This potentially life-threatening situation requires both nurse- and physician-prescribed interventions. The collaborative problem *PC: Respiratory related to thermal injury* would alert nurses that close monitoring for respiratory complications and management if they occur are indicated.
3. *Ineffective Airway Clearance related to decreased cough and gag reflexes secondary to anesthesia*
   The nursing focus for the above problem is on preventing aspiration through proper positioning and good oral hygiene, not on teaching effective coughing. Thus, the nurse should restate the diagnosis as *Risk for Aspiration related to decreased cough and gag reflexes secondary to anesthesia.*

KEY CONCEPTS
Generic Considerations

- Ventilation requires synchronous movement of the walls of the chest and abdomen. With *inspiration,* the diaphragm moves downward, the intercostal muscles contract, the chest wall lifts up and out, the pressure inside the thorax lowers, and air is drawn in. *Expiration* occurs as air is forced out of the lungs by the elastic recoil of the lungs and the relaxation of the chest and diaphragm. Expiration is diminished in older adults and those with chronic pulmonary disease, increasing the likelihood of CO_2 retention.
- Pulmonary function depends on
  - Adequate perfusion (passage of blood through pulmonary vessels)
  - Satisfactory diffusion (movement of oxygen and carbon dioxide across alveolar capillary membrane)
  - Successful ventilation (exchange of air between alveolar spaces and the atmosphere)

- Oxygenation depends on the ability of the lungs to deliver oxygen to the blood and on the ability of the heart to pump enough blood to deliver the oxygen to the microcirculation of the cells.
- With pulmonary dysfunction, pulmonary function tests (PFTs) are essential to determine the nature and extent of dysfunction caused by obstruction, restriction, or both. Airway resistance causes *obstructive* defects. A limitation in chest wall expansion causes *restrictive* defects. *Mixed* defects are a combination of obstructive and restrictive problems.
- Although arterial blood gases and oxygen saturation studies are very helpful in diagnosing problems with oxygenation, *vital signs* and *mental function* are key guides to determining the seriousness of the problem (some clients can tolerate oxygen problems better than others can).
- The effects of insufficient oxygenation (hypoxia or hypoxemia) on vital signs are as follows:

Vital Sign	Early Hypoxia/Hypoxemia	Late Hypoxia/Hypoxemia
Blood pressure	Rising systolic/falling diastolic	Falling
Pulse	Rising, bounding, arrhythmic	Falling, shallow, arrhythmic
Pulse pressure	Widening	Widened/narrowed
Respirations	Rapid	Slowed/rapid

- The effects of insufficient oxygenation on mental function are as follows:

Early Hypoxia/Hypoxemia	Late Hypoxia/Hypoxemia
Irritability	Seizures
Headache	Coma or brain tissue swelling
Confusion	
Agitation	

- A cough ("the guardian of the lungs") is accomplished by closure of the glottis and the explosive expulsion of air from the lungs by the work of the abdominal and chest muscles. Although most coughing serves a beneficial purpose, the following may be signs of a medical problem requiring medical intervention:
  - Coughs lasting longer than 2 weeks or associated with high fever
  - Coughs consistently triggered by something (may actually be allergic bronchial asthma)
  - Barking cough, especially in a child
- Breath holding can result in a Valsalva maneuver: a marked increase in intrathoracic and intraabdominal pressure, with profound circulatory changes (decreased heart rate, cardiac output, and blood pressure).
- The terms *tachypnea, hyperpnea, hyperventilation, bradypnea,* and *hypoventilation* are frequently confused.
  - *Tachypnea:* rapid, shallow respiratory rate
  - *Hyperpnea:* rapid respiratory rate with increased depth
  - *Hyperventilation:* increased rate or depth of respiration causing an alveolar ventilation that is above the body's normal metabolic requirements
  - *Bradypnea:* slow respiratory rate
  - *Hypoventilation:* decreased rate or depth of respiration, causing a minute alveolar ventilation that is less than the body's requirements
- Hypoxia and hypoxemia contribute to increased intracranial pressure, brain swelling, brain damage, and shock. Oxygen demand is greater during febrile illness, exercise, pain, and physical and emotional stress.
- Oxygen should be administered carefully (less than 3 mL/min) to people with a history of chronic CO_2 retention, because their drive to breathe is hypoxia.
- Suctioning or instillation of saline should not be used routinely; rather, their use should be based on assessment of individual needs.
  - Use the following as clinical indicators for need for endotracheal suctioning:
    - Secretions in the endotracheal tube
    - Frequent or sustained coughing
    - Adventitious breath sounds on auscultation (rhonchi, or upper airway gurgles)
    - Increased peak airway pressure
    - Decreasing pulse oximetry readings (SvO_2, PaO_2)
    - Sudden onset of respiratory distress whenever airway patency is questioned
  - Instill normal saline based on the client's response to suctioning (secretions sticking to tube or catheter, mucus plugging the airway, suction catheter not eliciting an acceptable cough). Instillation of saline benefits clients only when it causes vigorous cough.
  - Keep in mind that, although endotracheal suctioning is associated with several significant complications, insufficiently frequent or inadequate suction also carries substantial risks. Maintain a delicate balance to minimize all complications.

- The nurse can reduce risk of hypoxemia by using the following (Change, 1995):
  - Oxygen saturation and cardiac rhythm monitors during and immediately after suctioning
  - Intermittent suction for less than 15 s (prolonged, continuous suction causes microatelectasis)
  - Hyperinflation (increasing tidal volume to 1½ times preset ventilation volume using a resuscitation bag or the sigh function of the ventilator)
  - Preoxygenation (administering oxygen before suctioning)
  - Hyperoxygenation (administering oxygen at greater oxygen concentrations than the preset ventilator level)
  - Hyperventilation (increasing the respiratory rate without changing tidal volume)
- The use of harmonicas by pulmonary therapists to help people with lung disease exercise their lungs and learn how to control breathing during acute dyspnea shows promising results. Clients not only have fun, but they also improve their ability to control their breathing and maximize lung function.
- Nicotine is one of the most toxic and addicting of all poisonous substances. Education, preventive health practices, interventions to enhance tobacco cessation, nicotine dependence treatment, and relapse prevention should be standard nursing practice.* Nurses must be persistent in helping their clients to stop smoking by encouraging efforts to quit as often as indicated (in many cases, at each client encounter). Refer to *Ineffective Health Maintenance related to Insufficient Knowledge of Effects of Tobacco Use.*

Pediatric Considerations

- The characteristics of normal respiration in the newborn differ from those of older infants and children.
  - Respirations are irregular and abdominal; to be accurate, count respirations for 1 full minute (Wong, 2003).
  - The rate is between 30 and 50 breaths/min (Wong, 2003).
  - Periods of apnea, lasting less than 15 s, may occur (Wong, 2003).
  - Obligate nasal breathing occurs through the first 3 weeks of life (Wong, 2003).
- Characteristics of the respiratory system of the infant and young child include the following:
  - Abdominal breathing continues until the child is about 5 years of age (Wong, 2003).
  - Retractions are observed more often with respiratory illness because of increased chest wall compliance. Respiratory insufficiency may develop quickly in children (Hunsberger, 1989).
  - Smaller airway diameter increases the risk of obstruction.
  - Infants and small children swallow sputum when it is produced.
- Janson-Bjerklie et al. (1987) found that younger asthmatics appear to experience more intense dyspnea than older people at a given level of airway obstruction.
- Huckabay and Daderian (1989) noted that pediatric clients who were given a choice in the selection of color of water in blow bottles performed significantly more breathing exercises than those who were not given a choice.
- Studies show that the past common practice of placing infants on their stomach for sleep increases the incidence of sudden infant death syndrome (SIDS), making placement on back or side a safer option. Refer to *Risk for Sudden Infant Death Syndrome.*

Maternal Considerations

- Increased levels of estrogen and progesterone increase tidal volume by decreasing pulmonary resistance (Pillitteri, 2003).
- During pregnancy, oxygen consumption increases by 14%: half is for fetus development and the rest is for other increased needs (eg, uterus, breasts; Pillitteri, 2003).

---

* American Academy of Medical-Surgical Nursing Position Statement on Tobacco Use. Accessed from: *http://www. medsurgnurse.org/* 12/5/00.

> ### ⊙ Geriatric Considerations
>
> - Age-related changes in the respiratory system have little effect on function in healthy adults unless they interact with risk factors such as smoking, immobility, or compromised immune system (Miller, 2004).
> - The following age-related changes in the respiratory system are typical (Miller, 2004):
>   - No change in total volume
>   - 50% increase in residual volume
>   - Compromised gas exchange in lower lung regions
>   - Reduced compliance of bony thorax
>   - Decreased strength of respiratory muscles and diaphragm
> - Age-related kyphosis and diminished immune response compromise respiratory function and increase the risk of pneumonia and other respiratory infections.
> - Adults 65 years of age and older have a yearly death rate from pneumonia or influenza of 9 per 100,000. When smoking, exposure to air pollutants, or occupational exposure to toxic substances is present, the rate increases to 217 per 100,000. If two or more risk factors are present, the rate rises to 979 per 100,000 (Miller, 2004).

Focus Assessment Criteria

Subjective Data
Assess History of Symptoms (eg, Pain, Dyspnea, Cough).

Onset: Precipitated by what? Relieved by what?
Description: Relieved by what?
Effects on other body functions
    Gastrointestinal (nausea, vomiting, anorexia, constipation)
    Genitourinary (impotence, kidney function)
    Cardiovascular (angina, tachycardia/bradycardia, fluid retention)
    Neurosensory (thought processes, headache)
    Musculoskeletal (muscle fatigue, atrophy, use of accessory muscles)
Effects on lifestyle
    Occupation   Social/sexual functions
    Role functions   Financial status
Effects on activity/exercise

Assess for Related Factors.
Presence of contributing or causative factors
Smoking ("pack-years": number of packs per day times number of smoking years)
Smoking within the 8 weeks before anesthesia or surgery
Allergy (medication, food, environmental factors—dust, pollen, other)
Trauma, blunt or overt (chest, abdomen, upper airway, head)
Surgery/pain
    Incision of chest/neck/head/abdomen
    Recent intubation
Asthma/chronic obstructive pulmonary disease (COPD)/sinus problems
Environmental factors
    Toxic fumes (cleaning agents, smoke)
    Extreme heat or cold
    Daily inspired air, work and home (humid, dry, level of pollution, level of pollens)
Infection/inflammation

For infant, history of:

Placement on stomach to sleep	Prematurity	Low birth weight
Cesarean birth	Complicated delivery	Breast-feeding formula

Objective Data
Assess for Defining Characteristics.

Mental status
Respiratory status
Airway

Spontaneous nasal	Nasal endotracheal tube	Spontaneous mouth
Oral endotracheal tube	Oral airway	Tracheostomy
Nasal airway		

Description
Spontaneous, labored, or nonlabored
Controlled mechanical ventilation (CMV)
Spontaneous intermittent mechanical ventilations (SIMV)
Rate (per minute)
Rhythm
Depth
  Symmetric
Type

Splinted/guarded	Kussmaul	Use of accessory muscle
Cheyne-Stokes		

Cough
Effective (brings forth sputum and clears lungs)
Ineffective (does not bring forth mucus or clear lungs)
Triggered by what? Relieved by what?
Needs assistance with coughing
Sputum

Color	Character	Amount
Odor		

Breath sounds (detected by auscultation: compare right upper and lower lobes to left upper and lower lobes; listen to all four quadrants of the chest)

Circulatory status

Pulse	Blood pressure	Skin color

For more information on Focus Assessment Criteria, visit http://connection.lww.com.

Goal

 NOC Aspiration Control, Respiratory Status

The person will have a respiratory rate within normal limits compared with baseline.

Indicators

- Express willingness to be actively involved in managing respiratory symptoms and maximizing respiratory function.
- Relate appropriate interventions to maximize respiratory status (varies depending on health status).
- Have satisfactory pulmonary function, as measured by pulmonary function tests.

General Interventions

NIC Airway Management, Cough Enhancement, Respiratory Monitoring, Positioning

Determine Causative Factors.

Pain, lethargy
Medical order of bed rest
Neuromuscular impairment
Lack of motivation (to ambulate, to cough and deep breathe)
Decreased level of consciousness
Lack of knowledge
Medications (narcotics, muscle relaxants, other CNS depressants)
Inadequate humidity

Eliminate or Reduce Causative Factors, if Possible.

Assess for optimal pain relief with minimal periods of fatigue or respiratory depression.

Coordinate medication regimen with planned activities (eg, give PRN pain medication with least-sedating side effects 1 h before physical therapy).

Ensure adequate air humidity, providing additional humidification unless contraindicated by heart disease.

For nasal stuffiness, use saline nose drops; avoid other nose drops because of rebound effect.

Encourage ambulation as soon as consistent with medical plan of care.

> If client cannot walk, establish a regimen for being out of bed in a chair several times a day (eg, 1 h after meals and 1 h before bedtime).
>
> Increase activity gradually. Explain that respiratory function will improve and dyspnea will decrease with practice.

For neuromuscular impairment

> Vary the position of the bed, thereby gradually changing the horizontal and vertical position of the thorax, unless contraindicated.
>
> Assist client to reposition, turning frequently from side to side (hourly if possible).
>
> Encourage deep-breathing and controlled-coughing exercises five times every hour.
>
> Teach client to use blow bottle or incentive spirometer every hour while awake (with severe neuromuscular impairment, the person may have to be awakened during the night as well).
>
> For those with quadriplegia, teach person and caregivers the "quad cough" (caregiver places hand on client's diaphragm and thrusts upward and inward).
>
> For child, use colored water in blow bottle; have him or her blow up balloons.
>
> Ensure optimal hydration status.

For the person with a decreased level of consciousness

> Position from side to side with set schedule (eg, left side even hours, right side odd hours); do not leave person lying flat on back.
>
> Position client on right side after feedings (nasogastric tube feeding, gastrostomy) to prevent regurgitation and aspiration.
>
> Keep head of bed elevated 30 degrees unless contraindicated.
>
> See also *Risk for Aspiration.*

Prevent the complications of immobility.

See *Disuse Syndrome.*

Rationales

- Lying flat causes the abdominal organs to shift toward the chest, thereby crowding the lungs and making it more difficult to breathe.
- Interventions that can enhance pulmonary function include exercise conditioning to improve lung compliance, relaxation and breathing training, chest percussion, postural drainage, and psychosocial rehabilitation.
- Proper nutrition helps to
  - Maintain immunologic competence necessary to fight off respiratory infections.
  - Provide calories for the energy needed for the work of breathing (energy requirements are increased in COPD).
  - Nourish muscles used in breathing.
- Exercises and movement promote lung expansion and mobilization of secretions. Incentive spirometry promotes deep breathing by providing a visual indicator of the effectiveness of the breathing effort.
- Adequate hydration and humidity liquefy secretions, enabling easier expectoration and preventing stasis of secretions, which provide a medium for microorganism growth. Hydration also helps decrease blood viscosity, which reduces the risk of clot formation.

RISK FOR INEFFECTIVE RESPIRATORY FUNCTION

RELATED TO ALLERGIC RESPONSE

Goal

NOC Respiratory Status, Risk Control, Knowledge: Treatment

The person will report a decrease in allergic responses.

Indicators
- Explain how to prevent and manage allergic symptoms, including:
  - How to avoid allergens (eg, pollen, dust mites, animal dander), irritants (eg, smoke), and other triggers (eg, cold air, exercise, laughing, crying)
  - How to manage medication regimen, including appropriate use of inhalers and need to keep peak flowmeter diaries
  - How to use complementary strategies (eg, biofeedback, therapeutic exercise, and relaxation techniques) to manage symptoms
- Relate the importance of health maintenance visits to monitor pulmonary function and disease process.
- Discuss the need for immediate medical attention in cases of severe allergic response (eg, bee sting, severe asthma attack).
- Remain symptom-free and able to sleep through the night and perform usual activities, including going to work (if unable to be completely symptom-free, then other indicators include decreased symptoms, attacks, sick days, and trips to the primary caregiver or emergency room).

Interventions

NIC See *Ineffective Respiratory Function*

Determine Causative Factors.
Chronic allergy (known allergens such as molds, dust, pollen, food, others)
Stinging insect
Nonspecific (unknown) allergen

Provide the Following Health Teaching:
For Chronic Allergy to Molds:
Avoid barns, cut grass, leaves, weeds, decaying or rotting vegetation, firewood, houseplants, damp basements, attics, and crawl spaces.
Avoid eating marinated or aged foods (bread, flour, cheese, fruits, vegetables).
Keep household walls clean and dry.
    Be sure that house drainage is adequate to keep walls dry.
    Check walls for black or grayish-blue mold spots.
    Wash walls with chlorine bleach solution to remove mold.
Reduce environmental allergens, especially in the bedroom.*
    Empty room to the bare walls, including closets (store contents elsewhere if possible).
    Scrub woodwork and floors.
    Thereafter, dust and vacuum well daily and clean thoroughly once a week.
    Minimize bedroom furniture (preferably wood, rather than stuffed); avoid wall-to-wall carpets.

---

*It is difficult to keep one's home and work environment dust-free, but special efforts can readily be made to keep bedroom free of dust.

Choose waxed, hardwood floors (no carpets) if possible.
Use pull shades rather than Venetian blinds; do not use curtains or draperies.
Minimize closet use; keep it as dust-free as the bedroom, and keep the door closed.
Use bedroom for sleeping only; if it is a child's bedroom, encourage play elsewhere.
Do not use stuffed toys.
Keep animals with fur or feathers out of the area.
Do not use fuzzy blankets or feather comforters; cotton bedspreads are preferred.
Launder bed linens frequently.
Have air and heat ducts and carpets professionally cleaned yearly.
Keep dust down throughout the entire house.
Use steam or hot-water heat if available.
Maintain a clean filter in furnace; use air conditioning, if possible.
Cover hot-air furnace outlets with cheesecloth or have a filter installed; change filter frequently.
Avoid any room while it is being cleaned, and do not handle any objects that may be dust collectors (eg, books).
Wear a mask while cleaning.

For Chronic Allergy to Pollen:
Reduce exposure as much as possible to trees (April–May), grass (May–July), weeds (mid-May to first frost).
Use air conditioning with electrostatic filters.
Stay inside on windy days, avoiding drafts and cross-ventilation.
Use air conditioning in cars, and avoid extended rides.
Wear a dampened mask while cutting lawn.
Avoid strong odors (scents and perfumes).
Do not consume ice-cold beverages or food (can cause spasms).
Avoid granaries, barns, decaying materials, cut grass, weeds, dry leaves, and firewood.
Take vacations during the high-pollen season in a low-pollen area, such as the eastern seashore.
Be sure over-the-counter drugs (eg, antihistamines) are approved by a physician, because some may have the opposite of the intended effect.

To Avoid Stinging Insects (Bees, Wasps, Yellow Jackets, Hornets):
Do not wear brightly colored clothing. Choose colors such as white, light green, and khaki.
Keep hair short or tied back; avoid hair sprays, perfumes, and floppy clothing.
Wear shoes and socks.
Avoid riding horses or bicycles in areas where bees or wasps are plentiful (eg, fields of clover, flowers).
Avoid mowing lawns, trimming hedges, or pruning trees during the insect season.
Carry insect spray in the glove compartment and keep one handy at home (attempts to swat or kill insects must be well planned because a missed blow may infuriate the insect and make it more dangerous).
If a bee or wasp approaches in the open, stay still or move back very slowly.
Each spring, have home and garden searched for new hornets' or bees' nests and obtain professional assistance from an exterminator or fire department in eliminating them.

For a Severe Allergic Reaction in which Hives; Facial Swelling; Abnormal Sensations of Palate, Tongue, or Throat; or Any Respiratory Symptoms Appear, or If a Previous Reaction to Any Kind of Sting has Been Severe, Carry Out the Following Procedure:
Remove stinger immediately.
Keep as quiet as possible. Avoid panic.
Use emergency epinephrine injection if available.
Call emergency medical services.
Immediately apply ammonia or lemon to sting; follow with ice.

Discuss the Role of Medication in Reducing Allergies.
Point out that antihistamines prevent, but do not reverse, allergic responses; therefore, it is best to take them when expecting to encounter allergens or as soon as possible thereafter.
Explain that new over-the-counter allergy medications are available that do not cause drowsiness. Encourage the client to check with a pharmacist about them.
For those with more severe allergies, stress the need to see a physician (new, more effective medications with fewer side effects are now available by prescription).
Discuss the hazards of smoking and second-hand smoke exposure.

Discuss healthy living habits:
    Good nutrition
    Regular exercise
    Controlled breathing

For People with Asthma:

Explain asthma, airway response, and therapy goals.
Explain the rationale for the medication; evaluate the client's ability to use an inhaler and peak flowmeter.
Teach client how to use a peak flowmeter to manage symptoms.
    Teach proper technique and maintenance.
    Maintain daily chart of peak flows.
    Establish an evaluation system of peak flow readings and interventions needed (eg, medication, emergency room).
Explain the role of medications in managing asthma; clarify the need to avoid cigarette smoke and other triggers (eg, animals, dander, strong perfumes). Explain use of protective masks.
Clarify when primary provider should be contacted:
    Medications must be increased to control symptoms.
    Client has persistent cough or difficulty breathing with or without wheezing.
    Peak flows are less than 80% of normal.

Rationales

- Costing billions annually, asthma is responsible for about 500,000 hospitalizations,* 5,000 deaths,* and 134 million days[†] of restricted activity a year. Most of the problems that asthma causes could be averted if people with asthma and their health care providers manage the disease according to established guidelines. Effective asthma management involves four major components: controlling exposure to factors that trigger asthma episodes, adequately managing asthma with medicine, monitoring the disease by using objective measures of lung function, and educating clients with asthma to become partners in their own care.
- Although the cause of asthma is unknown, it tends to run in families. With asthma, the airways become narrow and blocked as a result of the shortening of muscle around them, swelling of the lining, and mucus inside them. Symptoms are cough, wheeze, and shortness of breath. In children with asthma, cough means asthma* (also true for adults).
- Death from asthma is two to six times more likely among African Americans and Hispanics than among whites. Although the number of deaths annually from asthma is low compared to other chronic diseases, the death rate for children 5 to 14 years of age and young adults 15 to 24 years of age doubled from 1979–1980 to 1993–1995 (from 1.5 to 3.7 deaths per million children 5 to 14 years of age and 2.8 to 6.3 deaths per million persons 15 to 34 years of age, respectively; Mannino et al., 1998).
- Treating clients with asthma without objective measurements of pulmonary function might be comparable to treating hypertension without first using a sphygmomanometer. Pulmonary function testing (spirometry) should be used to evaluate the degree of airway obstruction and to determine the presence of bronchial hyperresponsiveness (which, although closely associated with asthma, does not occur in all clients with this condition and may sometimes occur in those who do not have it; Owen, 1999).
- To control asthma, spirometric measurements of pulmonary function must be performed at least once a year in clients with well-controlled asthma and at any time medications fail to control symptoms (Owen, 1999).
- Adequate asthma management for both adults and children often depends on the client's willingness and ability to use a peak flowmeter to measure and record peak expiratory flow volume at various times throughout the day. Normal peak flow values are based on age, sex, height, and underlying lung disorder. Normal values range from 300 to 700 L/min and should be compared with baseline values.

---

*Accessed from: *http://hp2010.nhlbihin.net/as_frameset.htm* (National Heart, Lung, and Blood Institute Web Page) 12/5/00.

[†]Accessed from: *http://wellness.ucdavis.edu/child_health/special_needs/pediatric_asthma/index.html* 12/6/00.

Pediatric Interventions

Set asthma goals that children can relate to, including:
    No emergency room visits
    Staying out of the hospital
    Being able to keep up with friends during physical activity
    Sleeping through the night without waking[†]

The following factors can bring on or aggravate asthma:

Catching a cold	Laughing/crying	Cold air
Exercise	Smoke	Allergies

Explain the need to control environmental antigens (see previous Interventions).
Provide the child with age-appropriate explanations of antigens to avoid.
Teach parents to avoid over-the-counter drugs and to consult with a primary care professional.
Contract with parents to some level of smoking cessation.
    Complete smoking cessation
    No smoking in house, car, or when child is present
Consult with school nurse for coordination of treatment plan and school activities.
Include all family members in educational sessions if possible.
Encourage mothers to breast-feed for the first 6 months of life to reduce allergies in their child.

Rationales

- Card games such as *Slap the Smoker* (like *Slapjack,* but "No Smoking" cards are the jacks), *Old Lungs* (like *Old Maid,* but the "Old Lung" is the odd card), and *Go Fish* (like the traditional game of *Go Fish,* but groups of asthma-related cards must be gathered to win) can be an effective way to teach young children about managing asthma and avoiding smoking (for more information, visit www.theinspirationgame.com).
- Pregnant women (especially those with allergies) can reduce the chances of allergies in their children by controlling the environment for irritants such as tobacco smoke and allergens such as mites, molds, and animal dander; by avoiding common allergic triggers (eg, avoiding common allergic foods, such as eggs, peanuts, milk, fish, and wheat); and by breast-feeding exclusively for at least the first 6 months of the child's life (Schmierer, 2000).
- Participation in school-related activities should be encouraged, but evaluation is needed for duration and intensity (Wong, 2003).
- Certain drugs (eg, aspirin, cough syrup, nonsteroidal antiinflammatory agents, antihistamines) can exacerbate symptoms (Wong, 2003).
- Cigarette smoke is a known trigger of asthma attacks.

[†]Asthma Handbook for Children. Accessed from: *http://wellness.ucdavis.edu/child_health/special_needs/pediatric_asthma/goals.html* 12/5/00.

DYSFUNCTIONAL VENTILATORY WEANING RESPONSE

DEFINITION

Dysfunctional Ventilatory Weaning Response (DVWR): State in which a person cannot adjust to lowered levels of mechanical ventilator support, which interrupts and prolongs the weaning process

DEFINING CHARACTERISTICS

DVWR is a progressive state, and experienced nurses have identified three levels (Logan & Jenny, 1990): mild, moderate, and severe. The defining characteristics occur in response to weaning.

Mild

Major

Restlessness
Slight increase in respiratory rate from baseline

Minor

Expressed feelings of increased oxygen need, breathing discomfort, fatigue, warmth
Queries about possible machine dysfunction
Increased concentration on breathing

Moderate

Major

Slight increase in blood pressure = 20 mm Hg or less from baseline
Slight increase in heart rate = 20 beats/min or less from baseline
Increase in respiratory rate = 5 breaths/min or less from baseline

Minor

Hypervigilance to activities	Diaphoresis
Inability to respond to coaching	Eye-widening (wide-eyed look)
	Decreased air entry heard on auscultation
Inability to cooperate	Skin color changes: pale, slight cyanosis
Apprehension	Slight respiratory accessory muscle use

Severe

Major

Agitation
Significant deterioration in arterial blood gases from baseline
Increase in blood pressure greater than 20 mm Hg from baseline
Increase in heart rate greater than 20 beats/min from baseline
Rapid, shallow breathing greater than 25 breaths/min

Minor

Cyanosis	Full respiratory accessory muscle use
Shallow, gasping breaths	Profuse diaphoresis
Paradoxical abdominal breathing	Breathing uncoordinated with the ventilator
	Decreased level of consciousness
Adventitious breath sounds	

RELATED FACTORS
Pathophysiologic

Related to muscle weakness and fatigue secondary to:

Unstable hemodynamic status	Metabolic/acid–base abnormality	Anemia
		Infection

Decreased level of
  consciousness
Chronic neuromuscular
  disability

Severe disease process
Chronic respiratory disease
Multisystem disease
Fluid/electrolyte imbalance

Chronic nutritional deficit
Debilitated condition

Related to ineffective airway clearance

Treatment-Related
Related to obstructed airway
Related to muscle weakness and fatigue secondary to:
Excess sedation, analgesia   Uncontrolled pain

Related to inadequate nutrition (deficit in calories, excess carbohydrates, inadequate fats and protein intake)
Related to prolonged ventilator dependence (more than 1 week)
Related to previously unsuccessful ventilator weaning attempt(s)
Related to too-rapid pacing of the weaning process

Situational (Personal, Environmental)
Related to insufficient knowledge of the weaning process
Related to excessive energy demands (self-care activities, diagnostic and treatment procedures, visitors)
Related to inadequate social support
Related to insecure environment (noisy, upsetting events, busy room)
Related to fatigue secondary to interrupted sleep patterns
Related to inadequate self-efficacy
Related to moderate to high anxiety related to breathing efforts
Related to fear of separation from ventilator
Related to feelings of powerlessness
Related to feelings of hopelessness

⊙⊙ AUTHOR'S NOTE

DVWR is a specific diagnosis within the category of *Risk for Ineffective Respiratory Function. Ineffective Airway Clearance, Ineffective Breathing Patterns,* and *Impaired Gas Exchange* also can be encountered during weaning, either as indicators of lack of weaning readiness or as factors related to the onset of DVWR. DVWR is a separate client state. Its distinctive etiologies and treatments arise from the process of separating the client from the mechanical ventilator.

The process of weaning is an art and a science. Because weaning is a collaborative process, the nurse's ability to gain the client's trust and willingness to work is an important determinant of the weaning outcomes, especially with long-term clients. This trust is fostered by the knowledge and self-confidence nurses display, and by their ability to deal with clients' specific concerns (Jenny & Logan, 1991).

⊙⊙ ERRORS IN DIAGNOSTIC STATEMENTS

Dysfunctional Weaning Response related to increased blood pressure, heart rate, respiratory rate, and agitation during weaning

This diagnosis does not indicate the reasons for weaning problems. The related factors are evidence of *Dysfunctional Weaning Response,* not causative and contributing factors. The nurse should write the diagnosis with the related factors if they are known, or "unknown etiology" if not known.

Many of the following assessments and interventions apply to the prevention of moderate and severe responses as well as the treatment phases of managing the diagnosis.

KEY CONCEPTS
Generic Considerations

- *Weaning* is the process of assisting clients to breathe spontaneously without mechanical ventilation. Weaning success has been defined as spontaneous breathing for 24 h without ventilatory support, with or without an artificial airway.
- Ventilator weaning is a multidisciplinary effort in which the presence of knowledgeable nurses affects the outcomes positively. Experienced nurses agree that weaning is a collaborative process shared with the client that has both a physical and a psychological aspect. For ventilator-dependent clients, it can be a very stressful experience (Logan & Jenny, 1991). Recent works on clients' perceptions of ventilator weaning describe their concerns, which include physical discomfort, nurse caring behaviors, feelings of altered self, and the clients' physical, emotional, and cognitive work involved in weaning (Jenny & Logan, 1998).
- Ventilator-associated complications may occur with prolonged ventilation. A long period of intubation and mechanical ventilation places clients at risk for postoperative pulmonary complications. Systematic daily assessment of the oropharyngeal cavity is necessary for ventilated clients, especially those who are orally intubated, to detect or prevent lesions and infection (Treloar & Stechmiller, 1995). It is not recommended that normal saline instillation before suctioning be a routine practice but should be done only after assessing the need based on quality of secretions, quality of breath sounds, quality and effectiveness of cough, and oxygenation and ventilatory status.
- Various criteria have been proposed for determining weaning readiness. These criteria are measures of oxygenation, respiratory muscle strength, and the ability to ventilate sufficiently to maintain an adequate arterial carbon dioxide level ($PaCO_2$). Gaps exist, however, in our knowledge of client responses to ventilator weaning and in the prediction of outcomes. Goodnough Hanneman (1994) suggests that one reason that weaning predictors do not have adequate predictive power may be that the interrelationship of cardiopulmonary pathophysiologic determinants of outcomes is not reflected by independent predictive criteria (eg, pulmonary mechanics). The ongoing use of a systematic assessment tool may help tailor the process to the client's current status and prevent a premature weaning trial or a dysfunctional weaning response (Burns, Burns & Truwit, 1994).
- Outcomes after short-term mechanical ventilation differ from those after long-term ventilation. Psychological outlook, ventilatory drive, respiratory muscle strength and endurance, minute volume requirements, and nutritional status appear to have little bearing on short-term ventilator weaning (Morton et al., 2005).
- The physiologic inspiratory work of breathing includes three components (Porth, 2002):
  - Compliance work to expand the elastic forces of the lung
  - Tissue resistance work to overcome the viscosity of the lung and thoracic cage
  - Airway resistance work to overcome the resistance to the flow of air into and out of the lungs
- Mechanical ventilation increases the work of breathing by decreasing airway diameter and increasing its length, thus increasing resistance. During weaning, the clinician manipulates pressure/volume changes to promote reconditioning of the respiratory muscles without causing excessive fatigue (Morton et al., 2005).
- DVWR can involve respiratory inspiratory muscle fatigue, which can take up to 24 to 48 h for recovery. The fatigue increases dyspnea, which, in turn, creates anxiety, triggering more fatigue and increased breathlessness.

Focus Assessment Criteria

Subjective Data
Assess for Defining Characteristics.

Concerns about starting or continuing weaning process

Readiness	Previous experience	Expectations
Possibility of failure		

Feelings about comfort, rest, energy status

Knowledge of weaning process

Assess for Related Factors.

Medication history
Tobacco, alcohol use

Objective Data
Assess for Defining Characteristics.

Respiratory status: Complete respiratory assessment (see Focus Assessment Criteria in *Risk for Ineffective Respiratory Function*)

Level of consciousness	Use of accessory muscles	Vital signs
Secretions (type and amount)	Baseline skin color	Airway clearance
	Adventitious breath sounds	Arterial blood gases

Assess for Related Factors.

Respiratory disease, acute and chronic diseases
Mechanical ventilator information
    Ventilator settings and size of endotracheal or tracheostomy tube
    Ventilation history, including reason for ventilation
    Length of time on the ventilator
    Whether weaning has been attempted before, and if so, with what results
Current hemodynamic, nutritional, infection, and pain status

For more information on Focus Assessment Criteria, visit http://connection.lww.com.

Goal

> **NOC** Anxiety Control, Respiratory Status, Vital Signs Status, Knowledge: Weaning, Energy Conservation

The person will achieve progressive weaning goals.

Indicators

- Spontaneous breathing for 24 h without ventilatory support *or*
- Demonstrate a positive attitude toward the next weaning trial: collaborate willingly with the weaning plan, communicate comfort status during the weaning process, attempt to control the breathing pattern, and try to control emotional responses.
- Be tired from the work of weaning, but not exhausted.

General Interventions

> **NIC** Anxiety Reduction, Preparatory Sensory Information, Respiratory Monitoring, Ventilation Assistance, Presence, Endurance

If Applicable, Assess Causative Factors for Previous Unsuccessful Weaning Attempts.

Inadequate energy substrates: oxygen, nutrition, and rest
Inadequate comfort status
Excessive activity demands
Decreased self-esteem, confidence, feelings of control
Lack of knowledge of the client's role
Lack of trust in staff
Negative emotional state
Adverse weaning environment

Determine Readiness for Weaning (Burns, 1998; Morton et al., 2005).

Respiratory rate less than 25 breaths/min
Oxygen concentration of 40% or less on the ventilator
Negative inspiratory pressure less than −20
Positive expiratory pressure greater than +30
Spontaneous tidal volume greater than 5 mL/kg
Vital capacity greater than 10 to 15 mL/kg
Rested, controlled discomfort
Willingness to try weaning

If Readiness for Weaning is Present, Engage Client in Establishing the Plan.

Explain the weaning process.

Negotiate progressive weaning goals.

Create a visual display of goals that uses symbols to indicate progression (eg, bar or line graph to indicate increasing time off ventilator).

Explain that these goals will be reexamined daily with the client.

Refer to unit protocols for specific weaning procedures.

Explain Client's Role in the Weaning Process.

From initial intubation, promote the understanding that mechanical ventilation is temporary.

Share nurses' expectations of their collaborative work role when person is judged ready to wean.

Help person to understand the importance of communicating comfort status and trying to reach the current weaning goals, and that rest will be allowed throughout the process.

Strengthen Feelings of Self-Esteem, Self-Efficacy, and Control.

Reinforce self-esteem, confidence, and control through normalizing strategies such as grooming, dressing, mobilizing, and conversing socially about things of interest to the person.

Permit as much control as possible by informing person of the situation and his or her progress, permitting shared decision making about details of care, following client's preferences as far as possible, and improving comfort status.

Increase confidence by praising successful activities, encouraging a positive outlook, and reviewing positive progress to date. Explain that people usually succeed in weaning; reassure client that you will be with him or her every step of the way.

Demonstrate confidence in client's ability to wean.

Maintain client's confidence by adopting a weaning pace that ensures success and minimizes setbacks.*

Promote Trust in the Staff and Environment.

Establish a trust relationship by communicating interest and concern for the person's well-being.

Help client to get to know you by sharing information about yourself.

Demonstrate competence and confidence in your own ability to manage the weaning process.

Maintain a calm manner and a relaxed atmosphere.

Explain what you are doing and why, to reduce the person's vigilance and feelings of uncertainty.

Note concerns that hinder comfort and confidence (family members, topics of conversation, room events, previous weaning failures); discuss them openly. Reduce them, if possible.

Reduce Negative Effects of Anxiety and Fatigue.

Monitor status frequently to avoid undue fatigue and anxiety. Use a systematic, comprehensive tool. A pulse oximeter is a noninvasive and unobtrusive way to monitor oxygen saturation levels.

Provide regular periods of rest before fatigue advances.

  Reduce activities.

  Maintain or increase ventilator support and/or oxygen in consultation with a physician.

During a rest period, dim lights, post "do not disturb" signs, and play instrumental music with 60 to 80 beats/min. Allow client to select type of music (Chan, 1998).

Encourage calmness and breath control by reassuring client that he or she can and will succeed.

Consider use of alternative therapies such as music, hypnosis, and biofeedback.

If the client is becoming agitated, calm him or her down while remaining at the bedside, and coach him or her to regain breathing control. Monitor oxygen saturation and vital signs closely during this intervention.

If weaning trial is discontinued, address person's perceptions of weaning failure. Reassure client that the trial was good exercise and a useful form of training. Remind client that the work is good for the respiratory muscles and will improve future performance.

Create a Positive Weaning Environment that Increases Feelings of Security.

Provide a room with a quiet atmosphere, low activity, and no chatter within the person's hearing.

Delegate the most skilled staff to wean clients who have experienced moderate to severe responses or who are at high risk for doing so.

---

* May require a primary care professional's order.

Remain visible in the room to reinforce feelings of safety.

Reassure the person that help is immediately available, if needed.

Monitor visitors' effects on the client; help visitors understand how they can best assist.

Encourage supportive visitors when possible during the weaning process. Visits from people who upset the person should be postponed.

Ensure that clients are included in discussions that they are likely to overhear.

Promote Optimal Energy Resources.

Assist client to cough and deep breathe regularly, and use prescribed bronchodilators, humidification, and suctioning to improve air entry.

Ensure that nutritional support falls within current guidelines for ventilated and weaning clients.

Provide sufficient rest periods to prevent undue fatigue.

Use ventilator support at night if necessary to increase sleep time, and try to avoid unnecessary awakening.

Monitor the disease processes to determine the body systems' stability.

Control Activity Demands.

Coordinate necessary activities to promote adequate time for rest or relaxation.

Ensure that all staff follow the individualized care plan.

Coach client in breath control by regular demonstrations of slow, deep, rhythmic patterns of breathing. Help client to synchronize breathing with the ventilator.

If person's concentration starts to create tension and increase anxiety, provide distraction in the form of supportive visitors, radio, television, or conversation.

Optimize Comfort Status to Increase Participation.

Identify strengths and resources, such as supportive family members or friends or a sense of humor, that can be mobilized to enhance coping and weaning efforts.

Advocate for additional resources, such as analgesia, sedation, or room changes, that will increase client's comfort and willingness to work.

Coordinate analgesia schedule with the weaning schedule.

Wean client in a sitting or reverse Trendelenburg position, if not contraindicated.

Start weaning trial when the person is rested, usually in the morning after a night's sleep.

Use of a bedside fan may reduce feelings of dyspnea.

Negotiate Elements of the Weaning Process with Other Clinicians to Maximize the Probability of Success.

Starting time	Pace of weaning
Adherence to care plan	Diversional activities (eg, trips outside the unit)
Scheduling of activities and rest	

Rationales

- Successful weaning depends on adequate energy resources, careful use of available energy, and skilled withdrawal of the ventilator support within the limits of the person's ability to tolerate additional breathing work. Altered or depleted energy reserve enhances fatigue (Burns, 1991). Thus, energy-conservation techniques are crucial to all weaning approaches (Jenny & Logan, 1998; Logan & Jenny, 1990).

- Music with 60 to 80 beats/min decreases arousability of the CNS and exerts a hypnotic, relaxed state (Chan, 1998).

- To maintain adequate energy levels, nutritional support is necessary. It should avoid creating the complications of lipogenesis, overfeeding, and excessive carbohydrate loading to prevent excessive levels of carbon dioxide and respiratory acidemia (Higgins, 1998).

- As ventilator support is withdrawn, clients have to work harder. Their work of weaning involves controlling their breathing, communicating their comfort status, cooperating with the therapeutic regimen, and trying to control their emotional responses to feelings of fatigue and anxiety (Jenny & Logan, 1991).

- Weaning setbacks are common and require client support. During prolonged weaning, the client must be psychologically motivated to wean. Music therapy appears to have a beneficial effect in promoting relaxation in mechanically ventilated clients (Chlan, 1995). Feelings of powerlessness, hopelessness, and depression are combated with active decision making with the person, explanation of sensations experienced, positive feedback, and conveyance of hopefulness, encouragement, and support (Logan & Jenny, 1991). Additional optional interventions for weaning include use of active listening, humor, physical rest, spiritual support, and pressure ulcer prevention (McCloskey & Bulechek, 1996).

- Successful weaning is both an art and a science. The art depends on using subjective clinical judgment about the individual situation. The science involves the theories of oxygen exchange, carbon dioxide exchange, and mechanical efficiency (Henneman, 1991). Nurses are a critical factor in imparting a positive outlook, creating a secure environment, enhancing feelings of self-esteem and self-confidence, and helping clients deal with setbacks through their ability to combine the art and science of weaning (Jenny & Logan, 1994).

RISK FOR DYSFUNCTIONAL VENTILATORY WEANING RESPONSE

DEFINITION

Risk for Dysfunctional Ventilatory Weaning Response: State in which a person is at risk for experiencing an inability to adjust to lowered levels of mechanical ventilator support during the weaning process, related to physical and/or psychological unreadiness to wean

RISK FACTORS
Pathophysiologic
Related to airway obstruction
Related to muscle weakness and fatigue secondary to:

Impaired respiratory functioning	Decreased level of consciousness	Unstable hemodynamic status
Metabolic abnormalities	Fever	Acid–base abnormalities
Dysrhythmia	Anemia	Mental confusion
Fluid and/or electrolyte imbalance	Severe disease	Infection
	Multisystem disease	

Treatment-Related
Related to ineffective airway clearance
Related to excess sedation, analgesia
Related to uncontrolled pain
Related to fatigue
Related to inadequate nutrition (deficit in calories, excess carbohydrates, inadequate fats and protein intake)
Related to prolonged ventilator dependence (more than 1 week)
Related to previous unsuccessful ventilator weaning attempt(s)
Related to too-rapid pacing of the weaning process

Situational (Personal, Environmental)
Related to muscle weakness and fatigue secondary to:

Chronic nutritional deficit	Obesity	Ineffective sleep patterns

Related to knowledge deficit related to the weaning process
Related to inadequate self-efficacy related to weaning
Related to moderate to high anxiety related to breathing efforts
Related to fear of separation from ventilator
Related to feelings of powerlessness

Related to depressed mood
Related to feelings of hopelessness
Related to uncontrolled energy demands (self-care activities, diagnostic and treatment procedures, visitors)
Related to inadequate social support
Related to insecure environment (noisy, upsetting events, busy room)

◎ AUTHOR'S NOTE

See *Dysfunctional Ventilatory Weaning Response.*

◎ ERRORS IN DIAGNOSTIC CONSIDERATIONS

See *Dysfunctional Ventilatory Weaning Response.*

KEY CONCEPTS
Generic Considerations

- Clients at high risk for ventilator weaning are those who, for one reason or another, do not meet the traditional criteria for readiness to wean, such as:
  - Respiratory rate less than 25 breaths/min
  - Oxygen concentration of 40% or less on the ventilator
  - Negative inspiratory pressure less than –20
  - Positive expiratory pressure greater than +30
  - Spontaneous tidal volume greater than 5 mL/kg
  - Vital capacity greater than 10 to 15 mL/kg
  - Adequate arterial blood gases for client
  - Rested, controlled discomfort
- Although weaning as soon as possible is important to avoid muscle deconditioning and complications related to prolonged endotracheal intubation and tracheostomy, premature attempts may be counterproductive because of adverse physiologic and psychological effects.
- Because weaning is a collaborative process, the nurse's ability to gain the client's trust and willingness to work is an important determinant of outcomes, especially with long-term clients. This trust is fostered by the knowledge and self-confidence nurses display, and their ability to deal with the person's specific concerns (Jenny & Logan, 1991).
- Weaning collaboration involves specific roles for both the nurse and the client. The nurse must know the client, manage his or her energy, and assist with the work of weaning. The client's collaborative work requires a trust relationship, and the belief that he or she will be protected during weaning.
- Respiratory muscles must be stressed to a certain point of fatigue and then allowed to rest. The critical point of fatigue and duration of rest have not been documented in the literature, and this judgment depends on clinical expertise (Slutsky, 1993).
- Dysfunctional ventilatory weaning is usually multifactorial. Marini (1991) notes that, at the bedside, the subjective assessment of the weaning trial by an experienced clinician remains the most reliable predictor of weaning success or failure. Close monitoring of the client's weaning work is needed to prevent serious respiratory fatigue, which can require up to 24 to 48 h of recovery before the person can proceed.
- A dysfunctional weaning response to a weaning trial also can influence the client's motivation and self-efficacy, creating doubt about the ability to wean and weakening the resolve to work (Jenny & Logan, 1991).

Focus Assessment Criteria

See *Dysfunctional Ventilatory Weaning Response.*

Goals

NOC Refer to *Dysfunctional Ventilatory Weaning Response*

The person will:

* Demonstrate a willingness to start weaning.
* Demonstrate a positive attitude about ability to succeed.

Indicators

* Maintain emotional control.
* Collaborate with planning of the weaning.

General Interventions

NIC Refer to *Dysfunctional Ventilatory Weaning Response*

Assess for Causative and Contributory Factors of Inadequate Self-efficacy About Weaning Readiness.

Desire for continued need for ventilator support
Excuses for delaying the start of weaning
Concern about ability to adjust to lowered level of ventilator support or about the probability of success of weaning
Agitated when weaning is mentioned
Elevation of blood pressure, pulse, and respirations when weaning is discussed

Reduce Risk Factors.

Negotiate with the medical staff for a delayed start and a weaning plan with a slow pace that ensures success at each stage
See Interventions under *Dysfunctional Ventilatory Weaning Response.*

Rationales

* Experienced critical care nurses agree that weaning readiness involves both physical and psychological preparedness (Logan & Jenny, 1991). Despite ongoing research to evaluate objective criteria for weaning the "challenge to wean" client, consensus is growing that a more holistic evaluation of ventilator dependence is required (Curley & Fackler, 1998).
* A critical strategy in weaning at-risk clients is the development of a weaning plan that maximizes the chances of success in meeting progressive weaning goals and decreases the chances for failure. This plan is designed to eliminate or reduce the intensity of the risk factors, compensate for those factors that cannot be altered, or both.
* An initial step in the weaning plan is the careful preparation of clients. This includes teaching them about their collaborative weaning role, maximizing their energy resources and physical rest, enhancing their psychological willingness to proceed, and reinforcing their belief that they can perform the work of weaning (Jenny & Logan, 1994). Clients may have difficulty expressing their thoughts, so nurses must use multiple communication methods and persist until an effective method is found.

See also Rationale for *Dysfunctional Ventilatory Weaning Response.*

INEFFECTIVE AIRWAY CLEARANCE

DEFINITION

Ineffective Airway Clearance: State in which a person experiences a threat to respiratory status related to inability to cough effectively

DEFINING CHARACTERISTICS
Major (Must Be Present, One or More)

Ineffective or absent cough
Inability to remove airway secretions

Minor (May Be Present)

Abnormal breath sounds
Abnormal respiratory rate, rhythm, depth

RELATED FACTORS

See *Risk for Ineffective Respiratory Function.*

KEY CONCEPTS

See *Risk for Ineffective Respiratory Function.*

Focus Assessment Criteria

See *Risk for Ineffective Respiratory Function.*

Goal

NOC Aspiration Control, Respiratory Status

The person will not experience aspiration.

Indicators

- Demonstrate effective coughing and increased air exchange.
- Explain rationale for interventions to promote coughing.

General Interventions

NIC Cough Enhancement, Airway Suctioning, Positioning, Energy Management

The nursing interventions for the diagnosis *Ineffective Airway Clearance* represent interventions for any person with this nursing diagnosis, regardless of the related factors.

Assess for Causative or Contributing Factors.

Inability to maintain proper
  position
Pain or fear of pain
Fatigue, weakness,
  drowsiness

Ineffective cough
Viscous secretions (dehydration)
Chronic, nonrelieved cough

Reduce or Eliminate Factors, if Possible.

Inability to Maintain Proper Position
Assist with positioning frequently; monitor for *Risk for Aspiration* (see *High Risk for Aspiration*).

628

Ineffective cough

Instruct person on the proper method of controlled coughing:

Breathe deeply and slowly while sitting up as high as possible.

Use diaphragmatic breathing.

Hold the breath for 3 to 5 s and then slowly exhale as much of this breath as possible through the mouth (lower rib cage and abdomen should sink down).

Take a second breath, hold, slowly exhale, and cough forcefully from the chest (not from the back of the mouth or throat), using two short, forceful coughs.

Increase fluid intake if not contraindicated.

Pain or Fear of Pain Related to Surgery or Trauma

Assess present analgesic regimen.

Administer pain medications as needed.

Coordinate analgesic doses with coughing sessions (eg, give doses 30 to 60 min before coughing sessions)

Assess its effectiveness: Is the client too lethargic? Is he or she still in pain?

Note time when person appears to have best pain relief with optimal level of alertness and physical performance. This is the time for active breathing and coughing exercises.

Provide emotional support.

Explain the importance of coughing after pain relief.

Reassure that suture lines are secure and that splinting by hand or pillow will minimize pain of movement.

Use appropriate comfort measures for site of pain.

Splint abdominal or chest incisions with hand, pillow, or both.

For sore throat

Provide humidity unless contraindicated.

Consider warm saline gargle every 2 to 4 h.

Consider use of anesthetic lozenge or gargle, especially before coughing sessions.*

Examine throat for exudate, redness, and swelling; note if it is associated with fever.

Explain that a sore throat is common after anesthesia and should be a short-term problem.

Maintain good body alignment to prevent muscular pain and strain.

Acquire and use extra pillows on both sides, especially the affected side, for support.

Position client to prevent slouching and cramping positions of the thorax and abdomen; reassess positioning frequently.

Assess understanding of the use of analgesia to enhance breathing and coughing effort.

Teach during periods of optimal level of consciousness.

Continually reinforce rationale for plan of nursing care. ("I will be back to help you cough when the pain medicine is working and you can be most effective.")

Viscous (Thick) Secretions

Maintain adequate hydration (increase fluid intake to 2 to 3 quarts a day if not contraindicated by decreased cardiac output or renal disease).

Maintain adequate humidity of inspired air.

Fatigue, Weakness, Drowsiness

Plan and bargain for rest periods ("Work to cough well now; then I can let you rest.").

Vigorously coach and encourage coughing, using positive reinforcement ("You worked hard; I know it's not easy, but it is important.").

Be sure coughing session occurs at peak comfort period after analgesics, but not peak level of sleepiness.

Allow for rest after coughing and before meals.

For lethargy or decreased level of consciousness, stimulate person to breathe deeply hourly ("Take a deep breath.").

For Chronic, Nonrelieved Coughing:

Minimize irritants in the inspired air (eg, dust, allergens).

Provide periods of uninterrupted rest.

Administer prescribed medications—cough suppressant, expectorant—as ordered by physician (withhold food and drink immediately after administration of medications for best results).

Relieve mucous membrane irritation through humidity (inhaling steam from shower, or sitting over pot of steaming water with a towel over the head, loosens thick secretions and soothes the membranes).

---

* May require a primary care professional's order.

Rationales

- Uncontrolled coughing is tiring and ineffective and may contribute to bronchitis.
- Deep breathing dilates the airways, stimulates surfactant production, and expands the lung tissue surface, thus improving respiratory gas exchange. Coughing loosens secretions and forces them into the bronchus to be expectorated or suctioned. In some clients, "huffing" breathing may be effective and is less painful.
- Sitting upright shifts the abdominal organs away from the lungs, enabling greater expansion.
- Diaphragmatic breathing reduces the respiratory rate and increases alveolar ventilation.
- Increasing the volume of air in lungs promotes expulsion of secretions.
- Thick secretions are difficult to expectorate and can cause mucus plugs, leading to atelectasis.
- Good oral hygiene promotes a sense of well-being and prevents mouth odor.
- Secretions must be sufficiently liquid to enable expulsion.
- Pain or fear of pain can inhibit participation in coughing and breathing exercises. Adequate pain relief is essential.
- Coughing exercises are fatiguing and painful. Emotional support provides encouragement; warm water can aid relaxation.

♦ Pediatric Interventions

Instruct parents on the need for child to cough, even if painful.
Allow adult and older child to listen to lungs; describe if clear or if rales are present.
Consult with respiratory therapist for assistance, if needed.

Rationale

Explaining and demonstrating the benefits of coughing can increase parent and child cooperation.

INEFFECTIVE BREATHING PATTERNS

DEFINITION
Ineffective Breathing Patterns: State in which a person experiences an actual or potential loss of adequate ventilation related to an altered breathing pattern

DEFINING CHARACTERISTICS
Major (Must Be Present, One or More)
Changes in respiratory rate or pattern (from baseline)
Changes in pulse (rate, rhythm, quality)

Minor (May Be Present)

Orthopnea	Dysrhythmic respirations
Tachypnea, hyperpnea, hyperventilation	Splinted/guarded respirations

RELATED FACTORS
See *Risk for Ineffective Respiratory Function.*

(X) **AUTHOR'S NOTE**

See *Risk for Ineffective Respiratory Function.*

(X) **ERRORS IN DIAGNOSTIC STATEMENTS**

See *Risk for Ineffective Respiratory Function.*

KEY CONCEPTS
Generic Considerations

- Hyperventilation is overbreathing with reduced Pco_2 and respiratory alkalosis.
- Causes of hyperventilation syndrome are organic (drug effects, CNS lesions), physiologic (response to high altitude, heat, exercise), emotional (anxiety, hysteria, anger, depression), and habitual faulty breathing habits (rapid, shallow breathing; Porth, 2002).
- Symptoms of hyperventilation syndrome are headache, dyspnea, numbness and tingling, lightheadedness, chest pain, palpitations, and, occasionally, syncope (Porth, 2002).
- Panic can manifest with hyperventilation, and people with panic disorders can hyperventilate.
- All nurses involved in caring for clients with COPD must be skilled at teaching pursed-lip breathing, a critical survival skill that these clients must learn to maintain function (Truesdell, 2000). Studies show that pursed-lip breathing decreases respiratory rate, increases tidal volume, decreases arterial CO_2, increases arterial oxygen, and improves exercise performance (Truesdell, 2000).
- Teach the client to inhale through the nose, not too deeply. Breathe out through the mouth while holding the lips (except for a section in the center) together. Exhalation should be at least twice as long as inhalation and should be a steady stream of air without blowing too hard (Truesdell, 2000).

Goals

NOC Respiratory Status, Vital Signs Status, Anxiety Control

Indicators

- Have respiratory rate within normal limits, compared with baseline (8 to 24/min).
- Express relief of (or improvement in) feelings of shortness of breath.
- Relate causative factors and ways of preventing or managing them.

General Interventions

NIC Respiratory Monitoring, Progressive Muscle Relaxation, Teaching, Anxiety Reduction

Assess History of Symptoms and Causative Factors.

Previous episodes—when, where, circumstances
Causes
    Organic, physiologic
    Emotional
    Faulty breathing habits

Remove or Control Causative Factors.

Explain the cause.
Stay with person.
If fear or panic has precipitated the episode:
    Remove cause of fear, if possible.
    Reassure client that measures are being taken to ensure safety.
    Distract person from thinking about the anxious state by having him or her maintain eye contact with you (or perhaps with someone else he or she trusts); say, "Now look at me and breathe slowly with me like this."

Consider use of paper bag as means of rebreathing expired air (expired CO_2 will be reinspired, thereby slowing respiratory rate).
See *Fear*.
Reassure person he or she can control breathing; tell him or her that you will help.
Teach controlled breathing techniques (eg, pursed-lip breathing) or consult with respiratory therapist for training to overcome faulty breathing patterns.

Rationales

- Interventions focus on slowing breathing pattern and educating the person to control response.
- Calming a person with shortness of breath by telling him or her that actions are being taken to improve the situation (eg, "I'm here, and I will get you through this") is an essential intervention to reduce panic and decrease symptoms.

IMPAIRED GAS EXCHANGE

DEFINITION

Impaired Gas Exchange: State in which a person experiences an actual or potential decreased passage of gases (oxygen and carbon dioxide) between the alveoli of the lungs and the vascular system

DEFINING CHARACTERISTICS

Major (Must Be Present)

Dyspnea on exertion

Minor (May Be Present)

Tendency to assume three-point position (sitting, one hand on each knee, bending forward)
Pursed-lip breathing with prolonged expiratory phase
Confusion/agitation
Lethargy and fatigue
Increased pulmonary vascular resistance (increased pulmonary artery/right ventricular pressure)
Decreased gastric motility, prolonged gastric emptying
Decreased oxygen content, decreased oxygen saturation, increased Pco_2, as measured by blood gas analysis
Cyanosis

RELATED FACTORS

See *Risk for Ineffective Respiratory Function*.

> ### ⊚ AUTHOR'S NOTE
>
> Respiratory problems that nurses treat as nursing diagnoses are *Ineffective Airway Clearance, Ineffective Breathing Pattern, Risk for Ineffective Respiratory Function, Dysfunctional Ventilatory Weaning Response,* and *Activity Intolerance.* If these nursing diagnoses are treated, then it follows
> *(continued)*

AUTHOR'S NOTE (*Continued*)

that gas exchange should improve. If gas exchange does not improve, then the problem is a collaborative problem and should be labeled as such (eg, *PC: Hypoxemia* or *PC: Respiratory Insufficiency*). In this case, the nursing role is monitoring to detect changes in status. If respiratory status worsens, the nurse manages the situation using nurse- and physician-prescribed interventions.

 Some nurses are tempted to use *Impaired Gas Exchange* to describe the problem of COPD. Labeling COPD as *Impaired Gas Exchange* does not help in determining nursing interventions. What does the nurse do for *Impaired Gas Exchange*? The nurse helps the person by treating the *Ineffective Airway Clearance, Ineffective Breathing Patterns,* and *Activity Intolerance,* and preventing *Ineffective Respiratory Function*. The nurse also would assess for functional health patterns that decreased oxygenation has or may have affected, such as sleep, emotional status, and nutrition.

IMPAIRED SPONTANEOUS VENTILATION

DEFINITION

Impaired Spontaneous Ventilation: State in which a person is unable to maintain adequate breathing to support life. This is measured by deterioration of arterial blood gases, increased work of breathing, and decreasing energy.

DEFINING CHARACTERISTICS
Major (Must be Present, One or More)

Dyspnea   Increased metabolic rate

Minor

Increased restlessness   Decreased Po_2 Apprehension
Increased use of accessory   Increased Pco_2 Increased heart rate
 muscles   Decreased Sao_2 Decreased cooperation
Decreased tidal volume

AUTHOR'S NOTE

This diagnosis represents respiratory insufficiency with corresponding metabolic changes that are incompatible with life. This situation requires rapid nursing and medical management, specifically resuscitation and mechanical ventilation. Inability to sustain spontaneous ventilation is not appropriate as a nursing diagnosis—it is hypoxemia, a collaborative problem. Hypoxemia is insufficient plasma oxygen saturation because of alveolar hypoventilation, pulmonary shunting, or ventilation–perfusion inequality. As a collaborative problem, physicians prescribe the definitive treatments; however, both nurse- and physician-prescribed interventions are required for management. The nursing accountability is to monitor status continuously and to manage changes in status with the appropriate interventions, using protocols.

INEFFECTIVE ROLE PERFORMANCE

DEFINITION

Ineffective Role Performance: State in which a person experiences or is at risk of experiencing a disruption in the way he or she perceives his or her role performance

DEFINING CHARACTERISTICS
Major (Must Be Present)

Conflict related to role perception or performance

Minor (May Be Present)

Change in self-perception of role
Denial of role
Change in others' perception of role

Change in physical capacity to resume role
Lack of knowledge of role
Change in usual patterns of responsibility

 AUTHOR'S NOTE

The nursing diagnosis *Ineffective Role Performance* has a defining characteristic of "conflict related to role perception or performance." All people have multiple roles. Some are prescribed, such as gender and age; some are acquired, such as parent and occupation; and some are transitional, such as elected office or team member.

Various factors affect a person's roles, including developmental stage, societal norms, cultural beliefs, values, life events, illness, and disabilities. When a person has difficulty with role performance, it may be more useful to describe the effect of the difficulty on functioning, rather than to describe the problem as *Ineffective Role Performance*. For example, a person who has experienced a cerebrovascular accident (CVA) may undergo a change from being the primary breadwinner to becoming unemployed. In this situation, the nursing diagnosis *Grieving related to loss of role as financial provider secondary to effects of CVA* would be appropriate. In another example, if a woman could not continue her household responsibilities because of illness and other family members assumed these responsibilities, the situations that may arise would better be described as *Risk for Disturbed Self-Concept related to recent loss of role responsibility secondary to illness* and *Risk for Impaired Home Maintenance Management related to lack of knowledge of family members*.

A conflict in a family regarding others meeting role obligations or expectations can represent related factors for the diagnosis *Ineffective Family Processes related to conflict regarding expectations of members meeting role obligations*.

Until clinical research defines this diagnosis and the associated nursing interventions, use "ineffective role performance" as a related factor for another nursing diagnosis (eg, *Anxiety, Grieving, or Disturbed Self-Concept*).

Self-Care Deficit Syndrome*
Feeding Self-Care Deficit
Bathing/Hygiene Self-Care Deficit
Dressing/Grooming Self-Care Deficit
Toileting Self-Care Deficit
Instrumental Self-Care Deficit*

SELF-CARE DEFICIT SYNDROME

DEFINITION
Self-Care Deficit Syndrome: State in which a person experiences an impaired motor function or cognitive function, causing a decreased ability in performing each of the five self-care activities

DEFINING CHARACTERISTICS
Major (One Deficit Must Be Present in Each Activity)
Self-Feeding Deficits
Unable to cut food or open packages
Unable to bring food to mouth

Self-Bathing Deficits (Includes Washing Entire Body, Combing Hair, Brushing Teeth, Attending to Skin and Nail Care, and Applying Makeup)
Unable or unwilling to wash body or body parts
Unable to obtain a water source
Unable to regulate temperature or water flow
Unable to perceive need for hygienic measures

Self-Dressing Deficits (Including Donning Regular or Special Clothing, Not Nightclothes)
Impaired ability to put on or take off clothing
Unable to fasten clothing
Unable to groom self satisfactorily
Unable to obtain or replace articles of clothing

Self-Toileting Deficits
Unable or unwilling to get to toilet or commode
Unable or unwilling to carry out proper hygiene
Unable to transfer to and from toilet or commode
Unable to handle clothing to accommodate toileting
Unable to flush toilet or empty commode

Instrumental Self-Care Deficits

Difficulty using telephone	Difficulty shopping
Difficulty laundering, ironing	Difficulty accessing transportation
	Difficulty managing money
Difficulty preparing meals	Difficulty with medication administration

*This diagnosis is not currently on the NANDA list but has been included for clarity or usefulness.

635

RELATED FACTORS
Pathophysiologic
Related to lack of coordination secondary to (specify)
Related to spasticity or flaccidity secondary to (specify)
Related to muscular weakness secondary to (specify)
Related to partial or total paralysis secondary to (specify)
Related to atrophy secondary to (specify)
Related to muscle contractures secondary to (specify)
Related to visual disorders secondary to (specify)
Related to nonfunctioning or missing limb(s)
Related to regression to an earlier level of development
Related to excessive ritualistic behaviors
Related to somatoform deficits (specify)

Treatment-Related
Related to external devices (specify; casts, splints, braces, intravenous [IV] equipment)
Related to postoperative fatigue and pain

Situational (Personal, Environmental)

Related to cognitive deficits	*Related to fatigue*	*Related to pain*
	Related to confusion	*Related to disabling anxiety*
Related to decreased motivation		

Maturational
Older Adult
Related to decreased visual and motor ability, muscle weakness

---

◎ AUTHOR'S NOTE

Self-care encompasses the activities needed to meet daily needs, commonly known as activities of daily living (ADLs), which are learned over time and become lifelong habits. Self-care activities involve not only what is to be done (hygiene, bathing, dressing, toileting, feeding), but also how much, when, where, with whom, and how (Miller, 2004).

In every person, the threat or reality of a self-care deficit evokes panic. Many people report that they fear loss of independence more than death. A self-care deficit affects the core of self-concept and self-determination. For this reason, the nursing focus for self-care deficit should be not on providing the care measure, but on identifying adaptive techniques to allow the person the maximum degree of participation and independence possible.

The diagnosis *Total Self-Care Deficit* once was used to describe a person's inability to complete feeding, bathing, toileting, dressing, and grooming (Carpenito, 1983; Gordon, 1982). The intent of specifying "Total" was to describe a person with deficits in several ADLs. Unfortunately, sometimes its use invites, according to Magnan (1989, personal communication), "preconceived judgments about the state of an individual and the nursing interventions required." The person may be viewed as in a vegetative state, requiring only minimal custodial care. *Total Self-Care Deficit* has been eliminated because its language does not denote potential for growth or rehabilitation.

Currently not on the NANDA list, the diagnosis *Self-Care Deficit Syndrome* has been added here to describe a person with compromised ability in all five self-care activities. For this person, the nurse assesses functioning in each area and identifies the level of participation of which the person is capable. The goal is to maintain current functioning, to increase participation and independence, or both. The syndrome distinction clusters all five self-care deficits together to enable grouping of interventions when indicated, while also permitting specialized interventions for a specific deficit.

The danger of applying a Self-Care Deficit diagnosis lies in the possibility of prematurely labeling a person as unable to participate at any level, eliminating a rehabilitation focus. It is important that the nurse classify the person's functional level to promote independence. (Refer to the functional level classification scale in Focus Assessment Criteria.) Use this scale with the nursing diagnosis, eg, *Toileting Self-Care Deficit* (2). Continuous reevaluation also is necessary to identify changes in the person's ability to participate in self-care.

⊙⊙ **ERRORS IN DIAGNOSTIC STATEMENTS**

1. *Toileting Self-Care Deficit related to insufficient knowledge of ostomy care*
   The diagnosis *Toileting Self-Care Deficit* describes a person who cannot get to, sit on, or rise from the toilet, or perform clothing and hygiene activities related to toileting. Insufficient knowledge of ostomy care does not apply. Depending on the risk factors or signs and symptoms, the diagnosis of *Ineffective Management of Therapeutic Regimen related to insufficient knowledge of ostomy care* would apply.
2. *Dressing Self-Care Deficit related to inability to fasten clothing*
   Inability to fasten clothing represents a sign or symptom of *Dressing Self-Care Deficit,* not a related factor. Using a focus assessment, the nurse needs to determine the contributing factors (eg, insufficient knowledge of adaptive techniques needed).
3. *Self-Care Deficit Syndrome related to cognitive deficits*
   As a syndrome diagnosis, no related factors are indicated and, in fact, they are not very useful for treatment. Instead, the nurse should write the diagnosis as *Self-Care Deficit Syndrome: Feeding (1), Bathing (4), Dressing / Grooming (4), Toileting (5), Instrumental (2).* The number code indicates the present level of functioning needed. The goals or outcome criteria should represent improved or increased functioning.

KEY CONCEPTS
Generic Considerations

- The concept of self-care emphasizes each person's right to maintain individual control over his or her own pattern of living (this applies to both the ill person and the well person).
- It is acceptable to be dependent on others to provide basic physiologic and psychological needs for a limited time.
- Regression in ability to perform self-care activities may be a defense mechanism to threatening situations.
- Neglect of an extremity refers to the memory loss of the presence of an extremity (eg, a person who has had a stroke or brain injury resulting in partial paralysis may ignore the arm or leg on the affected side of the body).
- The following key elements promote relearning of self-care tasks:
  - Providing a structured, consistent environment and routine
  - Repeating instructions and tasks
  - Teaching and practicing tasks during periods of least fatigue
  - Maintaining a familiar environment and teacher
  - Using patience, determination, and a positive attitude (by both learner and teacher)
  - Practice, practice, practice
- Lubkin (1995) describes four principles to motivate:
  - Uncover hidden resources.
  - Increase underused abilities.
  - Initiate positive life patterns.
  - Flourish within existing limitations.

Endurance

- The endurance or ability of the person to maintain a given level of performance is influenced by the ability to use oxygen to produce energy (related to the optimal functioning of the heart and respiratory and circulatory systems) and the functioning of the neurologic and musculoskeletal systems. Thus, clients with alterations in these systems have increased energy demands or decreased ability to produce energy.
- Stress is energy-consuming; the more stressors a person has, the more fatigue he or she experiences. Stressors can be personal, environmental, disease-related, and treatment-related. Examples of possible stressors follow:

Personal	Environmental	Disease-Related	Treatment-Related
Age	Isolation	Pain	Walker
Support system	Noise	Anemia	Medications
Lifestyle	Unfamiliar setting	Diagnostic studies	

- Signs and symptoms of decreased oxygen in response to activity (eg, self-care, mobility) are as follows:
  - Sustained increased heart rate 3 to 5 min after ceasing the activity, or a change in the pulse rhythm
  - Failure of systolic blood pressure reading to increase with activity, or a decrease in value
  - Decrease or excessive increase in respiratory rate and dyspnea
  - Weakness, pallor, cerebral hypoxia (confusion, incoordination)

Refer to Key Concepts under *Activity Intolerance* for additional information.

Pediatric Considerations

- Infants and young children depend on caregivers for assistance with ADLs.
- Parents/caregivers can facilitate a child's mastery of self-care skills. The desired outcome is that the child participates in his or her care to the maximum of ability (Wong, 2003).
- The nurse should assess each child's unique ability to engage in self-care activities to promote control over self and environment.
- Children with cancer with higher self-concept scores performed more self-care practices and received less dependent care from their mothers (Mosher & Moore, 1998).
- When self-care requirements are met by oneself or others, self-concept is lower (Mosher & Moore, 1998).

Geriatric Considerations

- Age-related changes do not in themselves cause self-care deficits. Older adults do, however, have an increased incidence of chronic diseases that can compromise functional ability (eg, arthritis, cardiac disorders, visual impairment).
- Older adults with dementia have varying degrees of difficulty with self-care activities depending on memory deficits, ability to follow directions, and judgment (Miller, 2004).
- Sixty-three percent of older nursing home residents cannot perform basic ADLs because of cognitive impairment (Miller, 2004).
- Caregivers frequently promote excess disability and quicker deterioration in older adults because they believe independent behavior is atypical (Miller, 2004).

Transcultural Considerations

- In some cultures, family members may show their concern for the sick relative by doing as much as possible for him or her (eg, feeding, bathing). This practice may prevent the client from actively participating in a rehabilitation program (Andrews & Boyle, 2003).
- All cultures have rules, often unspoken, about who touches whom, when, and where (Andrews & Boyle, 2003).

Focus Assessment Criteria

Subjective and Objective Data
Evaluate Each ADL Using the Following Scale:

0 = Is completely independent
1 = Requires use of assistive device
2 = Needs minimal help
3 = Needs assistance and/or some supervision
4 = Needs total supervision
5 = Needs total assistance or unable to assist

Assess for Defining Characteristics.

Self-feeding abilities

Swallowing	Drinking from cup	Chewing
Using utensils and cutting food	Selecting foods	Opening cartons
	Seeing	

Self-bathing abilities

Undressing to bathe
Reaching water source
Differentiating water temperatures
Washing body parts
Performing oral care
Obtaining equipment (water, soap, towels)

Self-dressing/grooming abilities

Putting on or taking off clothing	Fastening clothing	Brushing teeth
Selecting appropriate clothing	Cleaning/trimming nails	Plugging in cord
Retrieving appropriate clothing	Washing and styling hair	Using deodorant
	Shaving	

Self-toileting abilities

Getting to toilet and undressing	Can use tampon/sanitary napkin	Sitting on toilet
Performing hygiene (washing hands)	Redressing	Cleaning self/flushing toilet
	Rising from toilet	

Instrumental ADLs

Telephone

Ability to dial	Ability to talk, hear	Ability to answer

Transportation

Ability to drive	Access to transportation

Laundry

Availability of washer	Ability to wash, iron	Ability to put away

Food procurement and preparation

Ability to cook	Ability to select foods	Ability to shop

Medications

Ability to remember	Ability to administer

Finances

Ability to write checks, pay bills
Ability to handle cash transactions (simple, complex)

Assess for Related Factors.

Ability to remember
Judgment
Ability to follow directions
Ability to identify/express needs
Ability to anticipate needs (food, laundry)
Social supports
    Support people
    Availability of help with transportation, shopping, money management, laundry, housekeeping, food preparation
    Community resources
Motivation
Endurance

For more information on Focus Assessment Criteria, visit http://connection.lww.com.

Goal

NOC See *Bathing/Hygiene, Feeding, Dressing, Toileting,* and/or *Instrumental Self-Care Deficit*

The person will participate in feeding, dressing, toileting, bathing activities.

Indicators

- Identify preferences in self-care activities (eg time, products, location).
- Demonstrate optimal hygiene after assistance with care.

General Interventions

> **NIC** See *Feeding, Bathing, Dressing, Toileting, and/or Instrumental Self-Care Deficit*

Assess for Causative or Contributing Factors.

Visual deficits	Impaired cognition	Decreased motivation
Impaired mobility	Lack of knowledge	Inadequate social support
Excessive ritualistic behavior	Disabling anxiety	Irrational fears
Developmental regression		

Promote Optimal Participation.

Assess present level of participation.

Determine areas for potentially increased participation in each self-care activity.

Explore the person's goals.

Allow ample time to complete activities without help. Promote independence, but assist when person cannot perform an activity.

Demonstrate how to perform an activity that is problematic.

Promote Self-esteem and Self-determination.

Determine preferences for:

Schedule	Products	Methods
Clothing selection	Hair styling	

During self-care activities, provide choices and request preferences.

Do not focus on disability.

Offer praise for independent accomplishments

Do not allow client to use a disability as a manipulative tool. Withdraw attention if person continues to focus on limitations.

Evaluate Client's Ability to Participate in Each Self-Care Activity (Feeding, Dressing, Bathing, Toileting).

Assign a number value to each activity (refer to the coding scale in Focus Assessment Criteria).

Reassess ability frequently and revise code as appropriate.

Refer to Interventions Under Each Diagnosis—Feeding, Bathing, Dressing, Toileting, and Instrumental Self-Care Deficit—as Indicated.

Rationales

- Enhancing a client's self-care abilities can increase his or her sense of control and independence, promoting overall well-being.
- Regardless of handicap, people should be given privacy and treated with dignity while performing self-care activities.
- Self-care does not imply allowing the person to do things for himself or herself as planned by the nurse, but encouraging and teaching the person to make his or her own plans for optimal daily living.
- Mobility is necessary to meet self-care needs and to maintain good health and self-esteem.
- Cleanliness is important for comfort, positive self-esteem, and social interactions.
- Inability to care for oneself produces feelings of dependency and poor self-concept. With increased ability for self-care, self-esteem increases.
- Disability often causes denial, anger, and frustration. These valid emotions must be recognized and addressed.
- Optimal education promotes self-care. To teach effectively, the nurse must determine what the learner perceives as his or her own needs and goals, determine what the nurse believes are the learner's needs and goals, and then work to establish mutually acceptable goals.
- Offering choices and including the client in planning care reduces feelings of powerlessness; promotes feelings of freedom, control, and self-worth; and increases the person's willingness to comply with therapeutic regimens.

FEEDING SELF-CARE DEFICIT

DEFINITION

Feeding Self-Care Deficit: State in which a person experiences an impaired ability to perform or complete feeding activities for himself or herself.

DEFINING CHARACTERISTICS

Unable to cut food or open food packages
Unable to bring food to mouth

RELATED FACTORS

See *Self-Care Deficit Syndrome.*

 AUTHOR'S NOTE

See *Self-Care Deficit Syndrome.*

 ERRORS IN DIAGNOSTIC STATEMENTS

See *Self-Care Deficit Syndrome.*

KEY CONCEPTS

See *Self-Care Deficit Syndrome.*

Focus Assessment Criteria

See *Self-Care Deficit Syndrome.*

Goal

| **NOC** | Nutritional Status, Self-Care: Eating, Swallowing Status |

The person will demonstrate increased ability to feed self or report that he or she needs assistance.

Indicators

- Demonstrate ability to make use of adaptive devices, if indicated.
- Demonstrate increased interest and desire to eat.
- Describe rationale and procedure for treatment.
- Describe causative factors for feeding deficit.

General Interventions

| **NIC** | Feeding, Self-Care Assistance: Feeding, Swallowing Therapy, Teaching, Aspiration Precautions |

Assess Causative Factors.

Visual deficits (blindness, field cuts, poor depth perception)
Affected or missing limbs (casts, amputations, paresis, paralysis)
Cognitive deficits (dementia, trauma, cerebrovascular accident [CVA])

Provide Opportunities to Relearn or Adapt to Activity.

Common Nursing Interventions for Feeding

Ascertain from person or family members what foods the person likes or dislikes.

Ensure client eats meals in the same setting with pleasant surroundings that are not too distracting.

Maintain correct food temperatures (hot foods hot, cold foods cold).

Provide pain relief, because pain can affect appetite and ability to feed self.

Provide good oral hygiene before and after meals.

Encourage person to wear dentures and eyeglasses.

Assist client to the most normal eating position suited to his or her physical disability (best is sitting in a chair at a table).

Provide social contact during eating.

See *Imbalanced Nutrition: Less Than Body Requirements.*

Specific Interventions for People with Sensory/Perceptual Deficits

Encourage client to wear prescribed corrective lenses.

Describe location of utensils and food on tray or table.

Describe food items to stimulate appetite.

For perceptual deficits, choose different-colored dishes to help distinguish items (eg, red tray, white plates).

Ascertain usual eating patterns and provide food items according to preference (or arrange food items in clocklike pattern); record on care plan the arrangement used (eg, meat, 6 o'clock; potatoes, 9 o'clock; vegetables, 12 o'clock).

Encourage eating of "finger foods" (eg, bread, bacon, fruit, hot dogs) to promote independence.

Avoid placing food to blind side of person with field cut, until visually accommodated to surroundings; then encourage him or her to scan entire visual field.

Specific Interventions for People with Missing Limbs

Provide for eating environment that is not embarrassing to client; allow sufficient time for eating.

Provide only the supervision and assistance necessary for relearning or adaptation.

To enhance independence, provide necessary adaptive devices:

 Plate guard to avoid pushing food off plate

 Suction device under plate or bowl for stabilization

 Padded handles on utensils for a more secure grip

 Wrist or hand splints with clamp to hold eating utensils

 Special drinking cup

 Rocker knife for cutting

Assist with set-up if needed, opening containers, napkins, condiment packages; cutting meat; and buttering bread.

Arrange food so person has enough space to perform the task of eating.

Specific Interventions for People with Cognitive Deficits

Provide isolated, quiet atmosphere until person can attend to eating and is not easily distracted from the task.

Supervise feeding program until there is no danger of choking or aspiration.

Orient person to location and purpose of feeding equipment.

Avoid external distractions and unnecessary conversation.

Place person in the most normal eating position he or she can physically assume.

Encourage person to attend to the task, but be alert for fatigue, frustration, or agitation.

Provide one food at a time in usual sequence of eating until person can eat the entire meal in normal sequence.

Encourage person to be tidy, to eat in small amounts, and to put food in unaffected side of mouth if paresis or paralysis is present.

Check for food in cheeks.

Refer to *Impaired Swallowing* for additional interventions.

For a Person Who is Not Eating Because of Fears of Being Poisoned:

Allow person to open cans of foods.

Serve food family style, so he or she can witness others eating.

Initiate Health Teaching and Referrals, as Indicated.

Ensure that both person and family understand the reason and purpose of all interventions.

Proceed with teaching as needed.

Maintain safe eating methods.

Prevent aspiration.

Use appropriate eating utensils (avoid sharp instruments).

Test temperature of hot liquids and wear protective clothing (eg, paper bib).

Teach use of adaptive devices.

Rationale

Eating has physiologic, psychological, social, and cultural implications. Providing control over meals promotes overall well-being.

BATHING/HYGIENE SELF-CARE DEFICIT

DEFINITION

Bathing/Hygiene Self-Care Deficit: State in which a person experiences an impaired ability to perform or complete bathing/hygiene activities for himself or herself

DEFINING CHARACTERISTICS

Self-bathing deficits (including washing entire body, combing hair, brushing teeth, attending to skin and nail care, and applying makeup)

Unable or unwilling to wash body or body parts

Unable to obtain a water source

Unable to regulate temperature or water flow

Inability to perceive need for hygienic measures

RELATED FACTORS

See *Self-Care Deficit Syndrome.*

AUTHOR'S NOTE

See *Self-Care Deficit Syndrome.*

ERRORS IN DIAGNOSTIC STATEMENTS

See *Self-Care Deficit Syndrome.*

KEY CONCEPTS

See *Self-Care Deficit Syndrome.*

Focus Assessment Criteria

See *Self-Care Deficit Syndrome.*

Goal

NOC Self-Care: Activities of Daily Living, Self-Care: Bathing, Self-Care: Hygiene

The person will perform bathing activity
at expected optimal level or report satisfaction with accomplishments despite limitations.

Indicators

- Relate feeling of comfort and satisfaction with body cleanliness.
- Demonstrate ability to use adaptive devices.
- Describe causative factors of bathing deficit.

General Interventions

NIC Self-Care Assistance: Bathing/Hygiene, Teaching: Individual

Assess Causative Factors.

Visual deficits (blindness, field cuts, poor depth perception)
Affected or missing limbs (casts, amputations, paresis, paralysis, arthritis)
Cognitive deficits (aging, trauma, CVA)

Provide Opportunities to Relearn or Adapt to Activity.

General Nursing Interventions for Inability to Bathe

Bathing time and routine should be consistent to encourage optimal independence.
Encourage person to wear prescribed corrective lenses or hearing aid.
Keep bathroom temperature warm; ascertain client's preferred water temperature.
Provide for privacy during bathing routine.
Keep environment simple and uncluttered.
Observe skin condition during bathing.
Provide all bathing equipment within easy reach.
Provide for safety in the bathroom (nonslip mats, grab bars).
When person is physically able, encourage use of either tub or shower stall, depending on which he or
  she uses at home (the person should practice in the hospital in preparation for going home).
Provide for adaptive equipment as needed.
    Chair or stool in bathtub or shower
    Long-handled sponge to reach back or lower extremities
    Grab bars on bathroom walls where needed to assist in mobility
    Bath board for transferring to tub chair or stool
    Safety treads or nonslip mat on floor of bathroom, tub, and shower
    Washing mitts with pocket for soap
    Adapted toothbrushes
    Shaver holders
    Hand-held shower spray
Provide for relief of pain that may affect ability to bathe self.*

Specific Interventions for Bathing for People with Visual Deficits

Place bathing equipment in location most suitable to individual.
Avoid placing bathing equipment to blind side if person has a field cut and is not visually accommo-
  dated to surroundings.
Keep call bell within reach if person is to bathe alone.
Give the person with visual impairment the same degree of privacy and dignity as any other person.
Announce yourself before entering or leaving the bathing area.
Observe the person's ability to locate all bathing utensils.
Observe the person's ability to perform mouth care, hair combing, and shaving.
Provide place for clean clothing within easy reach.

Specific Interventions for Bathing for People with Affected or Missing Limbs

Bathe early in morning or before bed at night to avoid unnecessary dressing and undressing.
Encourage client to use a mirror during bathing to inspect the skin of paralyzed areas.
Encourage the person with amputation to inspect remaining foot or stump for good skin integrity.

---

*May require a primary care professional's order.

For limb amputations, bathe stump twice a day and be sure it is dry before wrapping it or applying prosthesis.

Provide only the supervision or assistance necessary for relearning the use of extremity or adaptation to the handicap.

For lack of sensation, encourage use of the affected area in the bathing process (a person tends to forget the existence of body parts in which there is no sensation).

Specific Interventions for Bathing for People with Cognitive Deficits

Provide a consistent time for bathing as part of a structured program to help decrease confusion.

Keep instructions simple and avoid distractions; orient client to purpose of bathing equipment, put toothpaste on toothbrush.

If person cannot bathe the entire body, have him or her bathe one part until he or she does it correctly; give positive reinforcement for success.

Supervise activity until person can safely perform the task unassisted.

Encourage attention to the task, but be alert for fatigue that may increase confusion.

Apply firm pressure to the skin when bathing; it is less likely to be misinterpreted than a gentle touch.

Use a warm shower or bath to help a confused or agitated person to relax.

Initiate Health Teaching and Referrals, as Indicated.

Communicate to staff and family members the person's ability and willingness to learn.

Teach use of adaptive devices.

Ascertain bathing facilities at home and assist in determining if there is any need for adaptations; refer to occupational therapy or social service for help in obtaining needed home equipment.

Teach client to use tub or shower stall, depending on what is used at home.

If person is paralyzed, instruct client or family to demonstrate complete skin check on key areas for redness (buttocks, bony prominences).

Teach family to maintain a safe bathing environment.

Rationale

Inability to perform self-care produces feelings of dependency and poor self-concept. With increased ability for self-care, self-esteem increases (Maher et al., 1998).

DRESSING/GROOMING SELF-CARE DEFICIT

DEFINITION

Dressing/Grooming Self-Care Deficit: State in which a person experiences an impaired ability to perform or complete dressing and grooming activities for himself or herself.

DEFINING CHARACTERISTICS

Self-dressing deficits (including donning regular or special clothing, not nightclothes)

Impaired ability to put on or take off clothing

Unable to fasten clothing

Unable to groom self satisfactorily

Unable to obtain or replace articles of clothing

RELATED FACTORS

See *Self-Care Deficit Syndrome.*

AUTHOR'S NOTE

See *Self-Care Deficit Syndrome.*

ERRORS IN DIAGNOSTIC STATEMENTS

See *Self-Care Deficit Syndrome.*

KEY CONCEPTS
See *Self-Care Deficit Syndrome.*

Focus Assessment Criteria

See *Self-Care Deficit Syndrome.*

Goal

NOC Self-Care: Activities of Daily Living, Self-Care: Dressing, Self-Care: Grooming

The person will demonstrate increased ability to dress self or report the need to have someone else assist him or her to perform the task.

Indicators
- Demonstrate ability to use adaptive devices to facilitate independence in dressing.
- Demonstrate increased interest in wearing street clothes.
- Describe causative factors for dressing deficits.
- Relate rationale and procedures for treatments.

General Interventions

NIC Self-Care Assistance: Dressing/Grooming, Teaching: Individual, Dressing

Assess Causative Factors.

Visual deficits (blindness, field cuts, poor depth perception)
Affected or missing limbs (casts, amputations, arthritis, paresis, paralysis)
Cognitive deficits (aging, trauma, CVA)

Provide Opportunities to Relearn or Adapt to Activity.

General Nursing Interventions for Self-Dressing
Encourage person to wear prescribed corrective lenses or hearing aid.
Promote independence in dressing through continual and unaided practice.
Choose loose-fitting clothing with wide sleeves and pant legs and front fasteners.
Allow sufficient time for dressing and undressing, because the task may be tiring, painful, or difficult.
Plan for person to learn and demonstrate one part of an activity before progressing further.
Lay clothes out in the order in which the client will need them to dress.
Provide dressing aids as necessary (some commonly used aids include dressing stick, Swedish reacher, zipper pull, buttonhook, long-handled shoehorn, and shoe fasteners adapted with elastic laces, Velcro closures, or flip-back tongues; all garments with fasteners may be adapted with Velcro closures).
Encourage person to wear ordinary or special clothing rather than nightclothes.
Increase participation in dressing by medicating for pain 30 min before it is time to dress or undress, if indicated.*

---

* May require a primary care professional's order.

Provide for privacy during dressing routine.

Provide for safety by ensuring easy access to all clothing and by ascertaining person's performance level.

Specific Interventions for Dressing for People with Visual Deficits

Allow person to ascertain the most convenient location for clothing and adapt the environment to accomplish the task best (eg, remove unnecessary barriers).

Announce yourself before entering or leaving the dressing area.

If person has a field cut, avoid placing clothing to the blind side until he or she is visually accommodated to surroundings; then encourage him or her to turn head to scan entire visual field.

Apply adaptive devices (eg, hand splints) before dressing activity.

Consult or refer to physical or occupational therapy for teaching application of prosthetics to missing limbs.

Specific Interventions for Dressing for People with Cognitive Deficits (Miller, 2004)

Keep verbal communication simple.

    Ask yes/no questions.

    Use one-step requests (eg, "put your sock on").

    Praise after each step.

    Be specific and concise.

    Call by name.

    Use same word for same thing (eg, "shirt").

    Dress bottom half, then top half.

Prepare an uncluttered environment.

    Ensure good lighting.

    Make bed; minimize visual clutter.

    Lay clothes face down.

    Place clothes in order that they will be used.

    Allow resident a choice from only two pieces.

    Place matching clothes together on hangers.

    Remove dirty clothes from dressing area.

Provide nonverbal cues.

    Hand one clothing item at a time in correct order.

    Place shoes beside correct foot.

    Use gestures to explain.

    Point or touch body part to be used.

    If person cannot complete all the steps, always allow him or her to finish the dressing step, if possible—zipper pants, buckle belt.

    Decrease assistance gradually.

Initiate Health Teaching and Referrals, as Indicated.

Assess Understanding and Knowledge of Client and Family for Above Instructions and Rationale.

Proceed with Teaching as Needed.

Communicate to staff and family members the person's ability and willingness to learn.

Teach use of adaptive devices and techniques that are specific to each disability.

Teach client to maintain a safe dressing environment.

Attempt to be noncritical in correcting errors.

Rationale

Optimal personal grooming promotes psychological well-being (Tracey, 1992).

TOILETING SELF-CARE DEFICIT

DEFINITION

Toileting Self-Care Deficit: State in which a person experiences an impaired ability to perform or complete toileting activities for himself or herself

DEFINING CHARACTERISTICS

Unable or unwilling to get to toilet or commode
Unable or unwilling to carry out proper hygiene
Unable to transfer to and from toilet or commode
Unable to handle clothing to accommodate toileting
Unable to flush toilet or empty commode

RELATED FACTORS

See *Self-Care Deficit Syndrome.*

⊚ **AUTHOR'S NOTE**

See *Self-Care Deficit Syndrome.*

⊚ **ERRORS IN DIAGNOSTIC STATEMENTS**

See *Self-Care Deficit Syndrome.*

KEY CONCEPTS

See *Self-Care Deficit Syndrome.*

Focus Assessment Criteria

See *Self-Care Deficit Syndrome.*

Goal

NOC	Self-Care: Activities of Daily Living, Self-Care: Hygiene, Self-Care: Toileting

The person will demonstrate increased ability to toilet self or report the need to have someone assist him or her to perform the task.

Indicators

- Demonstrate ability to use adaptive devices to facilitate toileting.
- Describe causative factors for toileting deficit.
- Relate rationale and procedures for treatment.

General Interventions

NIC Self-Care Assistance: Toileting,
Self-Care Assistance: Hygiene,
Teaching: Individual, Mutual Goal Setting

Assess Causative Factors.

Visual deficits (blindness, field cuts, poor depth perception)

Affected or missing limbs (casts, amputations, paresis, paralysis)

Cognitive deficits (aging, trauma, CVA)

Provide Opportunities to Relearn or Adapt to Activity.

Common Nursing Interventions for Toileting Difficulties

Encourage client to wear prescribed corrective lenses or hearing aid.

Obtain bladder and bowel history from individual or significant other (see *Impaired Bowel Elimination* or *Impaired Urinary Elimination*).

Ascertain communication system person uses to express the need to toilet.

Maintain bladder and bowel record to determine toileting patterns.

Provide adequate fluid intake and balanced diet to promote adequate urinary output and normal bowel evacuation.

Promote normal elimination by encouraging activity and exercise within the person's capabilities.

Avoid development of "bowel fixation" by less frequent discussion and inquiries about bowel movements.

Be alert to possibility of falls when toileting person (be prepared to ease him or her to floor without injuring either of you).

Achieve independence in toileting by continual and unaided practice.

Allow sufficient time for the task of toileting to avoid fatigue (lack of sufficient time to toilet may cause incontinence or constipation).

Avoid use of indwelling and condom catheters to expedite bladder continence (if possible).

Specific Interventions for Toileting for People with Visual Deficits

Keep call bell easily accessible so person can quickly obtain help to toilet; answer call bell promptly to decrease anxiety.

If bedpan or urinal is necessary for toileting, be sure it is within person's reach.

Avoid placing toileting equipment to the blind side of a person with field cut (when he or she is visually accommodated to surroundings, you may suggest he or she search entire visual field for equipment).

Announce yourself before entering or leaving toileting area.

Observe person's ability to obtain equipment or get to the toilet unassisted.

Provide for a safe and clear pathway to toilet area.

Specific Interventions for Toileting for People with Affected or Missing Limbs

Provide only the supervision and assistance necessary for relearning or adapting to the prosthesis.

Encourage person to look at affected area or limb and use it during toileting tasks.

Encourage useful transfer techniques taught by occupational or physical therapy (the nurse become familiar with planned mode of transfer).

Provide the necessary adaptive devices to enhance independence and safety (commode chairs, spill-proof urinals, fracture bedpans, raised toilet seats, support siderails for toilets).

Provide for a safe and clear pathway to toilet area.

Specific Interventions for Toileting for People with Cognitive Deficits

Offer toileting reminders every 2 h, after meals, and before bedtime.

When person can indicate the need to toilet, begin toileting at 2-h intervals, after meals, and before bedtime.

Answer call bell immediately to avoid frustration and incontinence.

Encourage wearing ordinary clothes (many confused people are continent while wearing regular clothing).

Avoid the use of bedpans and urinals; if physically possible, provide a normal atmosphere of elimination in bathroom (the toilet used should remain constant to promote familiarity).

Give verbal cues as to what is expected of the person and positive reinforcement for success.

Work to achieve daytime continence before expecting nighttime continence (nighttime incontinence may continue after daytime continence has returned).

See *Impaired Urinary Elimination* for additional information on incontinence.

Initiate Health Teaching and Referrals, as Indicated.

Assess the Understanding and Knowledge of the Client and Significant Others of Foregoing Interventions and Rationales.

Communicate to staff and family members the person's ability and willingness to learn.

Maintain a safe toileting environment.

Reinforce knowledge of transferring techniques.

Teach use of adaptive devices.

Ascertain home toileting needs and refer to occupational therapy or social services for help in obtaining necessary equipment.

Rationales

- Inability to perform self-care produces feelings of dependency and poor self-concept. With increased self-care ability, self-esteem increases (Maher et al., 1998).
- The client's maximum involvement in toileting activities can reduce the embarrassment associated with needing assistance with toileting (Maher et al., 1998).

INSTRUMENTAL SELF-CARE DEFICIT

DEFINITION

Instrumental Self-Care Deficit: State in which a person experiences an impaired ability to perform certain activities or access certain services essential for managing a household

DEFINING CHARACTERISTICS

Observed or reported difficulty in one or more of the following:

Using a telephone
Accessing transportation
Laundering, ironing
Preparing meals
Shopping (food, clothes)
Managing money
Administering medication

RELATED FACTORS

See *Self-Care Deficit Syndrome.*

⊛ AUTHOR'S NOTE

Instrumental Self-Care Deficit is not currently on the NANDA list but has been added here for clarity and usefulness. This diagnosis describes problems in performing certain activities or accessing certain services needed to live in the community (eg, phone use, shopping, money management). This diagnosis is important to consider in discharge planning and during home visits by community nurses.

⊗⊗ **ERRORS IN DIAGNOSTIC STATEMENTS**

Instrumental Self-Care Deficit related to possible inability to plan meals and manage laundry
When a nurse suspects that a client or family may have compromised ability to engage in certain activities needed to live in and run a household, the nurse should label the diagnosis *Possible Instrumental Self-Care Deficit* and add related factors representing why he or she suspects the diagnosis (eg, *related to difficulty remembering routine tasks or related to poor planning skills*). The nurse detecting evidence of memory or judgment difficulties could interpret this as a risk factor for *Risk for Instrumental Self-Care Deficit.*

KEY CONCEPTS
Generic Considerations

- Brody (1985) found that, to live in the community, a person has to perform or have assistance with six ADLs as well as additional activities.
- Instrumental ADLs include housekeeping, preparing and procuring food, shopping, laundering, ability to self-medicate safely, ability to manage money, and access to transportation (Miller, 2004).
- Instrumental ADLs are more complex tasks than ADLs.
- Maintaining people in the community, rather than in nursing homes, has significant financial benefit. In 1981, 25% of all US health care expenditures for older adults went to nursing homes, but only 5% of older adults were receiving care in these facilities. Medicaid covers about 90% of public spending for nursing home care (Miller, 2004).
- Maintaining people in the community, rather than in nursing homes, also maintains autonomy, strengthens family life, and affirms the value of older adults in our society.

Focus Assessment Criteria

See *Self-Care Deficit Syndrome.*

Goal

NOC Self-Care Instrumental Activities of Daily Living (IADL)

The person or family will report satisfaction with household management.

Indicators

- Demonstrate use of adaptive devices (eg, phone, cooking aids).
- Describe a method to ensure adherence to medication schedule.
- Report ability to make calls and answer telephone.
- Report regular laundering by self or others.
- Report daily intake of at least two nutritious meals.
- Identify transportation options to stores, physician, house of worship, social activities.
- Demonstrate management of simple money transactions.
- Identify people who will assist with money matters.

General Interventions

NIC Teaching: Individual, Referral, Family Involvement Promotion

Assess for Causative and Contributing Factors.

Visual, hearing deficits	Impaired cognition	Impaired mobility
Lack of knowledge	Inadequate social support	

Assist Client to Identify Self-Help Devices.

Grooming/Dressing Aids
See *Impaired Physical Mobility.*

Kitchen/Eating Aids
Dishes with one side built up
Built-up handles on cutlery (use plastic foam curlers)
Bulldog clip to secure a straw in glass
Built-up corner of cutlery board to hold and anchor food or pot (eg, to butter toast, mash potatoes)

Mounted jar opener
Nonslip material applied under dishes (same strips used to prevent slipping in bathtub)
Two-sided suction holder to hold dishes in place

Communication/Security
Motion-activated lights near walkway/entrance
Nightlight for path to bathroom
Light next to bed
Specially adapted phones (amplified, big buttons)

Promote Self-Care and Safety for Person with Cognitive Deficit.

Evaluate Activities that are Achievable.

Teach Safety Techniques.
Turn lights on before dark.
Use nightlights.
Keep environment simple, uncluttered.
Use clocks and calendars as cues.
Mark on calendar (using picture symbols) reminders for shopping, laundry, cleaning, doctor's
   appointments, and the like.

For Laundry, Teach Client to:
Separate dark and light clothes.
Use pictures to illustrate steps for washing clothes.
Mark cup with line to indicate amount of soap needed.
Minimize ironing.
Use an iron with automatic shutoff mechanism.

Evaluate Client's Ability to Select, Procure, and Prepare Nutritious Food Daily.
Prepare a permanent shopping list with cues for essential foods, products.
Teach client to review list before shopping, check items needed, and, in the store, check off items
   selected. (Use a pencil that can be erased to reuse list.)
Teach client how to shop for single-person meals (refer to *Imbalanced Nutrition* for specific
   techniques).
If possible, teach client to use a microwave to reduce the risk of heat-related injuries or accidents.

Offer Hints to Improve Adherence to Medication Schedule.
Have someone place medications in a commercial pill holder divided into 7 days.
Take out exact amount of pills for the day. Divide them in small cups, each labeled with time of day.
If needed, draw a picture of the pills and the quantity on each cup.
Teach client to transfer pills from cup to small plastic bag when planning to be away from home.

Tell Client Whom to Call for Instructions if He or She Misses a Dose.

Determine Available Sources of Transportation.

Neighbors, relatives   Community center
Church group   Social service agency

Determine Available Sources of Social Support.

Discuss the possibility of bartering for services (eg, wash neighbor's clothes in exchange for
   shopping help).
Identify a person who can provide immediate help (eg, neighbor, friend, hotline).
Identify sources for help with laundry, shopping, and money matters.

Initiate Health Teaching and Referrals, as Indicated.

Discuss the importance of identifying the need for assistance.
Refer client to community agencies for assistance (eg, Department of Social Services, area agency on
   aging, senior neighbors, public health nursing).

Rationales

- Interventions focus on assisting the person and family to maintain as much functional independence as possible (Miller, 2004).
- Community resources can assist the person when caregivers are unavailable (Miller, 2004).

Disturbed Self-Concept*
Disturbed Body Image
Disturbed Personal Identity
Disturbed Self-Esteem
Chronic Low Self-Esteem
Situational Low Self-Esteem
Risk for Situational Low Self-Esteem

DISTURBED SELF-CONCEPT

DEFINITION

Disturbed Self-Concept: State in which a person experiences or is at risk of experiencing a negative state of change about the way he feels, thinks, or views himself. It may include a change in body image, self-esteem, or personal identity (Boyd, 2004).

DEFINING CHARACTERISTICS

Because a disturbed self-concept may include a change in any one or a combination of its three component parts (body image, self-esteem, personal identity), and because the nature of the change causing the alteration can be so varied, there is no typical response to this diagnosis. Reactions may include the following:

Refusal to touch or look at a body part
Refusal to look into a mirror
Unwillingness to discuss a limitation, deformity, or disfigurement
Inappropriate attempts or refusal to direct own treatment
Denial of the existence of a deformity or disfigurement
Increasing dependence on others
Signs of grieving: weeping, despair, anger
Self-destructive behavior (alcohol, drug abuse)
Displaying hostility toward the healthy
Showing change in ability to estimate relation of body to environment

RELATED FACTORS

A disturbed self-concept can occur as a response to a variety of health problems, situations, and conflicts. Some common sources follow.

Pathophysiologic
Related to change in appearance, lifestyle, role, response of others secondary to:

Chronic disease	Severe trauma	Loss of body parts
Pain	Loss of body functions	

Situational (Personal, Environmental)
Related to feelings of abandonment or failure secondary to:
Divorce, separation from or death of a significant other
Loss of job or ability to work

Related to immobility or loss of function
Related to unsatisfactory relationships (parental, spousal)

---

*These diagnoses are not currently on the NANDA list but have been included for clarity or usefulness.

Related to sexual preferences (homosexual, lesbian, bisexual, abstinent)
Related to teenage pregnancy
Related to gender differences in parental child rearing
Related to experiences of parental violence
Related to change in usual patterns of responsibilities

Maturational

Middle Aged
Loss of role and responsibilities

Older Adult
Loss of role and responsibilities

◯◯ AUTHOR'S NOTE

Self-concept reflects self-view, encompassing body image, esteem, role performance, and personal identity. Self-concept develops over a lifetime and is difficult to change. It is influenced by interactions with the environment and others, and by the person's perceptions of how others view him or her.

Disturbed Self-Concept represents a broad diagnostic category under which fall more specific nursing diagnoses. Initially, the nurse may not have sufficient clinical data to validate a more specific diagnosis, such as *Chronic Low Self-Esteem* or *Disturbed Body Image;* thus, he or she can use *Disturbed Self-Concept* until data can support a more specific diagnosis.

Self-esteem is one of the four components of self-concept. *Disturbed Self-Esteem* is the general diagnostic category. *Chronic Low Self-Esteem* and *Situational Low Self-Esteem* represent specific types of *Disturbed Self-Esteem* and thus involve more specific interventions. Initially, the nurse may not have sufficient clinical data to validate a more specific diagnosis, such as *Chronic Low Self-Esteem* or *Situational Low Self-Esteem*. Refer to the major defining characteristics under these categories for validation.

Situational Low Self-Esteem is an episodic event; repeated occurrence, continuous negative self-appraisals over time, or both can lead to *Chronic Low Self-Esteem* (Willard, 1990, personal communication).

◯◯ ERRORS IN DIAGNOSTIC STATEMENTS

1. *Disturbed Self-Concept related to substance abuse*

Although a relationship exists between negative self-concept and alcohol and/or drug abuse, listing substance abuse as a related factor does not describe the nursing focus. If the person acknowledged a substance abuse problem and expressed a desire for assistance, the diagnosis *Ineffective Coping related to inability to constructively manage stressors without alcohol or drugs* could be appropriate. If the person denied a problem, the diagnosis *Ineffective Denial related to lack of acknowledgment of substance abuse/dependency* would apply—if the nurse will address the denial. A nurse with data that suggest or confirm *Disturbed Self-Concept* should explore contributing factors (eg, guilt influenced by social stigma). The nurse can use "unknown etiology" until focus assessment identifies contributing factors.

2. *Disturbed Body Image related to mastectomy*

Mastectomy can produce various responses, including grief, anger, and negative feelings about self. A woman undergoing breast surgery for cancer is at high risk for both *Disturbed Body Image* and *Disturbed Self-Esteem*. Thus, the diagnosis *Risk for Disturbed Self-Concept related to perceived negative effects of changed appearance and diagnosis of cancer* would be most appropriate. A nurse with data to support *Disturbed Self-Concept* should record it as an actual diagnosis with these same related factors and including "as evidenced by" to specify signs and symptoms of or manifestations (eg, *Disturbed Self-Concept related to perceived negative effects of changed appearance and diagnosis of cancer, as evidenced by reports of negative feelings about "new self" and determination not to let husband see her*).

KEY CONCEPTS
Generic Considerations

- Both the client and the nurse have their own personal self-concept. To deal effectively with others, the nurse must be aware of his or her own behavior, feelings, attitudes, and responses.
- Self-concept involves a person's feelings, attitudes, and values and affects his or her reactions to all experiences.
- A person's self-concept evolves from infancy through old age. With aging, new skills and challenges emerge. Successful completion of developmental tasks contributes to a positive self-concept (Boyd, 2005).
- Interactions with others, the sociocultural milieu, and developmental task completion influence self-concept (Boyd, 2005).
- The concept of self includes components of body image, self-esteem, and personal identity (Boyd, 2005).
  - *Body Image:* The sum of the conscious and unconscious attitudes the person has toward his or her body. It includes present and past perceptions.
  - *Self-Esteem:* The individual's personal judgment of his or her own worth obtained by analyzing how well his or her behavior conforms to self-ideals. High self-esteem is rooted in unconditional acceptance of self, despite mistakes, defeats, and failures, as an innately worthy and important being.
  - *Personal Identity:* The organizing principle of the personality that accounts for the unity, continuity, consistency, and uniqueness of the individual. It connotes autonomy and includes self-perceptions of sexuality. Identity formation begins in infancy and proceeds throughout life, but is the major task of adolescence.
- Body image consists of three components: body reality, body ideal, and body presentation (Price, 1990).
  - *Body Reality:* The body as it really exists, constrained by the effects of human genetics and the wear and tear of life in the external environment (as it might be described in a formal physician's examination). It changes both as a result of the aging process and because we use and abuse it. Abrupt changes in body reality are associated with trauma, malignancy, infection, and malnutrition.
  - *Body Ideal:* This is the picture in our heads of how we would like the body to look and to perform. Influences include societal and cultural norms, advertising, and changing attitudes toward fitness and health. Changes in body reality threaten body ideal, but disorders of body ideal (eg, anorexia nervosa) also may affect the equilibrium directly.
  - *Body Presentation:* Body reality only rarely meets body ideal standards. In the effort to make these two balance, body presentation is used. This is how the body is literally presented to the outside environment: the way we dress, groom, walk, talk, pose limbs, and use props such as walking sticks or hearing aids. Equally, paralysis or loss of limb (body reality) also affects facility in body presentation. Much presentation is for public consumption, laden with symbolic value.
- Disturbances in the components of self-concept are described as follows:
  - *Body Image:* Viewing oneself differently as a result of actual or perceived changes in body structure or function
  - *Self-Ideal:* A change in self-expectations/striving
  - *Self-Esteem:* Lack of confidence in ability to accomplish that which is desired
  - *Role Performance:* Inability to perform those functions and activities expected of a particular role in a given society
  - *Personal Identity:* Disturbance in perception of self ("Who am I?")

Loss of Body Part/Function

- People have a concept of self that includes feelings about self-worth, attractiveness, lovableness, and capabilities. A physical injury assaults one's mental image of one's own body and person. This injury or loss involves the grieving process.
- Facial disfigurement causes the most changes in body image and self-concept.
- Bergamasco et al. (2002) identified two critical incidents in burned persons: noticing the changes in their bodies (eg, mirror) and noticing that others are aware of their scars.
- Factors that influence successful reimaging are the person's perspective on value of lost function, nature of change, prior life experiences, self-esteem, social support, and others' attitudes, and access to medical technology.
- The grieving process in response to a recent disability has been described as (Friedman-Campbell & Hart, 1984):

- Shock/denial
  - Denies injury or severity of the injury
  - Allows self to think of loss only minimally to protect self
  - Intellectually accepts the loss but denies it emotionally
- Developing awareness
  - Realizes the effects of the loss on self
  - Experiences acute somatic feelings of loss
  - Displaces anger
  - Is preoccupied with guilt and blaming
  - Mourns the loss and withdraws
  - Shuns change and clings to routines
- Managing loss of body function
  - Begins to deal with the effects of the loss on self
  - Frees self slowly from the bondage of the loss
  - Readjusts to changed environment
  - Invests in new relationships

Self-Esteem

- Self-esteem evolves from a comparison between self-concept and self-ideal. The greater the congruency, the higher is the self-esteem.
- Self-esteem derives from the person's own perceptions of competency and efficacy and from appraisals of others. In general, people hold positive self-enhancing beliefs about themselves, the world, and the future. These biased perceptions are considerably more positive than objective evidence indicates.
- As self-esteem declines, so does a person's belief that he or she can exert control over the environment. Likewise, as personal control is perceived to decrease, so does self-esteem. Attributing failure to a lack of ability (internal cause) leads to decreased expectations and motivation.
- In response to a threat to person's self-concept, three cognitive processes protect self-esteem:
  - Searching for meaning in the experience
  - Regaining mastery over the event; exerting personal control
  - Self-enhancement ("How am I managing compared with others?").
- The following behaviors are associated with low self-esteem: rigidity; procrastination; repetitive, unnecessary apologies; minimizing one's abilities; emphasizing deficits; expecting failure; self-destructive behaviors; approval-seeking behavior; inability to accept compliments; disregard for one's own opinions; difficulty in forming close relationships; and inability to say "no" when appropriate (Miller, 2004).
- Low self-esteem has been regarded as an important cause of violence; however, the opposite view is theoretically viable. Violence appears often as a result of threatened egotism (that is, highly favorable views of self that some person or circumstance disputes). This is the dark side of high self-esteem.

❖ Pediatric Considerations

- Self-concept is learned. A child's concept of self, for example, emerges as a result of changes during earlier developmental stages.
- To develop and maintain self-esteem, a child needs to feel worthwhile, different in some way, and superior to and more lovable than any other child (Wong, 2003).
- Self-esteem increases as a child develops meaningful relationships and masters developmental tasks. Early adolescence is a time of risk to self-esteem as the adolescent strives to define an identity and sense of self within a peer group (Boyd, 2005).
- Present and past perceptions of his or her body, physiologic functioning, developmental maturation, and responses from others influence a child's development of body image. Adolescence is probably the critical period of development for body image formation, as pubertal changes force alteration of the adolescent's body image. The development of a positive body image by age is charted below (Boyd, 2005):

◆ Pediatric Considerations (continued)

Age	Developmental Task
Birth to 1 year Learns to trust	Learns to tolerate small frustrations
1 to 3 years	Learns to like body
	Learns mastery of
	Motor skills
	Language skills
	Bowel training
3 to 6 years	Learns initiative
	Learns sex typing
	Identifies with parent models
	Increases skills (motor, language)
6 to 12 years	Develops a sense of industry
	Has a clear sex role identification
	Learns peer interaction
	Develops academic skills
Adolescence	Establishes self-identity and sexual role
	Uses abstract thought
	Develops personal value system

- Children learn to see themselves in the way that parents and significant others see them.
- To develop a healthy personality, a child needs a positive and accurate body image, realistic self-ideal, positive self-concept, and high self-esteem.
- Although experiences with and restrictions imposed by chronic illness or disability may interfere with development of healthy self-esteem, new research indicates contrary evidence. Although the population with disabilities may have lower self-concepts in social acceptance and athletic and job competence in comparison to the normative population, they did not have overall lower self-esteem. Comparing themselves to members of their own group rather than a nonstigmatized group, not heavily valuing things they were not good at, and attributing negative feedback to the fact that they belonged to a stigmatized group rather than to faults they personally possess are three strategies used to protect their self-esteem (Specht et al., 1998). It also should not be assumed that clients with mental illness always experience low self-esteem. Factors that influence quality of life, such as value of work, social relationships, and activities with family, have been measured and show that clients who experience these have high self-esteem (Van-Dongen, 1998).
- Although obese children and adolescents may be at particular risk for developing body image or self-esteem disturbance, lower self-esteem is more likely in children who believe they are responsible for their excess weight, as compared with those who attribute their excess weight to an external cause. Lower self-esteem is also found in those children who believe that their excess weight hinders their social interaction (Pierce & Wardle, 1997).
- Negative self-concepts have been associated with self-destructive health behaviors in children and adolescents, such as overeating, alcoholism, smoking, and drug abuse (Winkelstein, 1989).
- Mastery describes positive coping with stress. Successful coping enhances self-esteem.

⊙ Geriatric Considerations

- According to Miller (2004), self-esteem is "one of the characteristics most highly associated with both depression and happiness" in older adults.
- Self-esteem depends on interactions with others and on others' opinions. In Western societies, a generally negative view of aging can contribute to an older adult's decreased self-esteem.
- Many variables interact to produce a decline in self-esteem in older adults, including negative societal attitudes, decreased social interactions, and decreased power and control over the environment.

(continued)

ⓒ Geriatric Considerations (continued)

- Meisenhelder (1985) reported that the following people exert the most significant influence on self-esteem in older adults: spouse, peers (most important for men), authority figures (most important for women), people they live with, and people in the immediate social, work, and church environments.
- Environmental factors in long-term care facilities that can influence self-esteem of older residents include decor, social roles, choices available, architectural design, space, and privacy (Miller, 2004).
- Older adults with poor health, high degree of disability, and daily pain report the lowest self-esteem (Hunter, Linn & Harris, 1981–1982).

🌐 Transcultural Considerations

In the Latin culture, the man is the head of the household and has authority over his family. He must provide for and protect his family. Self-image and family image are intertwined. Anything that challenges his ability to provide for his family challenges his very core or self-concept (Andrews & Boyle, 2003).

Focus Assessment Criteria

Disturbed Self-Concept is manifested in a variety of ways. A person may respond with an alteration in another life process (see *Spiritual Distress, Fear, Ineffective Coping*). The nurse should be aware of this and use the assessment data to ascertain the dimensions affected.

It may be difficult for the nurse to identify the cues and make the inferences necessary to diagnose a self-concept disturbance. Each person reacts differently to loss, pain, disability, and disfigurement. Therefore, the nurse should determine a person's usual reactions to problems and feelings about himself or herself before attempting to diagnose a change.

Subjective Data
Assess for Defining Characteristics.

Self views
"Describe yourself."
"What do you like most/least about yourself?"
"What do you/others want to change about you?"
"What do you enjoy?"
"Has being ill affected how you see yourself?"

Identity
"What personal achievements have given you satisfaction?"
"What are your future plans?"

Role responsibilities
"What do you do for a living? Job responsibilities? Home responsibilities?"
"Are these satisfying?"
If the person has had a role change, how has it affected lifestyle and relationships?

Somatic problems
"Do you feel fearful, anxious, or nervous?"
"Ever feel like you are falling apart? Dizziness? Aches and pains? Shortness of breath? Palpitations? Urinary frequency? Nausea/vomiting? Sleep problems? Fatigue? Loss of sexual interest?"

Affect and mood
"How do you feel now?"
"How would you describe your usual mood?"
"What things make you happy/upset?"

Body image

"What do you like most/least about your body?"

"What limitations do you think will result?"

"How do you feel about this illness/disability?"

"Has it changed the way you feel about yourself or the way others respond to you?"

Children may be able to draw self-portraits.

Assess for Related Factors.

Stress management

"How do you manage stress?"

"To whom do you go for help with a problem?"

Support system

"Any problems in current relationships?"

"How does your family feel about your illness?" "Do they understand?"

"Does your family regularly discuss problems?"

"What other supports do you have? Spiritual? Social?"

Objective Data

Assess for Defining Characteristics.

General appearance

Facial expression

Body posture/language (eye contact, head and shoulder flexion, gait/stride)

Thought processes/content

Orientation

Suspicious

Homicidal/suicidal ideation

Rambling

Sexual preoccupation

Delusions (grandeur, persecution, reference, influence, or bodily sensations)

Difficulty concentrating

Slowed thought processes

Poor memory or may even be missing large portions of personal history

Impaired judgment

Anxiety

Behavior

School problems (truancy, low/drop in grades)

Problems on job (lateness, decreased productivity, accident-prone, burnout symptoms)

Social withdrawal

Sexual behavior (increase, decrease, promiscuity)

Communication patterns

With significant others

Relates well	Dependent
Hostile	Demanding

Nutritional status

Appetite

Eating patterns

Weight (gain/loss)

Rest–sleep pattern

Recent change

For more information on Focus Assessment Criteria, visit http://connection.lww.com.

Goal

 NOC Quality of Life, Depression Level, Self-Esteem, Coping

The person will demonstrate healthy adaptation and coping skills.

Indicators
- Appraise self and situations realistically without distortions.
- Verbalize and demonstrate increased positive feelings.

General Interventions

> **NIC** Hope Instillation, Mood Management, Values Clarification, Counseling, Referral, Support Group, Coping Enhancement

Nursing interventions for the various
problems that might be associated with a diagnosis of *Disturbed Self-Concept* are very similar.

Contact the Client Frequently and Treat Him or Her with Warm, Positive Regard.

Encourage the Client to Express Feelings and Thoughts About the Following:

| Condition | Progress | Prognosis |
| Effects on lifestyle | Support system | Treatment |

Provide Reliable Information and Clarify Any Misconceptions.

Explain the Process of Reimaging (Refer to Key Concepts—Loss of Body Parts or Functions).

Explain that reimaging oneself after a loss of appearance or function is distinct and unique.
Advise that the process takes at least 1 year.
Assist client to examine societal homophobia and its results, so it is not internalized. Link him or her to appropriate groups and organizations.
Provide maternal education and a sound supportive system, which includes alternatives for care of the infant when delivered.
Provide education and refer to support groups that promote empowerment and change of focus to assist in evaluating and raising quality of life.

Help Client to Identify Positive Attributes and Possible New Opportunities.

Assist with Hygiene and Grooming, as Needed.

Encourage Visitors.

Help Client Identify Strategies to Increase Independence and to Maintain Role Responsibilities.

Prioritizing activities
Using mobility aids and assistive devices, as needed

Discuss with Client's Support System the Importance of Communicating the Client's Value and Importance to Them.

Assess for Signs and Symptoms. Use the Focus Assessment Criteria to Isolate Signs and Symptoms. Refer to the Defining Characteristics of *Disturbed Self-Esteem, Disturbed Body Image,* and *Ineffective Role Performance.* After Confirmation, Use Interventions Under the Diagnosis.

Initiate Health Teaching, as Indicated.

Teach person what community resources are available, if needed (eg, mental health centers, self-help groups such as Reach for Recovery, Make Today Count).
Refer to specific health teaching issues under *Disturbed Body Image, Disturbed Self-Esteem* (*Chronic* and *Situational*).

Encourage Professional Counseling for Victims of Abuse, Violence, Cultism, or Unresolved Grief.

Rationales

- Frequent contact by the caregiver indicates acceptance and may facilitate trust. The client may be hesitant to approach the staff because of negative self-concept.
- Encouraging the client to share feelings can provide a safe outlet for fears and frustrations and can increase self-awareness.
- Misconceptions can increase anxiety and damage self-concept needlessly.
- The client may tend to focus only on the change in self-image and not on the positive characteristics that contribute to the whole concept of self. The nurse must reinforce these positive aspects and encourage the client to reincorporate them into the new self-concept.
- Participation in self-care and planning can aid positive coping.
- Frequent visits by support people can help the client feel that he or she is still a worthwhile, acceptable person, which should promote a positive self-concept.
- A strong component of self-concept is the ability to perform functions expected of one's role, thus decreasing dependency and reducing the need for others' involvement.
- Communication of the client's values enhances self-esteem and promotes adjustment.
- Optimism enhances social relationships and enables a person to make more effective use of social supports to maintain self-esteem. Supportive friends and family can bolster self-esteem by reinforcing a sense of personal control through suggestions and resources and a sense of confidence (Morse, 1997).
- Addressing spiritual issues within the counseling process involves an accurate assessment of spiritual functioning and relevant interventions used with discretion and respect for client beliefs.
- Nurses must receive adequate education and keep their knowledge updated. Nurses should receive regular clinical supervision and support to ensure that they can provide therapeutic care for patients with self-concept disturbances.

Pediatric Interventions

Allow the child to bring his or her own experiences into the situation (eg, "Some children say that an injection feels like an insect sting; some say they don't feel anything. After we do this, you can tell me how it feels"; Johnson, 1995).

Avoid using "good" or "bad" to describe behavior. Be specific and descriptive (eg, "You really helped me by holding still. Thank you for helping"; Johnson, 1995).

Connect previous experiences with the present one (eg, "The x-ray camera will look different from the last time. You will have to hold real still again. The table will move, too"; Johnson, 1995).

Convey optimism with positive self-talk (eg, "I am so busy today. I wonder if I will get all my work done? I bet I can." or "When you come back from surgery you will need to stay in bed. What would you like to do when you come back?").

Help the child plan playtime with choices. Encourage crafts that produce an end product.

Encourage interactions with peers and supportive adults.

Encourage child to decorate room with crafts and personal items.

Recommend and support policies that include divorce mediation, early referrals for family and sibling therapy, and school programs to identify and support these vulnerable clients.

When selecting a self-esteem measure, consider cognitive developmental level and chronologic age. During treatment, use a more reality-based evaluation with self-concept dimensions that include areas of competence, power, moral worth, and acceptance (Wong, 2003).

Rationales

- It is more helpful to be specific and descriptive when praising a child rather than describing behavior as "good" or "bad".
- Allowing the child to describe the experience supports that he or she is unique.
- The nurse can provide information that helps the child make sense of the situation by linking the present or future experience to past experience.
- Positive self-talk denotes optimism to the child.
- Allowing the child choices and productive play can enhance self-concept.
- Skill building and positive social relationships increase a child's sense of value and worth (Wong, 2003).

DISTURBED BODY IMAGE

DEFINITION
Disturbed Body Image: State in which a person experiences or is at risk to experience a disruption in the way he perceives one's body

DEFINING CHARACTERISTICS
Major (Must Be Present)
Verbal or nonverbal negative response to actual or perceived change in structure and/or function (eg, shame, embarrassment, guilt, revulsion)

Minor (May Be Present)
Not looking at body part
Not touching body part
Hiding or overexposing body part
Change in social involvement
Negative feelings about body; feelings of helplessness, hopelessness, powerlessness, vulnerability
Preoccupation with change or loss
Refusal to verify actual change
Depersonalization of part or loss
Self-destructive behaviors (eg, mutilation, suicide attempts, overeating/undereating)

RELATED FACTORS
Pathophysiologic
Related to changes in appearance secondary to

Chronic disease	Loss of body part	Loss of body function
Severe trauma	Aging	

Related to unrealistic perceptions of appearance secondary to

Psychosis	Anorexia nervosa	Bulimia

Treatment-Related
Related to changes in appearance secondary to

Hospitalization	Surgery	Chemotherapy
Radiation		

Situational (Personal, Environmental)
Related to physical trauma secondary to
Sexual abuse
Rape (perpetrator known or unknown)
Assault

Related to effects of (specify) on appearance

Obesity	Immobility	Pregnancy

> ⊙⊙ **AUTHOR'S NOTE**
>
> See *Disturbed Self-Concept.*

KEY CONCEPTS
See *Disturbed Self-Concept.*

Focus Assessment Criteria

See *Disturbed Self-Concept.*

Goals

NOC Body Image, Child Development: (specify age), Grief Resolution, Psychosocial Adjustment: Life Change, Self-Esteem

The person will implement new coping patterns and verbalize and demonstrate acceptance of appearance (grooming, dress, posture, eating patterns, presentation of self).

Indicators

- Demonstrate a willingness and ability to resume self-care/role responsibilities.
- Initiate new or reestablish contacts with existing support systems.

NIC Self-Esteem Enhancement, Counseling, Presence, Active Listening, Body Image Enhancement, Grief Work Facilitation, Support Group, Referral

General Interventions

Establish a Trusting Nurse–Client Relationship.

Encourage person to express feelings, especially about the way he or she feels, thinks, or views self.
Acknowledge feelings of hostility, grief, fear, and dependency; teach strategies for coping with emotions.
Explore belief system (eg, does pain, suffering, loss mean punishment?)
Encourage client to ask questions about health problem, treatment, progress, and prognosis.
Provide reliable information and reinforce information already given.
Clarify any misconceptions about self, care, or caregivers.
Avoid criticism.
Provide privacy and a safe environment.
Use therapeutic touch, with person's consent.
Encourage client to connect with spiritual beliefs and values regarding a higher power.

Promote Social Interaction.

Assist client to accept help from others.
Avoid overprotection, but limit the demands made.
Encourage movement.
Prepare significant others for physical and emotional changes.
Support family as they adapt.
Encourage visits from peers and significant others.
Encourage contact (letters, telephone) with peers and family.
Encourage involvement in unit activities.
Provide opportunity to share with people going through similar experiences.
Discuss the importance of communicating the client's value and importance to them with his or her support system.

Provide Specific Interventions in Selected Situations.

Loss of Body Part or Function
Assess the meaning of the loss for the person and significant others, as related to visibility of loss, function of loss, and emotional investment.
Explore and clarify misconceptions and myths regarding loss or ability to function with loss.

Expect the person to respond to the loss with denial, shock, anger, and depression.

Be aware of the effect of the responses of others to the loss; encourage sharing of feelings between significant others.

Validate feelings by allowing the person to express his or her feelings and to grieve.

Use role playing to assist with sharing; if person says, "I know my husband will not want to touch me with this colostomy," take the husband's role and discuss her colostomy, then switch roles so she can act out her feelings about her husband's response.

Explore realistic alternatives and provide encouragement.

Explore strengths and resources with person.

Assist with the resolution of a surgically created alteration of body image.

  Replace the lost body part with prosthesis as soon as possible.

  Encourage viewing of site.

  Encourage touching of site.

  Encourage activities that encompass new body image (eg, shopping for new clothes).

Teach about the health problem and how to manage.

Begin to incorporate person in care of operative site.

Gradually allow person to assume full self-care responsibility, if feasible.

Teach person to monitor own progress (Miller, 2004).

Refer to *Sexual Dysfunction* for additional information, if indicated.

Changes Associated with Chemotherapy (Camp-Sorrell, 2000)

Discuss the possibility of hair loss, absence of menses, temporary or permanent sterility, decreased estrogen levels, vaginal dryness, and mucositis.

Encourage client to share concerns, fears, and perception of the effects of these changes on life.

Explain where hair loss may occur (head, eyelashes, eyebrows, axillary, pubic, and leg hair).

Explain that hair will grow back after treatment, but may change in color and texture.

Encourage client to select and wear a wig before hair loss. Suggest consulting a beautician for tips on how to vary the look (eg, combs, clips).

Encourage the wearing of scarves or turbans when wig is not on.

Teach client to minimize the amount of hair loss by

  Cutting hair short

  Avoiding excessive shampooing, using a conditioner twice weekly

  Patting hair dry gently

  Avoiding electric curlers, dryers, and curling irons

  Avoiding pulling hair with bands, clips, or bobby pins

  Avoiding hair spray and hair dye

  Using wide-tooth comb, avoiding vigorous brushing

Refer client to American Cancer Society for information about new or used wigs. Inform the client that the wig is a tax-deductible item.

Discuss the difficulty that others (spouse, friends, coworkers) may have with visible changes.

Encourage client to initiate calls and contacts with others who may be having difficulty.

Encourage client to ask for assistance of friends, relatives. Ask person if the situation were reversed, what he or she would want to do to help a friend.

Allow significant others opportunities to share their feelings and fears.

Assist significant others to identify positive aspects of the client and ways this can be shared.

Provide information about support groups for couples.

Anorexia Nervosa, Bulimia Nervosa

Differentiate between body image distortion and body image dissatisfaction.

Refer individuals for psychiatric counseling.

Psychoses

Refer to *Disturbed Thought Process* for specific information and interventions.

Sexual Abuse

Refer to *Compromised Family Coping* for specific information and interventions.

Sexual Assault

Refer to *Rape Trauma Syndrome* for specific information and interventions.

Assault

Refer to *Post-Trauma Response* for specific information and interventions.

Initiate Health Teaching, as Indicated.

Teach what community resources are available, if needed (eg, mental health centers, self-help groups
such as Reach for Recovery, Make Today Count).

Teach wellness strategies (see *Health-Seeking Behaviors*).

Rationales

- Frequent contact by the caregiver indicates acceptance and may facilitate trust. The client may
  be hesitant to approach the staff because of negative self-concept; the nurse must reach out.
- Social interactions can reaffirm that the person is acceptable and that previous support system is
  still intact.
- Expressing feelings and perceptions increases the client's self-awareness and helps the nurse plan
  effective interventions to address his or her needs. Validating the client's perceptions provides
  reassurance and can decrease anxiety.
- Identifying personal attributes and strengths can help the client focus on the positive characteristics that contribute to the whole concept of self rather than only on the change in body image. The
  nurse should reinforce these positive aspects and encourage the client to reincorporate them into
  the new self-concept.
- Open, honest discussions—expressing that changes will occur but that they are manageable—
  promote feelings of control.
- Participation in self-care and planning promotes positive coping with the change.
- Professional counseling is indicated for a client with poor ego strengths and inadequate coping
  resources.
- Increased social interaction through involvement in groups enables a person to receive social and
  intellectual stimulation, which enhances self-esteem.

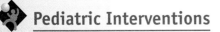 **Pediatric Interventions**

For Hospitalized Child:

Prepare child for hospitalization, if possible, with an explanation and a visit to the hospital to meet
personnel and examine the environment.

Provide familiarities/routines of home as much as possible (eg, favorite toy or blanket, story at
bedtime).

Provide nurturance (eg, hug).

Provide child with opportunities to share fears, concerns, and anger.

  Acknowledge the normality of these emotions.

  Correct misconceptions (eg, that the child is being punished; that parents are angry).

  Encourage family to stay with or visit child, despite the child's crying when they leave; teach them
  to provide accurate information about when they will return to reduce fears of abandonment.

  Allow parents to help with care.

  Ask child to draw a picture of self, and then ask for a verbal description.

Assist child to understand experiences.

  Provide an explanation ahead of time, if possible.

  Explain sensations and discomforts of condition, treatments, and medications.

  Encourage crying.

Maintain sense of intactness during periods of immobility.

  Encourage movement, no matter how slight.

  During bath, ask child to identify body parts: "Where is your leg?"

  Allow access to mirror to provide visualization of body.

Discuss with Parents How Body Image Develops and What Interactions Contribute to Their Child's Self-Perception.

Teach the names and functions of body parts.

Acknowledge changes (eg, height).

Allow some choices for what to wear.

For Adolescents:

Discuss with parents the adolescent's need to "fit in."

Do not dismiss concerns too quickly.

Be flexible and compromise when possible (eg, clothes are temporary, tattoos are not).

Negotiate a time period to think about options and alternatives (eg, 4 to 5 weeks).

Provide with reasons for denying a request. Elicit adolescent's reasons. Compromise if possible (eg, parents want curfew at 11:00; adolescent wants 12:00; compromise at 11:30).

Provide opportunities to discuss concerns when parents are not present.

Ask client to describe best features and those he or she dislikes.

Prepare for impending developmental changes.

Rationales

- Attempts to retain the normality of the child's world can help to increase security (Wong, 2003).
- Play therapy puts the child in control by providing opportunities to make choices (Wong, 2003).
- Interventions that provide expressive outlets for tension and fear can help maintain the child's integrity (Wong, 2003).
- Opportunities for choices and success enhance self-esteem and coping.

Maternal Interventions

Encourage the woman to share her concerns.

Attend to each concern, if possible, or refer her to others for assistance.

Discuss the challenges and changes that pregnancy and motherhood bring.

Encourage her to share expectations: her own and those of her significant others.

Assist her to identify sources for love and affection.

Provide anticipatory guidance to both parents-to-be concerning

Fatigue and irritability

Appetite swings

Gastric disturbances (nausea, constipation)

Back and leg aches

Changes in sexual desire and activity (eg, sexual positions as pregnancy advances)

Mood swings

Fear (for self, for unborn baby, of loss of attractiveness, of inadequacy as a parent)

Encourage sharing of concerns between spouses.

Rationales

- Open, honest discussions—expressing that changes will occur but that they are manageable—promote feelings of control.
- Support can be given more freely and more realistically if others are prepared.
- Pregnancy disrupts the adolescent from becoming comfortable with her body image.

DISTURBED PERSONAL IDENTITY

DEFINITION

Disturbed Personal Identity: State in which a person experiences or is at risk of experiencing an inability to distinguish between self and nonself

DEFINING CHARACTERISTICS

See Defining Characteristics for *Disturbed Self-Concept* or *Delayed Growth and Development*.

> **◯◯ AUTHOR'S NOTE**
>
> This nursing diagnosis is a subcategory under *Disturbed Self-Concept*. Until clinical research defines and differentiates it from others, refer to *Disturbed Self-Concept* or *Delayed Growth and Development* for assessment criteria and interventions.

DISTURBED SELF-ESTEEM

DEFINITION

Disturbed Self-Esteem: State in which a person experiences or is at risk of experiencing negative self-evaluation about self or capabilities

DEFINING CHARACTERISTICS (LEUNER ET AL., 1994; NORRIS & KUNES-CONNELL, 1987)
Major (Must be Present, One or More)

(Observed or reported)
Self-negating verbalization
Expressions of shame or guilt
Evaluates self as unable to deal with events
Rationalizes away or rejects positive feedback and exaggerates negative feedback about self
Lack of or poor problem-solving ability
Hesitant to try new things or situations
Rationalizes personal failures
Hypersensitivity to slight criticism

Minor

Lack of assertion
Overly conforming
Indecisiveness

Passive
Seeks approval or reassurance excessively
Lack of culturally appropriate body presentation (posture, eye contact, movements)
Denial of problems obvious to others
Projection of blame or responsibility for problems

RELATED FACTORS

Disturbed Self-Esteem can be either episodic or chronic. Failure to resolve a problem or multiple sequential stresses can result in chronic low self-esteem (CLSE). Those factors that occur over time and are associated with CLSE are indicated by "CLSE" in parentheses.

Pathophysiologic

Related to change in appearance secondary to
Loss of body parts
Loss of body functions
Disfigurement (trauma, surgery, birth defects)

Situational (Personal, Environmental)

Related to unmet dependency needs
Related to feelings of abandonment secondary to

Death of significant other	Separation from significant
Child abduction/murder	other

Related to feelings of failure secondary to

Loss of job or ability to work	Increase/decrease in weight	Unemployment
Financial problems	Premenstrual syndrome	Relationship problems
Marital discord	Separation	Stepparents
In-laws		

Related to assault (personal, or relating to the event of another's assault—eg, same age, same community)
Related to failure in school
Related to history of ineffective relationship with parents (CLSE)
Related to history of abusive relationships (CLSE)
Related to unrealistic expectations of child by parent (CLSE)
Related to unrealistic expectations of self (CLSE)
Related to unrealistic expectations of parent by child (CLSE)
Related to parental rejection (CLSE)
Related to inconsistent punishment (CLSE)
Related to feelings of helplessness and/or failure secondary to institutionalization

Mental health facility	Orphanage	Jail
Halfway house		

Related to history of numerous failures (CLSE)

Maturational

Infant/Toddler/Preschool
Related to lack of stimulation or closeness (CLSE)
Related to separation from parents/significant others (CLSE)
Related to continual negative evaluation by parents
Related to inadequate parental support (CLSE)
Related to inability to trust significant other (CLSE)

School-Aged
Related to failure to achieve grade-level objectives
Related to loss of peer group
Related to repeated negative feedback

Adolescent
Related to loss of independence and autonomy secondary to (specify)
Related to disruption of peer relationships
Related to scholastic problems
Related to loss of significant others

Middle-Aged
Related to changes associated with aging

Older Adult
Related to losses (people, function, financial, retirement)

◎ **AUTHOR'S NOTE**

See *Disturbed Self-Concept.*

◎ **ERRORS IN DIAGNOSTIC STATEMENTS**

See *Disturbed Self-Concept.*

KEY CONCEPTS
See *Disturbed Self-Concept.*

Focus Assessment Criteria

See *Disturbed Self-Concept.*

CHRONIC LOW SELF-ESTEEM

DEFINITION
Chronic Low Self-Esteem: State in which a person experiences a long-standing negative self-evaluation about self or capabilities

DEFINING CHARACTERISTICS (LEUNER ET AL., 1994; NORRIS & KUNES-CONNELL, 1987)
Major (80% to 100%)
Long-standing or chronic
Self-negating verbalization
Expressions of shame/guilt
Evaluates self as unable to deal with events
Rationalizes away/rejects positive feedback and exaggerates negative feedback about self
Hesitant to try new things/situations
Exaggerating negative feedback

Minor (50% to 79%)
Frequent lack of success in work or other life events
Overly conforming, dependent on others' opinions
Lack of culturally appropriate body presentation (eye contact, posture, movements)

Nonassertive/passive
Indecisive
Excessively seeks reassurance

RELATED FACTORS

See *Disturbed Self-Esteem.*

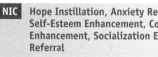

⊕ AUTHOR'S NOTE

See *Disturbed Self-Concept.*

⊕ ERRORS IN DIAGNOSTIC STATEMENTS

See *Disturbed Self-Concept.*

KEY CONCEPTS

See *Disturbed Self-Concept.*

Focus Assessment Criteria

See *Disturbed Self-Concept.*

Goals

NOC	Depression Level, Quality of Life, Self-Esteem

The person will identify positive aspects of self and report freedom from symptoms of depression.

Indicators

- Modify excessive and unrealistic self-expectations.
- Verbalize acceptance of limitations.
- Verbalize nonjudgmental perceptions of self.
- Cease self-abusive behavior.
- Begin to take verbal and behavioral risks.

General Interventions

NIC	Hope Instillation, Anxiety Reduction, Self-Esteem Enhancement, Coping Enhancement, Socialization Enhancement, Referral

Assist the Person to Reduce Present Anxiety Level.

Be supportive, nonjudgmental.
Accept silence, but let him or her know you are there.
Orient as necessary.
Clarify distortions; do not use confrontation.
Be aware of your own anxiety and avoid communicating it to the person.

Refer to *Anxiety* for further interventions.

Enhance the Person's Sense of Self.

Be attentive.
Respect personal space.
Validate your interpretation of what he or she is saying or experiencing ("Is this what you mean?").
Help him or her to verbalize what he or she is expressing nonverbally.
Assist client to reframe and redefine negative expressions (eg, not "failure," but "setback").

Use communication that helps to maintain his or her individuality ("I" instead of "we").

Pay attention to person, especially new behavior.

Encourage good physical habits (healthy food and eating patterns, exercise, proper sleep).

Provide encouragement as he or she attempts a task or skill.

Provide realistic positive feedback on accomplishments.

Teach person to validate consensually with others.

Teach and encourage esteem-building exercises (self-affirmations, imagery, mirror work, use of humor, meditation/prayer, relaxation).

Respect need for privacy.

Assist in establishing appropriate personal boundaries.

Provide consistency among staff (Miller, 2004).

Promote Use of Coping Resources.

Identify the client's areas of personal strength.

Sports, hobbies, crafts	Health, self-care	Work, training, education
Imagination, creativity	Writing skills, math	Interpersonal relationships

Share your observations with the person.

Provide opportunities for person to engage in the activities.

Assist Person to Express Thoughts and Feelings.

Use open-ended statements and questions.

Encourage expression of both positive and negative statements.

Use movement, art, and music as means of expression.

If person has impaired reality-testing ability, refer to *Disturbed Thought Processes* for further interventions.

Provide Opportunities for Positive Socialization.

Encourage visits/contact with peers and significant others (letters, telephone).

Be a role model in one-to-one interactions.

Involve in activities, especially when strengths can be used.

Do not allow person to isolate self (refer to *Social Isolation* for further interventions).

Involve client in supportive group therapy.

Teach social skills as required (refer to *Impaired Social Interaction* for further interventions).

Encourage participation with others sharing similar experiences.

Set Limits on Problematic Behavior Such as Aggression, Poor Hygiene, Ruminations, and Suicidal Preoccupation.

Refer to *Risk for Suicide* and/or *Risk for Violence* if these are assessed as problems.

Provide for Development of Social and Vocational Skills.

Reinforce confidence as person demonstrates new skills.

Refer for vocational counseling.

Involve client in volunteer organizations.

Encourage participation in activities with others of same age.

Arrange for continuation of education (eg, literacy class, vocational training, art/music classes).

Assist Client with Self-Exploration as Anxiety and Trust Permit.

Identify positive self-evaluation.

Assess self-appraisal.

Address unrealistic self-expectations (eg, "I should").

Encourage work on family of origin issues (healing) with one or combination of (Whitfield, 1990):

Professional counselor	Self-help workbooks	Self-help groups

Assist person with forgiveness issues (self, others, God).

Refer to *Situational Low Self-Esteem* for specific interventions.

Rationales

- People with low self-esteem are usually anxious, fearful people. Anxiety levels must be mild or moderate before other interventions can be effective (Mohr, 2003).

- Strategies focus on helping the person reexamine negative feelings about self and identifying positive attributes.
- Providing opportunities for the person to be successful increases self-esteem (Stuart & Sundeen, 1999).
- Client collaboration is necessary for him or her to assume ultimate responsibility for behavior (Stuart & Sundeen, 1999).
- Conveying acceptance of the person's feelings promotes self-acceptance.

SITUATIONAL LOW SELF-ESTEEM

DEFINITION

Situational Low Self-Esteem: State in which a person who previously had positive self-esteem experiences negative feelings about self in response to an event (loss, change)

DEFINING CHARACTERISTICS (LEVNER ET AL., 1994; NORRIS & KUNES-CONNELL, 1987)
Major (80% to 100%)

Episodic occurrence of negative self-appraisal in response to life events in a person with a previously positive self-evaluation
Verbalization of negative feelings about self (helplessness, uselessness)

Minor (50% to 79%)

Self-negating verbalizations
Expressions of shame/guilt
Evaluates self as unable to handle situations/events
Difficulty making decisions

RELATED FACTORS

See *Disturbed Self-Esteem.*

> ⊗ **AUTHOR'S NOTE**
>
> See *Disturbed Self-Concept.*

> ⊗ **ERRORS IN DIAGNOSTIC STATEMENTS**
>
> See *Disturbed Self-Concept.*

KEY CONCEPTS
Generic Considerations

- Qualities of a healthy personality are (Stuart & Sundeen, 2002)
  - Positive and accurate body image
  - Realistic self-ideal
  - Positive self-concept
  - High self-esteem

- Satisfying role performance
- Clear sense of identity
- People with healthy personalities can experience a change in their positive self-perception in response to a profound event or a series of negative experiences (Stuart & Sundeen, 2002).
- Responses to a situation that challenges a person's previously positive view of self are feelings of being weak, helpless, or hopeless; fear; vulnerability; and feelings of being fragile, incomplete, worthless, and inadequate (Stuart & Sundeen, 2002).

Goals

 NOC Decision-Making, Grief Resolution, Psychosocial Adjustment: Life Change, Self-Esteem

The person will express a positive outlook
for the future and resume previous level of functioning.

Indicators

- Identify source of threat to self-esteem and work through that issue.
- Identify positive aspects of self.
- Analyze his or her own behavior and its consequences.
- Identify one positive aspect of change.

General Interventions

NIC Active Listening, Presence, Counseling, Cognitive Restructuring, Family Support, Support Group, Coping Enhancement

Assist Client to Identify and to Express Feelings.

Be empathic, nonjudgmental.
Listen. Do not discourage expressions of anger, crying, and so forth.
Ask what was happening when he or she began feeling this way.
Clarify relationships between life events.
For an assault victim, encourage putting the traumatic event (assault) in context of life experiences as a whole while supporting common-sense safety precautions.

Assist Client to Identify Positive Self-Evaluations.

How has he or she handled other crises?
How does he or she manage anxiety—through exercise, withdrawal, drinking/drugs, talking?
Reinforce adaptive coping mechanisms.
Examine and reinforce positive abilities and traits (eg, hobbies, skills, school, relationships, appearance, loyalty, industriousness).
Help client accept both positive and negative feelings.
Do not confront defenses.
Communicate confidence in person's ability.
Involve person in mutual goal setting.
Have client write positive true statements about self (for his or her eyes only); have client read the list daily as a part of normal routine.
Reinforce use of esteem-building exercises (self-affirmations, imagery, meditation/prayer, relaxation, use of humor).

Explore Relation Between Behavior and Self-Appraisals.

Encourage examination of current behavior and its consequences (eg, dependency, procrastination, isolation).
Assist client to identify faulty perceptions.
Explore person's concept of success/failure and loss/punishment, and assist in putting things into proper perspective.
Assist client to identify unrealistic expectations.
Help client to identify negative automatic thoughts ("I will never be able to do this.").
Examine if person is overgeneralizing ("If I can't do this, then I'm a failure at everything.").
Assist person to identify own responsibility and control in a situation (eg, when continually blaming others for problems).

Assess and Mobilize Current Support System.

Does he or she live alone? Is he or she employed?
Does he or she have available friends and relatives?

Is religion a support?

Has he or she previously used community resources?

Refer client to vocational rehabilitation for retraining.

Support returning to school for further training.

Assist client to involve local volunteer organizations (senior citizens employment, foster grand-parents, local support groups).

Arrange continuation of school studies for students.

Assist Client to Learn New Coping Skills.

Practice self-talk (Murray, 2000).

> Write a brief description of the change and its consequence (eg, My spouse has had an affair. I am betrayed.).
>
> Write three things that may be useful about this situation.

Communicate that the person can handle the change.

Challenge the person to imagine positive futures and outcomes.

Encourage a trial of new behavior.

Reinforce the belief that the person does have control over the situation.

Obtain a commitment to action.

Assist Person to Manage Specific Problems.

Rape—refer to *Rape-Trauma Syndrome.*

Loss—refer to *Grieving.*

Hospitalization—refer to *Powerlessness* and *Parental Role Conflict.*

Ill family member—refer to *Interrupted Family Processes.*

Change or loss of body part—refer to *Disturbed Body Image.*

Depression—refer to *Ineffective Coping* and *Hopelessness.*

Domestic violence—refer to *Compromised Family Coping.*

Rationales

- See *Chronic Low Self-Esteem.*
- Self-talk does not imply that one likes the change; however, it helps one find potential benefits of the change (Murray, 2000).

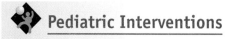 ## Pediatric Interventions

Provide opportunities for child to be successful and needed.

Personalize the child's environment with pictures, possessions, and crafts he or she made.

Provide structured and unstructured playtime.

Ensure continuation of academic experiences in the hospital and home. Provide uninterrupted time for schoolwork.

Rationales

See *Disturbed Self-Concept.*

Geriatric Interventions

Acknowledge person by name.

Use a tone of voice that you use for your peer group.

Avoid words associated with infants (eg, "diapers").

Ask about family pictures, personal items, and past experiences.

Avoid attributing disabilities to "old age."

Knock on door of bedrooms and bathrooms.

Allow enough time to accomplish tasks at own pace.

Rationale

Because self-esteem depends partially on the responses of others, caregivers must reflect respect for the aged as competent adults (Miller, 2004).

RISK FOR SITUATIONAL LOW SELF-ESTEEM

DEFINITION

Risk for Situational Low Self-Esteem: State in which a person who previously had a positive self-esteem is at risk to experience negative feelings about self in response to an event (loss, change)

RISK FACTORS

See *Situational Low Self-Esteem.*

AUTHOR'S NOTE

See *Situational Low Self-Esteem.*

ERRORS IN DIAGNOSTIC STATEMENT

See *Situational Low Self-Esteem.*

KEY CONCEPTS
See *Situational Low Self-Esteem.*

Goal

The person will continue to express a positive outlook for the future to identify positive aspects of self.

Indicators
- Identify threats to self-esteem.
- Identify one positive aspect of change.

General Interventions

See *Situational Low Self-Esteem.*

Risk for Self-Harm*
Risk for Self-Abuse
Self-Mutilation
Risk for Self-Mutilation
Risk for Suicide*

RISK FOR SELF-HARM

DEFINITION

Risk for Self-Harm: State in which a person is at risk for inflicting direct harm on himself. This may include one or more of the following: self-abuse, self-mutilation, suicide.

DEFINING CHARACTERISTICS
Major (Must Be Present, One or More)

Expresses desire or intent to harm self
Expresses desire to die or commit suicide
Past history of attempts to harm self

Minor

Reported or observed

Depression	Hopelessness	Poor self-concept
Helplessness	Hallucinations/delusions	Lack of support system
Substance abuse	Emotional pain	Poor impulse control
Hostility	Agitation	

RELATED FACTORS

Risk for Self-Harm can occur as a response to a variety of health problems, situations, and conflicts. Some sources are listed next.

Pathophysiologic

Related to feelings of helplessness, loneliness, or hopelessness secondary to:

Disabilities
Terminal illness
Chronic illness
Chronic pain
Chemical dependency
Substance abuse
New diagnosis of positive human immunodeficiency virus (HIV) status
Mental impairment (organic or traumatic)
Psychiatric disorder

Schizophrenia	Personality disorder	Bipolar disorder
Adolescent adjustment disorder	Post-trauma syndrome	Somatoform disorders

Treatment-Related

Related to unsatisfactory outcome of treatment (medical, surgical, psychological)

*These diagnoses are not currently on the NANDA list but have been included for clarity or usefulness.

Related to prolonged dependence on

Dialysis   Chemotherapy/radiation   Insulin injections
Ventilator

Situational (Personal, Environmental)

Related to:

Incarceration
Depression
Ineffective coping skills
Parental/marital conflict
Substance abuse in family
Child abuse
Real or perceived loss secondary to:

     Finances/job   Separation/divorce   Status/prestige
     Death of significant others   Threat of abandonment   Someone leaving home

Related to wish for revenge on real or perceived injury (body or self-esteem)

Maturational

Adolescent

Related to feelings of abandonment
Related to peer pressure
Related to unrealistic expectations of child by parents
Related to depression
Related to relocation
Related to significant loss

Older Adult

Related to multiple losses secondary to:

Retirement   Social isolation   Significant loss
Illness

⦾ AUTHOR'S NOTE

Risk for Self-Harm represents a broad diagnosis that can encompass self-abuse, self-mutilation, and/or risk for suicide. Although initially they may appear the same, the distinction lies in the intent. Self-mutilation and self-abuse are pathologic attempts to relieve stress temporarily, whereas suicide is an attempt to die to relieve stress permanently (Carscadden, 1992, personal communication). *Risk for Self-Harm* also can be a useful early diagnosis when insufficient data are present to differentiate one from the other.

    Risk for Suicide is not on the NANDA list but has been added here for clarity. *Risk for Violence to Self* is included under *Risk for Violence.* The term *violence* is defined as a swift and intense force or a rough or injurious physical force. As the reader knows, suicide can be either violent or nonviolent (eg, overdose of barbiturates). Using the term "violence" in this diagnostic context, unfortunately, can lead to nondetection of a person at risk for suicide because of the perception that the person is not capable of violence.

    Risk for Suicide clearly denotes a person at high risk for suicide and in need of protection. Treatment of this diagnosis involves validating the risk, contracting with the person, and providing protection. Treatment of the person's underlying depression and hopelessness should be addressed with other applicable nursing diagnoses (eg, *Ineffective Coping, Hopelessness*).

⦾ ERRORS IN DIAGNOSTIC STATEMENTS

1. *Risk for Suicide related to recent diagnosis of cancer*

    In this situation, the recent diagnosis of cancer in itself is not a risk factor for suicide. The person must be depressed, severely stressed, and exhibiting suicidal intentions. The nurse must not automatically label a person as suicidal based on a single crisis or severe physical disability. All *Risk for Self-Harm* diagnostic statements should contain both verbal and nonverbal cues to suicidal intent (eg, *Risk for Suicide related to remarks about life being unbearable and reports of giving belongings away*).

KEY CONCEPTS
Generic Considerations
- Violence, whether directed toward oneself or others, can elicit strong reactions from people. Nurses, whose profession encompasses caregiving, health promotion, and nurturance, must examine their own attitudes, responses, and behavior toward violence.
- Because much of the practice of self-harm is a "shame-based" problem, the condition is more likely to be underreported rather than overreported. Identification is difficult, because so many who engage in self-harm become extremely adept at hiding the causes of their injuries.
- Self-harm is found in people from all economic and educational backgrounds, and in both men and women. It usually appears in the early teenage years, although it may commence before adolescence. It frequently is associated with long-term effects of physical, psychological, and sexual abuse during childhood.
- Many people who harm themselves are given a psychiatric diagnosis of personality disorder or, more specifically, borderline personality disorder, although other psychiatric diagnoses may be associated with self-harm (see pathophysiologic section). An important consideration is that not all people with these diagnoses harm themselves, and not all self-injurers qualify for these diagnoses. Treatment will differ depending on the diagnosis (Carscadden, 1997).
- The person who has delusions or hallucinations (either schizophrenic or drug-induced) presents a different rationale for self-harm. Delusions and hallucinations must be brought under control. Meanwhile, the person's safety is essential. Self-harm also may be prevalent with mentally challenged people, and management in this particular population will differ again, owing to the cognition level of the self-injurer.
- Often repetitive and chronic in nature, self-harm frequently distorts or disrupts the client–therapist relationship and increases the need for and length of hospitalizations. These hospitalizations often further exacerbate the problem. Hospitalization usually increases the client's dependency and decreases his or her accountability.
- The following presents the basics of dysfunctional family dynamics:
  - *Characteristics*
    - Gives little nurturance
    - Avoids showing feelings
    - Maintains rigid rules
    - Is usually abusive (physical/psychological/sexual)
  - *Family members exhibit*
    - Denial
    - Need/expectation of perfection
    - Minimization
    - Need for control of self/others
    - Blame
  - *Child grows up with*
    - Fear of rejection
    - Fear of losing control
    - Fear of abandonment
    - Feelings of hopelessness and helplessness
  - *As a child and later as an adult, person will have difficulty in*
    - Trusting
    - Asking for wants and needs
    - Identifying and expressing feelings
    - Disregarding internalized messages that create poor self-concept

Self-Harm
- There are various levels or stages in impending self-harm. The transition from one level to another may be rapid or slowly progressive. The person may or may not be aware of the stages and the transition. Awareness of each stage and its characteristics facilitates intervention. The earlier the stage, the clearer the thinking, the less intense are the feelings, and the more control the person has. A person can easily identify stages once he or she learns the defining characteristics (Carscadden, 1993a).
- *Beginning Stage ("Thinking" Stage)*
  - Person often unaware of this stage.
  - Person may have been ruminating.

- Person may have encountered a "trigger," which set off memory or ignited a flashback.
- Advancement into this stage might produce
  - Change in concentration/attention
  - Mild heart palpitations
  - Small tremor
  - Slight tightening of muscles
  - Change in facial color
- *Climbing Stage ("Feeling" Stage)*
  - Stage many people become aware of first.
  - Feelings begin to intensify.
    - Tremor increases, may become a shake.
    - Muscles tense to fight or flight.
    - Person cannot concentrate.
    - Person may experience shortness of breath.
    - Heart begins to race.
    - Perspiration may occur.
- *Crisis Stage ("Behavior" Stage)*
  - Concentration will be extremely limited and focused on intent to relieve pent-up feelings.
    - Person may "numb out" or disassociate.
    - Agitation may increase or person may become extremely calm.
    - Moves are sudden, with flurried activity.
  - Person may perceive physical touch as a real threat.
  - Person often sees no alternative but self-harm at this point.
- *Postcrisis Stage*
  - Person may experience mixed emotions: whatever relief the self-harm provides, but also guilt, shame, or frustration at having failed expectations.
    - He or she may cry or withdraw.
    - This stage is often the worst for the person because of the negative response from others, including many caregivers.
- Although self-harm may create a sense of urgency, imminent disaster, and a strong and immediate sense of responsibility in the listener or observer, one must be careful not to be caught up in this and feel compelled to do something. (This excludes the psychotic and mentally challenged population.) The very act of trying to intervene or prevent the behaviors may increase the likelihood of more serious harm, including completed suicide. The risk increases because: (a) the more often intervention takes place, the more likely death by mistake will occur (wrong pills, too many, the expected rescue being thwarted); (b) there may be a need to use increasingly dangerous methods to get the same result; or (c) before long, countertransference hate sets in. In an empathic, yet matter-of-fact manner, the nurse must convey that the person's actions are in his or her hands alone and that no one can be his or her guardian or savior. This is the hardest thing for anyone to say; however, for the self-injurer to survive and mature, he or she must become responsible for his or her own actions. If someone else takes control, the self-injurer will not progress (Carscadden, 1998).
- In settings mandated to prevent, contain, or reduce self-harm, common practices are to use seclusion or a system of physical restraint, often a four-point restraint in which the person is tied to a mattress or bed with each arm and leg restrained separately. Statistics indicate that early sexual abuse appears to be a common experience for many self-injurers. The use of restraints, being held down or tied up, spreading the legs, or otherwise being at the complete mercy of another can represent the reenactment of sexual abuse or rape. Questions should be raised regarding the ethical use of this type of containment as well its effectiveness when records show that restraints or seclusion are used regularly (Carscadden, 1998).
- Families are often the forgotten sufferers in the self-harm syndrome. They are caught in the same shame-based system as the self-injurer, and this often precludes their reaching out for help with the bewilderment, frustration, and helplessness experienced in day-to-day living with the self-injurer. They need assistance in demystifying self-harm, identifying how it has affected them, and examining some coping methods for supporting themselves and the self-injurer on the road to recovery. Educational and support groups as well as family counseling are good ways to begin this process (Carscadden, 1997).

Suicide

- Self-harm ranges from injurious acts to reduce stress to direct acts of suicide. Self-abuse or mutilation behavior has the potential to be harmful and to result in death. Self-injurers are very aware that their actions have a potential of resulting in death if they miscalculate (eg, how many pills, how much cutting or burning; availability of help; their own degree of control to stop once started; Carscadden, 1993a). With direct self-destructive behavior, usually referred to as suicidal, the intent is death, and the person is aware of that.

- Suicidal behavior is an attempt to escape from intolerable life stressors that have accumulated over time. It is accompanied by intense feelings of hopelessness, little social support, and insufficient coping skills to manage extreme stressors that are present (Boyd, 2004).
- Lack of healthy coping skills and use of avoidant behaviors such as alcohol and drugs frequently are correlated with suicidal behavior.
- A suicidal crisis happens both to the person and to his or her support system. Suicide may be seen as a viable alternative both by the individual and by significant others.
- Depression, low self-esteem, helplessness, and hopelessness are positively related to suicide. The greater the degree of hopelessness, the greater is the risk for suicide. Loss clearly increases the risk of suicide. Cumulative losses increase the risk dramatically.
- People exhibiting poor reality testing, delusions, and poor impulse control are at high risk. Alcohol and drugs tend to lower impulse control.
- Changes in behavior (eg, giving away possessions) may signal an increase in risk. A person may appear to be better just before an attempt. This may result from feelings of relief after making a decision.
- Demographic factors can help identify people at high risk for suicide:
  - White men over 65 have the highest suicide rate in the United States. Risk increases linearly as the person ages (Boyd, 2005).
  - Adolescents also represent a high-risk group.
  - More women attempt suicide, but men complete suicide more often.
  - Unemployment and frequent job changes are associated with an increased risk.
  - Alcohol is associated with a high risk.
  - The greater the satisfaction with social relationships, the lower the risk will be; thus, divorce, separation, and widowhood increase the risk.
  - Previous attempts place people in a high-risk group because they are likely to repeat.
- The more resources that are available, the more likely it is that the crisis can be managed effectively. Resources include personal support systems, employment, physical and mental abilities, finances, and housing.
- Some people use suicide attempts as a way to cope with stress. The more frequent the attempts and the more lethal, the higher the current risk. Suicidal ideation moves from the general to the specific, with more detailed plans representing a higher risk. An event may precipitate an attempt. The difference between a negative life event and one that may lead to a suicide attempt is that with the latter, the person already has engaged in significant suicidal ideation.
- Long-term suicide risk exists for some people. This can be assessed best by evaluating:
  - Their coping strategies when confronted with stress
  - Their lifestyle—is it stable or unstable?
  - The specificity and lethality of the plan
- Lethality describes "the probability that a person will successfully complete suicide." It is determined by the "seriousness of the intent and the likelihood that the planned method of death will succeed" (Boyd, 2005, p. 860).
- Nurses should use verbal and nonverbal clues to assess risk, because seriously suicidal people may deny suicidal thoughts.
- Prediction of suicide risk is not an exact science. Some errors that can be made result from:
  - Overreliance on mood as an indicator; not all people who commit suicide are clinically depressed
  - Reliance on intuition; many people can totally conceal their intention
  - Failure to assess support system
  - Countertransference, particularly the failure of the therapist to acknowledge negative feelings that are aroused
- Levels of risk can be assessed as low or high. Not all of the following parameters are necessarily present in any one person (Varcarolis, 1998).

High

Adolescent or older than 45 years	Male
Divorced, separated, widowed	Isolated socially
Professional worker	Unemployed or lack of stable job history
Chronic or terminal illness	Severe depression
Delusions/hallucinations	Severe anxiety

Hopelessness/helplessness	Multiple attempts
Intoxicated or addicted	With a specific plan
Frequent or constant suicidal thoughts	Method is highly lethal
Means readily available	
Low	
25 to 45 years of age	Younger than 12 years
Married	Blue-collar worker
No serious medical problems	No specific plan, or plan with low lethality
Female	Socially active
Employed	Infrequent substance abuse
Fleeting thoughts (if plan is vague)	

- In an HIV-positive person, the risk for suicide is greatest "shortly after learning of one's infection and at the late stages of AIDS" (Siegel & Meyer, 1999, p. 53).
- The AIDS-related multiple losses that HIV-negative gay men may experience can result in repetitive overwhelming emotions, physical exhaustion, and spiritual demoralization. If coupled with shunning and isolation, despair is increased and chronic (Mallinson, 1999).

Pediatric Considerations

- The preteen and early adolescent years are often when self-harm begins to manifest itself. Adults must be in tune with changes in behavior and changes in apparel and be highly suspicious of multiple "accidents."
- Suicide is the second leading cause of death during adolescence. A significant trend is the rise among people in the younger age groups.
- Suicide in children (5 to 14 years of age) tends to be more impulsive than in other age groups. Hyperactivity also seems to contribute to the impulsive nature.
- Recognition of depression in adolescents is often difficult because they mask their feelings with bored and angry behavior. Some symptoms include being sad or blue, withdrawal from social activities, trouble concentrating, somatic complaints, changes in sleep or eating patterns, and feelings of guilt or inadequacy.
- Suicidal adolescents rarely have close friends and exhibit poor peer relationships.
- Gay youths are estimated to be two to three times more likely to attempt suicide than their heterosexual peers. As many as 30% of suicides annually are believed to be gay teens.
- Suicide is the leading cause of death among adolescents. A frequent factor is lack of or loss of a meaningful relationship (Mohr, 2003).
- Suicide attempts among Hispanic adolescent girls were reported to be 19.3%. Significant related factors included family history of suicide attempt, history of sexual or physical abuse, and environmental stress (Giger & Davidhazar, 2004).

Geriatric Considerations

- White men older than 65 years have twice the rate of suicide of all other age groups. They constitute 18.5% of the population but commit 23% of all suicides (Miller, 2004).
- Retirement, loss of vigor, and loss of a meaningful role negatively affect the self-esteem of older men.
- Older adults tend to complete suicide when they attempt it. The ratio of attempts to completion is 4:1, whereas for younger people it is approximately 200:1 (McIntosh, 1985).
- Alcohol contributes to depression. Depression increases alcohol use. Both are significant risk factors for suicide in older adults.
- Depressed older adults usually talk less about suicide than younger adults but use more violent means and are more often successful (Miller, 2004).

(continued)

⟲ Geriatric Considerations (continued)

- Suicide potential often is overlooked because of the prevalent view that older adults are generally passive and nonviolent. In addition, complaints about depression and hopelessness may be subtle and thus easily ignored in older adults (Miller, 2004).
- Older adults communicate their intentions less frequently and they use more lethal means (Mellick, Buckwalter & Stolley, 1992). Families, senior citizen centers, clergy, and physicians are the network that can most readily identify the potential problem.

🌐 Transcultural Considerations

- Acceptance of sudden, violent death is difficult for family members in most societies (Andrews & Boyle, 2003).
- Islamic law strictly forbids suicide. Some religions (eg, Catholicism) do not permit church funerals for suicide victims.
- The Northern Cheyenne Indians believe suicide or any violent death prevents the spirit from entering the spirit world (Andrews & Boyle, 2003).
- Suicide of elderly Eskimos, who could no longer contribute to the sustenance of the tribe, was expected (Giger & Davidhizar, 2004).

Focus Assessment Criteria

The nurse must be able to differentiate between the diagnoses of *Risk for Suicide* and *Risk for Self-Mutilation* or *Self-Abuse*. Although initially they may appear (in action) or sound (in statements) the same, the distinction lies in the intent. Self-mutilation and self-abuse are pathologic attempts to relieve stress (temporary reprieve), whereas suicide is an attempt to die (to relieve stress permanently). The nurse will be able in the assessment to gather data that enable him or her to distinguish which diagnosis is appropriate for the client. It is prudent to remember that some clients may become so self-harmful that they eventually die, even though they are not intentionally suicidal.

Subjective Data
Assess for Risk Factors.

Psychological status
Present concerns
Have you experienced a severe stressor recently?
How are you feeling?
Do you want to hurt yourself?
Can you tell me the reason?
Do you want to die or just have the pain (thoughts/feelings) go away?
Assess for a suicide plan.
    Method: Is there a specific plan (eg, pills, wrist-slashing, shooting)? Plans for rescue?
    Availability: Is the method accessible? Is access easy or difficult?
    Specificity: How specific is the plan?
    Lethality: How lethal is the method?
Feelings of

Hopelessness	Anger/hostility	Helplessness
Guilt/shame	Isolation/abandonment	Impulsivity

Chemical dependency / substance abuse
Assess if person is suffering from withdrawal or is under the influence. Chemical use lowers cognition ability and raises the level of impulsivity.
History of psychiatric problems
Previous history of self-harm

Methods	How recent	Ensures rescue will be made
Lethality	Number of times	

Outpatient follow-up support system

Medical status

Acute or chronic illness—how is it affecting life?

Prescribed drugs

    What is person using?

    Does he or she take it according to directions?

Sources of stress in past environment

Job change/loss

Failure in work/school

Threat of financial loss

Divorce/separation

Death of significant other

Illness/accident

Alcohol/drug use in family

Parental rejection

Dysfunctional family dynamics

Physical, psychological, sexual abuse

Unrealistic expectations

    Of child by parent

    Of parent by child

    Of self

Severe trauma

Sources of stress in current environment

Any of the above (past environment)

Threat of criminal prosecution

Alcohol/drug use by person

Role change/responsibilities

Any threat to self-concept (real or perceived)

Assessment of person's awareness of self-harm activities

Acknowledgment or denial—does the person admit self-harm or claim to have "accidents"?

What are the payoffs or reasons for self-harm?

    Is nonverbal communication—gains someone's attention and coerces others for their needs

    Makes others believe—physical evidence of pain

    Demonstrates the feeling of hopelessness

    Demonstrates outside what person feels like inside (ugly, scarred, garbage)

    Feels he or she deserves it—bad, ugly, evil, crazy

    Releases pain and anger—use of self-harm is a safety valve to prevent suicide

    (Re)establishes control over one's body

    Verifies there is still life—physical evidence of life in flow of blood

    Is sadomasochistic pleasure

    Is an addiction to near death

Can the person identify specifics in the process?

    Personal triggers

      Sensory input

      Situations

      Particular types of people or places

    Flashbacks or nightmares

    Does the person disassociate or "numb out"?

    Can person identify levels or stages before the act of self-harm?

Motivation to cease self-harm

    Wants to stop and is willing to work toward that end

    Wants emotional pain to stop, sees self-harm as part of that pain and is considering change

    Unwilling to give up self-harm behavior

Support system

Who is relied on during periods of stress?

    Are they available?

    What is their reaction to current situation?

Denial	Helplessness/frustration
Not receptive to helping	Concern and willingness to help
Anger/guilt	

Personal and financial resources

Employment	Housing	Finances

Objective Data
Assess for Risk Factors.

General appearance

Facial expression	Apparel	Posture

Behavior during interview

Agitated	Hostile	Restless
Cooperative	Withdrawn	Disassociated

Communication pattern

Hopeless/helpless (subjective)	Allusive	Denial
Suicidal expressions	Delusional	Indecisive
Hallucinates	Pressured speech	Misinterprets
Difficulty concentrating	Supersensitive (subjective)	

Nutritional status

Appetite	Bulimic behavior	Weight (anorectic, obese)

Sleep–rest pattern

Afraid of dark	Easily awakened	Difficulty falling asleep
Sleeps too much	Difficulty staying asleep	Nightmares

Physical manifestations

Tremors	Heart palpitations	Agitation
Tightness of chest	Hyperalertness	Buzzing in head
Shortness of breath	Fists clench	Perspiration
Aches and pains: stomach, head, muscles	Change in facial color	

Evidence of self-harm

Be highly suspicious if

There have been repeated accidents

Person wears long sleeves in hot weather

Person is reluctant to uncover parts of body

Look for

Scars	Lumps/bumps	Open cuts
Reddened, irritated areas	Sores	Burn marks
Areas that do not heal as expected	Clumps/patches of missing hair	

Body parts often affected

Wrists, arms, legs, feet	Head, face, eyes, neck	Chest, abdomen
Genitals		

Behaviors of self-mutilation

Cutting

Picking

Slashing

Gouging

Stabbing

Head smashing

Scratching

Hitting (eg, fists against walls)

Burning (cigarettes, lighters, matches, stove, clothes iron, curling iron)

Use of corrosives (eg, drain cleaner)

Behaviors of self-abuse

Head banging

Slapping

Picking

Scratching

Nonlethal use of drugs/poison

Anorectic/bulimic behaviors

Swallowing foreign objects (glass, needles, safety pins, straight pins, various hardware [eg, nails, screws])

Hair pulling

Excessive rubbing

Noncompliance with treatment for serious physical or medical conditions (eg, diabetes)

For more information on Focus Assessment Criteria, visit http://connection.lww.com.

Goal

NOC Aggression Control, Impulse Control

The person will choose alternatives that are not harmful.

Indicators

- Acknowledge self-harm thoughts.
- Admit to use of self-harm behavior if it occurs.
- Be able to identify personal triggers.
- Learn to identify and tolerate uncomfortable feelings.

General Interventions

NIC Presence, Anger Control, Environmental Management: Violence Prevention, Behavior Modification, Security Enhancement, Therapy Group, Coping Enhancement, Impulse Control Training, Crisis Intervention

Establish a Trusting Nurse–Client Relationship.

Demonstrate acceptance of client as a worthwhile person through nonjudgmental statements and behavior.

Ask questions in a caring, concerned manner.

Encourage expression of thoughts and feelings.

Actively listen or provide support by just being there if the person is silent.

Be aware of the client's supersensitivity.

Label the behavior, not the person.

Be honest in your interactions.

Assist client to recognize hope and alternatives.

Provide reasons for necessary procedures or interventions.

Maintain client's dignity throughout your therapeutic relationship.

Validate Reality.

Schizophrenia or Drug-Induced Psychosis

Tell the person "you are safe."

Use quiet, calming voice.

Use "talk downs" when client has taken a hallucinogenic drug. If agitation increases, stop immediately.

Orient client as required. Point out sensory/environmental misperceptions without belittling his or her fears or indicating disapproval of verbal expressions.

Reassure client that this will pass.

Watch for signs of increased delusional thinking and/or frightening hallucinations (increased anxiety, agitation, irritability, pacing, hypervigilance).

Post-Trauma or Dysfunctional

Tell the person "you are not bad, crazy, hopeless."

Say you believe him or her when he or she tells you personal history; many grew up in denial or minimization.

Let the person know he or she is not the only one.

Help Reframe Old Thinking/Feeling Patterns (Carscadden, 1993a).

Encourage the belief that change is possible.

Assist client to identify thought–feeling–behavior concept.

Help client assess payoffs and drawbacks to self-harm.

Rename words that have a negative connotation (eg, "setback," not "failure").

Encourage identification of personal triggers.

Assist client to explore viable alternatives.

Help client to examine feelings of ambivalence about recovery.

Encourage client to become comfortable with and to use feelings.

Facilitate the Development of New Behavior.

Validate good coping skills already in existence.

Serve as a role model in your own behavior and interactions.

Encourage the use of positive affirmations, meditation and relaxation techniques, and other esteem-building exercises.

Promote the concept of being helpful instead of helpless.

Encourage journaling, keeping a diary of triggers, thoughts, feelings, and alternatives that work or do not work.

Assist client to develop body awareness as a method of ascertaining triggers and determining levels of impending self-harm.

Assist with role playing to work on situations/relationships.

Promote development of healthy self-boundaries for the person.

Endorse an Environment that Demotes Self-Harm.

How much control or influence a professional exerts in this area will depend on the diagnosis, the environmental setting, and the policies of that setting (eg, a person's home, residential setting, treatment facility, or institution). If mandated by the setting's policies to intervene in self-harm attempts, then the following interventions should take place.

Structure the Client's Time and Activities.

Provide a scheduled day that meets the person's need for activity and rest.

Encourage assistance to and activities with others without competitiveness.

Relieve pent-up tension and purposeless hyperactivity with physical activity (eg, brisk walk, dance therapy, aerobics).

Reduce Excessive Stimuli.

Provide a quiet, serene atmosphere.

Establish firm, consistent limits while giving person as much control/choice as possible within those boundaries.

Intervene at earliest stages to assist person to regain control, prevent escalation, and allow treatment in the least restrictive manner.

Keep communication simple. Agitated people cannot process complicated communication.

Provide an area where the person can retreat to decrease stimuli (eg, time-out room, quiet room; person on hallucinogens needs a darkened, quiet room with a nonintrusive observer).

Remove potentially dangerous objects from environment (if in crisis stage).

Reduce Triggers as Much as Possible.

Assess problem areas and assist in problem solving with the client.

    Is person afraid of dark? Allow a small light on at night.

    Is person afraid of being alone? Put in a double room with roommate.

Promote the Use of Alternatives.

Stress that there are always alternatives.

Stress that self-harm is a choice, not something uncontrollable.

Allow opportunities for verbal expression of thoughts and feelings.

Provide acceptable physical outlets (eg, yelling, pounding pillow, tearing up newspapers, using clay or Play-Doh, taking a brisk walk).

Provide for less physical alternatives (eg, relaxation tapes, soft music, warm bath, diversional activities).

Determine Present Level of Impending Self-Harm if Indicated.

Beginning Stage (Thought Stage)

Provide soothing touch if permitted by person (predetermined).

Remind person that this is an "old tape" and to replace with new thinking and belief patterns.

Provide nonintrusive, calming alternatives.

Climbing Stage (Feeling Stage)

Remind person to consider alternatives.

Give as much control to the person as possible to support his or her accountability.

Are you in control?   How can I help?   Would you like me to assist?

Provide more intense interventions at this stage.

Encourage person to turn over any potential items of self-harm.

Crisis Stage (Behavior Stage)

Give positive feedback if person chooses an alternative and does not harm himself or herself.

Ask person to put down any object of harm if he or she possesses one.

Continue to emphasize there are always alternatives.

Restrain only if person becomes out of control.

Release from restraints as soon as possible to give responsibility back to person. "Are you in control now?" "Are you feeling safe?"

Remain calm and caring throughout the crisis period.

Attend to practical issues in a nonpunitive, nonjudgmental manner.

Postcrisis Stage

Give positive reinforcements if person did not harm himself or herself.

Assist client to problem-solve on how to divert self before crisis stage.

Assess degree of injury/harm if person did not choose alternative.

Provide assistance or medical care, as necessary.

Pay as little attention as possible to the act of self-harm and focus on prior stages (eg, "Can you remember what triggered you?" "What kinds of things were going through your mind?" "What do you think you might have done instead?").

Return person to normal activities/routine as soon as possible.

Initiate Support Systems to Community, When/Where Indicated.

Teach family

    Constructive expression of feelings

    How to recognize levels of impending self-harm

    How to assist with appropriate interventions

    How to deal with self-harm behavior/results

Supply Phone Number of 24-h Emergency Hotlines.

Provide referral to:

Individual therapist	Family counseling	Peer support group
Leisure/vocational counseling	Halfway houses	Other community resources

Rationales

- Frequent contact by the caregiver indicates acceptance and may facilitate trust. The client may be hesitant to approach staff because of negative self-concept; the nurse must reach out.
- Expressing feelings and perceptions increases the client's self-awareness and helps the nurse plan effective interventions to address his or her needs. Validating the client's perceptions provides reassurance and can decrease anxiety.
- The nurse must be aware that the person may express or exhibit ambivalence about stopping the self-harm behavior. This coping mechanism probably served a useful purpose. Often, unless the payoffs cease or until the payoffs for not harming are greater or more important, the behavior will continue.
- It is important not to reward the act of self-harm with reinforcements (negative or positive). Treatment of the injury should be done matter-of-factly, much like removing a splinter, but also provide the person with dignity. Returning to activities/schedules as quickly as possible restores responsibility to the person.
- Control of environment is a basic, but not to be discounted, intervention. A structured schedule provides boundaries and security, enhancing the sense of safety. A quiet environment reduces reactivity, enhances calm feelings, and decreases the likelihood of confusion and fear. Gross

motor activity in a protected environment can lessen aggressive drives, whereas rest periods promote opportunities for relaxation, calm the emergency response, and reconnect body/mind/heart.

- The therapeutic alliance promotes client responsibility for behavioral restraint while supplementing internal controls. Expression of feelings may assist in resolving them regardless of the discomfort involved and may decrease the need for physical action.
- Promise contracts contain things like "promise that you won't . . ." or "promise you'll come and tell me before you. . . ." They should never be used, because they reinforce the notion that the person is incompetent and impulse-driven, not in control. They also multiply the potential for distortions and make others, not the self-injurer, responsible for the behavior and its control. A no-harm contract is not a logical tool to use with psychotic, mentally challenged, or chemically impaired persons, who are not competent to enter into such agreements. With a depressed person, the intent might be misinterpreted. A contract might be more useful if used as boundaries (eg, results of self-harm are attended to before a therapy session, or details or specifics of self-harm are not discussed in group therapy so that other members are not triggered; Dawson & MacMillan, 1993; Egan et al., 1997).
- Maladaptive behaviors can be replaced with healthy ones to manage stress and anxiety (Stuart & Sundeen, 2002).
- Social isolation perpetuates feelings of low self-esteem and self-destructive behavior (Stuart & Sundeen, 2002).
- People who dissociate or are ungrounded or unsafe have difficulty when asked to "give up their body" or "close their eyes" in relaxation or visualization and should never be encouraged to do so until they are ready.

RISK FOR SELF-ABUSE

DEFINITION
Risk for Self-Abuse: State in which a person is at risk to perform a deliberate act on the self, without the intent to kill, that may or may not cause harm to the body

DEFINING CHARACTERISTICS
Major (Must Be Present, One or More)
Expresses a desire or intent to harm self
Evidence of self-abuse, including:
    Head banging
    Slapping
    Picking
    Scratching
    Nonlethal use of drugs/poison
    Anorectic/bulimic behaviors
    Swallowing foreign objects, (glass, needles, safety pins, straight pins, various hardware [eg, nails, screws])

RELATED FACTORS
See *Risk for Self-Harm.*

⊙⊙ **AUTHOR'S NOTE**

See *Risk for Self-Harm.*

⊙⊙ **ERRORS IN DIAGNOSTIC STATEMENTS**

See *Risk for Self-Harm.*

KEY CONCEPTS
See *Risk for Self-Harm.*

SELF-MUTILATION

DEFINITION

Self-Mutilation: State in which a person has performed a deliberate act on the self with the intent to injure, not kill, that produces immediate tissue damage

DEFINING CHARACTERISTICS

Expresses desire or intent to harm self
Past history of attempts to harm self, including:

Cutting	Scratching	Slashing
Picking	Stabbing	Gouging

RELATED FACTORS

See *Risk for Self-Harm.*

⊙⊙ **AUTHOR'S NOTE**

See *Risk for Self-Harm.*

⊙⊙ **ERRORS IN DIAGNOSTIC STATEMENTS**

See *Risk for Self-Harm.*

KEY CONCEPTS
See *Risk for Self-Harm.*

Focus Assessment

See *Risk for Self-Harm.*

General Interventions

See *Risk for Self-Harm.*

RISK FOR SELF-MUTILATION

DEFINITION

Risk for Self-Mutilation: State in which a person is at risk to perform a deliberate act on the self with the intent to injure, not kill, that produces immediate tissue damage

RELATED FACTORS

See *Risk for Self-Harm.*

 AUTHOR'S NOTE

See *Risk for Self-Harm.*

 ERRORS IN DIAGNOSTIC STATEMENTS

See *Risk for Self-Harm.*

KEY CONCEPTS
See *Risk for Self-Harm.*

General Interventions

See *Risk for Self-Harm.*

RISK FOR SUICIDE

DEFINITION

Risk for Suicide: State in which a person is at risk for killing himself or herself

DEFINING CHARACTERISTICS

Major (Must Be Present)

Suicidal ideation
Previous suicidal attempts

Minor

See *Risk for Self-Harm.*

RELATED FACTORS

See *Risk for Self-Harm.*

KEY CONCEPTS

See *Risk for Self-Harm.*

Focus Assessment Criteria

Refer to *Risk for Self-Harm*

Goal

NOC Impulse Control, Suicide Self-Restraint

The person will not commit suicide.

Indicators

- State the desire to live.
- Verbalize feelings of anger, loneliness, and hopelessness.
- Identify persons to contact if suicidal thoughts occur.
- Identify alternative coping mechanisms.

General Interventions

NIC Active Listening, Coping Enhancement, Suicide Prevention, Impulse Control Training, Behavior Management: Self Harm, Hope Instillation, Contracting, Surveillance: Safety

Assist the Person to Reduce His or Her Present Risk for Self-Destruction.

Assess Level of Present Risk (Table II.21).

High	Moderate	Low

Assess Level of Long-Term Risk.

Lifestyle	Lethality of plan	Usual coping mechanisms
Support available		

Provide a Safe Environment Based on Level of Risk.

Immediate management for high-risk person

Acutely suicidal people should be admitted to a closely supervised environment.

TABLE II.21 Assessing the Degree of Suicidal Risk

Behavior or Symptom	Intensity of Risk		
	Low	Moderate	High
Anxiety	Mild	Moderate	High, or panic state
Depression	Mild	Moderate	Severe
Isolation/withdrawal	Some feelings of isolation, no withdrawal	Some feelings of hopelessness, and withdrawal	Hopeless, withdrawn, and self-deprecating, isolation
Daily functioning	Effective	Moody	Depressed
	Good grades in school*	Some friends	Poor grades*
	Close friends	Prior suicidal thoughts	Few or no close friends
	No prior suicide attempt		Prior suicide attempts
	Stable job		Erratic or poor work history
Lifestyle	Stable	Moderately stable	Unstable
Alcohol/drug use	Infrequently to excess	Frequently to excess	Continual abuse
Previous suicide attempts	None or of low lethality (few pills)	One or more (pills, superficial wrist slash)	One or more (entire bottle of pills, gun, hanging)
Associated events	None, or an argument	Disciplinary action*	Relationship breakup
		Failing grades*	Death of a loved one
		Work problems	Loss of job
		Family illness	Pregnancy*
Purpose of act	None, or not clear	Relief of shame or guilt	Wants to die
		To punish others	Escape to join deceased
		To get attention	Debilitating disease
Family's reaction and structure	Supportive	Mixed reaction	Angry and unsupportive
	Intact family	Divorced/separated	Disorganized
	Good coping and mental health	Usually copes and understands	Rigid/abusive
	No history of suicide		Prior history of suicide in family
Suicide plan (method, location, time)	No plan	Frequent thoughts, occasional ideas about a plan	Specific plan

*Applies only to children and adolescents

Adapted from Hatton, C. L., & McBride, S. (1984). *Suicide: Assessment and intervention*. Norwalk, CT: Appleton-Century-Crofts; and Jackson, D. B., & Saunders, R. B. (1993). *Child health nursing*. Philadelphia: J. B. Lippincott.

Although it is impossible to create a completely safe environment, removal of dangerous objects and close observation convey a nonverbal message of concern. Restrict glass, nail files, scissors, nail polish remover, mirrors, needles, razors, soda cans, plastic bags, lighters, electric equipment, belts, hangers, knives, tweezers, alcohol, and guns.

Meals should be provided in a closely supervised area, usually on the unit or in person's room.
  Ensure adequate food and fluid intake.
  Use paper/plastic plates and utensils.
  Check to be sure all items are returned on the tray.

When administering oral medications, check to ensure that all medications are swallowed.

Designate a staff member to provide checks on the person as designated by institution's policy. Provide relief for the staff member.

Restrict the person to the unit unless specifically ordered by physician. When off unit, provide a staff member to accompany the person.

Instruct visitors on restricted items (eg, ensure they do not give person food in a plastic bag).

The person may use restricted items in presence of staff, depending on level of risk. Acutely suicidal people should not be allowed access to such items.

The acutely suicidal person may be required to wear a hospital gown to prevent him or her from leaving the facility. As risk decreases, client may be allowed own clothing.

Room searches should be done periodically according to institution policy.

Use seclusion and restraint if necessary (refer to *Risk for Violence* for discussion).

Notify police if the person leaves the facility and is at risk for suicide.

When the person is being constantly observed, he or she is not to be allowed out of sight, even though privacy is lost.

Notify All Staff that Person is at Risk for Self-Harm; Use Both Written and Oral Communication.

Make a No-Suicide Contract with the Person (Include Family if Person is at Home).
Use a written contract.
Mutual agreement
  "I will not kill myself"
  "I will not accidentally or intentionally take medicine except according to instructions."
  "I will talk to a staff member about my thoughts when suicidal ideas increase."

Help Build Self-Esteem.
Be nonjudgmental and empathic.
Be aware of own reactions to the situation.
Provide genuine praise.
Encourage interactions with others.
Divert attention to external world (eg, odd jobs).
Convey sense that he is not alone (use group or peer therapy).
Seek out person for interactions.
Set limits by informing of rules.
Use firm, consistent approach.
Provide planned daily schedules for people with low impulse control.

Assist Client to Identify and Contact Support System.
Inform family and significant others.
Enlist support.
Do not provide false reassurance that behavior will not recur.
Point out vague or unclear messages from person or support system.
Encourage an increase in social activity.

Assist Client to Develop Positive Coping Mechanisms.
Refer to *Anxiety, Ineffective Coping,* and *Hopelessness* for further interventions.
Encourage appropriate expression of anger and hostility.
Set limits on ruminations about suicide or previous attempts.
Assist client to recognize predisposing factors: "What was happening before you started having these thoughts?"
Facilitate examination of life stresses and past coping mechanisms.
Explore alternative behaviors.
Anticipate future stresses and assist in planning alternatives.
Use appropriate behavior modification techniques for noncompliant, resistive people.
Help client to identify negative thinking patterns and direct person to practice altering them.
Involve person in planning the treatment goals and evaluating progress.

Initiate Health Teaching and Referrals, When Indicated.

Provide teaching that prepares person to deal with life stresses (relaxation, problem-solving skills, how to express feelings constructively).

Refer for peer or group therapy.

Refer for family therapy, especially when child or adolescent is involved.

Teach family limit-setting techniques.

Teach family constructive expression of feelings.

Instruct significant others in how to recognize an increase in risk: change in behavior, verbal or non-verbal communication, withdrawal, signs of depression.

Supply phone number of 24-h emergency hotline.

Refer to vocational training if appropriate.

Refer to halfway house or other agencies, as appropriate.

Refer for ongoing psychiatric follow-up.

Refer to senior citizen centers or other agencies to increase leisure activities.

Initiate referral for family intervention after a completed suicide.

Rationales

- Suicidal behavior can be assessed by evaluating biologic, psychological, cognitive, and environmental risk factors; suicidal ideation; and precipitating events.
- Suicidal individuals are usually ambivalent about the decision. Staff can work with the positive goals to effect a change in attitude.
- To assess the risk for suicide, the caregiver must question the person directly with simple, straightforward questions. The more specific, more lethal, and more available the means, the higher the present risk. The most lethal methods in our culture are shooting and hanging. The least lethal is wrist-slashing.
- Interventions are based on the type of risk the person presents. Long-term treatment is often more difficult to institute than emergency care.
- Caregivers can become immobilized or drained by the acutely suicidal person. Feelings of hopelessness are often communicated to the caregiver.
- Making a contract with the person
  - Gets the subject out in the open
  - Conveys the attitude of acceptance of the person as a worthwhile individual
  - Presents element of choice, the possibility and importance of thinking through situations before acting
  - Provides person with some control, as he or she shares responsibility for own safety

 ## Pediatric Interventions

Take all suicide threats seriously.

Determine whether the child understands the finality of death (eg, "What does it mean to die?"; "Have you ever seen a dead animal on the road? Can it get up and run?").

Engage parents, friends, school personnel, and the person in behavior contracts to "keep safe."

Explore feelings and reason for suicidal feelings.

Consult with a psychiatric expert regarding the most appropriate environment for treatment.

Participate in programs in school to teach about the symptoms of depression and signs of suicidal behavior.

With adolescents, explore (Mohr, 2003):

   Family problems

   Mental status

   Strength of support systems

   Disruption of friendship or romantic relationship

   Seriousness of the attempt

   Presence of performance failure (eg, examination, course).

   Recent or upcoming change (change of school, relocation).

   Sexual orientation

Convey empathy regarding problems and/or losses.

Be alert for symptoms of a masked depression (eg, boredom, restlessness, irritability, difficulty concentrating, somatic preoccupation, excessive dependence on or isolation from others, especially adults; Mohr, 2003).

Rationales

- All threats or gestures to hurt oneself must be taken seriously regardless of the child's developmental age.
- Treatment strategies depend on child's living situation, psychiatric history, and support system available.
- Parents, friends, and school personnel should be enlisted to help.
- Suicidal threats and ideation signal a crisis that requires specific care.
- Suicide attempts or threats may not represent a true desire to die, but they definitely represent a cry for help.
- Children who attempt suicide may have marked depression (Varcarolis, 2002).
- Certain stressors are especially significant for adolescents, who are developmentally preoccupied with status, peers, and appearances (Varcarolis, 2002).

DISTURBED SENSORY PERCEPTION

DEFINITION

Disturbed Sensory Perception: State in which a person/group experiences or is at risk of experiencing a negative change in the amount, pattern, or interpretation of incoming stimuli

DEFINING CHARACTERISTICS

Major (Must Be Present)

Inaccurate interpretation of environmental stimuli and/or negative change in amount or pattern of incoming stimuli

Minor (May Be Present)

Disoriented in time or place	Disoriented about people
Altered ability to solve problems	Altered behavior or communication pattern
	Reports auditory or visual hallucinations
Restlessness	Anxiety
Fear	Irritability
Apathy	

RELATED FACTORS

Many factors can contribute to disturbed sensory perception. Some common factors are below.

Pathophysiologic (Sensory Organ Alterations)

Related to misinterpretations secondary to:

Sensory organ alterations
  Visual, gustatory, auditory, olfactory, and tactile deficits

Neurologic alterations

Cerebrovascular accident (CVA)	Tumors	Meningitis
	Neuropathies	Encephalitis

Metabolic alterations

Fluid and electrolyte imbalance	Alkalosis	Renal failure
	Acidosis	

Impaired oxygen transport

Cerebral	Cardiac	Respiratory
Anemia		

Related to mobility restrictions secondary to:

Paraplegia	Quadriplegia

Treatment-Related
Related to chemical changes secondary to:
Medications (eg, sedatives, tranquilizers, steroids, anticonvulsants, antihistamines, cardiac glyco-
    sides, anticholinergics)
Surgery (eg, glaucoma, cataract, detached retina)

Related to physical isolation (eg, reverse isolation, communicable disease, prison)
Related to immobility
Related to mobility restrictions (eg, bed rest, traction, casts, Stryker frame, CircOlectric bed)

Situational (Personal, Environmental)
Related to
Pain   Stress   Sleep interpretations

Related to environmental barriers
Noise   Lights   Lack of privacy
Constant changes   Excess activity   Frequent demands

Related to monotonous environment
Related to loss of socialization
Related to loss of control

○○ **AUTHOR'S NOTE**

Disturbed Sensory Perception describes a person with altered perception and cognition influenced
by physiologic factors (eg, pain, sleep deprivation, immobility, excessive or decreased meaningful environmental stimuli). Keep in mind that the diagnosis *Disturbed Thought Processes* also
can manifest with altered perception and cognition. To differentiate between the two diagnoses,
remember that *Disturbed Sensory Perception* applies when barriers or factors interfere with a
person's ability to interpret stimuli accurately; in contrast, when personality or mental disorders
interfere with this ability, *Disturbed Thought Processes* would be more accurate.

   Disturbed Sensory Perception encompasses six subcategories of diagnosis: *Visual, Auditory,
Kinesthetic, Gustatory, Tactile,* and *Olfactory.* Use of these subcategories can pose some problems
in clinical situations; for example, for a person with a visual deficit, how does the nurse intervene
with a diagnosis such as *Disturbed Sensory Perception: Visual related to effects of glaucoma?*
What would the goals be? The nurse should assess for the client's response to the visual loss and
specifically label the response, not the deficit.

   Disturbed Sensory Perception is more clinically useful without the addition of the sensory
deficit. Examples of responses to sensory deficits may be:

Visual:	*Risk for Injury*
	Self-Care Deficit
Auditory:	*Impaired Communication*
	Social Isolation
Kinesthetic:	*Risk for Injury*
Olfactory:	*Imbalanced Nutrition*
Tactile:	*Risk for Injury*
Gustatory:	*Imbalanced Nutrition*

○○ **ERRORS IN DIAGNOSTIC STATEMENTS**

1. *Disturbed Sensory Perception related to impairment of sensory tracts secondary to spinal
   cord injury*
      A person suffering spinal cord injury experiences several responses related to loss of
   sensation, which can be described and addressed by diagnoses such as *Risk for Injury, Deficient
   Diversional Activity,* and *Disturbed Sensory Perception.* If the nursing focus is to increase
   meaningful sensory input because of loss of sensation, immobility, and position restrictions, the
   (continued)

ⓞⓞ ERRORS IN DIAGNOSTIC STATEMENTS (*Continued*)

nurse should record the diagnosis as *Disturbed Sensory Perception related to decreased visual field when prone and inadequate tactile stimulation.*

2. *Disturbed Sensory Perception: Visual related to altered sensory reception*

   Visual deficits can contribute to various responses, including fear, high risk for injury, self-care deficits, and sensory deprivation. Using *Disturbed Sensory Perception* to rename a visual or hearing deficit fails to clarify a problem that the nurse can treat.

KEY CONCEPTS
Generic Considerations

- "Perception is the process of integrating, classifying, discriminating, and assigning meaning to stimuli. The individual is oriented to surroundings through the ability to receive and organize information. Stimuli are gathered through sensory receptors" (Drury & Akins, 1991, p. 369).
- Any situation or condition that compromises a person's senses or ability to interpret can cause sensory–perceptual alterations.
- "Behavioral characteristics of sensory–perceptual alterations develop suddenly, over 1–2 days of hospitalization, and usually last only hours to several weeks" (Wilson, 1993, p. 751). The number and severity of the behavioral manifestations may vary from mild disorientation to frank psychoses (Wilson, 1993).
- Manifestations of sensory–perceptual alterations may be continuous or have a diurnal pattern. For example, certain behaviors may occur only at night (Wilson, 1993).
- Changes in sensory perception affect a person's ability to interface with the environment.
- All people attempt to control the degree and variety of stimuli to a level that is comfortable for them.
- Clients need to experience change, complexity, and stimulus to:
  - Maintain the functions of attention, concentration, arousal, and consciousness.
  - Maintain internalized order and reality.
  - Promote cognitive activity and socialization.
- Immobility reduces the quality and quantity of available sensory information. In addition, the person has reduced ability to interact with the environment (Porth, 2002).
- Immobility in acute care settings also exposes the person to sensory overload with repetitive and meaningless sounds (eg, intercoms, monitors, hospital personnel; Porth, 2002).
- Sensory overload causes sensory bombardment and also blocks out meaningful stimuli, thus concurrently producing sensory deprivation.
- A disruption in the quality or quantity of incoming stimuli can affect a person's physiologic, emotional, cognitive, and affective domains.
- An illness state may decrease the efficiency of the sensory organs and thus alter a person's capacity for adequate reception and perception of information.

Refer to Key Concepts for *Disturbed Thought Processes* for additional information.

Pediatric Considerations

- The newborn has well-developed sensory abilities that greatly influence growth and development (Wong, 2003):
  - Newborns demonstrate discrimination between patterns, sizes, and shapes, but lack accommodation to distance.
  - Newborns respond to sound stimuli by alerting, crying, and the startle reaction.
  - Newborns differentiate between bitter and sweet tastes.
  - Newborns perceive tactile stimulation, particularly on the face (Wong, 2003).
- Piaget calls the first 2 years of life the sensorimotor period, characterized by integration and organization of information derived through sensorimotor experiences (Wong, 2003).
- Children with sensory–perceptual alterations have the same basic needs as other children. Their experiences must be adapted, however, to promote optimal development.

ⓖ Geriatric Considerations

- Older adults need more time to process visual information when in unfamiliar situations; they also need more light to identify and process the input, and take longer to respond to changes in illumination (Miller, 2004).
- Insufficient time to process auditory and visual input can lead to sensory overload.
- Older adults are more prone to development of sensory deprivation because of loneliness, physical isolation, and increased incidence of chronic disabilities during this life stage.
- There is a fourfold increase in the incidence of sensory–perceptual alteration after 40 years of age, with the highest occurrence among people older than 70 years (Miller, 2004).
- Wilson (1993) reported that the overall incidence of sensory–perceptual alterations in hospitalized older adults varied from 24% to 80%.

Focus Assessment Criteria

Subjective Data
Assess for Defining Characteristics.

History of symptoms
The person reports

Difficulty concentrating	Fatigue or irritability
Anxiety	Unusual sensations

Onset and description

Precipitated by?	Frequency?
Relieved by?	

Assess for Related Factors.

Recent surgery	Recent hospitalization	Neurologic impairment
Sensory organ deficit	Change in biorhythm pattern	Mobility restrictions
Substance abuse (drugs, alcohol)	Social isolation	Medications
		Environmental (noise, lights)

Objective Data
Assess for Related Factors.

Subjective and Objective Data
Assess Risk Level.

Refer to Table II.22.
Because all people in certain environments are at risk for disturbed sensory perception, the tool shown in Table II.23 identifies which people are at high risk. The higher the score, the higher the risk (Wilson, 1993).

For more information on Focus Assessment Criteria, visit http://connection.lww.com.

Goal

NOC	Cognitive Orientation, Distorted Thought Control

The person will demonstrate decreased symptoms of sensory overload, as evidenced by (specify).

Indicators
- Identify and eliminate the potential risk factors, if possible.
- Describe the rationale for the treatment modalities.

General Interventions

NIC	Cognitive Stimulation, Reality Orientation

Identify High-Risk Individuals.
See Focus Assessment Criteria.

TABLE II.22 Disturbed Sensory Perception Risk Assessment Tool

Prehospital Status	Current Status
A. Age greater than 80 Score A. ☐ ☐ No = 0 ☐ Yes = 1	A. Admission priority Score A. ☐ ☐ 1 = elective ☐ 2 = emergent or urgent
B. Gender Score B. ☐ ☐ 0 = female ☐ 1 = male	B. Predisposition Score B. ☐ ☐ 0 = home ☐ 1 = institutional setting
C. Documented history of cognitive impairment ☐ 0 = no impairment Score C. ☐ ☐ 1 = impaired	C. Cognitive status rating Score C. ☐ ☐ 0 = SPMSQ* score 0–2 or intact cognitive func- tion per assessment
D. Auditory function Score D. ☐ ☐ 0 = no impairment ☐ 1 = using corrective aid or assist device ☐ 3 = not using corrective aid or assist device Acute change—auditory ☐ No = 0 ☐ Yes = 1	☐ 1 = SPMSQ score 3–10 or impaired cognitive function per assessment SPMSQ score ☐
E. Vision Score E. ☐ ☐ 0 = no impairment ☐ 1 = using corrective aid or assist device ☐ 3 = not using corrective aid or assist device Acute change—vision ☐ No = 0 ☐ Yes = 1	D. Chemical agent variations Score D. ☐ 1. # chemicals before hospitalization (BH) ☐ 2. # of chemicals BH that are current ☐ 3. Difference 1 and 2 ☐ 4. # new chemicals since admission ☐ 5. Receiving narcotics ☐ No = 0 ☐ Yes = 1 ☐
F. Verbal ability Score F. ☐ ☐ 0 = no impairment ☐ 1 = using corrective aid or assist device ☐ 3 = not using corrective aid or assist device Acute change—verbal ☐ No = 0 ☐ Yes = 1	6. Receiving neuroleptics ☐ No = 0 ☐ Yes = 1 ☐ E. Blood chemistry Score E. ☐ ☐ 0 = within normal limits ☐ 1 = lab values out of normal range
G. Self-care ability Score G. ☐ ☐ 0 = independent ☐ 1 = requires assistance of another person Acute change—self-care ☐ No = 0 ☐ Yes = 1	F. Symptomatic infection Score F. ☐ ☐ No = 0 ☐ Yes = 1 G. Pain Score G. ☐ ☐ 0 = no pain ☐ 1 = controlled pain (rated 1–3 on scale of 0–10) ☐ 2 = uncontrolled pain (rated 4 or greater on scale of 0–10)
H. Mobility Score H. ☐ ☐ 0 = independent ☐ 1 = requires assist device ☐ 2 = requires human assistance Acute change—mobility ☐ No = 0 ☐ Yes = 1	H. Visitation by significant others Score H. ☐ ☐ 0 = continuous presence ☐ 1 = significant others visit 2–3 times a day ☐ 2 = Less than two visits per day
I. Fracture on admission Score I. ☐ ☐ No = 0 ☐ Yes = 1	I. Room type Score I. ☐ ☐ 0 = Window with view to outdoors and exposure to light changes
J. Elimination pattern Score J. ☐ ☐ 0 = normal or independent ☐ 1 = uncontrolled, incontinent, dependent Acute change—elimination pattern ☐ No = 0 ☐ Yes = 1	☐ 1 = Window with view into unit or outdoors walls or buildings ☐ 2 = No windows

Add the Prehospitalization and Current Status risk factor scores. Grand total risk score ☐

*SPMSQ = Short Portable Mental Status Questionnaire.

Lisa D. Brodersen, Copyright 1993 Revised 2/1/95. Used with author's permission. Cardio MAC Iowa Health Institute, Des Moines, IA.

Reduce or Eliminate Causative and Contributing Factors, When Possible.

Excessive Noise or Light

Cover nonessential blinking lights at bedside with tape.

Dim lights at night.

Encourage use of blindfolds.

Decrease noise output.

> Shut off nonessential alarms.
>
> Encourage use of earplugs.
>
> If possible, limit the use of flasher and similar equipment during sleep hours.
>
> Turn off unnecessary equipment.
>
> Position person away from direct source of noise, if possible.
>
> Curtail nonessential personnel conversation.
>
> Avoid loud noises.
>
> Discourage television after 10 PM.

Share with person the source of the noise.

Discuss the use of a radio with earplugs to provide soft, relaxing music.

Share with personnel the need to reduce noise and provide clients with uninterrupted sleep of at least 2 to 4 h duration.

Discuss the advantages of turning hearing aid off during high noise times.

Unfamiliar Environment

Attempt to reduce fears and concerns by explaining equipment, its purpose, and noises.

Encourage person to share his or her perceptions of noises.

Enlist the aid of an interpreter to explain the environment to person who does not speak English.

Promote Reorientation.

Orient Client to All Three Spheres (Person, Place, Time).

Address person by name.

Introduce yourself frequently.

Identify the place.

Identify the time.

> "Good morning, Mr. Jones. I am Mary Smith. I will be your nurse today."
> "Where are you, Mr. Jones? You are in the hospital."
> "Today is May sixth and it is eight-thirty in the morning."

Explain All Activities.

Offer simple explanations of each task.

Provide subjective and objective descriptions of sensations that will be experienced.

Allow person to handle equipment related to the task.

Allow client to participate in task, such as washing his or her face.

Acknowledge when you leave and when you will return.

Promote Movement.

Encourage client to remain out of bed as much as possible (eat meals in chair).

Teach client to perform isometric and isotonic exercises when in bed.

Encourage client to change position frequently, even if it is just lifting one side off a surface by rolling slightly.

To encourage walking, choose a destination to reach or give the walk a purpose (walking to the lounge for breakfast).

Use Measures to Prevent Injury.

Keep siderails in place and bed in lowest position.

Place call bell in convenient location.

Refer to *Risk for Injury* for additional interventions.

Assist Client to Differentiate Reality From Fantasy.

Refer to *Disturbed Thought Processes* for additional interventions.

Rationales

- Promoting regular and varied sensory stimulation can help prevent alterations from prolonged sensory deprivation.
- "Care givers should be aware that their actions and activity patterns may add to the environmental chaos or become a positive contribution to the therapeutic milieu" (Drury & Akins, 1991, p. 379).
- Immobility or confinement reduces the quality and quantity of sensory input.
- Explaining what sensory stimuli the person will experience before the experience reduces distress, tension, and confusion.
- Wearing hearing aids in an excessively noisy environment (eg, clinic, intensive care unit) also can cause sensory overload.

Ineffective Sexuality Patterns
 Related to Prenatal and Postpartum Changes
 Related to Fear of Pregnancy and/or Sexually Transmitted Diseases (STDs), Risk for
Sexual Dysfunction

INEFFECTIVE SEXUALITY PATTERNS

DEFINITION

Ineffective Sexuality Patterns: State in which a person experiences or is at risk of experiencing a change in sexual behaviors or sexual health

DEFINING CHARACTERISTICS
Major (Must Be Present)

Actual or anticipated negative changes in sexual behaviors, sexual health, sexual functioning, or sexual identity

Minor (May Be Present)

Expression of concern about sexual behaviors, health, functioning, or sexual identity
Expression of concern about impact a medical diagnosis or treatment for a medical condition may
  have on sexual functioning or sexual desirability
Inappropriate sexual verbal or nonverbal behavior
Changes in primary and/or secondary sexual characteristics

RELATED FACTORS

Ineffective sexual patterns can occur as a response to various health problems, situations, and conflicts. Some common sources are listed next.

Pathophysiologic
Related to biochemical effects on energy, libido secondary to:
Endocrine
  Diabetes mellitus   Hyperthyroidism
  Addison's disease   Decreased hormone production
  Myxedema   Acromegaly
Genitourinary
  Chronic renal failure
Neuromuscular and skeletal
  Arthritis
  Amyotrophic lateral sclerosis
  Multiple sclerosis
  Disturbances of nerve supply to brain, spinal cord, sensory nerves, or autonomic nerves
Cardiorespiratory
  Peripheral vascular   Cancer
    disorders   Myocardial infarction
  Congestive heart failure   Chronic respiratory disorders

Related to fears associated with (sexually transmitted diseases [STDs]) (specify)
Human immunodeficiency virus (HIV)/Acquired immunodeficiency syndrome (AIDS)
Human papilloma virus   Herpes   Gonorrhea
Chlamydia   Syphilis

Related to effects of alcohol on performance
Related to decreased vaginal lubrication secondary to (specify)
Related to fear of premature ejaculation
Related to pain during intercourse

Treatment-Related

Related to effects of:
Medications (Table II.23)
Radiation therapy

Related to altered self-concept from change in appearance (trauma, radical surgery)

Situational (Personal, Environmental)

Related to partner problem (specify)

Unwilling	Not available	Uninformed
Abusive	Separated, divorced	

Related to no privacy
Related to stressors secondary to:

Job problems	Value conflicts	Financial worries
Relationship conflicts		

TABLE II.23 Drugs That Impair Sexuality

Drug	Effect on Sexuality
Alcohol	In small amounts, may increase libido and decrease sexual inhibitions In large amounts, impairs neural reflexes involved in erection and ejaculation Chronic use causes impotence and sterility in men; decreased desire and orgasmic dysfunction in women
Amyl nitrate	Peripheral vasodilator reputed to cause intensified orgasms when inhaled at time of orgasm May cause loss of erection, hypotension, and syncope
Antidepressants	Peripheral blockage of nervous innervation to sex organs Significant percentage of impotence and ejaculatory dysfunction in men Decreased libido in both genders
Antihistamines	Block parasympathetic innervation of sex organs Sedative effect may decrease desire Decrease in vaginal lubrication
Antihypertensives	Libido may be decreased in both genders Some cause impotence and ejaculatory problems in up to 50% of men See specific class of medications.
Antispasmodics	Inhibit parasympathetic innervation of sex organs May cause impotence
Chemotherapeutics	Combination therapy may cause azoospermia or oligospermia in men and temporary or permanent menopause in women; fertility may be temporarily or permanently altered; libido may be decreased and body image altered.
Cocaine	Short-term use is reported to enhance sexual experience. Chronic use causes loss of desire and sexual dysfunction in both sexes.
Hormones	Estrogen suppresses sexual function in men. Testosterone may increase libido in both sexes but causes virilization in women. Chronic use of anabolic steroids causes testicular atrophy, decreased testosterone and decreased sperm production; may cause permanent sterility.
Marijuana	May decrease sexual inhibitions Chronic use may cause decreased libido and impotence.
Narcotics	Chronic use causes decreased libido in both sexes. Testosterone levels and amount of semen decreased Erectile and ejaculatory dysfunction common
Oral contraceptives	Remove fear of pregnancy May cause decreased libido
Sedatives/tranquilizers	Initially and in low doses may enhance sexual pleasure due to relaxation and decrease of inhibitions Long-term use decreases libido and may cause orgasmic dysfunction and impotence.
Diuretics	May cause erectile, ejaculatory, and libido problems, especially at higher doses
Anxiolytics	Altered libido in both genders; erectile problems and delayed ejaculation in men
Sildenafil citrate (Viagra)	Enhances erectile ability in men with impaired potency

Related to misinformation or lack of knowledge
Related to fatigue
Related to fear of rejection secondary to obesity
Related to pain
Related to fear of sexual failure
Related to fear of pregnancy
Related to depression
Related to anxiety
Related to guilt
Related to history of unsatisfactory sexual experiences

Maturational
Adolescent
Related to ineffective role models
Related to negative sexual teaching
Related to absence of sexual teaching

Adult
Related to adjustment to parenthood
Related to effects of menopause on libido
Related to values conflict
Related to effects of pregnancy on energy levels and body image
Related to effects of aging on energy levels and body image

⊗ AUTHOR'S NOTE

The diagnoses *Ineffective Sexuality Patterns* and *Sexual Dysfunction* are difficult to differentiate. *Ineffective Sexuality Patterns* represents a broad diagnosis, of which sexual dysfunction can be one part. *Sexual Dysfunction* may be used most appropriately by a nurse with advanced preparation in sex therapy. Until *Sexual Dysfunction* is well differentiated from *Ineffective Sexuality Patterns,* most nurses should not use it.

⊗ ERRORS IN DIAGNOSTIC STATEMENTS

1. *Ineffective Sexuality Patterns related to reports of absent libido*
   Report of absent libido represents a symptom of *Ineffective Sexuality Patterns*, not a "related to" statement. If further assessment revealed the person's dissatisfaction with present sexual patterns, the nurse could record the diagnosis *Ineffective Sexuality Patterns related to unknown etiology,* as evidenced by reports of absent libido. The use of "unknown etiology" in this diagnostic statement prompts focus assessments to determine contributing factors (eg, stress, medication side effects).
2. *Sexual Dysfunction related to impotence secondary to spinal cord injury*
   How would the nurse treat this diagnosis? A nurse planning to explore feelings and to provide information and referrals would not be treating sexual dysfunction. Instead, the nursing focus would be best described in the diagnosis *Anxiety related to effects of spinal cord injury on sexual function and insufficient knowledge of causes and community resources available.*

KEY CONCEPTS
Generic Considerations
- Sexual health is the integration of somatic, emotional, intellectual, and social aspects of a sexual being in ways that are enriching and that enhance personality, communication, and love.
- Sexual behaviors are the behaviors a person uses to communicate feelings and attitudes about sexuality. They include behaviors used in release of sexual tension, either alone or with another person to attain sexual satisfaction, or for procreation (Wilmoth, 1993).
- All people are sexual beings. Sexuality is an integral part of identity.

- Sexuality encompasses how a person feels about himself or herself and how a person interacts with others.
- Sexual function refers to psychological and physiologic ability to perform in a sexually satisfying manner, with or without a partner, old or young.
- Age, marital and/or relationship status, sexual orientation, personal value system, sexual knowledge, resources (social, economic, geographic), culture, physical health, and emotional health influence sexuality and sexual function (Katzun, 1990; Smith, 1993).
- Research shows that many people with a serious illness experience decreased sexual desire, decreased frequency of sexual activity, and/or decreased satisfaction with sexual function.
- The characteristics of a sexually healthy person are as follows (Reeder et al., 1997):
  - Positive body image despite the body's packaging
  - Acceptance of sexual and body functions as normal and natural
  - Accurate knowledge about human sexuality and sexual functioning
  - Recognition and acceptance of own sexual feelings
  - Capacity for intimacy in relationships
  - Acceptance of mistakes/imperfections in self and others
  - Prevention of pregnancy when it is not desired
  - Protection of self from STDs
- Sexual expression is not limited to sexual intercourse; it includes closeness and touch, as well as other forms of verbal and nonverbal communication.

Medications and Sexuality
- Drugs can influence sexual functioning positively and negatively (see Table II.24).
- The person has the right to be educated about all medication side effects, including those affecting sexuality.

The Nurse's Role in Discussing Sexuality
- The nurse must become educated regarding sexuality and sexual health through the life span. It is important for the nurse to examine his or her own beliefs and feelings concerning sexuality, sexual function, and what is considered sexually normal and abnormal.
- Many nurses have difficulty providing care in the area of sexuality and do not address sexual concerns unless the client asks specific questions. Research indicates, however, that many clients wish nurses and other health care professionals would initiate discussion of sexuality.
- The PLISSIT model (Annon, 1976) is helpful for the nurse generalist providing care in the area of sexuality:
  - **Permission:** Convey to person and significant others a willingness to discuss sexual thoughts and feelings (eg, "Some people with your diagnosis have concerns about how it will affect sexual functioning. Is this a concern for you or your partner?").
  - **Limited Information:** Provide the person and significant other with information on the effects certain situations (eg, pregnancy), conditions (eg, cancer), and treatments (eg, medications) can have on sexuality and sexual function.
  - **Specific Suggestions:** Provide specific instructions that can facilitate positive sexual functioning (eg, changes in coital positions).
  - **Intensive Therapy:** Refer people who need more help to an appropriate health care professional (eg, sex therapist, surgeon).
- Giving a person "permission" to discuss sexual concerns is by far the most important aspect of nursing care in the area of sexuality. The nurse should give permission by:
  - Including sexuality in the initial health history and addressing questions on sexuality in a manner similar to questions on bowel and bladder function. This helps the person see that nurses view sexuality as a routine part of human health.
  - Offering to discuss sexual concerns at appropriate times during the client's hospitalization/visit (Wilmoth, 1994a).
- The nurse should assure the person of the confidentiality of all data on sexuality and obtain permission from the person before making a referral for a sexual problem.

Contraception and STDs
- Research has shown that use of mechanical barrier methods (condom, diaphragm, vaginal sponge, cervical cap) and/or chemical barriers containing nonoxynol-9 (foam, jelly, cream) are effective in reducing the transmission of HIV and other STDs.
- Use of the intrauterine device, oral contraceptives, Norplant, Depo-Provera, or sterilization provides *no* protection from STDs. Clients using these methods must be counseled to use a chemical or mechanical barrier method to protect them from disease.

Pediatric Considerations

- Sex role identification begins in infancy and is determined by adolescence.
  - Infants can identify body parts by the end of the first year.
  - Toddlers learn gender differentiation.
  - Preschoolers frequently engage in masturbation and sex play with peers (eg, comparing genitals).
  - School-aged children continue to gain awareness about their sex role identity. Although masturbation and sex play are common in the young school-aged child, the older school-aged child becomes involved in purposeful sexual behavior (eg, hugging, kissing members of opposite sex; Wong, 2003).
  - Adolescents experience altered body image in response to the physical changes of puberty. The key developmental task of adolescence is identity formation, which is influenced by sexual maturation and assuming a sex role (Wong, 1999).
- Parents are the primary force in sex education in a child's life. This includes what is not said as well as what is said.
- Formal sex education, presented from a life span approach, is best offered during middle childhood. Topics should include sexual maturation and the process of reproduction (Wong, 1999).
- STDs continue to be a major cause of morbidity among adolescents and young adults. The highest rates of chlamydial infections in females occur in adolescents (Division of STD Prevention, 1997).
- Risky behavior by adolescents and young adults increases their vulnerability to STDs, pelvic inflammatory disease, infertility, AIDS, and chronic incurable conditions such as hepatitis B or C virus infection, human papilloma virus (HPV) infection, and genital herpes.
- Half of ninth through twelfth graders report having sexual intercourse (CDC, 2000).
- About 16% of high school students report having four or more sexual partners (CDC, 2000).
- Only 58% of high school students reported using a condom. Only 16% reported using birth control (CDC, 2000).

Maternal Considerations

- Pregnant women have varying degrees of sexual desire during pregnancy.
  - Some women are very sexually excitable.
  - Some women are not very desirous of sex.
  - Libido changes by large degrees during different stages of pregnancy.
  - A woman's body image affects her sexuality. (If thinness is an attribute, then many pregnant women are confused about changing size.)
  - A woman's attitude toward her body can influence her partner's sexual attraction toward her.
- The postpartum period is a time of self-doubt. For the first 6 weeks, a new mother feels lost, overwhelmed, tired, depressed, ignorant, and isolated. Her self-esteem as well as her sexuality may suffer.
- Polomeno (1999) found the postnatal sexual concerns of men and women to be (M, men; W, women):
  - Having time for each other (M, W)
  - Sexual intercourse the first time (M, W)
  - Separating oneself from baby (W)
  - Contraception (M, W)
  - Reactivating the passion, fun, romance (M, W)
  - To be desired (W)
  - Fatigue and its impact on sexual desire (W)
  - Postpartum depression (M)
  - Balancing intimacy and baby (W)
  - Time required for healing (W)
  - Fear of pain (M, W)
- His perception of her and her body (W)

Geriatric Considerations

- Older adults are psychologically and physically capable of engaging in sexual activity regardless of age-related changes in sexual anatomy and physiology.
- Sexual activity is often beneficial for older adults, reducing anxiety while providing intimacy and improving quality of life.
- Women experience decreased breast tone, thinning and loss of elasticity of the vaginal wall, decreased vaginal lubrication, and shortening of vaginal length from loss of circulating estrogen (Miller, 2004).
- Men experience decreased production of spermatozoa, decreased ejaculatory force, and smaller, less firm testicles. Direct stimulation may be required to achieve an erection; however, the erection may be maintained for a longer time (Miller, 2004).
- The need for intimacy and touch is especially important for older adults, who may be experiencing diminishing meaningful relationships.
- Past sexual function (enjoyment, interest, frequency) serves as a predictor of sexual activity in older adults. To be capable of sexual activity in old age, the person must participate in sexual activity throughout life.
- Adult children and caregivers commonly view sexual activities of older adults as immoral, inappropriate, and negative (Miller, 2004).
- The sexual functioning of older adults is most influenced by myths and misunderstanding. According to Miller (2004), because sex is so closely identified with youthfulness, the stereotype of "sexless seniors" is widely believed.

Transcultural Considerations

- People of some cultures (eg, Hispanic, Native American) are very hesitant to discuss sexuality.
- Horn (1993) reports that black women view child-bearing as a validation of their femaleness. White teenage girls approve of prevention of pregnancy; Indian teenage girls value pregnancy (Horn, 1993).
- Some cultures view the postpartum period as a state of impurity. Certain foods and practices are taboo (eg, intercourse). The woman may be secluded during postpartum bleeding. Some cultures end seclusion with a ritual bath (eg, Navajo, Hispanic, Orthodox Jewish; Andrews & Boyle, 2004).
- Native American women believe in the importance of monthly menstruation to maintain physical well-being and harmony (Andrews & Boyle, 2003).

Focus Assessment Criteria

Guidelines for Taking a Sexual History

Discuss sexuality in a private, relaxed setting to ensure confidentiality.

Do not judge the person by your own beliefs/practices.

Permit the person to refuse to answer.

Clarify vocabulary; use slang terms if needed to convey meaning.

Assess only those areas pertinent for this client at this time.

Strive to be open, warm, objective, unembarrassed, and reassuring.

Keep in mind that it is more appropriate to assume that the client has had some sexual experience than to assume none.

Several sessions may be necessary to complete the interview.

Subjective Data

Determine History:

Age, sex, marital/relationship status	Medications
	Communication patterns with significant others
Sexual orientation/preference	Quality of relationship with significant other

Number of children and siblings	Religious and cultural background
Sexual abuse	Job and financial status
Depression	Medical and surgical history
	Drug and alcohol use (present and past)

Assess Concerns and Sexuality Patterns.

How has your (health problem) affected your ability to function as a (wife/mother/partner/father/ husband; Wilmoth, 1994a)?

How has your (health problem) affected the way you feel about yourself as a (man/woman; Wilmoth, 1994a)?

How has your (health problem) affected your ability to function sexually (Wilmoth, 1994a)?

Sexual function

Usual pattern

Present pattern

Satisfaction (individual, partner)

Desire (individual, partner)

Erection problems for man (attaining, sustaining)

Ejaculation problems for man (premature, retarded, retrograde)

Decreased lubrication in woman

Decreased orgasm in woman

Sexual problem

Description

Onset (when, gradual/sudden)

Pattern over time (increased, decreased, unchanged)

Person's concept of cause

Knowledge of problem by others (partner, physician, others)

Expectations

School-aged child

Knowledge

"What is the difference between boys and girls?"

"What do you know about having babies?"

"Who taught you? At what age?"

Body changes

"Is your body changing in any way? How? Why?"

"How do you feel about these changes?"

Masturbation

"Almost everyone touches their body; how do you feel about this?"

Adolescent

Knowledge and attitudes

"What are your parents' attitudes toward sex, nudity, and touching?"

"How are subjects discussed in your home?"

"How does pregnancy occur?"

"What are some methods of birth control?"

"What do you know about sexually transmitted diseases?"

Body changes

"Is your body changing in any way? How? Why?"

"How do you feel about these changes?"

Sexual activity

"Some young people are sexually active and others choose not to be sexually active; what are your beliefs about this?"

"Are you sexually active? If so, describe the type of birth control and safe sex practices you use."

"Some teens are attracted to people of their gender; have you experienced these feelings?" (Smith, 1993)

Senior citizens

Knowledge

"How do you feel when you hear that older adults have little interest in sexuality?"

"What do you know about sexually transmitted diseases?"

Body changes

"How do you feel about the way your body has aged?"

"What do you do to make yourself feel good about yourself sexually?"

Sexual activity
"Do you feel loved, valued by others?"
"How are your needs for touching and intimacy met?"
"Have you been able to maintain your sexual activity?"

Assess for Related Factors.

See Related Factors.

For more information on Focus Assessment Criteria, visit http://connection.lww.com.

Goals

NOC	Body Image, Self-Esteem, Role Performance, Sexual Identity: Acceptance

The person will resume previous sexual
activity or engage in alternative satisfying sexual activity.

Indicators

- Identify effects of stressors, loss, or change on sexual functioning.
- Modify behavior to reduce stressors.
- Identify limitations on sexual activity caused by health problem.
- Identify appropriate modifications in sexual practices in response to these limitations.
- Report satisfying sexual activity.

General Interventions

NIC	Behavioral Management: Sexual, Counseling, Sexual Counseling, Emotional Support, Active Listening, Teaching: Sexuality

**Assess for Causative or
Contributing Factors (see Related Factors).**

Explore the Client's Patterns of Sexual Functioning.

Encourage him or her to share concerns; assume that all clients have had some sexual experience, and convey a willingness to discuss feelings and concerns.

**Discuss the Relationship Between Sexual Functioning and
Life Stressors.**

Clarify relation between stressors and problem in sexual functioning.
Explore options available for reducing the effects of the stressor on sexual functioning (eg, increase sleep, increase exercise, modify diet, explore stress reduction methods).

Reaffirm the Need for Frank Discussion Between Sexual Partners.

Explain how the client and partner can use role playing to discuss concerns about sex.
Reaffirm the need for closeness and expressions of caring through touching, massage, and other means.
Suggest that sexual activity need not always culminate in vaginal intercourse, but that the partner can reach orgasm through noncoital manual or oral stimulation.

With Acute or Chronic Illness:

**Eliminate or Reduce Causative or Contributing Factors, if Possible. Teach the Importance of
Adhering to Medical Regimen Designed to Reduce or Control Disease Symptoms.**

Provide Limited Information and Specific Suggestions.

Provide appropriate information to client and partner concerning actual limitations on sexual functioning caused by the illness (limited information).
Teach possible modifications in sexual practices to assist in dealing with limitations caused by illness (specific suggestions).

See Table II.24 for more details.

**Provide Opportunities for the Person to Discuss the Effects of Limited Activity Tolerance
on Sexuality.**

Promote an atmosphere of openness, understanding, and acceptance.
Some people with chronic obstructive pulmonary disease fear that sexual activity will increase dyspnea and, therefore, avoid sex. Others simply give up before or during sexual activity because of

TABLE II.24 Disorders That Alter Sexuality

Health Problem	Sexual Complication	Nursing Intervention
Diabetes mellitus	*Men:* Erectile difficulties due to diabetic neuropathies or microangiopathy *Women:* Decreased desire; decreased vaginal lubrication	LI: Encourage proper metabolic control. SS: Eventually may require penile implant; refer to urologist. LI: Encourage proper metabolic control; teach signs and symptoms of vaginitis. SS: Suggest use of water-soluble lubricating jelly.
Chronic obstructive pulmonary disease	Activity intolerance due to exertional dyspnea; coughing and expectoration Anxiety	LI: Teach controlled breathing; plan intercourse for time of peak effect from medications; avoid sex after large meal or physical exertion, or immediately after awakening; plan for nonhurried, relaxed, low-stress encounters, for losses. SS: Suggest positions that minimize chest pressure (sitting or side-lying); explain that waterbeds also help decrease exertion during sex.
Arthritis	 Pain, joint stiffness, fatigue Decreased libido from steroid medications	LI: Explain that arthritis has no effect on physiologic aspects of sexual functioning. SS: Suggest that the couple plan intercourse for time of peak medication effects; promote joint relaxation by taking warm bath/shower alone/with partner; perform mild range-of-motion exercises. LI: Teach that decreased desire is a common side effect of medication.
Transurethral resection of the prostate (TURP) to treat benign prostatic hypertrophy	Retrograde ejaculation due to damage to internal bladder sphincter	LI: Explain that erection and orgasm will still occur, but ejaculate will be decreased or absent; urine will be cloudy.
Cardiovascular disease	Anxiety, fear of performance, fear of chest pain, death, decreased desire, decreased arousal, decision of partner to stop sexual activity	LI: Explain that infarction has no direct effect on physiologic sexual functioning; activity usually is safe 5–8 weeks postinfarction, based on Index of Sexual Readiness (ability to take brisk walk, climb two flights of stairs without chest pain). Teach to avoid sexual activity after large meal, drinking alcohol, or in room with extremes in temperature. Point out that some medications may cause sexual dysfunction (see Table II.24). SS: Encourage nonsexual touching; suggest positions that conserve energy (side-to-side lying, supine lying position, or sitting in chair with partner on top); explore option of masturbation; assure that oral–genital sex does not place additional strain on heart. Warn to avoid anal sex, because anal penetration stimulates vagus nerve and decreases cardiac function.
Chronic renal failure (CRF)	Chronic/recurrent uremia can produce state of depression, decreased sexual desire and arousal Untreated CRF causes cessation of ovulation and menses in women and causes atrophy of testicles, decreased spermatogenesis, decreased plasma testosterone, and erectile dysfunction in men. Dialysis may restore ovulation and menses in women and return testosterone levels to normal in men; sexual desire may return to predisease levels with treatment.	LI: Acknowledge that stress of disease and dialysis may cause decreased desire; encourage nonsexual touching without pressure to perform. Reassure that these problems are usually reversible with dialysis. Warn that birth control should be continued because fertility may return. Explain that sexual dysfunction may be a product of emotional stress and the physiologic components of the disease. SS: Explain that measurement of nocturnal penile tumescence can distinguish between organic and psychological causes of sexual dysfunction in men.
Total abdominal hysterectomy with bilateral salpingo-oophorectomy	Loss of circulating estrogen	LI: Teach signs and symptoms of menopause, use of water-soluble vaginal lubricants. Encourage discussion with physician about estrogen replacement creams. Explain that in most cases intercourse may be resumed after 6-week post-operative visit.

(table continues on p. 710)

TABLE II.24 Disorders That Alter Sexuality (Continued)

Health Problem	Sexual Complication	Nursing Intervention
	Postoperative psychological adjustment or change in sexual identity, grieving, loss of reproductive capacity	Explore the meaning of uterine and ovarian loss to the woman. Assure her that the surgery will not change her ability to respond and function sexually.
Enterostomal surgery		
Anterior–posterior resection	*Women:* Loss of uterus and ovaries; shortening of vagina	LI: See above. SS: Suggest coital positions that decrease depth of penetration (eg, side-to-side lying, man on top with legs outside the woman's, woman on top).
	Men: Erectile dysfunction, decrease in amount/force of ejaculate or retrograde ejaculation due to interruption of sympathetic and parasympathetic nerve supply **Note:** Amount of rectal tissue removed appears to determine degree of dysfunction	LI: Explain that erectile dysfunction may be temporary or permanent. Encourage use of touch and other noncoital means of sexual communication.
Colostomy/ileostomy	Alteration in sexual self-concept, body image	LI: Allow person to express feelings about change in body appearance; encourage communication with partner.
	Decrease in desire, arousal, and orgasm	LI: Teach that fatigue and decreased desire are common after surgery. Discuss ways to increase sexual attractiveness; suggest wearing sexy lingerie or other clothing to hide appliance.
	Anxiety over spillage, odor	Teach to empty bag before sexual activity; encourage to maintain a sense of humor, because accidents will sometimes occur.
	Erectile dysfunction in men (varies with age and type of surgery)	Encourage alternative ways to express sexuality if intercourse is not possible.
Spinal cord injury	Sexual disability depends on level and type of cord injury: after injury, separation of genital sexual functioning and cerebral eroticism	LI: Discuss sexual options available depending on extent of injury (eg, a waterbed to amplify pelvic movements). Encourage continued use of contraceptives, as appropriate.
	Men with complete upper motor neuron injury may not be able to ejaculate.	SS: Discuss alternate positions (eg, partner on top). Encourage experimentation with vibrators, massage, and other means of sexual expression. May be a candidate for a penile implant. May have urinary tract infection. Refer to a urologist.

Note: Much information is available on the sexual implications of spinal cord injury. The reader is referred to available literature on this subject.

Cancer	Sexual implications depend on site of disease and treatment. May feel guilty about desiring touch, need for sexual activity	LI: Encourage expression of anxiety and fear; encourage grieving for losses. Assure that sexual expression, even when one has cancer, is natural, and that need for intimacy often increases during this time.
	Changes in role function and sexually defined gender roles	Encourage discussion between partners about this; encourage negotiation about role changes, which may be temporary.
	Fear of being contagious	Assure person and partner that the disease cannot be transmitted through sexual activity.
	Change in body image	Discuss purchase of wig, false eyelashes before hair loss; suggest sexy lingerie, other ways to pamper oneself to increase feelings of sexual desirability and attractiveness.
	Fatigue	Explain that severe fatigue may hinder sexual desire and that fatigue does not indicate rejection of partner. Encourage verbal and nonverbal communication between person and partner.

(table continues on p. 711)

TABLE II.24 Disorders That Alter Sexuality (Continued)

Health Problem	Sexual Complication	Nursing Intervention
Chemotherapy	*Alkylating agents, antimetabolites, and antitumor antibiotics:* Amenorrhea, oligospermia, azoospermia, decreased desire, ovarian dysfunction, erectile dysfunction *Vinca alkaloids:* Retrograde ejaculation, erectile dysfunction, decreased desire, ovarian dysfunction, temporary decrease in sexual desire/arousal	LI: Encourage discussion about changes in body appearance/function. Explore option of sperm banking. Urge to continue use of contraceptives. False-positive Pap smear possible. Encourage nonsexual touching; rest; avoidance of alcoholic beverages, narcotics, and sedatives before sexual activity; use of water-soluble lubricants to decrease vaginal irritation; avoidance of oral and anal sex during periods of neutropenia.
	Genetic teratogenicity and mutagenicity	Encourage the couple to seek genetic counseling before conception.
Radiation therapy	Most side effects are site-dependent; however, side effects such as fatigue, neutropenia, anorexia generally are present in all people.	LI: Teach to plan sexual activity after rest periods and to use positions that require less exertion for the patient. Encourage nonsexual touching and communication. Teach that patient is not radioactive during external treatment. Teach site-specific side effects and impact on sexual functioning.

LI = limited information; SS = specific suggestion.

shortness of breath and associated frustration. Providing some common-sense information may be all that is needed for people to resume satisfying sexual relations.

Explain that attempting lovemaking while fatigued, during a chest infection, after a large meal, or after drinking large amounts of alcohol increases the likelihood of failure.

Suggest that planned lovemaking during midday or early evening, when energy levels are highest, may be more satisfying than late-night relations when the person is already fatigued.

Facilitate Adaptation to Change in or Loss of Body Part.

Assess the stage of adaptation of the person and partner to the loss (denial, depression, anger, resolution; see *Grieving*).

Encourage adherence to the medical regimen to promote maximum recovery.

Encourage the couple to discuss the strengths of their relationship and to assess the influence of the loss on these strengths.

Clarify the relationship between loss or change and the problem in sexual functioning.

Teach Possible Modifications in Sexual Practices to Assist in Dealing with Limitations Caused by Illness (specific suggestions).

Modifications in positions
Use of pillows for comfort and/or balance
Techniques to control drainage or odor
Use of attractive lingerie to cover affected part

Provide Referrals as Indicated.

Enterostomal therapist   Physician
Nurse specialist   Sex therapist

Rationales

- Many clients are reluctant to discuss sexuality issues. The proper approach can encourage the client to share feelings and concerns.
- Explaining that impaired sexual functioning has a physiologic basis can reduce feelings of inadequacy and decreased self-esteem; this actually may help improve sexual function.
- Role playing helps a person gain insight by placing himself or herself in another's position, and allows more spontaneous sharing of fears and concerns.

- Both partners probably have concerns about sexual activity. Repressing these feelings hurts the relationship.
- Sexual pleasure and gratification are not limited to intercourse. Other expressions of caring may prove more meaningful.
- Sexual gratification is an individual matter. It is not limited to intercourse but includes closeness, touching, and giving pleasure to others, as well as self-pleasuring.
- Providing accurate information on the effect of cord injury on sexual functioning can prevent false hope or give real hope, as appropriate.
- Certain sexual problems necessitate continuing therapy and the advanced knowledge of specialists.

INEFFECTIVE SEXUALITY PATTERNS

RELATED TO PRENATAL AND POSTPARTUM CHANGES

Goal

NOC Self-Esteem, Body Image, Role Performance

The person will express increased satisfaction with sexual patterns.

Indicators
- Identify factors that can hinder sexuality.
- Share concerns.

Interventions

NIC Sexual Counseling, Anticipatory Guidance, Teaching: Sexuality, Body Image Enhancement, Support System Enhancement

Assess Sexual Patterns During and After Pregnancy (Reeder et al., 1997).

Prenatal
Has the pregnancy made many changes in your life and sexual relationship?
Are there any concerns or worries about your sexual relationship during pregnancy or afterward?
What has your physician said about sex during pregnancy?
How does the pregnancy make you feel? (Ask both partners.)
How do you feel about changes in appearance?
How do you feel about changes in emotions?
How do you feel about one another's experience of the pregnancy?
What are your feelings about sex during pregnancy? Cultural influences?
What have you heard about what you should or should not do sexually during pregnancy?
Have you experienced any physical difficulties with intercourse during pregnancy?
How do you think having a baby will change your life? How do you plan to manage these changes?
How do you feel physically?
What medications do you take?
Have you had any recent changes in your health?

Postpartum
Are you still bleeding?
Have you resumed sexual activity?
Are you concerned about conceiving again?
Has breast-feeding altered your sexual relationship?
How has having a baby affected your sexuality?

Is your episiotomy healed and comfortable during intercourse?
Have you experienced a lack of lubrication since delivery?
Do you ever have time alone with your partner?

Assess Contributing Factors.

Body changes
Change in sex drive
Fatigue
Emotional lability
   Anxieties about taking on parental responsibilities
   Grief about separating from childhood
   Anxiety about outcome of pregnancy
   Ambivalence about having a baby
   Guilt about desiring sex when pregnancy has been achieved (religious, social pressure)
   Fear of dependency
   Fear of loss of current status (career, freedom)
   Self-doubt
Fear of damaging fetus
Dyspareunia in pregnancy
Dyspareunia in postpartum
Guilt because of baby
   Afraid to let go and enjoy sex lest something happen to baby
   Woman may feel envious of all the care the infant receives. She may feel more infantile herself and
      less like a sexual woman.
Influence of others
   Relatives (mother, in-laws)
      Attitudes related to pregnancy and child care
      Cultural attitudes toward sex during pregnancy and toward mothers as sexual beings
   Partner: Intrusion on time together
   Baby: intrusion on time (nursing, care)
Fear of pregnancy (after delivery)
Breast-feeding
   The same hormones influence breast-feeding and orgasm. Nursing women often feel confused and
      ashamed at sensuous feelings aroused during nursing.
   See *Ineffective Breast-Feeding.*

Reduce or Eliminate Contributing Factors.

Body Changes

Provide literature or suggested reading list to establish knowledge about pregnancy and changes.
Refer to community resources.
Refer to early pregnancy classes.
Refer to childbirth preparation classes.
View video about sex during pregnancy.
Suggest alternative sexual positions for later pregnancy to prevent abdominal pressure.

Side-lying	Woman on hands and knees
Woman kneeling	Woman on top
Woman standing	Woman astride man

Discuss postpartum changes.
   Provide literature.
   Give reassurance about these changes.
      Episiotomy
      Lochia—how long it will last, how it will change
      Lubrication
      Uterine resolution
      Flabby abdominal musculature
      Breast engorgement
      Breast leakage during lovemaking
   Reassure that this state is temporary and will resolve in 2 to 3 months.
   Refer to postpartum exercise class.

Change in Sex Drive

Reassure that sexual attitudes change throughout pregnancy from feeling very desirous of sex to
   wanting only to be cuddled.

Support acceptance of whatever pleasuring may be desired. Encourage flexibility and alternative sexual patterns (eg, oral sex, mutual masturbation, fondling, stroking, massage, vibrators).

Encourage honest communication with partner concerning desires or changes in interest.

Fatigue

Acknowledge this as a factor, especially during first trimester and again during last month.

Fatigue can be a major contributor to postpartum sexual problems.

Encourage person to make time for her relationship, in sexual as well as other contexts.

Encourage client to ask for help, hire a sitter, and so forth.

Emotional Lability

Encourage woman and/or partner to discuss emotions.

>Postpartum emotional changes can be intense. They can be hormonally influenced but are aggravated by fatigue and loss of identity.

>Conflicting feelings are common. Woman and partner need opportunity to discuss.

>>Resentment of partner is common; this will certainly affect sexual rapport.

>>Resentment of infant can create intense guilt and may cause woman to cling more to child and reject others. Or she may become depressed and less responsive to infant and partner.

>>Expression and acceptance of their feelings are imperative.

Listen—allow time for person to elaborate on feelings.

Reassure that these feelings are normal.

Recommend reading material.

Refer to other pregnant couples for verification.

Relate your own experiences, if appropriate.

Refer to therapy, if indicated.

Fear of Damaging Fetus

Reassure that, unless problems exist (preterm labor, previous early loss, bleeding or rupture of membranes), intercourse is allowed until labor begins.

Refer to physician for reassurance.

Explore misinformation. Use anatomic charts to show protection of baby in uterus.

Inform that orgasm causes contractions that are not harmful and will subside.

Dyspareunia in Pregnancy

Explore what pain is experienced and when.

Suggest alternative positions:

>Woman on top   Posterior–vaginal entry   Side-lying

Suggest use of water-soluble lubricant.

Refer to physician if pain continues.

Dyspareunia Postpartum

Explore what pain is experienced and under what circumstances.

Assess healing of episiotomy.

>The incision heals on the surface after 1 week.

>Dissolvable stitches can take up to 1 month to resolve; there may be tenderness and swelling until then.

>Nerves can remain sensitive and tender for as long as 6 months.

Suggest varied positions.

Suggest use of water-soluble lubricant (nursing women report reduced vaginal lubrication during entire nursing experience).

Teach woman to identify her pelvic floor muscles and strengthen them with exercise.

>"For posterior pelvic floor muscles, imagine you are trying to stop the passage of stool, and tighten your anus muscles without tightening your legs or your abdominal muscles."

>"For anterior pelvic floor muscles, imagine you are trying to stop the passage of urine; tighten the muscles (back and front) for 4 seconds, and then release them; repeat ten times, four times a day" (can be increased to four times an hour if indicated).

Instruct person to stop and start the urinary stream several times during voiding.

Refer to physician if pain continues.

Guilt Over Baby

Encourage discussion; reassure that these feelings are normal; allow time to elaborate.

Expression of these feelings often creates a release and relaxation.

Include partner in discussion (both may have similar feelings they have not felt free to express to each other).

Refer to postpartum support groups.

Refer to psychological or social assistance if pathology is observed.

Encourage couple to allow themselves to get help in caring for infant. They need time alone. Arrange a "date" where they can be alone, with no threat of intrusion of a crying baby. They may then be able to rediscover or renew their intimacy.

Influence of Others

Encourage discussion of mother/woman relationship.

Does woman see her mother as a sexual being?

Does she now feel confused about her roles as mother versus sex partner?

Reassure that identity confusion is common.

Refer to postpartum discussion groups.

Allow client to express feelings concerning changes in life.

Include partner in discussion (perhaps at a later time)—let both parties talk about adjustment and pressures that interfere with relating sexually and otherwise.

Interview partners separately. (Opening up may be difficult with the other person present.)

Fear of Pregnancy

Encourage discussion.

Explore contraceptive choices.

Refer to nurse practitioner or gynecologist for contraception.

Inform client that breast-feeding does not provide effective contraception and that prepregnancy contraceptive devices may no longer fit.

Warn that, although some oral contraceptives can be used while nursing, they usually significantly reduce milk supply.

Techniques to Increase the Couple's Connectiveness (Polomeno, 1999)

Explore fears and anxieties (separately).

Discuss barriers to disclosing fears and anxieties.

Role play disclosure.

Encourage couple to share the "little things" that represent caring.

Instruct on "heart talks." One partner talks for 5 min with no interruption or arguing. The other partner then has a chance to talk. At the end, the couple hugs and says, "I love you" (Polomeno, 1999).

Instruct on "sexual conversation" (Gray, 1995). Useful questions are:

What do you like about having sex with me?

Would you like more sex?

Would you like more or less foreplay?

Is there a way that you would like me to touch you?

Talk regarding keeping romance alive.

Set aside regular time with each other.

Hold hands.

Send messages that partner is appreciated.

Initiate Health Teaching and Referrals.

Teach couples to abstain from intercourse and seek the advice of their health care provider if any of the following are present (Gilbert & Harmon, 1998):

Vaginal bleeding	Premature dilation
Multiple pregnancy	Engaged fetal head or lightening
Placenta previa	Rupture of membranes
History of premature delivery	History of miscarriage

If any of the above are present, the couple should not engage in *any* sex play. Orgasm even without intercourse is contraindicated in most circumstances. Couples should be instructed to ask *very specific* questions about what is allowed and what is not allowed.

Teach and encourage the use of safe sex practices throughout pregnancy if the woman is at risk for acquiring or transmitting an STD.

Refer to suggested references for printed material.

Refer to counselor if resolution is not achieved.

Rationales

- Barring complications, a pregnant woman is free to engage in sexual activity with her partner to the extent that it is comfortable and desired.
- Exploring sexual patterns, concerns, and fears can provide opportunities to correct misinformation and to open dialogue between partners.

- Pregnancy is a time of stress for both man and woman; to deny physical closeness at a time when both partners are struggling can add to tension and alienation.
- The woman may worry about her partner's acceptance; the man may be afraid of hurting the woman and needs to know that sexual activity does not harm the fetus.
- Fathers need to make their own adjustment, both pre- and postnatally. They may feel lost, displaced, or left out. They may have confusing feelings of resentment, especially as the infant suckles the breast (Barclay et al., 1996; Donoran, 1995).
- Intercourse and orgasm are safe for most women, except those with high-risk pregnancies. Semen contains prostaglandin, which may hasten cervical thinning (Gilbert & Harmon, 1998).
- Alternative sexual positions can prevent abdominal pressure or deep penetration.
- Preparation of the woman and her partner for the changes associated with pregnancy, labor, and delivery and postpartum can reduce anxiety.
- Helping the couple understand what factors affect libido (eg, fatigue) can reduce feelings of rejection.
- Communication problems are the most common type of marital problems. Couples are encouraged to share their sexual needs and preferences.
- For women, "little things" that represent caring have the same value, whether it is helping with household chores or planning a dinner out. For men, small acts earn small points whereas big gifts earn big points (Gray, 1995).
- "Romance is important in keeping love, passion and sex alive in a couple's relationship" (Polomeno, 1999, p. 15).
- Romance contributes to a woman that she is important and respected. When a woman appreciates her male partner's efforts, he feels more loved and is encouraged to be more romantic (Gray, 1995).

RISK FOR INEFFECTIVE SEXUALITY PATTERNS

 RELATED TO FEAR OF PREGNANCY AND/OR SEXUALLY TRANSMITTED DISEASES (STDs)

Goal

| NOC | Sexual Functioning, Risk Control: Sexually Transmitted Diseases |

The person will report satisfaction with contraceptive method and sexuality patterns.

Indicators

- Report proper use of contraceptive methods.
- Report use of methods to reduce risk of acquiring STDs.
- Not experience an unplanned pregnancy or acquire an STD.

General Interventions

| NIC | Behavior Modification, Infection Protection, Teaching: Safe Sex, Risk Identification |

Assess for Causative or Contributing Factors, Such as:

Lack of exposure to or understanding of information on contraception and STDs
Newly sexually active
Change in sexual partner
Multiple/sequential sexual partners
Intravenous drug use by self or partner

Eliminate or Reduce Causative or Contributing Factors, if Possible.

Stress genuine risk of pregnancy or STD with unprotected sexual activity.

   Clarify the confidentiality of your discussion.

   Directly ask, "Do you use condoms? Every time?"

   Emphasize that one sexual experience without a condom can transmit an STD.

   Clearly outline that some STDs are not curable (eg, HPV, HBV, HIV).

   Explain that many STDs produce no symptoms initially.

Encourage abstinence from sexual activity, or thoughtful consideration in choice and number of sexual partners.

   Discuss the hazards of casual sex.

   Role play with person on how to say no, how to discuss previous sexual partners, how to request condom use.

   Clarify that each sexual partner exposes one to all previous sexual partners of this person.

   Explain that herpes and HPV can be contracted even with condom use (eg, pubic contact).

Provide Limited Information and Specific Suggestions.

Discuss advantages and disadvantages of various contraceptive methods.

   Effectiveness of pregnancy prevention

   Effectiveness of disease prevention

Provide specific information on chosen contraceptive method, including written/graphic material and return demonstration if appropriate.

Teach client to abstain from sexual activity if partner has symptoms of an STD.

Teach danger of infertility, morbidity, or death from contracting an STD (see *Risk for Infection*).

Provide Referrals, as Indicated.

Physician	Nurse practitioners
Family planning clinic	Certified sex therapist

SEXUAL DYSFUNCTION

DEFINITION

Sexual Dysfunction: State in which a person experiences or is at risk of experiencing a change in sexual function that is viewed as unrewarding or inadequate

DEFINING CHARACTERISTICS
Major (Must Be Present, One or More)

Verbalization of problem with sexual function

Meets *DSM-IV* criteria for Sexual Dysfunction

Minor (May Be Present)

Fears future limitations on sexual performance

Misinformed about sexuality

Lacks knowledge about sexuality and sexual function

Value conflicts involving sexual expression (cultural, religious)

Altered relationship with significant other

Dissatisfaction with sex role (perceived or actual)

> ⊚ **AUTHOR'S NOTE**
>
> See *Ineffective Sexuality Patterns.*

DISTURBED SLEEP PATTERN

DEFINITION

Disturbed Sleep Pattern: State in which a person experiences or is at risk of experiencing a change in the quantity or quality of his rest pattern that causes discomfort or interferes with desired lifestyle

DEFINING CHARACTERISTICS
Major (Must be Present)
Adults
Difficulty falling or remaining asleep

Minor (May be Present)
Adults

Fatigue on awakening or during the day

Agitation

Dozing during the day

Mood alterations

Children
Sleep disturbances in children frequently are related to fear, enuresis, or inconsistent responses of parents to child's requests for changes in sleep rules, such as requests to stay up late.
Reluctance to retire
Persists in sleeping with parents
Frequent awakening during the night

RELATED FACTORS

Many factors can contribute to disturbed sleep patterns. Some common factors are listed below.

Pathophysiologic
Related to frequent awakenings secondary to:

Impaired oxygen transport

Angina	Respiratory disorders	Peripheral arteriosclerosis
Circulatory disorders		

Impaired elimination; bowel or bladder

Diarrhea	Retention	Constipation
Dysuria	Incontinence	Frequency

Impaired metabolism

Hyperthyroidism	Hepatic disorders	Gastric ulcers

Treatment-Related
Related to difficulty assuming usual position secondary to (specify)
Related to excessive daytime sleeping secondary to medications

Tranquilizers	Soporifics	Sedatives
Monoamine oxidase inhibitors	Hypnotics	Barbiturates
Antidepressants	Corticosteroids	Antihypertensives
Amphetamines		

Situational (Personal, Environmental)

Related to excessive hyperactivity secondary to:

Bipolar disorder   Attention-deficit disorder   Panic anxiety

Related to excessive daytime sleeping
Related to depression
Related to inadequate daytime activities
Related to pain
Related to anxiety response
Related to discomforts secondary to pregnancy
Related to lifestyle disruptions

Occupational   Emotional   Social
Sexual   Financial

Related to environmental changes (specify)

Hospitalization (noise, disturbing roommate, fear)
Travel

Related to fears
Related to circadian rhythm changes

Maturational

Children
Related to fear of dark

Adult Women
Related to hormonal changes (eg, perimenopausal)

⚭ AUTHOR'S NOTE

The inability to rest and sleep has been described as "one of the causes as well as one of the accompaniments of disease" (Henderson, 1969). Sleep disturbances can result from physiologic, psychological, social, environmental, and maturational changes or problems.

The nursing diagnosis *Disturbed Sleep Pattern* must be differentiated from sleep disorders, which are chronic conditions (eg, sleep apnea, narcolepsy) usually not treatable by a nurse generalist. *Disturbed Sleep Pattern* should be used to describe temporary changes in usual sleep patterns and/or those that a nurse can prevent or reduce (eg, disruptions for treatments, anxiety response).

⚭ ERRORS IN DIAGNOSTIC STATEMENTS

1. *Disturbed Sleep Pattern related to apnea*
   This diagnosis requires monitoring and comanagement by nurses and physicians; thus, the nurse should write it as the collaborative problem *PC: Sleep Apnea.*
2. *Disturbed Sleep Pattern related to hospitalization*
   This diagnosis does not reflect the treatment needed. The effects of hospitalization on sleep should be specified, such as in *Disturbed Sleep Pattern related to changes in usual sleep environment, unfamiliar noises, and interruptions for assessments.*

KEY CONCEPTS
Generic Considerations

- Sleep involves two distinct stages: rapid eye movement (REM) and non-rapid eye movement (NREM). NREM sleep constitutes about 75% of total sleep time; REM sleep accounts for the remaining 25% (Porth, 2002).
- The entire sleep cycle is completed in 70 to 100 min; this cycle repeats itself four or five times during the course of the sleep period.
- Sleep is a restorative and recuperative process that facilitates cellular growth and repair of damaged and aging body tissues. During NREM sleep, metabolic, cardiac, and respiratory rates

decrease to basal levels and blood pressure decreases. There is profound muscle relaxation, bone marrow mitotic activity, and accelerated tissue repair and protein synthesis. During REM sleep, the sympathetic nervous system accelerates, with erratic increases in cardiac output and heart and respiratory rate. Perfusion to gray matter doubles, and cognitive and emotional information is stored, filtered, and organized (Boyd, 2001).

- The active phase of the sleep cycle, REM sleep, is characterized by increased irregular vital signs, penile erections, flaccid musculature, and release of adrenal hormones. REM sleep occurs approximately four or five times a night and is essential to a person's sense of well-being. REM sleep is instrumental in facilitating emotional adaptation; a person needs substantially more REM sleep after periods of increased stress or learning (Blissitt, 2001).

- Percentage of time in bed at night actually spent asleep, or *sleep efficiency,* influences perception of the quality of sleep. Studies report that younger people typically report sleep efficiency of 80% to 95%, whereas older people report 67% to 70% (Hayashi & Endo, 1982).

- Sleep deprivation results in impaired cognitive functioning (memory, concentration, judgment) and perception, mental fatigue, reduced emotional control, and increased suspicion, irritability, depression, and disorientation. It also lowers the pain threshold and decreases production of catecholamines, corticosteroids, and hormones (Boyd, 2001; Dines-Kalinowski, 2000).

- The average amount of sleep needed according to age follows:

Age	Hours of Sleep
Newborn	14 to 18
6 months	12 to 16
6 months to 4 years	12 to 13
5 to 13 years	7 to 8.5
13 to 21 years	7 to 8.75
Adults younger than 60	6 to 9
Adults older than 60	7 to 8

- Hammer (1991) identified three subcategories of *Disturbed Sleep Pattern:* latency or difficulty falling asleep, interrupted, and early-morning awakening.

- People with depression report early-morning awakenings and inability to return to sleep. People with anxiety complain of insomnia and multiple awakenings (Boyd, 2001).

- Hypnotics contribute to sleep disturbances by (Abrams, 2004):
  - Requiring increasing dosage as a result of tolerance
  - Depressing central nervous system (CNS) function
  - Producing paradoxic effects (nightmares, agitation)
  - Interfering with REM and deep sleep stages
  - Causing daytime somnolence owing to a very long half-life
  - Sleep disturbances are reported by 50% to 100% of peri- and post-menopausal women. These sleep disturbances are caused by hot flashes and sweating caused by hormonal changes (Landis & Moe, 2004).
  - Sleep disturbances in peri- and post-menopausal women are caused by the re-regulation of neuroendocrine hypothalamic function and changes in the amount and type of sex steroid hormones. These changes affect mood, cognition, stress reactivity, body temperature, and sleep/wake cycles (Landis & Moe, 2004).

Pediatric Considerations

- Children exhibit wide variations in amount and distribution of sleep (Cureton-Lane & Fontaine, 1997).

Age	Hours of Sleep
Newborn	16 h
12 months	10 h, 3-h nap
24 months	11 h, 2-h nap
4 years	10.5 h
7 years	10 h
12 years	9 h
16 years	8 h

(continued)

> ### ❖ Pediatric Considerations (continued)
>
> - Sleep affects a child's growth and development as well as the family unit as a whole (Hunsberger, 1989).
> - As children mature, the number of hours spent in sleep decreases. Moreover, the quality of sleep changes with maturity. Sleep is characterized as being deep and restful 50% of the time in an infant versus 80% of the time in the older child (Wong, 2003).

> ### ⚕ Maternal Considerations
>
> - The activity of the fetus can interfere with sleep late in pregnancy. Dyspnea can occur if the mother is lying flat (Pillitteri, 2003).
> - The effects of maternal rest/sleep deprivation may negatively affect the woman's ability to acquire and sustain her new role (Larlein & Butler, 2000).

> ### ☺ Geriatric Considerations
>
> - Research has found that sleep efficiency declines with advancing age, so more time is needed in bed to achieve restorative sleep. Sleep time decreases with age (eg, 6 h by 70 years). Stages 3 and 4 and REM sleep decrease with aging (Hammer, 1991).
> - Sleep pattern disturbances are the most frequent complaint among older adults (Hammer, 1991).
> - Older adults have more difficulty falling asleep, are more easily awakened, and spend more time in the drowsiness stage and less time in the dream stages than do younger people (Miller, 2004).
> - Miller (2004) reports that approximately 70% of older adults complain of sleep disturbances, usually involving daytime sleepiness, difficulty falling asleep, and frequent arousals.

Focus Assessment Criteria

Subjective Data

Assess for Defining Characteristics.

Sleep patterns (present, past)
Rate sleep on a scale of 1 to 10 (10 = rested, refreshed)
Usual bedtime and arising time
Difficulty in getting to sleep, staying asleep, awakening

Sleep requirements
To establish the amount of sleep a person needs, have him or her go to bed and sleep until waking in the morning (without an alarm clock). The person should do this for a few days. Calculate the average of the total sleeping hours, subtracting 20 to 30 min, which is the time most people need to fall asleep.

History of symptoms
Complaints of

Sleeplessness	Fear (nightmares, dark,
Depression	maturational situations)
Anxiety	Irritability

Assess for Related Factors.

Refer to Related Factors.

Objective Data

Assess for Defining Characteristics.

Physical characteristics
Drawn appearance (pale, dark circles under eyes, puffy eyes)
Yawning
Dozing during the day
Decreased attention span
Irritability

For more information on Focus Assessment Criteria, visit http://connection.lww.com.

Goal

 NOC Rest, Sleep, Well-Being

The person will report an optimal balance of rest and activity.

Indicators

- Describe factors that prevent or inhibit sleep.
- Identify techniques to induce sleep.

General Interventions

NIC Energy Management, Sleep Enhancement, Environmental Management

Because various factors can disrupt sleep patterns, the nurse should consult the index for specific interventions to reduce certain factors (eg, pain, anxiety, fear). The following suggests general interventions for promoting sleep and specific interventions for selected clinical situations.

Identify Causative Contributing Factors.

Pain (see *Impaired Comfort*)
Fear (see *Fear*)
Stress or anxiety (see *Anxiety*)
Immobility or decreased activity
Pregnancy
Urinary frequency or incontinence (see *Impaired Urinary Elimination*)
Unfamiliar or noisy environment
Temperature (too hot/cold)
Insufficient daily stimulation or activity
Peri- and post-menopause

Reduce or Eliminate Environmental Distractions and Sleep Interruptions.

Noise
Close door to room.
Pull curtains.
Unplug telephone.
Use "white noise" (eg, fan; quiet music; tape of rain, waves).
Eliminate 24-h lighting.
Provide night lights.
Decrease the amount and kind of incoming stimuli (eg, staff conversations).
Cover blinking lights with tape.
Reduce the volume of alarms and televisions.
Place with compatible roommate, if possible.

Interruptions
Organize procedures to minimize disturbances during sleep period (eg, when person awakens for medication, also administer treatments and obtain vital signs).
Avoid unnecessary procedures during sleep period.
Limit visitors during optimal rest periods (eg, after meals).
If voiding during the night is disruptive, have person limit nighttime fluids and void before retiring.

Increase Daytime Activities, as Indicated.

Establish with person a schedule for a daytime program of activity (walking, physical therapy).
Discourage naps longer than 90 min.

Encourage naps in the morning.

Limit amount and length of daytime sleeping if excessive (ie, more than 1 h).

Encourage others to communicate with person and stimulate wakefulness.

Promote Sleep.

Assess with person, family, or parents the usual bedtime routine—time, hygiene practices, rituals (reading, toy)—and adhere to it as closely as possible.

Encourage or provide evening care.

    Bathroom or bedpan

    Personal hygiene (mouth care, bath, shower, partial bath)

    Clean linen and bedclothes (freshly made bed, sufficient blankets)

Use sleep aids.

    Warm bath

    Desired bedtime snack (avoid highly seasoned and high-roughage foods)

    Reading material

    Back rub or massage

    Milk

    Soft music or tape-recorded story

    Relaxation/breathing exercises

Use pillows for support (painful limb, pregnant or obese abdomen, back).

Ensure that the person has at least four or five periods of at least 90 min each of uninterrupted sleep every 24 h.

Document the amount of the person's uninterrupted sleep each shift.

Reduce the Potential for Injury During Sleep.

Use siderails, if needed.

Place bed in low position.

Provide adequate supervision.

Provide night lights.

Place call bell within reach.

Ensure that an adequate length of tubing is available for turning (intravenous [IV] tubing, Levin tube).

Provide Health Teaching and Referrals, as Indicated.

Teach an at-home sleep routine (Miller, 2004):

    Maintain a consistent daily schedule for waking, sleeping, and resting (weekdays, weekends).

    Arise at the usual time even after not sleeping well; avoid staying in bed when awake.

    Use bed only for activities associated with sleeping.

    If awakened and cannot return to sleep, get out of bed and read in another room for 30 min.

    Avoid caffeine-containing foods and beverages (eg, chocolate, tea, coffee) during afternoon and evening.

    Avoid alcohol.

    Try a bedtime snack of foods high in L-tryptophan (eg, milk, peanuts).

Teach the importance of regular exercise (walking, running, aerobic dance) for at least 30 min three times a week (if not contraindicated) to reduce stress and promote sleep.

Explain that hypnotic medications are not for long-term use owing to the risk for development of tolerance and interference with daytime functioning.

Explain to person and significant others the causes of sleep/rest disturbance and possible ways to avoid or minimize these causes.

Refer a person with a chronic sleep problem to a sleep disorders center.

For peri- and post-menopausal women, consult a primary care provider or women's health specialist for treatment.

Rationales

- Sleep cycle includes REM, NREM, and wakefulness. A person typically goes through four or five complete sleep cycles each night. Awakening during a cycle may cause him or her to feel poorly rested in the morning.
- Although many believe that a person needs 8 h of sleep each night, no scientific evidence supports this belief. Individual sleep requirements vary greatly. In general, a person who can relax and rest easily requires less sleep to feel refreshed. with age, total sleep time usually decreases—especially stage 4 sleep—and stage 1 sleep increases.
- Sleep is difficult without relaxation, which the unfamiliar hospital environment can hinder.

- To feel rested, a person usually must complete an entire sleep cycle (70 to 100 min) four or five times a night.
- Sedative and hypnotic drugs begin to lose their effectiveness after 1 week of use, requiring increasing dosages and leading to the risk of dependence.
- A familiar bedtime ritual may promote relaxation and sleep.
- Warm milk contains L-tryptophan, which is a sleep inducer (Hammer, 1991).
- Caffeine and nicotine are CNS stimulants that lengthen sleep latency and increase nighttime wakening (Miller, 2004).
- Alcohol induces drowsiness but suppresses REM sleep and increases the number of awakenings (Miller, 2004).
- Early-morning naps produce more REM sleep than do afternoon naps. Naps longer than 90 min long decrease the stimulus for longer sleep cycles in which REM sleep is obtained.
- Researchers have reported that the chief deterrents to sleep in critical care clients were activity, noise, pain, physical condition, nursing procedures, lights, vapor tents, and hypothermia.
- Environmental noise that cannot be eliminated or reduced can be masked with "white noise" (eg, fan, soft music, tape-recorded sounds [rain, ocean waves]; Miller, 2004).
- Irregular sleep patterns can disrupt normal circadian rhythms, possibly leading to sleep difficulties.

Pediatric Interventions

Explain night to the child (stars and moon).
Discuss how some people (nurses, factory workers) work at night.
Explain that when night comes for them, day is coming for other people elsewhere in the world.
If a nightmare occurs, encourage the child to talk about it, if possible. Reassure child that it is a dream, even though it seems very real. Share with child that you have dreams too.
Provide a night light or a flashlight to give child control over the dark.
Reassure child that you will be nearby all night.
Explain the possible problems of sleeping.
Ensure that infants and children in hospitals have complete sleep cycles for age (Cureton-Lane & Fontaine, 1997).

Rationales

- Sleep problems commonly are related to feeding, resistance to separation, and normal fears.
- Children need to understand nighttime and be assisted to prepare for it. Preparation for bedtime involves switching the child from activity to bedtime gradually. It is a time for calmness, reassurance, and closeness.
- Children should be helped to learn that their beds are safe places.
- REM sleep varies with developmental age (Cureton-Lane & Fontaine, 1997).

Maternal Interventions

Discuss reasons for sleeping difficulties during pregnancy (eg, leg cramps, backache, fetal movements).
Teach client how to position pillows in side-lying position (one between legs, one under abdomen, one under top arm, one under head).
Teach client to avoid caffeine and large meals within 2 to 3 h of bedtime.
Teach client to exercise daily and take a warm bath at bedtime.
Encourage an afternoon nap.
Attempt to arrange for assistance at home after delivery.

Rationales

- Interventions that reduce discomfort of enlarging uterus can promote sleep (Pillitteri, 2003).
- See Rationale for General Interventions.

Geriatric Interventions

Explain the effects of alcohol on sleep (eg, nightmares, frequent awakenings).
Explain that sleeping pills (prescribed or over-the-counter) are not effective after 1 month and that they interfere with the quality of sleep and daytime functioning.
Instruct client to avoid over-the-counter sleeping pills because of their antihistamine effects.
If client needs sleeping pills for a few days, advise him or her to consult primary care provider for a type with a short half-life.

Rationales

- Older adults have increased sensitivity to hypnotics and sleeping medications and experience more adverse effects (eg, constipation, confusion, and interference with quality of sleep).
- Alcohol and caffeine may cause insomnia, as do certain drugs such as steroids, theophylline, beta blockers, and chronic use of sedatives or hypnotics.

SLEEP DEPRIVATION

DEFINITION

Sleep Deprivation: State in which a person experiences prolonged periods of time without sustained, natural, periodic states of relative unconsciousness

> ### AUTHOR'S NOTE
>
> This diagnostic label represents a situation in which the client's sleep is insufficient. It is the most common type of sleep pattern disturbance and will probably be used for most clinical situations.

DEFINING CHARACTERISTICS

Refer to *Disturbed Sleep Pattern.*

RELATED FACTORS

Refer to *Disturbed Sleep Pattern.*

Goal

Refer to *Disturbed Sleep Pattern.*

General Interventions

Refer to *Disturbed Sleep Pattern.*

IMPAIRED SOCIAL INTERACTION

DEFINITION

Impaired Social Interaction: State in which a person experiences or is at risk of experiencing negative, insufficient, or unsatisfactory responses from interactions

DEFINING CHARACTERISTICS

Social isolation is a subjective state. Thus, the nurse must validate all inferences about a person's feelings of aloneness, because the causes vary and people show their aloneness in different ways.

Major (Must be Present, One or More)

Expresses feelings of aloneness, rejection
Desire for more contact with people
Reports insecurity in social situations
Describes a lack of meaningful relationships

Minor (May be Present)

Time passing slowly ("Mondays are so long for me.")
Inability to concentrate and make decisions
Feelings of uselessness
Feelings of rejection
Underactivity (physical or verbal)
Appearing depressed, anxious, or angry
Failure to interact with others nearby
Sad, dull affect
Uncommunicative
Withdrawn
Poor eye contact
Preoccupied with own thoughts and memories

RELATED FACTORS

Impaired social interactions can result from a variety of situations and health problems related to the inability to establish and maintain rewarding relationships. Some common sources are listed below.

Pathophysiologic

Related to embarrassment, limited physical mobility or energy secondary to:

Loss of body function	Loss of body part	Terminal illness

Related to communication barriers secondary to:

Hearing deficits	Speech impediments	Mental retardation
Chronic mental illness	Visual deficits	

Treatment-Related

Related to surgical disfigurement
Related to therapeutic isolation

Situational (Personal, Environmental)

Related to alienation from others secondary to:

Constant complaining	High anxiety	Rumination
Impulsive behavior	Overt hostility	Delusions
Manipulative behaviors	Hallucinations	Mistrust or suspicions
Disorganized thinking	Illogical ideas	Dependent behavior

Egocentric behavior

Depressive behavior

Strong unpopular beliefs

Aggressive responses

Emotional immaturity

Related to language/cultural barriers
Related to lack of social skills
Related to change in usual social patterns secondary to:

Divorce

Relocation

Death

Maturational
Child/Adolescent
Related to inadequate sensory stimulation
Related to altered appearance
Related to speech impediments

Adult
Related to loss of ability to practice vocation

Older Adult
Related to change in usual social patterns secondary to:

Death of spouse

Functional deficits

Retirement

ⓧ AUTHOR'S NOTE

Social competence refers to a person's ability to interact effectively with others. Interpersonal relationships assist a person through life experiences, both positive and negative. Positive relationships with others require positive self-concept, social skills, social sensitivity, and acceptance of the need for independence. To interact satisfactorily with others, a person must acknowledge and accept his or her limitations and strengths (Maroni, 1989).

A person without positive mental health usually does not have social sensitivity and, thus, is uncomfortable with the interdependence necessary for effective social interactions. A person with poor self-concept may constantly sacrifice his or her needs for those of others or may always put personal needs before the needs of others.

The diagnosis *Impaired Social Interaction* describes a person who exhibits ineffective interactions with others. If extreme and/or prolonged, this problem can lead to a diagnosis of *Social Isolation*. The nursing focus for *Impaired Social Interaction* is increasing the person's sensitivity to the needs of others and teaching reciprocity.

ⓧ ERRORS IN DIAGNOSTIC STATEMENTS

Impaired Social Interaction related to verbalized discomfort in social situations

In this diagnosis, the person's report of discomfort represents a diagnostic cue, not a related factor. The nurse performs a focus assessment to determine reasons for the person's discomfort; until he or she knows these reasons, the nurse can record the diagnosis *Impaired Social Interaction related to unknown etiology.*

KEY CONCEPTS
Generic Considerations

- Blumer described three premises of human conduct and interactions:
  - Life experiences have different meanings for each person. People respond toward situations and others on the basis of these meanings or significance.
  - People learn meanings from social interactions with others.
  - During encounters, people interpret and apply or modify their previous meanings.
- Social competence is a person's ability to interact effectively with his or her environment.

- Effective reality testing, ability to solve problems, and various coping mechanisms are necessary for the person to be socially competent.
- Both the person and the environment contribute to impaired functioning. A person may be able to function in one environment or situation but not in others.
- Adequate social functioning is associated most often with conjugal living and a stable occupation.

Chronic Mental Illness

- Chronic mental illness is characterized by recurring episodes over a long period. The extent to which role performance is impaired varies. The extent of impairment is related to social inadequacy.
- Disturbed thought processes may interfere with the person's ability to engage in appropriate social or occupational role behavior.
- Dependency is one of the most consistent features presented. It may be seen through multiple readmissions requiring a large amount of clinician's time, resistance to discharge, resistance to any change including medication, and refusal to leave home.
- The origins of impaired social interactions in people with chronic mental illness vary. For some, it is the result of poor reality testing. If a person cannot perceive reality accurately, it is difficult to manage everyday problems. For others, it may be the result of social isolation or the loss of interpersonal skills because of long-term institutionalization.
- The person with chronic mental illness usually has no friends, is socially isolated, and engages in little community activity (Varcarolis, 2002).
- Deinstitutionalization has decreased the number of institutionalized people and the median length of hospital stay, thus changing the character of today's chronically ill population. An emerging group of people 18 to 35 years of age is distinctly different from older institutionalized adults, in that their lives reflect a transient existence and multiple hospital admissions versus stable, long-term residence in a state hospital.
- People with chronic mental illness often lose their jobs, not because of an inability to do tasks but because of deficits in emotional and interpersonal functions. Research in social skills training has shown that skill-building programs improve posthospital adjustment.

Pediatric Considerations

- A child is significantly affected when a parent is emotionally disturbed. Emotionally disturbed parents may not be able to meet the physical or safety needs of their children.
- Young children depend on their parents to interpret the world for them. Parents with impaired social interaction, *Disturbed Thought Processes,* or both may not interpret experiences for the child accurately (Varcarolis, 2002).
- Impaired social interaction may result in *Social Isolation.* Also, see the nursing diagnosis *Impaired Parenting.*
- Adolescents with substance abuse problems use the substance to achieve popularity, to reduce stress, or both. Poor personal and social competence is also present (Johnson, 1995).
- Young people with chronic mental illness exhibit problems with impulse control (eg, suicidal gestures, legal problems, alcohol/drug intoxication), disturbances in affect (eg, anger, argumentativeness, belligerence), and poor reality testing, especially when under stress. the population varies from system-dependent, poorly motivated people to system-resistant people with low frustration tolerance and refusal to acknowledge problems (Varcarolis, 2002).
- Despite variations, children and adolescents with chronic mental illness share several factors (Varcarolis, 2002).
  - Difficulty maintaining stable, supportive relationships—most have transient, unstable relationships with marginally functional people.
  - Repeated errors in judgment—they seem unable to learn from their experiences or to transfer knowledge from one situation to another.
  - Vulnerability to stress—those experiencing stress are at greater risk for relapse.
  - Patterns of social interaction are demanding, hostile, and manipulative, producing negative reactions among caregivers.

Ⓖ **Geriatric Considerations**

- Effective social interactions depend on positive self-esteem. No data suggest that older adults have diminished self-esteem compared with younger adults (Miller, 2004).
- In older adults, common threats to self-esteem include devaluation, dependency, functional impairments, and decreased sense of control (Miller, 2004).
- Depression-related affective disturbances of daily life occur in 27% of older adults. Major depression occurs in 2% of community-living older adults and in 12% of older people living in nursing homes (Varcarolis, 2002).
- Depressed older adults lose interest in social activities and do not display positive interactions when they do interact.

Focus Assessment Criteria

Subjective Data

Assess for Defining Characteristics.

Relationships

Does he or she have friends, family?
Does he or she initiate friendships?
Does he or she initiate contact or wait for friends to make contact?
Is he or she satisfied with social interactions?
What is the reason for dissatisfaction with his social network?

Coping skills

How does the client respond to stress, conflict?

Substance abuse	Substance abuse (drugs, alcohol, food)
Aggression (verbal or physical)	Withdrawal
Suicidal ideation or gestures	

Legal history (arrests, convictions)

Assess for Related Factors.

Interaction patterns and skills

Job-related
Job-seeking and interviewing skills
   Can identify own job-related assets
   Dresses appropriately
   Asks appropriate questions
   Identifies employment sources
   Can complete an application
   Has realistic employment expectations
Employment history
   Length of employment
   Reasons for leaving (problems with coworkers or supervisors)
   Frequency of job changes
Interactions with coworkers
   Contacts outside work
Living arrangements
Residential patterns
   Where? (family, group home, boarding house, institution)
   How long?
   Frequency of relocation
   Reasons for relocation
Obstacles to community functioning

Poor personal hygiene	Legal problems
Expects self-reliance	Unemployed
Lacks leisure activities	Unstable, transient residences
Inappropriate behavior in public	Social isolation

Leisure / recreation
"What do you do with your free time?"
What interferes with participating in recreational activities?
Preference for individual or group activity

Objective Data
Assess for Related Factors.
General appearance
Facial expression (eg, sad, hostile, expressionless)
Dress (eg, meticulous, disheveled, seductive, eccentric)
Personal hygiene
    Cleanliness
    Clothes (appropriateness, condition)
    Grooming

Communication pattern
Content

Appropriate	Religiosity	Rambling
Worthlessness	Suspicious	Delusions
Denial of problem	Obsessions	Exaggerated
Homicidal or suicidal plans	Sexually preoccupied	

Pattern of speech

Appropriate	Indecisive	Neologisms
Circumstantial (cannot get to point)	Blocking (cannot finish idea)	Word salad
Jumps from one topic to another		

Rate of speech

Appropriate	Reduced	Excessive
Pressured		

Relationship skills
Can listen and respond appropriately
Has conversational skills
Is withdrawn/preoccupied with self
Shows dependency, passivity
Is demanding/pleading
Is hostile
Has barriers to satisfactory relationships

Social isolation	Thought disturbances	Severe depression
Chronic mental illness	Panic attacks	Preoccupation with illness

For more information on Focus Assessment Criteria, visit http://connection.lww.com.

Goal

NOC Family Environment: Internal, Social Interaction Skills, Social Involvement

The person/family will report increased satisfaction.

Indicators
- Identify problematic behavior that deters socialization.
- Substitute constructive behavior for disruptive social behavior (specify).
- Describe strategies to promote effective socialization.

NIC Anticipatory Guidance, Behavior Modification, Family Integrity: Promotion, Counseling, Behavior Management, Family Support, Self-Responsibility Facilitation

General Interventions

Provide Support to Maintain Basic Social Skills and Reduce Social Isolation (See *Social Isolation* for Further Interventions).

Provide an Individual, Supportive Relationship.
Assist person to manage life stresses.
Focus on present and reality.

Help client to identify how stress precipitates problems.
Support healthy defenses.
Help person to identify alternative courses of action.
Assist client to analyze approaches that work best.

Provide Supportive Group Therapy.
Focus on here and now.
Establish group norms that discourage inappropriate behavior.
Encourage testing of new social behavior.
Use snacks or coffee to decrease anxiety during sessions.
Model certain accepted social behaviors (eg, respond to a friendly greeting instead of ignoring it).
Foster development of relationships among members through self-disclosure and genuineness.
Use questions and observations to encourage people with limited interaction skills.
Encourage members to validate their perception with others.
Identify strengths among members and ignore selected weaknesses.
Activity groups, drop-in socialization centers can be used for some clients.

Monitor Medication Compliance.
Use small groups or scheduled individual sessions.
Question client about side effects and symptom exacerbation (do not expect person to self-monitor).

Be Assertive with People Who are Unmotivated or Passive.
Contact the person when he or she fails to attend a scheduled appointment, job interview, and so forth.
Do not wait for person to initiate participation.

Hold People Accountable for their Own Actions.
Treat as responsible citizens.
Allow decision making, but outline limits as necessary.
Do not allow them to use their illness as an excuse for their behavior.
Set consequences and enforce when necessary, including encounters with law.
Help to see how their behaviors or attitudes contribute to their frequent interpersonal conflicts.

Allow Person to be Dependent as Necessary.

Use a Wide Variety of Agencies and Services (Medical, Psychiatric, Vocational, Social, Residential).
One agency must coordinate services (person will not be able to coordinate for self).
Case managers have been successful in providing linkage.
Programs must be flexible and culturally relevant.

Decrease Problematic Behavior.
Impaired reality testing (see *Disturbed Thought Processes*)
Lack of leisure activities (see *Deficient Diversional Activity*)
    Companionship program
    Day treatment centers
Social isolation (see *Social Isolation*)
Hostility and violent outbursts (see *Anxiety* and *Risk for Violence*)
Suicidal threats or attempts (see *Risk for Suicide*)
Manipulation
    Use limit setting (refer to section on anger in *Anxiety*).
    Be aware of own reactions.

Provide for Development of Social Skills.
Identify the environment in which social interactions are impaired: living, learning, working.
Provide instruction in the environment where person is expected to function, when possible
  (eg, accompany to job site, work with person in own residence).
Develop an individualized social skill program. Examples of some social skills are grooming and personal hygiene, posture, gait, eye contact, beginning a conversation, listening, and ending a conversation. Include modeling, behavior rehearsal, and homework.
Combine verbal instructions with demonstration and practice.
Be firm in setting parameters of appropriate social behaviors, such as punctuality, attendance, managing illnesses with employers, and dress.
Use group as a method of discussing work-related problems.
Use sheltered workshops and part-time employment depending on level at which success can best be achieved.
Give positive feedback; make sure it is specific and detailed. Focus on no more than three behavioral connections at a time; too-lengthy feedback adds confusion and increases anxiety.

Convey a "can-do" attitude.

Role-play aspects of social interactions (McFarland et al., 1996):

How to initiate a conversation

How to continue a conversation

How to terminate a conversation

How to refuse a request

How to ask for something

How to interview for a job

How to ask someone to participate in an activity (eg, going to the movies)

Assist Family and Community Members in Understanding and Providing Support.

Provide facts concerning mental illness, treatment, and progress to family members. Gently help family accept the illness.

Validate family members' feelings of frustration in dealing with daily problems.

Provide guidance on overstimulating or understimulating environments.

Allow families to discuss their feelings of guilt and how their behavior affects the person. Refer to a family support group, if available.

Develop an alliance with family.

Arrange for periodic respite care.

Provide support to landlords, shopkeepers, and anyone else with whom person has contact.

Provide information on mental illness.

Teach relationship skills needed to manage person (eg, direct, firm, simple directions; use of modeling).

Give person name and number he or she can call when problems arise.

Provide this education as the need arises with specific individuals.

Explore Strategies for Handling Difficult Situations (eg, Disrupted Communications, Altered Thoughts, Alcohol and Drug Use; Stuart & Sundeen, 2001).

Discuss feelings among members.

Establish a cooperative plan.

Plan regular activities to strengthen marital–parental coalition.

Identify when stress reduction is needed.

Initiate Health Teaching and Referrals, as Indicated.

Teach the person (McFarland et al., 1996)

Responsibilities of role as client (making requests clearly known, participating in therapies)

To outline activities of the day and to focus on accomplishing them

How to approach others to communicate

To identify which interactions encourage others to give him or her consideration and respect

To identify how he or she can participate in formulating family roles and responsibility to comply

To recognize signs of anxiety and methods to relieve them

To identify positive behavior and to experience self-satisfaction in selecting constructive choices

Teach basic coping skills necessary to live independently (home management, personal hygiene, financial management, transportation skills).

Teach or refer for assertiveness skill training.

Teach or refer for anger management.

Teach basic conversational skills.

Teach job-seeking skills.

Teach parenting skills.

Refer to a variety of social agencies; however, one agency should maintain coordination and continuity.

Refer for supportive family therapy as indicated.

Refer families to local self-help groups.

Provide numbers for crisis intervention services.

Rationales

- The person needs continual encouragement to test new social skills and to explore new social situations.

- The nurse models appropriate social skills and uses group therapy as other examples of social skills.
- Effective social skills can be learned with guidance, demonstration, practice, and feedback (Stuart & Sundeen, 2001).
- Role playing provides an opportunity to rehearse problematic issues and to receive feedback. Consequences of responses can be explored safely (Stuart & Sundeen, 2001).
- Interventions for the family are very important for successful rehabilitation of a family member with chronic mental illness (Mohr, 2003).
- Both individuals and families are under stress. The person's behaviors that strain the family include excessively demanding behavior, social withdrawal, lack of conversation, and minimal leisure interests. The family also affects the person's ability to survive in the community by either supportive or nonsupportive behaviors.
- Passivity or lack of motivation is a part of the illness; thus, caregivers should not simply accept it. Caregivers must use an assertive approach in which the treatment is "taken to the person" rather than waiting for him or her to participate (Varcarolis, 2002).
- Helping the family learn strategies to handle problem behavior provides a sense of control over their lives (Stuart & Sundeen, 2001).

Pediatric Interventions

If Impulse Control is a Problem:

Set firm, responsible limits.
Don't lecture.
State limits simply and back them up.
Maintain routines.
Limit play to one playmate to learn appropriate play skills (eg, relative, adult, quiet child).
Gradually increase number of playmates.
Provide immediate and constant feedback.

Discuss Selective Parenting Skills.

Reward small increments of desired behavior.
Contract appropriate age-related consequences (eg, time-out, loss of activity [use of car, bicycle]).

Teach Parents To:

Avoid harsh criticism.
Not disagree in front of child.
Establish eye contact before giving instructions and ask child to repeat back what was said.
Teach older child to self-monitor target behaviors and to develop self-reliance.

If Antisocial Behavior is Present, Help to:

Describe behaviors that interfere with socialization.
Role-play alternative responses.
Limit social circle to a manageable size.
Elicit peer feedback for positive and negative behavior.

Assist the Adolescent to Decrease Social Deficits.

Assertiveness	Anger management
Problem solving	Refusal skills
Stress management	Values clarification

Rationales

- Failure to control impulses disrupts socialization (eg, family, peers, school; Johnson, 1995).
- Families can be helped to learn effective parenting skills to enhance the child's success (Wong, 2003).
- Skills that reduce social deficits can increase social acceptance, control, and self-esteem.

SOCIAL ISOLATION

DEFINITION

Social Isolation: State in which a person or group experiences or perceives a need or desire for increased involvement with others but is unable to make that contact

DEFINING CHARACTERISTICS

Social isolation is a subjective state. Thus, the nurse must validate all inferences concerning a person's feelings of aloneness, because the causes vary and people show their aloneness in different ways.

Major (Must be Present, One or More)

Expressed feelings of aloneness, rejection
Desire for more contact with people
Reports insecurity in social situations
Describes a lack of meaningful relationships

Minor (May be Present)

Time passing slowly ("Mondays are so long for me.")
Inability to concentrate and make decisions
Feelings of uselessness
Uncommunicative
Feeling of rejection
Withdrawn
Sad, dull affect
Poor eye contact
Preoccupied with own thoughts and memories
Underactivity (physical or verbal)
Appearing depressed, anxious, or angry
Failure to interact with others nearby

RELATED FACTORS

A state of social isolation can result from a variety of situations and health problems that are related to a loss of established relationships or to a failure to generate these relationships. Some common sources follow.

Pathophysiologic

Related to fear of rejection secondary to:
Obesity
Cancer (disfiguring surgery of head or neck, superstitions of others)
Physical handicaps (paraplegia, amputation, arthritis, hemiplegia)
Emotional handicaps (extreme anxiety, depression, paranoia, phobias)
Incontinence (embarrassment, odor)
Communicable diseases (acquired immunodeficiency syndrome [AIDS], hepatitis)
Psychiatric illness (schizophrenia, bipolar affective disorder, personality disorders)

Situational (Personal, Environmental)

Related to death of a significant other
Related to divorce
Related to disfiguring appearance
Related to fear of rejection secondary to:

Obesity	Hospitalization or terminal illness (dying process)
Extreme poverty	Unemployment

Related to moving to another culture (eg, unfamiliar language)
Related to loss of usual means of transportation
Related to history of unsatisfactory relationships secondary to:

Unacceptable social behavior	Drug abuse	Alcohol abuse
Delusional thinking	Immature behavior	

Maturational
Child
Related to protective isolation or a communicable disease

Older Adult
Related to loss of usual social contacts

> ◑ **AUTHOR'S NOTE**
>
> In 1994, NANDA added a new diagnosis, *Risk for Loneliness.* Although this diagnosis is only in stage I of a four-stage developmental process, it more accurately adheres to the NANDA definition of "response to." Social isolation is not a response but a cause or contributing factor to loneliness. In addition, a person can experience loneliness even with many people around. This author recommends deleting *Social Isolation* from clinical use and using *Loneliness* or *Risk for Loneliness.*

CHRONIC SORROW

DEFINITION
Chronic Sorrow: State in which a person experiences, or is at risk to experience, permanent pervasive psychic pain and sadness, variable in intensity, in response to a loved one forever changed by an event or condition and the ongoing loss of normalcy (Teel, 1991)

DEFINING CHARACTERISTICS
Major (Must be Present, One or More)
Lifelong episodic sadness to loss of a loved one or loss of normalcy in a loved one who is disabled
Variable intensity

Minor (May be Present)

Anger	Frustration	Fear
Helplessness		

RELATED FACTORS
Situational (Personal, Environmental)
Related to the chronic loss of normalcy secondary to a child's or adult child's condition

Autism	Severe scoliosis	Chronic psychiatric condition
Down syndrome	Mental retardation	Spina bifida
Sickle cell disease	Type I diabetes mellitus	Human immunodeficiency virus (HIV)

Related to lifetime losses associated with infertility
Related to ongoing losses associated with a degenerative condition (eg, multiple sclerosis, Alzheimer's disease)
Related to loss of loved one
Related to losses associated with caring for a child with fatal illness

---

◎ AUTHOR'S NOTE

Olchansky identified *Chronic Sorrow* in 1962. Chronic sorrow differs from grieving, which is time-limited and ends in adaptation to the loss. Chronic sorrow varies in intensity but persists as long as the person with the disability or chronic condition lives (Burke et al., 1992). Chronic sorrow also can accompany the loss of a child. It can also occur with an individual who suffers from a chronic disease that regularly impairs his or her ability to live a "normal life" (e.g., paraplegic, AIDS, sickle cell disease).

◎ ERRORS IN DIAGNOSTIC STATEMENTS

Chronic Sorrow related to recent death of sister
   Chronic Sorrow is related to ongoing losses secondary to loss of normalcy. This loss of normalcy can be related to a loved one with a condition that makes a certain relationship impossible. Death of a parent, sibling, or child can affect a person through his or her lifetime. The response to this loss initially can be grieving; however, over time the person may continue to experience pervasive psychic pain. This response can be either *Chronic Sorrow* or *Dysfunctional Grieving*. Careful assessment and discussion can help the nurse differentiate the two.

KEY CONCEPTS

- Chronic sorrow can be described as an "ongoing funeral," because there is no psychological closure or opportunity for resolution (Lindgren et al., 1992; Northington, 2000).
- Chronic sorrow is cyclic or recurrent. It is triggered by situations that bring to mind the person's losses, disappointments, or fears (Lindgren et al., 1992).
- Chronic mental illness produces a situation with no predictable end to the loss experience (Eakes, 1995; Mohr, 2003).
- Chronic sorrow is a functional coping response. It is normal, unlike pathologic grief or depression (Burke et al., 1992).
- Response to the death of a loved one could be chronic sorrow. For example, the death of a woman in her 30s could evoke a chronic sorrow response in a surviving sister.
- When a child is disabled, the initial response from the parent will be anxiety, family disorganization, denial, and grief. Then the parent will seek outside help. Unlike grief responses to death, which have some form of closure, parents with *Chronic Sorrow* reexperience the grief response periodically (Kearney & Griffin, 2001).
- When a loved one becomes inaccessible emotionally or cognitively, there are daily reminders of the lost relationship (Teel, 1991). Many situations can trigger recognition of the loss of a hoped-for relationship, such as a school play, school dances, family vacations, and dating.
- Mallow and Bechtel (1999) found mothers of disabled children responded with chronic sorrow, whereas fathers responded with resignation.
- Parents with children with a developmental disability experience joy and sorrow, hope and no hope, and defiance and despair (Kearney & Griffin, 2001).

Focus Assessment Criteria

Subjective Data

Assess for Defining Characteristics.

Perception/coping
Perception of child's abilities, language skills, motor skills, social skills, friendships, self-care abilities, past/recent illnesses (Melnyk et al., 2001)
Barriers to coping (Melnyk, et al., 2001)
Interfamily relationships
Social support
Financial issues, employment
Changes/stressors in family

For more information on Focus Assessment Criteria, visit http://connection.lww.com.

Goal

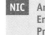 **NOC** Depression Control, Coping, Mood Management, Acceptance: Health Status,

The person will be assisted to anticipate developmental events that can trigger heightened sadness.

Indicators

- Express sadness.
- Discuss the losses periodically.

General Interventions

NIC Anticipatory Guidance, Coping Enhancement, Referral, Active Listening, Presence, Resiliency Promotion

Explain Chronic Sorrow.

Normal response
Focus on loss of normalcy
Not time-limited
Persists throughout life

Encourage Client to Share Feelings Since the Change (eg, Birth of Child, Accident).

Prepare client for subsequent crises over the life span.

Gently encourage client to share lost dreams or hopes.
Assist client to identify developmental milestones that will exacerbate the loss of normalcy (eg, school play, sports, prom, dating).
Clarify that feelings will fluctuate (intense, diminished) over the years, but the sorrow will not disappear.
Advise client that these crises may feel like the first response to the "news."

Encourage Participation in Support Groups with Others Experiencing Chronic Sorrow and Expression of Grief.

Stress the importance of maintaining support systems and friendships.
Share the difficulties of (Monsen, 1999):
   Living worried
   Treating child like other children
   Staying in the struggle

Acknowledge that Parent(s) is the Child's Expert Caregiver (Melnyk et Al., 2001).

Elicit routines from parent.
Prepare family for transition to another health care provider (eg, child to adult providers).
Educate parent about specific procedures.

Link the Family with Appropriate Services (eg, Home Health, Respite Counselor).

Refer to *Caregiver Role Strain* for Additional Interventions.

Rationales

- Families report that open, honest communication is beneficial. They need to know what to expect to help reduce life span crises (Eakes, 1995).
- Parents can learn successful coping mechanisms and prevent social isolation from other parents undergoing a similar experience.
- Monsen (1999) reported that parents of children with spina bifida had a pattern of coping that encompassed living worried, trying to treat the child like other children, and staying strong over the long haul.

Spiritual Distress
  Related to Conflict Between Religious or Spiritual Beliefs and Prescribed Health Regimen
  Related to (Specify), as Evidenced by Inability to Practice Spiritual Rituals
Risk for Spiritual Distress
Readiness for Enhanced Spiritual Well-Being
Impaired Religiosity
Risk for Impaired Religiosity

SPIRITUAL DISTRESS

DEFINITION
Spiritual Distress: State in which a person or group experiences a disturbance in the belief or value system that provides strength, hope, and meaning to life

DEFINING CHARACTERISTICS
Major (Must Be Present)
Experiences a disturbance in belief system

Minor (May Be Present)
Questions meaning of life, death, suffering
Questions credibility of belief system
Demonstrates discouragement or despair
Chooses not to practice usual religious rituals
Has ambivalent feelings (doubts) about beliefs
Expresses that he or she has no reason for living
Feels a sense of spiritual emptiness
Shows emotional detachment from self and others
Expresses concern—anger, resentment, fear—over meaning of life, suffering, death
Requests spiritual assistance for a disturbance in belief system

RELATED FACTORS
Pathophysiologic
Related to challenge to belief system or separation from spiritual ties secondary to:

Loss of body part or function	Pain	Terminal illness
Trauma	Debilitating disease	Miscarriage, stillbirth

Treatment-Related
Related to conflict between (specify prescribed regimen) and beliefs

Abortion	Isolation	Surgery
Amputation	Blood transfusion	Medications
Dietary restrictions	Medical procedures	

Situational (Personal, Environmental)
Related to death or illness of significant other
Related to embarrassment at practicing spiritual rituals
Related to barriers to practicing spiritual rituals

Restrictions of intensive care	Lack of privacy
Unavailability of special foods/diet	Confinement to bed or room

Related to beliefs opposed by family, peers, health care providers
Related to divorce, separation from loved one

⊙⊙ AUTHOR'S NOTE

Wellness represents a response to a person's potential for personal growth, involving use of all of a person's resources (social, psychological, cultural, environmental, spiritual, and physiologic). Nurses profess to care for the whole client, but several studies report that they commonly avoid addressing the spiritual dimension of clients, families, and communities (Kendrick & Robinson, 2000).

To promote positive spirituality with clients and families, the nurse must possess positive spirituality. for the nurse, self-evaluation must precede assessment of spiritual concerns, and assessment of spiritual health should be confined to the context of nursing. The nurse can assist people with spiritual concerns or distress by providing resources for spiritual help, by listening nonjudgmentally, and by providing opportunities for meeting spiritual needs (Stoll, 1984). The nurse should be cautioned against establishing practice patterns that routinely result in referring all spiritual needs of clients and families to religious or spiritual leaders.

Spirituality and religiousness are two different concepts. Burkhart and Solari-Twadell define spirituality as the "ability to experience and integrate meaning and self; others, art, music, literature, nature, or a power greater than oneself" (2001, p. 51). Religiousness is "the ability to exercise participation in the beliefs of a particular denomination of faith community and related rituals" (Burkhart & Solari-Twadell, 2001, p. 51). They can coexist and also exist separately.

Impaired Religiousness was approved by NANDA in 2004. This diagnosis can be used for *Spiritual Distress* when a person has a barrier to practicing his or her religious rituals that the nurse can assist by decreasing or removing. *Impaired Religiosity* would be appropriate.

If a person cannot practice his or her religious rituals, and the nurse cannot alter this situation, *Spiritual Distress* may be more appropriate.

⊙⊙ ERRORS IN DIAGNOSTIC STATEMENTS

Spiritual Distress related to critical illness and doubts about religious beliefs

Critical illness can challenge a person's spiritual beliefs and evoke feelings of guilt, anger, disappointment, and helplessness. Critical illness, however, does not represent a specific contributing factor or cue to spiritual distress. Until related factors are known, the nurse can record the diagnosis as *Spiritual Distress related to unknown etiology, as evidenced by expressions of doubt about religious beliefs.* The nursing focus will be on actively listening to the person's feelings and fears.

KEY CONCEPTS
Generic Considerations

- All people have a spiritual dimension, regardless of whether they participate in formal religious practices (Burkhardt, 1994; Carson, 1999). An individual is a spiritual person even when disoriented, confused, emotionally ill, irrational, or cognitively impaired.
- The nurse must consider the client's spiritual nature as part of total care, along with the physical and psychosocial dimensions. Research indicates that most clients feel religion is very important in times of crisis (Kendrick & Robinson, 2000).
- The spiritual may include, but is not limited to, religion; spiritual needs include religion, values, relationships, transcendence, and affective feeling and communication (Emblen & Halstead, 1993); creativity and self-expression also may be important to spirituality (Wald & Bailey, 1990). Other descriptions of spirituality include inner strength, meaning and purpose, and knowing and becoming (Burkhardt, 1994).
- Health care systems often give spiritual concerns low priority in care planning and delivery. This is less true in hospice organizations, where the spiritual component of care is more likely to be recognized and included (Millison, 1995).
- Religion influences attitudes and behavior related to right and wrong, family, child-rearing, work, money, politics, and many other functional areas.

- To deal effectively with a person's spiritual needs, the nurse must recognize his or her own beliefs and values, acknowledge that these values may not be applicable to others, and respect the client's beliefs when helping him or her to meet perceived spiritual needs.
- The value of prayers or spiritual rituals to the believer is not affected by whether they can be scientifically "proved" to be beneficial.
- Research indicates that many nurses feel inadequately prepared to provide spiritual care, and that fewer than 15% include spirituality in nursing care (Piles, 1990). "Among the reasons that nurses fail to provide spiritual care are the following: (1) They view religious and spiritual needs as a private matter concerning only an individual and his/her Creator; (2) they are uncomfortable about their own religious beliefs or deny having spiritual needs; (3) they lack knowledge about spirituality and the religious beliefs of others; (4) they mistake spiritual needs for psychosocial needs; and (5) they view meeting the spiritual needs of clients as a family or pastoral responsibility, not a nursing responsibility" (Andrews & Boyle, 2003, p. 402).
- To assist people in spiritual distress, the nurse must know certain beliefs and practices of various spiritual groups. Table II.25 provides information on the beliefs and practices that relate most directly to health and illness. It is intended as a reference only. Major religions, denominations, and spiritual groups are arranged alphabetically. Denominations with similar practices and restrictions are grouped together. No attempt is made to discuss the broad beliefs and philosophies of the selected groups; see References/Bibliography for texts supplying such in-depth information.

Pediatric Considerations

- Children's spiritual needs include love and relatedness, forgiveness, meaning, and purpose.
- Moral and cognitive development influence spiritual beliefs (Wong, 2003).
- Children learn faith and religion from the practices of parents/significant others (Wong, 2003).

Geriatric Considerations

- The White House Council on Aging in 1971 described spiritual concerns as "the human need to deal with sociocultural deprivations, anxieties and fears, death and dying, social alienation, and philosophy of life" (Moberg, 1984; Ryan, 1985).
- The National Interfaith Coalition on Aging describes spiritual well-being as the affirmation of life in a relationship with God, self, community, and environment that nurtures and celebrates wholeness (Ryan & Patterson, 1987).
- Factors that contribute to spiritual distress and put older adults at risk include questions concerning life after death as the person ages, separation from formal religious community, and a value–belief system that is continuously challenged by losses and suffering.
- About 75% of all older adults are members of religious organizations. This does not necessarily mean that they attend their formal services and meetings regularly (Miller, 2004).
- Older people tend to participate in formal religious groups more than younger people. Participation increases dramatically with age, and the desire to participate in church activities remains constant throughout their lives. Older people may find religious services difficult to attend and participate in owing to physical impairments. Factors such as lack of transportation, inaccessible toileting facilities, poor acoustics and sound systems for hearing-impaired, and small-print hymn books or prayer books can diminish active involvement in formal religious activities.
- Older adults must complete Erikson's developmental stage of Ego Integrity versus Despair to achieve life satisfaction. They may reflect on their lives, expressing contentment that they have lived in accordance with their value system. These behaviors demonstrate fulfillment of the need for meaning and purpose in life.
- Those who have not sought religion early in life will not automatically become more religious in later life.

(continued)

- A common coping method for older adults, prayer increases feelings of self-worth and hope by reducing sense of aloneness and abandonment. In addition to private prayer and meditation, television and radio often provide adjunct stimuli for spiritual life. Estimates indicate that 60% of viewers of religious television programs are older than 50 years and are primarily women (Bearon & Koenig, 1990).
- Older adults may rely on spiritual life more than most young people because of other limitations in their lives. The spiritual realm allows for satisfying connectedness with others. An older person can counterbalance some of the negative, isolating aspects of aging by identifying with tradition and institutional values. Private religion can help to motivate and provide purpose to life.
- Older adults commonly intertwine their religious beliefs with beliefs about health and illness. The nurse must assess these beliefs appropriately to facilitate the person's understanding of his illness in the context of his religion.

TABLE II.25 Overview of Religious Beliefs

Agnostic
Beliefs
It is impossible to know if God exists (specific moral values may guide behavior)

Amish
Illness
Usually taken care of within family

Texts
Bible; Ausbund (16th-century German hymnal)

Beliefs
Rejection of all government aid; rejection of modernization
Legally exempt from immunizations

Armenian
See Eastern Orthodox

Atheist
Beliefs
God does not exist (specific moral values may guide behavior)

Baha'i
Illness
Religion and science are both important
Usual hospital routines and treatments are usually acceptable

Death
Burial mandatory; interment near place of death

Beliefs
Purpose of religion is to promote harmony and peace
Education very important

Baptist, Churches of God, Churches of Christ, and Pentecostal (Assemblies of God, Foursquare Church)
Illness
Some practice laying on of hands, divine healing through prayer
May request Communion
Some prohibit medical therapy
May consider illness divine punishment or intrusion of Satan

Diet
No alcohol (mandatory for most); no coffee, tea, tobacco, pork, or strangled animals (mandatory for some)
Some fasting

Birth
Oppose infant baptism

Text
Bible

Beliefs
Some practice glossolalia (speaking in tongues)

Buddhism
Illness
Considered trial that develops the soul

(table continues on page 742)

(text continues on page 747)

TABLE II.25 Overview of Religious Beliefs (Continued)

May wish counseling by priest
May refuse treatment on holy days (1/1, 1/16, 2/15, 3/21, 4/8, 5/21, 6/15, 8/1, 8/23, 12/8, 12/31)

Diet
Strict vegetarianism (mandatory for some)
Use of alcohol, tobacco, and drugs discouraged

Death
Last-rite chanting by priest
Death leads to rebirth; may wish to remain alert and lucid

Texts
Buddha's sermon on the "eightfold path"; the Tripitaka, or "three baskets" of wisdom

Beliefs
Cleanliness is of great importance
Suffering is universal

Christian Science
Illness
Caused by errors in thought and mind
May oppose drugs; IV fluid; blood transfusions; psychotherapy; hypnotism; physical examinations; biopsies; eye, ear, and blood pressure screening; and other medical and nursing interventions
Accept only legally required immunizations
May desire support from a Christian Science reader or treatment by a Christian Science nurse or practitioner (a list of these nonmedical practitioners and nurses may be found in the *Christian Science Journal*)
Healing is spiritual renewal

Death
Autopsy permitted only in cases of sudden death

Text
Bible; *Science and Health With Key to the Scriptures* by Mary Baker Eddy

Church of Christ
See Baptist

Church of God
See Baptist

Confucian
Illness
The body was given by one's parents and should therefore be well cared for
May be strongly motivated to maintain or regain wellness

Beliefs
Respect for family and older people very important

Cults (Variety of Groups, Usually With Living Leader)
Illness
Most practice faith healing.
May reject modern medicine and condemn health personnel as enemies
Therapeutic compliance and follow-up are usually poor
Illness may represent wrong thinking or inhabitation by Satan

Beliefs
Expansion of cult through conversions important
May depend on cult environment for definition of reality

Eastern Orthodox (Greek Orthodox, Russian Orthodox, Armenian)
Illness
May desire Holy Communion, laying on of hands, anointing, or sacrament of Holy Unction
Most oppose euthanasia and favor every effort to preserve life
Russian Orthodox men should be shaved only if necessary for surgery

Diet
May fast Wednesdays, Fridays, during Lent, before Christmas, or for 6 hours before Communion (seriously ill are exempted)
May avoid meat, dairy products, and olive oil during fast (seriously ill are exempted)

Birth
Baptism 8–40 days after birth, usually by immersion (mandatory for some)
May be followed immediately by confirmation
    Greek Orthodox only: If death of infant is imminent, nurse should baptize infant by touching the forehead with a small amount of water three times

(*table continues on page 743*)

TABLE II.25 Overview of Religious Beliefs (Continued)

Death
Last rites and administration of Holy Communion (mandatory for some)
May oppose autopsy, embalming, and cremation

Texts
Bible; prayer book

Religious Articles
Icons (pictures of Jesus, Mary, saints) are very important
Holy water and lighted candles
Russian Orthodox wears cross necklace that should be removed only if necessary

Other
Greek Orthodox opposes abortion
Confession at least yearly (mandatory for some)
Holy Communion four times yearly: Christmas, Easter, 6/30, and 8/15 (mandatory for some)
Dates of holy days may differ from Western Christian calendar

Episcopal
Illness
May believe in spiritual healing; may desire confession and Communion

Diet
May abstain from meat on Fridays; may fast during Lent or before Communion

Birth
Infant baptism is mandatory (nurse may baptize infant when death is imminent by pouring water on forehead and saying, "I baptize you in the name of the Father, the Son, and the Holy Spirit")

Death
Last rites optional

Texts
Bible; prayer book

Friends (Quaker)
No minister or priests; direct, individual, inner experience of God is vital

Diet
Most avoid alcohol and drugs and favor practice of moderation

Death
Many do not believe in afterlife

Beliefs
Pacifism important; many are conscientious objectors to war

Greek Orthodox
See Eastern Orthodox

Hinduism
Illness
May minimize illness and emphasize its temporary nature
Viewed as result of karma (actions/fate) of previous life
Caused by body and spirit not being in harmony or by tension in interpersonal relationships
Belief in healing responses triggered by treatment
Strong belief in alternative healing practices (eg, herbal treatments, faith healing)

Diet
Various doctrines, many vegetarian; many abstain from alcohol (mandatory for some); beef and pork are forbidden; prefer fresh, cooked foods

Death
Believe in immortality of the soul
Seen as rebirth; may wish to be alert; chant prayer
Priest may tie sacred thread around neck or wrist, or body—do not remove
Water is poured into mouth, and family washes body
Cremation preferred—must be soon after death

Beliefs
Physical, mental, and spiritual discipline, and purification of body and soul emphasized
Believe in the world as a manifestation of *Brahman,* one divine being pervading all things

Texts

Vedas	Ramayana
Upanishads	Mahabharata
Bhagavad-Gita	Puranas

(table continues on page 744)

TABLE II.25 Overview of Religious Beliefs (Continued)

Worship
Daily prayers, usually in home; quiet meditation
Rituals may include use of water, fire, lights, sounds, natural objects, special postures, and gestures

Jehovah's Witness
Illness
Oppose blood transfusions and organ transplantation (mandatory)
May oppose other medical treatments and all modern science
Oppose faith healing; oppose abortion

Diet
Refuses foods to which blood has been added; may eat meats that have been drained

Text
Bible

Judaism
Illness
Medical care emphasized
Rabbinical consultation necessary for donation and transplantation of organs
May oppose surgical procedures on the Sabbath (sundown Friday to sundown Saturday); seriously ill are exempted
May prefer burial of removed organs or body tissues
May oppose shaving
May wear skull cap and socks continuously, believing head and feet should be covered

Diet
Fasting for 24 hours on holy days of Yom Kippur (in September or October) and Tishah-b'Ab (in August)
Matzo replaces leavened bread during Passover week (in March or April)
May observe strict Kosher dietary laws (mandatory for some) that prohibit pork, shellfish, and the eating of meat and dairy products at same meal or with same dishes (milk products, served first, can be followed by meat in a few minutes; reverse is not Kosher); seriously ill are exempted

Birth
Ritual circumcision 8 days after birth (mandatory for some); fetuses are buried

Death
Ritual burial; society members wash body
Burial as soon as possible
May oppose cremation
Many oppose autopsy and donation of body to science
Most do not believe in afterlife
Generally oppose prolongation of life after irreversible brain damage

Texts
Torah (first five books of Old Testament)
Talmud
Prayer book

Religious Articles
Menorah (seven-branched candlestick)
Yarmulke (skull cap, may be worn continuously)
Tallith (prayer shawl worn for morning prayers)
Tefillin, or phylacteries (leather boxes on straps containing scripture passages)
Star of David (may be worn around neck)

Beliefs
Observation of the Sabbath (Friday evening to Saturday evening) may require not writing, traveling, using electrical appliances, or receiving treatment

Krishna
Diet
Vegetarian diet; no garlic or onions
No drugs, alcohol; herbal tea only

Death
Cremation mandatory

Texts
Vedas
Srimad-Bhagavatam

Beliefs
Continual practice of mantra (chant)
Belief in reincarnation

(table continues on page 745)

TABLE II.25 Overview of Religious Beliefs (Continued)

Lutheran, Methodist, Presbyterian
Illness
May request Communion, anointing and blessing, or visitation by minister or elder
Generally encourages use of medical science

Birth
Baptism by sprinkling or immersion of infants, children, or adults

Death
Optional last rites or scripture reading

Texts
Bible; prayer book

Mennonite
Illness
Opposes laying on of hands; may oppose shock treatment and drugs

Texts
Bible; 18 articles of the Dondecht Confession of Faith

Beliefs
Shun modernization; no participation in government, pensions, or health plans

Methodist
See Lutheran

Mormon (Church of Jesus Christ of Latter-Day Saints)
Illness
May come through partaking of harmful substances such as alcohol, tobacco, drugs, and so forth
May be seen as a necessary part of the plan of salvation
May desire Sacrament of the Lord's Supper to be administered by a Church Priesthood holder
Divine healing through laying on of hands
Church may provide financial support during illness

Diet
Prohibits alcohol, tobacco, and hot drinks (tea and coffee); sparing use of meats

Birth
No infant baptism; infants are born innocent

Death
Cremation is opposed

Texts
Bible; Book of Mormon

Religious Articles
Special undergarment may be worn by both men and women and should not be removed except during serious illness, childbirth, emergencies, and so forth

Beliefs
Abortion is opposed
Vicarious baptism for deceased who were not baptized in life

Muslim (Islamic, Moslem) and Black Muslim
Illness
Opposes faith healing; favors every effort to prolong life
May be noncompliant because of fatalistic view (illness is God's will)
Group prayer may be helpful—no priests

Diet
Pork prohibited
May oppose alcohol and traditional black American foods (corn bread, collard greens)
Fasts sunrise to sunset during Ramadan (9th month of Muslim year—falls different time each year on Western calendar); seriously ill are exempted

Birth
Circumcision practiced with accompanying ceremony
Aborted fetus after 30 days is treated as human being

Death
Confession of sins before death, with family present if possible; may wish to face toward Mecca
Family follows specific procedure for washing and preparing body, which is then turned to face Mecca
May oppose autopsy and organ transplantation
Funeral usually within 24 hours after death

Texts
Koran (scriptures); Hadith (traditions)

(table continues on page 746)

TABLE II.25 Overview of Religious Beliefs (Continued)

Prayer
Five times daily—on rising, midday, afternoon, early evening, and before bed—facing Mecca and kneeling on prayer rug
Ritual washing after prayer

Beliefs
All activities (including sleep) restricted to what is necessary for health
Personal cleanliness very important
All Muslims: gambling and idol worship prohibited

Pentecostal
See Baptist

Presbyterian
See Lutheran

Quakers
See Friends

Roman Catholic
Illness
Allowed by God because of man's sins, but not considered personal punishment
May desire confession (penance) and Communion
Anointing of sick for all seriously ill patients (some patients may equate this with "Last Rites" and assume they are dying)
Donation and transplantation of organs permitted
Burial of amputated limbs (mandatory for some)

Diet
Fasting or abstaining from meat mandatory on Ash Wednesday and Good Friday (seriously ill are exempted); optional during Lent and on Fridays
Fasts from solid food for 1 hour and abstains from alcohol for 3 hours before receiving Communion (mandatory; seriously ill are exempted)

Birth
Baptism of infants and aborted fetuses mandatory (nurse may baptize in case of imminent death by sprinkling water on the forehead and saying, "I baptize you in the name of the Father, of the Son, and of the Holy Ghost")

Death
Anointing of sick (mandatory)
Extraordinary artificial means of sustaining life are unnecessary

Texts
Bible; prayer book

Religious Articles
Rosary, crucifix, saints' medals, statues, holy water, lighted candles

Other
Attendance at mass required (seriously ill are exempted) on Sundays or late Saturday and on holy days (1/1, 8/15, 11/1, 12/8, 12/25, and 40 days after Easter)
Sacrament of Penance at least yearly (mandatory); opposes abortion

Russian Orthodox
See Eastern Orthodox

Seventh-Day Adventist (Advent Christian Church)
Illness
May desire baptism or Communion
Some believe in divine healing
May oppose hypnosis
May refuse treatment on the Sabbath (sundown Friday to sundown Saturday)
Healthful diet and lifestyle are stressed

Diet
No alcohol, coffee, tea, narcotics, or stimulants (mandatory)
Some abstain from pork, other meat, and shellfish

Birth
Opposes infant baptism

Text
Bible, especially Ten Commandments and Old Testament

Shinto
Illness

(table continues on page 747)

TABLE II.25 Overview of Religious Beliefs (Continued)

May believe in prayer healing
Great concern for personal cleanliness
Physical health may be valued because of emphasis on joy and beauty of life
Family extremely important in giving care and providing emotional support

Beliefs
Worships ancestors, ancient heroes, and nature
Traditions emphasized; aesthetically pleasing area for worship important

Sikhism
Diet
Frequently vegetarian; may exclude eggs and fish

Religious Articles
Men may wear uncut hair, a wooden comb, an iron wrist band, a short sword, and short trousers. These symbols should not be disturbed.

Death
Cremation mandatory, usually within 24 hours after death

Text
Guru Grant Sahab

Taoist
Illness
Illness is seen as part of the health/illness dualism
May be resigned to and accepting of illness
May consider medical treatment as interference

Death
Seen as natural part of life; body is kept in house for 49 days
Mourning follows specific ritual patterns

Text
Tao-te-ching by Lao-tzu

Beliefs
Aesthetically pleasing area for meditation important

Unitarian Universalist
Illness
Reason, knowledge, and individual responsibility are emphasized, so may prefer not to see clergy

Birth
Most do not practice infant baptism

Death
Prefer cremation

Zen
Meditation using lotus position (many hours and years are spent in meditation and contemplation): goal is to discover simplicity

Illness
May wish consultation with Zen master

🌐 Transcultural Considerations

- Religious beliefs, an integral component of culture, may influence a client's explanation of the causes of illness, perception of its severity, and choice of healer. In times of crisis, such as serious illness and impending death, religion may be a source of consolation for the client and family and may influence the course of action believed to be appropriate (Andrews & Boyle, 2003).
- Belonging to a specific cultural group does not imply that the person subscribes to that culture's dominant religion. In addition, even when a person identifies with a particular religion, he or she may not accept all its beliefs or practices (Andrews & Boyle, 2003).
- The nurse's role is not "to judge the religious virtues of individuals but rather to understand" those aspects related to religion that are important to the client and family members (Andrews & Boyle, 2003, p. 142). Table II-26 was compiled with the intent to assist nurses with this understanding.

Focus Assessment Criteria

Subjective Data
Assess for Defining Characteristics.

What is your source of spiritual strength or meaning?
What is your source of peace, comfort, faith, well-being, hope, or worth?
How do you practice your spiritual beliefs?
Are any practices important for your spiritual well-being?
Do you have a spiritual leader?
Has being ill or hurt affected your spiritual beliefs?

Assess for Related Factors.

How can I help you maintain your spiritual strength (eg, contact spiritual leader, provide privacy at special times, request reading materials)?

Objective Data
Assess for Defining Characteristics.

Current practices
Any religious or spiritual articles (clothing, medals, texts)
Visits from spiritual leader
Visits to place of worship or meditation
Requests for spiritual counseling or assistance

Response to interview on spiritual needs

Grief	Doubt	Anxiety
Anger		

Participation in spiritual practices
Rejection or neglect of previous practices
Increased interest in spiritual matters

For more information on Focus Assessment Criteria, visit http://connection.lww.com.

Goal

 Hope, Spiritual Well-Being

The person will describe satisfaction with meaning and purpose of illness/suffering/death.

Indicators
- Express his or her feelings related to change in beliefs.
- Describe spiritual belief system positively.
- Express desire to perform religious/spiritual practices.

General Interventions

 Spiritual Growth Facilitation, Hope Instillation, Active Listening, Presence, Emotional Support, Spiritual Support

Assess for Causative and Contributing Factors.

Failure of spiritual beliefs to provide explanation or comfort during crisis of illness/suffering/impending death
Doubting quality or strength of own faith to deal with current crisis
Anger toward God or spiritual beliefs for allowing or causing illness/suffering/death

Eliminate or Reduce Causative and Contributing Factors, if Possible.

Feeling Threatened and Vulnerable Because of Symptoms or Possible Death
Inform clients and families about the importance of finding meaning in illness.
Suggest using prayer, imagery, and meditation to view selves as survivors rather than victims.

Failure of Spiritual Beliefs to Provide Explanation or Comfort During Crisis of Illness/Suffering/Impending Death
Communicate your concern seriously by being available to listen to feelings, questions, and so forth.

Give "permission" to discuss spiritual matters with nurse by bringing up subject of spiritual welfare, if necessary.

Use questions about past beliefs and spiritual experiences to assist person to put this life event into wider perspective.

Assist person to begin problem-solving process and move toward new spiritual understandings, if necessary.

Offer to contact usual or new spiritual leader.

Offer to pray/meditate/read with client if you are comfortable with this, or arrange for another member of health care team if more appropriate.

Provide uninterrupted quiet time for prayer/reading/meditation on spiritual concerns.

Doubting Quality of Own Faith to Deal with Current Illness/Suffering/Death

Be available and willing to listen when client expresses self-doubt, guilt, or other negative feelings.

Silence, touch, or both may be useful in communicating the nurse's presence and support during times of doubt or despair.

Suggest process of "life review" to identify past sources of strength or spiritual support.

Suggest guided imagery or meditation to reinforce faith/beliefs.

Offer to contact usual or new spiritual leader.

Anger Toward God or Spiritual Beliefs for Allowing or Causing Illness/Suffering/Death

Express to person that anger toward God is a common reaction to illness/suffering/death.

Help client recognize and discuss feelings of anger.

Allow client to problem solve to find ways to express and relieve anger.

Offer to contact usual spiritual leader.

Offer to contact other spiritual support person (eg, pastoral care, hospital chaplain) if person cannot share feelings with usual spiritual leader.

Engage in Spiritual Listening (Cameron 1998).

Avoid lecturing, criticizing, and giving advice.

Avoid using religious dogma as responses.

Use nondirective communication techniques.

Help person to determine what is right for them.

Rationales

- The client may view anger at God and a religious leader as "forbidden" and may be reluctant to initiate discussions of spiritual conflicts.
- Spirituality influences attitudes and behavior related to right and wrong, family, child-rearing, work, money, politics, and many other functional areas.
- According to Stoll (1984, p. 347), "prayer, private or with a significant other, is overwhelmingly reported as the most meaningful spiritual coping strategy and religious practice."
- The nature of the spiritual care a person receives may directly affect the speed and quality of recovery, or the quality of the dying experience.
- The physical environment often influences spirituality, so nurses should provide appropriate settings whenever possible, considering such aspects as quiet, nature, music, art, and the like.
- Research shows that people with higher levels of spiritual well-being tend to experience lower levels of anxiety. For many people, spiritual activities provide a direct coping action (Sodestrom & Martinson, 1987) and may improve adaptation to illness (Carson & Green, 1992).
- The nurse should function as an advocate in recognizing and respecting the client's spiritual needs, which other health professionals may sometimes overlook or ignore.
- Hinton (1999) found that a person's acceptance of impending death was related to the inevitability of death, faith and spiritual values, completing life, belief's diminishing rewards, and sharing.
- People with advanced human immunodeficiency virus (HIV) cleared their life of stressful and meaningless aspects and embraced those that strengthened their faith and defined personal meaning (Corbett, 1998).

Pediatric Interventions

Encourage children to maintain bedtime or before-meal prayer rituals.
If compatible with the child's religious beliefs:
>   Share religious picture book and other religious articles.
>   Consult with family for appropriate books or objects (eg, medals, statues).
>   Explore child's feelings regarding illness as punishment for wrongdoing (Wong, 2003).

Rationales

- Continuance of usual activities can help the child cope with threatening situations (Wong, 2003).
- Because US society has a Judeo-Christian orientation, the nurse must be sensitive to other religious backgrounds (eg, Buddhist, Hindu, Islamic).
- Often children view illness or injury as punishment for real or imagined wrongdoing (Wong, 2003).

SPIRITUAL DISTRESS

RELATED TO CONFLICT BETWEEN RELIGIOUS OR SPIRITUAL BELIEFS AND PRESCRIBED HEALTH REGIMEN

Goal

NOC See *Spiritual Distress*

The person will express religious or spiritual satisfaction.

Indicators

- Express decreased feelings of guilt and fear.
- Relate that he or she is supported in decisions about his or her health regimen.
- State that conflict has been eliminated or reduced.

General Interventions

NIC See *Spiritual Distress*

Assess for Causative and Contributing Factors (See Table II-26).

Lack of information about or understanding of spiritual restrictions
Lack of information about or understanding of health regimen
Informed, true conflict
Parental conflict concerning treatment of child
Lack of time for deliberation before emergency treatment or surgery

Eliminate or Reduce Causative and Contributing Factors, if Possible.

Lack of Information About Spiritual Restrictions

Have spiritual leader discuss restrictions and exemptions as they apply to those who are seriously ill or hospitalized.
Provide reading materials on religious and spiritual restrictions and exemptions.

Encourage person to seek information from and discuss restrictions with others in spiritual group. Chart results of these discussions.

Lack of Information About Health Regimen

Provide accurate information about health regimen, treatments, and medications.

Explain the nature and purpose of therapy.

Discuss possible outcomes without therapy; be factual and honest, but do not attempt to frighten or force person to accept treatment.

Informed, True Conflict

Encourage client and physician to consider alternative methods of therapy* (eg, use of Christian Science nurses and practitioners; special surgeons and techniques for surgery without blood transfusions).

Support client making informed decision—even if decision conflicts with own values.

Consult own spiritual leader.

Change assignment so a nurse with compatible beliefs can care for the person.

Arrange for discussions among health care team to share feelings.

Parental Conflict Over Treatment of Child

If parents refuse treatment of child, follow interventions under informed conflict above.

If parents still refuse treatment, physician or hospital administrator may obtain court order appointing temporary guardian to consent to treatment.

Call spiritual leader to support parents (and possibly child).

Encourage expression of negative feelings.

Emergency Treatment

Consult family if possible.

Delay treatment, if possible, until spiritual needs have been met (eg, receiving last rites before surgery)*; send spiritual leader to treatment room or operating room, if necessary.

Anticipate reaction and provide support when person chooses or is forced to accept spiritually unacceptable therapy.

Depression, withdrawal, anger, fear

Loss of will to live

Reduced speed and quality of recovery

Rationales

- The nurse's role is as an advocate for the family.
- Interventions focus on providing information about all alternatives and the consequences of each option.
- The nurse should be the link between the family and other members of the health care team.
- Court orders to save a child's life remove the parent's right to refuse (Wong, 2003).

---

*May require a primary care professional's order.

RISK FOR SPIRITUAL DISTRESS

DEFINITION

Risk for Spiritual Distress: State in which a person or group is at risk of experiencing a disturbance in their belief or value system that provides strength, hope, and meaning to life

RISK FACTORS

See *Spiritual Distress*.

⊗ AUTHOR'S NOTE

See *Spiritual Distress*.

⊗ ERRORS IN DIAGNOSTIC STATEMENTS

See *Spiritual Distress*.

KEY CONCEPTS

See *Spiritual Distress*.

Goal

NOC Hope, Spiritual Well-Being

The person will continue to express satisfaction with belief system.

Indicators

- Practice spiritual rituals.
- Express comfort with beliefs.

General Interventions

See *Spiritual Distress*.

READINESS FOR ENHANCED SPIRITUAL WELL-BEING

DEFINITION

Readiness for Enhanced Spiritual Well-Being: A person who experiences affirmation of life in a relationship with a higher power (as defined by the person), self, community, and environment that nurtures and celebrates wholeness

DEFINING CHARACTERISTICS (CARSON, 1999)

Inner strength that nurtures

Sense of awareness	Sacred source	Trust relationships
Inner peace	Unifying force	

Intangible motivation and commitment directed toward ultimate values of love, meaning, hope, beauty, and truth

Trust relations with or in the transcendent that provide bases for meaning and hope in life's experiences and love in one's relationships

Has meaning and purpose to existence

RISK FACTORS

Refer to Related Factors.

RELATED FACTORS

Because this is a diagnosis of positive functioning, the use of related factors is not warranted.

> ### 🔗 AUTHOR'S NOTE
>
> Refer to *Spiritual Distress.*

KEY CONCEPTS

- Growth in spirituality is a dynamic process in which an individual becomes increasingly aware of the meaning, purpose and values in life (Carson, 1999). Spiritual growth is a two-directional process: horizontal and vertical. The horizontal process increases the person's awareness of the transcendent values inherent in all relationships and activities of life (Carson, 1999). The vertical process moves the person into a closer relationship with a higher being, as conceived by the person. Carson illustrates that it is possible to develop spirituality through the horizontal process and not the vertical. For example, a person can define his or her spirituality in terms of relationships, art, or music without a relationship with a higher being, just as an individual can focus his or her spirituality on a higher being and may not express spirituality through other avenues.
- Faith is necessary for spiritual growth, particularly for a relationship to a higher being. Hope is also critical for spiritual development and integral to the horizontal and vertical processes (Carson, 1999).
- Research suggests that HIV-positive individuals who are spiritually well and who find meaning and purpose in life are also hardier (Carson & Green, 1992).
- Regardless of a person's religion or lack of belief in any, the process of spiritual growth is similar. The religious foundations that guide the growth are very different. When people are together on the level of spirituality, they meet on the level of the heart. On this level, all people are one. There is only one God, and it would seem logical that people's experiences of the transcendent would be

similar. When the experiences are reframed into religious dogma, that is when disagreements begin (Carson, 1999).
- Spirituality has been found especially important to caregivers of victims of chronic illness. Nurses can work to enhance spiritual well-being for them.

Focus Assessment Criteria

Subjective

Person Communicates.

A trust relationship with or in the transcendent that provides bases for meaning and hope in life's experiences
Meaning and purpose to existence
An inner strength that nurtures
An inner peace

For more information on Focus Assessment Criteria, visit http://connection.lww.com.

Goal

NOC Hope, Spiritual Well-Being

The person will express enhanced spiritual harmony and wholeness.

Indicators
- Maintain previous relationship with higher being.
- Continue spiritual practices not detrimental to health.

General Interventions

NIC Spiritual Support

Support the Person's Spiritual Practices.

Refer to Interventions to reduce barriers to spiritual practices under *Impaired Religiosity*.

IMPAIRED RELIGIOSITY

DEFINITION

Impaired Religiosity: State in which a person or group has an impaired ability to exercise reliance on beliefs of a particular denomination or faith community and to participate in related rituals

> ⊕ **AUTHOR'S NOTE**
>
> Refer to *Spiritual Distress*.

DEFINING CHARACTERISTICS

Individual experiences distress because of difficulty in adhering to prescribed religious rituals, for example:

Religious ceremonies
Dietary regulations
Certain clothing

Prayer

Request to worship

Holiday observances

Expresses emotional distress because of separation from faith community

Expresses emotional distress regarding religious beliefs and/or religious social network

Expresses a need to reconnect with previous belief patterns and customs

Questions religious belief patterns and customs

RELATED FACTORS

Pathophysiologic

Related to sickness/illness

Related to suffering

Related to pain

Situational

Related to personal crisis related to activity

Related to fear of death

Related to embarrassment at practicing spiritual rituals

Related to barriers to practicing spiritual rituals

Intensive care restrictions

Confinement to bed or room

Lack of privacy

Lack of availability of special foods/diets

KEY CONCEPTS

Refer to *Spiritual Distress.*

FOCUS ASSESSMENT CRITERIA

Refer to *Spiritual Distress.*

Goal

| NOC | Spiritual Well-Being |

The person will express satisfaction with spiritual condition.

Indicators

- Continue spiritual practices not detrimental to health.
- Express decreasing feelings of guilt and anxiety.

General Interventions

| NIC | Spiritual Support |

Explore Whether the Client Desires to Engage in an Allowable Religious or Spiritual Practice or Ritual; If So, Provide Opportunities To Do So.

Express Your Understanding and Acceptance of the Importance of the Client's Religious or Spiritual Beliefs and Practices.

Assess for Causative and Contributing Factors.

Hospital or nursing home environment

Limitations related to disease process or treatment regimen (eg, cannot kneel to pray owing to traction; prescribed diet differs from usual religious diet)

Fear of imposing on or antagonizing medical and nursing staff with requests for spiritual rituals

Embarrassment over spiritual beliefs or customs (especially common in adolescents)

Separation from articles, texts, or environment of spiritual significance

Lack of transportation to spiritual place or service

Spiritual leader unavailable because of emergency or lack of time

Eliminate or Reduce Causative and Contributing Factors, if Possible.

Limitations Imposed by the Hospital or Nursing Home Environment

Provide privacy and quiet as needed for daily prayer, visit of spiritual leader, and spiritual reading and contemplation.

Pull curtains or close door.

Turn off television and radio.

Ask desk to hold calls, if possible.

Note spiritual interventions on Kardex and include in care plan.

Contact spiritual leader to clarify practices and perform religious rites or services, if desired.

Communicate with spiritual leader concerning person's condition.

Address Roman Catholic, Orthodox, and Episcopal priests as "Father," other Christian ministers as "Pastor," and Jewish rabbis as "Rabbi."

Prevent interruption during visit, if possible.

Offer to provide table or stand covered with clean white cloth.

Chart visit and client's response.

Inform about religious services and materials available within the institution.

Limitations Related to Disease Process or Treatment Regimen

Encourage spiritual rituals not detrimental to health (see Table II.25).

Assist clients with physical limitations in prayer and spiritual observances (eg, help to hold rosary; help to kneeling position, if appropriate).

Assist in habits of personal cleanliness.

Avoid shaving if beard is of spiritual significance.

Allow client to wear religious clothing or jewelry whenever possible.

Make special arrangements for burial of resected limbs or body organs.

Allow family or spiritual leader to perform ritual care of body.

Make arrangements as needed for other important spiritual rituals (eg, circumcisions).

Maintain diet with spiritual restrictions when not detrimental to health (see Table II.25).

Consult with dietitian.

Allow fasting for short periods, if possible.*

Change therapeutic diet as necessary.*

Have family or friends bring in special food, if possible.

Have members of spiritual group supply meals to the person at home.

Be as flexible as possible in serving methods, times of meals, and so forth.

Fear of Imposing or Embarrassment

Communicate acceptance of various spiritual beliefs and practices.

Convey nonjudgmental, respectful attitude.

Acknowledge importance of spiritual needs.

Express willingness of health care team to help in meeting spiritual needs.

Provide privacy and ensure confidentiality.

Separation from Articles, Texts, or Environment of Spiritual Significance

Question person about missing religious or spiritual articles or reading material (see Table II.25).

Obtain missing items from clergy in hospital, spiritual leader, family, or members of spiritual group.

Treat these articles and books with respect.

Allow person to keep spiritual articles and books within reach as much as possible, or where they can be easily seen.

Protect from loss or damage (eg, medal pinned to gown can be lost in laundry).

Recognize that articles without overt religious meaning may have spiritual significance for person (eg, wedding band).

Use spiritual texts in large print, in Braille, or on tape when appropriate.

Provide opportunity for person to pray with others or be read to by members of own religious group or member of the health care team who feels comfortable with these activities.

Jews and Seventh-Day Adventists would find Psalms 23, 34, 42, 63, 71, 103, 121, and 127 appropriate.

Christians would also appreciate I Corinthians 13, Matthew 5:3–11, Romans 12, and the Lord's Prayer.

---

*May require a primary care professional's order.

Lack of Transportation

Take person to chapel or quiet environment on hospital grounds.

Arrange transportation to church or synagogue for person in home.

Provide access to spiritual programming on radio and television when appropriate.

Spiritual Leader Unavailable Because of Emergency or Lack of Time

Baptize critically ill newborn of Greek Orthodox, Episcopal, or Roman Catholic parents (see Table II.25).

Perform other mandatory spiritual rituals, if possible.

Rationales

- For a client who places a high value on prayer or other spiritual practices, these practices can provide meaning and purpose and can be a source of comfort and strength (Carson, 1999).
- Conveying a nonjudgmental attitude may help reduce the client's uneasiness about expressing his beliefs and practices.
- Privacy and quiet provide an environment that enables reflection and contemplation.
- The nurse—even one who does not subscribe to the same religious beliefs or values of the client—can still help him meet his spiritual needs.
- These measures can help the client maintain spiritual ties and practice important rituals.
- Many religions prohibit certain behaviors; complying with restrictions may be an important part of the client's worship.

RELIGIOSITY, RISK FOR IMPAIRED

DEFINITION

Risk for Impaired Religiosity: The state in which an individual is at risk for impaired ability to exercise reliance on beliefs of a particular denomination or faith community and to participate in related rituals

RELATED FACTORS

Refer to *Impaired Religiosity*.

Goal

NOC Spiritual Well-Being

The person will express continued satisfaction with religious activities.

Indicators

- Continue to practice religious rituals.
- Described increased comfort after assessment.

General Interventions

Refer to *Impaired Religiosity* for interventions.

RISK FOR SUDDEN INFANT DEATH SYNDROME

DEFINITION

Risk for Sudden Infant Death Syndrome: State in which an infant younger than 1 year old is at risk to experience sudden death, unexpected by history and unexplained by postmortem examination

RISK FACTORS

Presence of risk factors (refer to Related Factors)

RELATED FACTORS

(McMillan et al., 1999)

Pathophysiologic

Related to increased vulnerability secondary to:

Cyanosis	Hypothermia	Fever
Poor feeding	Irritability	Respiratory distress
Tachycardia	Tachypnea	*Low birth weight
*Small for gestational age	*Prematurity	Low Apgar score (<7)

History of diarrhea, vomiting, or listlessness 2 weeks before death

Related to increased vulnerability secondary to prenatal maternal:

*Anemia	Urinary tract infection	Poor weight gain

Sexually transmitted infections

Situational (Personal, Environmental)

Related to increased vulnerability secondary to maternal:

*Cigarette smoking	Drug use during pregnancy	*Lack of breast-feeding
*Inadequate prenatal care	*Low educational levels	*Single mother
Multiparity	*Young maternal age (<20)	*Young maternal age with first pregnancy

Related to increased vulnerability secondary to:

*Crowded living conditions	*Sleeping on stomach	Poor family financial status
Cold environment		

Related to increased vulnerability secondary to:

*Male gender	*Black/Native Americans	Multiple births

Previous sudden infant death syndrome (SIDS) death in family

○○ ERRORS IN DIAGNOSTIC STATEMENTS

Risk for Sudden Infant Death Syndrome related to low-income parents

Although poor living conditions have been linked to SIDS, the wording of this diagnosis is problematic. The following diagnosis would be more clinically useful: *Risk for Sudden Infant Death Syndrome related to insufficient knowledge of caregivers in causes and prevention of SIDS.*

---

*Widely accepted; general agreement among investigators.

KEY CONCEPTS

- SIDS is the leading single cause of death between 7 and 365 days of age (Wong, 2003).
- Incidence of SIDS has decreased approximately 40% since the American Academy of Pediatrics (AAP) advised sleeping position on the back for infants in 1996 (AAP, 2000).
- Although etiology is not known, autopsies show consistent pathologic findings as pulmonary edema and intrathoracic hemorrhages.
- There is no evidence that apnea monitors prevent SIDS (Sherratt, 1999).

Focus Assessment Criteria

Refer to Related Factors.

Goals

NOC Knowledge: Maternal-Child Health,
Risk Control: Tobacco Use, Risk Control,
Knowledge: Infant Safety

The caregiver will reduce or eliminate risk factors that are modifiable.

Indicators

- Position infant on back or side-lying.
- Eliminate smoking in the home, near the infant, and during pregnancy.
- Participate in prenatal and newborn medical care.
- Improve maternal health (eg, treat anemia, promote optimal nutrition).
- Enroll in drug and alcohol programs, if indicated.
- Avoid giving over-the-counter medications to infant.

General Interventions

NIC Teaching: Infant Safety,
Risk Identification

Explain SIDS to Caregivers and Identify Risk Factors Present.

Reduce or Eliminate Risk Factors That Can Be Modified.

Determine if Home Cardiorespiratory Monitoring Is Indicated. Consult with Pediatrician or Neonatal/Pediatric Nurse Practitioner (Wong, 2003).

Teach parents to focus on the infant when the alarm sounds, not on the machine.
Teach parents to assess:
    Infant's color (pink?)
    Infant's breathing

Teach Environmental Practices to Reduce SIDS.

Position infant on back.
Avoid overheating infant during sleep.
Avoid soft bedding (eg, mattresses).
Avoid pillows.
Avoid sleeping with infant (Anderson, 2000).
Avoid tobacco smoke.

Initiate Health Teaching and Referrals as Indicated.

Provide instructions on use of home monitor, CPR if appropriate.
Refer client to drug and alcohol treatment programs as indicated.
Discuss strategies to stop smoking (refer to index—SMOKING).
Provide emergency numbers as indicated.
Refer to social agencies as indicated.

Rationale

- To help the family cope with the numerous procedures they must learn, adequate preparation before discharge is critical.

- Sleeping on abdomen has been linked to SIDS (Wong, 2003).
- The primary focus of nursing with parents caring for an infant at risk for SIDS is emotional support.
- Maternal smoking during pregnancy and exposure to smoke after birth have been associated with SIDS (American Academy of Pediatrics, 2000).

DELAYED SURGICAL RECOVERY

DEFINITION

Delayed Surgical Recovery: State in which a person experiences, or is at risk to experience, an extension of the number of postoperative days required to initiate and perform self-care activities

---

ⓧ AUTHOR'S NOTE

This recently accepted diagnosis represents a person who has not achieved recovery from a surgical procedure within the expected time. Based on the defining characteristics from NANDA, some confusion exists regarding the difference between defining characteristics (signs and symptoms) and related factors. Those with an asterisk (*) are not defining characteristics but factors that can cause or contribute to *Delayed Surgical Recovery*. The diagnosis has not been developed sufficiently for clinical use. This author recommends using other nursing diagnoses, such as *Self-Care Deficit, Acute Pain,* or *Imbalanced Nutrition*.

DEFINING CHARACTERISTICS

Postpones resumption of activities (home, work)
Perceives that more time is needed to recover
Requires help to complete self-care
*Evidence of interrupted healing of surgical area
*Loss of appetite with or without nausea
*Difficulty moving about
*Reports pain or discomfort

---

* Refer to Author's Note for explanation.

DISTURBED THOUGHT PROCESSES

DEFINITION
Disturbed Thought Processes: State in which a person experiences a disruption in such mental activities as conscious thought, reality orientation, problem solving, judgment, and comprehension related to coping, personality, and/or mental disorder

DEFINING CHARACTERISTICS
Major (Must Be Present)
Inaccurate interpretation of stimuli, internal, external, or both

Minor (May Be Present)
Cognitive defects, including problem solving, abstraction, memory deficits

Suspiciousness	Delusions	Hallucinations
Phobias	Obsessions	Distractibility
Lack of consensual validation	Confusion/disorientation	Ritualistic behavior
Impulsivity	Inappropriate social behavior	

RELATED FACTORS
Pathophysiologic
Related to physiologic changes secondary to drug or alcohol withdrawal
Related to biochemical alterations
Related to acute primary brain pathology (eg, traumatic brain injury)
Related to degenerative brain pathology (eg, Alzheimer's dementia)

Situational (Personal, Environmental)
Related to emotional trauma
Related to abuse (physical, sexual, mental)
Related to torture
Related to childhood trauma
Related to repressed fears
Related to panic level of anxiety
Related to continued low levels of stimulation
Related to decreased attention span and ability to process information secondary to:

Depression	Anxiety	Fear
Grieving		

Maturational
Older Adult
Related to isolation, late-life depression

⊗ AUTHOR'S NOTE

Disturbed Thought Processes describes a person with alterations in perception and cognition that interfere with daily living. Causes are psychological disturbances (eg, depression, personality disorders, mood disorders). For this diagnosis, the focus of nursing is on reducing disturbed thinking, promoting reality orientation, or both.

The nurse is cautioned against using this diagnosis as a "waste basket" diagnosis for all clients with disturbed thinking or confusion. Frequently, confusion in an older adult is attributed erroneously to aging. Confusion in older adults can result from a single factor (eg, dementia, medication side effects, metabolic disorder) or from depression related to multiple factors associated with aging. Depression causes impaired thinking more frequently than does dementia in older adults (Miller, 2004). Refer to *Confusion* for additional information.

⊗ ERRORS IN DIAGNOSTIC STATEMENTS

1. *Disturbed Thought Processes related to depression*

When a person exhibits signs and symptoms of depression and impaired cognition, use of *Disturbed Thought Processes* would seem appropriate. The nurse should view the impaired cognition associated with depression, however, as a manifestation, not as a response to be treated. Depression is a state that represents ineffective coping; thus, the following diagnosis would be more clinically useful: *Ineffective Coping related to unknown etiology, as evidenced by slowed affect, reports of constant sadness, little motivation, and memory difficulties*. Because the central issue in depression is low self-esteem, the nurse uses a focus assessment to determine factors causing or contributing to low self-esteem (eg, disabilities, losses, feelings of rejection).

2. *Disturbed Thought Processes related to loss of memory*

Memory loss can occur in many situations (eg, depression, dementia, anxiety, sensory deprivation, psychiatric disorders, endocrine disorders). The nursing focus would vary, depending on the contributing factors. For example, loss of memory with head injuries usually is very anxiety-producing; thus, a diagnosis of *Anxiety* would be more useful. Loss of memory that poses a danger would be associated with *Risk for Injury*. If *Disturbed Thought Processes* were appropriate for this person, the nurse should restate the diagnosis as *Disturbed Thought Processes related to* (specify, eg, *effects of hypoxia secondary to cerebrovascular accident), as evidenced by loss of memory*.

KEY CONCEPTS

- Thought is a functioning process of the brain that integrates every person's daily living experiences. Cognitive processes are the mental processes related to reasoning, comprehension, judgment, and memory. Physiologic functions, environmental stimuli, and emotional state influence cognitive function (Porth, 2002).
- The person's current needs and interests, as well as his or her store of knowledge, influence the cognitive processes of remembering and perception.
- Development of cognitive abilities follows a systematic pattern of maturational experiences and requires varied perceptual stimulation.
- A disruption in the quality and quantity of incoming stimuli can affect thought processes.
- What a person thinks about an event influences both feelings and behavior. Any changes in thoughts, feelings, or behavior result in changes in the other two.
- People attempt to gain control over a situation by assigning meaning to it; sometimes, they assign a rational explanation, whereas other times, explanations are irrational. Over time, irrational beliefs lead to chronic dissatisfaction; the person's thinking patterns become characterized by "shoulds" and "musts."
- Suicide may be a risk for these clients because of the potential for multiple losses and disruptions to their life, such as loss of social supports through course of illness, low self-esteem enhancing delusions and hallucinations as illness recedes, hopelessness associated with a severe illness, and so forth.

Reality

- Reality testing is the objective evaluation and judgment of the world outside the self, differentiated from one's thoughts and feelings. It is determined by early life experiences and by significant others.
- Delusions—fixed false beliefs—and hallucinations originate during extreme emotional stress; they represent attempts to decrease panic (Varcarolis, 2002).
- Delusions include those of:
  - *Grandeur:* An exaggerated sense of importance of identity or ability
  - *Persecution:* A sense that one is being harassed
  - *Reference:* Belief that the behavior of others refers to oneself
  - *Influence:* Exaggerated sense of power over others
  - *Control:* Sense that one is being manipulated by others
  - *Bodily sensations:* Belief that one's organs are diseased, despite contrary evidence
  - *Infidelity:* Belief, as a result of pathologic jealousy, that one's lover is unfaithful
- Delusions arise when people attempt to alter reality. First, they deny their feelings, then they project those feelings onto the environment. Finally, they must explain this to others (Mohr, 2003).
- The fundamental feelings that suspicious and grandiose clients project are inadequacy and worthlessness.
- Hallucinations are perceptions that arise from within the person's own thoughts; the person actually hears, sees, feels, or tastes the phenomenon.
- Hallucinations meet underlying needs (eg, loneliness, anxiety, self-worth). Until a person can substitute other activities, he or she may be unwilling to "give these up" (Mohr, 2003). Hallucinations occur most frequently in the auditory mode.
- The person may spend much time in his or her fantasy world, which leads to a lack of consensual validation of language. Not only are the connections between words disturbed, but the words often have a different meaning to the person than is generally accepted.
- Disorganized thinking often leads to regression in behavior, disturbed communication, and difficulty in interactions with others.
- Illusions are mistaken or misinterpreted sensory perceptions. They occur most commonly in acute delirium and organic brain syndromes.

Focus Assessment Criteria

Acquire data from client and significant others.

Subjective Data

Assess the Client's History.

Lifestyle

Interests	Strengths and limitations
Work history	Coping patterns (past and present)
Education	Previous level of functioning and handling stress
Use of alcohol/drugs	

Support system (availability)

History of medical problems and treatments (medications)

Activities of daily living (ability and desire to perform)

Family

   Quality of relationships

   History of mental illness

   Beliefs about symptoms

   Involvement with cultural, religious, or ethnic groups

   Quality of support

   Beliefs about mental illness

Assess for Defining Characteristics.

Feelings of

Extreme sadness and worthlessness	Living in an unreal world
	Mistrust or suspiciousness of others
Guilt for past actions	Others making him or her do and say things

Apprehension in various situations

Excessive self-importance

Being rejected or isolated

Depersonalization

Fears

That others will harm him or her

Of being unable to cope

Of thoughts racing

Of falling apart

Of being held prisoner

That external agents are controlling mind

That body is rotting or not there

Hallucinations (visual, auditory, gustatory, olfactory, tactile—includes an objective component)

Circumstances

Positive or negative

Number/day, type, particulars, and details

Antecedents

Consequences

Frequency, time of day

Ability to control them

Duration

Depression (Miller, 2004)

Difficulties with memory

Consistent sadness

Lack of motivation

Apathetic responses

Inability to concentrate

Delusions

Fixed or fleeting

Thought broadcasting (others can hear person's thoughts)

Thought insertion (others putting thoughts into person's mind)

Physical complaints of fatigue, anorexia, constipation, insomnia, dysphagia

Delusions of foreboding gloom, diminished self-esteem, money, death, guilt

Orientation

Person, time, place

Problem-solving ability

"What would you do if the phone rang?"

"What is the difference between the doctor and the president?"

Memory

Objective Data (Includes a Subjective Component)
Assess for Defining Characteristics.

General appearance

Facial expression (alert, sad, hostile, expressionless)

Dress (meticulous, disheveled, seductive, eccentric)

Behavior during interview

Withdrawn	Quiet	Hostile
Negativism	Apathetic	Cooperative
Level of attention/ concentration	Level of anxiety	

Communication pattern

Content

Appropriate	Homicidal plans	Sexual preoccupations
Suicidal ideas	Rambling	Lacking content
Suspicious	Obsessions	Denying problem
Delusions	Religiousness	Worthlessness

Pattern of speech

Appropriate

Circumstantial (cannot get to point)

Loose connection of ideas

Cannot come to conclusion, be decisive

Blocking (cannot finish idea)

Echolalia

Jumps from one topic to another

Rate of speech

Appropriate	Reduced	Excessive
Pressured		

Affect

Blunted

Gestures, mannerisms, grimaces	Inappropriate to verbal content	Appropriate to verbal content
Congruent with content of speech	Bright	Flat
	Sad	Posture

Interaction Skills

With nurse

Inappropriate	Shows dependency	Relates well
Demanding/pleading	Withdrawn/preoccupied	Hostile

With significant others

Relates with all (some) family members

Does not seek interaction

Hostile toward one (all) members

Does not have visitors

Motor activity

Within normal limits	Agitated	Decreased/stuporous

For more information on Focus Assessment Criteria, visit http://connection.lww.com.

Goals

NOC Cognitive Ability, Cognitive Orientation, Concentration, Distorted Thought Control, Information Processing, Memory, Decision-Making

The person will maintain reality orientation and communicate clearly with others.

Indicators

- Recognize changes in thinking/behavior.
- Identify situations that precede hallucinations/delusions.
- Use coping strategies to deal effectively with hallucinations/delusions (specify).
- Participate in unit activities (specify).
- Express delusional material less frequently.

General Interventions

NIC Cognitive Stimulation, Dementia Management, Reality Orientation, Family Support, Decision-Making Support, Hallucination Management, Anxiety Reduction, Memory Training, Environmental Management Safety

Promote Communication that Enhances the Person's Sense of Integrity.

Encourage Open, Honest Dialogue.

Approach client in a calm, nurturing manner.

Persevere, be consistent, and be hopeful.

Be open and share with the person. Use his or her name throughout conversations.

Discuss expectations and demands.

Recognize when person is testing the trustworthiness of others.

Avoid making promises that cannot be fulfilled.

Offer set periods during each shift when you can meet; initial staff contact should be minimal and brief with a suspicious person. Increase time as suspiciousness decreases.

Explain if appointments cannot be kept.

Verify your interpretation of what the person is experiencing ("I understand you are fearful of others").

Be an attentive listener; note both verbal and nonverbal messages.

Help client verbalize what he or she indicates nonverbally.

Use terminology that is familiar and evokes little anxiety.

Speak clearly and audibly.

Recognize the importance of body posture, facial expression, and tone of voice.

Present information in a matter-of-fact way that is least likely to be misinterpreted; do not use humor or bantering with suspicious people.

Use communication that helps person maintain individuality (eg, "I" instead of "we").

Eliminate whispered comments or incomplete explanations that encourage fantasy interpretation.

Tell person about all the various meetings in which you will discuss his or her case with other health professionals.

Give brief explanations before doing any unfamiliar procedures (eg, medications, invasive procedures, treatments) with the person.

Maintain Client's Personal Space.

Do not touch the person until you have developed an ongoing trusting relationship.

Talk to the person in open space; avoid small rooms or offices.

Face client at a 45-degree angle.

Minimize Distress.

Reassure client that these symptoms are part of the illness but can recede as it improves.

Try to Understand the Client's Private World and What It Means.

Minimize Number of Staff Assigned to Care for Client to Help Establish Rapport.

Try to Maintain Client in Quiet, Well-Lit Areas.

Assist Client to Differentiate Between Own Thoughts and Reality.

Validate the Presence of Hallucinations.

Observe for verbal and nonverbal cues—inappropriate laughter, delayed verbal response, eye movements, lip movements without sound, increased motor movements, grinning.

> "Are you hearing/seeing something now?"
> "What's happening now?"

Assist client to observe thoughts and feelings as they relate to the underlying needs being met.

> "Has this happened before?" "You were lonely?"
> "What were you doing/thinking?"

Assist client to analyze the hallucinations.

> How often do they occur (*frequency*)?
> What is the intensity or clarity of the hallucinations (*intensity*)?
> How long do the episodes last (*duration*)?
> Where and when do the incidents occur; what happens just before them (*antecedents*)?
> What happens after the hallucinations (*consequences*)?
> Describe the hallucinations in detail.

Probe for any alternative hallucinations (eg, person may have different voices giving different messages).

Help Person to Self-Regulate or Control Hallucinations.

Identify triggers that increase anxiety.

Discuss the use of a control strategy.

> Keep a record—when, what, how they stopped.
> Reinforce what worked.

Focus on Here and Now.

Accept the person's experiences and perceptions of reality (Baker, 1995).

Understand the language the client uses to describe the experiences. Often, a variety of symbols and feelings are involved (Baker, 1995).

Encourage person to validate his or her thoughts by sharing them with significant others.

Avoid belittling the person when he or she misinterprets stimuli or is delusional; do not laugh or make fun.

Encourage person to identify and focus on strengths, not weaknesses.

Encourage differentiation of stimuli arising from inner sources from those from outside (eg, in response to "I hear voices," say: "Those are the voices of people on TV" or "I hear no one speaking now; they are your own thoughts").

Avoid giving the impression that you confirm or approve reality distortions; tactfully express doubt without arguing or debating.

Focus on feelings behind the reality distortions rather than the content.

Focus on reality-oriented aspects of the communication (eg, if person states, "The TV is controlling my mind," the nurse can say, "How does it make you feel when others try to control you?").

Set limits for discussing repetitive delusional material ("You've already told me about that; let's talk about something realistic.").

Teach person to relearn to focus attention on real things and people.

Identify the underlying needs being met by the delusions/hallucinations.

Help person become aware that he or she is expressing needs in fantasy; teach more appropriate ways to meet these needs (eg, aggression expressed through delusion of persecution can be put into constructive activity, such as hammering metal objects).

Do not dismiss physical complaints automatically; however, do not express undue concern.

Provide positive reinforcement when person talks about feelings and reality-based experiences.

When person is experiencing illusions, remove object causing the illusion; dismantle it, if possible, explaining in reassuring tones what it is, and allow person to examine it if he or she desires.

Minimize episodes of illusions by allowing person to have sense-related objects from home, providing a night light, explaining strange equipment/objects and allowing them to handle them, and matching surroundings to the person's sensory level (ie, reducing sensory overload or increasing sensory stimuli).

Assist Client with Decreasing Irrational Thoughts (Refer To *Anxiety*).

Explore Various Strategies that Help People Cope with Their Symptoms (ie, Hallucinations, Delusions).

Behavioral control strategies

Increasing or decreasing activity level

Postural change

Avoidance mechanisms

    Avoiding potentially unpleasant situations

    Using specific and restricted social withdrawal

Humming or singing quietly to self

Counting quietly

Reading out loud

Repeating a phrase (eg, "I'm okay")

Engaging in leisure activities

Reading	Shopping	Drawing
Hobbies	Yard work	

Monaural inclusion/single ear plug to reduce hallucinations

Listening to headphones	Gargling	Aversion self-therapy

Cognitive control strategies

Passive and active attention diversion

Actively suppressing disturbing thoughts and voices

Thought stopping

Challenging voices/thoughts

Dismissing the voices/thoughts

Problem solving

Distraction

Listening to radio	Singing	Watching TV
Praying		

Improving self-image

Rational self-talk

Positive affirmations

Physiologic control strategies

Drug or alcohol use	Sleep	Relaxation
Anxiety management	Exercise	Taking PRN medications

Avoid Chemicals that Worsen Hallucinations (Alcohol, Caffeine, Street Drugs, Antihistamines).

Encourage and Support Client to Participate Actively in the Treatment Program.

Initiate coping strategies.

Challenge symptoms.

Look for alternative views on how he or she interprets events, situations, and so forth.

Assist the Person with Disordered Thinking to Communicate More Effectively.

Ask for the meaning of what is said; do not assume that you understand.

Validate your interpretation of what is being said ("Is this what you mean?").

Clarify all global pronouns—we, they ("Who is *they?*").

Refocus when person changes the subject in the middle of an explanation or thought.

Tell the person when you are not following his or her train of thought.
Do not mimic or restate words or phrases that you do not understand.
Ask yes or no or multiple-choice questions.
Keep sentences short and clear.
Repeat sentences as often as needed.
Listen attentively.
When confronting the person about the behavior is necessary, use the components of DISC: *d*escribe the behavior of the person, *i*ndicate the desired behavior, *s*pecify nursing actions, and describe the positive and negative *c*onsequences. ("Your yelling is disrupting people. I suggest you spend some time alone in your room until you gain control. I'll check on you in 15 minutes. If you haven't gained control by then, I'll give you some medication to help you settle.")

Encourage a More Mature Level of Functioning.

Assist Person to Set Limits on His or Her Own Behavior.
Discuss alternative methods of coping (eg, taking a walk instead of crying).
Confront person with the attitude that regression is not acceptable behavior.
Help delay gratification (eg, "I want you to wait 5 minutes before you repeat your request for help in making your bed").
Encourage person to achieve realistic expectations.
Pace expectations to avoid frustration.

Encourage and Support Person in the Decision-Making Process.
Help person review options and the advantages and disadvantages of each option.
Assist in structuring daily living activities (eg, help schedule bath time before activity hour).
Compliment the person who assumes more responsibility.
Show patience and understanding when a mistake is made. Assist to develop a plan from which to learn from the mistake.
Provide opportunity for person to contribute to his or her own treatment plan.
Help establish future goals that are realistic; examine problems in achieving a goal and suggest various alternatives.

Assist Person to Differentiate Between Needs and Demands.

Explain the difference between needs and demands (eg, food and clothing are needs; expectations that others dress and feed the client, if he or she can do it, are demands).
Assist client to examine the effects of his or her behavior on others; encourage a change in behavior if it evokes negative responses.
Teach negotiation to achieve needs and goals.
Help person ask for what he or she wants and tell others how he or she feels.
Help person realize that failure of others to meet needs and demands is not always related to their regard for him or her.

Use Cognitive-Behavioral Therapy Either Individually or in Groups.
Help person to recognize that the symptoms are causing the problems and that he or she can do something about them.
Assist client to develop strategies to deal with symptoms.
Encourage the person to challenge symptoms.

Provide Person with Opportunities for Positive Socialization.

Help Client Share on a One-To-One Basis.
Be warm, honest, and sincere in interactions.
Demonstrate that you accept him or her.
Recognize that some people deny the need for close relationships.
Be sensitive to behaviors that indicate resistance to interpersonal involvement.
Help person know that you recognize his or her uneasiness in social situations ("It must be difficult for you.").
Use touch judiciously if person fears closeness.
Encourage discussion of reality-based issues and topics.

Help Person Recognize Behaviors that Stimulate Rejection.
Identify activities that reduce interpersonal anxiety (eg, exercise, controlled-breathing exercises).
Set limits firmly and kindly on destructive behavior.
Allow expression of negative emotions, verbally or in constructive activity.

Avoid argument or debate about delusional ideas or destructive behavior.
Help person accept responsibility for responses he or she elicits from others.
Encourage discussion of problems in relating after visits with family members.
Help person test new skills in relating to others in role-playing situations.

Refer To *Impaired Socialization* For Further Interventions.

Help Person Limit Delusional and Hallucinatory Activity to Private Situations.
When able to accomplish this, provide positive reinforcement of his or her ability for self-control.

Promote Physical Well-Being and Prevent Injury.

Explain and Monitor Medication Regimen.
Assess person's ability to remember to take medications.
Assist person to remember to take medications by color-coding each bottle with a sticker and writing out the times of the day to take medications, with the appropriate color of sticker next to the time.
Teach about the purpose of medications and their side effects.
Encourage client to report all physical symptoms.
Encourage client to take prescribed medication, especially antipsychotic (eg, lithium).
Check to ensure that the client swallowed the medication. if you have doubts about the client taking oral medications (eg, failure to improve), change to concentrate form. Extremely suspicious and hostile people should begin with concentrate form, so that you will not have to check mouth and increase distrust.
Do not mix medications with food.
Discuss dangers of mixing medications with alcohol.
Monitor for side effects, neuroleptic malignant syndrome, extrapyramidal side effects, and tardive dyskinesia.

Monitor Nutritional Intake.
Observe eating habits (amount, selection, frequency, food preferences and dislikes, appetite).
Note weight gain or loss.
Discuss adequate nutrition in relation to activity level.
Allow person to choose food he or she especially likes; contract with person who eats predominantly snack foods (eg, "If you eat one egg you can order a doughnut").
Note delusions regarding food or body that might interfere with nutritional intake.
Encourage increased calorie intake for hyperactive person.
Provide finger foods that can be eaten on-the-run (eg, sandwiches).
Allow choices in foods (may prefer to eat food brought in by family, in unopened packages, fruit, and the like).
Refer to *Imbalanced Nutrition* for additional interventions.

Assess Ability for Self-Care Activities.
Identify areas of physical care with which person needs assistance (sleep and rest, nutrition, bathing, dressing, elimination, exercise).
Note person's motivation and interest in appearance.
Teach skills required to assume responsibility for self-care.
Assist person in planning daily routines to foster independence and responsibility.
Monitor for sleep disturbances.
Provide a single room for extremely suspicious person.
Suggest leaving the light on.
Give nonstimulating drinks with a snack at bedtime.
Assess the need for a sleeping medication.
If appropriate, arrange to give last dose of antipsychotic medication at bedtime (eg, b.i.d. medication—give a.m. and h.s.).
Refer to *Self-Care Deficit* for additional interventions.

Assess Sleep–Rest Patterns (Disturbed Thought Processes Can Disrupt Sleep–Rest Patterns, and Disrupted Sleep–Rest Patterns Can Worsen Disturbed Thought Processes).
Structure times for sleep, rest, and diversional activities.
Explore techniques that may promote sleep (eg, warm milk, bath, reading).
Monitor sleep–rest patterns by graph until no longer a problem.

Monitor Stimuli and their Effects on the Person.

Teach client to gauge the effects stimuli have on his or her thoughts.

Explore strategies that mitigate the effects of the stimuli (distraction, physical activity, removing self from the stimuli).

Focus on one activity at a time.

Encourage Physical Activity.

Provide Hope. Refer to *Hopelessness* for Specific Interventions.

Reduce the Potential for Violence to Self and Others.

Provide a Minimally Stimulating Environment.

Reduce incidence of bright colors and loud noises.

Be short, concise, and matter-of-fact.

Be consistent.

Consider assigning staff responsible for developing trusting relationship.

Avoid large groups.

Provide Activities in Which Client will be Successful.

Avoid competitive sports.

Suspicious people are often good managers.

Involve client in activities of short duration.

Allow Expression of Hostility (As Long as It is Not Combative/Destructive).

Be nonjudgmental.

Do not personalize.

Assess for Signs Indicative of Aggression.

("Those Russian spies are going to attack me tonight.")

Refer to *Risk for Violence* for further interventions.

Identify Cues to Suicide.

Sudden changes in mood or behavior

Report of plan to harm self

Report of voices directing person to harm self or others

Observe closely for changes in behavior; increase vigilance.

Share with personnel the individual's potential for self-harm.

Refer to *Risk for Suicide* for further interventions.

Interview family and note approaches that have been beneficial in the past in controlling aggression.

Reduce anxiety and develop a sense of safety through a climate of care and concern.

Initiate Health Teaching and Referrals, as Indicated.

Anticipate difficulties in adjusting to community living; discuss concerns about returning to community and elicit family reaction to discharge.

Provide health teaching that prepares person to deal with life stresses (methods of relaxation, problem-solving skills, how to negotiate with others, how to express feelings constructively).

Review signs and symptoms of recurrent illness that indicate impending maladjustment.

Refer to other professionals for assistance:

    To occupational therapist to learn leisure activities

    To industrial therapist to improve or learn new job skills

    To social worker to discuss living arrangements, financial problems, or family negotiations

Supply telephone number and address of local mental health clinic.

Inform of social agencies that offer help in adjusting to community living.

    General social agencies

        Mental health and mental retardation centers

        Mental Health Association

        Family Service (family counseling)

        Drug rehabilitation centers

    Specific social agencies

Alcoholics Anonymous	Gray Panthers
Suicide Crisis	Synanon
Intervention Center	
Contact	

Educate family and significant others concerning person's illness and successful coping strategies.

  Support them emotionally.

Rationales

- Effective caregivers are self-confident, honest, flexible, hopeful, and tolerant of uncertainty, error, and irrational behavior (Mohr, 2003).
- Leaving a hallucinating person alone increases fear and deepens preoccupation (Mohr, 2003).
- The nurse provides a healthy role model with appropriate verbal and nonverbal responses (Mohr, 2003).
- Physiologic control strategies alter the physiologic state to reduce autonomic arousal.
- Cognitive control strategies involve mental processes to distract from symptoms.
- Behavioral control strategies are responses that can distract from the symptoms.
- The person can be helped to regain contact with reality by gently introducing conversation or activities that are oriented to the here-and-now (Mohr, 2003).
- Interventions that require the person to engage in active mental work (eg, must give a verbal response) are effective (Farrell et al., 1998).
- Helping the person identify what specific situations trigger hallucinations gives insight into possible prevention strategies.
- Honesty provides insight and discourages the person from discounting his or her feelings.
- Encouraging self-care promotes independence and increases self-esteem.
- Hostility can arise from therapeutic relationships because of the intensity of the closeness and fear of rejection (Mohr, 2003).
- Families can be helped to improve their interpersonal functioning and to handle behavior and feelings effectively (Varcarolis, 2002).
- Environmental stress increases anxiety and distorts reality (Varcarolis, 2002).

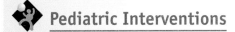 **Pediatric Interventions**

For children with thought disturbance, assess for signs of dissociative disorder (Mohr, 2003).
    Abuse history (physical, sexual)
    Amnestic periods
    Switching between personalities
    Affect disturbances
    Abrupt behavioral changes
Refer for multidisciplinary evaluation.

Rationale

Recognition, evaluation, and treatment of dissociative disorders are critical. The child is afforded proper treatment early and abuse is terminated. Family dysfunction can be addressed with a plan for family recovery (Mohr, 2003).

IMPAIRED MEMORY

DEFINITION

Impaired Memory: State in which a person experiences a temporary or permanent inability to remember or recall bits of information or behavioral skills

DEFINING CHARACTERISTICS
Major (Must Be Present, One or More)

Observed or reported experiences of forgetting
Inability to determine if a behavior was performed
Inability to learn or retain new skills or information
Inability to perform a previously learned skill
Inability to recall factual information
Inability to recall recent or past events

RELATED FACTORS
Pathophysiologic

Related to central nervous system changes secondary to:

Degenerative brain disease	Lesion	Head injury
Cerebrovascular accident		

Related to reduced quantity and quality of information processed secondary to:

Visual deficits	Hearing deficits	Poor physical fitness
Fatigue	Learning habits	Intellectual skills
Educational level		

Related to nutritional deficiencies (eg, vitamins C and B$_{12}$, folate, niacin, thiamine)

Treatment-Related
Related to effects of medication (specify) on memory storage

Situational (Personal, Environmental)
Related to self-fulfilling expectations
Related to excessive self-focusing and worrying secondary to:

Grieving	Anxiety	Depression

Related to alcohol consumption
Related to lack of motivation
Related to lack of stimulation
Related to difficulty concentrating secondary to:

Stress	Pain	Distractions
Lack of intellectual stimulation	Sleep disturbances	

(XX) AUTHOR'S NOTE

This diagnosis is useful when the person can be helped to function better because of improved memory. If the person's memory cannot be improved because of cerebral degeneration, this diagnosis is not appropriate. Instead, the nurse should evaluate the effects of impaired memory on functioning, such as *Self-Care Deficits* or *Risk for Injury*. The focus of interventions would be improving self-care or protection, not improving memory.

KEY CONCEPTS
Generic Considerations

- Memory is a continuum of processing. It ranges from shallow to deep levels, and the duration of particular memories depends on the depths of processing (Miller, 2004).
- There are three stages of memory (Miller, 2004):
  - *Sensory memory*—awareness of information obtained through vision, hearing, taste, smell, and touch, which lasts only a few seconds
  - *Short-term memory*—working memory, contains small amounts of information (eg, a telephone number)
  - *Long-term memory*—memory bank; can be retrieved whenever it is needed
- Memory function worries people more than any other cognitive function. When an older person forgets, it is interpreted as a sign of disease; when a younger person forgets, it is attributed to too many things being on one's mind.
- When concentration is difficult, relaxation and imagery have improved memory and learning (Miller, 2004).
- The most notable deficit in the first stage of Alzheimer's disease is the loss of recent memory (Maier-Lorentz, 2000).

Ⓖ Geriatric Considerations

- Short-term memory shows a slight decline with aging (Miller, 2004).
- Benign senescent forgetfulness involves minor degrees of memory loss; it is not progressive and does not produce dysfunction in daily living (Kane et al., 1994).
- If memory deficits progress and affect other areas of intellectual functioning, dementia should be considered (Kane et al., 1994).

Focus Assessment Criteria

Acquire from client and significant others.

Subjective Data
Assess for Defining Characteristics.

Remote events: "Where were you born?" "Where did you go to grade school?" "What was your first job?" "When were you married?"

Recent past events: "Do you live with anyone?" "Do you have any grandchildren?" "What are the names of your grandchildren?" "When was the last time you went to the doctor?"

Immediate memory, retention: State three unrelated facts and ask the person to repeat the information immediately and again after 5 min.

Immediate memory, general grasp, and recall: Have the person read a short story and then summarize the information.

Immediate memory, recognition: Ask a multiple-choice question and ask the person to choose the correct answer.

Ability to remember:

Self-care activities	To shop for necessities	To take medications
Appointments	To pay bills	

For more information on Focus Assessment Criteria, visit http://connection.lww.com.

Goal

NOC Cognitive Orientation, Memory

The person will report increased satisfaction with memory.

Indicators

- Identify three techniques to improve memory.
- Relate factors that deter memory.

General Interventions

 Reality Orientation, Memory Training, Environmental Management

Discuss the Person's Beliefs About Memory Deficits.

Correct misinformation.
Explain that negative expectations can result in memory deficits.

Explain that if One Wants to Improve One's Memory, Both the Intent to Remember and the Knowledge About Techniques for Remembering are Needed (Miller, 2004).

If the Person has Difficulty Concentrating, Explain the Favorable Effects of Relaxation and Imagery.

Teach the Person Two or Three of the Following Methods to Improve Memory Skills (Maier-Lorentz, 2000; Miller, 2004):

Write things down (eg, use lists, calendars, notebooks).
Use auditory cues (eg, timers, alarm clocks) in conjunction with written cues.
Use environmental cues (eg, you might remove something from its usual place, then return it to its normal location after it has served its purpose as a reminder).
Have specific places for specific items; keep items in their proper place (eg, keep keys on a hook near the door).
Put reminders in appropriate places (eg, place shoes to be repaired near the door).
Use visual images ("A picture is worth a thousand words"). Create a picture in your mind when you want to remember something; the more bizarre the picture, the more likely it is you will remember.
Use active observation—pay attention to details around you, and be alert to the environment.
Make associations or mental connections (eg, "Spring ahead and fall back" for changing clocks to and from daylight savings time).
Make associations between names and mental images (eg, Carol and Christmas carol).
Rehearse items you want to remember by repeating them aloud or writing them on paper.
Use self-instruction—say things aloud (eg, "I'm putting my keys on the counter so I remember to turn off the stove before I leave").
Divide information into small chunks that can be remembered easily (eg, to remember an address or a zip code, divide it into groups ["seven hundred sixty, fifty-five"]).
Organize information into logical categories (eg, shampoo and hair spray, toothpaste and mouthwash, soap and deodorant).
Use rhyming cues (eg, "In 1492, Columbus sailed the ocean blue").
Use first-letter cues and make associations (eg, to remember to buy carrots, apples, radishes, pickles, eggs, and tea bags, remember the word *carpet*).
Make word associations (eg, to remember the letters of your license plate, make a word, such as "camel" for CML).
Search the alphabet while focusing on what you're trying to remember (eg, to remember that someone's name is Martin, start with names that begin with "A" and continue naming names through the alphabet until your memory is jogged for the correct one).
Make up a story to connect things you want to remember (eg, if you have to go to the cleaners and post office, create a story about mailing a pair of pants).

When Trying to Learn or Remember Something:

Minimize distractions.
Do not rush.
Maintain some form of organization of routine tasks.
Carry a note pad or calendar or use written cues.

When Teaching (Miller, 2004):

Eliminate distractions.
Present information as concretely as possible.
Use practical examples.
Allow learner to pace the learning.
Use visual, auditory aids.
Provide advance organizers; outlines, written cues.

Encourage use of aids.
Make sure glasses are clean and lights are soft white.
Correct wrong answers immediately.
Encourage verbal responses.
Try to organize self-care activities in the same order and same time each day.

Rationales

- Many personal and environmental factors, such as level of education and expectations, influence memory significantly. For example, if society expects older people to be forgetful, it can become a self-fulfilling prophecy.
- Older adults can benefit from cognitive exercises to improve memory.
- Memory impairment can be improved when information is meaningful and logical rather than abstract.

⊙ Geriatric Interventions

Provide accurate information about age-related changes.
Explain the difference between age-related forgetfulness and dementia.

Rationales

- Clients and family members may equate any memory problems with Alzheimer's disease.
- Providing accurate information can allay fears.

INEFFECTIVE TISSUE PERFUSION (SPECIFY: RENAL, CEREBRAL, CARDIOPULMONARY, GASTROINTESTINAL)

DEFINITION

Ineffective Tissue Perfusion: State in which a person experiences or is at risk of experiencing a decrease in nutrition and respiration at the cellular level because of a decrease in capillary blood supply

---

⚭ AUTHOR'S NOTE

Tissue perfusion depends on many physiologic factors, both within body systems and at the cellular level. A person's response to ineffective tissue perfusion can disrupt some or all functional health patterns and can cause physiologic complications. for example, a person with chronic renal failure is at risk for fluid/electrolyte imbalances, acidosis, nutritional problems, edema, fatigue, pruritus, and disturbed self-concept. Does the diagnosis *Ineffective Renal Tissue Perfusion* describe these varied responses, or does it simply rename renal failure or renal calculi?

The use of any *Ineffective Tissue Perfusion* diagnosis other than *Peripheral* merely provides new labels for medical diagnoses, labels that do not describe the nursing focus or accountability. The following represent examples of *Ineffective Tissue Perfusion* diagnoses with associated goals from the literature:

- *Ineffective Tissue Perfusion related to hypovolemia secondary to GI bleeding*
  - *Goal:* Tissue perfusion improves, as evidenced by stabilized vital signs.
- *Ineffective Cerebral Tissue Perfusion related to increased intracranial pressure*
  - *Goal:* Intracranial pressure (ICP) is no greater than 15 mm Hg; clinical signs of ICP are decreased.
- *Ineffective Tissue Perfusion related to vaso-occlusive nature of sickling secondary to sickle cell crisis*
  - *Goal:* Client demonstrates improved tissue perfusion, as evidenced by adequate urine output, absence of pain, strong peripheral pulses.

All the above outcomes represent criteria that nurses use to assess the client's status to determine the appropriate nursing and medical interventions indicated. Thus, these situations represent the following collaborative problems, respectively: *PC: GI bleeding, PC: Increased ICP,* and *PC: Sickling crisis.*

NANDA approved the diagnosis *Ineffective Tissue Perfusion (Renal, Cerebral, Cardiopulmonary, Gastrointestinal)* in 1980. It does not conform to the NANDA definition approved in 1990 (refer to Chapter 2). When using these diagnoses, nurses cannot be accountable for prescribing the interventions for outcome achievement. Instead of using *Ineffective Tissue Perfusion,* the nurse should focus on the nursing diagnoses and collaborative problems applicable because of altered renal, cardiac, cerebral, pulmonary, or gastrointestinal (GI) tissue perfusion.

Ineffective Peripheral Tissue Perfusion can be a clinically useful nursing diagnosis if used to describe chronic arterial or venous insufficiency or potential thrombophlebitis. (In contrast, acute embolism and thrombophlebitis represent collaborative problems.) A nurse focusing on preventing thrombophlebitis in a postoperative client would write the diagnosis *Risk for Ineffective Peripheral Tissue Perfusion related to postoperative immobility and dehydration.*

ERRORS IN DIAGNOSTIC STATEMENTS

1. *Ineffective GI Tissue Perfusion related to esophageal bleeding varices*
    Because this diagnosis actually represents a situation that nurses monitor and manage with nursing and medical interventions, the diagnosis should be rewritten as the collaborative problem *PC: Esophageal bleeding varices.*
2. *Ineffective Cerebral Tissue Perfusion related to cerebral edema secondary to intracranial infections*
    This diagnosis represents merely a new label for encephalitis, meningitis, or abscess. Instead, the nurse should specify collaborative problems to clearly describe and designate the nursing accountability: *PC: Increased intracranial pressure* and *PC: Septicemia.* In addition, certain nursing diagnoses may be indicated (eg, *Risk for Infection Transmission, Impaired Comfort*).
3. *Ineffective Peripheral Tissue Perfusion related to deep vein thrombosis*
    Deep vein thrombosis is a medical diagnosis that evokes responses for which nurses are accountable: monitoring for and managing, with physician- and nurse-prescribed interventions, physiologic complications (eg, embolism, venous ulcers). This situation would be represented by collaborative problems such as *PC: Embolism.* In addition, the nurse would intervene independently to prevent complications of immobility and teach how to prevent recurrence, applying nursing diagnoses such as *Disuse Syndrome* and *Risk for Ineffective Health Maintenance related to insufficient knowledge of risk factors.*

INEFFECTIVE PERIPHERAL TISSUE PERFUSION

DEFINITION

Ineffective Peripheral Tissue Perfusion: State in which a person experiences or is at risk of experiencing a decrease in nutrition and respiration at the peripheral cellular level because of a decrease in capillary blood supply

DEFINING CHARACTERISTICS
Major (Must Be Present, One or More)

Presence of one of the following types (see Key Concepts for definitions):

Claudication (arterial)	Aching pain (arterial or venous)
Rest pain (arterial)	

Diminished or absent arterial pulses (arterial)
Skin color changes

Pallor (arterial)	Reactive hyperemia (arterial)
Cyanosis (venous)	

Skin temperature changes

Cooler (arterial)	Warmer (venous)

Decreased blood pressure (arterial)
Capillary refill longer than 3 s (arterial)

Minor (May Be Present)

Edema (venous)
Change in sensory function (arterial)
Change in motor function (arterial)
Trophic tissue changes (arterial)

Hard, thick nails	Loss of hair	Nonhealing wound

RELATED FACTORS
Pathophysiologic
Related to compromised blood flow secondary to:

Vascular disorders

Arteriosclerosis	Leriche's syndrome	Venous hypertension
Raynaud's disease/syndrome	Aneurysm	Varicosities
Arterial thrombosis	Buerger's disease	Deep vein thrombosis
Sickle cell crisis	Collagen vascular disease	Cirrhosis
Rheumatoid arthritis	Alcoholism	

Diabetes mellitus
Hypotension
Blood dyscrasias
Renal failure
Cancer/tumor

Treatment-Related
Related to immobilization
Related to presence of invasive lines
Related to pressure sites/constriction (elastic compression bandages, stockings, restraints)
Related to blood vessel trauma or compression

Situational (Personal, Environmental)
Related to pressure of enlarging uterus on pelvic vessels
Related to pressure of enlarged abdomen on pelvic vessels
Related to vasoconstricting effects of tobacco
Related to decreased circulating volume secondary to dehydration
Related to dependent venous pooling
Related to hypothermia
Related to pressure of muscle mass secondary to weight lifting

---

ⓧ **AUTHOR'S NOTE**

See *Ineffective Peripheral Tissue Perfusion.*

ⓧ **ERRORS IN DIAGNOSTIC STATEMENTS**

See *Ineffective Peripheral Tissue Perfusion.*

KEY CONCEPTS
Generic Considerations
- Cellular nutrition and respiration depend on adequate blood flow through the microcirculation.
- Adequate cellular oxygenation depends on the following processes (Porth, 2002):
  - The ability of the lungs to exchange air adequately (O_2–CO_2)
  - The ability of the pulmonary alveoli to diffuse oxygen and carbon dioxide across the cell membrane to the blood
  - The ability of the red blood cells (hemoglobin) to carry oxygen
  - The ability of the heart to pump with enough force to deliver the blood to the microcirculation
  - The ability of intact blood vessels to deliver blood to the microcirculation
- Hypoxemia (decreased oxygen content of the blood) results in cellular hypoxia, which causes cellular swelling and contributes to tissue injury.
- *Arterial* blood flow is enhanced by a *dependent* position and inhibited by an *elevated* position (gravity pulls blood downward, away from the heart).

- When an alteration in peripheral tissue perfusion exists, the nurse must consider its nature. the two major components of the peripheral vascular system are the arterial and the venous systems. Signs, symptoms, etiology, and nursing interventions are different for problems in each of these two systems and, therefore, are addressed separately.
- Changes in arterial walls increase the incidence of stroke and coronary artery disease (Porth, 2002).
- High levels of circulating lipids increase the risk of coronary heart disease, peripheral vascular disease, and stroke (Porth, 2002).

⊙ Geriatric Considerations

- Age-related vascular changes include stiffened blood vessels, which cause increased peripheral resistance, impaired baroreceptor functioning, and diminished ability to increase organ blood flow (Miller, 2004). These age-related changes cause the veins to become more dilated and less elastic. Valves of the large leg veins become less efficient. Age-related reductions in muscle mass and inactivity further reduce peripheral circulation (Miller, 2004).
- Physical deconditioning or lack of exercise accentuates the functional consequences of age-related cardiovascular changes. Contributing factors to deconditioning include acute illness, mobility limitations, cardiac disease, depression, and lack of motivation (Miller, 2004).

Focus Assessment Criteria

See Tables II.26 and II.27.

Subjective Data
Assess for Defining Characteristics.

Pain (associated with, time of day)	Pallor, cyanosis, paresthesias
Temperature change	Change in motor function

Assess for Related Factors.
Medical history
See Related Factors.

TABLE II.26 Arterial Insufficiency vs Venous Insufficiency: A Comparison of Subjective Data

Symptom	Arterial Insufficiency	Venous Insufficiency
Pain		
Location	Feet, muscles of legs, toes	Ankles, lower legs
Quality	Burning, shocking, prickling, throbbing, cramping, sharp	Aching, tightness
Quantity	Increase in severity with increased muscle activity or elevation	Varies with fluid intake, use of support hose, and decreased muscle activity
Chronology	Brought on predictably by exercise	Greater in evening than in morning
Setting	Use of affected muscle groups	Increases during course of day with prolonged standing or sitting
Aggravating factors	Exercise Extremity elevation	Immobility Extremity dependence
Alleviating factors	Cessation of exercise Extremity dependence	Extremity elevation Compression stockings or Ace wraps
Paresthesia	Numbness, tingling, burning, decreased touch sensation	No change unless arterial system or nerves are affected

Table II.27 Arterial Insufficiency vs Venous Insufficiency: A Comparison of Objective Data

Sign	Arterial Insufficiency	Venous Insufficiency
Temperature	Cool skin	Warm skin
Color	Pale on elevation, dependent rubor (reactive hyperemia)	Flushed, cyanotic Typical brown discoloration around ankles
Capillary filling	>3 seconds	Nonapplicable
Pulses	Absent or weak	Present unless there is concomitant arterial disease, or edema may obscure them
Movement	Decreased motor ability with nerve and muscle ischemia	Motor ability unchanged unless edema is severe enough to restrict joint mobility
Ulceration	Occurs on foot at site of trauma or at tips of toes (most distal to be perfused) Ulcers are deep with well-defined margins Surrounding tissue is shiny and taut with thin skin	Occurs around ankle (area of greatest pressure from chronic venous stasis due to valvular incompetence) Ulcers shallow with irregular edges Surrounding tissue edematous with engorged veins

Risk factors

Smoking (never, quit, years)

Immobility

History of phlebitis

Sedentary lifestyle

Family history of heart disease, vascular disease, stroke, kidney disease, or diabetes mellitus

Stress

Medications

Type   Side effects   Dosage

Objective Data

Assess for Defining Characteristics.

Skin

    Temperature (cool, warm)

    Color (pale, dependent rubor, flushed, cyanotic, brown discolorations)

    Ulcerations (size, location, description of surrounding tissue)

Bilateral pulses (radial, femoral popliteal, posterior tibial, dorsalis pedis)

    Rate, rhythm   Weak

    Volume   Normal, easily palpable

    Absent, nonpalpable   Aneurysmal

Paresthesia (numbness, tingling, burning)

Edema (location, pitting)

Capillary refill (normal less than 3 seconds)

Motor ability (normal, compromised)

For more information on Focus Assessment Criteria, visit http://connection.lww.com.

Goal

NOC Sensory Functions: Cutaneous, Tissue Integrity, Tissue Perfusion: Peripheral

The individual will report a decrease in pain.

Indicators

- Define peripheral vascular problem in own words.
- Identify factors that improve peripheral circulation.
- Identify necessary lifestyle changes.
- Identify medical regimen, diet, medications, activities that promote vasodilation.
- Identify factors that inhibit peripheral circulation.
- State when to contact physician or health care professional.

General Interventions

 NIC Peripheral Sensation Management,
Circulatory Care: Venous Insufficiency,
Circulatory Care: Arterial Insufficiency,
Positioning, Exercise Promotion

Assess Causative and Contributing Factors.

Underlying disease

Inhibited venous blood flow

Hypothermia or
vasoconstriction

Inhibited arterial blood flow

Fluid volume excess or deficit

Activities related to symptom/sign onset

Promote Factors that Improve Arterial Blood Flow.

Keep extremity in a dependent position.

Keep extremity warm (do not use heating pad or hot water bottle, because the person with a peripheral vascular disease may have a disturbance in sensation and will not be able to determine if the temperature is hot enough to damage tissue; the use of external heat also may increase the metabolic demands of the tissue beyond its capacity).

Reduce risk for trauma.
   Change positions at least every hour.
   Avoid leg crossing.
   Reduce external pressure points (inspect shoes daily for rough lining).
   Avoid sheepskin heel protectors (they increase heel pressure and pressure across dorsum of foot).
   Encourage range-of-motion exercises.
   Discuss smoking cessation (see *Ineffective Health Maintenance Related to Tobacco Use*).

Promote Factors that Improve Venous Blood Flow.

Elevate extremity above the level of the heart (may be contraindicated if severe cardiac or respiratory disease is present).

Avoid standing or sitting with legs dependent for long periods.

Consider the use of elastic compression bandages or below-knee elastic stockings to prevent venous pooling.

Reduce or remove external venous compression that impedes venous flow.
   Avoid pillows behind the knees or Gatch bed, which is elevated at the knees.
   Avoid leg crossing.
   Change positions, move extremities, or wiggle fingers and toes every hour.
   Avoid garters and tight elastic stockings above the knees.

Measure baseline circumference of calves and thighs if person is at risk for deep venous thrombosis, or if it is suspected.

Discuss the Implications of Condition and Choices.

Encourage client to share feelings, concerns, and understanding of risk factors, disease process, and effect on life.

Assist client to select lifestyle behaviors that he or she chooses to change (Burch et al., 1991).
   Avoid multiple changes.
   Consider personal abilities, resources, and overall health.
   Be realistic and optimistic.

Plan a Daily Walking Program.

Provide reasons for program.

Teach client to avoid fatigue.

Instruct client to avoid increase in exercise until assessed by physician for cardiac problems.

Reassure client that walking does not harm the blood vessels or the muscles; "walking into the pain," resting, and resuming walking improves the oxidative metabolic capacity of the muscle.

Start slowly.

Emphasize that it is not the speed or distance but the action of walking that is important.

Assist client to set goals and the steps to achieve them.
   Will walk 10 min daily.
   Will walk 10 min daily and 20 min three times a week.
   Will walk 20 min daily.
   Will walk 30 min three times a week.

Suggest a method to self-monitor progress (eg, graph, checklist).

Initiate Health Teaching, as Indicated.

Teach Client to

Avoid long car or plane rides (get up and walk around at least every hour).

Keep dry skin lubricated (cracked skin eliminates the physical barrier to infection).

Wear warm clothing during cold weather.

Wear cotton or wool socks.

Use gloves or mittens if hands are exposed to cold (including home freezers).

Avoid dehydration in warm weather.

Give special attention to feet and toes.

    Wash feet and dry well daily.

    Do not soak feet.

    Avoid harsh soaps or chemicals (including iodine) on feet.

    Keep nails trimmed and filed smooth.

Inspect feet and legs daily for injuries and pressure points.

Wear clean socks.

Wear shoes that offer support and fit comfortably.

Inspect the inside of shoes daily for rough lining.

Briefly Explain the Relation of Certain Risk Factors to the Development of Atherosclerosis.

Smoking

Vasoconstriction

Decreased oxygenation of the
  blood

Elevated blood pressure

Increased lipidemia

Increased platelet aggregation

Hypertension

Constant trauma of pressure causes damage to the vessel lining, which promotes plaque formation
  and narrowing.

Hyperlipidemia

Promotes atherosclerosis

Sedentary lifestyle

Decreases muscle tone and strength

Decreases circulation

Excess weight (>10% of ideal)

Fatty tissue increases peripheral resistance and claudication.

Fatty tissue is less vascular.

Teach Methods to Relieve Pain.

Assume dependent position for ischemic pain.

Elevate extremities for relief of venous aching.

Relieve phantom pain after an amputation by massaging or tapping stump or opposite limb.

Use other nursing measures such as relaxation or distraction to assist in pain relief.

If these methods do not relieve pain, refer to a physician or pain specialist.

Teach symptoms/signs of underlying disease and when to call the physician or health care professional.

Rationales

- *Venous* blood flow is enhanced by an *elevated* position and inhibited by a *dependent* position (gravity pulls blood downward, away from the heart).
- Immobility and venous stasis predispose to thrombus and embolus production.
- The effects of nicotine on the cardiovascular system contribute to coronary artery disease, stroke, hypertension, and peripheral vascular disease (Porth, 2002).
- Lack of exercise inhibits the pumping action of the muscles, which enhances circulation.
- Overweight status increases cardiac workload, causing hypertension (Porth, 2002).
- An older client may have lifestyle patterns of inactivity, smoking, and high-fat diet that are risk factors; he or she should be counseled to change.
- Attaining short-term goals can foster motivation to continue to change.
- Daily foot care can reduce tissue damage and help prevent or detect early further injury and infection.
- Properly fitted shoes help prevent injury to skin and underlying tissue.
- Tight garments and certain leg positions constrict leg vessels, further reducing circulation.
- Community resources can assist the client with weight loss, smoking cessation, diet, and exercise programs.

UNILATERAL NEGLECT

DEFINITION

Unilateral Neglect: State in which a person is unable to attend to or "ignores" the hemiplegic side of the body and/or, on the affected side, objects, persons, or sounds in the environment

DEFINING CHARACTERISTICS
Major (Must Be Present, One or More)

Neglect of involved body parts and/or extrapersonal space (hemispatial neglect), and/or
Denial of the existence of the affected limb or side of body (anosognosia)

Minor (May Be Present)

Difficulty with spatial–perceptual tasks
Hemiplegia (usually of the left side)

RELATED FACTORS
Pathophysiologic

Related to the impaired perceptual abilities secondary to:

Cerebrovascular accident   Brain injury/trauma
Cerebral aneurysms   Cerebral tumors

AUTHOR'S NOTE

Unilateral Neglect represents a disturbance in the reciprocal loop that occurs most often in the right hemisphere of the brain. This diagnosis also could be viewed as a syndrome diagnosis, *Unilateral Neglect Syndrome*. As mentioned in Chapter 3, syndrome diagnoses encompass a cluster of nursing diagnoses related to the situation. The nursing interventions for *Unilateral Neglect Syndrome* would focus on *Self-Care Deficit, Anxiety,* and *Risk for Injury.*

ERRORS IN DIAGNOSTIC STATEMENTS

Unilateral Neglect related to lack of grooming and hygiene for right side of face, head, and right arm
    Lack of grooming on one side of the body can be an indicator of *Unilateral Neglect* if neurologic disease or damage is present; it is not a related factor. When writing the diagnostic statement, the nurse should ask, "How does the nurse treat unilateral neglect?" Because the nursing focus is on teaching adaptive techniques, phrasing the diagnosis *Unilateral Neglect related to lack of knowledge of adaptive techniques* would be appropriate. If *Unilateral Neglect* were viewed as a syndrome diagnosis, the appropriate diagnostic statement would be *Unilateral Neglect Syndrome.* No "related to" is needed with a syndrome diagnosis because the label includes the etiology. The interventions would have the same focus, reducing neglect by using adaptive techniques.

KEY CONCEPTS
Generic Considerations

- Unilateral neglect is also called hemi-inattention, unilateral asomatognosia (unilateral spatial agnosia, Anton-Babinski syndrome), anosognosia, and atopognosia.
- The most common cause of unilateral neglect is right hemispheric brain damage; primarily, lesions in the right parietal lobe cause this defect. Lesions of the frontal lobe, inferior parietal lobe, thalamus, and striatum also can cause unilateral neglect (Lin, 1996).

- The right parietal lobe attends to stimuli presented to both the right and left sides; with a lesion of the left parietal lobe, the right parietal lobe could continue attending to the ipsilateral (same side) or contralateral (right-sided) stimuli. Because the left parietal lobe cannot attend to ipsilateral stimuli as well as the right parietal lobe can, however, lesions of the right parietal lobe are more likely to induce a profound contralateral sensory inattention than lesions of the left parietal lobe (Porth, 2002).
- Unilateral neglect is characterized by an unawareness or denial of the affected half of the body, often extending to the extrapersonal space.
- Homonymous hemianopsia (loss of vision on the contralateral side) usually occurs with unilateral neglect. Unilateral neglect and hemianopsia are two separate phenomena, and either can be present without the other. When they occur together, the person has more difficulty compensating for the loss (Porth, 2002).
- Anosognosia (ignorance of paralysis) and dressing apraxia may occur in lesions of either hemisphere but have been observed more frequently in lesions of the nondominant hemisphere.
- The person with a parietal lobe injury demonstrates problems with body schema, spatial judgment, and sensory interpretation.
- In addition, the person with this type of brain injury may exhibit some or all of the following characteristics that complicate the neglect syndrome:
  - Impulsiveness
  - Short attention span
  - Lack of insight into the extent of the disability
  - Diminished learning skills
  - Inability to recognize faces
  - Decrease in concrete thinking
  - Confusion
- Prognosis for recovery from many of the behavioral abnormalities associated with right hemisphere stroke is more favorable after hemorrhage as opposed to after infarction (Lin, 1996).
- Early recognition of the existence and extent of these syndromes allows more accurate planning of goals.

◆ Pediatric Considerations

Children at greatest risk for development of unilateral neglect are those with acquired hemiplegia (eg, from stroke). Strokes may occur in children with congenital heart disease, sickle cell anemia, meningitis, or head trauma.

◉ Geriatric Considerations

Most people who experience unilateral neglect are older adults, simply because the incidence of stroke is greatest in this population.

Focus Assessment Criteria

Subjective and Objective Data
Assess for Defining Characteristics.

Person's perception of the problem
Effects on activities of daily living (ADLs)
Bathing, grooming, and hygiene: Does the person

Wash the affected side of the body?	Put dentures in straight?
	Comb only part of the hair?
Shave both sides of the face?	Apply makeup to both sides of face?
	Put eyeglasses on straight?
Brush all his or her teeth?	

Feeding: Does the person
  Pocket food on the affected side of the mouth?
  Eat only half of his or her food (ie, eat only food on the unaffected side of plate/tray)?
Dressing: Does the person
  Dress the affected limbs?

Mobility/positioning

> When sitting in a wheelchair, does the person lean or tilt toward the unaffected side?
> Does the affected arm dangle off the lapboard?
> Are the head and eyes turned toward the unaffected side?
> When propelling the wheelchair or when ambulating, does the person bump or run into objects on affected side?

Safety: Does the person

> Attempt to walk or transfer out of the chair or bed when unable to ambulate?
> Have sensation in the affected limbs?
> Frequently injure the affected arm or hand (cuts, bumps, bruises)?
> Feel pain when injured?
> Realize when injury occurs?
> Scan the entire visual field?
> Turn head to the affected side to compensate?
> Respond to stimuli presented from the affected side?
> Does the affected arm dangle at the side and get caught in the wheelchair spokes, siderails, doorways, and so forth?

For more information on Focus Assessment Criteria, visit http://connection.lww.com.

Goal

NOC	Body Image, Body Positioning: Self-Initiated, Self-Care: Activities of Daily Living

The person will demonstrate an ability to
scan the visual field to compensate for loss of function/sensation in affected limbs.

Indicators

- Identify safety hazards in the environment.
- Describe the deficit and the rationale for treatment.

General Interventions

NIC	Unilateral Neglect Management, Self-Care Assistance

Assist Client to Recognize the Perceptual Deficit.

Initially adapt the environment to the deficit:

> Position person, call light, bedside stand, television, telephone, and personal items on the unaffected side.
> Position bed with unaffected side toward the door.
> Approach and speak to person from unaffected side.
> If you must approach person from affected side, announce your presence as soon as you enter the room to avoid startling the person.
> When working with the person's affected extremity, position the unaffected side near a wall to minimize distractions.

Gradually change the person's environment as you teach him or her to compensate and to learn to recognize the forgotten field; move furniture and personal items out of the visual field.

Provide a simplified, well-lit, uncluttered environment.

> Provide a moment between activities.
> Provide concrete cues: "You are on your side facing the wall."

Provide a full-length mirror to help with vertical orientation and to diminish the distortion of the vertical and horizontal plane, which manifests itself in the client leaning toward the affected side.

Use verbal instructions rather than mere demonstrations. Keep instructions simple.

For a person in a wheelchair, obtain a lapboard (preferably Plexiglas); position the affected arm on the lapboard with the fingertips at midline. Encourage person to look for the arm on the board.

For an ambulatory person, obtain an arm sling to prevent the arm from dangling and causing shoulder subluxation.

When the person is in bed, elevate affected arm on a pillow to prevent dependent edema.

Constantly cue to the environment.

Encourage client to wear a watch, favorite ring, or bracelet on affected arm to draw attention to it.

Assist Client with Adaptations Needed for Self-Care and Other ADLs.

Encourage Client to Wear Prescribed Corrective Lenses or Hearing Aids.
For Bathing, Dressing, and Toileting:
Instruct client to attend to affected extremity/side first when performing ADLs.

Instruct client always to look for affected extremity when performing ADL, to know where it is at all times.

Teach client to dress and groom in front of a mirror.

Suggest using color-coded markers sewn or placed inside shoes or clothes to help distinguish right from left.

Encourage client to integrate affected extremity during bathing and to feel extremity by rubbing and massaging it.

Use adaptive equipment as appropriate.

Refer to *Self-Care Deficit* for additional interventions.

For Feeding:

Set up meals with a minimum of dishes, food, and utensils.

Instruct client to eat in small amounts and place food on unaffected side of mouth.

Instruct client to use tongue to sweep out "pockets" of food from affected side after every bite.

After meals/medications, check oral cavity for pocketed food/medication.

Provide oral care t.i.d. and PRN.

Initially place food in the person's visual field; gradually move food out of field and teach person to scan entire visual field.

Use adaptive feeding equipment as appropriate.

Refer to *Self-Care Deficit: Feeding* for additional interventions.

Refer to *Imbalanced Nutrition: Less than Body Requirements related to swallowing difficulties* if person has difficulty chewing and swallowing food.

Teach Measures to Prevent Injury.

Retrain Person to Scan Entire Environment.

Instruct client to turn head past midline to view scene on the affected side.

Perform activities that require turning the head.

Remind client to scan when ambulating or propelling a wheelchair.

Use Tactile Sensation to Reintroduce Affected Arm/Extremity to the Person.

Have person stroke involved side with uninvolved hand and watch the arm or leg while stroking it.

Rub different-textured materials to stimulate sensations (hot, cold, rough, soft).

Instruct Client to Keep the Affected Arm and/or Leg in View.

Position arm on lapboard. (Plexiglas lapboards allow person to view affected leg, thereby helping to integrate the leg into the body schema.)

Provide an arm sling for an ambulatory person.

Instruct client to take extra care around sources of heat or cold and moving machinery or parts to protect affected side from injury.

Initiate Health Teaching and Referrals.

Ensure that both person and family understand the cause of unilateral neglect and the purpose of and rationale for all interventions.

Proceed with teaching as needed.

Explain unilateral neglect.

Instruct family on how to facilitate the person's relearning techniques (eg, cueing, scanning visual field).

Teach use of adaptive equipment, if appropriate.

Teach principles of maintaining a safe environment.

Rationales

- Adapting the environment minimizes sensory deprivation. Initially, however, attempts should be made to have the person attend to both sides.
- Reminders can help the client adapt to the environment.
- Rapid movements can precipitate anxiety.
- Cues can help with adjustment to position changes.
- Clients know that something is wrong but may attribute it to being "disturbed."
- Tactile stimulation of the affected parts promotes their integration into the whole body.
- Scanning can help prevent injury and increase awareness of entire space.
- Decreased sensation or motor function increases the vulnerability to injury.
- The client may need specific reminders to prevent him or her from ignoring nonfunctioning body parts.

Impaired Urinary Elimination
Maturational Enuresis*
Functional Incontinence
Reflex Incontinence
Stress Incontinence
Total Incontinence
Urge Incontinence
Urinary Retention

IMPAIRED URINARY ELIMINATION

DEFINITION

Impaired Urinary Elimination: State in which a person experiences or is at risk of experiencing urinary elimination dysfunction

DEFINING CHARACTERISTICS
Major (Must Be Present, One or More)

Reports or experiences a urinary elimination problem, such as:

Urgency	Dribbling	Frequency
Bladder distention	Hesitancy	Large residual urine volumes
Nocturia	Incontinence	Enuresis

RELATED FACTORS
Pathophysiologic

Related to incompetent bladder outlet secondary to congenital urinary tract anomalies
Related to decreased bladder capacity or irritation to bladder secondary to:

Infection	Glucosuria	Trauma
Carcinoma	Urethritis	

Related to diminished bladder cues or impaired ability to recognize bladder cues secondary to:

Cord injury/tumor/infection	Diabetic neuropathy	Brain injury/tumor/infection
Alcoholic neuropathy	Cerebrovascular accident	Tabes dorsalis
Demyelinating diseases	Parkinsonism	Multiple sclerosis

Treatment-Related

Related to effects of surgery on bladder sphincter secondary to:

Postprostatectomy	Extensive pelvic dissection

Related to diagnostic instrumentation
Related to decreased muscle tone secondary to:
General or spinal anesthesia
Drug therapy (iatrogenic)

Antihistamines	Immunosuppressant therapy	Epinephrine
Diuretics	Anticholinergics	Tranquilizers
Sedatives	Muscle relaxants	Post-indwelling catheters

*This diagnosis is not currently on the NANDA list but has been included for clarity or usefulness.

Situational (Personal, Environmental)
Related to weak pelvic floor muscles secondary to:

Obesity   Childbirth   Aging
Recent substantial weight loss

Related to inability to communicate needs
Related to bladder outlet obstruction secondary to fecal impaction/chronic constipation
Related to decreased bladder muscle tone secondary to dehydration
Related to decreased attention to bladder cues secondary to:

Depression
Delirium
Intentional suppression (self-induced deconditioning)
Confusion

Related to environmental barriers to bathroom secondary to:

Distant toilets   Poor lighting   Unfamiliar surroundings
Bed too high   Siderails

Related to inability to access bathroom on time secondary to:

Caffeine/alcohol use   Impaired mobility

Maturational
Child
Related to small bladder capacity
Related to lack of motivation

ⓧ AUTHOR'S NOTE

Impaired Urinary Elimination probably is too broad a diagnosis for effective clinical use. For this reason, the nurse should use a more specific diagnosis, such as *Stress Incontinence,* whenever possible. When the etiologic or contributing factors for incontinence have not been identified, the nurse could write a temporary diagnosis of *Impaired Urinary Elimination related to unknown etiology, as evidenced by incontinence.*

The nurse performs a focus assessment to determine whether the incontinence is transient, in response to an acute condition (eg, infection, medication side effects), or established in response to various chronic neural or genitourinary conditions (Miller, 2004). In addition, the nurse should differentiate the type of incontinence: functional, reflex, stress, urge, or total. The nurse should not use the diagnosis *Total Incontinence* unless all other types of incontinence have been ruled out.

ⓧ ERRORS IN DIAGNOSTIC STATEMENTS

1. *Impaired Urinary Elimination related to surgical diversion*
   This diagnosis represents a new label for urostomy and does not focus on the nursing accountability. The nurse should assess a person with a urostomy for its effect on functional patterns and physiologic functioning. For this person, the collaborative problems *PC: Stomal obstruction* and *PC: Internal urine leakage,* as well as nursing diagnoses such as *Risk for Disturbed Body Image* and *Risk for Impaired Health Maintenance,* could apply.
2. *Impaired Urinary Elimination related to renal failure*
   This nursing diagnosis renames renal failure and is inappropriate. For this reason, the diagnosis *Excess Fluid Volume related to acute renal failure* also would be incorrect. Renal failure causes or contributes to various actual or potential nursing diagnoses, such as *Risk for Infection* and *Risk for Imbalanced Nutrition,* and collaborative problems, such as *PC: Fluid/ electrolyte imbalances* and *PC: Metabolic acidosis.*
3. *Total Incontinence related to effects of aging*
   The physiologic effects of aging on the urinary tract system can influence functioning negatively when other risk factors (eg, mobility problems, dehydration, side effects of medications,

(continued)

⊙⊙ **ERRORS IN DIAGNOSTIC STATEMENTS** (*Continued*)

decreased awareness of bladder cues) also are present. This nursing diagnosis projects a biased view of anticipated incontinence in an older adult, with associated use of indwelling catheters, incontinence briefs, and/or bed pads. When this equipment is used, the nurse is not treating incontinence, but rather managing urine. The use of such equipment is a short-term solution. For these situations, *Risk for Infection* and *Risk for Impaired Skin Integrity* would apply. When an older adult has an incontinent episode, the nurse should proceed cautiously before applying the nursing diagnosis label of "incontinence." If factors exist that increase the likelihood of recurrence and the client is motivated, the diagnosis *Risk for Functional/Urge Incontinence related to* (specify—eg, dehydration, mobility difficulties, decreased bladder capacity) could apply. This diagnosis would focus nursing interventions on preventing incontinence, rather than expecting it as inevitable. For an older person with the combination of functional and urge incontinence, the nurse would focus on assisting him or her to increase bladder capacity and to reduce barriers to bathrooms, using the diagnosis *Functional/Urge Incontinence related to age-related effects on bladder capacity, self-induced fluid limitations, and unstable gait.*

KEY CONCEPTS
Generic Considerations

- The three components of the lower urinary tract that assist to maintain continence are as follows (Porth, 2002):
  - Detrusor muscle in the bladder wall, which allows bladder expansion to increase with volume of urine
  - Internal sphincter or proximal urethra, which, when contracted, prevents urine leakage
  - External sphincter, which by voluntary control provides added support during stressed situations (eg, overdistended bladder)
- Innervation of the bladder arises from the spinal cord at the levels of S2–S4. The bladder is under parasympathetic control. The cortex, midbrain, and medulla influence voluntary control over urination (Sampselle & DeLancey, 1998).
- The female urethra is 3 to 5 cm long. The male urethra is approximately 20 cm long. The urethra primarily maintains continence, but the cerebral cortex is the principal area for suppression of the desire to micturate.
- Capacity of the normal bladder (without experiencing discomfort) is 250 to 400 mL. The desire to void occurs when 150 to 250 mL of urine is in the bladder.
- The sitting position for the female and the standing position for the male allow optimal relaxation of the external urinary sphincter and perineal muscles.
- Bladder tissue tone can be lost if the bladder is distended to 1000 mL (atonic bladder) or continuously drained (Foley catheter).
- Mechanisms to stimulate the voiding reflex or Credé's method may be ineffective if the bladder capacity is less than 200 mL.
- Alcohol, coffee, and tea have a natural diuretic effect and are bladder irritants.
- Injury to the spinal cord above S2–S4 produces a spastic or reflex bladder tone. Injury to the spinal cord below S2–S4 produces a flaccid or atonic bladder.
- Lesions affecting inhibitory centers in the brain or the pathways transmitting inhibitory impulses to the bladder result in an uninhibited bladder.

Infection

- Stasis or pooling of urine contributes to bacterial growth. Bacteria can travel up the ureters to the kidney (ascending infection).
- Recurrent bladder infections cause fibrotic changes in the bladder wall, with a resultant decrease in bladder capacity.
- Urinary stasis, infections, alkaline urine, and decreased urine volume contribute to the formation of urinary tract calculi.

Incontinence

- Incontinence is transient in as many as 50% of people presenting with the problem. of the remaining group, about 66% can be cured or markedly improved with treatment (Resnick & Yalla, 1985). There are many effective corrective measures for the management of urinary tract disease in older adults, and a positive approach should be taken to minimize the incidence of urinary incontinence (Fanti et al., 1996).

- It is important to determine the natural history of the incontinent pattern. A new onset of incontinence is likely to be the result of a precipitating factor outside the urinary tract (eg, medications, acute illness, inaccessible toilets, impaired mobility that prevents getting to the toilet on time), which usually can be easily corrected. Incontinence can be either transient (reversible) or established (controllable).
  - Causes of transient incontinence include acute confusion, urinary tract infection, atrophic vaginitis, side effects of medications, metabolic imbalance, impaction, mobility problems, urosepsis, depression, and pressure sores.
  - Controllable incontinence cannot be cured, but urine removal can be planned (Fanti et al., 1996).
- Certain medications are associated with incontinence. Narcotics and sedatives diminish awareness of bladder cues. Adrenergic agents cause retention by increasing bladder outlet resistance. Anticholinergics (antidepressants, some antiparkinsonian medications, antispasmodics, antihistamines, antiarrhythmics, opiates) cause chronic retention with overflow. Diuretics rapidly increase urine volume and can cause incontinence if voiding cannot be delayed (Miller, 2004).
- People with diabetes mellitus, which can contribute to increased residual urine, frequency, and urgency, may have decreased awareness of bladder fullness.
- Social isolation of people with incontinence can be self-imposed because of fear and embarrassment, or imposed by others because of odor and aesthetics.
- Depression can prevent the person from recognizing or responding to bladder cues and, thus, contributes to incontinence.

Intermittent Catheterization

- This method maintains the tonicity of the bladder muscle, prevents overdistention, and provides for complete emptying of the bladder.
- The initial removal of more than 500 mL of urine from a chronically distended bladder can cause severe hemorrhage, which results when bladder veins, previously compressed by the distended bladder, rapidly dilate and rupture when bladder pressure is abruptly released. (After the initial release of 500 mL of urine, alternate the release of 100 mL of urine with 15-min catheter clamps.)
- The accumulation of more than 500 to 700 mL of urine in a bladder should not be permitted.
- In clients with spinal injuries at the T4 level or above, it is necessary to empty the bladder completely regardless of high volumes (>500 mL) owing to the risk of autonomic dysreflexia. Interruption of the sympathetic nervous system causes the veins not to dilate rapidly.

Total Incontinence

A cognitively impaired person with total incontinence requires caregiver-directed treatment. In institutional settings, indwelling and external catheters or disposal or washable incontinence briefs or pads are beneficial to the caregivers, but detrimental to the incontinent person. Aids and equipment should be considered only after other means have been attempted. In the home setting, the caregiver's needs may take precedence over the cognitively impaired person's. Urinary incontinence is cited as the major reason for seeking institutional care for people living at home (Miller, 2004).

◉ Geriatric Considerations

- Urinary incontinence affects 12% to 49% of older women and 7% to 22% of older men living in the community. Its prevalence increases to about 40% in hospitalized clients and 50% in institutionalized clients (Steeman & Defever, 1998). One of the major problems of incontinence in older adults is that it may be overlooked and not adequately evaluated by professionals; as a result, appropriate treatment is denied. Older clients may not admit to the problem because of attitudes about the inevitability of such complications.
- Age-related physiologic changes result in decreased bladder capacity, incomplete emptying, contractions during filling, and increased residual urine (Miller, 2004).
- Older adults can comfortably store 250 to 300 mL of urine, compared with a storage capacity of 350 to 400 mL in younger adults.

(continued)

> ### ⊙ Geriatric Considerations (continued)
>
> - The sensation to void is delayed in older adults, which shortens the interval between the initial perception of the urge and the actual need to void, resulting in urgency (Miller, 2004). Any factor that interferes with the older adult's perception to void (eg, medications, depression, limited fluid intake, neurologic impairments) or delays his or her ability to reach the toilet can cause incontinence.
> - Other physiologic components of aging that contribute to incontinence are the diminished ability of kidneys to concentrate urine, decreasing muscle tone of the pelvic floor muscles, and the inability to postpone urination.
> - Frequent voiding out of habit or limiting fluids may contribute to urgency by impairing the neurologic mechanisms that signal the need to void, because the bladder is rarely fully expanded.
> - The diminished vision, impaired mobility, and decreased energy level that may accompany aging mean that increased time is needed to locate the toilet, which also requires the person to be able to delay urination.
> - Older adults experience urgency owing to the bladder's limited capacity and their decreased ability to inhibit bladder contractions.

Focus Assessment Criteria

Subjective Data
Assess for Defining Characteristics.

"Do you have a problem with controlling your urine (or going to the bathroom)?"

History of symptoms

Lack of control	Pain or discomfort	Dribbling
Burning	Hesitancy	Change in voiding pattern
Urgency	Retention	Frequency

Onset and duration
Restrictions on lifestyle

Social	Sexual	Occupational
Role responsibilities		

Adult incontinence

History of continence

Is degree of continence acceptable	History of "weak" bladder
	Family history of incontinence
Age of attainment of continence	Previous history of enuresis

Onset and duration (day, night, just certain times)
Factors that increase incidence

Delay in getting to bathroom	Coughing	Laughing
When excited	Standing	Leaving bathroom
Turning in bed	Running	

Perception of need to void

Present	Absent	Diminished

Ability to delay urination after urge

Present (how long?)	Absent

Sensations before or during micturition

Difficulty starting stream	Need to force urine out	Difficulty stopping stream
Lack of sensation to void	Painful straining (tenesmus)	

Relief after voiding
Complete
Continued desire to void after emptying bladder
Use of catheters, incontinence briefs, bed pads

Childhood enuresis

Onset and pattern (day, night)
Toilet-training history

Family history of bed-wetting

Response of others to child (parents, siblings, peers)

Assess for Related Factors.

Physiologic risk factors

Fluid intake pattern (type and amount, especially before bedtime)

Dehydration (self-imposed, overuse of diuretics, caffeine, alcohol)

Prostatic hypertrophy

Bladder, vaginal infections

Chronic illnesses (eg, diabetes, alcoholism, Parkinson's disease, Alzheimer's disease, multiple sclerosis, cerebrovascular accident, vitamin B_{12} deficiency)

Metabolic disturbances (eg, hypokalemia, hypercalcemia)

Fecal impaction/severe constipation

Certain medications (diuretics, anticholinergics, antihistamines, sedatives, acetaminophen, amitriptyline, aspirin, barbiturates, chlorpropamide, clofibrate, fluphenazine, haloperidol, narcotics)

Multiple or difficult deliveries

Pelvic, bladder, or uterine surgery, disorders

Environmental barriers

Location of bathroom within 40 feet

Stairs, narrow doorways

Dim lighting

Ability to locate bathroom in social settings

Objective Data

Assess for Defining Characteristics.

Urination stream

Slow	Sprays	Small
Starts and stops	Drops	Slow or hard to start
Dribble		

Urine

Color, odor, appearance, specific gravity

Negative or positive for

Glucose	Bacteria	Protein
Red blood cells	Ketone	

Assess for Related Factors.

Voiding and fluid intake patterns

Record for 2 to 4 days to establish a baseline.

What is daily fluid intake?

When does incontinence occur?

Muscle tone

Abdomen firm, or soft and pendulous?

History of recent significant weight loss or gain?

Reflexes

Presence or absence of cauda equina reflexes

    Anal

    Bulbocavernosus

Bladder

Distention (palpable)

Can it be emptied by external stimuli? (Credé's method, gentle suprapubic tapping, or warm water over the perineum, Valsalva maneuver, pulling of pubic hair, anal stretch)

Capacity (at least 400 to 500 mL)

Residual urine

    None

    Present (in what amount?)

Functional ability

Get in/out of chair	Walk alone to bathroom	Maintain balance
Manipulate clothing		

Cognitive ability

Asks to go to bathroom

Expects to be incontinent

Initiates toileting with
reminders

Aware of incontinence

Assess for any

Constipation

Mobility disorders

Depression

Dehydration

Fecal impaction

Sensory disorders

For more information on Focus Assessment Criteria, visit http://connection.lww.com.

MATURATIONAL ENURESIS*

DEFINITION

Maturational Enuresis: State in which a child experiences involuntary voiding during sleep that is not pathophysiologic in origin

DEFINING CHARACTERISTICS

Major (Must Be Present)

Reports or demonstrates episodes of involuntary voiding during sleep

RELATED FACTORS

Situational (Personal, Environmental)

Related to stressors (school, siblings)

Related to inattention to bladder cues

Related to unfamiliar surroundings

Maturational

Child

Related to small bladder capacity

Related to lack of motivation

Related to attention-seeking behavior

⓪ AUTHOR'S NOTE

Enuresis can result from physiologic or maturational factors. Certain etiologies, such as strictures, urinary tract infection, constipation, nocturnal epilepsy, and diabetes, should be ruled out when enuresis is present. These situations do not represent nursing diagnoses.

When enuresis results from small bladder capacity, failure to perceive cues because of deep sleep, or inattention to bladder cues, or is associated with a maturational issue (eg, new sibling, school pressures), the nursing diagnosis *Maturational Enuresis* is appropriate. Psychological problems usually are not the cause of enuresis but may result from lack of understanding or insensitivity to the problem. Interventions that punish or shame the child must be avoided.

---

*This diagnosis is not on the NANDA list but has been added by this author for its clarity and usefulness.

⊗ **ERRORS IN DIAGNOSTIC STATEMENTS**

Maturational Enuresis related to stressors and conflicts

Rather than focus on etiology for maturational enuresis, the nurse should focus on teaching the child and parents management strategies. The nurse also should encourage parents to share their concerns and direct them away from punishing behaviors. Given this nursing focus, the nurse could restate the diagnosis as *Maturational Enuresis related to unknown etiology, as evidenced by reported episodes of bed-wetting.*

KEY CONCEPTS

- The newborn may void up to 20 times per day because of small bladder capacity. As the child grows, bladder capacity increases and frequency of urination decreases (Wong, 2003).
- Most children by 4 or 5 years of age have complete neuromuscular control of urination (Kelleher, 1997).
- Enuresis is defined as urinary incontinence at any age when urinary control would be expected.
- The etiology of enuresis is complex and not well understood. the following factors have been implicated:
  - Developmental/maturational delay (eg, small functional bladder capacity, deep sleep, mental retardation)
  - Organic factors (eg, infection, sickle cell anemia, diabetes, neuromuscular disorders)
  - Psychological/emotional factors (eg, stressors such as birth of sibling, hospitalization, divorce of parents; Kelleher, 1997)
- Children at risk for urinary retention include those who (Wong, 2003)
  - Have congenital anomalies of the urinary tract
  - Are neurologically impaired
  - Have undergone surgery
- Enuresis is primarily a maturational problem and usually ceases between 6 and 8 years of age. It is more common in boys. By adolescence, 99% become continent (Kelleher, 1997).
- There is a high frequency of bed-wetting in children whose parents or other near relatives were bed-wetters (Kelleher, 1997).
- High anxiety can impede the child's ability to master the skills necessary for the maintenance of continence (Morison, 1998).
- Most children with nocturnal enuresis have neither a psychiatric nor an organic illness (Kelleher, 1997).

Focus Assessment Criteria

Subjective Data

Assess for Defining Characteristics.

Onset
Pattern (day, night)
Number of episodes in month

Assess for Related Factors.

Toilet-training history
Family history of bed-wetting
Response of others (parents, peers, siblings)
Recent change or stressor

School	Relocation	Peers
Family problems	New sibling	

Inattention to bladder cues
Sexual abuse

For more information on Focus Assessment Criteria, visit http://connection.lww.com.

Goal

 NOC Urinary Continence, Knowledge: Enuresis, Family Functioning

The child will remain dry during the sleep cycle.

Indicator

The child and family will be able to list factors that decrease enuresis.

General Interventions

NIC Urinary Incontinence Care: Enuresis, Urinary Habit Training, Anticipatory Guidance, Family Support

Ascertain that Physiologic Causes of Enuresis Have Been Ruled Out.

Examples include infections, meatal stenosis, fistulas, pinworms, epispadias, ectopic ureter, and minor neurologic dysfunction (hyperactivity, cognitive delay).

Determine Contributing Factors.

Small bladder capacity
Sound sleeper
Response to stress (at school or at home, eg, new sibling)

Promote a Positive Parent–Child Relationship.

Explain the developmental nature of enuresis to parents and child, and that it has a high rate of spontaneous remission.
Explain to parents that disapproval (shaming, punishing) is useless in stopping enuresis but can make child shy, ashamed, and afraid.
Offer reassurance to child that other children wet the bed at night and that he or she is not bad or sinful.

Reduce Contributing Factors, if Possible.

Small Bladder Capacity
After child drinks fluids, encourage him or her to postpone voiding to help stretch the bladder.

Sound Sleeper
Have child void before retiring.
Restrict fluids at bedtime.
If child is awakened later (about 11 PM) to void, attempt to awaken child fully for positive reinforcement.

Too Busy to Sense a Full Bladder (If Daytime Wetting Occurs)
Teach child awareness of sensations that occur when it is time to void.
Teach child ability to control urination (have him or her start and stop the stream; have him or her "hold" the urine during the day, even if for only a short time).
Have child keep a record of how he or she is doing; emphasize dry days or nights (eg, stars on a calendar).
If child wets, have him or her explain or write down (if feasible) why he or she thinks it happened.

Initiate Health Teaching and Referrals, as Indicated.

For children with enuresis:
    Teach child and parents the facts about enuresis.
    Teach family techniques to control the adverse effects of enuresis (eg, plastic mattress covers, use of sleeping bag [machine-washable] when staying overnight away from home).
    Explain that the child cannot control bed-wetting but that bed-wetting can be controlled with intervention (Morison, 1998).
Seek opportunities to teach the public about enuresis and incontinence (eg, school and parent organizations, self-help groups).
Explain how the nocturnal enuresis alarm works.

Rationales

- Anger, punishment, and rejection by parents and peers contribute to feelings of shame, embarrassment, and low self-esteem (Carpenter, 1999).

- The use of an alarm intervention reduces nighttime bed-wetting in the majority of children both during and after treatment (Macaulay et al., 2004).
- Interventions for nocturnal enureses must focus on reducing social and emotional stigma (Macaulay, 2004).
- Explaining that enuresis is developmental reduces blaming of child and parental frustration (Morison, 1998).
- Behavioral reward system can enhance parent–child interactions related to toileting and decrease episodes of incontinence (Carpenter, 1999).
- Children who believe that they can be helped have the best chance of success (Morison, 1998).
- Self-concept improves in children treated for enuresis compared with those not treated (Longstaffe, 2000).

FUNCTIONAL INCONTINENCE

DEFINITION

Functional Incontinence: State in which a person experiences incontinence because of a difficulty or inability to reach the toilet in time

DEFINING CHARACTERISTICS
Major (Must Be Present)

Incontinence before or during an attempt to reach the toilet

RELATED FACTORS
Pathophysiologic

Related to diminished bladder cues and impaired ability to recognize bladder cues secondary to:

Brain injury/tumor/infection	Alcoholic neuropathy	Cerebrovascular accident
Parkinsonism	Demyelinating diseases	Progressive dementia
Multiple sclerosis		

Treatment-Related

Related to decreased bladder tone secondary to:

Antihistamines	Immunosuppressant therapy	Epinephrine
Diuretics	Anticholinergics	Tranquilizers
Sedatives	Muscle relaxants	

Situational (Personal, Environmental)

Related to impaired mobility
Related to decreased attention to bladder cues
Depression
Intentional suppression (self-induced deconditioning)
Confusion

Related to environmental barriers to bathroom

Distant toilets	Bed too high	Poor lighting
Siderails	Unfamiliar surroundings	

Maturational
Older Adult
Related to motor and sensory losses

Focus Assessment Criteria

See *Impaired Urinary Elimination.*

Goal

NOC Tissue Integrity, Urinary Continence, Urinary Elimination

The person will report no or decreased episodes of incontinence.

Indicators
- Remove or minimize environmental barriers at home.
- Use proper adaptive equipment to assist with voiding, transfers, and dressing.
- Describe causative factors for incontinence.

General Interventions

NIC Perineal Care, Urinary Incontinence Care, Prompted Voiding, Urinary Habit Training, Urinary Elimination Management, Teaching: Procedure/Treatment

Assess Causative or Contributing Factors.

Obstacles to Toilet
Poor lighting, slippery floor, misplaced furniture and rugs, inadequate footwear, toilet too far, bed too high, siderails up
Inadequate toilet (too small for walkers, wheelchair, seat too low/high, no grab bars)
Inadequate signal system for requesting help
Lack of privacy

Sensory/Cognitive Deficits
Visual deficits (blindness, field cuts, poor depth perception)
Cognitive deficits as a result of aging, trauma, stroke, tumor, infection

Motor/Mobility Deficits
Limited upper and/or lower extremity movement/strength (inability to remove clothing)
Barriers to ambulation (eg, vertigo, fatigue, altered gait, hypertension)

Reduce or Eliminate Contributing Factors, if Possible.

Environmental Barriers
Assess path to bathroom for obstacles, lighting, and distance.
Assess adequacy of toilet height and need for grab bars.
Assess adequacy of room size.
Provide a commode between bathroom and bed, if necessary.

Sensory/Cognitive Deficits
For a person with diminished vision:
Ensure adequate lighting.
Encourage person to wear prescribed corrective lens.
Provide clear, safe pathway to bathroom.
Keep call bell easily accessible.
If bedpan or urinal is used, make sure it is within easy reach in the same location at all times.
Assess person for safety in bathroom.
Assess person's ability to provide self-hygiene.

For a person with cognitive deficits:
Offer toileting reminders every 2 h, after meals, and before bedtime.
Establish appropriate means to communicate need to void.
Answer call bell immediately.
Encourage wearing of ordinary clothes.
Provide a normal environment for elimination (use bathroom, if possible).
Allow for privacy while maintaining safety.
Allow sufficient time for task.
Reorient client to where he or her is and what task he or she is doing.
Be consistent in your approach to person.
Give simple step-by-step instructions; use verbal and nonverbal cues.
Give positive reinforcement for success.
Assess person for safety in bathroom.
Assess need for adaptive devices on clothing to make dressing and undressing easier.
Assess person's ability to provide self-hygiene.

Motor/Mobility Deficits
For people with limited hand function:
Assess ability to remove and replace clothing. Loose clothing is easier to manipulate.
Provide dressing aids as necessary (eg, Velcro closures in seams for wheelchair patients, zipper pulls;
    all garments with fasteners may be adapted with Velcro closures).

Provide for Factors that Promote Continence.
Maintain Optimal Hydration.
Increase fluid intake to 2000 to 3000 mL/day, unless contraindicated.
Teach older adults not to depend on thirst sensations but to drink liquids even when not thirsty.
Space fluids every 2 h.
Decrease fluid intake after 7 PM; provide only minimal fluids during the night.
Reduce intake of coffee, tea, cola, alcohol, and grapefruit juice because of their diuretic effect.
Avoid large amounts of tomato and orange juice; they tend to make the urine more alkaline.
Encourage cranberry juice to acidify urine.

Maintain Adequate Nutrition to Ensure Bowel Elimination at Least Once Every 3 Days.
Monitor elimination pattern; check for fecal impaction if indicated.
Assess daily dietary intake for daily requirements of roughage, basic five food groups, and adequate
    fluids.
See *Imbalanced Nutrition* and *Constipation* for additional interventions.

Promote Micturition.
Ensure privacy and comfort.
Use toilet facilities, if possible, instead of bedpans.
Provide man with opportunity to stand, if possible.
Assist person on bedpan to flex knees and support back.
Teach postural evacuation (bend forward while sitting on toilet).
Ensure safe access to facilities.
    Provide access to urinal or bedpan.
    Provide call light.
    Reduce obstacles to toilet facilities (path that is well lighted and free of obstacles, bed at lowest level).
    Modify path to bathroom with rails.
    Modify bathroom with grab rails, elevated seats.
Stimulate the cutaneous surface to trigger the voiding reflex.
    Have person brush or stroke inner thigh or abdomen.
    Pour warm water over perineum.
    Give glass of water to drink while sitting on the toilet.

Promote Personal Integrity and Provide Motivation to Increase Bladder Control.
Encourage person to share feelings about incontinence and determine its effect on his or her social
    patterns.
Convey that incontinence can be cured or at least controlled to maintain dignity.
Expect client to be continent, not incontinent (eg, encourage street clothes, discourage use of bedpans).
Use protective pads or garments only after conscientious reconditioning efforts have been completely
    unsuccessful after 6 weeks.

Work to achieve daytime continence before expecting nighttime continence.
Encourage socialization.

    Encourage and assist person to groom self.

    If hospitalized, provide opportunities to eat meals outside bedroom (day room, lounge).

    If fear or embarrassment is preventing socialization, instruct person to use sanitary pads or briefs temporarily until control is established.

    Change clothes as soon as possible when wet to avoid indirectly sanctioning wetness.

    Advise the oral use of chlorophyll tablets to deodorize urine and feces.

    See *Social Isolation* and *Ineffective Coping* for additional interventions, if indicated.

Promote Skin Integrity.

Identify clients at risk for development of pressure ulcers.
Maintain acid pH of skin (Scardillo, 1999).
Avoid harsh soaps and alcohol products.
Keep moisture away from the skin.
See *Risk for Impaired Skin Integrity* for additional information.

Promote Personal Hygiene.

Encourage client to take showers rather than baths to prevent bacteria from entering urethra.
Instruct women to cleanse the perineum and urethra from front to back after each bowel movement.

Teach Prevention of Urinary Tract Infections.

Encourage regular, complete emptying of the bladder.
Ensure adequate fluid intake.
Keep urine acidic; avoid citrus juices, dark colas, and coffee.
Monitor urine pH.
Teach client to recognize abnormal changes in urine properties.

    Increased mucus and sediment

    Blood in urine (hematuria)

    Change in color (from normal straw-colored) or odor

Teach client to monitor for signs and symptoms of infection.

    Elevated temperature, chills, and shaking

    Changes in urine properties

    Suprapubic pain

    Painful urination

    Urgency

    Frequent small voids or frequent small incontinences

    Increased spasticity in spinal cord-injured individuals

    Increased urine pH

    Nausea/vomiting

    Lower back and/or flank pain

Explain Age-Related Effects on Bladder Function and that Urgency and Nocturia Do Not Necessarily Lead to Incontinence.

Initiate Health Teaching Referral, When indicated.

Refer to visiting nurse (occupational therapy department) for assessment of bathroom facilities at home.

Rationales

- Barriers can delay access to the toilet and cause incontinence if the client cannot delay urination. a few seconds' delay in reaching the bathroom can make the difference between continence and incontinence.
- Wearing normal clothing or nightwear helps simulate the home environment, where incontinence may not occur. A hospital gown may reinforce incontinence.
- A client with a cognitive deficit needs constant verbal cues and reminders to establish a routine and reduce incontinence (Fanti et al., 1996).
- Dehydration can prevent the sensation of a full bladder and can contribute to loss of bladder tone. Spacing fluids helps promote regular bladder filling and emptying.

- Coffee, tea, colas, and grapefruit juice act as diuretics, which can cause urgency.
- Dilute urine helps prevent infection and bladder irritation.
- Bacteria multiply rapidly in stagnant urine retained in the bladder. Moreover, overdistention hinders blood flow to the bladder wall, increasing the susceptibility to infection from bacterial growth. Regular, complete bladder emptying greatly reduces the risk of infection.
- Acidic urine deters the growth of most bacteria implicated in cystitis.
- Ammonia from urine makes the skin more alkaline and more vulnerable to irritants (Scardillo, 1999).

Geriatric Interventions

Emphasize that incontinence is not an inevitable age-related event.
Explain not to restrict fluid intake for fear of incontinence.
Explain not to rely on thirst as a signal to drink fluids.
Teach the need to have easy access to bathroom at night. If needed, consider commode chair or urinal.

Rationales

- Explaining the cause can motivate the person to participate.
- Dehydration can cause incontinence by eliminating the sensation of a full bladder (the signal to urinate) and also by reducing the person's alertness to the sensation.
- The older adult has an age-related decrease in thirst (Miller, 2004).

REFLEX INCONTINENCE

DEFINITION

Reflex Incontinence: State in which a person experiences predictable involuntary loss of urine with no sensation of urge, voiding, or bladder fullness

DEFINING CHARACTERISTICS
Major (Must Be Present)

Uninhibited bladder contractions
Involuntary reflexes producing spontaneous voiding
Partial or complete loss of sensation of bladder fullness or urge to void

RELATED FACTORS
Pathophysiologic

Related to impaired conduction of impulses above the reflex arc level secondary to:
Cord injury/tumor/infection

KEY CONCEPTS

- A lesion above the sacral cord segments (above T12) involving both motor and sensory tracts of the spinal cord results in a reflex bladder. Other common names for this type of bladder dysfunction are spastic, supraspinal, hypertonic, automatic, and upper motor neuron bladder.

- A lesion that does not completely transect the spinal cord can produce variable findings.
- Control from higher cerebral centers is removed in the reflex neurogenic bladder. Therefore, the person cannot start or stop micturition in a voluntary manner.
- The simple spinal reflex arc takes over the control of micturition.
- A positive bulbocavernosus reflex suggests that the voiding reflex (spinal reflex arc) is intact.
- If the opening of the urinary sphincter and the relaxation of the striated muscle surrounding the urinary sphincter are uncoordinated, there is a potential for large residual urine volumes after triggered voiding.
- Autonomic dysreflexia is an abnormal hyperactive reflex activity that occurs only in people with spinal cord injury with a lesion above T8. Most often, these clients have an upper motor neuron bladder (reflex incontinence). This is a life-threatening situation in which the blood pressure rises to lethal levels. Autonomic hyperreflexia is most often caused by stimuli resulting from an over-stretched bladder or bowel.

Focus Assessment Criteria

See *Impaired Urinary Elimination.*

Goal

NOC See *Functional Incontinence*

The person will report a state of dryness that is personally satisfactory.

Indicators
- Have a residual urine volume of less than 50 mL.
- Use triggering mechanisms to initiate reflex voiding.

General Interventions

NIC See also *Functional Incontinence,* Urinary Retention Care

Assess for Causative and Contributing Conditions.

Spinal cord lesion above T12	Traumatic injury	Infection
Tumor	Syringomyelia	Multiple sclerosis
Brown-Séquard syndrome	Transverse myelitis	Pernicious anemia

Explain Rationale for Treatments.

Develop a Bladder Retraining or Reconditioning Program (See Interventions Under *Total Incontinence*).

Teach Techniques to Stimulate Reflex Voiding.

Cutaneous triggering mechanisms
    Repeated deep, sharp suprapubic tapping (most effective)
    Instruct to:
        Place self in a half-sitting position.
        Tap directly at bladder wall at a rate of seven or eight times for 5 s (35 to 40 single blows).
        Use only one hand.
        Shift site of stimulation over bladder to find most successful site.
        Continue stimulation until a good stream starts.
        Wait approximately 1 min; repeat stimulation until bladder is empty.
        One or two series of stimulations without response signifies that nothing more will be expelled.
    If the preceding measures are ineffective, instruct client to perform each of the following for 2 to 3 min, waiting 1 min between attempts.
        Stroking glans penis
        Lightly punching abdomen above inguinal ligaments
        Stroking inner thigh
    Encourage person to void or trigger at least every 3 h.
    Indicate on intake and output sheet which mechanism was used to induce voiding.

People with abdominal muscle control should use the Valsalva maneuver during triggered voiding.
Teach person that if he or she increases fluid intake he or she also needs to increase the frequency
   of triggering to prevent overdistention.
Schedule intermittent catheterization program (see *Total Incontinence*).

Initiate Health Teaching, as Indicated.

Teach bladder-reconditioning program (see *Total Incontinence*).
Teach intermittent catheterization (see *Total Incontinence*).
Teach prevention of urinary tract infections (see *Total Incontinence*).
If at high risk for dysreflexia, see *Dysreflexia*.

Rationales

- Because the voiding reflex located in the sacral cord segments is spared, micturition can occur automatically after external cutaneous stimulation (manual triggering).
- Stimulating the reflex arc replaces the internal sphincter of the bladder, allowing urination. Stimulating the bladder wall or cutaneous sites (eg, suprapubic, pubic) can trigger the reflex arc.
- Clients with reflex neurogenic bladders can learn methods for stimulating the reflex arc to stimulate bladder emptying.
- Preferred cutaneous triggering methods are light, rapid suprapubic tapping, light pulling of pubic hairs, massage of the abdomen, and digital rectal stimulation.
- Use of Credé's maneuver should be avoided with a reflex bladder because the urethra may be damaged or vesicoureteral reflux may occur if the external sphincter is contracted.
- Contraction of abdominal muscles compresses the bladder to empty it.
- A regular voiding pattern can prevent incontinent episodes.

STRESS INCONTINENCE

DEFINITION

Stress Incontinence: State in which a person experiences an immediate involuntary loss of urine with an increase in intraabdominal pressure

DEFINING CHARACTERISTICS

Major (Must Be Present)

The person reports loss of urine (usually <50 mL) occurring with increased abdominal pressure from standing, sneezing, coughing, running, or lifting heavy objects.

RELATED FACTORS

Pathophysiologic

Related to incompetent bladder outlet secondary to congenital urinary tract anomalies
Related to degenerative changes in pelvic muscles and structural supports secondary to estrogen deficiency

Situational (Personal, Environmental)

Related to high intraabdominal pressure and weak pelvic muscles secondary to:

Obesity	Sex	Pregnancy
Poor personal hygiene		

Related to weak pelvic muscles and structural supports secondary to:

Recent substantial weight loss   Childbirth

Maturational

Older Adult
Related to loss of muscle tone

- Urinary continence is maintained by the junction of the bladder and the urethra, support from the perineal floor, and the muscle around the urethra.
- Stress incontinence is the leakage of small amounts of urine when the urethral outlet cannot control passage of urine in the presence of increased intraabdominal pressure.
- Menopausal decrease in elasticity usually worsens stress incontinence.
- A trial of vaginal estrogen cream in the postmenopausal woman who exhibits a pale, atrophic vaginal vault may help to reduce the incidence of incontinence.
- A stress test is used to help diagnose stress incontinence. It involves observation of the urethral meatus of a client with a full bladder in the standing position while she coughs or strains. Short spurts of urine escaping simultaneously with cough or strain suggest a probable diagnosis of stress incontinence.
- The client with pure stress incontinence has a normal cystometrogram.
- The degrees of stress incontinence are as follows:
  - Grade 1—Urine is lost with sudden increase in abdominal pressure, but never at night.
  - Grade 2—Lesser degrees of physical stress, such as walking, standing erect from a sitting position, or sitting up in bed, produce incontinence.
  - Grade 3—There is total incontinence, and urine is lost without any relation to physical activity or to position.

Maternal Considerations

Pressure of the uterus can cause stress incontinence, which can be misinterpreted as amniotic fluid.

Focus Assessment Criteria

See *Impaired Urinary Elimination.*

Goal

NOC See *Functional Incontinence*

The person will report a reduction or elimination of stress incontinence.

Indicator
Be able to explain the cause of incontinence and rationale for treatments.

General Interventions

NIC See also *Functional Incontinence,* Pelvic Muscle Exercise, Weight Management

Determine Contributing Factors.

Loss of tissue or muscle tone from:

Childbirth	Obesity	Aging
Recent weight loss	Cystocele	Rectocele
Atrophic vaginitis or urethritis	Prolapsed uterus	

History of surgery of the bladder and urethra with adhesions to the vaginal wall

Increased intraabdominal pressure from:
Overdistention between voidings
Pregnancy
Obesity

Explain the Effect of Incompetent Floor Muscles on Continence (See Key Concepts).

Teach Pelvic Muscle Exercises (Dougherty, 1998).

Teach How to Self-Assess Whether Exercises are Being Done Correctly.

Stand with one foot elevated on a stool, insert finger in vagina, and feel the strength of the contraction. Evaluate the strength of the contraction on a scale of 0 to 5 (Sampselle & DeLancey, 1998).

0 = No palpable contraction
1 = Very weak, barely felt
2 = Weak but clearly felt
3 = Good but not maintained when moderate finger pressure is applied
4 = Good but not maintained when intense finger pressure is applied
5 = Maximum strength with strong resistance

Use a mirror to observe whether the clitoris has downward movement and the anus tightens with contraction.

Consult an incontinence specialist for use of vaginal weights for pelvic floor strengthening (Perkins, 1998).

Provide Instructions for Pelvic Muscle Exercises.

For anterior pelvic floor muscles, imagine you are trying to stop the passage of urine, tighten the muscles (back and front) for 10 s, and then release them. Wait 10 s before the next contraction. Repeat ten times, four times a day. Stop and start the urine stream several times during voiding.

Use the urine stop test to measure the effectiveness of a contraction by the time it takes to stop voiding. Advise not to perform the urine stop test more than once a day.

Explain that pelvic muscle exercises are effective within 6 to 8 weeks with a 50% to 100% reduction in urine loss (Dougherty, 1998).

Advise that exercises should continue at least three times a week after optimal results are achieved (usually within 16 weeks; Dougherty, 1998).

Initiate Health Teaching for People Who Continue to Remain Incontinent After Attempts at Bladder Reconditioning or Muscle Retraining.

Promote personal integrity (see *Total Incontinence*).
Promote skin integrity (see *Total Incontinence*).
Schedule intermittent catheterization program, if appropriate (see *Total Incontinence*).

Rationales

- In stress incontinence, childbirth, trauma, menopausal atrophy, or obesity have weakened or stretched the pelvic floor muscles (pubococcygeus) and levator ani muscles.
- Pelvic muscle exercises strengthen and tone the muscles of the pelvic floor. They may provide enough augmentation or urethral pressure to prevent mild stress incontinence. They should be taught to all women as a preventive measure. Studies have shown that pelvic muscle exercises improve or completely control stress incontinence (Dougherty, 1998).

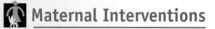 Maternal Interventions

For increased abdominal pressure during pregnancy:
Teach client to avoid prolonged standing.
Teach client the benefit of frequent voiding, at least every 2 h.
Teach pelvic muscle exercises after delivery.

Rationale

Pressure of the uterus on the bladder can cause involuntary loss of urine.

TOTAL INCONTINENCE

DEFINITION

Total Incontinence: State in which a person experiences continuous, unpredictable loss of urine without distention or awareness of bladder fullness

DEFINING CHARACTERISTICS
Major (Must Be Present, One or More)

Constant flow of urine without distention
Nocturia more than two times during sleep
Incontinence refractory to other treatments

Minor (May Be Present)

Unaware of bladder cues to void
Unaware of incontinence

RELATED FACTORS

Refer to *Impaired Urinary Elimination*.

KEY CONCEPTS

See *Impaired Urinary Elimination*.

Focus Assessment Criteria

See *Impaired Urinary Elimination*.

Goal

NOC See *Functional Incontinence*

The person will be continent (specify during day, night, 24 h).

Indicators

- Identify the cause of incontinence and rationale for treatments.
- Identify daily goal for fluid intake.

NIC See also *Functional Incontinence*, Environmental Management, Urinary Catheterization, Teaching: Procedure/Treatment, Tube Care: Urinary, Urinary Bladder Training

General Interventions

Develop a Bladder Retraining or Reconditioning Program, Which Should Include Communication, Assessment of Voiding Pattern, Scheduled Fluid Intake, and Scheduled Voiding Times.

Promote Communication Among All Staff Members and Among Individual, Family, and Staff.
Provide all staff with sufficient knowledge concerning the program planned.
Assess staff's response to program.

Assess the Person's Potential for Participation in a Bladder-Retraining Program.
Cognition
Desire to change behavior
Ability to cooperate
Willingness to participate

Provide Rationale for Plan and Acquire Client's Informed Consent.

Encourage Person to Continue Program by Providing Accurate Information Concerning Reasons for Success or Failure.

Assess Voiding Pattern
Monitor and record:
  Intake and output
  Time and amount of fluid intake
  Type of fluid
  Amount of incontinence; measure if possible or estimate amount as small, moderate, or large
  Amount of void, whether it was voluntary or involuntary
  Presence of sensation of need to void
  Amount of retention (amount of urine left in the bladder after an unsuccessful attempt at manual triggering or voiding)
  Amount of residual (amount of urine left in the bladder after either a voluntary or manual triggered voiding; also called a postvoid residual)
  Amount of triggered urine (urine expelled after manual triggering [eg, tapping, Credé's method])
Identify certain activities that precede voiding (eg, restlessness, yelling, exercise).
Record in appropriate column.

Schedule Fluid Intake and Voiding Times.
Provide fluid intake of 2000 mL each day unless contraindicated.
Discourage fluids after 7 PM.
Initially, bladder emptying is done at least every 2 h and at least twice during the night; goal is 2- to 4-h intervals.
If the person is incontinent before scheduled voids, shorten the time between voids.
If the person has a postvoid residual greater than 100 to 150 mL, schedule intermittent catheterization.

Reduce Incontinence-Related Irritant Dermatitis (Scardillo, 1999).
Decrease the alkalizing effect of urine on the skin:
  Use a no-rinse perineal cleanser.
  Avoid fragrances, alcohol, and alkaline agents (found in many commercial soaps).
  Apply moisturizer immediately after bathing, when pores are open.
  Select a moisturizer that is occlusive (white petroleum, lanolin, emollients).
Decrease injury with washing:
  Do not try to remove all of the ointment with cleansing.
  Gently wash skin, using very little soap.
  Dry skin very gently by patting, not rubbing.
  Use a moisture barrier product (eg, Curity Moisture Barrier Cream; No Sting Barrier Film).

Schedule Intermittent Catheterization Program (ICP), if Indicated.

Monitor intake and output.
Fluid intake should be at least 2000 mL/day.
Use sterile catheterization technique in the hospital, clean technique at home.
Desired catheter volumes are less than 500 mL.
Increase or decrease the interval between catheterizations to obtain the desired catheter volumes.
Usual catheterization times are every 4 to 6 h.
Urine volumes may increase at night; thus, it may be necessary to catheterize more frequently at night.
Encourage the client to attempt to void before scheduled catheterization time.
Initially obtain postvoid residuals at least every 6 h.
Terminate ICP when the bladder is consistently emptied voluntarily or by triggering with less than 50 mL residual urine after each void.

Teach ICP to Person and Family for Long-Term Management of Bladder (See Key Concepts).

Explain the reasons for the catheterization program.
Explain the relation of fluid intake and the frequency of catheterization.
Explain the importance of emptying the bladder at the prescribed time, regardless of circumstances, because of the hazards of an overdistended bladder (eg, circulation contributes to infection, and stasis of urine contributes to bacterial growth).

Teach the Client About the Bladder Reconditioning Program.

Explain rationale and treatments (see Key Concepts).

Explain the schedule of fluid intake, voiding attempts, manual triggering, and catheterization to control incontinence.

Teach person and family the importance of positive reinforcement and adherence to program for best results.

Refer to community nurses for assistance in bladder reconditioning if indicated.

If Bladder Retraining Fails, Consider Use of an Indwelling Catheter.

For men, use a catheter no larger than 16F.

For women, use up to 18F for routine use.

Teach care of indwelling catheter.

  Maintain 3000-mL fluid intake every day.

  Keep urine acidic.

  Change catheter at least every 2 weeks or when it does not drain properly.

  Tape catheter to prevent pulling.

    Men—to suprapubic abdominal area

    Women—to inner thighs

  Perform thorough cleaning of the meatus, distal catheter, and perineum at least twice a day.

  Maintain sterile drainage system at all times in the hospital; at home may use clean system.

  The urine collection system should drain by gravity.

  Do not lift collection bag above the level of the bladder without pinching off the tubing to prevent backflow.

  Connect the catheter to a leg bag drainage system during the day.

Initiate Health Teaching.

If appropriate, teach intermittent catheterization.

Instruct in prevention of urinary tract infection.

Teach how to change indwelling catheter.

For people living in the community, initiate a referral to the visiting nurse for follow-up and/or regular indwelling catheter changes.

Rationales

- Continence training programs are either self-directed or caregiver-directed. Self-directed programs of bladder training, retraining, and exercises are for motivated, cognitively intact clients. Caregiver-directed programs of scheduled toileting or habit training are appropriate for motivated caregivers of clients with cognitive impairment (Miller, 2004).
- The essential components of any continence training program (self-directed or caregiver-directed) include motivation, assessment of voiding and incontinence patterns, a regular fluid intake of 2000 to 3000 mL/day, timed voiding of 2- to 4-h intervals in an appropriate place, and ongoing assessment (Miller, 2004).
- Fecal impaction and an enlarged prostate gland can cause obstruction of the bladder neck that progresses to bladder distention and overflow (incontinence).
- Dehydration can cause incontinence by eliminating the sensation of a full bladder (the signal to urinate) and also by reducing the person's alertness to the sensation.
- Intermittent self-catheterization, periodic drainage of urine through the use of a catheter in the bladder, is indicated when a neurologic impairment alters bladder emptying.
- Intermittent catheterization, when performed in a health care facility, should follow aseptic technique, because the organisms present in such a facility are more virulent and resistant to drugs than organisms found outside. People at home can practice clean technique because of the lack of virulent organisms in the home environment.
- An overdistended bladder reduces blood flow to the bladder wall, making it more susceptible to infection from bacterial growth.
- Intermittent catheterization provides a decrease in morbidity associated with long-term use of indwelling catheters, increased independence, a more positive self-concept, and more normal sexual relations.
- Increased alkalinity of skin, moisture, friction, occlusive clothing, and heat cause incontinence-related irritant dermatitides (Scardillo, 1999).

URGE INCONTINENCE

DEFINITION
Urge Incontinence: State in which a person experiences an involuntary loss of urine associated with a strong, sudden desire to void

DEFINING CHARACTERISTICS
Major (Must Be Present)
Urgency followed by incontinence

RELATED FACTORS
Pathophysiologic
Related to decreased bladder capacity secondary to:

Infection	Cerebrovascular accident	Trauma
Demyelinating diseases	Urethritis	Diabetic neuropathy
Neurogenic disorders or injury	Alcoholic neuropathy	Brain injury/tumor/infection
Parkinsonism		

Treatment-Related
Related to decreased bladder capacity secondary to:

Abdominal surgery	Post-indwelling catheters

Situational (Personal, Environmental)
Related to irritation of bladder stretch receptors secondary to:

Alcohol	Caffeine	Excess fluid intake

Related to decreased bladder capacity secondary to frequent voiding

Maturational
Child
Related to small bladder capacity

Older Adult
Related to decreased bladder capacity

KEY CONCEPTS
- Urge incontinence is an involuntary loss of urine associated with a strong desire to void. It is characterized by loss of large volumes of urine and may be triggered by emotional factors, body position changes, or the sight and sound of running water. This type of incontinence is commonly called bladder detrusor instability or vesical instability.
- Detrusor instability is characterized by uninhibited detrusor contractions sufficient to cause urinary incontinence. Common causes include central nervous system disease, hyperexcitability of the afferent pathways, and deconditioned voiding reflexes.
- A person with an uninhibited neurogenic bladder has damage to the cerebral cortex (eg, cerebrovascular accident, Parkinson's disease, brain injury/tumor) affecting the ability to inhibit urination. Sensation of bladder fullness is also limited; this is manifested by urgency. There is little time between the sensation to void and the uninhibited contraction.
- Warning time is the time a person can delay urination after feeling the urge to void. Diminished warning time can cause incontinence if the person cannot reach a toilet in time.

Focus Assessment Criteria

See *Impaired Urinary Elimination.*

Goal

NOC Refer to *Functional Incontinence*

The person will report no or decreased episodes of incontinence (specify).

Indicators
- Explain causes of incontinence.
- Describe bladder irritants.

General Interventions

NIC Refer to *Functional Incontinence*

Assess for Causative or Contributing Factors.

Bladder Irritants
Infection
Inflammation
Alcohol, caffeine, or dark cola intake
Concentrated urine

Diminished Bladder Capacity
Self-induced deconditioning (frequent small voids)
Post-indwelling catheterization

Overdistended Bladder
Increased urine production (diabetes mellitus, diuretics)
Intake of alcohol and/or large quantities of fluids

Uninhibited Bladder Contractions from Neurologic Disorder
Cerebrovascular accident
Brain tumor/trauma/infection
Parkinson's disease

Assess Pattern of Voiding/Incontinence and Fluid Intake.

Maintain optimal hydration (see *Total Incontinence*).
Assess voiding pattern (see *Total Incontinence*).

Reduce or Eliminate Causative and Contributing Factors, When Possible.

Bladder Irritants
Infection/inflammation
    Refer to physician for diagnosis and treatment.
    Initiate bladder reconditioning program (see *Total Incontinence*).
    Explain the relation between incontinence and intake of alcohol, caffeine, and colas (irritants).
Explain the risk of insufficient fluid intake and its relation to infection and concentrated urine.

Diminished Bladder Capacity
Determine time between urge to void and need to void (record how long person can delay urination).
For a person with difficulty prolonging waiting time, communicate to personnel the need to respond rapidly to his request for assistance for toileting (note on care plan).
Teach client to increase waiting time by increasing bladder capacity.
    Determine volume of each void.
    Ask person to "hold off" urinating as long as possible.
    Give positive reinforcement.
    Discourage frequent voiding that is the result of habit, not need.
    Develop bladder reconditioning program (see *Total Incontinence*).

Overdistended Bladder

Explain that diuretics are given to help reduce the water in the body; they work by acting on the kidneys to increase the flow of urine.

Explain that in diabetes mellitus, insulin deficiency causes high levels of blood sugar. The high level of blood glucose pulls fluid from body tissues, causing osmotic diuresis and increased urination (polyuria).

Explain that because of the increased urine flow, regular voiding is needed to prevent overdistention of the bladder. Explain that overdistention can result in loss of bladder sensation, which increases incontinent episodes (diabetic neuropathy).

Assess voiding pattern (see *Total Incontinence*).

Check postvoid residual; if greater than 100 mL, include intermittent catheterization in bladder reconditioning program.

Initiate bladder reconditioning program (see *Total Incontinence*).

Uninhibited Bladder Contractions

Assess voiding pattern (see *Total Incontinence*).

Establish method to communicate urge to void (document on care plan).

Communicate to personnel the need to respond rapidly to a request to void.

Establish a planned-voiding pattern.

Provide an opportunity to void on awakening; after meals, physical exercise, bathing, and drinking coffee or tea; and before going to sleep.

Begin by offering bedpan, commode, or toilet every half hour initially, and gradually lengthen the time to at least every 2 h.

If person has incontinent episode, reduce the time between scheduled voidings.

Document behavior/activity that occurs with void or incontinence (see *Total Incontinence*).

Encourage person to try to "hold" urine until voiding time, if possible.

Consult primary care professional for pharmacological interventions.

Refer to *Total Incontinence* for additional information on developing a bladder reconditioning program.

Initiate Health Teaching.

Instruct person on prevention of urinary tract infections (see *Functional Incontinence*).

Rationales

- The essential components of any continence training program (self-directed or caregiver-directed) include motivation, assessment of voiding and incontinent patterns, a regular fluid intake of 2000 to 3000 mL/day, timed voiding of 2- to 4-h intervals in an appropriate place, and ongoing assessment (Miller, 2004).
- Deconditioning of the voiding reflex can result in incontinence through self-induced or iatrogenic causes. Frequent toileting (more than every 2 h) causes chronic low-volume voiding, which reduces bladder capacity and increases detrusor tone and bladder wall thickness, which, in turn, potentiate incontinent episodes.
- Iatrogenic causes include placing a person on the toilet after the incontinent episode or using uncomfortable equipment to make him continent.
- Factors that contribute to urgency include acute urinary tract infection, neurologic impairments, diuretics, diabetes mellitus, inadequate fluid intake, and habitual frequent voiding.
- Optimal hydration is needed to prevent urinary tract infection and renal calculi.

URINARY RETENTION

DEFINITION

Urinary Retention: State in which a person experiences a chronic inability to void followed by involuntary voiding (overflow incontinence)

DEFINING CHARACTERISTICS
Major (Must Be Present, One or More)

Bladder distention (not related to acute reversible etiology) or
Bladder distention with small, frequent voids or dribbling (overflow incontinence)
100 mL or more residual urine

Minor (May Be Present)

Report that it feels like the bladder is not emptying after voiding

RELATED FACTORS
Pathophysiologic

Related to sphincter blockage secondary to:

Strictures	Ureterocele	Bladder neck contractures
Prostatic enlargement	Perineal swelling	

Related to impaired afferent pathways or inadequacy secondary to:

Cord injury/tumor/infection	Brain injury/tumor/infection	Cerebrovascular accident
Demyelinating diseases	Multiple sclerosis	Diabetic neuropathy
Alcoholic neuropathy	Tabes dorsalis	

Treatment-Related

Related to bladder outlet obstruction or impaired afferent pathways secondary to drug therapy (iatrogenic)

Antihistamines	Theophylline	Epinephrine
Isoproterenol	Anticholinergics	

Situational (Personal, Environmental)

Related to bladder outlet obstruction secondary to fecal impaction
Related to detrusor inadequacy secondary to:

Deconditioned voiding	Association with stress or discomfort

KEY CONCEPTS

- Three entities can cause urinary retention: bladder outlet obstruction, detrusor inadequacy, and impaired afferent pathways.
- Detrusor inadequacy is characterized by the pressure of uninhibited detrusor contractions sufficient to cause urinary incontinence. One cause of detrusor inadequacy is deconditioned voiding reflexes characterized by anxiety or discomfort associated with voiding. Another cause is central nervous system diseases.
- Impaired afferent pathways occur when both the sensory and motor branches of the simple reflex arc are damaged. Therefore, there are no sensations to tell the person the bladder is full or no motor impulses for emptying the bladder. Thus, the person develops a neurogenic bladder (autonomous). With this type of neurogenic bladder, the person is likely to dribble urine when pressure in the bladder rises because of the bladder filling beyond its normal capacity or because of coughing, straining, or exercising.

- Other common names for this type of bladder are lower motor neuron, hypotonic, flaccid, cord, tabetic, and atonic bladder.
- External manual compression and abdominal straining are the most effective methods to empty a neurogenic bladder.

Focus Assessment Criteria

See *Impaired Urinary Elimination.*

Goal

 See *Functional Incontinence*

The person will achieve a state of dryness that is personally satisfactory.

Indicators

- Empty the bladder using Créde's or Valsalva maneuver with a residual urine of less than 50 mL if indicated.
- Void voluntarily.

General Interventions

NIC See also *Functional Incontinence,* Urinary Retention Care, Urinary Bladder Training

Assess for Causative or Contributing Factors.

Factors that Cause Impaired Afferent Pathways
Cerebrovascular accident
Demyelinating disease
Spinal cord injury/trauma/infection
Peripheral nerve damage
    Diabetic neuropathy   Pelvic fractures/extensive surgery
    Alcoholic neuropathy

Loss of Bladder Tone (Detrusor Weakness)
Benign prostatic hypertrophy (postoperative)
Spinal cord injury/tumor/infection
Cerebrovascular accident
Brain injury/tumor/infection
Medications
    Anticholinergics
    α-Adrenergics

Conditions Contributing to Bladder Neck Obstruction
Strictures/contracture/spasms
Edema (postsurgical, postpartum, vaginal or rectal packing)
Prostatic hypertrophy
Fecal impaction
Tumor
Congenital abnormalities

Conditions that Inhibit Micturition
Poor fluid intake
Anxiety

Explain Rationale for Treatment.

Develop a Bladder Retraining or Reconditioning Program (see *Total Incontinence*).

Instruct on Methods to Empty Bladder.

Assist to a Sitting Position.
Teach abdominal strain and Valsalva maneuver; instruct person to:
    Lean forward on thighs.
    Contract abdominal muscles, if possible, and strain or "bear down"; hold breath while straining
      (Valsalva maneuver).

Hold strain or breath until urine flow stops; wait 1 min, and strain again as long as possible.
Continue until no more urine is expelled.
Teach Credé's maneuver; instruct person to:
Place hands flat (or place fist) just below umbilical area.
Place one hand on top of the other.
Press firmly down and in toward the pelvic arch.
Repeat six or seven times until no more urine can be expelled.
Wait a few minutes and repeat to ensure complete emptying.
Teach anal stretch maneuver; instruct person to:
Sit on commode or toilet.
Lean forward on thighs.
Place one gloved hand behind buttocks.
Insert one to two lubricated fingers into the anus to the anal sphincter.
Spread fingers apart or pull to posterior direction.
Gently stretch the anal sphincter and hold it distended.
Bear down and void.
Take a deep breath and hold it while straining (Valsalva maneuver).
Relax and repeat the procedure until the bladder is empty.

Instruct Client to Try All Three Techniques or a Combination of Techniques to Determine Which is Most Effective in Emptying the Bladder.

Indicate on the Intake and Output Record which Technique was Used to Induce Voiding.

Obtain Postvoid Residuals After Attempts at Emptying Bladder; if Residual Urine Volumes are Greater than 100 mL, Schedule Intermittent Catheterization Program (see Total Incontinence).

Initiate Health Teaching.

Teach bladder reconditioning program (see *Total Incontinence*).
Teach intermittent catheterization (see *Total Incontinence*).
Instruct person on prevention of urinary tract infections (see *Total Incontinence*).

Rationales

- Reducing the pressure in the bladder and abdomen and strengthening the periurethral tissue often can reduce dribbling of urine.
- To increase comfort associated with voiding, the client must condition the voiding reflex by ingesting adequate fluids and inhibiting bladder contractions. Frequent toileting causes chronic low-volume voiding and increases detrusor activity. Resisting the urge to void may increase voiding intervals and reduce detrusor muscle activity.
- In many clients, Credé's maneuver can help empty the bladder. This maneuver is inappropriate, however, if the urinary sphincters are chronically contracted. In this case, pressing the bladder can force urine up the ureters as well as through the urethra. Reflux of urine into the renal pelvis may result in renal infection.
- External cutaneous stimulation can stimulate the voiding reflex.
- Valsalva maneuver contracts the abdominal muscles, which manually compresses the bladder.
- Anal sphincter stimulation can stimulate the voiding reflex.
- Clean intermittent self-catheterization (CISC) prevents overdistention, helps maintain detrusor muscle tone, and ensures complete bladder emptying. CISC may be used initially to determine residual urine after Credé's maneuver or tapping. As residual urine decreases, catheterization may be tapered. CISC may recondition the voiding reflex in some clients.
- If bladder emptying techniques are unsuccessful, other methods of managing incontinence are necessary.

RISK FOR VIOLENCE

DEFINITION
Risk for Violence: State in which a person has been, or is at risk to be, assaultive toward others or the environment

RISK FACTORS
Major (Must Be Present)
Presence of risk factors (see Related Factors)

RELATED FACTORS
Pathophysiologic
Related to history of aggressive acts and perception of environment as threatening secondary to:
or
Related to history of aggressive acts and delusional thinking secondary to:
or
Related to history of aggressive acts and manic excitement secondary to:
or
Related to history of aggressive acts and inability to verbalize feelings secondary to:
or
Related to history of aggressive acts and psychic overload secondary to:
Temporal lobe epilepsy
Head injury
Progressive central nervous system deterioration (brain tumor)
Hormonal imbalance
Viral encephalopathy
Mental retardation
Minimal brain dysfunction

Related to toxic response to alcohol or drugs
Related to organic brain syndrome

Treatment-Related
Related to toxic reaction to medication

Situational (Personal, Environmental)
Related to history of overt aggressive acts
Related to increase in stressors within a short period
Related to acute agitation
Related to suspiciousness
Related to persecutory delusions
Related to verbal threats of physical assault
Related to low frustration tolerance
Related to poor impulse control
Related to fear of the unknown
Related to response to catastrophic event
Related to response to dysfunctional family throughout developmental stages
Related to dysfunctional communication patterns
Related to drug or alcohol abuse

AUTHOR'S NOTE

The diagnosis *Risk for Violence* describes a person who has been assaultive or, because of certain factors (eg, toxic response to alcohol or drugs, hallucinations or delusions, brain dysfunction), is at high risk for assaulting others. In such a situation, the nursing focus is on decreasing violent episodes and protecting the person and others.

The nurse should not use this diagnosis to address underlying problems such as anxiety or poor self-esteem, but instead should refer to the diagnoses *Anxiety, Ineffective Coping,* or both to focus on the sources of the violence (spouse, child, older adult). When domestic violence is present or suspected, the nurse should explore the diagnosis *Disabled Family Coping.* A person at risk for suicide would warrant the diagnosis *Risk for Suicide.*

ERRORS IN DIAGNOSTIC STATEMENTS

1. *Risk for Violence related to reports of abuse by wife*

"Reports of abuse by a spouse" represents family dysfunction, which *Risk for Violence* does not cover. Spouse abuse is a complex situation necessitating individual and family therapy. The nursing diagnoses *Disabled Family Coping* and *Ineffective Coping* for the abuser and the victim would be more clinically useful.

2. *Risk for Violence related to poor management of agitation by staff*

This diagnostic statement is legally problematic and does not offer constructive strategies. When staff management of an agitated client is inappropriate, the nurse must treat this as a staff management problem, not a client problem. If staff members increased the client's agitation because of lack of knowledge, the nurse must outline specific do's and don'ts in the nursing care plan. In addition, an in-service program on identifying precursors to violence and agitation reduction strategies should be held for staff. for the client, the nurse could rewrite the diagnosis as *Risk for Violence related to mental dysfunction and persecutory delusions.*

KEY CONCEPTS
Generic Considerations

- A central theme in violent people is helplessness. Assaultive behavior is a defense against passivity and helplessness.
- Aggressive behavior is a defense against anxiety. This coping mechanism is reinforced because it reduces anxiety by increasing the person's sense of power and control. (Refer to Key Concepts, *Anxiety,* for further discussion of anger.) Interventions that encourage "acting out of anger" reinforce assaultiveness and, thus, are to be avoided.
- Violence is usually preceded by a predictable sequence of events (eg, a stressor or a series of stressors.
- When brain dysfunction is a prime or contributing factor to violent behavior, social and environmental variables still should be evaluated. Organic impairment may interfere with a person's ability to handle certain stresses. Exposure to or ingestion of toxic chemicals, such as lead and pesticides, can alter a person's normal behavior. Examples of violent behavior in brain dysfunction are biting, scratching, temper outbursts, and mood lability.
- Fear and anxiety can distort perceptions of the environment. Suspicious, delusional people often misinterpret stimuli. Alcohol and drugs also impair judgment and decrease internal controls over behavior.
- People who had a history of emotional deprivation in childhood are particularly vulnerable to attacks on their self-esteem.
- Although the individual may identify the person with whom he or she is angry, this may not be the real object of aggression. People often cannot allow themselves to express anger toward a person on whom they are dependent.
- Staff members frequently respond to violent clients with actual fear or overreactions. This can lead to punitive sanctions such as heavier medication, seclusion, or attempts to cope by avoidance and withdrawal from the client. Staff must identify their own reactions to violent individuals so

they can manage the situation more effectively. Staff should trust an intuition that the person is potentially violent (Farrell et al., 1998).

- In studies of clients' perception of seclusion, sense of powerlessness seemed to be the worst feeling, followed by fear, humiliation, loneliness, and shame (Norris & Kennedy, 1992).
- Physical aggression in long-term care, such as swearing, biting, kicking, spitting, and grabbing, may be in response to a loss of control over life. The more importance the person attaches to freedom and choice, the more forcefully he or she is likely to respond.

✦ Pediatric Considerations

- In 1994, there were 24,547 victims of violence in the United States; more than one third were younger than 25 years. Between 1985 and 1994, homicide rates for males 15 to 19 years of age increased 166% (Dowd, 1998).
- From 1985 to 1994, the percentage of gun-related homicides rose from 67% to 87% in people 15 to 24 years of age (Dowd, 1998).
- Homicide is the leading cause of death for African-American and Hispanic males 15 to 24 years of age (Dowd, 1998).
- Violent shaking of children, especially those younger than 6 months, can cause fatal intracranial trauma without signs of external head injury (Wong, 2003).
- The homicide rate in the United States is 4.3 times higher in children 0 to 4 years of age and 5.8 times higher in children 5 to 14 years of age than in 25 industrialized countries (Hennes, 1998).
- Children who are exposed to community violence experience more depression, anxiety, fear and aggressive acting-out behaviors than children not exposed (Veenema, 2001).

Focus Assessment Criteria

(Refer also to Focus Assessment Criteria for *Ineffective Coping, Compromised Family Coping, Disturbed Thought Processes,* and *Anxiety*).

Subjective Data
Assess for Risk Factors.

Medical history

Hormonal imbalance	Head injury
Brain disease	Drug abuse (amphetamines, PCP, marijuana, alcohol)

Psychiatric history

Previous hospitalizations	Outpatient therapy

History of emotional difficulties in client, family, or both

Mental retardation	Parental brutality
Cruelty to animals	Pyromania

Interaction patterns (note changes)

Family	Coworkers
Friends	Others

Coping patterns (past and present)
Sources of stress in current environment
Work/school history

How does client function under stress?	Fights in school
	Stable employment
Level of education attained	Frequency of job changes
Learning disabilities	Periods of unemployment

Legal history
Arrests and convictions for violent crimes
Juvenile offenses for violent behavior

History of violence

Assess recency, severity, and frequency

"What is the most violent thing you have ever done?"

"What is the closest you have ever come to striking someone?"

"In what kinds of situations have you hit someone or destroyed property?"

"When was the last time this happened?"

"How often does this occur?"

"Were you using drugs or alcohol during these episodes?"

Present thoughts about violence

Identify possible victim and weapon

"How do you feel after an incident?"

"Are you currently having thoughts about harming someone?"

"Is there anyone in particular you think about harming?" (Identify the victim and the person's access to victim.)

"Do you have a specific plan for how you might accomplish this?" (Identify plan, type of weapon, and availability of weapon.)

Thought content

Helplessness

Suspiciousness or hostility

Perceived intention (eg, "He meant to hit me" in response to a slight bump)

Fear of loss of control

Persecutory delusions

Disorientation

Child–adolescent

Conflict management—impulse control

How does child respond to conflict?

History of fights

History of being victim of bullying

Relationships

Has he or she experienced pushing, hitting, being afraid, being hurt, or being forced to have sexual contact?

Safety

"Do you feel safe?"

"Are you afraid of someone you know?"

"Have you talked with an adult about this situation?"

If abuse is suspected, refer to *Compromised Family Coping.*

Objective Data
Assess for Risk Factors.

Body language

Posture (relaxed, rigid)

Hands (relaxed, rigid, clenched)

Facial expression (calm, annoyed, tense)

Motor activity

Within normal limits	Pacing	Immobile
Agitation	Increased	

Affect

Within normal limits	Flat	Labile
Inappropriate	Controlled	

For more information on Focus Assessment Criteria, visit http://connection.lww.com.

Goal

NOC	Abuse Cessation, Abusive Behavior Self-Control, Aggression Control, Impulse Control

The person will have fewer violent responses.

Indicators

- Show control of behavior with assistance from others.
- Describe causation and possible preventive measures.
- Explain rationales for interventions.

General Interventions

 NIC Abuse Protection Support, Anger Control Assistance, Environmental Management: Violence Prevention, Impulse Control Training, Crisis Intervention, Seclusion, Physical Restraint

The nursing interventions for *Risk for Violence* apply to any person who is potentially violent, regardless of related factors.

Promote Interactions that Increase the Person's Sense of Trust.

Acknowledge the client's feelings (eg, "You are having a rough time").
    Be genuine and empathic.
    Tell person that you will help him or her to control behavior and not do anything destructive.
    Be direct and frank ("I can see you are angry").
    Be consistent and firm.
Set limits when person poses a risk to others. Refer to *Anxiety* for further interventions on limit-setting.
Offer choices and options. At times, it is necessary to give in to some demands to avoid a power struggle.
Encourage person to express anger and hostility verbally instead of "acting out."
Encourage walking or exercise as activities that may diffuse aggression.
Maintain client's personal space.
    Do not touch the individual.
    Avoid feelings of physical entrapment of individual or staff.
Be aware of your own feelings and reactions.
    Do not take verbal abuse personally.
    Remain calm if you are becoming upset; leave the situation to others, if possible.
    After a threatening situation, discuss your feelings with other staff.
Observe for cues to increasing anger (Boyd, 2005):
    Reports of numbness, nausea, vertigo
    Choking sensation, chills, prickly sensations
    Increased muscle tone, clenched fists, set jaw, eyebrows lower and drawn together
    Lips pressed together to form a thin line
    Flushing or paleness
    "Goose bumps"
    Twitching
    Sweating

Initiate Immediate Management of High-Risk Person.

Allow the client with acute agitation space that is five times greater than that for a person who is in control. Do not touch the person unless you have a trusting relationship.
Avoid physical entrapment of individual or staff.
Convey empathy by acknowledging the person's feelings. Let the client know you will not let him or her lose control. Remind the client of previous successes at self-control.
Do not approach a violent individual alone. Often, the presence of three or four staff members is enough to reassure the person that you will not let him or her lose control. Use a positive tone; do not demand or cajole.
Give the client control by offering alternatives (eg, walking, talking).
Set limits on actions, not feelings. Use concise, easily understood statements.
Maintain eye contact, but do not stare. Stand at a friendly angle (45 degrees); keep an open posture if person is standing, sit when the person sits.
Do not make promises you cannot keep.
Avoid using "always" and "never."
When assault is imminent, quick, coordinated action is essential.
Approach client in a calm, self-assured manner so as not to communicate your anxiety or fear.
Avoid using force in giving intramuscular injections, when possible, because it increases the person's sense of powerlessness. Use only when a clear danger to others or self exists.
If the person has a weapon, do not attempt to grab it. Instruct the person to put it down. Attempt to calm the person without risking bodily harm to yourself.

Establish an Environment that Reduces Agitation (Farrell et al., 1998).

Decrease noise level.

Give short, concise explanations.

Control the number of persons present at one time.

Provide single or semiprivate room.

Allow individual to arrange personal possessions.

Be aware that darkness can increase disorientation and enhance suspiciousness.

Decrease situations in which the person is frustrated.

Provide music if person is receptive.

Assist Client to Maintain Control Over His or Her Behavior (Bauer & Hill, 1994).

Establish the expectation that he or she can control behavior, and continue to reinforce the expectation. Explain exactly which behavior is inappropriate and why.

Give three options: two offer a choice, whereas the third is the consequence of violent behavior.

Allow time for person to make choice.

Provide positive feedback when person is able to exercise restraint.

Enforce consequences when indicated.

Reassure client that you will provide control if he or she cannot ("I am concerned about you. I will get [more staff, medications] to keep you from doing anything impulsive.").

Set firm, clear limits when a client presents a danger to self or others ("Put the chair down").

Call person by name in a calm, quiet, respectful manner.

Avoid threats; refer to yourself, not policies, rules, or supervisors.

Allow appropriate verbal expressions of anger. Give positive feedback.

Set limits on verbal abuse. Do not take insults personally. Support others (clients, staff) who may be targets of abuse.

Do not give attention to person who is being verbally abusive. Tell the person what you are doing and why.

Assist with external controls, as necessary.

   Maintain observation every 15 to 30 min.

   Remove items that the client could use as weapons (eg, glass, sharp objects).

   Assess client's ability to tolerate off-unit procedures.

   If person is acutely agitated, be cautious with items such as hot coffee.

Plan for Unpredictable Violence.

Monitor for cues to potential aggression (Alvarey, 1998).

Verbal

Morose silence	Loud, demanding remarks	Illogical responses
Negative response to requests	Demeaning remarks	Overt hostility
Threats	Sarcasm	Mistrust

Nonverbal, Facial Expression

Tense jaw	Staring	Clenched teeth
Dilated pupils	Lip biting	Pulsing carotid

Nonverbal, Body Language

Hand twisting	Stony withdrawal	Aggression toward objects (slamming doors)
Confrontational stance	Fist clenching, unclenching	
Pounding, kicking	Pacing	

Ensure availability of staff before potential violent behavior (never try to assist person alone when physical restraint is necessary).

Determine who will be in charge of directing personnel to intervene in violent behavior if it occurs.

Ensure protection for self (door nearby for withdrawal, pillow to protect face).

Use Seclusion and/or Restraint, if Indicated.

Remove person from situation if environment is contributing to aggressive behavior, using the least amount of control needed (eg, ask others to leave, and take individual to quiet room).

Reinforce that you are going to help the client control himself or herself.

Repeatedly tell the person what is going to happen before external control begins.

Protect person from injuring self or others through use of restraints or seclusion.*
When using seclusion, institutional policy provides specifics; the following are general.
    Observe client at least every 15 min.
    Search client before secluding to remove harmful objects.
    Check seclusion room to see that safety is maintained.
    Offer fluids and food periodically (in nonbreakable containers).
    When approaching an individual to be secluded, have sufficient staff present.
    Explain concisely what is going to happen ("You will be placed in a room by yourself until you can better control your behavior"); give person a chance to cooperate.
    Assist with toileting and personal hygiene (assess client's ability to be out of seclusion; a urinal or commode may need to be used).
    If person is taken out of seclusion, someone must be present continually.
    Maintain verbal interaction during seclusion (provides information necessary to assess person's degree of control).
    When person is allowed out of seclusion, a staff member needs to be in constant attendance to determine whether person can handle additional stimulation.
When using restraint, institutional policy provides specifics. The following are general measures.
    A person in a four-point or two-point restraint must be in seclusion or with one-on-one nursing care for protection. Seclusion guidelines should be followed.
    Restraints must be loosened every hour (one limb at a time).
    Waist restraints must allow enough arm movement to enable eating/smoking and self-protection against falling.
    Restraints should be padded.
    Restraints never should be attached to siderails, but rather to the bed frame.
Provide an opportunity to clarify the rationale for seclusion and to discuss the person's reactions after the seclusion period is over.

Convene a Group Discussion After a Violent Episode on an Inpatient Unit.

Include all those who witnessed the episode (client, staff).
Include individual(s) exhibiting the violent behavior, if possible.
Discuss what happened, the consequences, and the feelings of the community.

If the Client Has Assaulted Another Client or Staff Member:

Reintegrate the client with the assaulted individual when the client has regained control, but before release from seclusion.

Assist Client to Develop Alternative Coping Strategies When Crisis Has Passed and Learning Can Occur.

Explore what precipitates the person's loss of control ("What was happening before you began to feel like hitting her?").
Assist the person to recall the physical symptoms associated with anger.
Help person to evaluate where in the chain of events change was possible.
    Use role playing to practice communication techniques.
    Discuss how issues of control interfere with communication.
    Help the person recognize negative thinking patterns associated with low self-esteem.
Help client to practice negotiation skills with significant others and people in authority.
Encourage increased recreational activities.
Use group therapy to decrease sense of aloneness and increase communication skills.
    Instruct or refer for assertiveness training.
    Instruct or refer for negotiation skills development.

Rationales

- The client is in an agitated/mentally compromised state. Environmental stimuli unnecessarily increase this state and can send the client "over the edge."

---

*May require a primary care professional's order.

- Violence can have a pattern. Detecting and changing the pattern can eliminate the violence.
- The presence of four or five staff members reassures the client that you will not let him or her lose control. The focus is respect, concern and safety.
- Assaultive behavior tends to occur when conditions are crowded, are without structure, and involve staff-"demanded" activity (Farrell et al., 1998).
- Staff activities may be counterproductive to managing aggressive behavior. Recognition and replacement of attitudes such as "I must be calm and relaxed at all times" with "No matter how anxious I feel, I will keep thinking and decide on the best approach" often prevent escalation of aggression (Davies, 1989).
- Although people may verbalize hostile threats and take a defensive stance, most fear losing control and want assistance to maintain their control (Alvarey, 1998).
- A habitually violent person exhibits a wider-than-average body buffer zone (Davies, 1989).
- Eye contact can increase arousal and be misinterpreted as hostility; the best approach is to maintain short periods of eye contact with no staring (Davies, 1989).
- Maintain the same physical level (eg, both people either sitting or standing prevents feelings of intimidation; Alvarey, 1998). The least aggressive stance is at a 45-degree angle to the person, rather than face-to-face (Davies, 1989).
- Crisis management techniques can help prevent escalation of aggression and help the person achieve self-control. The least restrictive safe and effective measure should be used (Alvarey, 1998).
- Seclusion and restraint are options for a person exhibiting serious, persistent aggression. The nurse must protect the person's safety at all times. Use of the least restrictive measures allows the person the most opportunity to regain self-control (Farrell et al., 1998).
- The nurse and the client collaborate to find solutions and alternatives to aggression (Boyd, 2005).
- The nurse practices from the perspective of acknowledging that the person has solved problems before and is in need of help periodically (Boyd, 2005).
- After a violent act, leading a group discussion of the event, outcome, and feelings can decrease anxiety and increase understanding of violence.
- Setting limits clarifies rules, guidelines, and standards of acceptable behavior and establishes the consequences of violating the rules (Alvarey, 1998).
- Physical activity can help reduce muscle tension (Alvarey, 1998).
- Diversions that require a short attention span are useful, because high anxiety causes scattered thinking (Alvarey, 1998).

Pediatric Interventions

Discuss with parents methods of disciplining child. Refer to *Compromised Family Coping* for more information on child abuse if indicated.

Discuss the risks of firearms in the home. Explore the storage of firearms and protective devices (eg, lockboxes, trigger locks).

Explore various sources of media violence (eg, television, video games, music, movies).

Explain strategies to prevent adverse effects of media violence (Willis & Strasburger, 1998).

  Watch television and videos with children.

  If possible, avoid programs that emphasize violence.

  Creatively illustrate when violent acts are punished.

  Explore alternatives to violence (eg, "What could the man have done besides shooting?")

  When selecting programs, consider:

    Are good characters violent?

    Is the violence justified?

    Are there negative consequences of violence?

  Consider the child's age when selecting television programs and movies.

  Engage the child and peers in a nonthreatening manner to discuss age-related violence (eg, hitting, bullying, throwing objects, date rape).

  Consult with school personnel to explore programs focusing on conflict resolution and impulse control.

  Role play high-risk situations, such as:

    Finding a gun in a friend's house

    Bullying a victim

    Refusing sexual advances

Rationales

- Violence is a learned behavior. If it is learned, then prosocial behavior can also be taught as an alternative (Davies & Flannery, 1998).
- Parents can model appropriate problem-solving strategies.
- Discussions that correlate with the actual viewing of violent behavior are more meaningful (Davies & Flannery, 1998).
- Children with impulse control and positive coping skills have good social skills, effective problem-solving abilities, strong autonomy, and a strong sense of purpose and future (Edari & McManus, 1998).
- Environments (families, schools, communities) that provide caring and support, have high expectations, and provide opportunities for children to participate in discussions can increase children's hardiness and invulnerability to violence (Edari & McManus, 1998).

WANDERING

DEFINITION

Wandering: State in which a person with dementia has meandering, aimless, or repetitive locomotion that exposes the person to harm

DEFINING CHARACTERISTICS

Person with dementia who (Algase, 1999; Ederly & Donovick, 1998):

 Ambulates in an aimless, endless manner
 Has repetitive locomotion in a circular pattern
 Paces repeatedly
 Exceeds or transgresses environmental limits into hazardous or unauthorized locations
 Has spatial disorientation or navigational deficits
 Cannot find what he or she is seeking

RELATED FACTORS
Pathophysiologic

Related to impaired cerebral function secondary to:*

Cerebrovascular accident	Mental retardation	Alzheimer's dementia

Related to physiologic urge (eg, hunger, thirst, pain, urination, constipation)

Situational (Personal, Environmental)

Related to increased frustration, anxiety, boredom, depression, or agitation
Related to over/understimulating environment
Related to separation from familiar people and places

Maturational

Older Adult
Related to faulty judgments secondary to motor and sensory deficits, medications

---

*This related factor must be present. Other related factors also can be present concurrently.

⊕ AUTHOR'S NOTE

This recently approved NANDA diagnosis is more useful than *Risk for Injury,* which was previously used. *Risk for Injury* focuses on strategies to protect a person from injury. *Wandering* directs interventions to protect the person from injury in addition to addressing the reasons for the wandering behavior, if possible.

⊕ ERRORS IN DIAGNOSTIC STATEMENTS

Wandering related to repetitive episodes of "being lost" in neighborhood

This diagnosis as written does not have related factors. These related factors are signs of *Wandering.* If the contributing factors to *Wandering* are not known, the nurse can write the diagnosis as *Wandering related to unknown etiology, as evidenced by repetitive episodes of "being lost" in the neighborhood.*

KEY CONCEPTS

- Wandering behavior is thought to result from frontal and parietal lobe damage that causes cognitive problems (Maier-Lorentz, 2000). Severity and duration of the dementia correlate with the wandering (Algase, 1999).
- It is uncertain why people wander. Some possible causes are as follows (Brown et al., 1999):
  - Feeling lost
  - Searching for something/someone
  - Overstimulation
  - Anxiety
  - Boredom
  - Needing exercise
- Wandering is the most frequent reason for admission to a nursing home. It is reported as the second most frequent problem behavior in nursing homes (the first is physical aggression) (Algase, 1999).
- Wandering causes significant caregiver distress. People who wander can become lost or injured or even die from related injuries or exposure (Logsdon et al., 1998).

Focus Assessment Criteria

Subjective Data
Assess for Related Factors.

Emotional, coping patterns
See *Ineffective Coping.*

Objective Data
Assess for Defining Characteristics.

Reported episodes of getting lost	Trespassing	Persistent locomotion
Pacing	Following caregiver	Hyperactivity
Locomotion with no apparent destination		

For more information on Focus Assessment Criteria, visit http://connection.lww.com.

Goals

NOC Risk Control, Environmental Management: Safety, Support Groups, Family Mobilization

The person will not elope or get lost.

Indicators (Person, Family)
- Ambulate safely.
- Identify factors that contribute to wandering behaviors.
- Anticipate wandering behaviors.

General Interventions

NIC Surveillance: Safety, Environmental Management: Safety, Referral, Risk Identification

Assess for Contributing Factors.

Anxiety
Confusion
Frustration
Boredom
Agitation
Separation from familiar people and places
Faulty judgments
Physiologic urge (hunger, thirst, pain, urination, constipation)

Reduce or Eliminate Contributing Factors, if Possible.

Anxiety/Agitation
Refer to *Anxiety* for interventions.

Unfamiliar Environment
Select a familiar picture to exhibit on the client's door.
Redirect client if he or she is lost.
Provide a safe route for walking.
Encourage activities that involve exercise (eg, sweeping, raking).
Create nature scenes in hallways (Cohen-Mansfield, 1998).
Mark exit door with big signs.
Place horizontal stripes on exit door or use a cloth panel across the width of the door.

Physiologic Urges
Anticipate need for toileting with a schedule.
Schedule times for fluids and food.
Evaluate for any pain.

Promote a Safe Environment.

Install locks on doors and windows.
Install electronic devices with buzzers on doors and property boundaries.
Use pressure-sensitive alarms (doormats, bed sensor, chair sensor).
Provide regular opportunities for client to walk with a companion or in a safe area.

Notify Others (Neighbors, Police, Others in Residence, Staff, Community Resources) About Person's Wandering Behaviors.

Explain the use of electronic devices (Altus, 2000).
Instruct them to notify provider if they see the person wandering.
Supply them with a recent photograph and current identification information (age, height, weight, hair color, description of clothes, identifying characteristics) of the client.
Contact local Alzheimer's Association for safety programs.

Rationales

- Research has shown that horizontal configurations on doors reduce elopement (Algase, 1999).
- People with cognitive impairments need external controls for protection.
- Modifying the environment rather than using restraints can decrease stress and agitation (Logsdon et al., 1998).
- Safe paths within or on the outside of a unit can provide a release for the need to wander (Logsdon et al., 1998).
- When an environment is enhanced with murals, pictures, and so forth, people with dementia trespass and exit less (Cohen-Mansfield, 1998).

Manual of Collaborative Problems

INTRODUCTION

This Manual of Collaborative Problems presents 52 specific collaborative problems grouped under nine generic collaborative problem categories. These problems have been selected because of their high incidence or morbidity. Information on each generic collaborative problem is presented under the following subheads:

- Definition
- Author's Note: Discussion of the problem to clarify its clinical use
- Significant Laboratory/Diagnostic Assessment Criteria: Laboratory findings useful in monitoring

  Discussions of the 52 specific collaborative problems cover the following information:

- Definition
- High-Risk Populations
- Nursing Goals: A statement specifying the nursing accountability for the collaborative problem
- General Interventions and Rationales: These specifically direct the nurse to:
  - Monitor for onset or early changes in status
  - Initiate physician- or advanced practice nurse-prescribed interventions as indicated
  - Initiate nurse-prescribed interventions as indicated
  - Evaluate the effectiveness of these interventions

A statement in parentheses and italics explains why a sign or symptom is present or gives the scientific explanation for why an intervention produces the desired response

Keep in mind that for many of the collaborative problems in Section III, associated nursing diagnoses also can be predicted to be present. For example, a client with diabetes mellitus would receive care under the collaborative problem *PC: Hypo/Hyperglycemia* along with the nursing diagnosis *Risk for Ineffective Health Maintenance related to insufficient knowledge of (specify);* a client with renal calculi would be under the collaborative problem *PC: Renal Calculi* and also the nursing diagnosis *Risk for Ineffective Therapeutic Regimen Management related to insufficient knowledge of prevention of recurrence, dietary restrictions, and fluid requirements.*

Potential Complication: Cardiac/Vascular
PC: Decreased Cardiac Output
PC: Dysrhythmias
PC: Pulmonary Edema
PC: Deep Vein Thrombosis
PC: Hypovolemia
PC: Compartmental Syndrome
PC: Pulmonary Embolism

POTENTIAL COMPLICATION: CARDIAC/VASCULAR

DEFINITION

PC: Cardiac/Vascular: Describes a person experiencing or at high risk to experience various cardiac and/or vascular dysfunctions

---

AUTHOR'S NOTE

The nurse can use this generic collaborative problem to describe a person at risk for several types of cardiovascular problems. For example, for a client in a critical care unit vulnerable to cardiovascular dysfunction, using *PC: Cardiac/Vascular* would direct nurses to monitor cardiovascular status for various problems, based on focus assessment findings. Nursing interventions for this client would focus on detecting and diagnosing abnormal functioning.

For a client with a specific cardiovascular complication, the nurse would add the applicable collaborative problem to the client's problem list, along with specific nursing interventions for that problem. For example, a Standard of Care for a client after myocardial infarction could contain the collaborative problem *PC: Cardiac/Vascular,* directing nurses to monitor cardiovascular status. If this client later experienced a dysrhythmia, the nurse would add *PC: Dysrhythmia* to the problem list, along with specific nursing management information (eg, *PC: Dysrhythmia related to myocardial infarction*). When the risk factors or etiology is not directly related to the primary medical diagnosis, the nurse still should add them, if known (eg, *PC: Hypo/Hyperglycemia related to diabetes mellitus* in a client who has sustained myocardial infarction).

For information on Focus Assessment Criteria, visit http://connection.lww.com.

Significant Laboratory/Diagnostic Assessment Criteria

Cardiac enzymes (elevated with cardiac tissue damage [eg, in myocardial infarction])
    Creatinine phosphokinase, isoenzymes (eg, CK-MB, Troponin)
    Lactic dehydrogenase (LDH), isoenzymes
Serum potassium (fluctuates with diuretic therapy, parenteral fluid replacement)
Serum calcium, magnesium, phosphate
White blood cell count (elevated with inflammation)
Erythrocyte sedimentation rate (elevated with inflammation, tissue injury)
Arterial blood gas (ABG) values (lowered SaO_2 indicates hypoxemia; elevated pH, alkalosis; lowered pH, acidosis)
Coagulation studies (elevated with anticoagulant and/or thrombolytic therapy or coagulopathies)

Hemoglobin and hematocrit (elevated with polycythemia, lowered with anemia)
Doppler ultrasonic flowmeter
Cardiac catheterization
Electrocardiograph with stress test
Nuclear magnetic resonance
Echocardiography with stress test
Transesophageal echocardiography

PC: DECREASED CARDIAC OUTPUT

DEFINITION

PC: Decreased Cardiac Output: Describes a person experiencing or at high risk to experience inadequate blood supply for tissue needs because of insufficient blood pumping by the heart

High-Risk Populations

- Acute myocardial infarction
- Aortic or mitral valve disease
- Cardiomyopathy
- Cardiac tamponade
- Hypothermia
- Septic shock
- Coarctation of the aorta
- Chronic obstructive pulmonary disease (COPD)
- Congenital heart disease
- Hypovolemia (eg, due to severe bleeding or burns)
- Bradycardia
- Tachycardia
- Congestive heart failure
- Cardiogenic shock
- Hypertension

Nursing Goals

The nurse will monitor and manage episodes of decreased cardiac output.

General Interventions and Rationales

- Monitor for signs and symptoms of decreased cardiac output/index:
  - Increased, decreased, and/or irregular pulse rate
  - Increased respiratory rate
  - Decreased blood pressure, increased blood pressure
  - Abnormal heart sounds
  - Abnormal lung sounds (crackles)
  - Decreased urine output (<30 mL/h)
  - Changes in mentation
  - Cool, moist, cyanotic, mottled skin

- Delayed capillary refill time
- Neck vein distention
- Weak peripheral pulses
- Abnormal pulmonary artery pressures
- Abnormal renal artery pressures
- Decreased mixed venous oxygen saturation
- Electrocardiogram (ECG) changes
- Dysrhythmias
- Decreased SaO_2
- Decreased SvO_2

(*Decreased cardiac output/index leads to insufficient oxygenated blood to meet the metabolic needs of tissues. Decreased circulating volume can result in hypoperfusion of the kidneys and decreased tissue perfusion with a compensatory response of decreased circulation to extremities and increased pulse and respiratory rates. Changes in mentation may result from cerebral hypoperfusion. Vasoconstriction and venous congestion in dependent areas [eg, limbs] produce changes in skin and pulses.*)

- Initiate appropriate protocols or standing orders, depending on the underlying etiology of the problem affecting ventricular function. (*Nursing management differs based on etiology [eg, measures to help increase preload for hypovolemia and to decrease preload for impaired ventricular contractility].*)
- Position the client with the legs elevated, unless ventricular function is impaired. (*This position can help increase preload and enhance cardiac output.*)
- During acute episodes, maintain absolute bed rest and minimize all controllable stressors. Administer intravenous (IV) morphine PRN according to protocol. Use with caution if client is hypotensive. (*These measures decrease metabolic demands.*)
- Assist client with measures to conserve strength, such as resting before and after activities (eg, meals, baths). (*Adequate rest reduces oxygen consumption and decreases the risk of hypoxia.*)
- Monitor intake and output and weight. (*Changes can indicate fluid retention.*)
- In a client with impaired ventricular function, cautiously administer IV fluids. Consult with physician or advanced practice nurse if ordered rate exceeds 125 mL/h. Be sure to include any additional IV fluids (eg, antibiotics) when calculating hourly allocation. (*A client with poorly functioning ventricles may not tolerate increased blood volumes.*)
- If decreased cardiac output results from hypovolemia, septic shock, or dysrhythmia, refer to the specific collaborative problem in this section.
- Administer inotropic and vasoactive agents (eg, digoxin, dopamine, dobutamine) as prescribed to improve contractility.
- Assist with insertion and/or maintenance of mechanical cardiac assist devices as indicated (eg, intraaortic balloon pump, hemapump, ventricular assist devices).

PC: DYSRHYTHMIAS

DEFINITION

PC: Dysrhythmias: Describes a person experiencing or at high risk to experience a disorder of the heart's conduction system that results in an abnormal heart rate, abnormal rhythm, or a combination of both

High-Risk Populations

- Myocardial infarction
- Congestive heart failure

- Hypoendocrine or hyperendocrine status
- Increased intracranial pressure
- Electrolyte imbalance (calcium, potassium, magnesium, phosphorus)
- Atherosclerotic heart disease
- Medication side effects (eg, aminophylline, dopamine, stimulants, digoxin, beta blockers, dobutamine, lidocaine, procainamide, quinidine, diuretics)
- COPD
- Cardiomyopathy, valvular heart disease
- Anemia
- Postoperative cardiac surgery

Nursing Goals

The nurse will manage and minimize dysrhythmic episodes.

General Interventions and Rationales

- Monitor for signs and symptoms of dysrhythmias.
  - Abnormal rate, rhythm
  - Palpitations, chest pain, syncope, fatigue
  - Decreased SaO_2
  - ECG changes
  - Hypotension
  (Ischemic tissue is electrically unstable, causing dysrhythmias. Certain congenital cardiac conditions, electrolyte imbalances, and medications also can cause disturbances in cardiac conduction.)
- Initiate appropriate protocols depending on the type of dysrhythmia; this may include:
  - Supraventricular tachycardia: vagal stimulation (direct or indirect), IV calcium channel blockers, digoxin (IV), adenosine, synchronized cardioversion, overdrive pacing
  - Atrial fibrillation: digitalization, electrical cardioversion, anticoagulant therapy
  - Premature ventricular contractions, ventricular tachycardia: IV lidocaine, IV procainamide, IV bretylium, oxygen
  - Ventricular tachycardia: oxygen, lidocaine, procainamide, bretylium, amiodarone, synchronized cardioversion, precardial thump if witnessed
  - Bradycardia or heart blocks: atropine, pacing, dopamine infusion, epinephrine infusion
  - Ventricular fibrillation: cardiopulmonary resuscitation (CPR), defibrillation, epinephrine, lidocaine, bretylium
  - Pulseless electrical activity: CPR, epinephrine (diagnose and treat the cause)
  - Asystole: CPR, epinephrine, atropine, pacing
- Administer supplemental oxygen, if indicated. *(It increases circulating oxygen levels and decreases cardiac workload.)*
- Monitor oxygen saturation (SaO_2) with pulse oximetry and ABGs as necessary.
- Monitor serum electrolyte levels (eg, sodium, potassium, calcium, magnesium). *(High or low electrolyte levels may exacerbate a dysrhythmia.)*
- Monitor pacemaker and automatic implantable cardioverter defibrillator therapy.

PC: PULMONARY EDEMA

DEFINITION

PC: Pulmonary Edema: Describes a person experiencing or at high risk to experience insufficient gas exchange because of accumulation of fluid related to left-sided heart failure or fluid overload

High-Risk Populations

- Hypertension
- Dysrhythmias
- Myocardial infarction
- Congestive heart failure
- Cardiomyopathy
- Coronary artery disease
- Aortic or mitral cardiac valve disease
- Diabetes mellitus
- Inhalation of toxins
- Drug overdose
- Smoking
- Congenital heart defects
- Neurologic trauma

Nursing Goals

The nurse will manage and minimize episodes of pulmonary edema.

General Interventions and Rationales

- Monitor for signs and symptoms of pulmonary edema:
  - Dyspnea, cyanosis
  - Tachypnea
  - Adventitious breath sounds, crackles
  - Persistent cough or productive cough with frothy, pink-tinged sputum
  - Abnormal ABGs
  - Decreased O_2 saturation by pulse oximetry
  - Decreased cardiac output/cardiac index
  - Elevated pulmonary artery pressure
  - Tachycardia
  - Abnormal heart sounds (S_3)

  (Impaired pumping of left ventricle accompanied by decreased cardiac output and increased pulmonary venous pressure and pulmonary artery pressure produce pulmonary edema. Hypoxia produces increased capillary, causing fluid to enter pulmonary tissue and triggering signs and symptoms.)
- If indicated, administer oxygen as prescribed.
- Initiate appropriate treatments according to protocol, which may include
  - Diuretics *(to decrease preload)*
  - Vasodilators *(to decrease afterload)*
  - Positive inotropics (eg, digitalis; *to enhance ventricular contractions)*
  - Morphine *(to decrease anxiety, preload and afterload, and metabolic demands)*

- Monitor urine hemodynamic parameters, specific gravity, intake/output, weight, and serum osmolality values. *(These values can help evaluate hydration.)*
- Take steps to maintain adequate hydration while avoiding overhydration. *(Adequate hydration helps liquefy pulmonary secretions; overhydration can increase preload and worsen pulmonary edema.)*
- Change client's position every 2 h with chest physical therapy. Determine which position provides optimum oxygenation by analyzing PaO_2 from pulse oximetry and/or ABG values with the client in various positions. *(Limiting time the client spends in positions that compromise oxygenation improves PaO_2.)*
- Place the client in high Fowler's position with legs dependent if dyspnea is severe. Encourage client to be out of bed and in a chair for meals. *(This positioning helps decrease venous return, increase venous pooling, and decrease preload.)*
- Encourage use of incentive spirometer, cough, and deep breathing every 2 h.
- Minimize controllable stressors (eg, noise, long tests and procedures, strenuous activity); explain all procedures and treatments. *(These measures may reduce anxiety, which can help decrease metabolic demands.)*
- Continue monitoring cardiovascular status—vital signs, ABG values, cardiac output, fluid balance, weight, pulse-oximeter. *(This monitoring helps evaluate response to treatment.)*

PC: DEEP VEIN THROMBOSIS

DEFINITION

PC: Deep Vein Thrombosis: Describes a person experiencing venous clot formation because of blood stasis, vessel wall injury, or altered coagulation

High-Risk Populations (Porter, 2002)

- Immobility > 72 h
- Fractures
- Chemical irritation of vein
- Blood dyscrasias
- Orthopedic, urologic, or gynecologic surgery
- History of venous insufficiency
- Obesity
- Estrogen use (high dose)
- Cancer
- Heart failure
- Varicose veins
- Inflammatory bowel disease
- Pregnant postpartum
- Severe COPD
- History of deep vein thrombosis (DVT) or pulmonary embolism
- Surgery greater than 30 min
- Over 40 years of age

Nursing Goals

The nurse will manage and minimize complications of DVT.

General Interventions and Rationales

- Monitor the status of venous thrombosis, noting
  - Diminished or absent peripheral pulses *(Insufficient circulation causes pain and diminished peripheral pulses.)*
  - Unusual warmth and redness or coolness and cyanosis *(Unusual warmth and redness point to inflammation; coolness and cyanosis indicate vascular obstruction.)*
  - Increasing leg pain *(Leg pain results from tissue hypoxia.)*
  - Sudden, severe chest pain, increased dyspnea, tachypnea *(These findings may indicate mobilization of thrombi to the lungs.)*
  - Positive Homans' sign *(In a positive Homans' sign, dorsiflexion of the foot causes pain because of insufficient circulation.)*
  - Consult physician for use of below-knee antiembolic stockings or sequential pressure devices, low-dose dextran, or anticoagulant therapy for high-risk clients. *(These assist to reduce venous stasis.)*
- Refer to High-Risk Populations.
- Evaluate hydration status based on urine specific gravity, intake/output, weights, and serum osmolality. Take steps to ensure adequate hydration. *(Increased blood viscosity and coagulability and decreased cardiac output may contribute to thrombus formation.)*
- Encourage client to perform isotonic leg exercises. *(They promote venous return.)*
- Ambulate as soon as possible with at least 5 min of walking each waking hour. Avoid prolonged chair sitting with legs dependent. *(Walking contracts leg muscles, stimulates the venous pump, and reduces stasis.)*
- Elevate the affected extremity above the level of the heart. *(This positioning can help reduce interstitial swelling by promoting venous return.)*
- Discourage smoking. *(Nicotine can cause vasospasms.)*
- Administer anticoagulant therapy as the physician or advanced practice nurse prescribes, and monitor blood coagulation results daily. *(Anticoagulant therapy prevents extension of a thrombosis by delaying the clotting time of blood.)*
- For a client receiving anticoagulant therapy, monitor for early signs of abnormal bleeding (eg, hematuria, bleeding gums, ecchymoses, petechiae, epistaxis). *(Prolonged clotting time can increase the risk of bleeding.)*
- Administer analgesics for leg pain as prescribed.
- Explain the importance of external compression devices (graded compression below-knee elastic stockings, intermittent external pneumatic compression [IEPC] impulse boots). *(Venous return is increased; pooling is decreased. IPC and impulse boots increase the rate and velocity of venous flow and decrease hypercoagulability [Byrne, 2002].)*

PC: HYPOVOLEMIA

DEFINITION

PC: Hypovolemia: Describes a person experiencing or at high risk to experience inadequate cellular oxygenation and inability to excrete waste products of metabolism secondary to decreased fluid volume (eg, from bleeding, plasma loss, prolonged vomiting, or diarrhea)

High-Risk Populations

- Intraoperative status
- Postoperative status
- Anaphylactic shock
- Trauma
- Bleeding

- Diabetic ketoacidosis
- Prolonged vomiting or diarrhea
- Infants, children, elderly
- Acute pancreatitis
- Major burns
- Disseminated intravascular coagulation
- Rupture of esophageal varices
- Dissecting aneurysms
- Prolonged pregnancy
- Trauma in pregnancy
- Diabetes insipidus
- Ascites
- Peritonitis
- Intestinal obstruction

Nursing Goals

The nurse will manage and minimize hypovolemic episodes.

General Interventions and Rationales

- Monitor fluid status; evaluate
  - Intake (parenteral and oral)
  - Output and other losses (urine, drainage, and vomiting), nasogastric tube
- *(Early detection of fluid deficit enables interventions to prevent shock.)*
- Monitor the surgical site for bleeding, dehiscence, and evisceration. *(Careful monitoring allows early detection of complications.)*
- Teach client to splint the surgical wound with a pillow when coughing, sneezing, or vomiting. *(Splinting reduces stress on suture line by equalizing pressure across the wound.)*
  - Monitor for signs and symptoms of shock:
  - Increased pulse rate with normal or slightly decreased blood pressure, narrowing pulse pressure
  - Urine output less than 20 mL/h
  - Restlessness, agitation, decreased mentation
  - Increased respiratory rate, thirst
  - Diminished peripheral pulses
  - Cool, pale, moist, or cyanotic skin
  - Decreased oxygenation saturation (SaO_2, SvO_2), pulmonary artery pressures
  - Decreased hemoglobin/hematocrit, decreased cardiac output/index
  - Decreased central venous pressure
  - Decreased right atrial pressure
  - Decreased wedge pressure
  (The compensatory response to decreased circulatory volume aims to increase oxygen delivery through increased heart and respiratory rates and decreased peripheral circulation [manifested by diminished peripheral pulses and cool skin]. Decreased oxygen to the brain alters mentation. Decreased circulation to the kidneys leads to decreased urine output. Hemoglobin and hematocrit values decline if bleeding is significant.)
- If shock occurs, place client in the supine position unless contraindicated (eg, head injury). *(This position increases blood return [preload] to the heart.)*
- Insert an IV line; use a large-bore catheter if blood replacement is anticipated. Initiate appropriate protocols for shock (eg, vasopressor therapy). Refer also to *PC: Acidosis* or *PC: Alkalosis,* if indicated, for more information. *(Protocols aim to increase peripheral resistance and elevate blood pressure.)*
- Collaborate with physician or advanced practice nurse to replace fluid losses at a rate sufficient to maintain urine output greater than 0.5 mL/kg/h (eg, saline or Ringer's lactate). *(This measure promotes optimal renal tissue perfusion.)*
- Restrict client's movement and activity. *(This helps decrease tissue demands for oxygen.)*
- Provide reassurance, simple explanations, and emotional support to help reduce anxiety. *(High anxiety increases metabolic demands for oxygen.)*
- Administer oxygen as ordered.

PC: COMPARTMENTAL SYNDROME

DEFINITION

PC: Compartmental Syndrome: Describes a person experiencing increased pressure in a limited space, such as a fascial envelope, which compromises circulation and function, usually in the forearm or leg (Bryant, 1998). Risk factors can either cause internal compression or external compression (Tumbarello, 2000).

High-Risk Populations

Internal Factors

* Fractures
* Musculoskeletal surgery
* Injuries (crush, electrical, vascular)
* Allergic response (snake, insect bites)
* Excessive edema
* Thermal injuries
* Vascular obstruction
* Intramuscular bleeding

External Factors

* Casts
* Prolonged use of tourniquet
* Tight dressings
* Tight closure of fascial detects
* Positioning during surgery
* Lying on limb for extended periods

Nursing Goals

The nurse will manage and minimize compartmental syndrome.

General Interventions and Rationales

* Refer to nursing diagnosis *Risk for Peripheral Neurovascular Dysfunction* for specific extremity assessment techniques and prevention of compartmental syndrome.
* Monitor for signs of compartmental syndrome:

Early Signs
  * Unrelieved or increasing pain
  * Pain with passive stretch movement or flexion of toes or fingers
  * Mottled or cyanotic skin
  * Excessive swelling
  * Delay in capillary refill
  * Paresthesia
  * Inability to move toes or fingers

(Pain and paresthesia indicate compression of nerves and increasing pressure within muscle compartment. Passive stretching of muscles decreases muscle compartment, thus increasing pain. Delayed capillary refill or mottled or cyanotic skin indicates obstructed capillary blood flow.)

Late Signs
- Pallor
- Diminished or absent pulse
- Cold skin

(Arterial occlusion produces these late signs.)
- Assess neurovascular function at least every hour for first 24 h. *(Peripheral neurovascular compromise may be the first sign [Tumbarello, 2000].)*
- Instruct client to report unusual, new, or different sensations (eg, tingling, numbness, and/or decreased ability to move toes or fingers). *(Early detection of compromise can prevent serious impairment [Pellino et al., 1998].)*
- If signs of compartmental syndrome occur, notify physician or advanced practice nurse and
  - Discontinue elevation and ice applications.
  - Loosen circumferential dressings, splints, casts per protocol. *(Elevation will impede perfusion.)*
- If invasive compartmental monitoring system is used, follow procedure for use.
- Monitor and document compartmental pressures according to protocol. Report elevated pressures promptly.
- Carefully maintain hydration. *(Hypovolemia can result from fluid volume shift.)*
- Evaluate cardiovascular and renal status; pulse, respiration, blood pressure and urine output. *(Eight liters of fluid can extravasate into a limb, causing hypovolemia, decreased renal function, and shock [Pellino et al., 1998].)*
- Notify the physician or advanced practice nurse of any early signs and symptoms of neurovascular compromise. *(The physician or advanced practice nurse will evaluate the cause and determine the necessary treatment, such as cast-splitting, removal of medical antishock trousers [MAST], removal of intraaortic balloon pump, surgery [eg, fasciotomy].)*

PC: PULMONARY EMBOLISM

DEFINITION

PC: Pulmonary Embolism: Describes a person experiencing or at high risk to experience obstruction of one or more pulmonary arteries from a blood clot or air or fat embolus

High-Risk Populations

- Infection
- Prolonged immobilization
- Prolonged sitting/traveling
- Varicose veins
- Vascular injury
- Tumor
- Increased platelet count (eg, from polycythemia, splenectomy)
- Thrombophlebitis
- Vascular disease
- Presence of foreign bodies (eg, IV or central venous catheters)
- Heart disease (especially congestive heart failure)
- Surgery or trauma (especially of hip, pelvis, spine, lower extremities)
- Postoperative state
- Pregnancy
- Postpartum state

- Diabetes
- COPD
- History of previous pulmonary embolism or thrombophlebitis
- Obesity
- Oral contraceptive use, estrogen therapy
- Leg, pelvic fractures, injuries
- Increased coagulability (eg, cancer)
- Sickle cell disease
- Thermal injuries
- Polycythemia
- Acute spinal cord injury
- Thrombus formation in heart from cardioversion, bacterial endocarditis, atrial fibrillation, or myocardial infarction

For air embolism

- Central line insertion or removal
- Central line tubing changes, manipulation, or disconnection

Nursing Goals

The nurse will manage and minimize complications of pulmonary embolism.

General Interventions and Rationales

- Consult with physician or advanced practice nurse for low-dose heparin therapy for a high-risk client until ambulatory (see Anticoagulant Therapy in PC: Medication Therapy Adverse Effects). *(Heparin therapy decreases blood viscosity and platelet adhesiveness, reducing the risk of embolism.)*
- Refer to the nursing diagnosis *Risk for Ineffective Peripheral Tissue Perfusion* in Section II for information on preventing DVT.
- Monitor for signs and symptoms of pulmonary embolism:
  - Acute, sharp chest pain
  - Dyspnea, restlessness, cyanosis, decreased mental status
  - Decreased oxygen saturation (SaO_2, SvO_2)
  - Tachycardia
  - Neck vein distention
  - Hypotension
  - Acute right ventricular dilation without parenchymal disease (on chest x-ray)
  - Confusion
  - Cardiac dysrhythmias
  - Low-grade fever
  - Productive cough with blood-tinged sputum
  - Pleural friction rub
  - Crackles
  (Occlusion of pulmonary arteries impedes blood flow to the distal lung, producing a hypoxic state.)
- If these manifestations occur, promptly initiate protocols for shock.
  - Establish an IV line (for medication and fluid administration).
  - Administer fluid replacement therapy according to protocol.
  - Insert indwelling urinary (Foley) catheter (to monitor circulatory volume through urine output).
  - Initiate ECG monitoring and invasive hemodynamic monitoring (to detect dysrhythmias and guide therapy).
  - Administer vasopressors to increase peripheral resistance and raise blood pressure.
  - Administer sodium bicarbonate as indicated (to correct metabolic acidosis).
  - Administer digitalis glycosides and IV diuretics and antiarrhythmic agents, as indicated.
  - Administer small IV doses of morphine (to reduce anxiety and decrease metabolic demands).
  - Refer to *PC: Hypovolemic Shock* for additional interventions.
  - Prepare for angiography and/or perfusion lung scans (to confirm diagnosis and detect the extent of atelectasis).
  (Because death from massive pulmonary embolism commonly occurs in the first 2 h after onset, prompt intervention is crucial.)

- Initiate oxygen therapy through nasal cannula; monitor oxygen saturation. *(This measure rapidly increases circulating oxygen levels.)*
- Monitor serum electrolyte levels, ABG values, blood urea nitrogen, and complete blood count results. *(These laboratory tests help determine perfusion and volume status.)*
- Initiate thrombolytic therapy (eg, urokinase, streptokinase) per orders. *(Thrombolytics can cause lysis of emboli and increase pulmonary capillary perfusion.)*
- When prescribed after thrombolytic infusion, initiate heparin therapy (continuous IV infusion or intermittent). Monitor clotting times during heparin therapy. *(Heparin can slow or halt the underlying thrombotic process, helping prevent clot extension or recurrence.)*
- For a client receiving thrombolytics and/or anticoagulant therapy, monitor for signs of abnormal bleeding (eg, hematuria, bleeding gums, ecchymosis, petechiae, epistaxis).

For PC: Air Embolism

- Before central line catheter insertion and tubing changes, place client in Trendelenburg's position and instruct him or her to perform Valsalva maneuver during the procedure. *(These measures increase intrathoracic pressure and help prevent air from entering the catheter.)*
- Follow instruction policies for central lines.
- Before IV catheter removal, place client in Trendelenburg's position and instruct to perform Valsalva maneuver or at least hold breath during the procedure. After removal, immediately apply direct pressure to the catheterization site, then apply a sterile nonpermeable dressing. Leave dressing in place for 24 to 48 h. *(These measures help prevent air entry.)*
- Monitor for signs and symptoms of air embolism during dressing and IV tubing changes and after any accidental separation of IV connections:
  - Sucking sound on insertion
  - Dyspnea
  - Tachypnea
  - Wheezing
  - Substernal chest pain
  - Anxiety

  (Air embolism can occur with IV tubing changes, with accidental tubing separation, and during catheter insertion and disconnection. [For example, a client can aspirate as much as 200 mL of air from a deep breath during subclavian line disconnection.] Entry of air into the pulmonary arterial system can obstruct blood flow, causing bronchoconstriction of the affected lung area.)
  - If air embolism is suspected
  - Place client in steep Trendelenburg's position on left side. *(This position displaces air away from pulmonary valve and prevents more air from entering.)*
  - Administer oxygen through face mask according to protocol. *(This promotes diffusion of nitrogen, which compresses an air embolism in about 80% of cases.)*
  - Initiate protocols for respiratory or cardiac arrest if indicated.

For PC: Fat Embolism

- Monitor for sign and symptoms of fat embolism:
  - Tachypnea more than 30/min
  - Sudden onset of chest pain or dyspnea
  - Restlessness, apprehension
  - Confusion
  - Elevated temperature above 103°F
  - Increased pulse rate more than 140/min
  - Petechial skin rash (12 to 96 h postoperative)

  (These changes are the result of hypoxemia. Fatty acids attack red blood cells and platelets to form microaggregates, which impair circulation to vital organs, such as the brain. Fatty globules passing through the pulmonary vasculature cause a chemical reaction that decreases lung compliance and ventilation/perfusion ratio and raises body temperature. Rash results from capillary fragility. Common sites are conjunctiva, axilla, chest, and neck [Pellino et al., 1998].)
- Minimize movement of a fractured extremity for the first 3 days after the injury. *(Immobilization minimizes further tissue trauma and reduces the risk of embolism dislodgement [Pellino et al., 1998].)*
- Ensure adequate hydration. *(Optimal hydration dilutes the irritating fatty acids through the system [Pellino et al., 1998].)*
- Monitor intake/output, urine color, and specific gravity. *(These data reflect hydration status.)*

Potential Complication: Respiratory
PC: Hypoxemia
PC: Atelectasis, Pneumonia
PC: Tracheobronchial Constriction
PC: Pneumothorax

POTENTIAL COMPLICATION: RESPIRATORY

DEFINITION

PC: Respiratory: Describes a person experiencing or at high risk to experience various respiratory problems

---

⊘⊘ AUTHOR'S NOTE

The nurse uses the generic collaborative problem *PC: Respiratory* to describe a person at risk for several types of respiratory problems and to identify the nursing focus—monitoring respiratory status for detection and diagnosis of abnormal functioning. Nursing management of a specific respiratory complication is then described under the appropriate collaborative problem for that complication. For example, a nurse using *PC: Respiratory* for a client in whom hypoxemia later develops would then add *PC: Hypoxemia* to the client's problem list. If the risk factors or etiology were not related directly to the primary medical diagnosis, the nurse would add this information to the diagnostic statement (eg, *PC: Hypoxemia related to COPD* in a client with chronic obstructive pulmonary disease [COPD] who experiences respiratory problems after gastric surgery).

For a person vulnerable to respiratory problems because of immobility or excessive tenacious secretions, the nurse should apply the nursing diagnosis *Risk for Ineffective Respiratory Function related to immobility* rather than *PC: Respiratory*.

For information on Focus Assessment Criteria, visit http://connection.lww.com.

Significant Laboratory/Diagnostic Assessment Criteria

Blood pH (elevated in alkalosis, lowered in acidosis)
Arterial blood gas (ABG) values
    pH (elevated in alkalemia, lowered in acidemia)
    PCO_2 (elevated in pulmonary disease, lowered in hyperventilation)
    PO_2 (lowered in pulmonary disease)
    CO_2 content (elevated in COPD, lowered in hyperventilation)
Sputum stain and culture
Chest x-ray
Ventilation/perfusion scanning
Pulse oximetry
Capnography

PC: HYPOXEMIA

DEFINITION

PC: Hypoxemia: Describes a person experiencing or at high risk to experience insufficient plasma oxygen saturation (PO_2 less than normal for age) because of alveolar hypoventilation, pulmonary shunting, or ventilation–perfusion inequality

High-Risk Populations

- COPD
- Pneumonia
- Atelectasis
- Pulmonary edema
- Adult respiratory distress syndrome
- Central nervous system depression
- Medulla or spinal cord disorders
- Guillain-Barré syndrome
- Myasthenia gravis
- Muscular dystrophy
- Obesity
- Compromised chest wall movement (eg, trauma)
- Drug overdose
- Head injury
- Near-drowning
- Multiple trauma

Nursing Goals

The nurse will manage and minimize complications of hypoxemia.

General Interventions and Rationales

- Monitor for signs of acid–base imbalance:
  - ABG analysis: pH < 7.35, $PaCO_2$ > 48 mm Hg (*ABG analysis helps evaluate gas exchange in the lungs. In mild to moderate COPD, the client may have a normal $PaCO_2$ level as chemoreceptors in the medulla respond to increased $PaCO_2$ by increasing ventilation. In severe COPD, however, the client cannot sustain this increased ventilation, and the $PaCO_2$ value gradually increases.*)
- Increased and irregular pulse, and increased respiratory rate initially, followed by decreased rate. (Respiratory acidosis develops as a result of excessive CO_2 retention. A client with respiratory acidosis from chronic disease at first experiences increased heart rate and respirations in an attempt to compensate for decreased oxygenation. After a while, the client breathes more slowly and with prolonged expiration. Eventually, the respiratory center may stop responding to the higher CO_2 levels, and breathing may stop abruptly.)
- Changes in mentation (somnolence, confusion, irritability; *Changes in mentation result from cerebral tissue hypoxia.*)
- Decreased urine output (<5 mL/kg/h); cool, pale, or cyanotic skin. (*The compensatory response to decreased circulatory oxygen aims to increase blood oxygen by increasing heart and respiratory*

rates and to decrease circulation to the kidneys and extremities [marked by decreased pulses and skin changes].)

- Administer low-flow (2 L/min) oxygen as needed through a mask or nasal cannula, if indicated. *(Oxygen therapy increases circulating oxygen levels. High flow rates increase CO_2 retention in people with COPD. Using a cannula rather than a mask may help reduce the client's fears of suffocation.)*
- Evaluate the effects of positioning on oxygenation, using ABG values as a guide. Change client's position every 2 h, avoiding positions that compromise oxygenation. *(This measure promotes optimal ventilation.)*
- Ensure adequate hydration. Teach client to avoid dehydrating beverages (eg, caffeinated drinks, grapefruit juice). *(Optimal hydration helps liquefy secretions.)*
- Teach client effective coughing technique. *(Effective coughing moves mucus from the lower airways to the trachea for expectoration.)*
- If client cannot expectorate secretions, use coughing, chest physiotherapy, or both to move secretions up from the trachea for suctioning. *(Suctioning is effective only at the tracheal level.)*
- Administer supplemental oxygen before and after suctioning. *(This measure helps prevent decreased PO_2 as a result of suctioning.)*
- Obtain a sputum sample for culture and sensitivity and Gram stain testing. *(Sputum culture and sensitivity determine whether an infection is contributing to symptoms.)*
- Eliminate smoke and strong odors from the client's room. *(Irritation of the respiratory tract can exacerbate symptoms.)*
- Monitor the electrocardiogram for dysrhythmias secondary to altered oxygenation. *(Hypoxemia may precipitate cardiac dysrhythmias.)*
- Monitor for signs of right-sided congestive heart failure:
  - Elevated diastolic pressure
  - Distended neck veins
  - Edema
  - Elevated central venous pressure
  (The combination of arterial hypoxemia and respiratory acidosis acts locally as a strong vasoconstrictor of pulmonary vessels. This leads to pulmonary arterial hypertension, increased right ventricular systolic pressure, and, eventually, right ventricular hypertrophy and failure.)
- Refer to the nursing diagnosis *Activity Intolerance* in Section II for specific adaptive techniques to teach a client with chronic pulmonary insufficiency.

PC: ATELECTASIS, PNEUMONIA

DEFINITION

PC: Atelectasis, Pneumonia: Describes a person experiencing impaired respiratory functioning because of alveolar collapse, which can result in pneumonia*

High-Risk Populations

- Pulmonary edema
- Postoperative status (abdominal or thoracic surgery)

---

*The nurse should use the nursing diagnosis *Risk for Ineffective Respiratory Function* for people at high risk for atelectasis and pneumonia, to focus on prevention. The collaborative problem *PC: Atelectasis, Pneumonia* is applicable only if the condition occurs.

- Immobilization
- Decreased level of consciousness
- Nasogastric feedings
- Chronic lung disease (COPD, bronchiectasis, cystic fibrosis)
- Debilitation
- Decreased surfactant production
- Compression of lung tissue (eg, from cancer, abdominal distention, obesity, pneumothorax)
- Airway obstruction

Nursing Goals

The nurse will manage and minimize complications of atelectasis or pneumonia.

General Interventions and Rationales

- Monitor respiratory status and assess for signs and symptoms of inflammation:
  - Increased respiratory rate
  - Fever and chills (sudden or insidious)
  - Productive cough
  - Diminished or absent breath sounds
  - Pleuritic chest pain
  - Tachycardia
  - Marked dyspnea
  - Cyanosis
  - Lethargy
  (Tracheobronchial inflammation, impaired alveolar capillary membrane function, edema, fever, and increased sputum production disrupt respiratory function and compromise the blood's oxygen-carrying capacity. Reduced chest wall compliance in older adults affects the quality of respiratory effort. In older adults, tachypnea [>26 respirations/min] is an early sign of pneumonia, often occurring 3 to 4 days before a confirmed diagnosis. Delirium or mental status changes are often seen early in pneumonia in older adults [Porth, 2002].)
- Monitor for signs and symptoms of infection:
  - Fever of 101°F (39.4°C) or higher
  - Chills
  - Tachycardia
  - Manifestations of shock: restlessness or lethargy, confusion, decreased systolic blood pressure
  (Endogenous pyrogens are released and reset the hypothalamic set point to febrile levels. The body temperature is sensed as "too cool"; shivering and vasoconstriction result to generate and consume heat. Core temperature rises to the new level of the set point, resulting in fever. White blood cells are released to destroy some pathogens. The impaired respiratory system cannot compensate; tissue hypoxia results [Porth, 2002].)
- If fever occurs, provide cooling measures (eg, reduced clothing and bed linen, tepid baths, increased fluids, hypothermia blanket). *(Reducing body temperature is necessary to lower metabolic rate and reduce oxygen consumption.)*
- Monitor for signs and symptoms of septic shock:
  - Altered body temperature (>38°C or <36°C)
  - Hypotension
  - Decreased level of consciousness
  - Weak, rapid pulse
  - Rapid, shallow respirations or CO_2 less than 32
  - Cold, clammy skin
  - Oliguria
  (Septic shock is a systemic inflammatory response syndrome [SIRS] associated with infection because of microorganisms resulting in hypotension and perfusion abnormalities despite fluid resuscitation or vasopressors.)
- Evaluate the effectiveness of cough suppressants and expectorants. *(A dry, hacking cough interferes with sleep and affects energy. Cough suppressants should be used judiciously, however,*

because complete depression of the cough reflex can lead to atelectasis by hindering movement of tracheobronchial secretions.)

- Maintain oxygen therapy, as prescribed, and monitor its effectiveness. *(Oxygen therapy may help prevent dyspnea and also reduce the risk of pulmonary edema.)*
- Provide respiratory physiotherapy (eg, chest percussion, postural drainage) to move thick, tenacious secretions along the tracheobronchial tree. *(Exudate in the alveoli and bronchospasms linked to increased bronchopulmonary secretions can decrease ventilatory effort and impair gas exchange.)*
- Teach client how to do diaphragmatic breathing. *(This technique increases tidal volume by maximizing diaphragmatic descent.)*
- Refer to PC: *Hypoxemia* for additional interventions.

PC: TRACHEOBRONCHIAL CONSTRICTION

DEFINITION

PC: Tracheobronchial Constriction: Describes a person experiencing or at high risk to experience air flow limitations through the tracheobronchial tree because of asthma, bronchitis, emphysema, and/or allergic reaction

High-Risk Populations

- COPD
- Allergies
- Asthma
- Chronic bronchitis
- Viral infections (<6 months of age)
- Cystic fibrosis

Nursing Goals

The nurse will manage and minimize episodes of tracheobronchial constriction.

General Interventions and Rationales

- Monitor respiratory status continuously during acute exacerbation; evaluate:
  - Use of accessory muscles
  - Respiratory rate, pulse rate, blood pressure
  - Breath sounds (eg, wheezing)
  - ABG values
  - Peripheral perfusion (skin color, pulses)
  - Level of consciousness
  (A client's respiratory status can change rapidly, with specific changes depending on response to treatments, level of fatigue, and severity of the episode.)
- Administer oxygen through nasal cannula at 2 to 3 L/min. *(Oxygen therapy reduces hypoxemic effects; cannula rather than mask may help minimize feelings of suffocation.)*

- Ensure adequate hydration either orally or intravenously. *(Good hydration status helps prevent tenacious, impacted mucus.)*
- During acute episodes, stay with client and have him or her breathe using pursed-lip or diaphragmatic breathing. *(A panicky, dyspneic client needs a nurse's constant presence to help gain control over his or her breathing.)*
- Maintain client in upright position. *(It promotes optimal lung expansion.)*
- Initiate interventions as prescribed by physician or advanced practice nurse, which may include anti-inflammatory agents, β_2-agonists, theophylline preparations, or corticosteroids (systemic or inhaled).
- Consult with physician or advanced practice nurse for possible intubation if work of breathing becomes increasingly difficult for the client. *(Exhaustion brought on by excessive respiratory effort can lead to pulmonary arrest.)*
- When indicated, initiate health teaching, using the nursing diagnosis *Risk for Ineffective Health Maintenance related to insufficient knowledge of (specify).*

Pediatric Interventions and Rationales

- Refer also to General Interventions.
- Monitor respiratory status:
  - Pulse rate, respiratory rate
  - Use of accessory respiratory muscles, retractions, nasal flaring
  - Diaphoresis, cyanosis
  - Wheezing, cough

  (Increased pulse and respiratory rate indicate hypoxia. Asthma often manifests as a cough rather than wheezing.)
- Assess for signs of dehydration. *(Children with dyspnea may refuse fluids.)*
- Ensure adequate hydration. *(Good hydration helps prevent tenacious, impacted mucus.)*
- Evaluate child's and parents' understanding of condition, triggers, monitoring, and treatment.
- Ask child and/or parent to demonstrate use of inhaler, spacer, or nebulizer. *(Many drug failures result from improper use of equipment.)*
- Teach how to monitor peak expiratory flow rates (PEFR) twice daily, before and after treatments, in a diary.
  - Determine the child's personal-best values.
  - Instruct to increase medications if PEFR falls below 50% to 80% of personal best.
  - Instruct to use bronchodilator immediately if rate is below 50%, and seek emergency treatment if not improved immediately.

  (PEFR monitoring is critical to effective prevention of acute exacerbations in children with moderate or severe asthma.)

PC: PNEUMOTHORAX

DEFINITION

PC: Pneumothorax: Describes a person experiencing or at high risk to experience accumulation of air in the pleural space because of lung injury

High-Risk Populations

- Severe blunt or penetrating chest injury
- Postoperative status (cardiac or thoracic surgery)
- Mechanically ventilated with positive end-expiratory pressure
- Interstitial lung disease
- Insertion of central venous catheter
- Transbronchial biopsy
- Thoracentesis

Nursing Goals

The nurse will manage and minimize complications of pneumothorax.

General Interventions and Rationales

- Monitor for signs and symptoms of pneumothorax (Holloway & Harris, 2000):
  - Acute pleuritic chest pain
  - Dyspnea, tachypnea, tachycardia
  - Hyperresonant percussion sounds with loss of breath sounds over the affected side
  - Shifting of trachea
  (Early detection and prompt intervention are necessary to prevent serious complications.)
- Administer oxygen, if indicated. If chronic CO_2 retention occurs, limit the flow rate to no more than 2 L/min. *(Higher flow rates can depress ventilatory drive.)*
- Prepare for stat chest x-ray, ABGs, possible chest tube placement.
- Evaluate the need for analgesics to manage thoracic pain. *(Pain interferes with lung expansion on inspiration, compromising oxygenation.)*
- Reposition client every 2 h, keeping the unaffected lung in the dependent position. *(This position limits pain and improves oxygenation by better equalizing ventilation and perfusion.)*
- Explain and supervise deep breathing with sustained maximum inspiration. *(Deep breathing expands lungs and evacuates air from pleural space into chest drainage system [if present].)*
- Instruct person to avoid coughing except when necessary to clear secretions. *(Coughing increases pain.)*
- Minimize environmental stimuli, provide emotional support, and offer simple explanations for all procedures. *(These measures may help reduce anxiety, increasing respiratory rate.)*
- If use of a chest drainage system is indicated, follow institutional protocols for set-up, assessment, and maintenance.

Potential Complication: Metabolic/Immune/Hematopoietic
PC: Hypo/Hyperglycemia
PC: Negative Nitrogen Balance
PC: Electrolyte Imbalances
PC: Sepsis
PC: Acidosis (Metabolic, Respiratory)
PC: Alkalosis (Metabolic, Respiratory)
PC: Allergic Reaction
PC: Thrombocytopenia
PC: Opportunistic Infections
PC: Sickling Crisis

POTENTIAL COMPLICATION: METABOLIC/IMMUNE/HEMATOPOIETIC

DEFINITION

PC: Metabolic/Immune/Hematopoietic: Describes a person experiencing or at high risk to experience various endocrine, immune, or metabolic dysfunctions

---

AUTHOR'S NOTE

The nurse can use this generic collaborative problem to describe a person at risk for several types of metabolic and immune system problems. For example, for a client with pituitary dysfunction who is at risk for various metabolic problems, using *PC: Metabolic* directs nurses to monitor endocrine system function for specific problems, based on focus assessment findings. Under this collaborative problem, nursing interventions would focus on monitoring metabolic status to detect and diagnose abnormal functioning. If the client developed a specific complication, the nurse would add the appropriate specific collaborative problem, along with nursing management information, to the client's problem list. For a client with diabetes mellitus, the nurse would add the diagnostic statement *PC: Hypo/Hyperglycemia*. For a client receiving chemotherapy, the nurse would use *PC: Immunodeficiency,* a collaborative problem that encompasses leukopenia, thrombocytopenia, and erythrocytopenia. If thrombocytopenia were an isolated problem, it would warrant a separate diagnostic statement (ie, *PC: Thrombocytopenia*).

For a client with a condition or undergoing a treatment that produces immunosuppression (eg, acquired immunodeficiency syndrome [AIDS], graft-versus-host disease, immunosuppressant therapy), the collaborative problem *PC: Immunosuppression* would be appropriate. When conditions have or possibly could have affected coagulation (eg, chronic renal failure, alcohol abuse, anticoagulant therapy), a collaborative problem such as *PC: Hemolysis* or *PC: Erythrocytopenia* would be indicated. If the risk factors or etiology were not directly related to the primary medical diagnosis, they could be added (eg, *PC: Immunosuppression related to chronic corticosteroid therapy* in a client who has sustained a myocardial infarction).

For information on Focus Assessment Criteria, visit http://connection.lww.com.

Significant Laboratory/Diagnostic Assessment Criteria

Serum amylase (elevated in acute pancreatitis, lowered in chronic pancreatitis)
Serum albumin (lowered in malnutrition)

Lymphocyte count (lowered in malnutrition)
Serum calcium (elevated in hyperparathyroidism, certain cancers, and acute pancreatitis, lowered in hypoparathyroidism)
Blood pH (elevated in alkalosis, lowered in acidosis)
Serum glucose (elevated in diabetes mellitus and pancreatic insufficiency, lowered in pancreatic islet cell tumors)
Serum glycosylated hemoglobin (reflects mean glucose levels for preceding 2 to 3 months)
Urine acetone, urine glucose (present in diabetes mellitus)
Urine ketone bodies (present in uncontrolled diabetes)
Platelets (elevated in polycythemia and chronic granulocytic leukemia, lowered in anemia and acute leukemia)
Immunoglobins (elevated in autoimmune disease)
Coagulation tests (elevated in thrombocytopenia, purpura, and hemophilia)
Prothrombin time (elevated in anticoagulant therapy, cirrhosis, and hepatitis)
Red blood cell (RBC) count (lowered in anemia, leukemia, and renal failure)

PC: HYPO/HYPERGLYCEMIA

DEFINITION

PC: Hypo/Hyperglycemia: Describes a person experiencing or at high risk to experience a blood glucose level that is too low or too high for metabolic function*

High-Risk Populations

- Diabetes mellitus
- Parenteral nutrition
- Sepsis
- Enteral feedings
- Corticosteroid therapy
- Neonate of diabetic mother
- Small-for-gestational-age neonate
- Neonate of narcotic-addicted mother
- Thermal injuries (severe)
- Pancreatitis (hyperglycemia), cancer of pancreas
- Addison's disease (hypoglycemia)
- Adrenal gland hyperfunction
- Liver disease (hypoglycemia)

Nursing Goals

The nurse will manage and minimize episodes of hypoglycemia or hyperglycemia.

---

* If the person is not at risk for both, the diagnosis should specify the problem (eg, *PC: Hyperglycemia related to corticosteroid therapy*).

General Interventions and Rationales

For Hypoglycemia

- Monitor serum glucose level at the bedside before administering hypoglycemic agents and/or before meals and hour of sleep. (*Serum glucose is a more accurate parameter than urine glucose, which is affected by renal threshold and renal function.*)
- Monitor for signs and symptoms of hypoglycemia:
  - Blood glucose level below 60 mg/dL
  - Pale, moist, cool skin
  - Tachycardia, diaphoresis
  - Jitteriness, irritability
  - Hypoglycemia unawareness
  - Incoordination
  - Drowsiness, confusion

  (*Hypoglycemia [insufficient glucose levels] can result from excessive insulin, insufficient food intake, or excessive physical activity. A rapid drop in blood glucose level stimulates the sympathetic system to produce adrenaline, which causes diaphoresis, cool skin, tachycardia, and jitteriness.*)
- If client can swallow, give him or her ½ cup of orange juice, cola, or ginger ale every 15 min until blood glucose level exceeds 69 mg/dL. (*Simple carbohydrates are metabolized quickly.*)
- If client cannot swallow, administer glucagon hydrochloride subcutaneously or 50 mL of 50% glucose in water intravenously (IV), according to protocol. (*Glucagon causes glycogenolysis in the liver when glycogen stores are adequate. In a client in critical condition who has been in a coma for some time, glycogen stores likely have already been used up, and IV glucose is the only effective treatment.*)
- Recheck blood glucose level 1 h after an initial blood glucose reading of greater than 69 mg/dL. (*Regular monitoring detects early signs of high or low levels.*)
- If indicated, consult with a dietitian to provide a complex carbohydrate snack at bedtime. (*This measure can help prevent hypoglycemia during the night.*)

For Hyperglycemia

- Monitor for signs and symptoms of diabetic ketoacidosis:
  - Blood glucose level greater than 300 mg/dL
  - Positive plasma ketone, acetone breath
  - Headache
  - Kussmaul's respirations
  - Anorexia, nausea, vomiting
  - Tachycardia
  - Decreased blood pressure
  - Polyuria, polydipsia
  - Decreased serum sodium, potassium, and phosphate levels

  (*When insulin is unavailable, blood glucose levels rise and the body metabolizes fat for energy-producing ketone bodies. Excessive ketone bodies cause headaches, nausea, vomiting, and abdominal pain. Respiratory rate and depth increase to help increase CO_2 excretion and reduce acidosis. Glucose inhibits water resorption in the renal glomerulus, leading to osmotic diuresis with severe loss of water, sodium, potassium, and phosphates. Diabetic ketoacidosis occurs in type I diabetes.*)
- If ketoacidosis occurs, initiate appropriate protocols to reverse dehydration, restore the insulin–glucagon ratio, and treat circulatory collapse, ketoacidosis, and electrolyte imbalance.
- Continue to monitor hydration status every 30 min; assess skin moisture and turgor, urine output and specific gravity, and fluid intake. (*Accurate assessments are needed during the acute stage [first 10–12 h] to prevent overhydration or underhydration.*)
- Continue to monitor blood glucose levels according to protocol. (*Careful monitoring enables early detection of medication-induced hypoglycemia or continued hyperglycemia.*)
- Monitor serum potassium, sodium, and phosphate levels. (*Acidosis causes hyperkalemia and hyponatremia. Insulin therapy promotes potassium and phosphate return to the cells, causing serum hypokalemia and hypophosphatemia*).
- Monitor neurologic status every hour. (*Fluctuating glucose levels, acidosis, and fluid shifts can affect neurologic functioning.*)

- Carefully protect client's skin from microorganism invasion, injury, and shearing force; reposition every 1 to 2 h. *(Dehydration and tissue hypoxia increase the skin's vulnerability to injury.)*
- Do not allow a recovering client to drink large quantities of water. Give a conscious client ice chips to quench thirst. *(Excessive fluid intake can cause abdominal distention and vomiting.)*
- Monitor for signs and symptoms of hyperosmolar hyperglycemic nonketotic (HHNK) coma:
  - Blood glucose 600 to 2000 mg/dL
  - Serum sodium, potassium normal or elevated
  - Elevated hematocrit, blood urea nitrogen (BUN)
  - Nausea, vomiting
  - Hypotension, tachycardia
  - Dehydration, weight loss, poor skin turgor
  - Lethargy, stupor, coma
  - Elevated urine glucose (>2+)
  - Urine ketones negative or <2+
  - Polyuria
  (HHNK results from relative insulin deficiency. Hyperglycemia and hyperosmolality are present, but these are an absence of significant ketones. HHNK coma can be a response to acute stress [eg, from myocardial infarction, burns, severe infection, dialysis, or hyperalimentation]. People with type II insulin-resistant diabetes who experience marked dehydration are especially at risk. Glucose inhibits water resorption in the renal glomerulus, leading to osmotic diuresis with loss of water, sodium, potassium, and phosphates. Cerebral impairment results from intracellular dehydration in the brain [Porth, 2002].)
- Monitor cardiac function and circulatory status; evaluate:
  - Rate, rhythm (cardiac, respiratory)
  - Skin color
  - Capillary refill time, central venous pressure
  - Peripheral pulses
  - Serum potassium
  (Severe dehydration can cause reduced cardiac output and compensatory vasoconstriction. Cardiac dysrhythmias can result from potassium imbalances.)
- Follow protocols for ketoacidosis, as indicated.
- Investigate for causes of ketoacidosis or hypoglycemia, and teach prevention and early management, using the nursing diagnosis *Risk for Ineffective Therapeutic Regimen Management related to insufficient knowledge of (specify)* (see Section II).

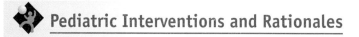

Pediatric Interventions and Rationales

Refer also to General Interventions.

Consult with dietitian for nutritional management. *(The goal is a consistent, well-balanced diet to ensure normal growth and development.)*

Evaluate child's growth and development. *(Poor control of glucose levels affects growth.)*

Teach about condition, insulin therapy, self-monitoring of glucose, nutrition, exercise, and prevention of complications. Consult with school nurse for management at school. *(Effective management is a team effort.)*

PC: NEGATIVE NITROGEN BALANCE

DEFINITION

PC: Negative Nitrogen Balance: Describes a person experiencing or at risk to experience catabolism, when more nitrogen is excreted from tissue breakdown than is replaced by intake

High-Risk Populations

- Severe malnutrition
- Prolonged NPO state
- Elderly with chronic disease
- Uncontrolled diabetes
- Digestive disorders
- Prolonged use of glucose or saline IV therapy
- Inadequate enteral replacement
- Excessive catabolism (eg, due to cancer, infection, burns, surgery, excess stress)
- Anorexia nervosa, bulimia
- Critical illness
- Chemotherapy
- Sepsis

Nursing Goals

The nurse will manage and minimize negative nitrogen balance.

General Interventions and Rationales

- Establish the client's optimum weight for height. *(This establishes baseline goals.)*
- Weigh client daily at same time, wearing same amount of clothes, same scale, and same bedding. *(Monitoring weight helps detect excessive catabolism.)*
- Monitor for signs of negative nitrogen balance:
  - Weight loss
  - 24-h urine nitrogen balance below zero
  (Cachexia results from increased metabolic demands, insufficient replacement, and anorexia. Impaired carbohydrate metabolism causes increased metabolism of fats and protein, which—especially with metabolic acidosis—can lead to negative nitrogen balance and weight loss.)
- Monitor for signs and symptoms of hypoalbuminemia, which can have a rapid or insidious onset:
  - Emotional depression, fatigue *(These effects result from decreased energy supplies.)*
  - Muscle wasting *(This results from insufficient protein available for tissue repair.)*
  - Poorly healing wounds *(This results from insufficient protein available for tissue repair.)*
  - Edema *(Edema results from a plasma-to-interstitial fluid shift because of insufficient vascular osmotic pressure.)*
- Monitor laboratory values:
  - Serum prealbumin and transferring *(These values evaluate visceral protein. Prealbumin is a precursor to albumin and a much more sensitive measure of visceral protein.)*
  - BUN *(This value measures kidney clearance ability.)*

- 24-h urine nitrogen *(Because the glomerulus reabsorbs 99% of what is filtered, measurement of urea nitrogen, a waste product of protein metabolism, gives data to calculate the nitrogen balance.)*
  - Electrolytes, osmolality *(These values help assess kidney function.)*
  - Total lymphocyte count *(Lymphocyte production requires protein.)*
- Continually reevaluate the client's energy/protein requirements. Consult with a registered dietitian for evaluation (eg, indirect calorimetry test, anthropometric measures). *(The person's calorie/protein requirements will change depending on metabolic demands [eg, from stress, fever, or infection].)*
- Administer total parenteral solutions, intralipid fat emulsions, and/or enteral formulas as prescribed by the physician or advanced practice nurse and in accordance with appropriate procedures and protocols. *(This client's increased caloric requirements for tissue repair cannot be met with routine IV therapy.)*
- For specific nursing interventions to increase oral nutrient intake, refer to the nursing diagnosis *Imbalanced Nutrition: Less Than Body Requirements* (see Section II).

PC: ELECTROLYTE IMBALANCES*

- ○ *PC:* **Hypokalemia**
- ○ *PC:* **Hyperkalemia**
- ○ *PC:* **Hyponatremia**
- ○ *PC:* **Hypernatremia**
- ○ *PC:* **Hypocalcemia**
- ○ *PC:* **Hypercalcemia**
- ○ *PC:* **Hypophosphatemia**
- ○ *PC:* **Hyperphosphatemia**
- ○ *PC:* **Hypomagnesemia**
- ○ *PC:* **Hypermagnesemia**
- ○ *PC:* **Hypochloremia**
- ○ *PC:* **Hyperchloremia**

DEFINITION
PC: Electrolyte Imbalances: Describes a person experiencing or at risk to experience a deficit or excess of one or more electrolytes

High-Risk Populations

For Hypokalemia
- Crash dieting (diabetic ketoacidosis)
- Metabolic or respiratory alkalosis
- Excessive intake of licorice
- Diuretic therapy
- Loss of gastrointestinal (GI) fluids (through excessive nasogastric suctioning, nausea, vomiting, or diarrhea)
- Steroid use
- Estrogen use
- Hyperaldosteronism

---

* For a person experiencing or at high risk to experience a deficit or excess in a single electrolyte, the diagnostic statement should specify the problem (eg, *PC: Hypokalemia related to diuretic therapy*).

- Severe burns
- Decreased potassium intake
- Liver disease with ascites
- Renal tubular acidosis
- Malabsorption
- Severe catabolism
- Salt depletion
- Hemolysis
- Hypoaldosteronism
- Rhabdomyolysis
- Laxative abuse
- Villous adenoma
- Hyperglycemia
- Severe magnesium depletion

For Hyperkalemia
- Renal failure
- Excessive potassium intake (oral or IV)
- Cell damage (eg, from burns, trauma, surgery)
- Crushing injuries
- Potassium-sparing diuretic use
- Adrenal insufficiency
- Lupus
- Sickle cell disease
- Post-transplant
- Chemotherapy
- Metabolic acidosis
- Transfusion of old blood
- Internal hemorrhage
- Hypoaldosteronism
- Acidosis

For Hyponatremia
- Water intoxication (oral or IV)
- Renal failure
- Gastric suctioning
- Vomiting, diarrhea
- Burns
- Potent diuretic use
- Excessive diaphoresis
- Excessive wound drainage
- Congestive heart failure
- Hyperglycemia
- Malabsorption syndrome
- Cystic fibrosis
- Addison's disease
- Psychogenic polydipsia
- Oxytocin administration
- Syndrome of inappropriate antidiuretic hormone (resulting from central nervous system [CNS] disorders, major trauma, malignancies, or endocrine disorders)
- Adrenal gland insufficiency
- Chronic illness (eg, cirrhosis)
- Hypothyroidism (moderate, severe)

For Hypernatremia
- Elderly, infants
- Inadequate fluid intake
- Heat stroke
- Diarrhea
- Severe insensible fluid loss (eg, through hyperventilation or sweating)

- Diabetes insipidus
- Excessive sodium intake (oral, IV, medications)
- Hypertonic tube feeding
- Coma
- High protein feeding with inadequate H_2O intake

For Hypocalcemia

- Renal failure (increased phosphorus)
- Protein malnutrition (eg, due to malabsorption)
- Inadequate calcium intake
- Diarrhea
- Burns
- Malignancy
- Hypoparathyroidism
- Vitamin D deficiency
- Osteoblastic tumors

For Hypercalcemia

- Chronic renal failure
- Sarcoidosis and granulomatous disease
- Excessive vitamin D intake
- Hyperparathyroidism
- Decreased hypophosphatemia
- Bone tumors
- Cancers (Hodgkin's disease, myeloma, leukemia, neoplastic bone disease)
- Prolonged use of thiazide diuretics
- Paget's disease
- Parathyroid hormone-secreting tumors (eg, lung, kidney)
- Hemodialysis
- Multiple fractures
- Prolonged immobilization
- Excessive calcium-containing antacids

For Hypophosphatemia

- Diabetic ketoacidosis
- Prolonged use of IV dextrose solutions
- Malabsorption disorders
- Renal wasting of phosphorus
- Low-phosphate diet (oral, total parenteral nutrition)
- Rickets
- Excessive use of phosphate binders
- Osteomalacia
- Alcoholism

For Hyperphosphatemia

- Excessive vitamin D intake
- Renal failure
- Healing fractures
- Bone tumors
- Hypoparathyroidism
- Hypocalcemia
- Phosphate laxatives
- Excessive IV or PO phosphate
- Chemotherapy
- Catabolism
- Lactic acidosis

For Hypomagnesemia

- Malnutrition
- Prolonged diuretic use

- Chronic alcoholism
- Excessive lactation
- Severe diarrhea, nasogastric suctioning
- Cirrhosis
- Severe dehydration
- Ulcerative colitis
- Toxemia
- Burns
- Cisplatinum use
- Hyperthyroidism/Cushing's disease
- Prolonged IV therapy without magnesium

For Hypermagnesemia

- Addison's disease
- Renal failure
- Severe dehydration with oliguria
- Excessive intake of magnesium-containing antacids, laxatives
- Thiazide use

For Hypochloremia

- Loss of GI fluids (eg, through vomiting, diarrhea, suctioning)
- Metabolic alkalosis
- Diabetic acidosis
- Prolonged use of IV dextrose
- Excessive diaphoresis
- Excessive diuretic use
- Ulcerative colitis
- Fever
- Acute infections
- Severe burns

For Hyperchloremia

- Metabolic acidosis
- Severe diarrhea
- Excessive parenteral isotonic saline solution infusion
- Urinary diversion
- Renal failure
- Cushing's syndrome
- Hyperventilation
- Eclampsia
- Anemia
- Cardiac decompensation

Nursing Goals

The nurse will manage and minimize episodes of electrolyte imbalance(s).

General Interventions

Identify the electrolyte imbalance(s) for which the client is vulnerable, and intervene as follows. (Refer to High-Risk Populations under the specific imbalance.)

PC: Hypo/Hyperkalemia

- Monitor for signs and symptoms of hyperkalemia:
  - Weakness to flaccid paralysis
  - Muscle irritability
  - Paresthesias
  - Nausea, abdominal cramping, or diarrhea

- Oliguria
- Electrocardiogram (ECG) changes: tall, tented T waves, ST segment depression, prolonged PR interval (>0.2 s), first-degree heart block, bradycardia, broadening of the QRS complex, eventual ventricular fibrillation, and cardiac standstill (Porth, 2002)

  (Hyperkalemia can result from the kidney's decreased ability to excrete potassium or from excessive potassium intake. Acidosis increases the release of potassium from cells. Fluctuations in potassium level affect neuromuscular transmission, producing cardiac dysrhythmias, and reducing action of GI smooth muscle.)

- For a client with hyperkalemia
  - Restrict potassium-rich foods, fluids, and IV solutions with potassium. *(High potassium levels necessitate a reduction in potassium intake.)*
  - Provide range-of-motion (ROM) exercises to extremities. *(ROM improves muscle tone and reduces cramps.)*
  - Per orders or protocols, give medications to reduce serum potassium levels, such as:
    - IV calcium *(To block effects on the heart muscle temporarily)*
    - Sodium bicarbonate, glucose, insulin *(To force potassium back into cells)*
    - Cation-exchange resins (eg, Kayexalate, hemodialysis; *To force excretion of potassium)*
- Monitor for signs and symptoms of hypokalemia:
  - Weakness or flaccid paralysis
  - Decreased or absent deep tendon reflexes
  - Hypoventilation, change in consciousness
  - Polyuria
  - Hypotension
  - Paralytic ileus
  - ECG changes: U wave, low-voltage or inverted T wave, dysrhythmias, and prolonged QT interval
  - Nausea, vomiting, anorexia

  (Hypokalemia results from losses associated with vomiting, diarrhea, or diuretic therapy, or from insufficient potassium intake. Hypokalemia impairs neuromuscular transmission and reduces the efficiency of respiratory muscles. Kidneys are less sensitive to antidiuretic hormone and thus excrete large quantities of dilute urine. GI smooth muscle action also is reduced. Abnormally low potassium levels also impair electrical conduction of the heart [Porth, 2002].)

- For a client with hypokalemia:
  - Encourage increased intake of potassium-rich foods. *(An increase in dietary potassium intake helps ensure potassium replacement.)*
  - If parenteral potassium replacement (always diluted) is instituted, do not exceed 10 mEq/h in adults. Monitor serum potassium levels during replacement. *(Excessive levels can cause cardiac dysrhythmias.)*
  - Observe the IV site for infiltration. *(Potassium is very caustic to tissues.)*

PC: Hypo/Hypernatremia

- Monitor for signs and symptoms of hyponatremia:
  - CNS effects ranging from lethargy to coma, headache
  - Weakness
  - Abdominal pain
  - Muscle twitching or convulsions
  - Nausea, vomiting, diarrhea
  - Apprehension

  (Hyponatremia results from sodium loss through vomiting, diarrhea, or diuretic therapy; excessive fluid intake; or insufficient dietary sodium intake. Cellular edema, caused by osmosis, produces cerebral edema, weakness, and muscle cramps.)

- For a client with hyponatremia, initiate IV sodium chloride solutions and discontinue diuretic therapy, as ordered. *(These interventions prevent further sodium losses.)*
- Monitor for signs and symptoms of hypernatremia with fluid overload:
  - Thirst, decreased urine output
  - CNS effects ranging from agitation to convulsions
  - Elevated serum osmolality
  - Weight gain, edema
  - Elevated blood pressure
  - Tachycardia

(Hypernatremia results from excessive sodium intake or increased aldosterone output. Water is pulled from the cells, causing cellular dehydration and producing CNS symptoms. Thirst is a compensatory response to dilute sodium.)

- For a client with hypernatremia:
  - Initiate fluid replacement in response to serum osmolality levels, as ordered. *(Rapid reduction in serum osmolality can cause cerebral edema and seizures.)*
  - Monitor for seizures. *(Sodium excess causes cerebral edema.)*
  - Monitor intake and output, weight. *(This evaluates fluid balance.)*

PC: Hypo/Hypercalcemia

- Monitor for signs and symptoms of hypocalcemia:
  - Altered mental status
  - Numbness or tingling in fingers and toes
  - Muscle cramps
  - Seizures
  - ECG changes: prolonged QT interval, prolonged ST segment, and dysrhythmias
  - Chvostek's or Trousseau's sign
  - Tetany

(Hypocalcemia can result from the kidney's inability to metabolize vitamin D [needed for calcium absorption]. Retention of phosphorus causes a reciprocal drop in serum calcium level. A low serum calcium level produces increased neural excitability, resulting in muscle spasms [cardiac, facial, extremities] and CNS irritability [seizures]. It also causes cardiac muscle hyperactivity, as evidenced by ECG changes.)

- For a client with hypocalcemia:
  - Per orders for acute hypocalcemia, administer calcium by way of IV bolus infusion.
  - Consult with the dietitian for a high-calcium, low-phosphorus diet. *(Lower serum calcium level necessitates dietary replacement.)*
  - Assess for hyperphosphatemia or hypomagnesemia. *(Hyperphosphatemia inhibits calcium absorption; in hypomagnesemia, the kidneys excrete calcium to retain magnesium.)*
  - Monitor for ECG changes: prolonged QT interval, irritable dysrhythmias, and atrioventricular conduction defects. *(Calcium imbalances can cause cardiac muscle hyperactivity.)*
- Monitor for signs and symptoms of hypercalcemia:
  - Altered mental status
  - Anorexia, nausea, vomiting, constipation
  - Numbness or tingling in fingers and toes
  - Muscle cramps, hypotoxicity
  - Deep bone pain
  - AV blocks (ECG)

(Insufficient calcium level reduces neuromuscular excitability, resulting in decreased muscle tone, numbness, anorexia, and mental lethargy.)

- For a client with hypercalcemia:
  - Initiate normal saline IV therapy and loop diuretics, as ordered; avoid thiazide diuretics. *(IV fluids dilute serum calcium. Loop diuretics enhance calcium excretion; thiazide diuretics inhibit calcium excretion.)*
  - Per order, administer phosphorus preparations and mithramycin (contraindicated in clients with renal failure). *(These increase bone deposition of calcium.)*
  - Monitor for renal calculi (see *PC: Renal Calculi*).

PC: Hypo/Hyperphosphatemia

- Monitor for signs and symptoms of hypophosphatemia:
  - Muscle weakness, pain
  - Bleeding
  - Depressed white cell function
  - Confusion
  - Anorexia

(Phosphorus deficiency impairs cellular energy resources and oxygen delivery to tissues and also causes decreased platelet aggregation.)

- For a client with hypophosphatemia, per order, replace phosphorus stores slowly by oral supplements, and discontinue phosphate binders. *(This helps prevent precipitation with calcium.)*
- Monitor for signs and symptoms of hyperphosphatemia:

- Tetany
- Numbness or tingling in fingers and toes
- Soft tissue calcification
- Chvostek's and Trousseau's signs
- Coarse, dry skin

(Hyperphosphatemia can result from the kidneys' decreased ability to excrete phosphorus. Elevated phosphorus does not cause symptoms in itself, but contributes to tetany and other neuromuscular symptoms in the short term and to soft tissue calcification in the long term.)

- For a client with hyperphosphatemia, administer phosphorus-binding antacids, calcium supplements, or vitamin D, and restrict phosphorus-rich foods. *(Supplements are needed to overcome vitamin D deficiency and to compensate for a calcium-poor diet. High phosphate decreases calcium, which increases parathyroid hormone [PTH]. PTH is ineffective in removing phosphates due to renal failure, but causes calcium reabsorption from bone and decreases tubular reabsorption of phosphate.)*

PC: Hypo/Hypermagnesemia

- Monitor for hypomagnesemia:
  - Dysphagia, nausea, anorexia
  - Muscle weakness
  - Facial tics
  - Athetoid movements (slow, involuntary twisting movements)
  - Cardiac dysrhythmias, flat or inverted T waves, prolonged QT intervals, tachycardia, depressed ST segment
  - Confusion

(Magnesium deficit causes neuromuscular changes and hyperexcitability.)

- For a client with hypomagnesemia, initiate magnesium sulfate replacement (dietary for mild deficiency, parenteral for severe deficiency), as ordered.
- Initiate seizure precautions. *(This protects from injury.)*
- Monitor for hypermagnesemia:
  - Decreased blood pressure, bradycardia, decreased respirations
  - Flushing
  - Lethargy, muscle weakness
  - Peaked T waves

(Magnesium excess causes depression of central and peripheral neuromuscular function, producing vasodilation.)

- If respiratory depression occurs, consult with the physician for possible hemodialysis. *(Magnesium-free dialysate causes excretion.)*

PC: Hypo/Hyperchloremia

- Monitor for hypochloremia:
  - Hyperirritability
  - Slow respirations
  - Decreased blood pressure

(Hypochloremia occurs with metabolic alkalosis, resulting in loss of calcium and potassium, which produces the symptoms.)

- For a client with hypochloremia, see *PC: Alkalosis* for interventions.
- Monitor for hyperchloremia:
  - Weakness
  - Lethargy
  - Deep, rapid breathing

(Metabolic acidosis causes loss of chloride ions.)

- For a client with hyperchloremia, see *PC: Acidosis* for interventions.

PC: SEPSIS

DEFINITION

PC: Sepsis: Describes a person experiencing or at high risk to experience a systemic response to the presence of pathogenic bacteria, viruses, fungi, or their toxins. The microorganisms may or may not be present in the bloodstream.

High-Risk Populations

- Extreme age
- Drug dependency, alcoholism
- Burns, multiple trauma
- Infection (urinary, respiratory, wound)
- Immunosuppression
- Invasive lines (urinary, arterial, or central venous catheter)
- AIDS
- Disseminated intravascular coagulation
- Pressure ulcers
- Extensive slow-healing wounds
- Surgical procedures (GI, thoracic, cardiac)
- Diabetes mellitus
- Malnutrition
- Cancer
- Cirrhosis, pancreatitis
- Transplants

Infants/Children
- Viral upper respiratory infection
- Bacterial enteritis
- Burns
- Urinary tract infections
- Bite wounds (eg, dog, human)
- Craniofacial surgery
- Compromised host defenses

Nursing Goals

The nurse will manage and monitor the complications of sepsis.

General Interventions and Rationales

- Monitor for signs and symptoms of sepsis (AACP/SCCM Consensus Conference Committee, 1992):
  - Temperature >38°C or <36°C
  - Heart rate >90 beats/min
  - Respiratory rate >20 breaths/min or $PaCO_2$ <32 torr (<4.3 kPa)
  - White blood cell (WBC) count >12,000 cells/mm³, <4000 cells/mm³, or >10% immature (band) forms
- Monitor older adults for changes in mentation; weakness, malaise; normothermia or hypothermia; and anorexia. *(These clients do not exhibit the typical signs of infection. Usual presenting findings—*

fever, chills, tachypnea, tachycardia, and leukocytosis—frequently are absent in older adults with significant infection.)
- Per orders, initiate anti-infectives, monitoring and management of oxygen consumption and delivery, immunomodulation, and nutritional support. *(These four areas in the management of septic clients show promise in reducing morbidity and mortality.)*
- If indicated, refer to *PC: Hypovolemic Shock* for more information.

Pediatric Interventions and Rationales

- Monitor temperature (temperature >41°C [105.8°F] implies bacteremia). Very young infants can be hypothermic.
- Monitor for behavior changes:
  - Quality of cry
  - Response to parental stimulation
  - State variation
  - Response to social stimulation
  (These changes reflect compromised cerebral circulation.)
- Monitor respiratory pattern. *(Tachypnea and acrocyanosis may reflect poor peripheral perfusion.)*
- Monitor blood pressure, peripheral pulses, and capillary refill times. *(Circulatory inadequacy can be present even with normal blood pressures.)*
- Monitor for cutaneous changes. *(Petechiae, ecchymoses of distal extremities, and diffuse erythroderma can manifest with sepsis.)*
- Monitor oxygen saturation. *(Pulse oximetry measures oxygen levels.)*

PC: ACIDOSIS (METABOLIC, RESPIRATORY)*

DEFINITION
PC: Acidosis: Describes a person experiencing or at high risk for experiencing an acid–base imbalance due to increased production of acids or excessive loss of base

High-Risk Populations

For Respiratory Acidosis
- Hypoventilation
- Acute pulmonary edema
- Airway obstruction
- Pneumothorax
- Sedative overdose
- Severe pneumonia
- Chronic obstructive pulmonary disease
- Asthma

*When indicated, the nurse should specify the diagnosis as either *PC: Metabolic Acidosis* or *PC: Respiratory Acidosis.*

- CNS lesions
- Disorders of respiratory system, muscle and chest wall (myasthenia gravis, amyotrophic lateral sclerosis, Guillain-Barré syndrome)

For Metabolic Acidosis

- Diabetes mellitus
- Lactic acidosis
- Late-phase salicylate poisoning
- Uremia
- Methanol or ethylene glycol ingestion
- Diarrhea
- Intestinal fistulas, malabsorption
- Intake of large quantities of isotonic saline or ammonium chloride
- Renal failure (acute or chronic)
- Massive rhabdomyolysis
- Poisoning
- Drug toxicity

Nursing Goals

The nurse will manage and minimize complications of acidosis.

General Interventions and Rationales

For Metabolic Acidosis

- Monitor for signs and symptoms of metabolic acidosis:
  - Rapid, shallow respirations
  - Headache, lethargy, coma
  - Nausea and vomiting
  - Low plasma bicarbonate and pH of arterial blood
  - Behavior changes, drowsiness
  - Increased serum potassium
  - Increased serum chloride
  - PCO_2 less than 35 to 40 mm Hg
  - Decreased HCO_3

  (*Metabolic acidosis results from the kidney's inability to excrete hydrogen ions, phosphates, sulfates, and ketone bodies. Bicarbonate loss results when the kidney reduces its resorption. Hyperkalemia, hyperphosphatemia, and decreased bicarbonate levels aggravate metabolic acidosis. Excessive ketone bodies cause headaches, nausea, vomiting, and abdominal pain. Respiratory rate and depth increase to increase CO_2 excretion and reduce acidosis. Acidosis affects the CNS and can increase neuromuscular irritability because of the cellular exchange of hydrogen and potassium.*)
- For a client with metabolic acidosis:
  - Initiate IV fluid replacement as ordered, depending on the underlying etiology. (*Dehydration may result from gastric and urinary fluid losses.*)
  - If the etiology is diabetes mellitus, refer to *PC: Hypo / Hyperglycemia* for interventions.
  - Assess for signs and symptoms of hypocalcemia, hypokalemia, and alkalosis as acidosis is corrected. (*Rapid correction of acidosis may cause rapid excretion of calcium and potassium and rebound alkalosis.*)
  - Correct, per orders, any electrolyte imbalances. Refer to *PC: Electrolyte Imbalances* for specific interventions for each type of electrolyte imbalance.
  - Monitor arterial blood gas (ABG) values, urine pH. (*These values help evaluate the effectiveness of therapy.*)

For Respiratory Acidosis

- Monitor for signs and symptoms of respiratory acidosis:
  - Tachycardia, dysrhythmias, bounding pulses
  - Blurred vision, papilledema

- Diaphoresis
- Nausea and/or vomiting
- Restlessness, headaches
- Dyspnea, hypoventilation
- Increased respiratory effort
- Decreased respiratory rate
- Increased PCO_2
- Normal or decreased PO_2
- Increased serum calcium
- Decreased sodium chloride
- Decreased reflexes
- Decreased level of consciousness
- *(Respiratory acidosis can occur when an impaired respiratory system cannot remove CO_2, or when compensatory mechanisms that stimulate increased cardiac and respiratory efforts to remove excess CO_2 are overtaxed. Elevated $PaCO_2$ is the chief criterion. Elevated $PaCO_2$ increases cerebral blood flow, which decreases perfusion to heart, kidneys, and GI tract.)*
- For a client with respiratory acidosis:
  - Improve ventilation by
    - Positioning with head of bed up *(To promote diaphragmatic descent)*
    - Coaching in deep-breathing with prolonged expiration *(To increase exhalation of CO_2)*
    - Aiding expectoration of mucus followed by suctioning, if needed *(To improve ventilation–perfusion)*
  - Consult with physician or advanced practice nurse for possible use of mechanical ventilation if improvement does not occur after the preceding interventions.
  - Administer oxygen after the client is breathing better. *(Use of oxygen is of no value if the client is not breathing effectively.)*
  - Promote optimal hydration. *(This helps liquefy secretions and prevent mucous plugs.)*
  - Limit use of sedatives and tranquilizers. *(Both can cause respiratory depression.)*
  - Initiate the first five interventions for respiratory acidosis to correct metabolic acidosis.

PC: ALKALOSIS (METABOLIC, RESPIRATORY)*

DEFINITION

PC: Alkalosis: Describes a person experiencing or at high risk for experiencing an acid–base imbalance due to excessive bicarbonate or loss of hydrogen ions

High-Risk Populations

For Respiratory Alkalosis

- Pulmonary disease
- CNS disorders/lesions
- Hyperventilation
- Severe infection, fever
- Asthma
- Overly vigorous mechanical ventilation
- Restricted diaphragmatic movement (eg, due to obesity, pregnancy)

---

*When indicated, the nurse should specify the diagnosis as either *PC: Metabolic Acidosis* or *PC: Respiratory Acidosis*.

- Inadequate oxygen in inspired air
- Congestive heart failure
- Alcohol intoxication
- Cirrhosis
- Thyrotoxicosis
- Paraldehyde, epinephrine, early salicylate overdose
- Overrapid correction of metabolic acidosis

For Metabolic Alkalosis

- Prolonged vomiting, gastric suctioning, diarrhea
- Use of potent diuretics (eg, thiazides), with resultant hydrogen and potassium loss
- Corticosteroid therapy
- IV replacement with potassium-free IV solutions
- Primary and secondary hyperaldosteronism
- Adrenocortical hormone disease
- Prolonged hypercalcemia or hypokalemia
- Excessive correction of metabolic acidosis

Nursing Goals

The nurse will manage and minimize complications of alkalosis.

General Interventions and Rationales

For Metabolic Alkalosis

- Monitor for early signs and symptoms of metabolic alkalosis:
  - Tingling of fingers, dizziness
  - Hypertonic muscles (tremors)
  - Hypoventilation (to conserve carbonic acid)
  - Increased HCO_3
  - Slightly increased PCO_2
  - Decreased serum chloride, serum potassium, serum calcium
  - Hypoventilation
  - Polydipsia

  (*A decrease in ionized calcium produces most symptoms.*)
- For a client with metabolic alkalosis:
  - Initiate order for parenteral fluids. (*To correct sodium, water, chloride deficits*)
  - Monitor carefully the administration of ammonium chloride if ordered. (*Ammonium chloride increases circulating hydrogen ions, which results in decreased pH. Treatment can cause too-rapid decrease in pH and hemolysis of RBCs.*)
  - Evaluate renal and hepatic function before administration of ammonium chloride. (*Impaired renal or hepatic function cannot accommodate increased hemolysis.*)
  - Administer sedatives and tranquilizers cautiously, if ordered. (*Both depress respiratory function.*)
  - Monitor ABG values, urine pH, serum electrolyte levels, and BUN. (*These values help evaluate response to treatment and detect rebound metabolic acidosis resulting from too-rapid correction.*)

For Respiratory Alkalosis

- Monitor for respiratory alkalosis:
  - Lightheadedness
  - Numbness, tingling
  - Carpopedal spasm
  - Muscle weakness
  - Normal or decreased HCO_3
  - Decreased PCO_2
  - Decreased serum potassium
  - Increased serum chloride

- Decreased serum calcium
(Decrease in plasma carbonic acid content causes vasoconstriction, decreased cerebral blood flow, and decreased ionized calcium.)
- For a client with respiratory alkalosis:
  - Determine the cause of hyperventilation. *(Different etiologies warrant different interventions [eg, anxiety versus incorrect mechanical ventilation].)*
  - Calm the anxious person by maintaining eye contact and remaining with him or her. *(Anxiety increases respiratory rate and CO_2 retention.)*
  - Instruct the person to breathe slowly with you. *(This increases CO_2 retention.)*
  - Alternatively, have the anxious person breathe into a paper bag and rebreathe from the bag. *(This increases $PaCO_2$ as the person rebreathes his or her own exhaled CO_2.)*
  - If anxiety is causative, refer to the nursing diagnoses *Anxiety* and *Ineffective Breathing Patterns* in Section II for additional interventions.
  - Consult with physician or advanced practice nurse for use of sedation as necessary. *(Sedation can help reduce respiratory rate and anxiety.)*
  - Monitor ABG values and electrolyte levels (eg, potassium, calcium). *(Monitoring these values helps evaluate the client's response to treatment.)*
  - As necessary, refer to *PC: Electrolyte Imbalances* for specific management of electrolyte imbalance.

PC: ALLERGIC REACTION

DEFINITION

PC: Allergic Reaction: Describes a person experiencing or at high risk to experience hypersensitivity and release of mediators to specific substances (antigens)

High-Risk Populations

- History of allergies
- Asthma
- Immunotherapy
- Individuals exposed to high-risk antigens:
  - Insect stings (eg, bee, wasp, hornet, ant)
  - Animal bites/stings (eg, stingray, snake, jellyfish)
  - Radiologic iodinated contrast media (eg, used in arteriography, intravenous pyelography)
  - Transfusion of blood and blood products
- High-risk individuals exposed to:
  - High-risk medications (eg, aspirin, antibiotics, opiates, local anesthetics, animal insulin, chymopapain)
  - High-risk foods (eg, peanuts, chocolate, eggs, seafood, shellfish, strawberries, milk)
  - Chemicals (eg, floor waxes, paint, soaps, perfume, new carpets)

Nursing Goals

The nurse will manage and minimize complications of allergic reactions.

General Interventions and Rationales

- Carefully assess for history of allergic responses (eg, rashes, difficulty breathing). *(Identifying a high-risk client allows precautions to prevent anaphylaxis.)*
- If the client has a history of allergic response, consult with physician or advanced practice nurse regarding skin tests, if indicated. *(Skin testing can confirm hypersensitivity.)*
- Monitor for signs and symptoms of localized allergic reaction:
  - Wheals, flares (due to histamine release)
  - Itching
  - Nontraumatic edema (perioral, periorbital)
  (These early manifestations can indicate the beginning of a continuum of localized reaction to systemic reaction to anaphylactic shock.)
- At the first sign of hypersensitivity, consult with physician or advanced practice nurse for pharmacologic intervention, such as antihistamines. *(Antihistamines are commonly used to treat mild localized reactions by inhibiting histamine release.)*
- Monitor for signs and symptoms of systemic allergic reaction and anaphylaxis:
  - Lightheadedness, skin flushing, and slight hypotension (resulting from histamine-induced vasodilation)
  - Throat or palate tightness, wheezing, hoarseness, dyspnea, and chest tightness (from smooth muscle contraction from prostaglandin release)
  - Irregular, increased pulse and decreased blood pressure (from leukotriene release, which constricts airways and coronary vessels)
  - Decreased level of consciousness, respiratory distress, and shock (resulting from severe hypotension, respiratory insufficiency, and tissue hypoxia)
  (Within minutes, such reactions can progress to severe hypotension, decreased level of consciousness, and respiratory distress, and can prove rapidly fatal.)
- Promptly initiate emergency protocol for anaphylaxis and/or stat page physician or advanced practice nurse.
  - Start an IV line. *(For rapid medication administration)*
  - Administer epinephrine IV or endotracheally. *(To produce peripheral vasoconstriction, which raises blood pressure and acts as a β agonist to promote bronchial smooth muscle relaxation, and to enhance inotropic and chronotropic cardiac activity)*
  - Administer oxygen; establish a patent airway if indicated. Have suction available. Oropharyngeal intubation may be required. *(Laryngeal edema interferes with breathing.)*
- Administer other medications, as ordered, which may include:
  - Corticosteroids *(To inhibit enzyme and WBC response to reduce bronchoconstriction)*
  - Aminophylline *(To produce bronchodilation)*
  - Vasopressins *(To counter profound hypotension)*
  - Diphenhydramine *(To prevent further antigen–antibody reaction)*
- Frequently evaluate response to therapy; assess:
  - Vital signs
  - Level of consciousness
  - Lung sounds, peak flows
  - Cardiac function
  - Intake and output
  - ABG values
  (Careful monitoring is necessary to detect complications of shock and identify the need for additional interventions.)
- After recovery, discuss with the client and family preventive measures for anaphylaxis and the need to carry an anaphylaxis kit, which contains injectable epinephrine and oral antihistamines for use in self-treating allergic reaction.

PC: THROMBOCYTOPENIA

DEFINITION

PC: Thrombocytopenia: Describes a person experiencing or at high risk to experience insufficient circulating platelets (less than 150,000). This decrease can be caused by a reduction in platelet production, a change in platelet distribution, platelet destruction, or vascular dilution.

High-Risk Populations

Decreased Platelet Production From

- Chemotherapy
- Radiation therapy
- Bone marrow invasion by tumor
- Leukemia
- Heparin therapy
- Toxins
- Severe infection
- Alcoholism
- Aplastic anemia
- Human immunodeficiency virus (HIV)

Increased Platelet Destruction From

- Antibodies
- Aspirin
- Alcohol
- Quinine, quinidine
- Digoxin
- Sulfonamides
- Entrapment in large spleen
- Infections (bacteremia, postviral infections)
- Renal disease
- Post-transfusion status
- Hypertension
- Hypothermia
- Viral infection (eg, Epstein-Barr)
- HIV

Increased Platelet Utilization From

- Disseminated intravascular coagulation
- Thrombotic thrombocytopenic purpura
- Liver disease
- Administration of several units of non–platelet-containing fluids

Nursing Goals

The nurse will manage and minimize complications of decreased platelets.

General Interventions and Rationales

- Monitor complete blood count (CBC), hemoglobin, coagulation tests, and platelet counts. *(These values help evaluate response to treatment and risk for bleeding. Platelet count <20,000/mm³ indicates a high risk for intracranial bleeding.)*
- Assess for other factors that may lower platelet count in addition to the primary cause:
  - Abnormal hepatic function
  - Abnormal renal function
  - Infection, fever
  - Anticoagulant use
  - Alcohol use
  - Aspirin use
  - Administration of several units of non–platelet-containing fluids (eg, packed RBCs)
  (Assessment may identify factors that could be controllable.)
- Monitor for signs and symptoms of spontaneous or excessive bleeding:
  - Spontaneous petechiae, ecchymoses, hematomas
  - Bleeding from nose or gums
  - Prolonged bleeding from invasive procedures such as venipunctures or bone marrow aspiration
  - Hematemesis or coffee-ground emesis
  - Hemoptysis
  - Hematuria
  - Vaginal bleeding
  - Rectal bleeding
  - Gross blood in stools
  - Black, tarry stools
  - Change in vital signs
  - Change in neurologic status (blurred vision, headache, disorientation)
  - Urine, feces, and emesis positive for occult blood
  - High pad count for menstruating women
  (Constant monitoring is needed to ensure early detection of bleeding.)
- Assess for systemic signs of bleeding and hypovolemia:
  - Increased pulse, increased respirations, decreased blood pressure
  - Changes in neurologic status (eg, subtle mental status changes, blurred vision, headache, disorientation; *Changes in circulatory oxygen levels produce changes in cardiac, vascular, and neurologic functioning.)*
- If hemorrhage is suspected, refer to *PC: Hypovolemic Shock* for specific interventions.
- Anticipate platelet transfusion.
- Apply direct pressure for 5 to 10 min, then a pressure dressing, to all venipuncture sites. Monitor carefully for 24 h. *(These measures promote clotting and reduce blood loss.)*
- Treat nausea aggressively to prevent vomiting. *(Severe vomiting can cause GI bleeding.)*
- Minimize rectal probing. *(This avoids injury to rectal tissue and bleeding.)*
- Using the nursing diagnosis *Risk for Injury related to bleeding tendency* (see Section II), implement nursing interventions and teaching to reduce the risk of trauma.

PC: OPPORTUNISTIC INFECTIONS

DEFINITION

PC: Opportunistic Infections: Describes a person experiencing or at high risk to experience an infection by an organism capable of causing disease only when immune system dysfunction is present

High-Risk Populations

- Immunosuppressive therapy (chemotherapy, antibiotics)
- Malignancy
- Sepsis
- AIDS
- Nutritional deficits
- Burns
- Trauma
- Extensive pressure ulcers
- Radiation therapy (long bones, skull, sternum)
- Elderly with chronic illness
- Drug/alcohol addiction

Nursing Goals

The nurse will manage and minimize complications of immunodeficiency.

General Interventions and Rationales

- Monitor CBC, WBC differential (neutrophils, lymphocytes), and absolute neutrophil count (WBC × neutrophil). *(These values help evaluate response to treatment.)*
- Monitor for signs and symptoms of primary or secondary infection:
  - Slightly increased temperature
  - Chills
  - Dysphagia
  - Adventitious breath sounds
  - Cloudy or foul-smelling urine
  - Complaints of urinary frequency, urgency, or dysuria
  - WBCs and bacteria in urine
  - Redness, change in skin temperature, swelling or unusual drainage in any area of disrupted skin integrity, including previous and current puncture sites
  - Irritation or ulceration of oral mucous membrane
  - Complaints of perineal or rectal pain and any unusual vaginal or rectal discharge
  - Increased hemorrhoidal pain, redness, or bleeding
  - Painful, pruritic skin lesions (herpes zoster), particularly in cervical or thoracic area
  - Change in WBC count, especially increased immature neutrophils
  (In a client with severe neutropenia, usual inflammatory responses may be decreased or absent.)
- Obtain culture specimens (eg, urine, vaginal, rectal, mouth, sputum, stool, blood, skin lesions, indwelling lines) as ordered. *(Testing determines the type of causative organism and guides treatment.)*
- Monitor for signs and symptoms of sepsis. *(Gram-positive and gram-negative organisms can invade open wounds, causing septicemia. A debilitated client is at increased risk. Sepsis produces*

massive vasodilation, resulting in hypovolemia and subsequent tissue hypoxia. Hypoxia leads to decreased renal function and cardiac output, triggering a compensatory response of increased respirations and heart rate in an attempt to correct hypoxia and acidosis. Bacteria in urine or blood indicates infection [Morton et al., 2005].)

- Monitor for therapeutic and nontherapeutic effects of antibiotics.
- Monitor for signs and symptoms of opportunistic protozoal infections:
  - *Pneumocystis carinii* pneumonia: dry, nonproductive cough, low-grade fever, gradual to severe dyspnea
  - *Toxoplasma gondii* encephalitis: headache, lethargy, seizures
  - *Cryptosporidium* enteritis: watery diarrhea, nausea, abdominal cramps, malaise
  (Clients with immunodeficiency are at risk for secondary diseases of opportunistic infections; protozoal infections are the most common and serious.)
- Monitor for signs and symptoms of opportunistic viral infections:
  - Herpes simplex oral or perirectal abscesses: severe pain, bleeding, rectal discharge
  - Cytomegalovirus retinitis, colitis, pneumonitis, encephalitis, or other organ disease
  - Progressive multifocal leukoencephalopathy: headache, decreased mentation
  - Varicella zoster, disseminated (shingles)
- Monitor for signs and symptoms of opportunistic fungal infections:
  - *Candida albicans* stomatitis and esophagitis: exudate, complaints of unusual taste in mouth
  - *Cryptococcus neoformans* meningitis: fever, headaches, blurred vision, stiff neck, confusion
- Monitor for signs and symptoms of opportunistic bacterial infections, which commonly affect the pulmonary system:
  - *Mycobacterium avium* (intracellular disseminated)
  - *Mycobacterium tuberculosis* (extrapulmonary and pulmonary)
- Emphasize the need to report symptoms promptly. *(Early treatment of adverse manifestations often can prevent serious complications [eg, septicemia] and also increases the likelihood of a favorable response to treatment.)*
- Explain the need to balance activity and rest and to consume a nutritious diet. *(Rest and a nutritious diet give energy for healing and enhancement of the body's defense system.)*
- Avoid or minimize invasive procedures (eg, urinary catheterization, arterial or venous punctures, injections, rectal tubes, suppositories). *(This precaution helps prevent introduction of microorganisms.)*
- Explain the importance of adhering to medication regimen (prophylaxis and antiviral).
- Refer to the nursing diagnosis *Risk for Infection* in Section II for interventions to prevent introduction of microorganisms and to increase resistance.

PC: SICKLING CRISIS

DEFINITION

PC: Sickling Crisis: Describes a person with sickle cell disease experiencing vascular occlusion by the sickled cells, which damages cells and tissue and causes hemolytic anemia, massive splenomegaly, and hypovolemic shock, acute chest syndrome, cerebrovascular accidents (Jenkins, 2002)

High-Risk Populations

People With Sickle Cell Disease With Precipitating Factors, eg:

- High altitude (>7000 feet above sea level)
- Unpressurized aircraft
- Dehydration (eg, diaphoresis, diarrhea, vomiting)

- Strenuous physical activity
- Cold temperatures (eg, iced liquids)
- Infection (eg, respiratory, urinary, vaginal) parvovirus
- Ingestion of alcohol
- Cigarette smoking

Nursing Goals

The nurse will manage and minimize the sickling crisis.

General Interventions and Rationales

- Monitor for signs and symptoms of anemia:
  - Lethargy
  - Weakness
  - Fatigue
  - Increased pallor
  - Dyspnea on exertion

  (Because anemia is common with most of these clients, and low hemoglobins are relatively tolerated, changes should be described in reference to person's baseline or acute symptoms [Rausch & Pollard, 1998].)
- Monitor laboratory values, including CBC with reticulocyte count. *(Reticulocyte [normal level about 1%] elevation represents active erythropoiesis. Lack of elevation with anemia may represent a problem [Newcombe, 2002].)*
- Monitor for signs and symptoms of acute chest syndrome:
  - Fever
  - Acute chest pain

  (Acute chest syndrome is the term used to represent the group of symptoms—acute pleuritic chest pain, fever, leukocytosis, and infiltrates on chest x-ray—seen in sickle cell disease [Rausch & Pollard, 1998]. This medical emergency may be caused by "sickling" leading to pulmonary infarction.)
- Monitor for signs and symptoms of infection:
  - Fever
  - Pain
  - Chills
  - Increased WBCs

  (Bacterial infection is a major cause of morbidity and mortality. Decreased spleen function [asplenia] results from sickle cell anemia. The loss of the spleen's ability to filter and destroy various infectious organisms increases the risk of infection [Porth, 2002].)
- Monitor for changes in neurologic function:
  - Speech disturbances
  - Sudden headache
  - Numbness, tingling

  (Cerebral infarction and intracranial hemorrhage are complications of sickle cell disease. Occlusion of nutrient arteries to major cerebral arteries causes progressive wall damage and eventual occlusion of the major vessel. Intracerebral hemorrhage may be secondary to hypoxic necrosis of vessel walls [Rausch & Pollard, 1998].)
- Monitor for splenic dysfunction. *(The spleen is responsible for filtering blood to remove old bacteria. Sluggish circulation and increased viscosity of sickled cells causes splenic blockage. The normal acidotic and anoxic environment of the spleen stimulates sickling, which increases blood flow obstruction [Porth, 2002].)*
- Monitor for splenic sequestration crisis:
  - Sudden onset of lassitude
  - Very pale, listless
  - Rapid pulse
  - Shallow respirations
  - Low blood pressure

  (Increased obstruction of blood from the spleen together with rapid sickling can cause sudden pooling of blood into the spleen. This causes intravascular hypovolemia and hypoxia, progressing to shock [Rausch & Pollard, 1998].)

- Instruct client to report the following:
  - Any acute illness
  - Severe joint or bone pain
  - Chest pain
  - Abdominal pain
  - Headaches, dizziness
  - Gastric distress
  - Priapism
  - Recurrent vomiting

  (These symptoms may indicate vaso-occlusion in varied sites as a result of sickling. Some illnesses may predispose the client to dehydration [Rausch & Pollard, 1998].)
- Initiate therapy per physician or nurse practitioner prescription (eg, antisickling agents, analgesics, transfusions).
- Provide:
  - Bed rest
  - Fluids and foods high in folic acid
  - Warm compresses to areas of pain
- Refer to the nursing diagnosis *Acute Pain* (see Section II) for interventions to manage the pain associated with a sickling crisis.

POTENTIAL COMPLICATION: RENAL/URINARY

DEFINITION

PC: Renal/Urinary: Describes a person experiencing or at high risk to experience various renal or urinary tract dysfunctions.

⊚ AUTHOR'S NOTE

The nurse can use this generic collaborative problem to describe a person at risk for several types of renal or urinary problems. For such a client (eg, a client in a critical care unit, who is vulnerable to various renal/urinary problems), using *PC: Renal/Urinary* directs nurses to monitor renal and urinary status, based on the focus assessment, to detect and diagnose abnormal functioning. Nursing management of a specific renal or urinary complication would be addressed under the collaborative problem applying to the specific complication. For example, a standard of care for a client recovering from coronary bypass surgery could contain the collaborative problem *PC: Renal/Urinary,* directing the nurse to monitor renal and urinary status. If urinary retention developed in this client, the nurse would add *PC: Urinary Retention* to the problem list, along with specific nursing interventions to manage this problem. If the risk factors or etiology were not directly related to the primary medical diagnosis, the nurse still would specify them in the diagnostic statement (eg, *PC: Renal Insufficiency related to chronic renal failure* in a client who has sustained a myocardial infarction).

Keep in mind that the nurse must differentiate those problems in bladder function that nurses can treat primarily as nursing diagnoses (eg, incontinence, chronic urinary retention) from those that nurses manage using both nurse-prescribed and physician-prescribed interventions (eg, acute urinary retention).

Significant Laboratory/Diagnostic Assessment Criteria

Blood
Prealbumin, albumin (lowered in renal disease)
Amylase (elevated with renal insufficiency)
pH, base excess, bicarbonate (lowered in metabolic acidosis, elevated in metabolic alkalosis)
Calcium (lowered in uremic acidosis)
Chloride (elevated with renal tubular acidosis)
Creatinine (elevated with kidney disease)
Magnesium (lowered in chronic nephritis)
Phosphorus (elevated with chronic glomerular disease, lowered with renal tubular acidosis)
Potassium (elevated in renal failure, lowered with chronic diuretic therapy, renal tubular acidosis)
Proteins (total, albumin, globulin) (lowered in nephritic syndrome)
Sodium (elevated with nephritis, lowered with chronic renal insufficiency)
Blood urea nitrogen (BUN) (elevated in acute or chronic renal failure)
Uric acid (elevated with chronic renal failure)
White blood cell (WBC) count (elevated, lowered with acute and chronic infections)
Urine (clean catch)
Blood (present with hemorrhagic cystitis, renal calculi, renal, bladder tumors)
Creatinine (elevated in acute/chronic glomerulonephritis, nephritis, lowered in advanced degeneration of kidneys)
pH (elevated with metabolic acidosis, lowered with metabolic alkalosis)
Specific gravity (elevated with dehydration, lowered with overhydration, renal tubular disease)
WBC count (elevated with urinary tract infections)
Myoglobin
Culture and sensitivity
24-hour urine creatinine clearance
Renal ultrasound, magnetic resonance imaging
Kidneys, ureters, bladder x-ray

PC: ACUTE URINARY RETENTION

DEFINITION

PC: Acute Urinary Retention: Describes a person experiencing or at high risk to experience an acute abnormal accumulation of urine in the bladder and the inability to void due to a temporary situation (eg, postoperative status) or to a condition reversible with surgery (eg, prostatectomy) or medications.

High-Risk Populations

- Postoperative status (eg, surgery of the perineal area, lower abdomen)
- Postpartum status
- Anxiety
- Prostate enlargement, prostatitis
- Medication side effects (eg, atropine, antidepressants, antihistamines)
- Postarteriography status
- Bladder outlet obstruction (infection, tumor)
- Impaired detrusor contractility

Nursing Goals

The nurse will manage and minimize acute urinary retention episodes.

General Interventions and Rationales

- Monitor a postoperative client for urinary retention. *(Trauma to the detrusor muscle and injury to the pelvic nerves during surgery can inhibit bladder function. Anxiety and pain can cause spasms of the reflex sphincters. Bladder neck edema also can cause retention. Sedatives and narcotics can affect the CNS and effectiveness of smooth muscles [Porth, 2002].)*
- Monitor for urinary retention by palpating and percussing the suprapubic area for signs of bladder distention (overdistention, etc.). Instruct client to report bladder discomfort or inability to void. *(These problems may be early signs of urinary retention.)*
- Monitor for urinary retention in postpartum women. *(Labor and delivery can slacken the tone of the bladder wall temporarily, causing urinary retention.)*
- Encourage client to void within 6 to 8 hours after delivery. *(Desire to void may be diminished because of increased bladder capacity related to reduced intraabdominal pressure after delivery.)*
- In a postpartum client, differentiate between bladder distention and uterine enlargement:
  - A distended bladder protrudes above the symphysis pubis.
  - When the nurse massages the uterus to return it to its midline position, the bladder protrudes further.
  - Percussion and palpation can distinguish between a rebounding bladder (from fluid) and a firm uterus.
  (A distended bladder can push the uterus up and to the side and cause uterine relaxation.)
- If client does not void within 8 to 10 hours after surgery or complains of bladder discomfort, take the following steps:
  - Warm the bedpan.
  - Encourage client to get out of bed to use the bathroom, if possible.
  - Instruct a man to stand when urinating, if possible.
  - Run water in the sink as client attempts to void.
  - Pour warm water over client's perineum.
  (These measures help promote relaxation of the urinary sphincter and facilitate voiding.)
- After the first voiding postdelivery or postsurgery, continue to monitor and to encourage client to void again in 1 hour or so. *(The first voiding usually does not empty the bladder completely.)*
- If the client still cannot void after 10 hours, follow protocols for straight catheterization, as ordered by physician/advanced practice nurse. *(Straight catheterization is preferable to indwelling catheterization because it carries less risk of urinary tract infection from ascending pathogens.)*
- For a client with chronic urinary retention, refer to the nursing diagnosis *Urinary Retention* in Section II.
- If person is voiding small amounts, use straight catheterization; if postvoid residual is >200 mL, leave catheter indwelling. Notify physician or advanced practice nurse.

PC: RENAL INSUFFICIENCY

DEFINITION

PC: Renal Insufficiency: Describes a person experiencing or at high risk to experience a decrease in glomerular filtration rate that results in oliguria or anuria.

High-Risk Populations

- Renal tubular necrosis from ischemic causes
  - Excessive diuretic use
  - Pulmonary embolism
  - Burns
  - Intrarenal thrombosis
  - Renal infections
  - Renal artery stenosis/thrombosis
  - Peritonitis
  - Sepsis
  - Hypovolemia
  - Hypotension
  - Congestive heart failure
  - Myocardial infarction
  - Aneurysm
  - Aneurysm repair
- Renal tubular necrosis from toxicity (Lancaster, 2001)
  - Nonsteroidal anti-inflammatory drugs
  - Gout (hyperuricemia)
  - Hypercalcemia
  - Certain street drugs (eg, PCP)
  - Gram-negative infection
  - Radiocontrast media
  - Aminoglycoside antibiotics
  - Antineoplastic agents
  - Methanol, carbon tetrachloride
  - Snake venom, poison mushroom
  - Phenacetin-type analgesics
  - Heavy metals
  - Insecticides, fungicides
  - Aminoglycosides
- Diabetes mellitus
- Primary hypertensive disease
- Hemolysis (eg, from transfusion reaction)

Nursing Goals

The nurse will manage and minimize complications of renal insufficiency.

General Interventions and Rationales

- Monitor for early signs and symptoms of renal insufficiency:
  - Sustained elevated urine specific gravity, elevated urine sodium levels

- Sustained insufficient urine output (<5 mL/kg/hour), elevated blood pressure
- Elevated BUN, serum creatinine, potassium, phosphorus, and ammonia; decreased creatinine clearance
- Dependent edema (periorbital, pedal, pretibial, sacral)
- Nocturia
- Lethargy
- Itching
- Nausea/vomiting

(Hypovolemia and hypotension activate the renin–angiotensin system, increasing renal vasculature resistance, which decreases renal plasma flow and glomerular filtration rate. Decreased glomerular filtration rate eventually causes insufficient urine output and stimulates renin production, elevating the blood pressure in an attempt to increase blood flow to the kidney. Decreased excretion of urea and creatinine in the urine elevates BUN and creatinine levels. Dependent edema results from increased plasma hydrostatic pressure, salt and water retention, and/or decreased colloid osmotic pressure from plasma protein losses [Porth, 2002].)

- Weigh the client daily at a minimum; more often, if indicated. Ensure accurate findings by weighing at the same time each day, on the same scale, and with the client wearing the same amount of clothing. *(Daily weights and intake and output records help evaluate fluid balance and guide fluid intake recommendations.)*
- Maintain strict intake and output records; determine the net fluid balance and compare with daily weight loss or gain for correlation. (A 1-kg [2.2-lb] weight gain correlates with excess intake of 1 L.)
- Explain prescribed fluid management goals. *(Client and family understanding may enhance cooperation.)*
- Adjust client's daily fluid intake so it approximates fluid loss plus 300–500 mL/day. *(Careful replacement therapy is necessary to prevent fluid overload.)*
- Distribute fluid intake fairly evenly throughout the entire day and night. It may be necessary to match fluid intake with loss every 8 hours or even every hour if the client is critically imbalanced. *(Maintaining a constant fluid balance, without major fluctuations, is essential. Allowing toxins to accumulate because of poor hydration can cause complications such as nausea and sensorium changes.)*
- Encourage client to express feelings and frustrations; give positive feedback. *(Fluid and diet restrictions can be extremely frustrating. Emotional support can help reduce anxiety and may improve compliance with the treatment regimen.)*
- Consult with a dietitian regarding the fluid and diet plan. *(Important considerations in fluid management, requiring a specialist's attention, include the fluid content of nonliquid food, appropriate amount and type of liquids, liquid preferences, and sodium content.)*
- Administer oral medications with meals whenever possible. If medications must be administered between meals, give with the smallest amount of fluid necessary. *(This measure avoids using parts of the fluid allowance unnecessarily.)*
- Avoid continuous IV fluid infusion whenever possible. Dilute all necessary IV drugs in the smallest amount of fluid that is safe for IV administration. Use small IV bags and an IV controller or pump, if possible, to prevent accidental infusion of a large volume of fluid. *(Extremely accurate fluid infusion is necessary to prevent fluid overload.)*
- Monitor for signs and symptoms of metabolic acidosis:
  - Rapid, shallow respirations
  - Headaches
  - Nausea and vomiting
  - Low plasma pH
  - Behavioral changes, drowsiness, lethargy

(Acidosis results from the kidney's inability to excrete hydrogen ions, phosphates, sulfates, and ketone bodies. Bicarbonate loss results from decreased renal resorption. Hyperkalemia, hyperphosphatemia, and decreased bicarbonate levels aggravate metabolic acidosis. Excessive ketone bodies cause headaches, nausea, vomiting, and abdominal pain. Respiratory rate and depth increase in an attempt to increase CO_2 excretion and thus reduce acidosis. Acidosis affects the CNS and can increase neuromuscular irritability because of the cellular exchange of hydrogen and potassium [Lancaster, 2001].)

- For a client with metabolic acidosis, ensure adequate caloric intake while limiting fat and protein intake. Consult with a dietitian for an appropriate diet. *(Restricting fats and protein helps prevent accumulation of acidic end products.)*

- Assess for signs and symptoms of hypocalcemia, hypokalemia, and alkalosis as acidosis is corrected. (*Rapid correction of acidosis may cause rapid excretion of calcium and potassium and result in rebound alkalosis.*)
- Consult with the primary provider to initiate bicarbonate/acetate dialysis if the preceding measures do not correct metabolic acidosis:
  - Bicarbonate dialysis for severe acidosis: dialysate – $NaHCO_3$ = 100 mEq/L
  - Bicarbonate dialysis for moderate acidosis: dialysate – $NaHCO_3$ = 60 mEq/L
  (*The acetate anion, which the liver converts to bicarbonate, is used in dialysate to combat metabolic acidosis. Bicarbonate dialysis is indicated for clients with liver impairment, lactic acidosis, or severe acid–base imbalance.*)
- Monitor for signs and symptoms of hypernatremia with fluid overload:
  - Extreme thirst
  - CNS effects ranging from agitation to convulsion
  (*Hypernatremia results from excessive sodium intake or increased aldosterone output. Water is pulled from the cells, causing cellular dehydration and producing CNS symptoms. Thirst is a compensatory response aimed at diluting sodium.*)
- Maintain prescribed sodium restrictions. (*Hypernatremia must be corrected slowly to minimize CNS deterioration.*)
- Monitor for electrolyte imbalances:
  - Potassium
  - Calcium
  - Phosphorus
  - Sodium
  - Magnesium
  (Refer to *PC: Electrolyte Imbalance* for specific signs and symptoms and interventions. *Renal dysfunction can cause hyperkalemia, hypernatremia, hypocalcemia, hypermagnesemia, or hyperphosphatemia. Diuretic therapy can cause hypokalemia or hyponatremia.*)
- Monitor for gastrointestinal (GI) bleeding. (Refer to *PC: GI Bleeding* for more information and specific interventions. *The poor platelet aggregation and capillary fragility associated with high serum levels of nitrogenous wastes may aggravate bleeding. Heparinization required during dialysis in cases of gastric ulcer disease also may precipitate GI bleeding.*)
  - Monitor for manifestations of anemia:
  - Dyspnea
  - Fatigue
  - Tachycardia, palpitations
  - Pallor of nail beds and mucous membranes
  - Low hemoglobin and hematocrit levels
  - Easy bruising
  (*Chronic renal failure results in decreased red blood cell production and survival time because of elevated uremic toxins.*)
- Avoid unnecessary collection of blood specimens. (*Some blood loss occurs with every blood collection.*)
- Instruct client to use a soft toothbrush and to avoid vigorous nose blowing, constipation, and contact sports. (*Trauma prevention reduces the risk of bleeding and infection.*)
- Demonstrate the pressure method to control bleeding should it occur. (*Applying direct, constant pressure on a bleeding site can help prevent excessive blood loss.*)
- Monitor for manifestations of hypoalbuminemia:
  - Serum albumin level less than 3.5 g/dL; proteinuria (<100–150 mg protein/24 hours)
  - Edema formation: pedal, facial, sacral
  - Hypovolemia
  - Increased hematocrit and hemoglobin levels.
  (Refer to *PC: Negative Nitrogen Balance* for more information and interventions. *When albumin leaks into the urine because of changes in the glomerular electrostatic barrier or because of peritoneal dialysis, the liver responds by increasing production of plasma proteins. When the loss is great, the liver cannot compensate, and hypoalbuminemia results.*)
- Monitor for hypervolemia. Evaluate daily:
  - Weight
  - Fluid intake and output records
  - Circumference of the edematous parts
  - Laboratory data: hematocrit, serum sodium, and plasma protein in specific serum albumin
  (*As glomerular filtration rate decreases and the functioning nephron mass continues to diminish, the kidneys lose the ability to concentrate urine and to excrete sodium and water, resulting in hypervolemia.*)

- Monitor for signs and symptoms of congestive heart failure and decreased cardiac output:
  - Gradual increase in heart rate
  - Increasing dyspnea
  - Diminished breath sounds, rales
  - Decreased systolic blood pressure
  - Presence of or increase in S_3 and/or S_4 heart sounds
  - Gallop rhythm
  - Peripheral edema
  - Distended neck veins

  (Congestive heart failure can result from increased cardiac output, hypervolemia, dysrhythmias, and hypertension, reducing the ability of the left ventricle to eject blood, with subsequent decreased cardiac output and increased pulmonary vascular congestion.)
- Encourage adherence to strict fluid restrictions: 800–1000 mL/24 hours, or 24-hour urine output plus 500 mL. *(Fluid restrictions are based on urine output. In an anuric client, restriction usually is 800 mL/day, which accounts for insensible losses from metabolism, the GI tract, perspiration, and respiration.)*
- Collaborate with physician, advanced practice nurse, or dietitian to plan an appropriate diet. Encourage adherence to a low-sodium diet (2–4 g/day). *(Sodium restrictions should be adjusted based on urine sodium excretion.)*
- If hemodialysis or peritoneal dialysis is initiated, follow institutional protocols.

Pediatric Interventions and Rationales

- Assess for signs and symptoms unique to children with renal failure (Kohaut, 1999):
  - Growth failure
  - Bone deformities
  - Abnormal tooth development
  - Unexplained dehydration
  - Salt craving

  (Children with renal insufficiency present differently from adults.)
- Explore with parents child's response to exercise. *(Lethargy and reduced exercise tolerance are two early signs of renal insufficiency [Wong, 2003].)*
- Per orders, initiate treatment for anemia, hypertension, acidosis, and renal osteodystrophy. *(These represent the key nondialytic therapy goals.)*
- Consult with dietitian. *(Children with renal dysfunction present a challenge for obtaining adequate protein for growth and development and to prevent worsening of renal function [Wong, 2003].)*

PC: RENAL CALCULI

DEFINITION

PC: Renal Calculi: Describes a person with or at high risk for development of a solid concentration of mineral salts in the urinary tract.

High-Risk Populations

- History of renal calculi
- Urinary infection
- Urinary stasis, obstruction

- Immobility
- Hypercalcemia (dietary)
- Conditions that cause hypercalcemia
  - Hyperparathyroidism
  - Renal tubular acidosis
  - Myeloproliferative disease (leukemia, polycythemia vera, multiple myeloma)
- Excessive excretion of uric acid
- Inflammatory bowel disease
- Gout
- Dehydration

Nursing Goals

The nurse will manage and minimize complications of renal calculi.

General Interventions and Rationales

- Monitor for signs and symptoms of calculi:
  - Increased or decreased urine output
  - Sediment in urine
  - Flank or loin pain
  - Hematuria
  - Abdominal pain, distention, nausea, diarrhea
  (Stones in the urinary tract can cause obstruction, infection, and edema, manifested by loin / flank pain, hematuria, and dysuria. Stones in the renal pelvis may raise urine production. Calculi-stimulating renointestinal reflexes can cause GI symptoms.)
- Send urine for culture and sensitivity; send 24-hour urine for calcium oxalate, phosphorus, and uric acid. *(Tests are needed to determine type of stone and infection.)*
- Strain urine to obtain a stone sample; send samples to the laboratory for analysis. *(Acquiring a stone sample confirms stone formation and enables analysis of stone constituents.)*
- If the client complains of pain, consult with the physician or advanced practice nurse for aggressive therapy (eg, narcotics, antispasmodics). *(Calculi can produce severe pain from spasms and proximity of the nerve plexus.)*
- Track the pain by documenting location, any radiation, duration, and intensity (using a rating scale of 0–10). *(This measure helps evaluate movement of calculi.)*
- Instruct the client to increase fluid intake, if not contraindicated. *(Increased fluid intake promotes increased urination, which can help facilitate stone passage and flush bacteria and blood from the urinary tract.)*
- Prepare person for KUB x-ray, excretory urography, and/or renal ultrasound.
- Monitor for signs and symptoms of pyelonephritis:
  - Fever, chills
  - Costovertebral angle pain (a dull, constant backache below the 12th rib)
  - Leukocytosis
  - Bacteria, blood, and pus in urine
  - Dysuria, frequency
  (Urinary stasis or irritation of tissue by calculi can cause urinary tract infections. Signs and symptoms reflect various mechanisms. Bacteria can act as pyrogens by raising the hypothalamic thermostat through the production of endogenous pyrogen, which may be mediated through prostaglandins. Chills can occur when the temperature set-point of the hypothalamus changes rapidly. Costovertebral angle pain results from distention of the renal capsule. Leukocytosis reflects increased leukocytes to fight infection through phagocytosis. Bacteria and pus in urine indicate a urinary tract infection. Bacteria can irritate bladder tissue, causing spasms and frequency [Porth, 2002].)
- Monitor for early signs and symptoms of renal insufficiency. (Refer to *PC: Renal Insufficiency.*)

Potential Complication: Neurologic/Sensory
PC: Increased Intracranial Pressure
PC: Seizures
PC: Increased Intraocular Pressure
PC: Neuroleptic Malignant Syndrome
PC: Alcohol Withdrawal

POTENTIAL COMPLICATION: NEUROLOGIC/SENSORY

DEFINITION

PC: Neurologic/Sensory: Describes a person experiencing or at high risk to experience various neurologic or sensory dysfunctions

---

⊕ AUTHOR'S NOTE

The nurse can use this generic collaborative problem to describe a person at risk for several types of neurologic or sensory problems (eg, a client recovering from cranial surgery or who has sustained multiple trauma). For such a person, using *PC: Neurologic / Sensory* directs nurses to monitor neurologic and sensory function based on focus assessment findings. Should a complication occur, the nurse would add the applicable specific collaborative problem (eg, *PC: Increased Intracranial Pressure*) to the client's problem list to describe nursing management of the complication. If the risk factors or etiology were not related directly to the primary medical diagnosis or treatment, the nurse could add this information to the diagnostic statement. For example, for a client with a seizure disorder admitted for abdominal surgery, the nurse would add *PC: Seizures related to epilepsy* to the problem list.

In addition to the collaborative problem, the nurse should assess for other actual or potential responses that can compromise functioning. Some of these responses may represent nursing diagnoses (eg, *Risk for Injury related to poor awareness of environmental hazards secondary to decreased sensorium*).

For information on Focus Assessment Criteria, visit http://connection.lww.com.

Significant Laboratory/Diagnostic Assessment Criteria

Cerebrospinal Fluid

Protein (increased in meningitis)
White blood cell (WBC) count (increased in meningitis)
Albumin (elevated with brain tumors)
Glucose (decreased with bacterial meningitis)

Blood

WBC count (elevated with bacterial infection, decreased in viral infection)
Alcohol level
Glucose calcium
Mercury, lead levels if indicated

Radiologic/Imaging
Skull, spine x-rays
Computed tomography (CT)
Magnetic resonance imaging (MRI)
Cerebral angiography
Myelography

Other
Doppler
Lumbar puncture
Electroencephalography (EEG)
Continuous bedside cerebral blood flow monitoring

PC: INCREASED INTRACRANIAL PRESSURE

DEFINITION
PC: Increased Intracranial Pressure: Describes a person experiencing or at high risk to experience increased pressure (>15 mm Hg) exerted by cerebrospinal fluid within the brain's ventricles or the subarachnoid space

High-Risk Populations

- Intracerebral mass (lesions, hematomas, tumors, abscesses)
- Blood clots
- Blockage of venous outflow
- Head injuries
- Reye's syndrome
- Meningitis
- Premature birth
- Cranial surgery

Nursing Goals

The nurse will manage and minimize episodes of increased intracranial pressure (ICP).

General Interventions and Rationales

- Monitor for signs and symptoms of increased ICP.
  - Assess the following:
    - Best eye opening response: spontaneously, to auditory stimuli, to painful stimuli, or no response
    - Best motor response: obeys verbal commands, localizes pain, flexion–withdrawal, flexion–decorticate, extension–decerebrate, or no response
    - Best verbal response: oriented to person, place, and time; confused conversation; inappropriate speech; incomprehensible sounds; or no response
    (Deficiencies of cerebral blood supply resulting from hemorrhage, hematoma, cerebral edema, thrombus, or emboli compromise cerebral tissue. These responses evaluate the client's ability to

integrate commands with conscious and involuntary movement. The nurse can assess cortical function by evaluating eye opening and motor response. No response may indicate damage to the midbrain.)

- Assess for changes in vital signs:
  - Pulse changes: slowing rate to 60 beats/min or lower or increasing rate to 100 beats/min or higher *(Bradycardia is a late sign of brain stem ischemia. Tachycardia may indicate hypothalamic ischemia and sympathetic discharge.)*
  - Respiratory irregularities: slowing rate with lengthening apneic periods *(Respiratory patterns vary depending on the site of impairment. Cheyne-Stokes breathing [a gradual increase followed by a gradual decrease, then a period of apnea] points to damage in both cerebral hemispheres, midbrain, and upper pons. Central neurogenic hyperventilation occurs with midbrain and upper pontine lesions. Ataxic breathing [irregular with random sequence of deep and shallow breaths] indicates pontine dysfunction. Hypoventilation and apnea occur with medullary lesions.)*
  - Rising blood pressure and/or widening pulse pressure
  - Bradycardia, increased systolic blood pressure, and increased pulse pressure *(These are late signs of brain stem ischemia leading to cerebral herniation.)*
- Assess pupillary responses. *(Changes indicate pressure on oculomotor or optic nerves.)*
  - Inspect the pupils with a bright pinpoint light to evaluate size, configuration, and reaction to light. Compare both eyes for similarities and differences. *(The oculomotor nerve [cranial nerve III] in the brain stem regulates pupil reactions.)*
  - Evaluate gaze to determine whether it is conjugate (paired, working together) or if eye movements are abnormal. *(Conjugate eye movements are regulated from parts of the cortex and brain stem.)*
  - Evaluate the ability of the eyes to adduct and abduct. *(Cranial nerve VI, or the abducens nerve, regulates abduction and adduction of the eyes. Cranial nerve IV, or the trochlear nerve, also regulates eye movement.)*
- Note any other signs and symptoms:
  - Vomiting *(Vomiting results from pressure on the medulla, which stimulates the brain's vomiting center.)*
  - Headache: constant, increasing in intensity, or aggravated by movement
  - Straining *(Compression of neural tissue increases ICP and causes pain.)*
  - Subtle changes (eg, lethargy, restlessness, forced breathing, purposeless movements, changes in mentation; *These signs may be the earliest indicators of cranial pressure changes.)*
- Elevate the head of the bed 30 to 45 degrees unless contraindicated. *(Slight head elevation can aid venous drainage to reduce cerebrovascular congestion, thereby decreasing ICP.)*
- Avoid the following situations or maneuvers, which can increase ICP (Porth, 2002):
  - Carotid massage *(This slows the heart rate and reduces systemic circulation, which is followed by a sudden increase in circulation.)*
  - Neck flexion or extreme rotation *(This inhibits jugular venous drainage, which increases cerebrovascular congestion and ICP.)*
  - Digital anal stimulation, breath-holding, straining *(These can initiate the Valsalva maneuver, which impairs venous return by constricting the jugular veins, thus increasing ICP.)*
  - Extreme flexion of the hips and knees *(Flexion increases intrathoracic pressure, which inhibits jugular venous drainage, increasing cerebrovascular congestion and, thus, ICP.)*
  - Rapid position changes
- Teach client to exhale during position changes. *(This helps prevent the Valsalva maneuver.)*
- Consult with the physician or nurse practitioner for stool softeners, if needed. *(Stool softeners prevent constipation and straining during defecation, which can trigger the Valsalva maneuver.)*
- Maintain a quiet, calm, softly lit environment. Schedule several lengthy periods of uninterrupted rest daily. Cluster necessary procedures and activities to minimize interruptions. *(These measures promote rest and decrease stimulation, both of which can help decrease ICP.)*
- Avoid sequential performance of activities that increase ICP (eg, coughing, suctioning, repositioning, bathing). *(Research has validated that such sequential activities can cause a cumulative increase in ICP [Porth, 2002].)*
- Monitor temperature. As indicated, initiate external hypothermia or hyperthermia measures per orders and institutional protocol. *(Impaired hypothalamic function can interfere with temperature regulation, necessitating intervention. Hypothermia may reduce ICP, whereas hyperthermia may increase it.)*

- Limit suctioning time to 10 s at a time; hyperoxygenate and hyperventilate client both before and after suctioning. *(These measures help prevent hypercapnia, which can increase cerebral vasodilation and raise ICP, and prevent hypoxia, which may increase cerebral ischemia.)*
- Consult with physician or advanced practice nurse about administering prophylactic lidocaine before suctioning. *(This measure may help prevent acute intracranial hypertension [Thelan et al., 1998].)*
- Maintain optimal ventilation through proper positioning and regular suctioning. *(These measures help prevent hypoxemia and hypercapnia.)*
- Monitor arterial blood gas (ABG) values. *(ABG values help evaluate gas exchange in the lungs and determine circulating oxygen level and arterial CO_2. It is recommended that arterial O_2 be between 90 and 100 torr, and that arterial CO_2 be between 25 and 30 mm Hg, to prevent cerebral ischemia and cerebrovascular congestion, which increase ICP.)*
- If indicated, initiate protocols or collaborate with physician or advanced practice nurse for drug therapy, which may include the following (Thelan et al., 1998):
  - Sedation, barbiturates *(These drugs reduce cerebral metabolic rate, contributing to decreased ICP.)*
  - Anticonvulsants *(These agents help prevent seizures, which increase cerebral metabolic rate.)*
  - Osmotic diuretics *(These agents draw water from brain tissue to the plasma to reduce cerebral edema.)*
  - Nonosmotic diuretics *(These agents draw sodium and water from edematous areas to reduce cerebral edema.)*
  - Steroids *(These drugs can reduce capillary permeability, limiting cerebral edema.)*
- Carefully monitor hydration status; evaluate fluid intake and output, serum osmolality, and urine specific gravity and osmolality. *(Dehydration from diuretic therapy can cause hypotension and decreased cardiac output.)*
- If intravenous (IV) fluid therapy is prescribed, carefully administer IV fluids with an infusion pump. *(Careful IV fluid administration is necessary to prevent overhydration, which increases ICP.)*
- If using an ICP monitoring device, refer to the procedure manual for guidelines (eg, ventriculostomy, subarachnoid bolt, epidural monitor).

PC: SEIZURES

DEFINITION

PC: Seizures: Describes a person experiencing or at high risk to experience paroxysmal episodes of involuntary muscular contraction (tonus) and relaxation (clonus)

High-Risk Populations

- Perinatal injuries
- Family history of seizure disorder
- Cerebral cortex lesions
- Head injury
- Infectious disorder (eg, meningitis)
- Cerebral circulatory disturbance (eg, cerebral palsy, stroke)
- Brain tumor
- Alcohol overdose or withdrawal
- Drug overdose or withdrawal (eg, theophylline)
- Electrolyte imbalances (eg, hypocalcemia, pyridoxine deficiency)
- Hypoglycemia
- High fever
- Eclampsia

- Metabolic abnormalities (renal, hepatic, electrolyte)
- Poisoning (mercury, lead, carbon monoxide)

Nursing Goals

The nurse will manage and minimize seizure episodes.

General Interventions and Rationales

- Determine whether the client senses an aura before onset of seizure activity. If so, reinforce safety measures to take during an aura (eg, lie down, pull car over to roadside and shut off ignition).
- If seizure activity occurs, observe and document the following (Hickey, 2002):
  - Where seizure began
  - Type of movements, parts of body involved
  - Changes in pupil size or position
  - Urinary or bowel incontinence
  - Duration
  - Unconsciousness (duration)
  - Behavior after seizure
  - Weakness, paralysis after seizure
  - Sleep after seizure (postictal period)

  (Progression of seizure activity may assist in identifying its anatomic focus.)
- Provide privacy during and after seizure activity. *(To protect the client from embarrassment)*
- During seizure activity, take measures to ensure adequate ventilation (eg, loosen clothing). **Do not** try to force an airway or tongue blade through clenched teeth. *(Strong clonic/tonic movements can cause airway occlusion. Forced airway insertion can cause injury.)*
- During seizure activity, gently guide movements to prevent injury. Do not attempt to restrict movements. *(Physical restraint could result in musculoskeletal injury.)*
- If the client is sitting when seizure activity occurs, ease him or her to the floor and place something soft under his or her head. *(These measures help prevent injury.)*
- After seizure activity subsides, position client on the side. *(This position helps prevent aspiration of secretions.)*
- Allow person to sleep after seizure activity; reorient on awakening. *(The person may experience amnesia; reorientation can help him or her regain a sense of control and can help reduce anxiety.)*
- If person continues to have generalized convulsions, notify physician or advanced practice nurse and initiate protocol:
  - Establish airway.
  - Suction PRN.
  - Administer oxygen through nasal catheter.
  - Initiate an IV line.

  (Status epilepticus is a medical emergency with a 10% mortality rate. Impaired respiration can cause systemic and cerebral hypoxia. IV administration of a rapid-acting anticonvulsant [eg, diazepam] is indicated [Hickey, 2002].)
- Keep the bed in a low position with the siderails up, and pad the siderails with blankets. *(These precautions help prevent injury from fall or trauma.)*
- If the client's condition is chronic, evaluate the need for teaching self-management techniques. Use the nursing diagnosis *Risk for Ineffective Therapeutic Regimen Management related to insufficient knowledge of condition, medication regimen, safety measures, and community resources* (see Section II).

PC: INCREASED INTRAOCULAR PRESSURE

DEFINITION

PC: Increased Intraocular Pressure: Describes a person experiencing or at high risk to experience increased aqueous humor production or resistance to outflow, which can cause compression of nerve fibers and blood vessels in the optic disc (Schremp 1995a)

High-Risk Population

- Glaucoma
- Corneal transplant
- Radiation therapy
- Eye trauma
- Ophthalmic surgery

Nursing Goals

The nurse will manage and minimize increased intraocular pressure.

General Interventions and Rationales

- Reinforce prescribed postoperative activity restrictions, which may include avoiding the following:
  - Bending at the waist
  - Making sudden head movements
  - Valsalva maneuver (eg, straining during bowel movements)
  (These activities can increase intraocular pressure.)
- Reinforce the need to wear eye protection (patch and shield). *(These protect the eye from trauma.)*
- Monitor for bleeding, dehiscence, and evisceration. *(Ocular tissue is vulnerable to these problems because of its high vascularity and fragile vessels.)*
- Monitor for signs and symptoms of increased intraocular pressure:
  - Eyebrow pain
  - Nausea
  - Halos around lights
  (Intraocular pressure may increase in response to surgery or owing to medications, such as steroid eye drops [Schremp, 1995b].)
- Administer an antiemetic if nausea develops. *(Vomiting increases intraocular pressure and must be avoided.)*
- Monitor visual acuity and note any changes (eg, halos around lights). *(Factors that can alter vision include blood in the vitreous or from the incision, infection, dislocation of the lens implant, redetachment of the retina, and increased intraocular pressure.)*
- Position client on the back with the head elevated; turn on the unaffected side. *(This positioning can help reduce pressure in the affected eye.)*
- Maintain a quiet environment; limit external stimuli and activities. *(These measures can help reduce stress and may promote a decrease in intraocular pressure.)*

PC: NEUROLEPTIC MALIGNANT SYNDROME

DEFINITION

PC: Neuroleptic Malignant Syndrome (NMS): Describes a person experiencing or at high risk to experience an acute, life-threatening reaction to neuroleptic medication. The pathophysiology of NMS is poorly understood, but like other forms of extrapyramidal symptoms, there appear to be neuroleptic-induced dopaminergic blockade and dopamine depletion in the CNS, particularly in the basal ganglia and hypothalamus, which causes the various symptoms. It is most often characterized by the rapid onset of severe muscular rigidity, autonomic instability, hyperthermia, and deteriorating mental state. It occurs in 1% of clients receiving neuroleptic agents.

High-Risk Populations

- Use of neuroleptics, especially the higher-potency drugs haloperidol, fluphenazine, and chlorpromazine
- Use of long-acting depot neuroleptics
- Use of neuroleptic medications in combination with:
  - Concurrent lithium therapy
  - Physiologic stress
  - Nutritional deficiencies
  - Concurrent organic brain syndrome
  - Physical exhaustion
  - Dehydration
  - Acquired immunodeficiency syndrome (AIDS)
  - Restraints
  - Anticholinergic drugs
  - Agitation
  - Mood disorders
  - High temperature and humidity
- High doses of neuroleptics
- Concurrent use of two or more neuroleptics
- Previous history of NMS
- Male gender, younger than 40 years of age (80% of cases)
- Undergoing "rapid neuroleptization," especially if administered by injections
- Initial 2 weeks of therapy, although it can occur at any point in neuroleptic therapy (eg, 16% within 24 h of administration)
- Discontinuation of antiparkinsonian drugs

Nursing Goals

The nurse will manage and minimize NMS episodes.

General Interventions and Rationales

- Hold doses of all neuroleptic drugs and drugs with anticholinergic properties, and notify physician.
- Maintain airway. Provide a calm environment. *(Any client with altered level of consciousness is at risk for airway compromise and hypoventilation. Chest wall muscle rigidity also contributes.)*

- Recognize and treat promptly cardiac dysrhythmias and blood pressure instabilities as necessary.
- Monitor for signs and symptoms.
  - Severe extrapyramidal symptoms:
    - Muscular rigidity
    - Dysarthria
    - Dysphagia (difficulty swallowing)
    - Excess salivation
    - Myoglobinuria (urine turning red)
    - Akinesis
    - Cogwheel rigidity
    - Muteness
    - Waxy flexibility
    - Exaggerated deep tendon reflexes
  - Autonomic dysfunction:
    - Tachycardia
    - Diaphoresis
    - Urinary incontinence
    - Labile or sustained hypertension
    - Hypotension (abnormal blood pressure)
    - Dyspnea
    - Tachypnea
    - Pallor
    - Cardiac dysrhythmias
  - Fever above 100°F
  - Behavioral changes or fluctuations (eg, confusion, delirium, agitation, coma, catatonic-like posturing, combativeness)
  - Dehydration
  - Malnutrition

  (The underlying pathophysiology is not well understood but appears to be related to the blockage or depletion of the CNS neurotransmitter dopamine. Signs and symptoms of NMS appear to be related to the degree and sites of involvement of dopamine blockade. For example, dopamine blockade in the nigrostriatal pathway appears to cause muscular rigidity; dopamine impairment in the preoptic anterior hypothalamus, which regulates temperature, appears to cause fever; dopamine disturbance in the spinal cord may cause autonomic dysfunction.)

- Monitor for abnormal laboratory findings:
  - Elevated creatine phosphokinase
  - Elevated WBC count
  - Elevated liver functions
  - ABG
  - Electrolytes

  (As the body reacts to dopamine depletion, WBC count rises, creatine phosphokinase is elevated because of micronecrosis of the skeletal muscles, and hepatic enzymes are elevated. Blood gas determinations measure the degree of autonomic instability. Electrolytes measure the effect of autonomic instability and micronecrosis on the body systems.)

- Assess vital signs frequently (blood pressure; temperature, pulse, respiration; and electrocardiogram) for signs of respiratory and cardiovascular decompensation.
- Monitor degree of rigidity through deep tendon reflexes. If rigidity is worsening, further measures must be taken because it can affect the muscles of the vital organs. *(Deep tendon reflexes indicate objectively whether the rigidity is worsening or improving.)*
- Institute seizure precautions.
- Monitor fluid intake and output and for signs of renal decompensation. *(Excessive muscle breakdown [micronecrosis] can cause myoglobinuria and renal failure.)*
- Auscultate and evaluate lungs for pulmonary stasis and embolus. *(Dysphagia can lead to aspiration pneumonia. Immobility places a person at risk for pulmonary stasis or embolus.)*
- If dantrolene is ordered to help decrease muscle rigidity, remain alert for:
  - Liver toxicity
  - Phlebitis and tissue damage (if administered IV)

  (Dantrolene, a skeletal muscle relaxant, acts at the level of the sarcoplasmic reticulum, complementing the effects of a dopaminergic agent.)
- Apply cooling blankets, antipyretic medications, and cool sponge baths (to control fever).

- If dysphagia is present:
  - Monitor food intake closely.
  - Provide soft or liquid diet.
  - Tube feedings or total parenteral nutrition if nutritional status continues to decline
  - Refer also to *Impaired Swallowing.*
- Refer to *Risk for Impaired Skin Integrity* to prevent pressure ulcers. *(Profuse diaphoresis, dehydration, urinary incontinence, and contracted limbs set the stage for skin breakdown.)*
- Provide mouth care and suctioning as needed. *(Dysphagia can cause increased salivation.)*
- Apply eye patches and lubricants as needed. *(These prevent exposure keratitis secondary to inadequate blinking.)*
- After recovery:
  - Teach client and significant others the importance of maintaining proper nutrition, sleep, and exercise. *(Physiologic depletion predisposes the person to NMS.)*
  - Review manifestations of NMS and teach client and significant others to seek immediate medical help if stiffness, fever, excess sweating, and racing pulse occur. *(Early detection can prevent serious complications; NMS has an 11.6% mortality rate.)*
- Institute seizure precautions.

PC: ALCOHOL WITHDRAWAL

DEFINITION

PC: Alcohol Withdrawal: Describes a person experiencing or at high risk to experience the complications of alcohol withdrawal (eg, delirium tremens, autonomic hyperactivity, seizures, alcohol hallucinosis, and hypertension)

High-Risk Populations

Alcoholics

Nursing Goals

The nurse will manage and minimize alcohol withdrawal complications.

General Interventions and Rationales

- Carefully attempt to determine if the client abuses alcohol. Consult with the family regarding their perception of alcohol consumption. Explain why accurate information is necessary. *(It is critical to identify high-risk people so potentially fatal withdrawal symptoms can be prevented.)*
- Obtain history of previous withdrawals.
  - Delirium tremens:
    - Time of onset
    - Manifestation
  - Seizures:
    - Time of onset
    - Type

(Withdrawal occurs 6 to 96 h after drinking ends. Withdrawal can occur in people who are considered "social drinkers" [6 oz of alcohol daily for a period of 3 to 4 weeks]. Withdrawal patterns may resemble those of previous episodes. Seizure patterns unlike previous episodes may indicate another underlying pathology.)

- Obtain a complete history of prescription and nonprescription drugs taken. *(Benzodiazepine or barbiturate withdrawal may mimic alcohol withdrawal and complicate the picture.)*
- Consult with the primary provider regarding the risk of the client and initiation of benzodiazepine therapy, with dosage determined by assessment findings. *(Benzodiazepine requirements in alcohol withdrawal are highly variable and client specific. Fixed schedules may oversedate or undersedate.)*
- Observe for the desired effects of benzodiazepine therapy:
    - Relief from withdrawal symptoms
    - Peaceful sleep but rousable

(Benzodiazepines are the drugs of choice in controlling withdrawal symptoms. Neuroleptics cause hypotension and lower seizure threshold. Barbiturates may effectively control symptoms of withdrawal but have no advantages over benzodiazepines.)

- Monitor for indicators of a drop in blood alcohol level and determine the time of onset:
    - Anxiety
    - Insomnia
    - Mild tachycardia
    - Tremors
    - Sensory hyperacuity
    - Low-grade fever
    - Disorientation
    - Dehydration

(Once a level drops 100 mg/dL below the person's normal, withdrawal typically occurs. These symptoms can last up to 5 days. Withdrawal results in a hypermetabolic state from adrenergic excess and possible alteration of prostaglandin E_1 levels.)

- Monitor for withdrawal seizures.
    - Determine time of onset.
    - Refer also to *PC: Seizures.*

(Withdrawal seizures can occur 6 to 96 h after drinking ends. They are usually nonfocal and grand mal, last minutes or less, and occur singly or in clusters of two to six.)

- Monitor for and intervene promptly in cases of status epilepticus. Follow institution's emergency protocol. *(Status epilepticus is life-threatening if not controlled immediately with IV diazepam.)*
- Monitor for delirium tremens.
    - Delirium component (vivid hallucinations, confusion, extreme disorientation, and fluctuating levels of awareness)
    - Extreme hyperadrenergic stimulation (tachycardia, hypertension or hypotension, extreme tremor, agitation, diaphoresis, and fever)

(Delirium tremens appears on either the 4th or 5th day after cessation of drinking and resolves within 5 days.)

- Monitor and determine onset of alcohol hallucinosis, which involves visual, auditory, and tactile hallucinations (however, the person senses that the hallucinations are not real and is aware of surroundings). *(Alcohol hallucinosis occurs 6 to 96 h after abstinence and can last up to 3 days.)*
- Monitor vital signs every 2 h:
    - Temperature, pulse, and respiration
    - Blood pressure

(Clients in withdrawal have elevated heart rate, respirations, and fever. Clients experiencing delirium tremens can be expected to have a low-grade fever. Rectal temperature greater than 37.7°C (99.9°F) is a clue to possible infection.)

- Maintain the client's IV running continuously. *(This is necessary for fluid replacement and dextrose, thiamine bolus, benzodiazepine, and magnesium sulfate administration. Chlordiazepoxide and diazepam should not be given IM because of unpredictable absorption.)*
- Refer to the nursing diagnosis *Ineffective Denial* for interventions for substance abuse.

POTENTIAL COMPLICATION: GASTROINTESTINAL/HEPATIC/BILIARY

DEFINITION

PC: Gastrointestinal/Hepatic/Biliary: Describes a person experiencing or at high risk to experience compromised function in the gastrointestinal (GI), hepatic, or biliary systems. (*Note:* These three systems are grouped together for classification purposes. In a clinical situation, the nurse would use either *PC: Gastrointestinal, PC: Hepatic,* or *PC: Biliary* to specify the applicable system.)

◎ AUTHOR'S NOTE

The nurse can use these generic collaborative problems to describe a person at risk for various problems affecting the GI, hepatic, or biliary systems. Doing so focuses nursing interventions on monitoring GI, hepatic, or biliary status to detect and diagnose abnormal functioning. Should a complication develop, the nurse would add the applicable specific collaborative problem (eg, *PC: GI Bleeding, PC: Hepatic Dysfunction*) to the problem list, specifying appropriate nursing management.

In most cases, along with these collaborative problems, the nurse treats other associated responses, using nursing diagnoses (eg, *Impaired Comfort related to accumulation of bilirubin pigment and bile salts*).

For information on Focus Assessment Criteria, visit http://connection.lww.com.

Significant Laboratory/Diagnostic Assessment Criteria

Serum albumin (lowered in chronic liver disease)
Serum amylase (elevated in biliary tract disease)
Bilirubin (elevated in hepatic disease, newborn hyperbilirubinemia)
Potassium (lowered in liver disease with ascites, vomiting, diarrhea)
Blood urea nitrogen (BUN; increased in hepatic failure)
Prothrombin time (elevated in cirrhosis, hepatitis)
Hemoglobin, hematocrit (decreased with bleeding)
Sodium (decreased with dehydration)
Platelets (decreased with liver disease or bleeding)
Abdominal x-ray
Urinalysis
Colonoscopy, barium enema
Endoscopy, upper GI series

PC: PARALYTIC ILEUS

DEFINITION

PC: Paralytic Ileus: Describes a person experiencing or at high risk to experience neurogenic or functional bowel obstruction

High-Risk Populations

- Thrombosis or embolus to mesenteric vessels
- Postoperative status (bowel, retroperitoneal, or spinal cord surgery)
- Electrolyte imbalances (eg, hypokalemia)
- Hypokalemia
- Postshock status
- Hypovolemia
- Post-trauma (eg, spinal cord injury)
- Strangulated hernias
- Congenital bowel deformities
- Uremia
- Spinal cord lesion

Nursing Goals

The nurse will manage and minimize complications of paralytic ileus.

General Interventions and Rationales

- In a postoperative client, monitor bowel function, looking for:
  - Bowel sounds in all quadrants returning within 24 to 48 h of surgery
  - Flatus and defecation resuming by the second or third postoperative day
  (Surgery and anesthesia decrease innervation of the bowel, reducing peristalsis and possibly leading to transient paralytic ileus [Porth, 2002].)
- Do not allow client any fluids until bowel sounds are present. When indicated, begin with small amounts. Monitor client's response to resumption of fluid and food intake, and note the nature and amount of any emesis or stools. *(The client will not tolerate fluids until bowel sounds resume.)*
- Monitor for signs of paralytic ileus—primarily pain, typically localized, sharp, and intermittent; hiccups; nausea/vomiting; constipation; distended abdomen; rebound tenderness. *(Intraoperative manipulation of abdominal organs and the depressive effects of narcotics and anesthetics on peristalsis can cause paralytic ileus, typically developing between the third and fifth postoperative day.)*
- If paralytic ileus is related to hypovolemia, refer to *PC: Hypovolemia* for more information and specific interventions.

PC: GI BLEEDING

DEFINITION

PC: GI Bleeding: Describes a person experiencing or at high risk to experience GI bleeding

High-Risk Populations

- Disorders of GI, hepatic, and biliary systems
- Transfusion of 5 U (or more) of blood
- Recent stress (eg, trauma, sepsis), prolonged mechanical ventilation
- Esophageal varices
- Peptic ulcer
- Colon cancer
- Platelet deficiency
- Coagulopathy
- Shock, hypotension
- Major surgery (>3 h)
- Head injury
- Severe vascular disease
- Burns (>35% of body)
- Daily use of aspirin or nonsteroidal anti-inflammatory drugs (NSAIDs)

Infants/Children (Wong, 2003)
- Neonate (*swallowed maternal blood, *hemorrhagic disease, anal fissure, stress ulcers, enterocolitis, vascular malformations)
- 6 months (same as above except [*], intussusception, lymphonodular hyperplasia)
- 6 months to 5 years (same as above, epistaxis, esophagitis, varices, gastritis, Meckel's diverticulum, Henoch-Schönlein purpura, polyps)
- 5 to 18 years (same as above, Mallory-Weiss tear, peptic ulcer, chronic ulcerative colitis, Crohn's disease, hemorrhoids)

Nursing Goals

The nurse will manage and minimize complications of GI bleeding.

General Interventions and Rationales

- Monitor for signs and symptoms of GI bleeding:
  - Nausea
  - Hematemesis
  - Blood in stool
  - Decreased hematocrit or hemoglobin
  - Hypotension, tachycardia
  - Diarrhea or constipation
  - Anorexia

  (Clinical manifestations depend on the amount and duration of GI bleeding. Early detection enables prompt intervention to minimize complications.)
- Monitor for occult blood in gastric aspirates and bowel movements.

- Monitor gastric pH every 2 to 4 h. *(Maintenance of gastric pH <5 has decreased bleeding complications by 89%.)*
  - Use pH paper that has a range from 0 to 7.5. Use good light to interpret the color on the pH paper.
  - Position client on the left side lying down. *(The left side down position allows the tip of the nasogastric (NG) or gastrostomy tube to move into the greater curvature of the stomach and usually below the level of gastric fluid.)*
  - Use two syringes (>30 mL) to obtain the aspirate. Aspirate a gastric sample and discard. Use aspirate in the second syringe for testing. *(The first aspirate clears the tube of antacids and other substances that can alter the pH of the sample.)*
- Evaluate for other factors that affect the pH reading:
  - Medications (eg, cimetidine)
  - Tube feeding
  - Irrigations
  (False-positive and false-negative findings can result when aspirate contains certain substances. Most investigators recommend a range of 3.5 to 5.0.)
- Monitor vital signs often, particularly blood pressure and pulse. *(Careful monitoring can detect early changes in blood volume.)*
- Consult with physician/advanced practice nurse for the specific prescription for titration ranges of pH and antacid administration.
- If NG intubation is prescribed, use a large-bore (18-gauge) tube and follow protocols for insertion and client care. *(An NG tube can remove irritating gastric secretions, blood, and clots and can reduce abdominal distention.)*
- Follow the protocol for gastric lavage, if ordered. *(Lavage provides local vasoconstriction and may help control GI bleeding.)*
- Monitor hemoglobin, hematocrit, red blood cell count, platelets, prothrombin time, partial thromboplastin time, type blood and cross match, and blood urea nitrogen (BUN) values. *(These values reflect the effectiveness of therapy.)*
- If hypovolemia occurs, refer to *PC: Hypovolemia* for more information and specific interventions.
- Prepare for transfusion per physician/advanced practice nurse order. *(Doing so can reestablish volume status.)*

PC: HEPATIC DYSFUNCTION

DEFINITION

PC: Hepatic Dysfunction: Describes a person experiencing or at high risk to experience progressive liver dysfunction

High-Risk Populations

Infections

- Hepatitis A, B, C, D, E, non-A, non-B, non-C
- Herpes simplex virus (types 1 and 2)
- Epstein-Barr virus
- Varicella zoster
- Dengue fever virus
- Rift Valley fever virus

Drugs/Toxins

- Industrial substances (chlorinated hydrocarbons, phosphorus)
- *Amanita phalloides* (mushrooms)
- Aflatoxin (herb)
- Medications (isoniazid, rifampin, halothane, methyldopa, tetracycline, valproic acid, monoamine oxidase inhibitors, phenytoin, nicotinic acid, tricyclic antidepressants, isoflurane, ketoconazole, cotrimethoprim, sulfasalazine, pyrimethamine, octreotide, antivirals)
- Acetaminophen toxicity
- Cocaine
- Alcohol

Hypoperfusion

- Venous obstructions
- Budd-Chiari syndrome
- Veno-occlusive disease
- Ischemia

Metabolic Disorders

- Hyperbilirubinemia
- Wilson's disease
- Tyrosinemia
- Heat stroke
- Galactosemia
- Nutritional deficiencies

Surgery

- Jejunoileal bypass
- Partial hepatectomy
- Liver transplant failure

Other

- Reye's syndrome
- Acute fatty liver of pregnancy
- Massive malignant infiltration
- Autoimmune hepatitis
- Rh incompatibility
- Ingestion of raw contaminated fish
- Thalassemia

Nursing Goals

The nurse will manage and minimize the complications of hepatic dysfunction.

General Interventions and Rationales

- Monitor for signs and symptoms of hepatic dysfunction:
  - Anorexia, indigestion *(GI effects result from circulating toxins.)*
  - Jaundice *(Yellowed skin and sclera result from excessive bilirubin production.)*
  - Petechiae, ecchymoses *(These skin changes reflect impaired synthesis of clotting factors.)*
  - Clay-colored stools *(This can result from decreased bile in stools.)*
  - Elevated liver function tests (eg, serum bilirubin, serum transaminase) *(Elevated values indicate extensive liver damage.)*
  - Prolonged prothrombin time *(This reflects reduced production of clotting factors.)*
- With hepatic dysfunction, monitor for hemorrhage. *(The liver has a central role in hemostasis. Decreased platelet count results from impaired production of new platelets from the bone marrow. Decreased clearance of old platelets by the reticuloendothelial system also results. In addition, synthesis of coagulation factors [II, V, VII, IX, and X] is impaired, resulting in bleeding. The most frequent site is the upper GI tract. Other sites include the nasopharynx, lungs, retroperitoneum, kidneys, and intracranial and skin puncture sites [Porth, 2002].)*

- Teach client to report any unusual bleeding (eg, in the mouth after brushing teeth). *(Mucous membranes are prone to injury because of their high surface vascularity.)*
- Monitor for portal systemic encephalopathy by assessing:
  - General appearance and behavior
  - Orientation
  - Speech patterns
  - Laboratory values: blood pH and ammonia level
  (Profound liver failure results in accumulation of ammonia and other toxic metabolites in the blood. The blood–brain barrier permeability increases, and both toxins and plasma proteins leak from capillaries to the extracellular space, causing cerebral edema.)
- Monitor for signs and symptoms of (refer to the index under each electrolyte for specific signs and symptoms):
  - Hypoglycemia *(Hypoglycemia is caused by loss of glycogen stores in the liver from damaged cells and decreased serum concentrations of glucose, insulin, and growth hormones.)*
  - Hypokalemia *(Potassium losses occur from vomiting, NG suctioning, diuretics, or excessive renal losses.)*
  - Hypophosphatemia *(The loss of potassium ions causes the proportional loss of magnesium ions. Increased phosphate loss, transcellular shifts, and decreased phosphate intake contribute to hypophosphatemia.)*
- Monitor for acid–base disturbances. Hepatocellular necrosis can result in accumulation of organic anions, resulting in metabolic acidosis. *(People with ascites often have metabolic alkalosis from increased bicarbonate levels resulting from increased sodium/hydrogen exchange in the distal tubule.)*
- Assess for side effects of medications. Avoid administering narcotics, sedatives, and tranquilizers and exposing the client to ammonia products. *(Liver dysfunction results in decreased metabolism of certain medications [eg, opiates, sedatives, tranquilizers], increasing the risk of toxicity from high drug blood levels. Ammonia products should be avoided because of the client's already high serum ammonia level.)*
- Monitor for signs and symptoms of renal failure. (Refer to *PC: Renal Failure* for more information.) *(Obstructed hepatic blood flow results in decreased blood to the kidneys, impairing glomerular filtration and leading to fluid retention and decreased urinary output.)*
- Monitor for hypertension. *(Fluid retention and overload can cause hypertension.)*
- Teach client and family to report signs and symptoms of complications, such as:
  - Increased abdominal girth *(It may indicate worsening portal hypertension.)*
  - Rapid weight loss or gain *(Weight loss points to negative nitrogen balance; weight gain points to fluid retention.)*
  - Bleeding *(Unusual bleeding indicates decreased prothrombin time and clotting factors.)*
  - Tremors *(They can result from impaired neurotransmission because of failure of the liver to detoxify enzymes that act as false neurotransmitters.)*
  - Confusion *(This can result from cerebral hypoxia caused by high serum ammonia levels resulting from the liver's impaired ability to convert ammonia to urea.)*

PC: HYPERBILIRUBINEMIA

DEFINITION

PC: Hyperbilirubinemia: Describes a neonate with or at high risk for development of excessive serum bilirubin levels (>0.15 mg/dL)

High-Risk Neonates

- ABO incompatibility
- Rh-negative mother
- Polycythemia
- Small for gestational age
- Preterm status
- Large for gestational age
- Diabetic mother
- Isoimmune hemolytic disease
- Hypothyroidism
- Biliary obstruction
- Use of oxytocin or bupivacaine during labor
- Traumatic delivery
- Bacterial infection
- Breast-feeding

Nursing Goals

The nurse will manage and minimize complications of hyperbilirubinemia.

General Interventions and Rationales

- Prevent cold stress. *(Metabolism of brown adipose tissue releases nonesterified free fatty acids, which compete with bilirubin for albumin-binding sites.)*
- Ensure adequate hydration and intake. *(Optimal fluid and feedings facilitate bilirubin excretion.)*
- Differentiate physiologic jaundice from pathologic jaundice. Physiologic jaundice requires no treatment, whereas pathologic jaundice does.
  - Physiologic jaundice:
    - Benign
    - Onset 3 to 6 days (breast-feeding jaundice)
    - Onset 5 to 15 days (breast milk jaundice)
  - Pathologic jaundice:
    - Rapidly rises
    - Onset first 24 h of life
- Screen for high-risk infants.
  - Evaluate for presence of jaundice.
    - Face (early sign of bilirubin level >5 mg/dL)
    - Trunk/sternum (seen with levels >10 mg/dL)
    - Lower body (seen with levels >15 mg/dL)
  - Assess for ecchymoses, abrasions, or petechiae. *(Extravasated hemoglobin in the tissue will add to normal hemoglobin breakdown and increase bilirubin production.)*

- Monitor for bilirubin-induced neurologic dysfunction. *(Bilirubin deposits in the basal ganglia and at nerve terminals cause encephalopathy in 25% of preterm infants and 2% of healthy term infants.)*
  - Behavior change: lethargy, somnolence progressing to convulsions and coma
  - Muscle tone abnormalities
  - Shrill, high-pitched cry
  - Poor sucking
- Initiate phototherapy according to protocol, if indicated. *(Phototherapy breaks down bilirubin into water-soluble products that can be excreted.)*
- If phototherapy is performed, ensure optimal hydration. Weigh infant daily to assess fluid status. *(Phototherapy increases fluid loss through diaphoresis.)*
- Protect infant's eyes during phototherapy treatment. Use Plexiglas shields; ensure that lids are closed before applying shields. Provide periods out of light with eye shields removed. *(These precautions help ensure safe treatment.)*
- Monitor for eye discharge, excessive pressure on lids, and corneal irritation. *(These complications may result from use of eye shields.)*
- Turn infant frequently during phototherapy. *(Any areas not exposed to light will remain jaundiced.)*
- Monitor temperature, checking it at least every 4 h. *(A nude infant is vulnerable to hypothermia; use of radiant warmers increases the risk of hyperthermia.)*
- Prepare parents for home phototherapy. *(Term infants older than 48 h with bilirubin levels >14 mg/dL but <18 mg/mL are candidates.)*
- Explain procedure.
  - Teach warning signs of neurotoxicity.
  - Provide written instructions.
  - Arrange for daily home health nurse visits.

POTENTIAL COMPLICATION: MUSCULAR/SKELETAL

DEFINITION

PC: Muscular/Skeletal: Describes a person experiencing or at high risk to experience various musculo-skeletal problems

---

⦾ AUTHOR'S NOTE

The nurse can use this generic collaborative problem to describe people at risk for several types of musculoskeletal problems (eg, all clients who have sustained multiple trauma). This collaborative problem focuses nursing management on assessing musculoskeletal status to detect and to diagnose abnormalities.

For a client exhibiting a specific musculoskeletal problem, the nurse would add the applicable collaborative problem (eg, *PC: Pathologic Fractures*) to the problem list. If the risk factors or etiology were not related directly to the primary medical diagnoses, the nurse would add this information to the diagnostic statement (eg, *PC: Pathologic Fractures related to osteoporosis*).

Because musculoskeletal problems typically affect daily functioning, the nurse must assess the client's functional patterns for evidence of impairment. Findings may have significant implications—for instance, a casted leg that prevents a woman from assuming her favorite sleeping position and impairs her ability to perform housework. After identifying any such problems, the nurse should use nursing diagnoses to address specific responses of actual or potential altered functioning.

For information on Focus Assessment Criteria, visit http://connection.lww.com.

Significant Laboratory/Diagnostic Assessment Criteria

Laboratory

Serum calcium (decreased in osteoporosis)
Serum phosphorus (decreased in osteoporosis)
Sedimentation rate (increased in inflammatory disorders)

Diagnostic

X-ray
Computed tomography (CT) scan
Magnetic resonance imaging (MRI)
Bone scan
Aspiration

PC: PATHOLOGIC FRACTURES

DEFINITION

PC: Pathologic Fractures: Describes a person experiencing or at high risk to experience a fracture unrelated to trauma because of defects in bone structure

High-Risk Populations

- Osteoporosis
- Cushing's syndrome
- Malnutrition
- Long-term corticosteroid therapy
- Osteogenesis imperfecta
- Bone tumors (primary or metastatic)
- Paget's disease
- Prolonged immobility
- Irradiation fraction
- Rickets
- Osteomalacia
- Hyperparathyroidism
- Multiple myeloma
- Lymphatic leukemia
- Cystic bone disease
- Infection

Nursing Goals

The nurse will manage and minimize complications of pathologic fractures.

General Interventions and Rationales

- Monitor for signs and symptoms of pathologic fractures:
  - Localized pain that is continuous and unrelenting (back, neck, or extremities)
  - Visible bone deformity
  - Crepitation on movement
  - Loss of movement or use
  - Localized soft tissue edema
  - Skin discoloration

  (Detection of pathologic fractures enables prompt intervention to prevent or minimize further complications.)
- In a client with osteoporosis, monitor for signs and symptoms of vertebral, hip, and wrist fractures, such as:
  - Pain in the lower back, neck, or wrist
  - Localized tenderness
  - Pain radiating to abdomen and flank
  - Spasm of paravertebral muscles

  (Progressive osteoporosis more readily affects bones with high amounts of trabecular tissue [eg, hip, vertebrae, wrist].)

- Promote weight-bearing activities as soon as possible. *(Weight-bearing prevents bone demineralization.)*
- Teach measures to help prevent injury and promote weight bearing, such as:
  - Using smooth movements to avoid pulling or pushing on limbs
  - Supporting the extremities when turning in bed
  - Lifting the buttocks up slightly when sitting to provide weight bearing to the legs and arms
- Monitor x-ray results and serum calcium levels. *(These diagnostic findings help evaluate the client's risk for fractures.)*
- If a fracture is suspected, maintain proper alignment and immobilize the site using pillows or a splint; notify the physician or advanced practice nurse promptly. *(Timely, appropriate intervention can prevent or minimize soft tissue damage.)*
- Teach client and family measures to prevent or delay bone demineralization, using the nursing diagnosis *Health-Seeking Behaviors: Management of osteoporosis.*

PC: JOINT DISLOCATION

DEFINITION

PC: Joint Dislocation: Describes a person experiencing or at high risk to experience displacement of a bone from its position in a joint

High-Risk Populations

- Total hip replacement
- Total knee replacement
- Fractured hip, knee, shoulder

For Infants/Children
- Birth trauma (eg, breech, firstborn)
- Sports
- Cerebral palsy (hip)

Nursing Goals

The nurse will manage and minimize complications of joint dislocation.

General Interventions and Rationales

- Maintain correct positioning.
  - Hip: Maintain the hip in abduction, neutral rotation, or slight external rotation.
  - Hip: Avoid hip flexion over 60 degrees.
  - Knee: Slightly elevated from hip; avoid using bed knee gatch or placing pillows under the knee (to prevent flexion contractures). Place pillows under the calf.
  (Specific positions are used to prevent prosthesis dislocation.)
- Assess for signs of joint (hip, knee) dislocation:
  - *Hip*
    - Acute groin pain in operative hip
    - Shortening of leg with external rotation

- *Hip, Knee, Shoulder*
  - "Popping" sound heard by client
  - Bulge at surgical site
  - Inability to move
  - Pain with mobility

(Until the surrounding muscles and joint capsule heal, joint dislocation may occur if positioning exceeds the limits of the prosthesis, as in flexing or hyperextending the knee or abducting the hip >45 degrees.)

- Maintain bed rest as ordered. Keep the affected joint in a neutral position with rolls, pillows, or specified devices. *(Bed rest typically is ordered for 1 to 3 days after surgery to allow stabilization of the prosthesis.)*
- The client may be turned toward either side unless contraindicated. Always maintain an abduction pillow when turning; limit the use of Fowler's position. *(If proper positioning is maintained, including the abduction pillow, clients may safely be turned toward the operative and nonoperative side. This promotes circulation and decreases the potential for pressure ulcer formation as a result of immobility. A prolonged Fowler's position can dislocate the prosthesis.)*
- Monitor for shoulder joint dislocation/subluxation. *(Total shoulder arthroplasty has a higher risk of joint dislocation/subluxation because the shoulder is capable of movement in three planes [flexion/extension, abduction/adduction, internal/external rotation.)*

❖ Pediatric Interventions and Rationales

- Evaluate newborn for developmental dysplasia of the hip (Sponsellar, 1999).
  - "Clunk" sound of subluxation or dislocation (Barlow test)
  - Abducting and lifting hip back in place (Ortolani test)

(These maneuvers test for instability.)

- For infants older than 6 months, assess for (Sponsellar, 1999):
  - Asymmetry
  - Abduction and full extension limitations
  - Shortened flexed thigh length on dysplasic side

(After 6 months, the Barlow and Ortolani tests are often falsely negative because of diminished laxity.)

Potential Complication: Reproductive
PC: Prenatal Bleeding
PC: Preterm Labor
PC: Pregnancy-Associated Hypertension
PC: Fetal Distress
PC: Postpartum Hemorrhage

POTENTIAL COMPLICATION: REPRODUCTIVE

DEFINITION

PC: Reproductive: Describes a person experiencing or at high risk to experience a problem in reproductive system functioning

---

⊗ AUTHOR'S NOTE

This generic collaborative problem provides a category under which to classify more specific collaborative problems affecting the reproductive system. Unlike the other generic collaborative problems (eg, *PC: Respiratory, PC: Cardiac*), it is of little clinical use by itself. So, instead of adding this generic collaborative problem to a client's problem list, the nurse should use the appropriate specific collaborative problem, such as *PC: Fetal Distress* or *PC: Postpartum Hemorrhage*.

For information on Focus Assessment Criteria, visit http://connection.lww.com.

Significant Laboratory/Diagnostic Assessment Criteria

Culture for gonorrhea and chlamydia
Gram's stain for diplococci
Rapid plasma reagin test (RPR; positive in syphilis)
Cervical, urethral smears (positive in infections)
Pap smear (positive in dysplasia, carcinoma)
Fetal pH (lowered in hypoxia)
Western blot test (positive for human immunodeficiency virus [HIV])

PC: PRENATAL BLEEDING

DEFINITION

PC: Prenatal Bleeding: Describes a woman experiencing or at high risk to experience bleeding during pregnancy

High-Risk Populations

- Incompetent cervix
- Spontaneous therapeutic abortion
- Ectopic pregnancy
- Gestational trophoblastic disease (hydatidiform mole)
- Disseminated intravascular coagulation

For Placenta Previa (Late Pregnancy)
- Multiparity
- Previous placenta previa
- Uterine abnormalities
- Increased maternal age
- Multiple gestation
- Previous cesarean section
- Endometritis

For Abruptio Placentae (Late Pregnancy)
- Shortened umbilical cord
- Trauma
- Precipitous labor
- Uterine abnormalities
- Hypertension
- Folic acid deficiency
- Compression of vena cava
- History of abruption
- High multiparity
- Oxytocin induction
- Second born of multiple births (eg, twins, triplets)
- Increased maternal age
- Cocaine/amphetamine use
- Cigarette smoking
- Excessive alcohol consumption

Nursing Goals

The nurse will manage and minimize complications of prenatal bleeding.

General Interventions and Rationales

- Teach the client to report unusual bleeding immediately.
- If bleeding occurs, notify physician or midwife and monitor:
  - Amount, character, color

- Cramps, contractions, pain, or tenderness
- Vital signs, hematocrit
- Urine output
- Start and maintain intravenous (IV) if hypovolemic, according to protocol.
- Monitor fetal heart tones (refer to *PC: Fetal Distress* for specific guidelines).
- Do not perform vaginal or rectal examinations if placenta previa is suspected.
- *(These procedures can tear the placenta, causing life-threatening hemorrhage.)*
- Maintain client in a supine position. *(This position reduces compression on the vena cava, which increases perfusion to the fetus.)*
- Administer oxygen by face mask at a rate of 8 L/min, as indicated. *(Supplemental oxygen therapy increases maternal circulating oxygen to the fetus.)*
- If signs of shock occur, refer to *PC: Hypovolemic shock* for more information on nursing management.
- Refer to the nursing diagnosis *Grieving* for interventions to provide support.

PC: PRETERM LABOR

DEFINITION

PC: Preterm Labor: Describes a woman experiencing or at high risk to experience expulsion of a viable fetus before the 37th week of gestation

High-Risk Populations (Mandeville & Troiano, 2002)

- Age (younger than 19 years or older than 40 years)
- Low socioeconomic status
- Maternal medical conditions (eg, infection, renal disease, hypertension, anemia, heart disease)
- Premature membrane rupture
- Multifetal gestation
- Previous premature birth
- Previous second-trimester abortion
- Uterine anomalies
- Cervical incompetency
- Closely spaced pregnancies
- Low-weight, small-stature mother
- Heavy work outside home
- Hydramnios
- Poor weight gain
- Tobacco use, substance abuse
- Physical abuse/battery
- Premature bleeding
- Reproductive tract infection
- Cervical dilation more than 2 cm by 32 weeks
- Diethylstilbestrol exposure in utero

Nursing Goals

The nurse will manage and minimize complications of premature labor.

General Interventions and Rationales

- Teach client to watch for and report (Reeder et al., 1997):
  - Menstrual-like cramps, abdominal tightening
  - Low backache
  - Pelvic pressure
  - Change in character of vaginal secretions
  - Diarrhea
  - Vaginal spotting or bleeding
  - Urinary tract infection

  (Early detection of impending premature labor enables interventions to ensure successful delivery and decrease the risk of complications.)
- Once labor begins, stay with the client and provide emotional support. *(Reassurance and support can help the client prepare for and cope with premature birth.)*
- Maintain constant bed rest. *(Bed rest is thought to reduce pressure of the fetal presenting part on the cervix, thus improving uterine blood flow.)*
- Ensure optimal hydration (oral and/or IV). *(Studies indicate that hydration inhibits the antidiuretic hormone and suppresses uterine activity [Mandeville & Troiano, 2002].)*
- Monitor fetal heart rate and rhythm.
- If IV tocolytic therapy (eg, magnesium sulfate, ritodrine, nifedipine, indomethacin) is prescribed, refer to protocol for preparation (eg, baseline laboratory tests, electrocardiogram [ECG]) and administration.
- During IV tocolytic therapy (Mandeville & Troiano, 2002):
  - Establish a baseline and then assess pulse, respirations, blood pressure, and breath sounds every 15 min during loading doses, with dosage increases, or with unstable vital signs and every hour during maintenance. *(Cardiopulmonary complications of tocolytic therapy can be fatal; close monitoring is essential.)*
  - With magnesium sulfate, assess deep tendon reflexes and level of consciousness every hour and ensure antidote calcium gluconate is available at bedside. *(Hypermagnesemia can cause central nervous system [CNS] depression.)*
  - Evaluate uterine activity every hour. *(This information is necessary to evaluate the effectiveness of the therapy.)*
  - With ritodrine, assess urine for ketones hourly or with every void; auscultate breath sounds and assess for cough, chest pain, or shortness of breath every 2 h.
  - Maintain NPO status and hourly intake and output during infusion.
  - Maintain bed rest in lateral recumbent position. *(This position increases uterine perfusion.)*
- Notify physician or midwife if the following occur (Mandeville & Troiano, 2002):
  - Respiratory rate less than 12/min or more than 24/min
  - Abnormal breath sounds, signs and symptoms of dyspnea, or mild coughing
  - Pulse rate greater than 120 beats/min, systolic pressure less than 90 mm Hg or diastolic pressure less than 50 mm Hg or greater than 90 mm Hg
  - Decreasing deep tendon reflexes or level of consciousness
  - Fetal heart rate above 160 beats/min or nonreassuring
  - Six or more uterine contractions per minute
  - ECG changes
  - Suspected $MgSO_4$ toxicity
  - Symptoms of placental abruption
  - $SaO_2 < 95\%$

PC: PREGNANCY-ASSOCIATED HYPERTENSION

DEFINITION

PC: Pregnancy-Associated Hypertension: Describes a woman experiencing or at high risk to experience a multisystem disease with vasoconstriction, hypertension (systolic pressure 130 mm Hg or higher or a diastolic pressure 85 mm Hg or higher), proteinuria, and edema during pregnancy

High-Risk Populations

- Younger than 21 years of age
- Older than 35 years of age
- Pre-existing renal disease
- Diabetes mellitus
- Vascular disease
- Multifetal pregnancy
- Hydatidiform mole
- Chronic hypertensive disease
- History of pregnancy-associated hypertension

Nursing Goals

The nurse will manage and minimize complications of hypertension.

General Interventions and Rationales

- Monitor blood pressure and compare readings to those taken earlier in the pregnancy. *(Midway through pregnancy, blood pressure commonly is lower than the woman's usual reading; thus, any elevation—even if readings still are within normal limits—may be significant [Reeder et al., 1997].)*
- Monitor daily weights. *(Sudden weight gain of 2 lb or more can indicate tissue or occult edema.)*
- Monitor for edema, particularly in the ankles, fingers, and face. *(Edema results from sodium retention related to decreased glomerular filtration.)*
- Monitor laboratory results for proteinuria. *(Peripheral arterial vasoconstriction leads to decreased glomerular filtration.)*
- Assess for and teach client to report (Mandeville & Troiano, 2002):
  - Edema
  - Visual disturbances
  - Dyspnea
  - Decreased urine output
  - Headache
  - Blurred vision
  - Nausea and vomiting
  - Change in level of consciousness
  - Epigastric pain

  (These are indicators of cerebral edema, pulmonary edema, and gastrointestinal [GI], renal, or hepatic impairments.)
- Teach a client exhibiting mild hypertension with minimal or no edema or proteinuria to:
  - Restrict activities and rest in bed most of the day.
  - Increase dietary protein intake to compensate for losses in urine.
  - Measure and record intake, output, and weight daily.

- For a client with progressive or severe hypertension and/or proteinuria, hospitalization may be indicated with:
  - Complete bed rest in left lateral position
  - Daily weight, intake and output monitoring
  - Daily urinalysis for protein and casts
  - Liver function tests
  - Magnesium sulfate therapy, sedation
- Ensure that the client gets as much undisturbed rest as possible. *(Adequate rest promotes relaxation and may help reduce hypertension and decrease the risk of seizure activity.)*
- Assess deep tendon reflexes of biceps and quadriceps and compare responses on each side (Reeder et al., 1997). *(CNS irritability increases the reflex response.)*
- Assess for signs and symptoms of impending convulsion:
  - Epigastric or right upper quadrant pain
  - Increasing hyperreflexia
  - Development or worsening of clonus (alternating contraction and relaxation [eg, twitching]) *(Convulsions are a sign of cerebral hemorrhage.)*
- Assess fetal heart tones for incidence of late decelerations, absent long-term variability, or bradycardia. *(Decreased placental perfusion causes late deceleration; hypoxia causes bradycardia [Mandeville & Troiano, 2001].)*
- Consult with physician or advanced practice nurse regarding low-dose aspirin therapy or calcium supplements for high-risk women during pregnancy. *(Studies have shown these therapies to reduce pregnancy-associated hypertension in high-risk women.)*
- If seizures occur, refer to *PC: Seizures* for nursing interventions.
- Refer to *PC: Preterm Labor* for nursing interventions with magnesium sulfate therapy.

PC: FETAL DISTRESS

DEFINITION

PC: Fetal Distress: Describes a fetus experiencing or at high risk to experience a disruption of the physiologic exchange of nutrients, oxygen, and metabolites

High-Risk Populations

Fetal Factors

- Prematurity
- Intrauterine growth retardation
- Atresia of umbilical cord
- Cord compression
- Placental insufficiency
- Infection
- Multiple gestation
- Congenital anomalies
- Dysmaturity
- Acute hemolytic crisis
- Prolonged labor
- Prolonged rupture of membranes
- Rh disease

Maternal Factors

- Chronic hypertension
- Pregnancy-associated hypertension
- Diabetes mellitus
- Third-trimester bleeding
- Maternal hypoxia (eg, respiratory insufficiency)
- Seizures, hypotension
- Prolonged uterine activity
- Abruptio placentae
- Cardiovascular disease
- Substance abuse
- Malnutrition

Nursing Goals

The nurse will manage and minimize episodes of fetal distress.

General Interventions and Rationales

- Determine baseline fetal heart tones and evaluate as reassuring if:
  - Rate of 120 to 160 beats/min
  - Presence of beat-to-beat variation (normal fetal rate has a fine irregularity of more than 5 to 10 beats/min)
  - Early decelerations (transient slowing of fetal heart rate with compression of the contraction causing parasympathetic stimulation)
- Monitor for nonreassuring fetal heart rate or rhythm, including:
  - Decreased variability (<6 beats/min)
  - Tachycardia (>160 beats/min)
  - Bradycardia (<110 beats/min)
  - Late decelerations (a drop in fetal heart rate of 15 to 45 beats/min after the contraction)
  - Variable decelerations, caused by compression of the umbilical cord
  - Sinusoidal pattern (repetitive undulation of baseline)
  (Fetal hypoxia, maternal drugs, maternal anemia, or dysrhythmias can cause changes in fetal heart rate [Merenstein & Gardner, 1998].)
- If tachycardia occurs, assess
  - Maternal temperature *(Fetal tachycardia occurs when maternal core temperature rises. It may increase before the mother's temperature can be measured orally or rectally.)*
  - Maternal intake, output, and urine specific gravity *(Maternal dehydration can cause fetal tachycardia.)*
  - Maternal anxiety level *(Severe anxiety can increase fetal heart rate.)*
  - Maternal medication use *(Certain medications used by the mother can cause increased fetal heart rate [eg, atropine, ritodrine hydrochloride, scopolamine].)*
  - Increase maternal hydration *(Maternal dehydration can cause fetal tachycardia.)*
- Notify the physician or advanced practice nurse of the situation and your assessment findings.
- Position the mother on her left side. *(This position decreases occlusion of the inferior vena cava by the uterus, promoting venous return to the heart.)*
- If decreased variability occurs, evaluate possible causes, which can include:
  - Sleeping fetus
  - Effects of narcotics or sedatives
  - Fetal hypoxia
  - Maternal position
- If nonreassuring fetal heart patterns continue, notify the physician or advanced practice nurse and take the following steps:
  - Keep the mother in a left side-lying position.
  - Administer oxygen by face mask at a flow rate of 8 L/min, according to protocol. *(This increases oxygen delivery to the fetus.)*
  - Acquire a fetal scalp blood sample according to protocol. *(To evaluate fetal pH and metabolic status)*

- If fetal scalp monitoring is not immediately available, perform fetal scalp stimulation with a gloved finger. *(Immediate fetal heart rate accelerations indicate a well-oxygenated brain and fetal reserve [Merenstein & Gardner, 1998].)*
- Discontinue oxytocin infusion, if indicated, according to protocol.
- Initiate electronic fetal monitoring according to protocol, if indicated.
- Remain with the mother and partner, provide information, and give them opportunities to share concerns and fears. *(This ensures constant monitoring and also may help reduce the mother's anxiety.)*
- If the mother's condition worsens or if fetal pH is 7.2 or below, anticipate a cesarean section and assist as indicated.
- If mild variable decelerations occur, change the mother's position from supine to lateral or from one side to the other. *(Position shifts may relieve cord compression.)*
- If severe variable decelerations occur, take the following steps:
  - Notify the physician or advanced practice nurse.
  - Discontinue oxytocin infusion per protocol.
  - Perform a vaginal examination to assess for cord prolapse.
  - Shift the mother's position to left side lying and evaluate fetal heart rate; if not improved, turn the mother on her right side.
  - If these position changes do not improve fetal heart rate, or if cord is prolapsed, help the mother assume a knee–chest position. *(This reduces pressure on the cord and increases perfusion to the fetus.)*
  - Administer oxygen by face mask at a rate of 8 to 12 L/min, according to protocol. *(This increases oxygen delivery to the fetus.)*
  - Assess for improvement in fetal heart rate within 1 min.
- Anticipate an emergency vaginal delivery or cesarean section if the mother's condition worsens, if cord prolapse occurs, and/or if fetal pH is 7.2 or lower.

PC: POSTPARTUM HEMORRHAGE

DEFINITION

PC: Postpartum Hemorrhage: Describes a woman who is experiencing or is at high risk to experience acute blood loss greater than 500 mL within the first 24 h postpartum or occurring after 24 h and before the 6th week postpartum

High-Risk Populations

- Problematic third stage of labor
- Overdistended uterus (eg, due to hydramnios, large fetus, multiple gestation)
- Prolonged labor
- Precipitous labor
- Oxytocin induction
- Multiparity
- Maternal exhaustion
- Instrument delivery
- History of uterine atony
- Uterine fibroids
- Prior postpartum hemorrhage
- Excessive analgesic or anesthesia use

- Pregnancy-associated hypertension
- Retained placental fragments
- Maternal systemic disease (leukemia, thrombocytopenia, blood dyscrasia)

Nursing Goals

The nurse will manage and minimize postpartum bleeding.

General Interventions and Rationales

- Assess the uterine fundus every 5 min for the first hour postpartum and PRN thereafter for the first 24 h; evaluate:
  - Height (normally should be at the level of the umbilicus after delivery)
  - Size (when contracted, should be about the size of an apple)
  - Consistency (should feel firm)
  (A boggy or relaxed uterus will not control bleeding by compression of the uterine muscle fibers.)
- If the uterus is relaxed or relaxing, massage it with firm but gentle circular strokes until it contracts. *(Massage stimulates the uterine muscle to contract.)*
- Avoid routine massage or overmassaging the uterus. *(Unnecessary massage can cause pain and muscle fatigue, with subsequent uterine relaxation.)*
- Monitor blood pressure and pulse every 15 min for 1 h, then every 30 min for the next hour, and then once every hour until the mother's condition stabilizes. *(Careful vital sign monitoring provides accurate evaluation of hemodynamic status.)*
- Monitor perineal blood loss. Keep a record of the number of pads used and the amount of saturation. *(Continuous seepage of blood with a firm uterus can indicate cervical or vaginal lacerations. Bleeding after the first 24 h can indicate retained placental fragments or subinvolution.)*
- Obtain hemoglobin and hematocrit levels. Report a decrease to the physician or midwife. *(A decrease in the hemoglobin value of 1.0 to 1.5 g/dL and a four-point drop in hematocrit indicate a blood loss of 450 to 500 mL.)*
- Monitor bladder size and urine output with the same frequency as for vital signs. *(A distended bladder can displace the uterus and increase uterine atony.)*
- If bleeding becomes excessive, if the uterus fails to contract, or if vital sign changes occur, notify the physician or advanced practice nurse.
- If the woman exhibits signs of shock, refer to *PC: Hypovolemic Shock* for nursing interventions.

Potential Complication: Medication Therapy Adverse Effects
PC: Anticoagulant Therapy Adverse Effects
PC: Antianxiety Therapy Adverse Effects
PC: Adrenocorticosteroid Therapy Adverse Effects
PC: Antineoplastic Therapy Adverse Effects
PC: Anticonvulsant Therapy Adverse Effects
PC: Antidepressant Therapy Adverse Effects
PC: Antiarrhythmic Therapy Adverse Effects
PC: Antipsychotic Therapy Adverse Effects
PC: Antihypertensive Therapy Adverse Effects

POTENTIAL COMPLICATION: MEDICATION THERAPY ADVERSE EFFECTS*

DEFINITION

PC: Medication Therapy Adverse Effects: Describes a client experiencing or at high risk to experience potentially serious effects or reactions related to medication therapy

 AUTHOR'S NOTE

The nurse can use these collaborative problems to describe a client who has experienced or who is at risk for adverse effects of medication therapy. In contrast to side effects, which are troublesome and annoying but rarely serious, adverse effects are unusual, unexpected, and potentially serious reactions. Adverse drug reactions are drug-induced toxic reactions (Arcangelo & Peterson, 2001). Examples of adverse effects include dysrhythmias, gastric ulcers, blood dyscrasias, and anaphylactic reactions; examples of side effects include drowsiness, dry mouth, nausea, and weakness. Side effects usually can be managed by changing the dose, form, route of administration, or diet, or by using preventive measures with continuation of the medication (Arcangelo & Peterson, 2001). Adverse effects may require discontinuation of the medication. A care plan will not contain a collaborative problem for every medication that the client is taking. Nurses routinely teach clients about side effects of medications and monitor for side effects as part of the standard of care for every client. These collaborative problems are indicated for clients who are at high risk for adverse effects or reactions because of the duration of the therapy, high predictability of their occurrence, the potential seriousness if they occur, and previous history of an adverse response. Students may add these collaborative problems to care plans. Practicing nurses could have access to standardized plans for *Medication Therapy Adverse Effects* for major medications.

High-Risk Populations

- Prolonged medication therapy
- History of hypersensitivity

---

*This section is intended as an overview of the nursing accountability for adverse effects of medication therapy. It is not intended to provide the reader with complete information on individual drugs, which can be found in pharmacology texts or manuals.

910

- History of adverse reactions
- High single or daily doses
- Multiple medication therapy
- Mental instability
- Hepatic insufficiency
- Renal insufficiency
- Disease or condition that increases the risk of a specific adverse response (eg, history of gastric ulcer)

PC: ANTICOAGULANT THERAPY ADVERSE EFFECTS

High-Risk Populations for Adverse Effects

- Diabetes mellitus
- Hypothyroidism
- Gastrointestinal (GI) bleeding
- Bleeding tendency
- Hyperlipidemia
- Elderly women
- Vitamin K deficiency
- Debilitation
- Congestive heart failure
- Children
- Mild hepatic or renal dysfunction
- Tuberculosis
- Pregnancy
- Immediately postpartum

Nursing Goals

The nurse will manage or assist the client and family to manage and minimize adverse effects.

General Interventions and Rationales

- Refer also to a pharmacology text for specific information on the individual drug.
- Assess for contraindications to anticoagulant therapy:
  - History of hypersensitivity
  - Wounds
  - Presence of active bleeding
  - Blood dyscrasias
  - Anticipated or recent surgery
  - GI ulcers
  - Subacute bacterial endocarditis
  - Pericarditis
  - Severe hypertension
  - Impaired renal function
  - Impaired hepatic function
  - Hemorrhagic cerebrovascular accident
  - Use of drugs that affect platelet formation (eg, salicylates, dipyridamole, nonsteroidal anti-inflammatory drugs [NSAID])

- Presence of drainage tubes
- Eclampsia
- Hemorrhagic tendencies
- Threatened abortion
- Ascorbic acid deficiency
- Spinal puncture
- Regional anesthesia
- Pregnancy (coumadin)
- Explain possible adverse effects:
  - *Systemic*
    - Hypersensitivity (fever, chills, runny nose, headache, nausea, vomiting, rash, itching, tearing)
    - Bleeding, hemorrhage
  - *Gastrointestinal*
    - Vomiting
    - Diarrhea
  - *Cardiovascular*
    - Hypertension
    - Chest pain
  - *Renal*
    - Impaired renal function
- Monitor for and reduce the severity of adverse effects.
  - Monitor laboratory results of activated partial thromboplastin time (APTT) for heparin therapy and prothrombin time (PT) and international normalized ratio (INR) for oral therapy. Report values over target for therapeutic range. *(The therapeutic range for PT is 1.3 to 1.5 × control or INR of 2.0 to 3.0 [Arcangelo & Peterson, 2001].)*
  - Monitor for signs of bleeding (eg, bleeding gums, skin bruises, dark stools, hematuria, epistaxis).
  - For a client receiving heparin therapy, have protamine sulfate available during administration. For warfarin, the antidote is vitamin K. *(Protamine sulfate is the antidote to reverse the effects of heparin.)*
  - Carefully monitor older adult clients. *(They are more sensitive to the effects of anticoagulants [Arcangelo & Peterson, 2001].)*
  - Consult with the pharmacist about medications that can potentiate (eg, antibiotics, cimetidine, salicylates, phenytoin, acetaminophen, antifungals, NSAIDS) or inhibit (eg, barbiturates, dicloxacillin, carbamazepine, nafcillin) anticoagulant action.
- Monitor for signs and symptoms of heparin-induced thrombocytopenia (fever, weakness difficulty speaking, seizures, yellowing of skin/eyes, dark or bloody urine, petechiae). *(Antibodies directed against platelet membrane are produced in the presence of heparin, causing increased platelet consumption [Arcangelo & Peterson, 2001].)*
- Reduce hematomas and bleeding at injection sites.
  - Use small-gauge needles.
  - Do not massage sites.
  - Rotate sites.
  - Use subcutaneous route.
  - Apply steady pressure for 1 to 2 min.
  (These techniques reduce the trauma to tissues and avoid highly vascular areas [eg, muscles].)
- Instruct client to avoid use of razors or to use electric razors.
- Instruct client to avoid pregnancy while on therapy. *(Warfarin is toxic to fetuses.)*
- Teach client and family how to prevent or reduce the severity of adverse effects.
  - Instruct them to monitor for and report signs of bleeding.
  - Tell them to inform physicians, dentists, and other health care providers of anticoagulant therapy before invasive procedures. *(Precautions may be needed to prevent bleeding.)*
  - Instruct them to contact physician or advanced practice nurse immediately after the onset of a fever or rash. *(These can indicate an infection or allergic response.)*
  - Tell them that it takes 2 to 10 days for PT levels to return to normal after warfarin (Coumadin) is stopped.
  - Explain that certain medications can inhibit or potentiate anticoagulant effect, and advise them to consult with a pharmacist before taking any prescribed or over-the-counter drug (eg, aspirin, antibiotics, ibuprofen, diuretics). Teach them to avoid foods high in vitamin K; such foods include turnip greens, asparagus, broccoli, watercress, cabbage, beef liver, lettuce, and green tea. *(Vitamin K decreases anticoagulant action.)*

- Teach client to avoid alcohol, which potentiates the effects of the anticoagulant if hepatic disease is also present.
- Instruct client to wear Medic-Alert identification.
- Stress the importance of regular follow-up care.
- Instruct the client and family to report the following (Porter, 2002):

• Bleeding	Dark stools
• Fever	Chills
• Sore throat, difficulty speaking	Itching Yellowing of skin or eyes
• Dark urine	Severe headache
• Mouth sores	Major illness
• New rash	Episode of fainting
• Persistent abdominal pain	

PC: ANTIANXIETY THERAPY ADVERSE EFFECTS

High-Risk Populations for Adverse Effects

- Children
- Older adults
- Impaired liver or kidney function
- Psychosis
- Depression
- Pregnancy or breast-feeding
- Severe muscle weakness
- Limited pulmonary reserves

Nursing Goals

The nurse will manage or assist the client and family to manage and minimize adverse effects.

General Interventions and Rationales

- Refer also to a pharmacology text for specific information on the individual drug.
- Assess for contraindications to antianxiety therapy:
  - Hypersensitivity
  - Impaired consciousness
  - Compromised respiratory function
  - Shock
  - Porphyria
  - History of drug or alcohol (for benzodiazepines) abuse
  - Undiagnosed neurologic disorders
  - Glaucoma, paralytic ileus, prostatic hypertrophy (for benzodiazepines)
  - Pregnancy or breast-feeding
  - Alcohol use
  - Severe, uncontrolled pain
  - Narrow-angle glaucoma

- Explain possible adverse effects:
  - *Systemic*
    - Hypersensitivity (pruritus, rash, hypotension)
    - Hair loss
    - Drug dependency
    - Sleep disturbances
  - *Cardiovascular*
    - Decreased heart rate, blood pressure
    - Transient tachycardia, bradycardia
    - Edema
  - *Central Nervous System*
    - Impaired judgment
    - Paradoxical excitement
    - Excessive drowsiness
    - Tremors
    - Dizziness
    - Slurred speech
    - Confusion
    - Dysphagia
    - Headache
  - *Respiratory*
    - Respiratory depression
  - *Hematologic*
    - Leukopenia
  - *Ophthalmic*
    - Blurred vision
  - *Genitourinary*
    - Urine retention
  - *Hepatic*
    - Jaundice
- Monitor for and reduce the severity of adverse effects.
  - Evaluate the client's mental status before drug administration. Consult the physician or advanced practice nurse if the client exhibits confusion or excessive drowsiness.
  - Evaluate the client's risk for injury; see *Risk for Injury* for more information.
  - Monitor for signs of overdose (eg, slurred speech, continued somnolence, respiratory depression, confusion).
  - Monitor for signs of tolerance (eg, increased anxiety, wakefulness).
- Teach client and family how to prevent or reduce the severity of adverse effects.
  - Instruct client never to discontinue taking the medication abruptly after long-term use. *(Abrupt cessation can cause vomiting, tremors, and convulsions.)*
  - Teach family or significant others the signs of overdose (eg, slurred speech, continued somnolence, respiratory depression, confusion).
  - Remind client and family that alcohol and other sedatives potentiate the action of the medication.
  - Instruct client to avoid driving and other hazardous activities when drowsy.
  - Discuss the possibility of drug tolerance and dependence with long-term use.
- Instruct the client and family to report the following signs or symptoms:

Slurred speech	Vivid dreams
Continued somnolence	Euphoria
Confusion	Hallucinations
Respiratory insufficiency	Sore throat
Hostility, rage	Fever
Muscle spasms	Mouth ulcers

PC: ADRENOCORTICOSTEROID THERAPY ADVERSE EFFECTS

High-Risk Populations for Adverse Effects

- Acquired immunodeficiency syndrome (AIDS)
- Thrombophlebitis
- Congestive heart failure
- Diabetes mellitus
- Hypothyroidism
- Glaucoma
- Osteoporosis
- Myasthenia gravis
- Bleeding ulcers
- Seizure disorders or mental illness
- Older adults
- Pregnancy or breast-feeding
- Severe stress, trauma, or illness

Nursing Goals

The nurse will manage or assist the client and family to manage and minimize adverse effects.

General Interventions and Rationales

- Refer also to a pharmacology text for specific information on the individual drug.
- Assess for contraindications to steroid therapy:

History of hypersensitivity	Hypertension
Active tuberculosis	Active peptic ulcer disease
Herpes	Active fungus infection
	Cardiac disease

- Explain possible adverse effects:
  - *Systemic*
    Hypersensitivity (rash, hives, hypotension, respiratory distress, anaphylaxis)
    Increased susceptibility to infection
    Acute adrenal insufficiency (response to abrupt cessation after 2 weeks of therapy)
    Hypokalemia
    Delayed wound healing
    Hypertriglyceridemia
  - *Central Nervous System*

Hallucinations	Psychosis
Headaches	Papilledema
Depression	

  - *Ophthalmic*

Glaucoma	Cataracts

  - *Cardiovascular*

Thrombophlebitis	Hypertension
Embolism	Edema
Dysrhythmias	

  - *Gastrointestinal*

Bleeding	Pancreatitis
Ulcers	

- *Musculoskeletal*

Osteoporosis	Growth retardation in children
Muscle wasting	Buffalo hump

- Monitor for adverse effects.
  - Establish baseline assessment data.

Weight	Serum potassium
Complete blood count (CBC)	Blood glucose
	Serum sodium
Blood pressure	

  - Monitor:

Weight	Blood glucose
CBC	Serum sodium
Blood pressure	Stool for guaiac
Serum potassium	

  - Report changes in monitored data.
- Teach the client and family how to prevent or reduce the severity of adverse effects.
  - Instruct to take the medication with food or milk. *(This reduces gastric distress.)*
  - Advise to weigh self daily at the same time and wearing the same clothes each time. *(Weight gain may indicate fluid retention.)*
  - Instruct to avoid people with infections. *(The client's compromised immune system increases his or her vulnerability to infection.)*
  - Advise to consult with a physician, advanced practice nurse, or pharmacist before taking any over-the-counter drugs. *(Serious drug interactions can occur.)*
  - Instruct to inform physicians, advanced practice nurse, dentists, and other health care providers of therapy before any invasive procedure. *(Precautions should be taken to prevent bleeding.)*
  - Instruct to contact the physician or advanced practice nurse if signs of infection occur.
  - Teach to take anticoagulant medication in the morning. *(This can help reduce adrenal suppression.)*
  - Instruct to wear Medic-Alert identification. *(He or she may need more medication in an emergency.)*
  - Warn never to discontinue the medication without consulting the physician or advanced practice nurse about side effects. *(Adrenal function needs a gradual return time.)*
  - Limit sodium intake to 6 g a day. *(Excess sodium will increase fluid retention.)*
  - Discuss the possible problems of weight gain and sodium retention (refer to *Imbalanced Nutrition: More Than Body Requirements* and *Excess Fluid Volume* for more information).
  - Explain possible drug-induced appearance changes (eg, moon face, hirsutism, abnormal fat distribution).
  - Encourage client to establish a system to prevent dosage omission or double dosage (eg, check sheet, prefilled daily dose containers).
  - Explain the risk for hyperglycemia. *(Steroids interfere with glucose metabolism.)*
- Instruct the client and family to report the following signs and symptoms:
  - Gastric pain
  - Darkened stool color
  - Unusual weight gain
  - Vomiting
  - Sore throat, fever
  - Adrenal insufficiency (fatigue, anorexia, palpitations, nausea, vomiting, diarrhea, weight loss, mood swings)
  - Menstrual irregularities
  - Change in vision, eye pain
  - Persistent, severe headache
  - Leg pain, cramps
  - Excessive thirst, hunger, urination
  - Diarrhea
  - Change in mental status
  - Dizziness
  - Palpitations
  - Fatigue, weakness

PC: ANTINEOPLASTIC THERAPY ADVERSE EFFECTS

High-Risk Populations for Adverse Effects

- Debilitation
- Bone marrow depression
- Malignant infiltration of kidney
- Malignant infiltration of bone marrow
- Liver dysfunction
- Renal insufficiency
- Older adult
- Children

Nursing Goals

The nurse will manage or assist the client and family to manage and minimize adverse effects.

General Interventions and Rationales

- Refer also to a pharmacology text for specific information on the individual drug.
- Assess for contraindications to antineoplastic therapy:
  - Hypersensitivity to the drug
  - Radiation therapy within the previous 4 weeks
  - Severe bone marrow depression
  - Breast-feeding
  - First trimester of pregnancy
- Explain possible adverse effects:
  - *Systemic*
    Hypersensitivity (pruritus, rash, chills, fever, difficulty breathing, anaphylaxis)
    Immunosuppression
    Alopecia
    Fever
  - *Cardiovascular*
    Congestive heart failure
    Dysrhythmias
  - *Respiratory*
    Pulmonary fibrosis
  - *Central Nervous System*

Confusion	Depression
Headaches	Dizziness
Weakness	Neurotoxicity

  - *Hematologic*

Leukopenia	Anemia
Bleeding	Hyperuricemia
Thrombocytopenia	Electrolyte imbalances
Agranulocytosis	

  - *Gastrointestinal*

Diarrhea	Enteritis
Anorexia	Intestinal ulcers
Vomiting	Paralytic ulcer
Mucositis	

- *Hepatic*
  Hepatotoxicity
- *Genitourinary / Reproductive*
  Renal failure   Decreased sperm count
  Amenorrhea   Hemorrhagic cystitis
  Sterility   Renal calculi
- Take steps to reduce extravasation of vesicant medications (agents that cause severe necrosis if they leak from blood vessels into tissue). Examples of vesicant medications are amsacrine, bisantrene, dactinomycin, dacarbazine, daunorubicin, estramustine, nitrogen mustard, plicamycin, vinblastine, vincristine, and vindesine.
- Preventive measures are as follows:
  - Avoid infusing vesicants over joints, bony prominences, tendons, neurovascular bundles, or the antecubital fossa (Goodman et al., 2001).
  - Avoid multiple punctures of the same vein within 24 h.
  - Administer the drug through a long-term venous catheter.
  - Do not administer the drug if edema is present or blood return is absent.
  - If peripheral intravenous (IV) site is used, evaluate its status and whether it is less than 24 h old.
  - Observe the infusion continuously if it is peripheral.
  - Provide infusion through a central line and check every 1 to 2 h.
  - Infuse vesicant before any other medications, even antiemetics.
- Monitor during drug infusion.
  - Assess patency of IV infusion line.
  - Observe tissue at the IV site every 30 min for the following:
    - Swelling (most common)
    - Leakage
    - Burning/pain (not always present)
    - Inflammation
    - Erythema (not seen initially)
    - Hyperpigmentation
- If extravasation occurs, take the following steps:
  - Stop administration of drug.
  - Leave needle in place.
  - Gently aspirate residual drug and blood in tubing or needle.
  - Avoid applying direct pressure on site.
  - Give antidote as ordered by physician or institutional policy.
  - If plant alkaloid extravasation, apply warm compresses 15 to 20 min q.i.d. for 24 h.
  - If anthracycline extravasation, apply ice for 15 to 20 min every 3 to 4 h for 24 to 48 h.
  - Instruct on local care:
    - Elevate limb for 48 h.
    - After 48 h, encourage to use limb normally.
- Monitor for and reduce the severity of adverse effects.
  - Document a baseline assessment of vital signs, cardiac rhythm, and weight. Monitor daily. *(This facilitates subsequent assessments for adverse reactions.)*
  - Ensure that baseline electrolyte, blood chemistry, bone marrow, and renal and hepatic function studies are done before administering the first dose. *(This enables monitoring for adverse reactions.)*
  - Ensure adequate hydration, at least 2 L/day. *(Good hydration can help prevent kidney damage from rapid destruction of cells.)*
  - Monitor for early signs of infection. *(Bone marrow suppression increases the risk of infection.)*
  - Monitor for sodium, potassium, magnesium, phosphate, and calcium imbalances. *(Electrolyte imbalances are commonly precipitated by renal injury, vomiting, and diarrhea.)*
  - Monitor for renal insufficiency: insufficient urine output, elevated specific gravity, elevated urine sodium levels. *(Certain antineoplastics have toxic effects on renal glomeruli and tubules.)*
  - Monitor for renal calculi: flank pain, nausea, vomiting, abdominal pain; refer to *PC: Renal Calculi* if it occurs. *(Rapid lysis of tumor cells can produce hyperuricemia.)*
  - Monitor for neurotoxicity: paresthesias, gait disturbance, disorientation, confusion, foot drop or wrist drop, fine motor activity disturbances. *(Some antineoplastics impair neural conduction.)*
- Teach the client and family how to prevent or reduce the severity of adverse effects.
  - Stress the importance of follow-up assessments and laboratory tests. *(This can help detect adverse effects early.)*

- Instruct to avoid crowds and people with infectious diseases. *(A client receiving antineoplastic therapy is very susceptible to infectious diseases.)*
- Teach to monitor weight and intake and output daily. *(Regular monitoring can detect adverse effects early.)*
- Instruct to consult with primary health care provider before taking any over-the-counter drugs. *(Serious drug interactions can occur.)*
- Advise to avoid vaccines. *(A compromised immune system increases the risk for onset of disease.)*
- Refer to appropriate nursing diagnoses for selected responses (eg, *Imbalanced Nutrition, Impaired Oral Mucous Membranes*).
- Instruct the client and family to report the following signs and symptoms:
  - Fever (>100°F)
  - Chills, sweating
  - Diarrhea
  - Severe cough
  - Sore throat
  - Unusual bleeding
  - Burning on urination
  - Muscle cramps
  - Flulike symptoms
  - Pain, swelling at IV site
  - Abdominal pain
  - Confusion, dizziness
  - Decreased urine output

PC: ANTICONVULSANT THERAPY ADVERSE EFFECTS

High-Risk Populations for Adverse Effects

- Hepatic insufficiency
- Renal insufficiency
- Coagulation problems
- Hyperthyroidism
- Diabetes mellitus
- Older adults
- Debilitation
- Cardiac dysfunction
- Glaucoma
- Myocardial insufficiency

Nursing Goals

The nurse will manage or assist the client and family to manage and minimize adverse effects.

General Interventions and Rationales

- Refer also to a pharmacology text for specific information on the individual drug.
- Assess for contraindications to anticonvulsant therapy (Arcangelo & Peterson, 2001):
  - Hypersensitivity

- Bone marrow depression
- Heart block, sinus bradycardia (Dilantin)
- Pregnancy
- Hepatic insufficiency (Depakote)
- Blood dyscrasias
- Respiratory obstruction
- Explain possible adverse effects:
  - *Systemic*

  | Hypersensitivity (excessive side effects, rashes) | Lupuslike reactions Folate deficiency |
  - *Central Nervous System*

Depression	Personality changes
Irritability	Tremors
Ataxia	Cognitive impairment
  - *Hematologic*

  | Leukopenia | Anemias |
  | Bone marrow suppression | Thrombocytopenia |
  - *Gastrointestinal*

  Gingival hyperplasia (with hydantoin)
  - *Hepatic*

  Hepatitis
  - *Genitourinary*

  | Albuminuria | Impotence |
  | Urine retention | Renal calculi |
- Monitor for and reduce the severity of adverse effects.
  - Document baseline information on seizures: type, frequency, usual time, presence of aura, precipitating factors.
  - Administer medication at regular intervals. *(Regular administration helps prevent fluctuating serum drug levels.)*
  - Keep a flow record of serum drug levels; report levels outside the therapeutic range. *(Seizures can occur with lower levels; higher levels can cause toxicity.)*
  - Monitor hepatic and blood count studies. *(These studies can detect blood dyscrasias and hepatic dysfunction.)*
  - Monitor for sore throat, persistent fatigue, fever, and infections. *(These signs and symptoms can indicate blood dyscrasias.)*
  - Take vital signs before and after parenteral drug administration. *(Vital signs demonstrate the drug's effect on cardiac function.)*
  - When administering the drug IV, monitor vital signs closely and give the drug slowly. *(Close monitoring can enable early detection of bradycardia, hypotension, and respiratory depression.)*
- Teach the client and family how to prevent or reduce the severity of adverse effects.
  - Stress not to alter the dosage or abruptly discontinue the medication. *(Changing the regimen can precipitate severe seizures.)*
  - Emphasize the importance of taking the medication on time, around-the-clock if needed. *(Regular administration helps maintain therapeutic drug levels.)*
  - Instruct to consult with a pharmacist before taking any medications (eg, aspirin, oral contraceptives, folic acid). *(Certain medications reduce the effects of anticonvulsants.)*
  - Stress the importance of maintaining a proper diet; encourage to consult with a physician or advanced practice nurse to determine the need for supplements. *(Some anticonvulsants interfere with vitamin and mineral absorption.)*

PC: ANTIDEPRESSANT THERAPY ADVERSE EFFECTS

High-Risk Populations for Adverse Effects

- Increased ocular pressure
- Impaired renal function
- Impaired hepatic function
- Urine retention
- Diabetes mellitus
- Seizure disorder
- Hyperthyroidism
- Parkinson's disease
- Pregnancy or breast-feeding
- Electroconvulsive therapy
- Cardiovascular disease
- Schizophrenia, psychosis
- Older adults

Nursing Goals

The nurse will manage or assist the client and family to manage and minimize adverse effects.

General Interventions and Rationales

- Refer also to a pharmacology text for specific information on the individual drug.
- Assess for contraindications to antidepressant therapy:
  - Hypersensitivity
  - Narrow-angle glaucoma
  - Acute recovery phase after myocardial infarction
  - Severe renal impairment
  - Severe hepatic impairment
  - Prostatic hypertrophy
  - Cerebrovascular disease
  - Cardiovascular disease
  - Schizophrenia (for monoamine oxidase [MAO] inhibitors)
  - Anesthesia administration within the past 1 to 2 weeks (for MAO inhibitors)
  - Hypertension (for MAO inhibitors)
  - Concomitant use of MAO inhibitors and tricyclics
  - Seizure disorder (for tricyclics)
  - Ingestion of foods containing tyramine (for MAO inhibitors)
  - Concomitant use of MAO inhibitors, sympathomimetics, narcotics, sedatives, hypnotics, barbiturates, phenothiazides, alcohol, street drugs, and antihypertensives
- Explain possible adverse effects:
  - *Systemic*
    Hypersensitivity (rash, petechiae, urticaria, photosensitivity)
    Diaphoresis
  - *Central Nervous System*

Nightmares	Tremors
Ataxia	Delusions
Seizures	Agitation

Paresthesias
Extrapyramidal
   symptoms
- *Cardiovascular*
Orthostatic
   hypotension (MAO
   inhibitors)
Hypertension crisis
   (MAO inhibitors)
- *Hematologic*
Blood dyscrasias
Bone marrow suppression
- *Gastrointestinal*
Paralytic ileus
Vomiting
Diarrhea
- *Hepatic*
Hepatotoxicity
- *Genitourinary*
Urine retention
Prostatic
   hypertrophy
Acute renal failure
- *Endocrine*
Altered blood glucose levels

Hypomania
Confusion
Hallucinations

Tachycardia
Dysrhythmias (MAO inhibitors)

Impotence
Nocturia
Priapism (MAO inhibitors)

- Monitor for and reduce the severity of adverse effects.
- Consult with a pharmacist regarding potential interactions with the client's other medications. *(MAO inhibitors cause many adverse interactions.)*
- Document baseline pulse, cardiac rhythm, and blood pressure. *(Antidepressants can seriously affect cardiac function; baseline assessment enables accurate monitoring during drug therapy.)*
- Ensure that baseline blood, renal, and hepatic function studies are done. *(Baseline values allow monitoring for changes.)*
- Record signs and symptoms of depression before initiating therapy. *(This information facilitates evaluation of the client's response to therapy.)*
- Monitor weight and intake and output, and assess for edema. *(Some antidepressants can cause fluid retention and anorexia.)*
- Teach the client and family how to prevent or reduce the severity of adverse effects.
- Stress that alcohol potentiates medication effects.
- Instruct the client to consult a pharmacist before taking any over-the-counter drugs. *(Many medications interact with antidepressants.)*
- Warn the client not to adjust dosage or discontinue medication without consulting a physician or nurse.
- For a client taking an MAO inhibitor, stress the importance of avoiding certain foods containing tyramine, such as avocados, bananas, fava beans, raisins, figs, aged cheeses, sour cream, red wines, sherry, beer, yeast, yogurt, pickled herring, chicken liver, aged meats, fermented sausages, chocolate, caffeine, soy sauce, licorice. *(These foods have a pressor effect, which may cause a hypertensive reaction.)*
- Instruct the client to continue to avoid hazardous foods and medications for several weeks after the medication is discontinued. *(MAO enzyme regeneration takes several weeks.)*
- Advise family members to watch for and report signs of hypomania or exaggerated symptoms in the client.
- Explain that MAO inhibitors must be discontinued 1 week before anesthesia administration. *(MAO inhibitors can have serious interactions with anesthetics and narcotics.)*
- For diaphoresis-related electrolyte depletion associated with selective serotonin reuptake inhibitors, instruct to:
  - Avoid caffeine.
  - Avoid activity in hot weather.
  - Drink 8 oz of fluids with electrolytes every 30 min.
- Instruct the client to report the following signs and symptoms:
  - Hypertensive reaction (headache, neck stiffness, palpitations, sweating, nausea, photophobia)

- Visual disturbances
- Yellowed skin or eyes
- Rash
- Abdominal pain
- Pruritus
- Urinary problems
- Seizures
- Changes in mental status

PC: ANTIARRHYTHMIC THERAPY ADVERSE EFFECTS

High-Risk Populations for Adverse Effects

- Hypertension
- Diabetes mellitus
- Children
- Older adults
- Impaired hepatic function
- Impaired renal function
- Cardiomegaly
- Pulmonary pathology
- Thyrotoxicosis
- Peripheral vascular disease
- Atrioventricular conduction abnormalities
- Congestive heart failure
- Hypotension
- Digitalis intoxication
- Potassium imbalance

Nursing Goals

The nurse will manage or assist the client and family to manage and minimize adverse effects.

General Interventions and Rationales

- Refer also to a pharmacology text for specific information on the individual drug.
- Assess for contraindications to antiarrhythmic therapy: (Arcangelo & Peterson, 2001)

  Hypersensitivity
  Ventricular fibrillation (digoxin)
  Thrombocytopenia purpura

  Myasthenia gravis
  Cardiac, renal, or hepatic failure
  Heart block (diltiazem, metoprolol, propranolol)
  Ventricular tachycardia (digoxin)
- Explain possible adverse effects:
  - *Systemic*
    Hypersensitivity (rash, difficulty breathing, heightened side effects)
    Lupuslike reaction

- *Cardiovascular*
  Worsening or new dysrhythmia
  Hypotension
  Cardiotoxicity (widened QRS complex >25%, ventricular extrasystoles, absent P waves)
- *Central Nervous System*
  Dizziness
  Apprehension
- *Hematologic*
  Agranulocytosis
- Monitor for and reduce the severity of adverse effects.
  - Establish a baseline assessment of blood pressure, heart rate, respiratory rate, peripheral pulses, lung sounds, and intake and output. *(Baseline assessment facilitates evaluation for adverse reactions to drug therapy.)*
  - Report any electrolyte imbalance, acid–base imbalance, or oxygenation problems. *(Dysrhythmias are aggravated by these conditions.)*
  - Withhold the dose and consult the physician or advanced practice nurse if the client experiences a significant drop in blood pressure, bradycardia, worsening dysrhythmia, or a new dysrhythmia after receiving the medication. *(These signs may indicate an adverse reaction.)*
  - During parenteral administration, have emergency drugs (eg, vasopressors, cardiac glycosides, diuretics) available and resuscitation equipment on hand; use microdrip infusion equipment to ensure close regulation of IV flow rate.
- Teach the client and family how to prevent or reduce the severity of adverse effects.
  - Stress the importance of ongoing follow-up with the primary health care provider.
  - Emphasize the need to take the medication on time and to avoid "doubling up" on doses. *(A regular schedule prevents toxic blood levels.)*
  - Instruct to take the medication with food. *(This can help minimize GI distress.)*
  - Teach to monitor pulse and blood pressure daily. *(Careful monitoring can detect early signs of adverse effects.)*
  - Advise to consult a pharmacist before taking any over-the-counter drugs. *(Possible drug interactions may alter cardiac stability.)*
- Instruct the client and family to report the following signs and symptoms:
  - Dizziness, faintness
  - Palpitations
  - Visual disturbances
  - Hallucinations
  - Confusion
  - Headache
  - 1- to 2-lb weight gain
  - Coldness and numbness in extremities

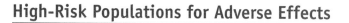

PC: ANTIPSYCHOTIC THERAPY ADVERSE EFFECTS

High-Risk Populations for Adverse Effects

- Glaucoma
- Prosthetic hypertrophy
- Epilepsy
- Diabetes mellitus
- Severe hypertension
- Ulcers

- Cardiovascular disease
- Chronic respiratory disorders
- Hepatic insufficiency
- Pregnancy or breast-feeding
- Exposure to extreme heat, phosphorus insecticides, or pesticides

Nursing Goals

The nurse will manage or assist the client and family to manage and minimize adverse effects.

General Interventions and Rationales

- Refer also to a pharmacology text for specific information on the individual drug.
- Assess for contraindications to antipsychotic therapy:
  - Bone marrow suppression
  - Blood dyscrasias
  - Parkinson's disease
  - Hepatic insufficiency
  - Renal insufficiency
  - Cerebral arteriosclerosis
  - Coronary artery disease
  - Circulatory collapse
  - Mitral insufficiency
  - Severe hypotension
  - Alcoholism, drug abuse
  - Subcortical brain damage
  - Comatose states
- Explain possible adverse effects:
  - *Systemic*
    Hypersensitivity (rash, abdominal pain, jaundice, blood dyscrasias)
    Photosensitivity
    Fever
  - *Cardiovascular*
    Hypertension   Orthostatic hypotension
    Palpitations
  - *Central Nervous System*
    Extrapyramidal (acute dystonia, akathisia, pseudoparkinsonism)
    Hyperreflexia   Tardive dyskinesia
    Cerebral edema   Neuroleptic malignant syndrome
    Sleep disturbances   Bizarre dreams
  - *Gastrointestinal*
    Constipation
    Paralytic ileus
    Fecal impaction
  - *Hematologic*
    Agranulocytosis   Thrombocytopenia
    Leukopenia   Purpura
    Leukocytosis   Pancytopenia
    Anemias
  - *Ophthalmic*
    Ptosis   Lens opacities
    Pigmentary retinopathy
  - *Respiratory*
    Laryngospasm   Dyspnea
    Bronchospasm
  - *Genitourinary*
    Urine retention   Incontinence
    Enuresis   Impotence

- *Endocrine*

Gynecomastia	Glycosuria
Altered libido	Hyperglycemia
Amenorrhea	

- Monitor for and reduce the severity of adverse effects.

  Document a baseline assessment of blood pressure (sitting, standing, and lying), pulse, and temperature. *(Baseline assessment facilitates monitoring for adverse reactions.)*

  Ensure that baseline bone marrow, renal, and hepatic function studies are done before administering the first dose. *(Results of these studies enable monitoring for changes.)*

  After parenteral administration, keep the client flat and monitor blood pressure. *(These measures help reduce hypotensive effects.)*

  Monitor blood pressure during initial treatment. *(Blood pressure monitoring detects early hypotensive effects.)*

  Assess bowel and bladder functioning. *(Anticholinergic and antiadrenergic effects decrease sensory stimulation to the bowel and bladder.)*

  Observe for fine, wormlike movements of the tongue. *(Early detection of tardive dyskinesia enables prompt intervention and possible reversal of its course.)*

  Monitor for acute dystonic reactions, neck spasms, eye rolling, dysphagia, convulsions. *(Early detection of these signs may indicate the need for dose reduction.)*

  Ensure optimal hydration; evaluate urine specific gravity regularly. *(Dehydration increases susceptibility to dystonic reactions.)*

  Monitor for signs and symptoms of blood dyscrasias: decreased white cells, platelets, and red cells; sore throat; fever; malaise. *(Antipsychotic medication can cause bone marrow suppression.)*

  Monitor weight. *(Antipsychotic medication can cause hypothyroidism, commonly marked by weight gain.)*

  Monitor for neuroleptic malignant syndrome; refer to *PC: Neuroleptic Malignant Syndrome* for interventions. *(Neuroleptic malignant syndrome is a potentially dangerous adverse effect of antipsychotic drug therapy.)*

- Teach the client and family how to prevent or reduce the severity of adverse effects.

  - Instruct to consult a pharmacist before taking any over-the-counter drugs. *(Serious drug interactions can occur with various over-the-counter medications.)*
  - Stress the need to continue the medication regimen as prescribed and never abruptly stop taking it. *(Abrupt cessation can cause vomiting, tremors, and psychotic behavior.)*
  - Caution the client to protect himself from sun exposure with clothing, hat, sunglasses, and sunscreen. *(Photosensitivity is a common side effect of antipsychotic therapy.)*
  - Warn against using alcohol, barbiturates, or sedatives. *(Their effects are potentiated in combination with antipsychotic medication.)*

- Instruct the client and family to report the following signs and symptoms:

Urine retention	Fine, wormlike tongue movements
Visual disturbances	Neck spasms
Fever	Dysphagia
Sore throat	Eye rolling
Signs of infection	Involuntary chewing, puckering
Tremors	Puffing movements
Abdominal pain	

PC: ANTIHYPERTENSIVE THERAPY ADVERSE EFFECTS

- β-Adrenergic Blocker Therapy Adverse Effects
- Calcium Channel Blocker Therapy Adverse Effects
- Angiotensin-Converting Enzyme Inhibitor Therapy Adverse Effects

> ## 🔗 AUTHOR'S NOTE
>
> Antihypertensive medications are classified into nine groups: central adrenergic agents, ganglionic blockers, peripherally acting catecholamine depleters, α-adrenergic blockers, calcium channel blockers, β-adrenergic blockers, vascular smooth muscle relaxants, angiotensin-converting enzymes, and diuretics. Because their sites of action differ greatly, it is not useful to present a generic collaborative problem of *PC: Antihypertensive Therapy Adverse Effects*. Instead, three classifications are addressed: β-adrenergic blockers, calcium channel blockers, and angiotensin-converting enzymes. For information on other classifications, consult a pharmacology text.

PC: β-ADRENERGIC BLOCKER THERAPY ADVERSE EFFECTS

High-Risk Populations for Adverse Effects

- Diabetes mellitus
- Severe liver disease
- Pregnancy or breast-feeding
- Chronic bronchitis, emphysema
- Peripheral vascular insufficiency
- Allergic rhinitis
- Renal insufficiency
- Hepatic insufficiency
- Myasthenia gravis

Nursing Goals

The nurse will manage or assist the client and family to manage and minimize adverse effects.

General Interventions and Rationales

- Refer also to a pharmacology text for specific information on the individual drug.

- Assess for contraindications to β-adrenergic blockers (Arcangelo & Peterson, 2001):
  - Hypersensitivity
  - Sinus bradycardia
  - Second- or third-degree heart block
  - PR interval greater than 0.24 s on electrocardiogram (ECG)
  - Heart (except carvedilol, metoprolol)
  - Cardiogenic shock
  - MAO inhibitor or tricyclic antidepressant therapy
  - Asthma (for nonselective β-adrenergic blockers)
  - Diabetes
  - Hyperlipidemia
  - Peripheral
  - Arterial insufficiency
  - Pregnancy 1st trimester
- Explain possible adverse effects:
  - *Systemic*
    Hypersensitivity (rash, pruritus)
    Increased triglycerides
    Decreased high-density lipoproteins (HDL)
  - *Central Nervous System*

Depression	Memory loss
Paresthesias	Bizarre dreams
Insomnia	Hallucinations
Behavior changes	Catatonia
Vertigo	

  - *Cardiovascular*

Bradycardia	Cerebrovascular accident
Edema	Tachycardia
Hypotension	Peripheral arterial insufficiency
Congestive heart failure	

  - *Hematologic*
    Agranulocytosis
    Thrombocytopenia
    Eosinophilia
  - *Gastrointestinal*

Diarrhea	Vomiting
Ischemic colitis	Gastric pain

  - *Hepatic*
    Hepatomegaly
  - *Respiratory*

Bronchospasm	Dyspnea
Rales	

  - *Endocrine*
    Hypoglycemia or hyperglycemia
  - *Genitourinary*
    Difficulty urinating
    Elevated blood urea nitrogen and serum transaminase
- *Ophthalmic*
  Blurred vision
- Monitor for and reduce the severity of adverse effects.
  - Establish a baseline assessment of pulse, blood pressure (lying, sitting, standing), lung fields, and peripheral pulses. *(Baseline assessment facilitates monitoring for adverse reactions.)*
  - Ensure that baseline renal, hepatic, glucose, and blood studies are done before drug therapy begins. *(Results of these studies enable monitoring for changes.)*
  - Establish with the physician or advanced practice nurse the parameters (blood pressure, pulse) that call for withholding the medication. *(Hypotension and bradycardia can reduce cardiac output.)*
  - Monitor intake, output, and weight and assess for edema. *(Reduced cardiac output can cause fluid accumulation.)*
  - Monitor for congestive heart failure. *(β-Adrenergic blockers can compromise cardiac function.)*

- Monitor for hypoglycemia in a client with diabetes. *(β-Adrenergic blockers interfere with the conversion of glycogen to glucose by occupying β-adrenergic receptor sites.)*
- Teach the client how to prevent or reduce the severity of adverse effects.
  - Stress the importance of continuing the medication regimen as prescribed, and warn client never to discontinue the drug abruptly. *(Abrupt cessation may precipitate dysrhythmias or angina.)*
  - Emphasize the need to monitor pulse and blood pressure daily. Explain the pulse and blood pressure values that indicate the need to withhold the medication.
  - Instruct to weigh self daily, at the same time each day and wearing the same clothes every time; tell client to report any weight gain of 1 lb or more. *(Weight gain may indicate fluid retention resulting from decreased cardiac output.)*
  - Explain the need to protect hands and feet from prolonged exposure to cold. *(β-Adrenergic blockers decrease circulation in the skin and extremities.)*
  - Instruct to consult with primary health care provider before exercising. *(The medication impedes the body's adaptive response to stress.)*
  - Stress the importance of follow-up laboratory tests. *(Significant abnormalities in liver or renal function studies and blood count may be seen.)*
- Instruct the client and family to report the following signs and symptoms:
  - To 2-lb weight gain
  - Edema
  - Difficulty breathing
  - Pulse or blood pressure above or below pre-established parameters
  - Dark urine
  - Difficult urination
  - Visual disturbances
  - Sore throat
  - Fever
  - Sleep disturbances
  - Memory loss
  - Mental changes
  - Behavioral changes

PC: CALCIUM CHANNEL BLOCKER THERAPY ADVERSE EFFECTS

High-Risk Populations for Adverse Effects

- Renal insufficiency
- Hepatic insufficiency
- Hypotension
- Decreased left ventricular function
- Pregnancy or breast-feeding
- Digitalis therapy
- β-Adrenergic blocker therapy

Nursing Goals

The nurse will manage or assist the client and family to manage and minimize adverse effects.

General Interventions and Rationales

- Refer also to a pharmacology text for specific information on the individual drug.
- Assess for contraindications to calcium channel blocker therapy:
  - Severe left ventricular dysfunction
  - Sick sinus syndrome
  - Second- or third-degree heart block
  - Cardiogenic shock
  - Acute myocardial infarction (with diltiazem)
  - IV use of verapamil and β-adrenergic blockers
  - Symptomatic hypotension
  - Advanced congestive heart failure
- Explain possible adverse effects:
  - *Systemic*
    Hypersensitivity (rash, pruritus, extreme hypotension)
    Hair loss
    Sweating, chills
  - *Central Nervous System*

Tremors	Insomnia
Confusion	Headache
Mood changes	

  - *Cardiovascular*

Palpitations	Heart failure
Myocardial	Bradycardia
infarction	Third-degree heart block (with verapamil)
Hypotension	

  - *Gastrointestinal*

Diarrhea	Cramping

  - *Hepatic*
    Elevated liver enzymes
  - *Respiratory*

Dyspnea	Pulmonary edema
Wheezing	

  - *Musculoskeletal*

Muscle cramping	Inflammation
Joint stiffness	

  - *Genitourinary*

Impotence	Menstrual irregularities

- Monitor for and reduce the severity of adverse effects.
  - Establish a baseline assessment of pulse, blood pressure, cardiac rhythm, and lung fields. *(Baseline data facilitate detection of adverse reactions.)*
  - Ensure that baseline hepatic function studies are performed before starting drug therapy. *(Calcium channel blockers can cause liver enzyme elevation.)*
  - Carefully monitor blood pressure and heart rate during initial stages of therapy. *(Bradycardia and hypotension may occur.)*
  - Monitor for congestive heart failure. *(Decreased cardiac output can compromise heart function.)*
  - Establish with the physician or advanced practice nurse the parameters (blood pressure, pulse) for withholding the medication. *(Hypotension and bradycardia can reduce cardiac output.)*
  - Monitor intake and output and weight, and assess for edema. *(Reduced cardiac output can cause fluid accumulation.)*
- Teach the client and family how to prevent or reduce the severity of adverse effects. Refer to *PC: β-Adrenergic Blocker Therapy Adverse Effects* for specific interventions.
- Instruct the client and family to report the following signs and symptoms:
  - 1- to 2-lb weight gain
  - Edema
  - Difficulty breathing
  - Pulse or blood pressure above or below pre-established parameters
  - Sleep disturbances
  - Mental changes
- Instruct not to stop or miss medication doses. *(Withdrawal hypertension can occur.)*
- Instruct not to chew, divide, or crush. *(Medication will be absorbed too quickly.)*

PC: ANGIOTENSIN-CONVERTING ENZYME INHIBITOR THERAPY ADVERSE EFFECTS

High-Risk Populations for Adverse Effects

- Severe renal dysfunction
- Systemic lupuslike syndrome
- Reduced white blood cell count
- Valvular stenosis
- Diabetes mellitus
- Pregnancy or breast-feeding
- Autoimmune disease (for captopril)
- Coronary disease (for captopril)
- Cerebrovascular disease (for captopril)
- Medication therapy that causes leukopenia or agranulocytosis
- Collagen vascular disease (for enalapril)

Nursing Goals

The nurse will manage or assist the client and family to manage and minimize adverse effects.

General Interventions and Rationales

- Refer also to a pharmacology text for specific information on the individual drug.
- Assess for contraindications to angiotensin-converting enzyme inhibitor therapy:
  - History of adverse effects
  - Renal stenosis (bilateral, unilateral)
  - Previous hypersensitivity
  - Pregnancy
- Explain possible adverse effects:
  - *Systemic*
    Hypersensitivity (urticaria; rash; angioedema of face, throat, and extremities; difficulty breathing; stridor)
    Photosensitivity
    Alopecia
  - *Central Nervous System*
    Vertigo   Insomnia
    Fainting   Headache
  - *Cardiovascular*
    Tachycardia   Angina pectoris
    Congestive heart   Chest pain
      failure   Palpitations
    Hypotension   Flushing
    Pericarditis   Raynaud's disease
  - *Gastrointestinal*
    Loss of taste   Diarrhea
    Vomiting   Peptic ulcer
    Anorexia
  - *Hematologic*
    Neutropenia   Eosinophilia
    Agranulocytosis Hyperkalemia
    Hemolytic anemia

- *Musculoskeletal*
  Joint pain
- *Genitourinary*
  Proteinuria   Urinary frequency
  Polyuria   Renal insufficiency
  Oliguria
- *Respiratory*
  Cough
- Monitor for and reduce the severity of adverse effects.
  - Establish a baseline assessment of pulse, blood pressure (lying, sitting, and standing), cardiac rhythm, and lung fields. *(Baseline assessment data are vital to evaluating response to therapy and identifying adverse reactions.)*
  - Ensure that baseline electrolyte, blood, and renal and hepatic function studies are performed. *(The medication can cause liver enzyme elevation and hypokalemia.)*
  - Carefully monitor blood pressure and heart rate during initial stages of therapy. *(Bradycardia and hypotension may occur.)*
  - Monitor for congestive heart failure. *(Decreased cardiac output can compromise heart function.)*
  - Establish with the physician or advanced practice nurse the parameters (blood pressure, pulse) for withholding the medication. *(Hypotension and bradycardia can reduce cardiac output.)*
  - Monitor intake and output and weight, and assess for edema. *(Reduced cardiac output can cause fluid accumulation.)*
- Teach the client and family how to prevent or reduce the severity of adverse effects.
  - Refer to *PC: β-Adrenergic Blocker Therapy Adverse Effects.*
  - Stress the importance of follow-up laboratory tests. *(Significant abnormalities in urinary protein and blood counts can occur.)*
- Instruct the client and family to report the following signs and symptoms:
  - 1- to 2-lb weight gain
  - Edema
  - Difficulty breathing
  - Pulse or blood pressure above or below pre-established parameters
  - Dark urine
  - Difficult urination
  - Visual disturbances
  - Sore throat
  - Fever
  - Sleep disturbances
  - Memory loss
  - Mental changes
  - Behavioral changes

NURSING DIAGNOSES GROUPED UNDER
FUNCTIONAL HEALTH PATTERNS*

1. *Health Perception–Health Management*
   Falls, Risk for
   Growth and Development, Delayed
      Adult Failure to Thrive
      Growth, Risk for Altered
      Development, Risk for Altered
   Health Maintenance, Impaired
      †Surgical Recovery, Delayed
   Health-Seeking Behaviors
   Lifestyle, Sedentary
   Effective Therapeutic
      Regimen
   Ineffective Therapeutic
      Regimen

   Ineffective Therapeutic
      Regimen:
      Community
   Ineffective Therapeutic
      Regimen: Family
   †Management of Therapeutic Regimen,
      Readiness for Enhanced
   Noncompliance
   Risk for Injury
      Risk for Suffocation
      Risk for Poisoning
      Risk for Trauma
   Injury, Risk for
      Perioperative Positioning
      †Wandering
   †Sudden Infant Death Syndrome, Risk for

2. *Nutritional–Metabolic*
   Body Temperature, Risk for Imbalanced
      Hypothermia
      Hyperthermia
      Thermoregulation, Ineffective
   Deficient Fluid Volume
   Excess Fluid Volume
   Deficient Fluid Volume, Risk for
   †Fluid Balance, Readiness for Enhanced
   Infection, Risk for
   ‡Infection Transmission, Risk for
   Latex Allergy
   Latex Allergy, Risk for
   Nutrition, Imbalanced: Less Than Body
      Requirements
      Breastfeeding, Effective

   Breastfeeding, Ineffective
   Breastfeeding, Interrupted
   Dentition, Impaired
   Feeding Pattern, Ineffective Infant
   Swallowing, Impaired
   Nutrition, Imbalanced: More Than Body
      Requirements
   Nutrition, Imbalanced: Risk for More Than
      Body Requirements
   †Nutrition, Readiness for Enhanced
   Protection, Ineffective
      Tissue Integrity, Impaired
         Oral Mucous Membrane, Altered
         Skin Integrity, Impaired

3. *Elimination*
   Constipation
   Constipation, Risk for
   Perceived Constipation
   Diarrhea
   Bowel Incontinence
   Urinary Elimination, Impaired
   †Urinary Elimination, Readiness
      for Enhanced

   Urinary Retention
   Total Urinary Incontinence
   Functional Urinary Incontinence
   Reflex Urinary Incontinence
   Urge Urinary Incontinence
   Urge Urinary Incontinence, Risk for
   Stress Urinary Incontinence
   ‡Maturational Enuresis

---

*The Functional Health Patterns were identified in Gordon, M. (1982). *Nursing diagnosis: Process and application.*
New York: McGraw-Hill, with minor changes by the author.
†These diagnoses were accepted by the North American Nursing Diagnosis Association in 2003.
‡These diagnoses are not currently on the NANDA list but have been included for clarity and usefulness.

4. *Activity–Exercise*
Activity Intolerance
Adaptive Capacity, Intracranial Decreased
Cardiac Output, Decreased
Disuse Syndrome
Deficient Diversional Activity
Home Maintenance, Impaired
Infant Behavior, Disorganized
Infant Behavior, Risk for Disorganized
Infant Behavior, Readiness for Enhanced
    Organized
Mobility, Impaired Physical
    Bed Mobility, Impaired
    Walking, Impaired
    Wheelchair Mobility, Impaired
    Wheelchair Transfer Ability, Impaired

Peripheral Neurovascular Dysfunction, Risk for
‡Respiratory Function, Risk for Impaired
    Dysfunctional Ventilatory Weaning Response
    Ineffective Airway Clearance
    Ineffective Breathing Patterns
    Impaired Gas Exchange
    Ventilation, Inability to Sustain Spontaneous
‡Self-Care Deficit Syndrome (Specify):
    (‡Instrumental, Feeding, Bathing/Hygiene,
    Dressing/Grooming, Toileting)
Tissue Perfusion, Ineffective (Specify Type):
    (Cerebral, Cardiopulmonary, Renal,
    Gastrointestinal, Peripheral)

5. *Sleep–Rest*
Disturbed Sleep Pattern
    Sleep Deprivation
†Sleep, Readiness for Enhanced

6. *Cognitive–Perceptual*
Comfort, Impaired
    Acute Pain
    Chronic Pain
    Nausea
Confusion
    Acute Confusion
    Chronic Confusion
Decisional Conflict
Dysreflexia
Dysreflexia, Risk for Autonomic
Environmental Interpretation Syndrome,
    Impaired

Deficient Knowledge (specify)
†Knowledge, Readiness for Enhanced (specify)
Risk for Aspiration
Disturbed Sensory Perception: (Specify):
    (Visual, Auditory, Kinesthetic, Gustatory,
    Tactile, Olfactory)
Thought Processes, Disturbed Memory,
    Impaired
Unilateral Neglect

7. *Self-Perception*
Anxiety
    Death Anxiety
Fatigue
Fear
Hopelessness
Powerlessness
Powerlessness, Risk for

‡Disturbed Self-Concept
    Disturbed Body Image
    Disturbed Personal Identity
        Disturbed Self-Esteem
            Chronic Low Self-Esteem
            Situational Low Self-Esteem
            Situational Low Self-Esteem, Risk for
†Self-Concept, Readiness for Enhanced

8. *Role–Relationship*
‡Communication, Impaired
    Communication, Impaired Verbal
†Communication, Readiness for Enhanced
Family Processes, Interrupted
    Family Processes, Dysfunctional:
    Alcoholism
†Family Processes, Readiness for Enhanced
‡Grieving
    Grieving, Anticipatory
    Grieving, Dysfunctional
    †Chronic Sorrow

Loneliness, Risk for
Parent–Infant Attachment, Risk for Impaired
Parenting, Impaired
†Parenting, Readiness for Enhanced
Parental Role Conflict
Role Performance, Ineffective
Social Interaction, Impaired
Social Isolation

†These diagnoses were accepted by the North American Nursing Diagnosis Association in 2003.
‡These diagnoses are not currently on the NANDA list but have been included for clarity and usefulness.

9. *Sexuality–Reproductive*
   Sexual Dysfunction
   Sexuality Patterns, Altered

10. *Coping–Stress Tolerance*
    Adjustment, Impaired
    Caregiver Role Strain
    Coping, Ineffective
      Defensive Coping
      Ineffective Denial
    Coping: Compromised, Family
    Coping: Readiness for Enhanced Family
    Coping: Ineffective Community

    †Coping, Readiness for Enhanced
    Coping, Readiness for Enhanced Community
    Disabled Family Coping
    Disturbed Energy Field
    Post-trauma Response
      Rape Trauma Syndrome
    Post-trauma Syndrome, Risk for
    Relocation Stress Syndrome
    Relocation Stress Syndrome, Risk for
    ‡Self-Harm, Risk for
      Self-Abuse, Risk for
      Self-Mutilation
      Self-Mutilation, Risk for
    Suicide, Risk for
    Violence, Risk for

11. *Value–Belief*
    Spiritual Distress
    Spiritual Distress, Risk for
    Spiritual Well-Being, Readiness for
        Enhanced
      Religiosity, Impaired
      Religiosity, Risk for Impaired

---

†These diagnoses were accepted by the North American Nursing Diagnosis Association in 2003.
‡These diagnoses are not currently on the NANDA list but have been included for clarity and usefulness.

HEALTH-PROMOTION/WELLNESS DIAGNOSES

NANDA International's Diagnostic Review Process in 2002–2003 resulted in twelve new nursing diagnoses. Three diagnoses—*Nausea, Risk for Sudden Infant Death Syndrome,* and *Readiness for Enhanced Family Coping*—are found in the main body of this text. Nine of the diagnoses are health-promotion/wellness diagnoses and are contained in this appendix.

There is still considerable debate regarding the clinical usefulness of this type of diagnosis. This author takes the position that some of these health states can be strengthened and are clinically useful, for example, *Readiness for Enhanced Parenting.* Others are questionable to be clinically useful, for example, *Readiness for Enhanced Fluid Balance, Readiness for Enhanced Urinary Elimination,* and other similar diagnoses. If a person has a pattern of equilibrium between fluid volume and the chemical composition of body fluids that is sufficient for meeting physical needs, how can this be strengthened? Is this not an assessment conclusion? Given the multiple needs of clients, is this a reasonable use of nursing resources? In contrast, *Readiness for Enhanced Parenting* describes family functioning that is sufficient to support the well-being of family members. This could be strengthened.

Clinically, data that represent strengths can be important for nurses to know. These strengths can assist the nurse in selecting interventions to reduce or prevent a problem in another health pattern. If nurses want to designate a strength, delete "Readiness for" and use "Enhanced (insert pattern)." If the client desires assistance in promoting a higher level of function, "Readiness for Enhanced (specify)" could be useful. Interested clinicians can utilize these health-promotion/wellness diagnoses and are invited to share their work with NANDA and this author.

Readiness for Enhanced Family Processes (2002, LOE 2.1)

DEFINITION

A pattern of family functioning that is sufficient to support the well-being of family members and can be strengthened

DEFINING CHARACTERISTICS

- Expresses willingness to enhance family dynamics
- Family functioning meets physical, social, and psychological needs of family members
- Activities support the safety and growth of family members
- Communication is adequate
- Relationships are generally positive; interdependent with community; family task are accomplished
- Family roles are flexible and appropriate for developmental stages
- Respect for family members is evident
- Family adapts to change
- Boundaries of family members are maintained
- Energy level of family supports activities of daily living
- Family resilience is evident
- Balance exists between autonomy and cohesiveness

References

Bryan, A. A. (2000). Enhancing parent-child interaction with a prenatal couple intervention. *The American Journal of Maternal/Child Nursing, 25*(3), 139–145.

Carruth, A. K., & Tate, U. S. (1997). Reciprocity, emotional well-being, and family functioning as determinants of family satisfaction in caregivers of elderly parents. *Nursing Research, 46*(2), 93–100.

Edelman, C. L., & Mandle, C. L. (2002). Health promotion of the family [Chapter 7]. In *Health promotion throughout the lifespan* (5th ed., pp. 169–198). St. Louis, MO: Mosby.

Readiness for Enhanced Fluid Balance (2002, LOE 2.1)

DEFINITION

A pattern of equilibrium between fluid volume and chemical composition of body fluids that is sufficient for meeting physical needs and can be strengthened

DEFINING CHARACTERISTICS

- Expresses willingness to enhance fluid balance
- Stable weight
- Moist mucous membranes
- Food and fluid intake adequate for daily needs
- Straw-colored urine with specific gravity within normal limits
- Good tissue turgor
- No excessive thirst
- Urine output appropriate for intake
- No evidence of edema or dehydration

References

Dabinett, J. A., Reid, K., & James, N. (2001). Educational strategies used in increasing fluid intake and enhancing hydration status in field hockey players preparing for competition in a hot and humid environment: A case study. *International Journal of Sport Nutrition and Exercise Metabolism, 11*(3), 334–348.

Holben, D. H., Hassell, J. T., Williams, J. L., & Helle, B. (1999). Fluid intake compared with established standards and symptoms of dehydration among elderly residents of a long-term-care facility. *Journal of the American Dietetic Association, 99*(11), 1447–1450.

Kleiner, S. M. (1999). Water: An essential but overlooked nutrient. *Journal of the American Dietetic Association, 99*(2), 200–206.

Readiness for Enhanced Knowledge (Specify) (2002, LOE 2.1)

DEFINITION

The presence or acquisition of cognitive information related to a specific topic is sufficient for meeting health-related goals and can be strengthened

DEFINING CHARACTERISTICS

- Expresses an interest in learning
- Explains knowledge of the topic
- Behaviors congruent with expressed knowledge
- Describes previous experiences pertaining to the topic

References

Crosby, R. A., & Yarber, W. L. (2001). Perceived versus actual knowledge about correct condom use among U.S. adolescents: Results from a national study. *Journal of Adolescent Health, 28*(5), 415–420.

Meischke, H., Kuniyuki, A., Yasui, Y., Bowen, D. J., Anderson, R., & Urban, N. (2002). Information women receive about heart attacks and how it affects their knowledge, beliefs and intentions to act in a cardiac emergency. *Health Care for Women International, 23,* 149–162.

Taylor, K. L., Turner, R. O., Davis, J. L., Johnson, L., Schwartz, M. D., Kerner, J., & Leak, C. (2001). Improving knowledge of the prostate cancer screening dilemma among African American men: An academic-community partnership in Washington, DC. *Public Health Reports, 116*(6), 590–598.

Readiness for Enhanced Nutrition (2002, LOE 2.1)

DEFINITION

A pattern of nutrient intake that is sufficient for meeting metabolic needs and can be strengthened

DEFINING CHARACTERISTICS

- Expresses willingness to enhance nutrition
- Eats regularly
- Consumes adequate food and fluid
- Expresses knowledge of healthy food and fluid choices
- Follows an appropriate standard for intake (eg, the food pyramid or America Diabetic Association guidelines)

- Safe preparation and storage for food and fluids
- Attitude toward eating and drinking is congruent with health goals

References
Long, V. A., Martin, T., & Janson-Sand, C. (2002). The great beginnings program: Impact of a nutrition curriculum on nutrition knowledge, diet quality, and birth outcomes in pregnant and parenting teens. *Journal of the American Dietetic Association, 102*(3 Suppl. 1), S86–89.
Murphy, P. W., Davis, T. C., Mayeaux, E. J., Sentell, T., Arnold, C., & Rebouche, C. (1996). Teaching nutrition education in adult learning centers: Linking literacy, health care, and the community. *Journal of Community Health Nursing, 13*(3), 149–158.
Satia, J. A., Kristal, A. R., Curry, S., & Trudeau, E. (2001). Motivations for healthful dietary change. *Public Health Nutrition, 4*(5), 953–959.

Readiness for Enhanced Parenting (2002, LOE 2.1)

DEFINITION

A pattern of providing an environment for children or other dependent person(s) that is sufficient to nurture growth and development and can be strengthened

DEFINING CHARACTERISTICS

- Expresses willingness to enhance parenting
- Children or other dependent person(s) express satisfaction with home environment
- Emotional and tacit support of children or dependent person(s) is evident; bonding or attachment evident
- Physical and emotional needs of children/dependent person(s) are met
- Realistic expectations of children/dependent person(s) exhibited

References
Bell, R. P., & McGrath, J. M. (1996). Implementing a research-based kangaroo care program in the NICU. *Nursing Clinics of North America, 31*(2), 387–403.
Gielen, A. C., McDonald, E. M., & Wilson, M. E. (2002). Effects of improved access to safety counseling, products, and home visits on parents' safety practices: Results of a randomized trial. *Archives of Pediatric Adolescent Medicine, 156*(1), 33–45.
Long, A., McCarney, S., & Smyth, G. (2001). The effectiveness of parenting programmes facilitated by health visitors. *Journal of Advanced Nursing, 34*(5), 611–620.

Readiness for Enhanced Self-Concept (2002, LOE 2.1)

DEFINITION

A pattern of perceptions or ideas about the self that is sufficient for well-being and can be strengthened

DEFINING CHARACTERISTICS

- Expresses willingness to enhance self-concept
- Expresses satisfaction with thoughts about self, sense of worthiness, role performance, body image, and personal identity
- Actions are congruent with expressed feelings and thoughts
- Expresses confidence in abilities
- Accepts strengths and limitations

References
Carnevale, F. A. (1999). Toward a cultural conception of the self. *Journal of Psychosocial Nursing Mental Health Service, 37*(8), 26–31.
Cole, D. A., Maxwell, S. E., Martin, J. M., Peeke, L. G., Seroczynski, A. D., Tran, J. M., Hoffman, K. B., Ruiz, M. D., Jacquez, F., & Maschman, T. (2001). The development of multiple domains of child and adolescent self-concept: A cohort sequential longitudinal design. *Child Development, 72*(6), 1723–1746.
Walter, R., Davis, K., & Glass, N. (1999). Discovery of self: exploring, interconnecting and integrating self (concept) and nursing. *Collegian, 6*(2), 12–15.

Readiness for Enhanced Sleep (2002, LOE 2.1)

DEFINITION

A pattern of natural, periodic suspension of consciousness that provides adequate rest, sustains a desired lifestyle, and can be strengthened

DEFINING CHARACTERISTICS

- Expresses willingness to enhance sleep
- Amount of sleep and REM sleep is congruent with developmental needs
- Expresses a feeling of being rested after sleep
- Follows sleep routines that promote sleep habits
- Occasional or infrequent use of medications to induce sleep

References

Floyd, J. A., Falahee, M. L., & Fhobir, R. H. (2000). Creation and analysis of a computerized database of interventions to facilitate adult sleep. *Nursing Research, 49*(4), 236–241.

Mead-Bennett, E. (1990). Sleep promotion: An important dimension of maternity nursing. *Journal of National Black Nurses Association, 4*(2), 9–17.

Stockert, P. A. (2001). Sleep, health promotion. In P. A. Potter & A. G. Perry (Eds.), *Fundamentals of nursing* (5th ed., pp. 1268–1273). St. Louis, MO: Mosby.

Readiness for Enhanced Therapeutic Regimen Management (2002, LOE 2.1)

DEFINITION

A pattern of regulating and integrating into daily living a program(s) for treatment of illness and its sequelae that is sufficient for meeting health-related goals and can be strengthened

DEFINING CHARACTERISTICS

- Expresses desire to manage the treatment of illness and prevention of sequelae
- Choices of daily living are appropriate for meeting the goals of treatment or prevention
- Expresses little to no difficulty with regulation/integration of one or more prescribed regimens for treatment of illness or prevention of complications
- Describes reduction of risk factors for progression of illness and sequelae
- No unexpected acceleration of illness symptoms

References

Bakken, S., Holzemer, W. L., Brown, M., Powell-Cope, G. M., Turner, J. G., Inouye, J., Nokes, K. M., & Corless, I. B. (2000). Relationship between perception of engagement with health care provider and demographic characteristics, health status, and adherence to therapeutic regimen in persons with HIV/AIDS. *AIDS Patient Care and STDs, 14*(4), 189–197.

Dodge, J. A., Janz, N. K., & Clark, N. M. (1994). Self management of the health care regimen: A comparison of nurses' and cardiac patients' perceptions. *Patient Education and Counseling, 23*(2), 73–82.

Schumann, A., Nigg, C. R., Rossi, J. S., Jordan, P. J., Norman, G. J., Garber, C. E., Riebe, D., & Benisovich, S. V. (2002). Construct validity of the stages of change of exercise adoption for different intensities of physical activity in four samples of differing age groups. *American Journal of Health Promotion, 16*(5), 280–287.

Readiness for Enhanced Urinary Elimination (2002, LOE 2.1)

DEFINITION

A pattern of urinary functions that is sufficient for meeting eliminatory needs and can be strengthened

DEFINING CHARACTERISTICS

- Expresses willingness to enhance urinary elimination
- Urine is straw colored with no odor
- Specific gravity is within normal limits
- Amount of output is within normal limits for age and other factors
- Positions self for emptying of bladder
- Fluid intake is adequate for daily needs

References

Kilpatrick, J. A. (2001). Urinary elimination, health promotion. In P. A. Potter and A. G. Perry (Eds.), *Fundamentals of nursing* (5th ed., pp. 1408–1411). St. Louis, MO: Mosby.

Palmer, M. H., Czarapata, B. J. R., Wells, T. J., & Newman, D. K. (1997). Urinary outcomes in older adults: Research and clinical perspective. *Urologic Nursing, 17*(1), 2–9.

Pfister, S. M. (1999). Bladder diaries and voiding patterns in older adults. *Journal of Gerontological Nursing, 25*(3), 36–41.

BIBLIOGRAPHY

GENERAL REFERENCES

Abdellah, F. G., & Levine, E. (1965). *Better patient care through nursing research.* New York: Macmillan.

Abrams, A. C. (2004). *Clinical drug therapy* (8th ed.). Philadelphia: Lippincott Williams & Wilkins.

Alfaro-LeFevre, R. (2001). *Applying nursing process: A step-by-step guide* (5th ed.). Philadelphia: Lippincott Williams & Wilkins.

Allender, J., & Spradley, B. (2001). *Community health nursing* (4th ed.). Philadelphia: Lippincott Williams & Wilkins.

American Nurses Association. (1980). *ANA social policy statement.* Washington, DC: Author.

American Psychiatric Association. (2000). *DSM IV-TR: Diagnostic and statistical manual of mental disorders* (4th ed., text revision). Washington, DC: Author.

Andrews, M., & Boyle, J. (2003). *Transcultural concepts in nursing* (4th ed.). Philadelphia: Lippincott Williams & Wilkins.

Aspinall, M. J., & Tanner, C. (1981). *Decision-making in patient care.* New York: Appleton-Century-Crofts.

Bellack, J. P. (1984). *Nursing assessment: A multidimensional approach.* Monterey, CA: Wadsworth.

Bennett, J. V., & Brachman, P. S. (Eds.). (1995). *Hospital infections* (3rd ed.). Boston: Little, Brown.

Bickley, B. (2003). *A guide to physical examination and history taking* (8th ed.). Philadelphia: Lippincott Williams & Wilkins.

Block, G. J., & Nolan, J. W. (1986). *Health assessment for professional nursing: A developmental approach* (2nd ed.). New York: Appleton-Century-Crofts.

Bower, C. (1993, September). *Patient outcomes and nursing diagnosis: Expanding the value of critical paths.* Workshop. Pasadena, California.

Boyd, M. A. (2005). *Psychiatric nursing: Contemporary practice* (3rd ed.). Philadelphia: Lippincott Williams & Wilkins.

Bulechek, G. M., & McCloskey, J. C. (Eds.). (1985). *Nursing interventions: Treatments for nursing diagnoses.* Philadelphia: W. B. Saunders.

Bulechek, G., & McCloskey, J. (1989). Nursing interventions: Treatments for potential nursing diagnoses. In R. M. Carroll-Johnson (Ed.), *Classification of nursing diagnoses: Proceedings of the eighth national conference.* Philadelphia: J. B. Lippincott.

Carnevali, D., & Thomas, M. (1993). *Diagnostic reasoning and treatment decision making in nursing.* Philadelphia: J. B. Lippincott.

Carpenito, L. J. (2004). *Nursing care plans and documentation: Nursing diagnoses and collaborative problems* (4th ed.). Philadelphia: Lippincott Williams & Wilkins.

Carpenito, L. J. (1995). *Nurse practitioner and physician discipline specific expertise in primary care.* Unpublished manuscript.

Clemen-Stone, E., Eigasti, D. G., & McGuire S. L. (1997). *Comprehensive family and community health nursing* (5th ed.). St. Louis: Mosby Year Book.

Curtin, L., & Flaherty, M. J. (1982). *Nursing ethics.* Bowie, MD: Brady Communications.

Dudek, S. (2006). *Nutrition handbook for nursing practice* (5th ed.). Philadelphia: Lippincott Williams & Wilkins.

Giger, J., & Davidhizar, R. (2004). *Transcultural nursing: Assessment and intervention* (5th ed.). St. Louis: Mosby Yearbook.

Gordon, M. (1994). *Nursing diagnosis: Process and application.* St. Louis: Mosby Yearbook.

Gordon, M. (1982). Historical perspective: The National Group for Classification of Nursing Diagnoses. In M. J. Kim & D. A. Moritz (Eds.), *Classification of nursing diagnoses:* Proceedings of the fourth national conference. New York: McGraw-Hill.

Grondin, L., Lussier, R., Phaneuf, M., & Riopelle, L. (1990). *Planification des soins infirmiers.* Montreal: Les Editions de la Cheneliere.

Henderson, U., & Nite, G. (1960). *Principles and practice of nursing* (5th ed.). New York: Macmillan.

Hickey, J. (2002). *The clinical practice of neurological and neurosurgical nursing* (5th ed). Philadelphia: Lippincott Williams & Wilkins.

Jackson, D. B., & Saunders, R. B. (1993). *Child health nursing.* Philadelphia: J. B. Lippincott.

Johnson, B. S. (1995). *Child, adolescent and family psychiatric nursing.* Philadelphia: J. B. Lippincott.

Kritek, P. (1986). Development of a taxonomic structure for nursing diagnosis. In M. Hurley (Ed.), *Classification of nursing diagnoses: Proceedings of sixth NANDA national conference.* St. Louis: C. V. Mosby.

Lubkin, J. M. (1995). *Chronic illness: Impact and interventions* (3rd ed.). Boston: Jones & Bartlett.

Luis, M. T. (1995). *Diagnostico de enfermeria* (2nd ed.). Barcelona: Doyma.

Matteson, M. A., & McConnell, E. S. (1988). *Gerontological nursing: Concepts and practices.* Philadelphia: W. B. Saunders.

May, K. A., & Mahlmeister, L. R. (1994). *Maternal and neonatal nursing: Family-centered care* (3rd ed.). Philadelphia: J. B. Lippincott.

McCafferty, M. (1980). *Nursing management of the patient with pain* (2nd ed.). Philadelphia: J. B. Lippincott.

McCafferty, M., & Beebe, A. (1989). *Pain: Clinical management for nursing practice.* St. Louis: C. V. Mosby.

McCafferty, M., & Pasera, C. (1999). *Pain: Clinical manual.* St. Louis: C. V. Mosby.

McCourt, A. (1991). Syndromes in nursing. In R. M. Carroll-Johnson (Ed.), *Classification of nursing diagnoses: Proceedings of the ninth NANDA national conference.* Philadelphia: J. B. Lippincott.

McMillan, J., De Angelis, C., Feigin, R., & Waishaw, J. (1999). *Oski's pediatrics.* Philadelphia: Lippincott Williams & Wilkins.

Miller, C. (2004). *Nursing for wellness in older adults* (4th ed.). Philadelphia. Lippincott Williams & Wilkins.

Mohr, W. K. (2003). *Psychiatric–mental health nursing: Adaptation and growth* (5th ed). Philadelphia: Lippincott Williams & Wilkins.

Morton, P., Fontaine, D., Hudak, C., & Gallo, B. (2005). *Critical care nursing* (8th ed.). Philadelphia: Lippincott Williams & Wilkins.

Norris, J., & Kunes-Connell, M. (1987). Self-esteem disturbance: A clinical validation study. In A. McLane (Ed.), *Classification of nursing diagnoses: Proceedings of the seventh NANDA national conference.* St. Louis: C. V. Mosby.

North American Nursing Diagnosis Association (2002). *Nursing diagnosis: Definitions and classification 2001–2002.* Philadelphia: Author.

North American Nursing Diagnosis Association. (1992). *Taxonomy of nursing diagnoses.* Philadelphia: Author.

Oski, F. (1999). *Principles and practice of pediatrics* (3rd ed.) Philadelphia: Lippincott Williams & Wilkins.

Pillitteri, A. (2003). *Maternal and child health nursing* (4th ed.). Philadelphia: Lippincott Williams & Wilkins.

Popkess-Vawter, S. (1984). Strength-oriented nursing diagnoses. In M. J. Kim, G. McFarland, & A. McLane (Eds.), *Classification of nursing diagnoses.* St. Louis: C. V. Mosby.

Porth, C. (2002). *Pathophysiology* (6th ed.). Philadelphia: Lippincott Williams & Wilkins.

Reeder, S. J., Martin, L. L., & Koniak, D. (1997). *Maternity nursing: Family, newborn and women's health care* (18th ed.). Philadelphia: J. B. Lippincott.

Smeltzer, S., & Bare, B. (2004). *Brunner and Suddarth's textbook of medical–surgical nursing* (10th ed.). Philadelphia: Lippincott Williams & Wilkins.

Stolte, K. M. (1996). *Wellness: Nursing diagnosis for health promotion.* Philadelphia: J. B. Lippincott.

Stuart, G. W., & Sundeen, S. (2002). *Principles and practice of psychiatric nursing* (6th ed.). St. Louis: Mosby–Year Book.

Taylor, C., Lillis, C., & LeMone, P. (2001). *Fundamentals of nursing: The art and science of nursing care* (4th ed.). Philadelphia: Lippincott Williams & Wilkins.

Varcarolis, E. (2002). *Foundations of psychiatric mental health nursing* (4th ed.). Philadelphia: W. B. Saunders.

Weber, J., & Kelley, J. (2003). *Health assessment in nursing* (2nd ed.). Philadelphia: Lippincott Williams & Wilkins.

Wilson, H. S., & Kneisel, C. R. (1996). *Psychiatric nursing* (5th ed.). Redwood City, CA: Addison-Wesley Nursing.

Wong, D. (2003). *Nursing care of infants and children* (7th ed.). St. Louis: Mosby-Year Book.

SECTION ONE

Carlson-Catalino, J. (1998). Nursing diagnosis and interventions for post-acute-phase battered woman. *Nursing Diagnosis, 9,* 101–110.

Clark, J., & Lang, N. (1992). Nursing's next advance: An international classification for nursing practice. *International Nursing Review, 39*(4), 109–112.

Florida Board of Nursing. (1988). *Administrative policies pertaining to certification of advanced registered nurse practitioners.* Rule chapter 210–11, pp. 15–17.

Fry, V. S. (1953). The creative approach to nursing. *American Journal of Nursing, 53,* 301–302.

Gleit, C., & Tatro, S. (1981). Nursing diagnoses for healthy individuals. *Nursing Health Care, 2,* 456–457.

Gordon, M. (1990). Towards theory-based diagnostic categories. *Nursing Diagnoses, 1*(1), 5–11.

Leininger, M. (1990). Issues, questions, and concerns related to the nursing diagnosis cultural movement from a transcultural nursing perspective. *Journal of Transcultural Nursing, 2,* 23–32.

Levin, R. F., Krainovitch, B. C., Bahrenburg, E., & Mitchell, C. A. (1989). Diagnostic content validity of nursing diagnoses. *Image: The Journal of Nursing Scholarship, 21*(1), 40–44.

Miskowski, C., & Nielson, B. (1985). A cancer nursing assessment tool. *Oncology Nursing Forum, 12*(6), 37–42.

Mitchell, G. J. (1991). Nursing diagnosis: An ethical analysis. *Image: The Journal of Nursing Scholarship, 23,* 99–103.

Nelms, B. C. (1991). Nursing diagnosis: Opinions please [editorial]. *Journal of Pediatric Health Care, 5,* 1.

Pearson, L. (2001). Annual update of how each state stands on legislative issues affecting advanced practice. *Nurse Practitioner, 26*(1), 26, 47–57.

Seahill, L. (1991). Nursing diagnosis vs. goal oriented treatment planning in inpatient child psychiatry. *Image: The Journal of Nursing Scholarship, 23,* 95–97.

Wallace, D., & Ivey, J. (1989). The bifocal clinical nursing model: Descriptions and application to patients receiving thrombolytic or anticoagulant therapy. *Journal of Cardiovascular Nursing, 4*(1), 33–45.

ACTIVITY INTOLERANCE

Cohen, J., Gorenberg, B., & Schroeder, B. (2000). A study of functional status among elders at two academic nursing centers. *Home Care Provider, 5*(3), 108–112.

Corcoran, P. J. (1991). Use it or lose it—The hazards of bed rest and inactivity. *Western Journal of Medicine, 154,* 536–538.

Magnan, M. A. (1987, September). *Activity intolerance: Toward a nursing theory of activity.* Paper presented at the Fifth Annual Symposium of the Michigan Nursing Diagnosis Association, Detroit, Michigan.

Sarna, L. & Bialous, S. A. (2004). Why tobacco is a women's health issue. *Nursing Clinics of North America, 39*(1), 165–180.

Pulmonary

Bauldoff, G., Hoffman, L., Sciurba, F., & Zullo, T. (1996). Home based upper arm exercises training for patients with chronic obstructive pulmonary disease. *Heart and Lung, 25*(4), 288–294.

Breslin, E. H. (1992). Dyspnea-limited response in chronic obstructive pulmonary disease: Reduced unsupported arm activities. *Rehabilitation Nursing, 17,* 12–20.

Klesges, R. C., Eck, L. H., Mellon, M. W., Fulliton, W., Somes, G. W., & Hanson, C. L. (1989). The accuracy of self-reports of physical activity. *Medicine and Science in Sports and Exercise, 22,* 690–697.

Martinez, F. K., Couser, J. I., & Celli, B. R. (1989). Respiratory mechanics and ventilatory muscle recruitment during arm elevation in subjects with severe chronic airflow obstruction. *American Review of Respiratory Disease, 139,* A292.

Cardiac

Day, N. R. (1984). *After your heart attack.* Daly City, CA: Krames Communications.

Froelicher, V. F. (1987). *Exercise and the heart: Clinical concepts.* Chicago: Year Book Medical Publishers.

Gulanick, M. (1991). Is phase 2 cardiac rehabilitation necessary for early recovery of patients with cardiac disease? A randomized, controlled study. *Heart and Lung, 20,* 9–15.

Guyatt, G. H., Sullivan, M. J., & Thompson, P. J. (1985). The 6-minute walk: A new measure of exercise capacity in patients with chronic heart failure. *Canadian Medical Association Journal, 132,* 919–923.

Jenkins, L. S. (1987). Self-efficacy: New perspectives in caring for patients recovering from myocardial infarction. *Progress in Cardiovascular Nursing, 2,* 32–35.

Jillings, C. R. (Ed.). (1988). *Cardiac rehabilitation nursing.* Rockville, MD: Aspen Publications.

Kavanagh, T. Exercise and coronary artery disease. In J. V. Basmajian (Ed.). *Therapeutic exercise.* Baltimore: Williams & Wilkins.

Lemanski, K. M. (1990). The use of self-efficacy in cardiac rehabilitation. *Progress in Cardiovascular Nursing, 5,* 114–117.

McAuley, E., Courneya, K. S., & Lettunich, J. (1991). Effects of acute and long-term exercise on self-efficacy responses in sedentary, middle-aged males and females. *The Gerontologist, 31,* 534–542.

Parmley, W. W. (1986). Position report on cardiac rehabilitation. *Journal of the American College of Cardiology, 7,* 451–453.

Sanderson, R. G., & Kurth, C. L. (1983). *The cardiac patient: A comprehensive approach.* Philadelphia: W. B. Saunders.

Deconditioning

Brandstater, M. E., & Basmajian, J. V. (Eds.). (1987). *Stroke rehabilitation.* Baltimore: Williams & Wilkins.

Corcoran, P. J. (1991). Use it or lose it—The hazards of bed rest and inactivity. *Western Journal of Medicine, 154,* 536–538.

Fisher, S. V., & Gullickson, G. (1978). The energy costs of ambulation in health and disability: A literature review. *Archives of Physical Medicine and Rehabilitation, 59*(3), 124–133.

Greenleaf, J. E., Wade, C. E., & Leftheriotis, G. (1989). Orthostatic responses following 30-day bed rest deconditioning with isotonic and isokinetic exercise training. *Aviation, Space and Environmental Medicine, 6,* 537–542.

Harper, C. M., & Lyles, Y. M. (1988). Physiology and complications of bed rest. *Journal of the American Geriatric Society, 36,* 1047–1054.

LeBlanc, A., Gogia, P., & Schneider, V. (1988). Calf muscle area and strength changes after five weeks of horizontal bed rest. *American Journal of Sports Medicine, 16,* 624–629.

Rubin, M. (1988). The physiology of bed rest. *American Journal of Nursing, 88*(1), 50–58.

Sandler, H., Popp, R. L., & Harrison, D. (1988). The hemodynamic effects of repeated bed rest exposure. *Aviation, Space and Environmental Medicine, 11,* 1047–1054.

ANXIETY

Blanchard, C. M., Courneya, K. S. & Larng, D. (2001). Effects of acute exercise on state anxiety in breast cancer survivors. *Oncology Nursing Forum, 28*(10) 1617–21.

Brant, J. M. (1998). The art of palliative care: Living with hope, dying with dignity. *Oncology Nursing Forum, 25*(6), 995–1004.

Christman, N., & Kirchhoff, K. (1992). Preparatory sensory information. In G. Bulechek & J. McCloskey (Eds.), *Nursing interventions.* Philadelphia: W. B. Saunders.

Courts, N. F., Barba, B. E. & Tesh, A. (2001). Family Caregivers attitudes towards aging, caregiving, and nursing home placement. *Journal of gerontological Nursing, 27*(8) 44–52.

DeMarco-Sinatra, J. (2000). Relaxation Training as a holistic nursing intervention. *Holistic Nursing Practice, 14*(3), 30–39.

DeVito, A. (1990). Dyspnea during hospitalization for acute phase of illness as recalled by patients with chronic obstructive pulmonary disease. *Heart and Lung, 19,* 186–191.

Grainger, R. (1990). Anxiety interrupters. *American Journal of Nursing, 90*(2), 14–15.

Grealish, L., Lomasney, A., & Whiteman, B. (2000). Foot massage. A nursing intervention to modify the distressing symptoms of pain and nausea in patients hospitalized with cancer. *Cancer Nursing, 23,* 237–243.

Hunt, B, Rosenthal, D. (2000). Rehabilitation counselors' experiences with client death and death anxiety. Journal of Rehabilitation 66(4). 44–50.

Jones, P. E., & Jakob, D. F. (1984). Anxiety revisited from a practice perspective. In M. J. Kim, G. K. McFarland, & A. M. McLane (Eds.). *Classification of nursing diagnoses: Proceedings of the fifth national conference.* St. Louis: C. V. Mosby.

Keegan, L. (2000). Protocols for practice: Applying research at the bedside. Alternative and complimentary modalities for managing stress and anxiety. *Critical Care Nurse, 20*(3), 93–96.

Krietemeyer, B. C., & Heiney, S. P. (1992). Storytelling as a therapeutic technique in a group for school-aged oncology patients. *Children's Health Care, 21,* 14–19.

Lancaster, K. A. (1997). Care of the pediatric patient in ambulatory surgery. *Nursing Clinics of North America, 32*(2), 441–456.

Leske, J. (1993). Anxiety of elective surgical patients, family members. *AORN Journal, 57,* 1091–1103.

Lugina, H. I., Christenson, K., et al. (2001). Change in maternal concerns during midwifery 6 weeks postpartum period. *Journal of Midwifery and Women's Health, 46*(4), 248–257.

Lyon, B.A. (2002). Cognitive self-care skills: A model for managing stressful lifestyles. *Nursing Clinics of North America, 37*(2), 285–294.

May, R. (1977). *The meaning of anxiety.* New York: W. W. Norton.

Maynard, C. K. (2004). Assess and manage somatization. *Holistic Nursing Practice, 18*(2), 54–60.

Nelson, K. A., Walsh, D., Behrens, C., Zhukovsky, D. S., Lipnickey, V., & Brady, D. (2000). The dying cancer patient. *Seminars in Oncology, 27*(1), 84–89.

Redman, B., & Thomas, S. (1992). Patient teaching. In G. Bulechek & J. McCloskey (Eds.). *Nursing interventions: Essential nursing interventions* (2nd ed.). Philadelphia: W. B. Saunders.

Stephenson, N. L., Weinrich, S. P., & Tavakoli, A. S. (2000). The effects of foot reflexology on anxiety and pain in patients with breast and lung cancer. *Oncology Nursing Forum, 27,* 67–72.

Tarsitano, B. P. (1992). Structured preoperative teaching. In G. Bulechek & J. McCloskey (Eds.). *Nursing interventions: Essential nursing interventions.* Philadelphia: W. B. Saunders.

Taylor, E. J. (2000). Spiritual and ethical end-of-life concerns. In C. H. Yarbro, M. H. Frogge, M. Goodman, & S. L. Groenwald. *Cancer nursing: Principles and practice* (5th ed.). Boston: Jones and Bartlett.

Taylor-Loughran, A., O'Brien, M., LaChapelle, R., & Rangel, S. (1989). Defining characteristics of the nursing diagnoses fear and anxiety: A validation study. *Applied Nursing Research, 2,* 178–186.

Tusaie, K. & Dyer, J. (2004). Resilience: A historical review of construct. *Holistic Nursing Practice, 18*(1), 3–8.

Whitley, G. (1994). Concept analysis in nursing diagnosis research. In R. Carroll-Johnson & M. Paquette. *Classification of Nursing Diagnosis: Proceedings of the tenth conference.* Philadelphia: J. B. Lippincott.

Wong, H. L. C., Lopez-Nahas, V. & Molassiotis, A. (2001). Effects of Music Therapy on anxiety in venulator dependent patients. Heart Lung Journal of Acute Cutical Care. 30(5) 376–87.

Yokom, C. J. (1984). The differentiation of fear and anxiety. In M. J. Kim, G. K. McFarland, & A. M. McLane (Eds.). *Classification of nursing diagnoses: Proceedings of the fifth national conference.* St. Louis: C. V. Mosby.

RISK FOR IMBALANCED BODY TEMPERATURE

Andrews, A. (1990). Inadvertent hypothermia: A complication of postoperative cholecystectomy patients. *AORN Journal, 52,* 987–991.

Bernthal, E. (1999). Inadvertent hypothermia prevention: The anaesthetic nurse's role. *British Journal of Nursing, 8*(1), 17–18, 20–25.

Carroll, S. M. (1989). Nursing diagnosis: Hypothermia. In R. M. Carroll-Johnson (Ed.). *Classification of nursing diagnoses: Proceedings of the eighth conference.* Philadelphia: J. B. Lippincott.

DeFabio, D. C. (2000). Fluid and nutrient maintenance before, during and after exercise. *Journal of Sports Chiropractic and Rehabilitation, 14*(2), 21–24, 42–43.

Erickson, R., & Yount, S. (1991). Comparison of tympanic and oral temperatures in surgical patients. *Nursing Research, 40*(2), 90–93.

Giuliano, K. K., Giuliano, A. J., Scott, S. S., et al. (2000). Temperature measurement in critically ill adults: A comparison of tympanic and oral methods. *American Journal of Critical Care, 9*(4), 254–261.

Howell, R., Macrae, L., Sanjines, S., Burke, J., & DeStefano, P. (1992). Effects of two types of head coverings in the rewarming of patients after coronary artery bypass graft surgery. *Heart and Lung, 21,* 1–6.

Hunsberger, M. (1989). Principles and skills adapted to the care of children. In R. L. Foster, M. M. Hunsberger, & J. J. T. Anderson (Eds.). *Family-centered nursing care of children.* Philadelphia: W. B. Saunders.

Johnson, S. (1989). Alteration in temperature regulation: Hypothermia. In R. M. Carroll-Johnson (Ed.). *Classification of nursing diagnoses: Proceedings of the eighth conference.* Philadelphia: J. B. Lippincott.

Lorin, M. (1995). Pathogenesis of fever and treatment. In F. Oski (Ed.). *Principles and practices of pediatrics* (2nd ed.). Philadelphia: J. B. Lippincott.

Mahoney, C. B., & Odom, J. (1999). Maintaining intraoperative normothermia: A meta-analysis of outcomes with costs. *AANA Journal, 67*(2), 155–164.

Robbins, A. S. (1989). Hypothermia and heat stroke: Protecting the elderly patient. *Geriatrics, 44*(1), 73–79.

Sallis, R. & Chassy, C. M. (1999). Recognizing and treating common cold-induced injury in outdoor sports. *Medical Science & Sports Exercise, 31*(10), 1367–1373.

Summers, S., Dudgeon, N., Byram, K., & Zingsheim, K. (1991). Validation of the nursing diagnosis hypothermia. In R. M. Carroll-Johnson (Ed.). *Classification of nursing diagnoses: Proceedings of the ninth conference.* Philadelphia: J. B. Lippincott.

Ineffective Thermoregulation

Hunter, L. (1991). Measurement of axillary temperature in neonate. *Western Journal of Nursing Research, 13*(3), 324.

Peterec, S. (1999). The premature newborn. In F. Oski (Ed.). *Principles and practices of pediatrics* (3rd ed.). Philadelphia: Lippincott Williams & Wilkins.

Varda, K. E., & Behnke, R. S. (2000). The effect of timing of initial bath on newborn temperature. *JOGNN, 29*(1), 27–32.

BOWEL INCONTINENCE

Chassagne, P., Jego, A., & Gloc, P. (2000). Does treatment of constipation improve fecal incontinence in institutionalized elderly patients? *Aging, 29*(2), 159–164.

Demata, E. (2000). Faecal incontinence. *Journal of Wound Care and Enterostomal Therapy, 19*(4), 6–11.

Maas, M., & Specht, J. (1991). Bowel incontinence. In M. Maas, K. Buckwalter, & M. Hardy (Eds.). *Nursing diagnoses and interventions for the elderly.* Redwood City, CA: Addison-Wesley Nursing.

McLane, A., & McShane, R. (1991). Constipation. In M. Maas, K. Buckwalter, & M. Hardy (Eds.). *Nursing diagnoses and interventions for the elderly.* Redwood City, CA: Addison-Wesley Nursing.

Weeks, S. K., Hubbartt, E., & Michaels, T. K. (2000). Keys to bowel success. *Rehabilitation Nursing, 25*(2), 66–69.

EFFECTIVE AND INEFFECTIVE BREASTFEEDING

Auerbach, K. G. (1990). Assisting the employed breastfeeding mother. *Journal of Nurse Midwifery, 35*(11), 26–34.

Bell, K. & Rawlings, N. (1998). Promoting breastfeeding by managing common lactation problems. *Nurse Practitioner, 23*(6), 102, 104, 106, 109, 114, 119–123.

Ortiz, J., McGilligan, K. & Kelly, P. (2004). Duration of breast milk expression among working mother's enrolled in an employer-sponsored location program. *Pediatric Nursing, 30*(2), 111–119.

Shirago, L., & Bocar, D. (1990). The infant's contribution to breastfeeding. *Journal of Obstetric, Gynecologic and Neonatal Nursing, 19,* 209–215.

CAREGIVER ROLE STRAIN

Clipp, E., & George, L. (1990). Caregiver needs and patterns of social support. *Journal of Gerontology, 45*(3; Suppl), 102–111.

Corcaran, M. A., & Gitlin, L. N. (2001). Family caregiver acceptance and use of environmental strategies provided in an occupational therapy intervention. *Physical Occupational Therapy in Geriatrics,* 1911–1920.

Flaskerud, J. H., Carter, P. A., & Lee, P. (2000). Distressing emotions in female caregivers of people with AIDS, age-related dementias and advanced stage cancers. *Perspectives in Psychiatric Care, 36*(4), 121–130.

Gaynor, S. (1990). The effects of home care on caregivers. *Image: The Journal of Nursing Scholarship, 22,* 208–212.

Hagen, B. (2001). Nursing home placement. *Journal of Gerontological Nursing, 27*(2), 44–53.

Irvin, B., & Acton, G. (1997). Stress, hope and well-being of women caring for family member with Alzheimer's disease. *Holistic Nursing Practice, 11*(2), 69–79.

Lazarus, R. S., & Folkman, S. (1984). *Stress, appraisal and coping.* New York: Springer.

Miller, B., & McFall, S. (1991). Stability and change in the informal task support network of frail older persons. *The Gerontologist, 31,* 735–745.

O'Connor, P., Vander Plaats, S., & Betz, C. L. (1992). Respite care services to caretakers of chronically ill children in California. *Journal of Pediatric Nursing, 7,* 269–275.

Pearlin, L., Mullan, J., Semple, S., & Skaff, M. (1990). Caregiving and the stress process: An overview of concepts and their measures. *The Gerontologist, 30,* 583–594.

Pruchno, R., Kleban, M., Michaels, J. E., & Dempsey, N. (1990). Mental and physical health of care giving spouses: Development of a causal model. *Journal of Gerontology, 45*(5), 192–199.

Shields, C. (1992). Family interaction and caregivers of Alzheimer's disease patients: Correlates of depression. *Family Process, 31*(3), 19–32.

Smith, G., Smith, M., & Toseland, R. (1991). Problems identified by family caregivers in counseling. *The Gerontologist, 31*(1), 15–22.

Tusaie, K. & Dyer, J. (2004). Resilence: A historical review of construct. *Holistic Nursing Practice, 18*(1), 3–8.

Winslow, B., & Carter, P. (1999). Patterns of Burden in wives who care for husbands with dementia. *Nursing Clinics of North America, 34*(2), 275–287.

Wong, D. L. (1991). Transition from hospital to home for children with complex medical care. *Journal of Pediatric Oncology, 8*(1), 3–9 www.alz.org.

Young, M. G. (2001). Providing care for the caregiver. *Patient Care for the Nurse Practitioner, 2,* 36–47.

Resources for the Consumer

Alzheimer's Disease and Related Disorders, Inc., National Headquarters, 70 East Lake Street, Chicago, IL 60601-5997 (800-621-0379).

American Association of Retired Persons, 1909 K Street NW, Washington, DC 20049.

Children of Aging Parents (CAPS), 2761 Trenton Road, Levittown, PA 19056.

National Association for Home Care, 519 C Street, NE, Stanton Park, Washington, DC 20002.

National Association of Area Agencies on Aging, 600 Maryland Avenue, SW, Suite 208, Washington, DC 20024 www.patientcarenp.com (information on caregiving).

IMPAIRED COMFORT

Agency for Health Care Policy and Research. (1992). *Acute pain management: Operative or medical procedures and trauma.* Rockville, MD: Author.

Agency for Health Care Policy and Research. (1994). *Management of cancer pain.* Rockville, MD: Author.

Beyer, J. E. (1984). *Ultra: A user manual and technical report.* Evanston, IL: Hospital Play Equipment Co.

Clinton, P., & Eland, J. A. (1991). Pain. In M. Maas, K. Buckwalter, & M. Hardy (Eds.). *Nursing diagnoses and interventions for the elderly.* Redwood City, CA: Addison-Wesley Nursing.

Davis, D. C. (1996). The discomforts of pregnancy. *JOGNN, 25*(1), 73–81.

DeWitt, S. (1990). Nursing assessment of skin and dermatological lesions. *Nursing Clinics of North America, 25*(1), 235–245.

Eckert, R. M. (2001). Understanding anticipatory nausea. *Continuing Education, 28*(10) 1553–1560.

Eland, J. (1988). Pain management and comfort. *Journal of Gerontology Nursing, 14*(4) 10–15.

Eland, J. M. (1981). Minimizing pain associated with prekindergarten intramuscular injections: Issues in comprehension. *Pediatric Nursing, 5,* 361–372.

Ezzone, S., Baker, C., Rosselet, R., & Terepka, E. (1998). Music as an adjunct to antiemetic therapy. *Oncology Nursing Forum, 25*(9), 1551–1556.

Ferrell, B. R. (1995). The impact of pain on quality of life. *Nursing Clinics of North America, 30,* 609–624.

Field, T., Peck, M., Hernandez Reif, M., et al. (2000). Postburn itching, pain and psychological symptoms are reduced with massage therapy. *Journal of Burn Care Rehabilitation, 21*(3), 189–193.

Foltz, A. T., Gaines, G., & Gullatte, M. (1996). Recalled side effects and self-care actions of patients receiving inpatient chemotherapy. *Oncology Nursing Forum, 23*(4), 679–683.

Gaston-Johansson, F. (2000). The effectiveness of the comprehensive coping strategy program on clinical outcomes in breast cancer autologous bone marrow transplantation. *Cancer Nursing, 23*(4), 277–285.

Grealish, L., Lomasney, A., & Whiteman, B. (2000). Foot massage. A nursing intervention to modify the distressing symptoms of pain and nausea in patients hospitalized with cancer. *Cancer Nursing, 23*(3), 237–243.

Hester, N. (1979). The preoperational child's reaction to immunization. *Nursing Research, 28,* 250–255.

Ieiorio, C. (1988). The management of nausea and vomiting in pregnancy. *Nurse Practitioner, 13*(5), 23–28.

Ladd, L. A. (1999). Symptom management: Nausea in palliative care. *Journal of Hospice and Palliative Nursing, 1*(2), 67–70.

Lowe, N. K. (1996). The pain and discomfort of labor and birth. *JOGNN, 25*(1), 82–92.

Ludwig-Beymer, P. (1989). Transcultural aspects of pain. In J. Boyle & M. Andrews (Eds.). *Transcultural concepts in nursing.* Glenview, IL: Scott, Foresman.

Malseed, R., Goldstein, F., & Balkan, N. (1995). *Pharmacology: Drug therapy and nursing considerations* (4th ed.). Philadelphia: J. B. Lippincott.

McGuire, D., Sheidler, V., & Polomano, R. C. (2000). Pain. In S. Groenwald, M. Frogge, M. Goodman, & C. Yarbo (Eds.). *Cancer nursing: Principles and practice* (5th ed.). Boston: Jones and Bartlett.

Perry, S., & Heidrich, G. (1981). Placebos. *American Journal of Nursing, 81,* 721–725.

Phillips, W. G. (1992). Pruritus: What to do when itching won't stop. *Postgraduate Medicine, 92*(7), 34–56.

Porter, J., & Jick, H. (1980). Addiction rate in patients treated with narcotics. *New England Journal of Medicine, 302,* 123.

Rhodes, V. (1990). Nausea, vomiting and retching. *Nursing Clinics of North American, 24,* 885–890.

Rounseville, C. (1992). Phantom limb pain: The ghost that haunts the amputee. *Orthopedic Nursing, 11*(2), 67–71.

Seiz, A. M., & Yarbro, C. H. Pruritus. In S. L. Groenwald, M. Goodman, M. H. Frogge, & C. H. Yarbro (Eds.). (1996a). *Cancer symptom management.* Boston: Jones & Bartlett.

Seiz, A. M. & Yarbro, C. H. Pruritus: A self-care guide. In S. L. Groenwald, M. Goodman, M. H. Frogge, & C. H. Yarbro (Eds.). (1996b). *Cancer symptom management.* Boston: Jones & Bartlett.

Sherman, R. (1989). Stump and phantom limb pain. *Neurological Clinics, 1,* 249–263.

Sloman, R. (1995). Relaxation and relief of cancer pain. *Nursing Clinics of North America, 30,* 697–709.

Thorns, A., & Edmonds, P. (2000). The management of pruritus in palliative care patients. *European Journal of Palliative Care, 7*(1), 9–12.

Voda, A., & Randall, M. (1982). Nausea and vomiting of pregnancy. In C. Norris (Ed.). *Concept clarification in nursing.* Rockville, MD: Aspen Systems.

Weber, S. E. (1996). Cultural aspects of pain in childbearing women. *JOGNN, 25*(1), 67–72.

Williamson, V. (1998). Amputation. In A. Maher, S. W. Salmond, & T. Pellino. *Orthopedic nursing* (2nd ed.). Philadelphia: W. B. Saunders.

Zborowski, M. (1952). Cultural components in response to pain. *Journal of Social Issues, 8,* 16–30.

Children

Berde, C. (1989). Pediatric postoperative pain management. *Pediatric Clinics of North America, 36,* 921–940.

Chapman, L. (1991). Searching: Expectant fathers' experiences during labor and birth. *Journal of Perinatal and Neonatal Nursing, 4*(4), 21–29.

Eland, J. M., & Anderson, J. (1977). The experience of pain in children. In A. K. Jacox (Ed.). *Pain: A source book for nurses and other health professionals.* Boston: Little, Brown.

Hymovich, D. P., & Hagopian, G. A. (1992). *Chronic illness in children and adults: A psychological approach.* Philadelphia: W. B. Saunders.

O'Brien, S., & Konsler, G. (1988). Alleviating children's postoperative pain. *Maternal-Child Nursing Journal, 13,* 183–186.

Schechter, N. (Ed.). (1989a). Acute pain in children. *Pediatric Clinics of North America, 36,* 781–794.

Schechter, N. (1989b). Undertreatment of pain in children: An overview. *Pediatric Clinics of North America, 36,* 795–1045.

IMPAIRED COMMUNICATION

Iezzoni, L. F., O'Day, B., Keleen, M. A., & Harker, H. (2004). Improving patient care: Communicating about health care: Observations from persons who are deaf or hard of hearing. *Annals of Internal Medicine, 140*(5), 356–362.

Koester, L. S., Karkowski, A. M., & Traci, M. A. (1998). How do deaf and hearing-impaired mothers regain eye contact when their infants look away? *American Annals of the Deaf, 143*(1), 5–13.

Lindeblade, P. O., & McDonald, M. (1995). Removing communication barriers for the hearing-impaired elderly. *Med-Surg Nursing, 4*(5), 379–385.

Underwood, C. (2004). How can we best deliver an inclusive health service? *Primary Health Care, 14*(9), 20–21.

CONFUSION

Anderson, C. (1999). Delirium and confusion are not interchangeable terms [letter to editor]. *Oncology Nursing Forum, 26*(3), 497–498.

Alzheimer's disease and related disorders. (1988). In *Special care for Alzheimer's patients.* Chicago: Alzheimer's Disease and Related Disorders Association, Inc.

Blazer, D. G. (1986). Depression: Paradoxically a cause for hope. *Generations, 10*(3), 21–23.

Burnside, I., & Haight, B. (1994). Reminiscence and life review: Therapeutic interventions for older people. *Nurse Practitioner, 19*(4), 55–60.

Dellasega, C. (1998). Assessment of cognition in the elderly. *Nursing Clinics of North America, 33*(3), 395–406.

Dennis, H. (1984). Remotivation therapy groups. In I. M. Burnside (Ed.). *Working with the elderly group: Process and techniques* (2nd ed.). Monterey, CA: Jones & Bartlett.

Feil, N. (1992). Validation therapy. *Geriatric Nursing, 13*(3), 129–133.

Foreman, M. D., Mion, L. C. Tyrostad, L., & Flitcher, K. (1999). Standard of practice protocol: Acute confusion/delirium. *Geriatric Nursing, 20*(3), 147–152.

Gerdner, L. (1999). Individualized music intervention protocol. *Journal of Gerontological Nursing, 25*(10), 10–16.

Hall, G. R. (1988). Care of the patient with Alzheimer's disease living at home. *Nursing Clinics of North America, 23,* 31–46.

Hall, G. R. (1991). Altered thought processes: Dementia. In M. Maas, K. Buckwalter, & M. Hardy (Eds.). *Nursing diagnoses and interventions for the elderly.* Menlo Park, CA: Addison-Wesley.

Hall, G. R. (1994). Caring for people with Alzheimer's disease using the conceptual model of progressively lowered stress threshold in the clinical setting. *Nursing Clinics of North America, 29,* 129–141.

Hall, G. R., & Buckwalter, K. C. (1987). Progressively lowered stress threshold: A conceptual model for care of adults with Alzheimer's disease. *Archives of Psychiatric Nursing, 1,* 399–406.

Janssen, J., & Giberson, D. (1988). Remotivation therapy. *Journal of Gerontological Nursing, 14*(6), 31–34.

Katzman, R. (1988). *Alzheimer's disease as an age dependent disorder, research and the aging population* (CIBA Foundation Symposium 1334). New York: John Wiley & Sons.

Ludwick, R. (1999). Clinical decision making: Recognition of confusion and application of restraints. *Orthopedic Nursing, 18*(1), 65–72.

Parmelee, P. A., Katz, I. R., & Lawton, M. P. (1989). Depression among institutionalized aged: Assessment and prevalence estimation. *Journal of Gerontology: Medical Sciences, 44,* M22–M29.

Quinn, C. (1994). The four A's of restraint reduction: Attention, assessment, anticipation, avoidance. *Orthopaedic Nursing, 13*(2), 11–19.

Rasin, J. (1990). Confusion. *Nursing Clinics of North America, 25,* 909–918.

Rateau, M. R. (2000). Confusion and aggression in restrained elderly persons undergoing hip repair surgery. *Applied Nursing Research, 13*(1), 50–54.

Roberts, B. L. (2001). Managing delirium in adult intensive care patients. *Critical Care Nurse, 21*(1), 48–55.

Smith, B. (1990). *Role of orientation therapy and reminiscence therapy: Alzheimer's disease.* St. Louis: C. V. Mosby.

Stolley, J., & Buckwalter, K. (1992). Confusion management. In G. Gulechek & J. McCloskey (Eds.). *Nursing interventions* (2nd ed.). Philadelphia: W. B. Saunders.

Wolanin, M., & Phillips, L. (1981). *Confusion: Prevention and care.* St. Louis: C. V. Mosby.

Young, M. G. (2001). Providing care for the caregiver. *Patient Care for the Nurse Practitioner,* 36–48.

Resources for the Consumer

Alzheimer's Association (ADRDA), 919 North Michigan Avenue, Suite 100, Chicago, IL 60611; Tel. (800) 272-3900
- 24-hour hotline to provide information about Alzheimer's disease
- Free publications and newsletter
- Information about local chapters of the Alzheimer's Association

Alzheimer's Disease Education and Referral (ADEAR) Center, P.O. Box 8250, Silver Spring, MD 20907-8250; Tel. (301) 495-3311

CONSTIPATION

Braun, M. K., & Everett, I. (1990). Gentle bowel fitness with fiber. *Geriatrics Nursing, 11*(1), 26–27.

Christopherson, R. D. (1991). Toileting problems in children. *Pediatric Annual, 20,* 240–244.

DiPiro, J., Talbert, R., Hayes, P., Yee, G., Matzke, G., & Posey, L. M. (2001). *Pharmacotherapy* (4th ed.). Norwalk, CT: Appleton & Lange.

Evans, K. (1990). Pediatric management problems: Chronic constipation. *Pediatric Nursing, 16,* 590–591.

Hardy, M. A. (1991). Normal changes with aging. In M. Maas, K. Buckwalter, & M. Hardy (Eds.). *Nursing diagnoses and interventions for the elderly.* Redwood City, CA: Addison-Wesley Nursing.

Lara, L. L. (1990). The risk of urinary tract infection in bowel incontinent men. *Journal of Gerontological Nursing, 16*(5), 24–26, 40–41.

Maas, M., & Specht, J. (1991). Bowel incontinence. In M. Maas, K. Buckwalter, & M. Hardy (Eds.). *Nursing diagnoses and interventions for the elderly.* Redwood City, CA: Addison-Wesley Nursing.

McLane, A., & McShane, R. (1991). Constipation. In M. Maas, K. Buckwalter, & M. Hardy (Eds.). *Nursing diagnoses and interventions for the elderly.* Redwood City, CA: Addison-Wesley Nursing.

McShane, R., & McLane, A. (1988). Constipation: Impact of etiological factors. *Journal of Gerontological Nursing, 14*(4), 31–34.

Murray, F. E., & Bliss, C. M. (1991). Geriatric constipation: Brief update on a common problem, *Geriatrics, 46*(3), 64–68.

Schaefer, D. & Cheskin, L. (1998). Constipation in the elderly. *American Family Physician, 58*(4), 907–914.

Shua-Haim, J. Sabo, M., & Ross, J. (1999). Constipation in the elderly: A practical approach. *Clinical Geriatrics, 7*(12), 91–99.

Weeks, S. K., Hubbartt, E., & Michaels, T. K. (2000). Keys to bowel success. *Rehabilitation Nursing, 25*(2), 66–80.

Yakabowich, M. (1990). Prescribe with care: The role of laxatives in the treatment of constipation. *Journal of Gerontological Nursing, 16*(7), 4–11, 42–43.

Zernike, W., & Henderson, A. (1999). *International Journal of Nursing Practice, 25*(5), 106–109.

INEFFECTIVE COPING

Arrendondo, R., Weddige, R., Justice, C., & Fitz, J. (1987). Alcoholism in Mexican-Americans: Intervention and treatment. *Hospital and Community Psychiatry, 38,* 180–183.

Barry, K.L. (1999). *Brief interventions and brief therapies for substance abuse.* Center for Substance Abuse Treatment Protocol (TIP) Series 34. Rockville, MD: Dept. of Health & Human Services.

Byrne, C., & Hunsberger, M. (1989). Concepts of illness: Stress, crisis, and coping. In R. L. Foster, M. M. Hunsberger, & J. J. T. Anderson (Eds.). *Family-centered nursing care of children.* Philadelphia: W. B. Saunders.

Calarco, M., & Krone, K. (1991). An integrated nursing model of depressive behavior in adults. *Nursing Clinics of North America, 26,* 573–583.

Captain, C. (1989). Family recovery from alcoholism. *Nursing Clinics of North America, 24,* 55–67.

Comfort, M., Sockloff, A., Loverro, J., & Kaltenbach, K. (2003). Multiple predictors of substance abuse, women's treatments and outcomes: A prospective longitudal study. *Addiction Behavior, 28*(2), 199–224.

Depression Guideline Panel. (1993, April). *Depression in primary care: Detection, diagnosis and treatment quick reference guide for clinicians, no. 5.* AHCPR Pub. No. 93-0552. Rockville, MD: U.S. Department of Health Care Policy and Research.

Finkelman, A. W. (2000). Self-management for psychiatric patient at home. *Home Care Provider, 5*(6), 95–101.

Flaskerud, J. H. (1984). A comparison of perceptions of problematic behavior by six minority groups and mental health professionals. *Nursing Research, 33,* 190–197.

Folkman, S., Lazarus, R., Pimley, S., & Novacek, J. (1987). Age differences in stress and coping processes. *Psychology and Aging, 2,* 171–184.

Hamburg, D. A., & Adams, J. E. (1953). A perspective on coping behavior. *Archives of General Psychiatry, 17,* 1–20.

Henderson, G., & Primeaux, M. (1981). *Transcultural health care reading.* Boston: Addison-Wesley.

Kovalesky, A. (2004). Women with substance abuse concerns. *Nursing Clinics of North America, 39*(1), 97–115.

Lazarus, R. (1985). The costs and benefits of denial. In A. Monat & R. Lazarus (Eds.). *Stress and coping: An anthology* (2nd ed.). New York: Columbia.

Lazarus, R., & Folkman, S. (1984). *Stress, appraisal and coping.* New York: Springer.

Lyon, B. L. (2002). Cognitive self-care skills: A model for managing stressful lifestyles. *Nursing Clinics of North America, 37*(2), 285–294.

Miller, P. (1983). Family health and psychosocial response to cardiovascular diseases. *Health Values, 7*(6), 10–15.

Monat, A., & Lazarus, R. (Eds.). (1985). *Stress and coping: An anthology.* New York: Columbia.

Nyamathi, A. (1989). Comprehensive health seeking and coping paradigm. *Journal of Advanced Nursing, 14,* 281–290.

Potocki, E., & Everly, G. (1989). Control and the human stress response. In G. Everly (Ed.). *A clinical guide to treatment of human stress response.* New York: Plenum Press.

Selye, H. (1974). *Stress without distress.* Philadelphia: J. B. Lippincott.

Simons, R. L., & West, G. E. (1984). Life changes, coping resources and health among the elderly. *International Journal of Aging and Human Development, 20,* 173–189.

Tweed, S. H. (1989). Identifying the alcoholic client. *Nursing Clinics of North America, 24*(1), 13–32.

Vincent, K. G. (1985). The validation of a nursing diagnosis. *Nursing Clinics of North America, 20,* 631–639.

Willis, L., Thomas, P., Garry, P.J., & Goodwin, J. (1987). A prospective study of response to stressful life events in initially healthy elders. *Journal of Gerontology, 42,* 627–630.

Substance Abuse

Chychula, M. M. (1990). The cocaine epidemic: A comprehensive review of use, abuse and dependence. *Nurse Practitioner, 15*(7), 31–39.

Ewing, J. A. (1984). Detecting alcoholism: The CAGE questionnaire. *Journal of the American Medical Association, 252,* 1905–1907.

Flagler, S., Hughes, & Kovalesky, A. (1997). Toward understanding of addiction. *JOGNN, 26*(4), 441–448.

Kappas-Larson, P., & Lathrop, L. (1993). Early detection and intervention for hazardous ethanol use. *Nurse Practitioner, 18*(7), 50–55.

Lynch, C. S., & Phillips, M. W. (1989). Nursing diagnosis: Ineffective denial. In R. M. Carroll-Johnson (Ed.). *Classification of nursing diagnoses: Proceedings of the eighth conference.* Philadelphia: J. B. Lippincott.

Metzger, L. (1988). *From denial to recovery: Counseling problem drinkers, alcoholics, and their families.* San Francisco: Jossey-Bass.

Miller, W. R. (1989). Evaluation and motivation. In R. K. Hester & W. R. Miller (Eds.). *Handbook of alcoholism treatment approaches: Effective alternatives.* New York: Pergamon Press.

Smith-DiJulio, K. (1998). People who depend on alcohol. In E. M. Varcarolis (Ed.). *Foundations of psychiatric mental health nursing* (3rd ed). Philadelphia: W. B. Saunders.

Tweed, S. H. (1989). Identifying the alcoholic client. *Nursing Clinics of North America, 24,* 13–32.

DISABLED FAMILY COPING

Aiken, M. M. (1990). Documenting sexual abuses in prepubertal girls. *American Journal of Maternal–Child Nursing, 15,* 176–177.

Blair, K. (1986). The battered woman: Is she a silent partner? *Nurse Practitioner, 11*(6), 38.

Browne, K. (1989). The health visitor's role in screening for child abuse. *Health Visitor, 62*(3), 275–277.

Bullock, L. F., & McFarlane, J. (1989). Higher prevalence of low birthweight infants born to battered women. *American Journal of Nursing, 89,* 1153–1155.

Bullock, L. F., McFarlane, J., Bateman, L., & Miller, V. (1989). Characteristics of battered women in a primary care setting. *Nursing Practitioner, 14,* 47–55.

Centers for Disease Control and Prevention. (2003). Male batterers. www.edc.gov/ncipc/factsheets/malebat.htm.

Campbell, J. C. (1989). A test of two explanatory models of women's responses to battering. *Nursing Research, 38,* 18–24.

Campbell, J., Poland, M., Waller, J., & Ager, J. (1992). Correlates of battering during pregnancy. *Research in Nursing and Health, 15,* 219–226.

Captain, C. (1989). Family recovery from alcoholism. *Nursing Clinics of North America, 24,* 55–67.

Carlson-Catalano, J. (1998). Nursing Diagnoses and interventions for post–acute phase battered women. *Nursing Diagnosis, 9*(3), 101–109.

Chescheir, N. (1996). Violence against women; response from clinicians. *Journal of Emergency Medicine, 27,* 766–768.

Cowen, P. S. (1999). Child neglect: Injuries of omission. *Pediatric Nursing, 25*(4), 401–418.

Else, L., et al. (1993). Personality characteristics of men who physically abuse women. *Hospital and Community Psychiatry, 44*(10), 54–62.

Greany, G. (1984). Is she a battered woman? A guide for emergency response. *American Journal of Nursing, 84,* 725–727.

Johnstone, H., & Marcinak, J. (1997). Sibling abuse: Another component of domestic violence. *Journal of Pediatric Nursing, 12*(1), 51–54.

Lyon, B. L. (2002). Cognitive self-care skills: A model for managing stressful lifestyles. *Nursing Clinics of North America, 37*(2), 285–294.

Novello, A. C., & Soto-Torres, L. E. (1992). Women and the hidden epidemics: HIV/AIDS and domestic violence. *The Female Patient, 17,* 17.

O'Malley, T. A., Everitt, D. F., O'Malley, H., & Campion, E. (1983). Identifying and preventing family mediated abuse and neglect of elderly. *Annals of Internal Medicine, 93,* 998–1004.

Patterson, M. M. (1998). Child abuse: Assessment and interventions. *Orthopedic Nursing, 17*(1), 49–56.

Sammons, L. (1981). Battered and pregnant. *Maternal-Child Nursing Journal, 6,* 246–250.

Shapiro, R. (1984). Therapy with violent families. In S. Saunders, A. Anderson, C. Hart, C., et al. (Eds.). *Violent individuals and families: A handbook for practitioners.* Springfield, IL: Charles C. Thomas.

Smith-DiJulio, K., & Holzapfel, S. K. (1998). Families in crises: Family violence. In E. M. Varcarolis (Ed.). *Foundations of psychiatric mental health nursing* (3rd ed). Philadelphia: W. B. Saunders.

Spector, R. (1993). Culture, ethnicity and nursing. In P. Potter & A. Perry (Eds.). *Fundamentals of nursing* (pp. 95–115). St. Louis: C. V. Mosby.

Stringham, P. (1999). Domestic violence. *Primary Care, 26*(2), 373–384.

Willis, D. & Porche, D. (2004). Male battering of intimate partners: Theoretical underpinnings, approaches and interventions. *Nursing Clinics of North America, 39*(1), 271–282.

Child Abuse

Besharov, D. J. (1990, Spring). Gaining control over child abuse reports: Public agencies must address both under reporting and over reporting. *Public Welfare,* 34–40.

Heindl, C. (1979). *The nurse's role in the prevention and treatment of child abuse and neglect.* Publication No. 79-30202. Washington, DC: U.S. Department of Health, Education and Welfare.

Helfer, R. E., & Kempe, C. H. (1972). *Helping the battered child and his family.* Philadelphia: J. B. Lippincott.

Hurwitz, A., & Castells, S. (1987). Misdiagnosed child abuse and metabolic diseases. *Pediatric Nursing, 13,* 33–36.

Kauffman, C. K., Neill, M. K., & Thomas, J. N. (1986). The abusive parent. In S. H. Johnson (Ed.). *High-risk parenting: Assessment and nursing strategies for families at risk.* Philadelphia: J. B. Lippincott.

National Center on Child Abuse and Neglect. (1995). *A coordinated response to child abuse and neglect: A basic manual.* Washington, DC: NCCAN.

Seditus, C., & Mock, D. (1988). Interrupting the cycle of child abuse. *Maternal–Child Nursing Journal, 13,* 196–198.

Wissow, L. (1994). Child maltreatment. In F. Oski (Ed.). *Principles and practice of pediatrics* (2nd ed.). Philadelphia: J. B. Lippincott.

Wong, D. L. (1987). False allegations of child abuse: The other side of the tragedy. *Pediatric Nursing, 13,* 329–333.

Elder Abuse/Neglect

Anetzberger, G. J. (1987). *The etiology of elder abuse by adult offspring.* Springfield, IL: Charles C. Thomas.

Fulmer, T. & Paveza, G. (1998). Neglect in the elderly. *Nursing Clinics of North America, 33*(3), 457–466.

Steinmetz, S. K. (1988). *Duty bound: Elder abuse and family care.* Newberry Park, CA: Sage.

Winslow, B. W. (1998). Family caregiving and the use of formal community support services: A qualitative case study. *Issues in Mental Health Nursing, 19*(1), 11–27.

INEFFECTIVE COMMUNITY COPING

Allender, J., & Spradley, B. (2005). *Community health nursing* (6th ed.). Philadelphia: Lippincott Williams & Wilkins.

Aroskar, M. (1979). Ethical issues in community health nursing. *Nursing Clinics of North America, 14,* 35–44.

Fruger, A. (1993). Factors involving ethical decision-making in the home setting. *Home Health Care Nurse, 10*(2), 16–20.

White, M. S. (1982). Construct for public health nursing. *Nursing Outlook, 30,* 527–530.

Williams, C. (1977). Community health nursing—what is it? *Nursing Outlook, 25,* 250–254.

READINESS FOR ENHANCED COMMUNITY COPING

Archer, S. E. (1983). Marketing public health nursing services. *Nursing Outlook, 31,* 49–53.

Bushy, A. (1990). Rural determinants in family health: Considerations for community nurse. *Family and Community Health, 12*(4), 89–94.

DECISIONAL CONFLICT

Bailey, J. T., & Hendricks, D. E. (1987). Decisions made easy. *Nursing Life, 7*(4), 18–19.

Beaver, K. et al. (1996). Treatment decision making in women newly diagnosed with breast cancer. *Cancer Nursing, 19*(1), 8–19.

Bille, D. A. (1987). Locus of decision making in patient and family education: Its effects on promoting wellness. *Nursing Administration Quarterly, 2*(3), 62–65.

Blackhall, L. J., Murphy, S. T. Frank, G., Michel, V., & Azen, S. (1995). Ethnicity and attitudes toward patient autonomy. *JAMA, 74*(3); 1820–1825.

Brady, T. J. (1990). Point: Patient control of treatment is essential. *Arthritis Care and Research, 3,* 163–166.

Brunnquell, D. (1990, May). *Difficult decisions: Overcoming factors which make discussion of ethical issues difficult.* Paper presented at the meeting of the

Association for the Care of Children's Health, Washington, DC.

Burke, G. (1980). Ethics and medical decision-making. *Primary Care, 7*, 615–624.

Caress, A. (1997). Patient roles in decision-making. *Nursing Times, 93*(31), 45–48.

Cicirelli, V., & MacLean, A. P. (2000). Hastening death: A comparison of two end-of-life decisions. *Death Studies, 24*(3), 401–419.

Davis, A. J. (1989). Clinical nurses' ethical decision making in situations. *Advanced Nursing Science, 11*(3), 63–69.

Davison, B. J. & Degner, L. F. (1998). Promoting patient decision making in life-and-death situations. *Seminars in Oncology Nursing, 14*(2), 129–136.

Degner, L. F. & Beaton, J. I. (1987). *Life–death decisions in health care*. Washington, DC: Hemisphere Publishing Corporation.

Degner, L. F. & Russell, C. A. (1998). Preferences for treatment control among adults with cancer. *Research in Nursing and Health, 11*(6), 367–374.

Degner, L. F. & Sloan, J. A. (1992). Decision making during serious illness: What role do patients really want to play? *Journal of Clinical Epidemiology, 45*, 944–950.

Degner, L. F., Sloan, J. A., & Venkatesh, P. (1997). The control preferences scale. *Canadian Journal of Nursing Research, 29*(3), 21–43.

Dellasega, C., & Mastrian, K. (1995) The process and consequences of institutionalizing an elder. *Western Journal of Nursing Research, 17*, 133–140.

Doukus, D. J., & McCullough, L. B. (1991) The values history: The evaluation of the patient's values and advance directives. *Journal of Family Practice, 32*, 145–153.

Erlen, J. A. (1998). Treatment decision making: Who should decide? *Orthopaedic Nursing, 17*(4), 60–64.

Gallagher, S. M. (1998). Ethics: Paternalism in health-care decision making. *Ostomy Wound Management, 44*(4), 24–25.

Geary, C. M. B. (1987). Nursing grand rounds: The patient with viral cardiomyopathy. *Journal of Cardiovascular Nursing, 2*(1), 48–52.

Hiltunen, E. (1987). Decisional conflict: A phenomenological description from the points of view of the nurse and the client. In A. M. McLane (Ed.). *Classification of nursing diagnosis: Proceedings of the seventh conference*. St. Louis: C. V. Mosby.

Hiltunen, E. (1989). Nursing diagnosis: Decisional conflict (specify). In R. M. Carroll-Johnson (Ed.). *Classification of nursing diagnoses: Proceedings of the eighth conference*. Philadelphia: J. B. Lippincott.

Hiltunen, E. (1994). Validation of decisional conflict by critical care nurses. In R. M. Carroll-Johnson & Paquette M. (Eds.). *Classification of nursing diagnoses: Proceedings of the tenth conference*. Philadelphia: J. B. Lippincott.

Janis, I. L., & Mann, L. (1977). *Decision making: A psychological analysis of conflict, choice, and commitment*. New York: The Free Press.

Jezewski, M. A. (1993). Consenting to DNR: Critical care nurses' interactions with patients and family members. *American Journal of Critical Care, 2*, 302–309.

Jezewski, M. A. (1994). Do-not-resuscitate status: Conflict and culture brokering in critical care units. *Heart and Lung: Journal of Critical Care, 23*(6), 458–465.

Kelly-Powell, M. L. (1997). Personalizing choices: Patients' experiences with making treatment decisions. *Research in Nursing and Health, 20*(3), 219–227.

Kohnke, M. F. (1980). The nurse as advocate. *American Journal of Nursing, 80*, 2038–2040.

Lancaster, W., & Lancaster, J. (1982). Rational decision making: Managing uncertainty. *Journal of Nursing Administration, 12*(2), 23–28.

Low, M. B. (1992). Personal values and contraceptive choices. *NAACOG's Clinical Issues in Perinatal and Women's Health Nursing, 3*(2), 193–198.

Marsh, F. L. (1986). Refusal of treatment. *Clinical Geriatric Medicine, 2*, 511–520.

McDevitt-Graham, S. M. (1987). Decision-making: The multi-attribute model. *Nursing Management, 18*(3), 18–19.

Minogue, J. P., & Reedy, N. J. (1988). Companioning parents in perinatal decision making. *Journal of Perinatal and Neonatal Nursing, 1*(3), 25–35.

Nugent, P. S. (1982). Management and modes of thought. *Journal of Nursing Administration, 12*(2), 19–25.

O'Connor, A. M. (1995). Validation of a decisional conflict scale. *Medical Decision Making, 15*(1), 25–30.

Pinch, W. J., & Spielman, M. L. (1990). The parent's perspective: Ethical decision making in neonatal intensive care. *Journal of Advanced Nursing, 15*, 712–719.

Raines, D. A. (1993). Values: A guiding force. *AWHONNS Clinical Issues in Perinatal and Women's Health Nursing, 4*, 533–541.

Roberts, S. J., Krouse, H. J., & Michaud, P. (1995). Negotiated and nonnegotiated nurse–patient interactions: Enhancing perceptions of empowerment. *Clinical Nursing Research, 4*(1), 67–77.

Scott, P. N. (1989). Families with adolescents. In R. L. Foster, M. M. Hunsberger, & J. J. T. Anderson (Eds.). *Family-centered nursing care of children*. Philadelphia: W. B. Saunders.

Sims, S. L., Boland, D. L., & O'Neill, C. A. (1992). Decision making in home health care. *Western Journal of Nursing Research, 14*, 186–200.

Simon, S. B., Howe, L. W., & Kirschenbaum, H. (1978). *Values clarification: A handbook of practical strategies for teachers and students*. New York: A & W Publishers.

Soholt, D. (1990). *A life experience: Making a health care treatment decision*. Unpublished master's thesis, South Dakota State University, Brookings.

Taylor, E. J. (1993). Managing cancer pain at home: The decisions and ethical conflicts of patients, family caregivers, and homecare nurses. *Oncology Nursing Forum, 20*, 919–927.

Valanis, B. G., & Rumpler, C. H. (1985). Helping women to choose breast cancer treatment alternatives. *Cancer Nursing, 8*, 167–175.

Zotti, M. E. (1987). Nursing intervention to assist patients' decision making with respect to family planning. *Public Health Nursing, 4*(3), 146–150.

DIARRHEA

Bennett, R. (2000). Acute gastroenteritis and associated conditions. In L. R. Barker, J. Burton, & P. Zieve (Eds.). *Principles of ambulatory medicine*. Baltimore: Williams & Wilkins.

Brown, K. C. (1991). Dietary management of acute childhood diarrhea: Optimal timing of feeding and appropriate use of milk and mixed diets. *Journal of Pediatrics, 118*, S92–S98.

Duggan, C., Lasche, J., McCarty, C. et al. (1999). Oral rehydration solution for acute diarrhea prevents subsequent unscheduled follow-up visits. *Pediatrics, 102*(104), 55–63.

Fuhrman, M. P. (1999). Diarrhea and tube feeding. *Nutritional Clinical Practice, 14*(2), 83–84.

Goepp, J., & Santosham, M. (2001). Oral rehydration therapy. In F. Oski (Ed.). *Principles and practice of pediatrics*. Philadelphia: J. B. Lippincott.

Larson, C. E. (2000). Evidence-based practice. Safety and efficacy of oral rehydration therapy for treatment of diarrhea and gastroenteritis in pediatrics. *Pediatric Nursing, 26*(2), 177–179.

DISUSE SYNDROME

Caswell, D. (1993). Thromboembolic phenomena. *Critical Care Nursing Clinics of North America, 5,* 489–497.

Chen, D., Apple, D. F., Hudson, L. M., & Bode, R. (1999). Medical complications during acute rehabilitation following spinal cord injury. *Archives of Physical Medical Rehabilitation, 80*(11), 1397–1401.

Christian, B. J. (1982). Immobilization: Psychosocial aspects. In C. Norris (Ed.). *Concept clarification in nursing.* Rockville, MD: Aspen Publications.

Maher, A. Salmond, S., & Pellino, T. (1998). *Orthopedic nursing* (2nd ed.). Philadelphia: W. B. Saunders.

Maklebust, J., & Sieggreen, M. (1996). *Pressure ulcers: Guidelines for prevention and nursing management* (2nd ed.). Springhouse, PA: Springhouse.

McKinley, W. O., Jackson, A. B., Cardenas, D. D., & Devivo, M. J. (1999). Long-term medical complications after traumatic spinal cord injury. *Archives of Physical Medical Rehabilitation, 80*(11) 1402–1410.

Tyler, M. (1984). The respiratory effects of body positioning and immobilization. *Respiratory Care, 29,* 472–481.

Whitbourne, S. K. (1985). Appearance and movement. In S. K. Whitbourne (Ed.). *The aging body.* New York: Springer-Verlag.

Wright, S. (1989). Nursing strategies: Altered musculoskeletal function. In R. L. Foster, M. M. Hunsberger, & J. J. T. Anderson (Eds.). *Family-centered nursing care of children.* Philadelphia: W. B. Saunders.

Zubek, J. P., & McNeil, M. (1967). Perceptual deprivation phenomena: Role of the recumbent position. *Journal of Abnormal Psychology, 72,* 147.

DEFICIENT DIVERSIONAL ACTIVITY

Buckle, J. (1998). Clinical aromatherapy and touch: Complementary therapies for nursing practice. *Critical Care Nurse, 18*(5), 54–55.

Dossey, B. (1998). Holistic modalities and healing moments. *American Journal of Nursing, 98*(6), 44–47.

Kuntz, N., Adams, J., Zahr, L., Killen, R., Cameron, K., & Wasson, H. (1996). Therapeutic play and bone marrow transplantation. *Journal of Pediatric Nursing: Nursing Care of Children and Families, 11*(6), 359–367.

Longino, C. F., & Kart, C. S. (1982). Explicating activity theory: A formal replication. *Journal of Gerontology, 37,* 713–722.

McPherson, B., & Guppy, N. (1979). Preretirement lifestyle and the degree of planning for retirement. *Journal of Gerontology, 34,* 254–263.

Rantz, M. (1991). Diversional activity deficit. In M. Maas, K. Buckwalter, & M. Hardy (Eds.). *Nursing diagnoses and interventions for the elderly.* Redwood City, CA: Addison-Wesley Nursing.

Roenke, L., & Mulligan, S. (1998). The therapeutic value of the human–animal connection. *Occupational Therapy in Health Care, 11*(2), 27–43.

Scipien, G. M., Chard, M. A., Howe, J., & Barnard, M. U. (1990). *Pediatric nursing care.* St. Louis: C. V. Mosby.

DYSREFLEXIA

Black, K., & DeSantis, N. (1999). Medical complications common to spinal-cord injury and brain injured patients. *Topics in Spinal Cord Injury Rehabilitation, 5*(2), 47–75.

Bennett, C. (2003). Urgent urological management of the paraplegic/quadriplegic patient. *Urologic Nursing, 23*(6), 436–437.

Eisenhauer, L., Nichois, L., Spencer, R., et al. (1997). *Clinical pharmacology and nursing management* (5th ed.). Philadelphia: J. B. Lippincott.

Johnson, K. M. S. (1991). Growing up with a spinal cord injury. *SCI Nursing, 8*(1), 11–19.

Kavchak-Keyes, M. A. (2000). Autonomic hyperreflexia. *Rehabilitation Nursing, 25*(1), 31–35.

McClain, W., Shields, C., & Sixsmith, D. (1999). Autonomic dysreflexia presenting as a severe headache. *American Journal of Emergency Medicine, 17*(3), 238–240.

Silver, J. R. (2000). Early autonomic dysreflexia. *Spinal Cord, 38,* 229–233.

Teasell, R., Arnold, J., & Delaney, G. (1996). Sympathetic nervous system dysfunction in high level spinal cord injuries. *Physical Medicine and Rehabilitation, 10*(1), 37–55.

Travers, P. (1999). Autonomic dysreflexia: A clinical rehabilitation problem. *Rehabilitation Nursing, 24*(1), 9–23.

ENERGY FIELD DISTURBANCE

Bradley, D. B. (1987). Energy fields: Implications for nurses. *Journal of Holistic Nursing, 5*(1), 32–35.

Denison, B. (2004). Touch the pain away. *Holistic Nursing Practice, 18*(3), 142–151.

Dossey, B. M., Keegan, L., Guzzetta, C. E., & Kolmeier, L. G. (1995). *Holistic nursing: A handbook for practice* (2nd ed.). Rockville, MD: Aspen Publishers.

Krieger, D. (1975). Therapeutic touch: The imprimatur of nursing. *American Journal of Nursing, 75,* 784–787.

Krieger, D. (1979). *The therapeutic touch: How to use your hands to help or to heal.* Englewood Cliffs, NJ: Prentice-Hall.

Krieger, D. (1981). *Foundations of holistic health nursing practices: The Renaissance nurse.* Philadelphia: J. B. Lippincott.

Krieger, D. (1987). *Living the therapeutic touch: Healing as a lifestyle.* New York: Dodd, Mead.

Lionberger, H. J. (1986). Therapeutic touch: A healing modality or a caring strategy. In P. Chinn (Ed.). *Nursing research methodology: Issues and implementation.* Rockville, MD: Aspen Publishers.

Macrae, J. (1988). *Therapeutic touch: A practical guide.* New York: Knopf.

Meehan, T. C. (1991). Therapeutic touch. In G. Bule-chek & J. McCloskey (Eds.). *Nursing interventions: Essential nursing treatments.* Philadelphia: W. B. Saunders.

Meehan, T. C. (1998). Therapeutic touch as nursing intervention. *Journal of Advanced Nursing, 28*(1), 117–125.

Quinn, J. F. (1989). Therapeutic touch as energy exchange: Replication and extension. *Nursing Science Quarterly, 2*(2), 79–87.

Quinn, J., & Strelkauskas, A. (1993). Psychoimmunologic effects of therapeutic touch on practitioners and recently bereaved recipients: A pilot study. *Advances in Nursing Science, 15*(4), 13–26.

Straneva, J. A. (2000). Therapeutic touch coming of age. *Holistic Nursing Practice, 14*(3), 1–13.

Umbreit, A. W. (2000). Healing touch: Applications in the acute care setting. *ACCN Clinical Issues of Advanced Practice in Acute Critical Care, 11*(1), 105–119.

INTERRUPTED FAMILY PROCESSES

Burgess, E. S., Dratar, D., Taylor, H. G., et al. (1999). The family burden of injury interview: Reliability and validity studies. *Journal of Head Trauma Rehabilitation, 14*(4), 394–405.

Clark, J., & Gwin, R. (2001). Psychological responses of the family. In S. Groenwald, M. Frogge, M. Goodman, & C. Yarbo (Eds.). *Cancer nursing: Principles and practice* (3rd ed.). Boston: Jones and Bartlett.

Craft, M. J., & Craft, J. L. (1989). Perceived changes in siblings of hospitalized children: A comparison of sibling and hospitalized and parent reports. *Children's Health Care, 18*(1), 42–48.

Duvall, E. M. (1977). *Marriage and family development* (5th ed.). Philadelphia: J. B. Lippincott.

Fife, B. L. (1985). A model for predicting the adaptation of families to medical crisis: An analysis of role integration. *Image: Journal of Nursing Scholarship, 18*(4), 108–112.

Harkulich, J., & Calamita, B. (1986). *A manual for caregivers of Alzheimer's disease clients in long-term care* (2nd ed.). Beachwood, OH: Nursing Home Training Center, Menorah Park Center for the Aged.

Hashizume, S., & Takano, J. (1983). Nursing care of Japanese American patients. In M. S. Orque, B. Bloch, & L. S. A. Monroy (Eds.). *Ethnic nursing care: A multicultural approach.* St. Louis: C. V. Mosby.

Kurnat, E., & Moore, C. (1999). The impact of a chronic condition on the families of children with asthma. *Pediatric Nursing, 25*(3), 288–292.

Nugent, K., Hughes, R., Ball, B., & Davis, K., (1992). A practice model for pediatric support groups. *Pediatric Nursing, 18*(1), 11–16.

Orque, M. S., Bloch, B., & Monroy, L. S. A. (Eds.). (1983). *Ethnic nursing care: A multicultural approach.* St. Louis: C. V. Mosby.

Smith-DiJulio, K. (1998). Families in crisis: Family violence. In E. M. Varcarolis (Ed.). *Foundations of psychiatric mental health nursing* (3rd ed.). Philadelphia: W. B. Saunders.

Alcoholism

Captain, C. (1989). Family recovery from alcoholism. *Nursing Clinics of North America, 24*, 55–67.

Collins, R. L., Leonard, K., & Searles, J. (1990). *Alcohol and the family: Research and clinical perspectives.* New York: Guilford Press.

Grisham, K., & Estes, N. (1982). Dynamics of alcoholic families. In N. Estes & M. E. Heinemann (Eds.). *Alcoholism: Development, consequences and interventions.* St. Louis: Mosby–Year Book.

Kellett, S. K. (2000). Do women carry more emotional baggage? Gender difference in contact length to a community alcohol treatment alcohol treatment service. *Journal of Substance Use, 5*(3) 211–7.

Lindeman, M., Hokanson, J., & Bartek, J. (1994). The alcoholic family. *Nursing Diagnoses, 5*(2), 65–73.

North American Nursing Diagnosis Association. (1992). *NANDA nursing diagnosis: Definitions and classifications.* Philadelphia: Author.

Smith-DiJulio, K. (1998). People who depend on alcohol. In E. M. Varcarolis (Ed.). *Foundations of psychiatric mental health nursing* (3rd ed.). Philadelphia: W. B. Saunders.

Starling, B. P., & Martin, A. C. (1990). Adult survivors of parental alcoholism: Implications for primary care. *Nursing Practice, 15*(7), 16–24.

Vanicelli, M. (1987). Treatment of alcoholic couples in outpatient group therapy. *Group 11, 4,* 247–257.

Wegscheider, S. (1981). *Another chance.* Palo Alto, CA: Science and Behavior Books.

Wing, D. M. (1991). Goal setting and recovery from alcoholism. *Archives of Psychiatry in Nursing, 5,* 178–184.

Wing, D. M. (1994). Understanding alcoholism relapse. *Nurse Practitioner, 19*(4), 67–69.

Resources for the Consumer

Beattie, M. (1992). *Codependent no more—how to stop controlling others and start caring for yourself.* Center City: Hazelden.

Peele, S., & Brodsky, A. (1992). *The truth about addiction and recovery.* New York: Simon & Schuster.

Woititz, J. G. (1990). *Adult children of alcoholics.* Deerfield Beach, CA: Health Communications, Inc.

FATIGUE

Aaronson, L. S., Teel, C. S., Cassmeyer, V. et al. (1999). Defining and measuring fatigue. *Image: Journal of Nursing Scholarship, 31*(1), 45–50.

Adinolfi, A. (2001). Assessment and treatment of HIV-related fatigue. *Journal of the Association of Nurses in AIDS Care, 12*(Suppl.), 33–39.

Badger, T. A. (2001). Depression burden, self-help interventions, and side effect experience in women receiving treatment for breast cancer. *Badger, 28*(3), 567–574.

Beck, A. T. (1984). Cognitive approaches to stress. In R. F. Woolfolk & P. M. Lehrer (Eds.). *Principles and practice of stress management.* New York: Guilford Press.

Braden, C. J. (1990). A test of the self-help model: Learned response to chronic illness experience. *Nursing Research, 39*(1), 42–47.

Crosby, L. (1991). Factors which contribute to fatigue associated with rheumatoid arthritis. *Journal of Advanced Nursing, 16,* 974–981.

Dzurec, L. C. (2000). Fatigue and relativeness experiences of inordinately tired women: Fourth quarter. *Journal of Nursing Scholarship, 32*(4), 339–345.

Gardner, D. L. (1992). Fatigue in postpartum women. *Applied Nursing Research, 4*(5), 57–62.

Gardner, D. L., & Campbell, B. (1991). Assessing postpartum fatigue. *Maternal–Child Nursing Journal, 16,* 264–266.

Greenberg, D., Sawicka, J., Eisenthal, S., & Ross, D. (1992). Fatigue syndrome due to localized radiation. *Journal of Pain and Symptom Management, 7*(1), 38–45.

Hargreaves, M. (1977). The fatigue syndrome. *Practitioner, 218,* 841–843.

Hart, L., Freel, M., & Milde, F. (1990). Fatigue. *Nursing Clinics of North America, 25,* 967–976.

Houde, S. C., & Kampfe-Leacher, R. (1997). Chronic fatigue syndrome: An update for clinicians in primary care. *Nurse Practitioner, 22*(7), 30, 35–40, 42–48.

Jiricka, M. K. (2002). Alterations in activity tolerance. In C. M. Porth (Ed.), *Pathophysiology: Concepts of altered health states* (6th ed.). Philadelphia: Lippincott Williams & Wilkins.

Longino, C. F., & Kart, C. S. (1982). Explicating activity theory: A formal replication. *Journal of Gerontology, 37,* 713–722.

Nail, L., & Winningham, M. (1997). Fatigue. In S. Groenwald, M. Frogge, M. Goodman, & C. Yarbo (Eds.). *Cancer nursing: Principles and practice* (4th ed.). Boston: Jones and Bartlett.

Rhoten, D. (1982). Fatigue and the postsurgical patient. In C. Norris (Ed.). *Concept clarification in nursing.* Rockville, MD: Aspen Systems.

Stuifburgen, A. K., & Rogers, S. (1997). The experience of fatigue and strategies of self-care among persons with multiple sclerosis. *Applied Nursing Research 10*(1), 2–10.

Tilden, V. P., & Weinert, C. (1987). Social support and the chronically ill individual. *Nursing Clinics of North America, 22,* 613–620.

Winningham, M. L. (1992). How exercise mitigates fatigue: Implications for people receiving cancer therapy. In R. M. Johnson (Ed.). *The biotherapy of cancer: V.* Pittsburgh: Oncology Nursing Press.

FEAR

Broome, M. E., Bates, T. A., Lillis, P. P., & McGahee, T. W. (1990). Children's medical fears, coping behaviors, and pain perceptions during a lumbar puncture. *Oncology Nursing Forum, 17,* 361–367.

Cesarone, D. (1991). Fear. In M. Maas, K. Buckwalter, & M. Hardy (Eds.). *Nursing diagnoses and interventions for the elderly.* Redwood City, CA: Addison-Wesley Nursing.

Kuntz, N., Adams, I., Zahr, I., et al. (1996). Therapeutic play and bone marrow transplantation. *Journal of Pediatric Nursing, 11*(6), 359–367.

Nicastro, E., & Whetsell, M. V. (1999). Children's fears. *Journal of Pediatric Nursing, 14*(6), 392–402.

DEFICIENT AND EXCESS FLUID VOLUME

Compher, C., Kim, J., & Bader, J. (1998). Nutritional requirements of an aging population with emphasis on subacute care. *AACN Clinical issues: Advanced Practice in Acute and Critical Care, 9*(3), 441–445.

Cravens, C. (1998). The boiling point. *Occupational Health and Safety, 67*(7), 26–28.

Davis, D. (1996). The discomforts of pregnancy. *JOGNN, 25*(1), 73–81.

Fischback, F. (1995). *A manual of laboratory & diagnostic tests.* Philadelphia: J. B. Lippincott.

Gershan, J. (1990). Fluid volume deficit: Validating indicators. *Heart and Lung, 19,* 152–156.

Harvey, R. (1997). Body check. Eat, drink, and rehydrate. *Health and You, 133*(2), 14–15.

House, N. (1992). The hydration question: Hydration or dehydration for terminally ill patients. *Professional Nurse, 8*(1), 10–23.

Maughan, R., Leiper, J., & Shirreffs, S. (1997). Factors influencing the restoration of fluid and electrolyte balance after exercise in the heat. *British Journal of Sports Medicine, 31*(3), 175–182.

Parkash, R., & Burge, F. (1997). The family's perspective on issues of hydration in terminal care. *Journal of Palliative Care, 13*(4), 23–27.

Powell, A., & Armstrong, M. (1997). Peripheral edema. *American Family Physician, 55*(5), 1721–1726.

Sansevero, A. (1997). Dehydration in the elderly: Strategies for prevention and management. *Nurse Practitioner: American Journal of Primary Health Care, 22*(4), 41–42, 51–52, 54–57.

Sergent, E., Strauss, C., Jaffe, M., Majewsky, E., & Mitchell, C. (1991). Diagnostic content validity of fluid volume excess: A construct replication. In R. Carroll-Johnson (Ed.). *Classification of nursing diagnoses: Proceedings of the ninth conference.* Philadelphia: J. B. Lippincott.

Steiner, N., & Bruera, E. (1998). Methods of hydration in palliative care patients. *Journal of Palliative Care, 14*(2), 6–18.

Terry, M., O'Brien, S., & Derstein, M. (1998). Lower-extremity edema: Evaluation and diagnosis. *Wounds: A Compendium of Clinical Research and Practice, 10*(4), 118–124.

Zembruski, C. (1997). GN management. A three-dimensional approach to hydration of elders: Administration, clinical staff, and in-service education. *Geriatric Nursing: American Journal of Care for the Aging, 18*(1), 20–26.

GRIEVING

Andrews, M., & Hansen, P. (2004). Religious beliefs: Implications for nursing practice. In M. Andrews & J. Boyle (Eds.), *Transcultural concepts in nursing* (4th ed.). Philadelphia: Lippincott Williams & Wilkins.

Bateman, A. L. (1999). Understanding the process of grieving and loss: A critical social thinking perspective. *Journal of American Psychiatric Nurses Association, 5*(5), 139–149.

Bourne, V., & Meier, J. (1988). What happens now? A book to be read to children who have lost a loved one. *Oncology Nursing Forum, 15*(1), 81–85.

Caserta, M. S., Lund, D. A., & Dimond, M. F. (1985). Assessing interviewer effects in a longitudinal study of bereaved elderly adults. *Journal of Gerontology, 40,* 637–640.

Cutcliffe, J. R. (2004) The inspiration of hope in bereavement counseling. *Issues in Mental Health Nursing, 25*(2), 165–190.

Engle, G. (1964) Grief and grieving. *American Journal of Nursing, 64,* 93–97.

Gallagher, D. E., Breckenridge, J. N., Thompson, L. W., & Peterson, J. A. (1983). Effects of bereavement on indicators of mental health in elderly widows and widowers. *Journal of Gerontology, 38,* 565–571.

Haylor, M. (1987). Human response to loss. *Nurse Practitioner, 12*(5), 63.

Hull, M. M. (1992). Coping strategies of family caregivers in hospice home care. *Oncology Nursing Forum, 19,* 1179–1187.

Kahn, A. M. (1995) Coping with fear and grieving. In J. M. Lubkin (Ed.). *Chronic illness: Impact and interventions* (3rd ed.). Boston: Jones & Bartlett.

Kaprio, J., & Koskenvuo, R. H. (1987). Mortality after bereavement: A prospective study of 95,647 widowed persons. *American Journal of Public Health, 77,* 283–287.

Kübler-Ross, E. (1975). *Death: The final stage of growth.* Englewood Cliffs, NJ: Prentice-Hall.

Kübler-Ross, E. (1983). *On children and death.* New York: Macmillan.

Mallinson, R. K. (1999). The lived experience of AIDS-related multiple losses by HIV-negative gay men. *Journal of the Association of Nurses in AIDS Care, 10*(5), 22–31.

Martinez, J., & Wagner, S. (2001). Hospice care. In S. L. Greenwald, M. Goodman, M. H. Frogge, & C. Yarbo (Eds.). *Cancer nursing: Principles and practice* (5th ed.). Boston: Jones & Bartlett.

Mina, C. (1985) A program for helping grieving parents. *Maternal–Child Nursing Journal, 10,* 118–121.

Pallikkathayil, L., & Flood, M. (1991). Adolescent suicide. *Nursing Clinics of North America, 26*(3), 623–630.

Rando, T. A. (1984). *Grief, dying, and death: Clinical interventions for caregivers.* Champaign, IL: Research Press.

Ransohoff-Adler, M., & Berger, C. S. (1989). When newborns die: Do we practice what we preach? *Journal of Perinatal, 9,* 311–316.

Vanezis, M. & McGee, A. (1999). Mediating factors in the grieving process of the suddenly bereaved. *British Journal of Nursing, 8*(14), 932–937.

Vickers, J. L. & Carlisle, C. (2000). Choices and control: Parental experiences in pediatric terminal home care. *Journal of Pediatric Oncology Nursing, 17*(1), 12–21.

Worden, W. (2002). *Grief counseling and grief therapy* (3rd ed.). New York: Springer.

Zisook, S., & Schochter, C. (1992). Depression through the first year after the death of a spouse. *American Journal of Psychiatry, 148*(10), 1346–1352.

DELAYED GROWTH AND DEVELOPMENT

Bergland, Adel (2001). Thriving-a useful theoretical perspective to capture the experience of well-being among frail elderly in nursing homes? *Journal of Advanced Nursing* 36(3), 426–432.

Haight, Barbara K. (2002). Thriving: A life span theory. *Journal Of Gerontological Nursing* 14–22.

Kimball, M. J., & Williams-Burgess, C. (1995). Failure to thrive: The silent epidemic of the elderly. *Archives of Psychiatric Nursing, 9*(2), 99–105.

Newbern, V. B., & Krowchuk, H. V. (1994). Failure to thrive in elderly people: A conceptual analysis. *Journal of Advanced Nursing,* 840–849.

Wagnild, G. & Young H. M. (1990) Resilience among older women. *Image: Journal of Nursing Scholarship* 22,252–255.

INEFFECTIVE HEALTH MAINTENANCE

Allen, K. M., & Phillips, J. M. (1997). *Women's health across the life span.* Philadelphia: J. B. Lippincott.

Belloc, N., & Breslow, L. (1972). The relation of physical health status and health practice. *Preventive Medicine, 1,* 409–421.

Dunn, H. L. (1959). What high-level wellness means. *Canadian Journal of Public Health, 50,* 447–457.

Edelman, C. L., & Mandle, C. L. (2001). *Health promotion throughout the lifespan* (5th ed.). St. Louis: Mosby-Year Book.

Hanson, S. M., & Boyd, S. T. (1996). *Family health care nursing: Theory, practice and research.* Philadelphia: W. B. Saunders.

Moore, S. M., & Charvat, J. M. (2002). Using the CHANGE intervention to enhance long-term exercise. *The Nursing Clinics of North America, 37*(2), 273–281.

Rankins, S., & Stallings, K. D. (2001). *Patient education: Issues, principles, practices* (4th ed.). Philadelphia: Lippincott Williams & Wilkins.

U.S. Department of Health and Human Services, Public Health Service. *Healthy people 2000.* Washington, DC: U.S. Government Printing Office.

U.S. Department of Health and Human Services. (1994). *Clinician's handbook of preventive services.* Washington, DC: U.S. Government Printing Office.

Gerontologic

Allison, M., & Keller, C. (1997). Physical activity in the elderly: Benefits and intervention strategies. *Nurse Practitioner, 22*(8), 53–54, 56, 58, 63, 64.

U.S. Department of Health and Human Services. (1987). *Current estimates for the national health interview survey.* Hyattsville, MD: Author.

Tobacco Use

Andrews, J. (1998). Optimizing smoking cessation strategies. *Nurse Practitioner, 23*(8), 47–48, 51–52, 57, 61, 64, 67.

Ash, C. R. (1987). Smoking and lung cancer. *Cancer Nursing, 10*(4), 171.

Centers for Disease Control and Prevention (2000). Selected cigarette smoking initiation and quitting behaviors among high school students–US. *MMWR, 47,* 386.

Centers for Disease Control and Prevention. (2004). www.cdc.gov/health/tobacco.htm.

Cinelli, B., & Glover, E. (1988). Nurses' smoking in the work-place: Causes and solutions. *Journal of Community Health Nursing, 5,* 255–261.

DuRant, R., & Smith, J. (1999). Adolescent tobacco use and cessation. *Primary Care, 26*(3), 553–576.

Koepke, D., Flay, B., & Johnson, C. A. (1990). Health behaviors in minority families: The case of cigarette smoking. *Family and Community Health, 13,* 35–43.

McAndrew, M. (1998). People who depend on substances other than alcohol. In E. M. Varcarolis (Ed.). *Foundations of psychiatric–mental health nursing.* (3rd ed.). Philadelphia: W. B. Saunders.

Mitchell, B., Sobel, H. L., & Alexander, M. H. (1999). The adverse health effects of tobacco and tobacco-related products. *Primary Care, 26*(3), 463–498.

Mullen, P. D. (1999). Maternal smoking during pregnancy and evidence-based intervention to promote cessation. *Primary Care, 26*(3), 557–590.

Pletsch, P. K. (2002). Reduction of primary and secondary smoke exposure for low-income black pregnant women. *The Nursing Clinics of North America, 37*(2), 315–326.

U.S. Department of Health and Human Services. (1994). *Preventing tobacco use among young people: A report of the surgeon general.* Washington, DC: U.S. Government Printing Office.

Obesity

Bal, D. G., & Foester, S. B. (1991). Changing the American diet: Impact on cancer prevention policy recommendations and program implications for the American Cancer Society. *Cancer, 67,* 2671–2680.

Buiten, C., & Metzger, B. (2000). Childhood obesity and risk of cardiovascular disease: A review of the science. *Pediatric Nursing 26*(1), 13–18.

Dennis, K. (2004). Weight management in women. *Nursing Clinics in North America, 39*(14), 231–241.

Fleury, J. D. (1991). Empowering potential: A theory of wellness motivation. *Nursing Research, 40,* 286–291.

Jeffery, R. W. (1991). Population perspectives on the prevention and treatment of obesity in minority populations. *American Journal of Clinical Nutrition, 53*(6 Suppl), 1621S–1624S.

Keller, C., & Stevens, K. (1996). Assessment, etiology and intervention in obesity in children. *Nurse Practitioner, 21*(9), 31–32, 34–36, 38, 41.

Moran, R. (1999). Evaluation and treatment of childhood obesity. *American Family Physician, 59*(4), 861–868.

Myers, S., & Vargas, J. K. (2000). Parental perceptions of the preschool obese child. *Pediatric Nursing, 26*(1), 23–31.

Pencak, M. (1991). Workplace health promotion programs: An overview. *Nursing Clinics of North America, 26,* 233–240.

Roberts, S. O. (2000). The role of physical activity in the prevention and treatment of childhood obesity. *Pediatric Nursing, 26*(1), 33–43.

Wiereng, M. E., & Oldham, K. K. (2002). Weight control: a lifestyle-modification model for improving health. *The Nursing Clinics of North America, 37*(2), 303–311.

Osteoporosis

Bellantoni, M. F., & Blackman, M. R. (1988). Osteoporosis: Diagnostic screening and its place in current care. *Geriatrics, 43*(2), 63–70.

Eastell, R., Boyle, I., Compston, J., et al. (1998). Management of male osteoporosis: Report of UIC Consensus Group. *Quarterly Journal of Medicine, 91*(2), 71–92.

Lindsay, R. (1989). Osteoporosis: An updated approach to prevention and management. *Geriatrics, 44*(1), 45–54.

Woodhead, G., & Moss, M. (1998). Osteoporosis: Diagnosis and prevention. *Nursing Practitioner, 23*(11), 18, 23–24, 26–27, 31–32, 34–35.

Pediatric

Hunsberger, M. (1989). Impact of acute illness. In R. L. Foster, M. M. Hunsberger, & J. J. T. Anderson (Eds.). *Family-centered nursing care of children.* Philadelphia: W. B. Saunders.

Internet Resources

www.cdc.gov/tobacco
www.endsmoking.org
www.tobaccofreekids.org
www.tobacco.org

HEALTH-SEEKING BEHAVIORS

See also References/Bibliography for *Ineffective Health Maintenance*.

American Heart Association. (1990). *Help your heart: Children and cholesterol.* Philadelphia: American Heart Association.

Fleury, J. D. (1991). Empowering potential: A theory of wellness motivation. *Nursing Research, 40,* 286–291.

Leon, L. (2002). Smoking cessation—Developing a workable program. *Nursing Spectrum, FL9*(18), 12–13.

Neale, A., Singleton, S., Dupius, M., & Hess, J. Correlates of adherence to behavioral contracts for cholesterol reduction. *Journal of Nutrition Education, 21,* 221–225.

Nyamathi, A. (1989). Comprehensive health seeking and coping paradigm. *Journal of Advanced Nursing, 14,* 281–290.

Torisky, C., Hertzler, A., Johnson, J., Keller, J., Hodges, P., & Mifflin, B. (1990). Virginia EFNEP homemakers' dietary improvement and relation to selected family factors. *Journal of Nutrition Education, 21,* 249–257.

Tusaie, K. & Dyer, J. (2004). Resilience: A historical review of construct. *Holistic Nursing Practice, 18*(1), 3–8.

Woodhead, G. (1996). The management of cholesterol in coronary heart disease. *Nurse Practitioner, 21*(9), 45, 48, 51, 53.

Pediatric

Cox, C. L. (1990). The health self-determinism index for children. *Research in Nursing and Health, 13,* 237–246.

Manworren, R. C. B., & Woodring, B. (1998). Evaluating children's literature as a source for patient education. *Pediatric Nursing, 24*(6), 548–553.

IMPAIRED HOME MAINTENANCE

Arling, G. (1987). Strain, social support and distress in old age. *Journal of Gerontology, 42,* 107–113.

Green, K. (1998). *Home care survival guide.* Philadelphia: Lippincott.

Holzapfil, S. (1998). The elderly. In E. Varcarolis (Ed.). *Foundations of psychiatric mental health nursing* (3rd ed.). Philadelphia: W. B. Saunders.

Schank, M. J., & Lough, M. A. (1990). Profile: Frail elderly women, maintaining independence. *Journal of Advanced Nursing, 15,* 674–682.

U.S. Department of Health and Human Services. (1987). *Current estimates for the national health interview survey.* Hyattsville, MD: Author.

Wong, D. L. (1991). Transition from hospital to home for children with complex medical care. *Journal of Pediatric Oncology Nursing, 8*(1), 3–9.

HOPELESSNESS

Christman, N. J. (1990). Uncertainty and adjustment during radiotherapy. *Nursing Research, 39*(1), 17–20, 47.

Coulter, M. A. (1989). The needs of family members of patients in intensive care units. *Intensive Care Nursing, 5,* 4–10.

Davies, H. N. (1993). Hope as a coping strategy for the spinal cord injured individual. *Axone, 15*(2), 40–45.

Drew, B. L. (1990). Differentiation of hopelessness, helplessness and powerlessness using Erikson's "Roots of Virtue." *Archives of Psychiatric Nursing, 14,* 332–337.

Engel, G. (1989). A life setting conducive to illness: The giving up–given up complex. *Annals of Internal Medicine, 69,* 293–300.

Fromm, E. (1968). *The evolution of hope.* New York: Harper.

Herth, K. (1993). Hope in the family caregiver of terminally ill people. *Journal of Advanced Nursing, 18,* 538–547.

Hickey, S. S. (1986). Enabling hope. *Cancer Nursing, 9,* 133–137.

Hinds, P. (1988). Adolescent hopefulness in illness and health. *Advances in Nursing Science, 10*(3), 79–88.

Hinds, P., Martin, J., & Vogel, R. (1987). Nursing strategies to influence adolescent hopefulness during oncologic illness. *Journal of the Association of Pediatric Oncology Nurses, 4*(1/2), 14–23.

Jackson, B. S. (1993). Hope and wound healing. *Journal of Enterostomal Therapy in Nursing, 20*(2), 73–77.

Jennings, P. (1997). The aging spirit. Faith and hope—therapeutic tools for case managers. *Aging Today, 18*(2), 17.

Johnson, L. H., Roberts, S. L., & Cheffer, N. D. (1996). A hope and a hopelessness model applied to the family of multi-trauma injury patient. *Journal of Trauma Nursing, 3*(3), 72–85.

Korner, I. N. (1970). Hope as a method of coping. *Journal of Consultation and Clinical Psychology 34,* 134–139.

Kübler-Ross, E. (1975). *Death: The final stage of growth.* Englewood Cliffs, NJ: Prentice-Hall.

LeGresley, A. (1991). Validation of hopelessness: Perceptions of the critically ill. In R. M. Carroll-Johnson (Ed.). *Classification of nursing diagnoses: Proceedings of the ninth conference.* Philadelphia: J. B. Lippincott.

Leininger, M. (1978). *Transcultural nursing: Concepts, theories, and practices.* New York: John Wiley & Sons.

McGill, J. S. (1992). Functional status as it relates to hope in elders. *Kentucky Nurse, 40*(4), 6.

Miller, J. F. (1989). Hope inspiring strategies of the critically ill. *Applied Nursing Research, 2*(1), 23–29.

Notewotney, M. L. (1989). Assessment of hope in patients with cancer: Development of an instrument. *Oncology Nursing Forum, 16,* 57–61.

Owen, D. C. (1989). Nurses' perspectives on the meaning of hope in patients with cancer: A qualitative study. *Oncology Nursing Forum, 16,* 75–79.

Parse, R. R. (1990). Parse's research methodology within an illustration of the lived experience of hope. *Nursing Science Quarterly, 3*(3), 9–17.

Plummer, E. M. (1988). Measurement of hope in the elderly hospitalized institutionalized person. *New York State Nurses' Association, 19*(3), 8–11.

Poncar, P. J. (1994). Inspiring hope in the oncology patient. *Journal of Psychosocial Nursing, 32*(1), 33–38.

Reed, P. G. (1986). Developmental resources and depression in the elderly. *Nursing Research, 35,* 368–373.

Schmale, A. H., & Iher, H. P. (1966). The affect of hopelessness and the development of cancer. *Psychosomatic Medicine, 28,* 714–721.

Stotland, E. (1969). *The psychology of hope.* San Francisco: Jossey-Bass.

Watson, J. (1979). *Nursing: The philosophy and science of caring.* Boston: Little, Brown.

Yates, P. (1993). Towards a reconceptualization of hope for patients with a diagnosis of cancer. *Journal of Advanced Nursing, 18,* 701–706.

DISORGANIZED INFANT BEHAVIOR

Acute Pain Management Guideline Panel (1992a). *Acute pain management in infants, children, and adolescents: Operative and medical procedures.* Quick Reference Guide for Clinicians, AHCPR Pub. No. 92-0020.

Rockville, MD: Agency for Health Care Policy and Research, Public Health Service, U.S. Department of Health and Human Services.

Acute Pain Management Guideline Panel (1992b). *Acute pain management: Operative or medical procedures and trauma.* Clinical Practice Guideline, AHCPR Pub. No. 92-0032. Rockville, MD: Agency for Health Care Policy and Research, Public Health Service, U.S. Department of Health and Human Services.

Als, H. (1986). A synactive model of neonatal behavioral organization: Framework for the assessment of neurobehavioral development in the premature infant and for the support of infants and parents in the neonatal intensive care environment. *Physical and Occupational Therapy in Pediatrics, 6,* 3–53.

Bill, S. G. (1994). The national pain management guideline: Implications for neonatal intensive care. *Neonatal Network, 13*(3), 9–17.

Blackburn, S. (1993). Assessment and management of neurologic dysfunction. In C. Kenner, A. Brueggemeyer, & L. Gunderson (Eds.). *Comprehensive neonatal nursing.* Philadelphia: W. B. Saunders.

Blackburn, S., & Vandenberg, K. (1993). Assessment and management of neonatal neurobehavioral development. In C. Kenner, A. Brueggemeyer, & L. Gunderson (Eds.). *Comprehensive neonatal nursing.* Philadelphia: W. B. Saunders.

Bozzette, M. (1993). Observations of pain behavior in the NICU: An exploratory study. *Journal of Perinatal and Neonatal Nursing, 7*(1), 76–87.

Broome, M. E., & Tanzillo, H. (1990). Differentiating between pain and agitation in premature neonates. *Journal of Perinatal and Neonatal Nursing, 4*(1), 33–62.

Cole, J., & Frappier, P. (1985). Infant stimulation reassessed. *Journal of Obstetrical, Gynecological, and Neonatal Nursing, 14,* 471–477.

Collins, S. K., & Kuck, K. (1991). Music therapy in the neonatal intensive care unit. *Neonatal Network, 9*(6), 23–26.

Flandermyer, A. A. (1993). The drug-exposed neonate. In C. Kenner, A. Brueggemeyer, & L. Gunderson (Eds.). *Comprehensive neonatal nursing.* Philadelphia: W. B. Saunders.

Grunau, R., & Craig, K. (1987). Pain expression in neonates: Facial action and cry. *Pain, 28,* 395–410.

Harrison, L., et al. (1996). Effects of gentle human touch on preterm infants: Pilot study results. *Neonatal Network, 15*(2), 35–41.

Hill, A., & Rath, L. (1993). The care and feeding of low birth weight infant. *Journal of Perinatal and Neonatal Nursing, 6*(4), 56–68.

Johnson-Crowley, N. (1993). Systematic assessment and home follow-up. In C. Kenner, A. Brueggemeyer, & L. Gunderson (Eds.). *Comprehensive neonatal nursing.* Philadelphia: W. B. Saunders.

Korner, A. F. (1986). The use of waterbeds in the care of preterm infants. *Journal of Perinatology, 6,* 142–147.

Merenstein, G. B., & Gardner, S. L. (1998). *Handbook of neonatal intensive care* (4th ed.). St. Louis: Mosby–Year book.

Thomas, K. A. (1989). How the NICU environment sounds to a preterm infant. *MCN: American Journal of Maternal–Child Nursing, 14,* 249–251.

Vandenberg, K. (1990). The management of oral nippling in the sick neonate, the disorganized feeder. *Neonatal Network, 9*(1), 9–16.

Williamson, P. S., & Williamson, M. L. (1983). Physiologic stress reduction by local anesthetic during newborn circumcision. *Pediatrics, 7,* 36–40.

Yecco, G. J. (1993). Neurobehavioral development and developmental support of premature infants. *Journal of Perinatal and Neonatal Nursing, 7*(1), 56–65.

RISK FOR INFECTION/ INFECTION TRANSMISSION

Bertin, M. L. (1999). Communicable diseases: Infection prevention for nurses at work and at home. *Nursing Clinics of North America, 34*(2), 509–526.

Centers for Disease Control and Prevention. (2000). Guidelines for prevention of transmission of human immunodeficiency virus and hepatitis B virus to health-care and public safety workers. *MMWR, 49,* 5–15.

Centers for Disease Control and Prevention. (1995). Guidelines for handwashing and hand antisepsis in health care settings. *MMWR, 44,* 1–17.

Centers for Disease Control and Prevention: HIV/AIDS Surveillance. (2001). *U.S. HIV and AIDS cases reported through December 2001.* Atlanta, GA: Department of Health and Human Services.

Crossley, K. B. (1985). Infection control practices in Minnesota nursing homes. *Journal of the American Medical Association, 254,* 2918–2921.

Goldschmidt, R. H., & Dong, B. J. (1995) Current report—HIV: Treatment of AIDS and HIV-related conditions. *Journal of the American Board of Family Practice, 8,* 139–162.

Kovach, T. (1990) Nip it in the bud: Controlling wound infection with preoperative shaving. *Today's O.R. Nurse, 9,* 23–26.

Mandell, A., Bennett, G. H., & Dolin, L. (1995). *Principles and practices of infectious diseases* (4th ed). Los Angeles: Churchill Livingstone.

Owen, M., & Grier, M. (1987). *Infection risk assessment guide.* Orange, CA: Unpublished.

Sharbaugh, R. J. (1999). The risk of occupational exposure and infection with infectious disease. *Nursing Clinics of North America, 34*(2), 493–508.

Stamm, W. E. (1991). Catheter-associated urinary tract infections: Epidemiology, pathogenesis, and prevention. *American Journal of Medicine, 91,* 65S–71S.

U.S. Department of Health and Human Services. (1991). Rules and regulations. *Federal Register, 56*(235), 47632–47649.

U.S. Department of Health and Human Services. (1994). Draft guidelines for isolation precautions in hospitals. *Federal Register, 59*(214), 55552–55570.

U.S. Department of Health and Human Services and Centers for Disease Control and Prevention. (1994). *Core curriculum on tuberculosis: What the clinician should know* (3rd ed.). Washington, DC: Public Health Service.

U.S. Department of Health and Human Services. (1994). Guidelines for preventing the transmission of *Mycobacterium* tuberculosis in health-care facilities: Notice. *Federal Register, 59*(208), 54242–54303.

Weinstein, R. A. (1991). Epidemiology and control of nosocomial infections in adult intensive care units. *American Journal of Medicine, 91,* 179S–184S.

Wenzel, R. P. (1997). *Prevention and control of nosocomial infections.* Baltimore: Williams & Wilkins.

Internet Resources

www.cdc.gov—Centers for Disease Control and Prevention

www.apic.org—Association for Professionals in Infection Control

www.cdc.gov/ncidod/nicid.htm—National Center for Infectious Disease

RISK FOR INJURY

Baumann, S. L. (1999). Defying gravity and fears: The prevention of falls in community-dwelling older adults. *Clinical Excellence for Nurse Practitioners, 3*(5), 254–261.

Green, P. M. (1989). Potential for injury. In G. McFarland & E. McFarlane (Eds.). *Nursing diagnosis and interventions.* St. Louis: C. V. Mosby.

Lipsitz, L. A., & Fullerton, K. J. (1986). Postprandial blood pressure reduction in health elderly. *Journal of the American Geriatrics Society, 34,* 267–270.

Moss, A. B. (1992). Are the elderly safe at home? *Journal of Community Health Nursing, 9*(1), 13–19.

National Center for Health Statistics. (1993). *Monthly vital statistics report, 1991.* Hyattsville, MD: U.S. Public Health Service Publications.

Schoenfelder, D. P. (2000). A fall prevention program for elderly individuals. *Journal of Gerontological Nursing, 26*(3), 43–45.

Child Safety

American Medical Association Board of Trustees. (1991). Use of infant walkers. *American Journal of Diseases of Children, 145,* 933–934.

Guyer, B., & Ellers, B. (1990). Childhood injuries in the United States. *American Journal of Diseases of Children, 144,* 649–652.

Retsky, J. (1991). Skateboarding injuries in children: A second wave. *American Journal of Diseases of Children, 145,* 188–193.

U.S. Public Health Services (1998). *Clinician handbook of preventative services* (2nd ed.). Washington, DC: U.S. Government.

Weiss, B. D. (1992). Trends in bicycle helmet use by children: 1985 to 1990. *Pediatrics, 89,* 78–80.

Perioperative

Fairchild, S. (1993). *Perioperative nursing: Principles and practice.* Boston: Jones and Bartlett.

Fuller, J. (1994). *Surgical technology: Principles and practice.* Philadelphia: W. B. Saunders.

Murphy, E. (1987). Cases involving ulnar nerve injuries demonstrate precautions nurses can and should take. *AORN Journal, 46,* 762–763, 768.

Rothrock, J. (1996). *Perioperative nursing care planning.* (11th ed.). St. Louis: Mosby-Year Book.

Smith, K. (1990). Positioning principles. *AORN Journal, 52,* 1196–1198, 1200–1202.

Stanley, M., & Beare, P. G. (1995). *Gerontological nursing.* Philadelphia: F. A. Davis.

LATEX ALLERGY RESPONSE

Bernstein, M. L. (1998). Latex-safe emergency cart products list. *Journal of Emergency Nursing, 24*(1), 58–61. (This source has a comprehensive list of latex-free equipment [*e.g.,* vials, syringes].)

Kim, K. T., Graves, P. B., Safadi, G., & Metcalfe, J. (1998). Implementation recommendations for making health care facilities latex safe. *AORN, 67*(3), 615–631.

Kinnaird, S., McClure, N., & Wilham, S. (1995). Latex allergy: An emergency problem in health care. *Neonatal Network, 14*(7), 33–38.

Kleinbeck, S., English, L., Sherley, M. A., & Howes, J. (1998). A criterion-referenced measure of latex allergy knowledge. *AORN, 68*(3), 384–392.

Reddy, S. (1998). Latex allergy. *American Family Physician, 57*(1), 93–100.

Tarlo, S. (1998). Latex allergy: A problem for both health care professionals and patients. *Ostomy / Wound Management 14*(8), 80–88.

RISK FOR LONELINESS

Bender, S. J. (1990). Anxiety and isolation in siblings of pediatric cancer patients: The need for prevention. *Social Work in Health Care, 14*(3), 17–35.

Bidwell, R. J., & Deisher, R. W. (1991). Adolescent sexuality: Current issues. *Pediatric Annals, 20,* 293–302.

Davis, B. (1990). Loneliness in children and adolescents. *Issues in Comprehensive Pediatric Nursing, 13*(1), 59–69.

Drew, N. (1991). Combating the social isolation of chronic mental illness. *Journal of Psychosocial Nursing and Mental Health Services, 29*(6), 14–17.

Durham, R. (1983). Long-stay psychiatric patients in hospital. In S. Spence & G. Shepherd (Eds.). *Development in social skills training.* New York: Academic Press.

Elsen, J., & Blegen, M. (1991). Social isolation. In M. Maas, K. Buckwalter, & M. Hardy (Eds.). *Nursing diagnoses and interventions for the elderly.* Redwood City, CA: Addison-Wesley Nursing.

Folden, S. L. (1990). On the inside looking out: Perceptions of the homebound. *Journal of Gerontological Nursing, 16*(1), 9–15.

Hillestad, E. A. (1984). Toward understanding of loneliness. In *Proceedings of conference on spirituality.* Milwaukee, WI: Marquette University.

Kelly, J. H., & Cavan Frisch, N. (1994). A transcultural concept analysis of social isolation. In R. Carrol-Johnson & Paquette, M. (Eds.). *Classification of nursing diagnosis: Proceedings of the tenth conference.* Philadelphia: J. B. Lippincott.

Leiderman, P. H. (1969). Loneliness: A psychodynamic interpretation. In E. S. Scheidman & M. J. Ortega (Eds.). *Aspects of depression: International psychiatric clinics.* Boston: Little, Brown.

Lien-Gieschen, T. (1993). Validation of social isolation related to maturational age: Elderly. *Nursing Diagnosis, 4*(1), 37–44.

Longino, C. F., & Karl, C. S. (1982). Explicating activity theory: A formal replication. *Journal of Gerontology, 37,* 713–722.

Lynch, J. J. (1979). *The broken heart: The medical consequences of loneliness.* New York: Basic Books.

Mallinson, R. K. (1999). The lived experience of AIDS-related multiple losses by HIV-negative gay men. *Journal of Association of Nurses in AIDS Care, 10*(5), 22–31.

Maslow, A. H. (1968). *Towards a psychology of being* (2nd ed.). New York: Van Nostrand.

Stanley, M., & Beare, P. G. (1994). *Gerontological nursing.* Philadelphia: W. B. Saunders.

Warren, B. J. (1993). Explaining social isolation through concept analysis. *Archives of Psychiatric Nursing, 7*(5), 270–276.

Weiss, R. S. (1973). *Loneliness: The experience of emotional and social isolation.* Cambridge, MA: MIT Press.

INEFFECTIVE THERAPEUTIC REGIMEN MANAGEMENT

Bandura, A. (1982). Self-efficacy mechanism in human agency. *American Psychology, 37*(3), 122–147.

Edelman, C. L., & Mandle, C. L. (2001). *Health promotion throughout the lifespan.* (5th ed.). St. Louis: Mosby-Year Book.

Grainger, R. (1990). Anxiety interruptors. *American Journal of Nursing, 90,* 14–15.

Leske, J. (1993). Anxiety of elective surgical patients, family members. *AORN Journal, 57,* 1091–1103.

Prochasaska, J., DiClemente, C. C., & Norcross, J. C. (1992). In search of how people change. *American Psychology, 47*(8), 1102–1104.

Rakel, B. (1991). Knowledge deficit. In M. Maas, K. Buckwalter, & M. Hardy (Eds.). *Nursing diagnoses and interventions for the elderly.* Redwood City, CA: Addison-Wesley Nursing.

Rakel, B. A. (1992). Interventions related to teaching. In G. Bulechek & J. McCloskey (Eds.). *Nursing interventions* (2nd ed.). Philadelphia: W. B. Saunders.

Redman, B., & Thomas, S. (1996). Patient teaching. In G. Bulechek & J. McCloskey (Eds.). *Nursing interventions* (3rd ed.). Philadelphia: W. B. Saunders.

Zerwich, J. (1992). Laying the groundwork for family self-help: Locating families, building trust and building strength. *Public Health Nursing, 9*(1), 15–21.

Zimmerman, G., Olsen, C. & Bosworth, M. (2000). A "Stages of Change" approach to helping patients change behavior. *American Family Physicians, 61*(5), 1409–1416.

Community

Allender, J., & Spradley, B. (2005). *Community health nursing* (6th ed.). Philadelphia: Lippincott Williams & Wilkins.

Edelman, C. L., & Mandle, C. L. (2001). *Health promotion throughout the lifespan.* (5th ed.). St. Louis: Mosby-Year Book.

Kriegler, N., & Harton, M. (1991). Community health assessment tool: A patterned approach to data collection and diagnosis. *Journal of Community Health Nursing, 9*, 229–234.

IMPAIRED PHYSICAL MOBILITY

Addams, S. & Clough, J. A. (1998) Modalities for mobilization. In A. B. Mahler, S. Salmond, & T. Pellino (Eds.). *Orthopedic nursing.* Philadelphia: W. B. Saunders.

Christian, B. J. (1982). Immobilization: Psychosocial aspects. In C. Norris (Ed.). *Concept clarification in nursing.* Rockville, MD: Aspen Publications.

Hogue, C. (1985). Mobility. In E. Schneider (Ed.). *The teaching nursing home: A new approach to geriatric research, education, and clinical care.* New York: Raven Press.

Kasper, C. E. (1993). Alterations in skeletal muscle related to impaired physical mobility: An empirical model. *Research and Nursing Health, 16*, 265–273.

Levin, R. F., Krainovitch, B. C., Bahrenburg, E., & Mitchell, C. A. (1989). Diagnostic content validity of nursing diagnoses. *Image, 21*(1), 40–44.

Maas, M. (1991). Impaired physical mobility. In M. Maas, K. Buckwalter, & M. Hardy (Eds.). *Nursing diagnoses and interventions for the elderly.* Redwood City, CA: Addison-Wesley Nursing.

Pellino, T., Polacek, L. P., Preston, A., Bell, N., & Evans, R. (1998). Complications of orthopedic disorders and orthopedic surgery. In A. Maher, S. Salomond, & T. Pellino (Eds.). *Orthopaedic nursing* (2nd ed.). Philadelphia: W. B. Saunders.

Simpson, W. (1986). Exercise: Prescriptions for the elderly. *Geriatrics, 41*(1), 95–100.

Whitbourne, S. K. (1985). Appearance and movement. In S. K. Whitbourne (Ed.). *The aging body.* New York: Springer-Verlag.

NONCOMPLIANCE

Blevins, D., & Lubkin, J. (1999). Compliance. In J. Lubkin (Ed.). *Chronic illness: Impact and interventions* (4th ed.). Boston: Jones & Bartlett.

Campbell, M. K., DeVillis, B., Stretcher, V., Ammerman, A., Devillis, R., & Sandler, R. (1994). Improving dietary behavior: The effectiveness of tailored messages in primary care settings. *American Journal of Public Health, 84*, 783–787.

Cassells, J. M., & Redman, B. K. (1989). Preparing students to be moral agents in clinical nursing practice. *Nursing Clinics of North America, 24*, 463–473.

Charonko, C. (1992). Cultural influences in "noncompliant" behavior and decision making. *Holistic Nursing Practice, 6*(3), 73–78.

DeGreest, S., Von Renteln-Kruse, W., Steeman, E., Degraeve, S., & Abraham, I. (1998). Compliance issues with the geriatric population: Complexity with aging. *Nursing Clinics of North America, 33*(3), 467–480.

Dracup, K. A., & Meleis, A. I. (1982). Compliance: An interactionist approach. *Nursing Research, 31*, 32–35.

Elpern, E. H., & Girzardas, A. M. (1993). Tuberculosis update: New challenges of an old disease. *Medical-Surgical Nursing, 2*, 176–183.

Fleury, J. (1992). The application of motivational theory to cardiovascular risk reduction. *Image, 24*, 229–239.

Hussey, L., & Gilliland, K. (1989). Compliance, low literacy and locus of control. *Nursing Clinics of North America, 24*, 605–611.

Kavanagh, D. J., & Gooley, S. (1993). Prediction of adherence and control in diabetes. *Journal of Behavioral Medicine, 16*, 509–522.

Redland, A. R., & Stuifbergen, A. K. (1993). Strategies for maintenance of health-promoting behaviors. *Nursing Clinics of North America, 28*, 427–442.

Scipien, G. M., Chard, M. A., Howe, J., & Barnard, M. U. (1990). *Pediatric nursing care.* St. Louis: C. V. Mosby.

Whatley, J. H. (1991). Effects of health locus of control and social network on adolescent risk taking. *Pediatric Nursing, 17*(2), 239–240.

Wysocki, T., & Wayne, W. (1992). Childhood diabetes and the family. *Practical Diabetology, 11*(2), 29–32.

IMBALANCED NUTRITION: LESS THAN BODY REQUIREMENTS

Evans-Stoner, N. (1997). Nutrition assessment. *Nursing Clinics of North America, 32*(4), 637–650.

Folsom, A. R., Kaye, S. A., & Sellers, T. A. (1993). Body fat distribution and 5-year risk of death in older women. *Journal of the American Medical Association, 269*, 483–487.

Foltz, A. (2001). Nutritional disturbances. In S. Groenwald, M. Frogge, M. Goodman, & C. Yarbo (Eds.). *Cancer nursing: Principles and practices* (4th ed.). Boston: Jones and Bartlett.

Human Nutrition Information Service. (1992). *Food guide pyramid: A guide to daily food choices.* Leaflet No. 572. Washington, DC: U.S. Department of Agriculture.

Keller, C., & Stevens, K. (1996). Assessment, etiology and intervention in obesity in children. *Nurse Practitioner, 21*(9), 31–32, 34–36, 41.

Lo, C. (1995). Nutritional requirements of women. In P. L. Carr, K. M. Freud, & S. Somati (Eds.). *The medical care of women.* Philadelphia: J. B. Lippincott.

Mahan, L. K., & Arlin, M. T. (1996). *Food, nutrition and diet therapy* (9th ed.). Philadelphia: W. B. Saunders.

National Research Council, Committee on Diet and Health of Food and Nutrition Board. (1989). Diet and health: Implications for reducing chronic disease risk. *Nutrition Reviews, 47*, 142–149.

Overfield, T. (1985). *Biologic variation in health and illness: Race, age, and sex differences.* Menlo Park, CA: Addison-Wesley.

Rajcevich, K., & Wakefield, B. (1991). Altered nutrition: Less than body requirements. In M. Maas, K. Buckwalter, & M. Hardy (Eds.). *Nursing diagnoses and interventions for the elderly.* Redwood City, CA: Addison-Wesley Nursing.

Rhodes, V. (1990). Nausea, vomiting and retching. *Nursing Clinics of North America, 25,* 885–890.

U.S. Department of Health and Human Services. (1989). *Healthy People 2000.* Washington, DC: Government Printing Office.

Varella, L., & Utermohlen, U. (1993). Nutritional support for the patient with renal failure. *Critical Care Nursing Clinics of North America, 5*(1), 79–96.

White, R., & Ashworth, A. (2000). How drug therapy can affect, threaten and compromise nutritional status. *Journal Human Nutrition and Dieting, 13,* 119–129.

Wilson, M. H. (1994) Feeding the healthy child. In F. Oski (Ed.). *Principles and practice of pediatrics* (2nd ed.). Philadelphia: J. B. Lippincott.

Impaired Swallowing

DiIorio, C., & Price, M. (1990). Swallowing: An assessment guide. *American Journal of Nursing, 90*(7), 38–48.

Emick-Herring, B., & Wood, P. (1990). A team approach to neurologically based swallowing disorders. *Rehabilitation Nursing, 15,* 126–132.

Grober, M. (Ed.). (1984). *Dysphagia.* Oxford, UK: Butterworth-Heinemann.

Ter Matt, M., & Tandy, L. (1991). Impaired swallowing. In M. Maas, K. Buckwalter & M. Hardy (Eds.). *Nursing diagnoses and interventions for the elderly.* Redwood City, Ca: Addison-Wesley Nursing.

Ineffective Infant Feeding Pattern

Hazinski, M. F. (1992). *Nursing care of the critically ill child.* St. Louis: C. V. Mosby.

McCain, G. (1992). Facilitating inactive awake states in preterm infants: A study of three interventions. *Nursing Research, 41,* 157–160.

Shaker, C. S. (1991). Nipple feeding premature infants: A different perspective. *Neonatal Network, 8*(5), 9–17.

VandenBerg, K. (1991). Nippling management of the sick neonate in the NICU: The disorganized feeder. *Neonatal Network, 9*(1), 9–16.

IMPAIRED PARENTING

Alexander, D., Powell, G. M., Williams, P., White, M., & Conlon, M. (1988). Anxiety levels of rooming-in and non-rooming-in parents of young hospitalized children. *Maternal–Child Nursing Journal, 17*(2), 79–98.

Christopherson, E. R. (1992). Discipline. *Pediatric Clinics of North America, 39,* 395–411.

Herman-Staab, B. (1994). Screening, management and appropriate referral for pediatric behavior problems. *Nurse Practitioner, 19*(7), 40–49.

Klaus, M., & Kennell, J. (1976). *Maternal-infant bonding.* St. Louis: C.V. Mosby.

Koepke, J., Anglin, S., Austin, J., & Delesalle, J. (1991). Becoming parents: Feelings of adoptive mothers. *Pediatric Nursing, 17*(4), 337–340.

Merenstein, G., & Gardner, S. (1998). *Handbook of neonatal intensive care* (4th ed.). St. Louis. Mosby-Year Book.

Attachment

Brown, W., Pearl, L., & Carrasco, R. (1991). Evolving models of family-centered services in neonatal intensive care. *Children's Health Care, 20,* 50–52.

Goulet, C., Bell, L., & Tribble, D. (1998). A concept analysis of parent–infant attachment. *Journal of Advanced Nursing, 28*(5), 1071–1081.

Mercer, R., & Ferketich S. (1990). Predictors of parental attachment during early parenthood. *Journal of Advanced Nursing, 15*(3), 268–280.

Zahr, L. (1991). Correlates of mother–infant interaction in premature infants from low socioeconomic background. *Pediatric Nursing, 17*(3), 259–263.

Parental Role Conflict

Baker, N. A. (1994). Avoid collisions with challenging families. *Maternal–Child Nursing Journal, 19,* 97–101.

Chan, J. M., & Leff, P. T. (1982). Parenting the chronically ill child in the hospital: Issues and concerns. *Children's Health Care, 11,* 9–16.

Clements, D., Copeland, L., & Loftus, M. (1990). Critical times for families with a chronically ill child. *Pediatric Nursing, 16*(2), 157–161.

Dunst, C. J., Trivette, C. M., Davis, M., & Wheeldreyer, J. C. (1988). Enabling and empowering families of children with health impairments. *Children's Health Care, 17,* 71–81.

Gallo, A. (1991). Family adaptation in childhood chronic illness. *Journal of Pediatric Health Care, 5,* 78–85.

Jay, S. (1977). Pediatric intensive care: Involving parents in the care of their child. *Maternal–Child Nursing Journal, 6,* 195–204.

Jay S., & Youngblut, J. (1991). Parent stress associated with pediatric critical care nursing: Linking research and practice. *AACN Clinical Issues, 2,* 278–283.

Knafl, K., & Dixon, D. (1984). The participation of fathers in their children's hospitalization. *Issues in Comprehensive Pediatric Nursing, 7,* 269–281.

Melnyk, B. (1991). Changes in parent–child relationships following divorce. *Pediatric Nursing, 17,* 337–340.

Melnyk, B., Feinstein, N., Moldenhouer, Z., & Small, L. (2001). Coping in parents of children who are chronically ill. *Pediatrics, 27*(6), 548–558.

Mott, S. (1990). *Nursing care of children and families: A holistic approach* (2nd ed.). Redwood City, CA: Addison-Wesley.

Newton, M. S. (2000). Family-centered care: Current realities in parent participation. *Pediatric Nursing, 26*(2), 164–168.

Ogden-Burke, S., Castello, E. A., & Handley-Derry, M. H. (1989). Maternal stress and repeated hospitalizations of children who are physically disabled. *Children's Health Care, 18,* 82–90.

Pass, M., & Pass, C. (1987). Anticipatory guidance for parents of hospitalized children. *Journal of Pediatric Nursing, 2,* 250–258.

Schepp, K. (1991). Factors influencing the coping effort of mothers of hospitalized children. *Nursing Research, 40,* 42–45.

Smith, L. (1999). Family-centered decision-making: A model for parent participation. *Journal of Neonatal Nursing, 5*(6), 31–33.

Thurman, K. (1991). Parameters for establishing family-centered neonatal intensive care services. *Children's Health Care, 20*(1), 34–40.

RISK FOR PERIPHERAL NEUROVASCULAR DYSFUNCTION

Bourne, R. B., & Rorabeck, C. H. (1989). Compartmental syndrome of the lower leg. *Clinical Orthopaedics and Related Research, 240,* 97–104.

Fahey, V., & Milzarek, A. (1999). Extra-anatomic bypass surgery. *Journal of Vascular Nursing, 17*(3), 71–75.

Kracun, M. D., & Wooten, C. L. (1998). Crush injuries: A case of entrapment. *Critical Care Nursing Quarterly, 21*(2), 81–86.

Peck, S. (1991). Crush syndrome. *Orthopaedic Nursing, 9*(3), 33–40.

Pellino, T., Polacek, L. P., Preston, A., Bell, N., & Evans, R. (1998). Complications of orthopedic disorders and orthopedic surgery. In A. Maher, S. Salomond, &

T. Pellino (Eds.). *Orthopaedic nursing* (2nd ed.). Philadelphia: W. B. Saunders.

Ross, D. (1991). Acute compartmental syndrome. *Orthopaedic Nursing, 10*(2), 33–38.

POST-TRAUMA SYNDROME

Bender, S. (1995). Crisis Intervention. In G. Stuart & S. Sundeen (Eds.). *Principles and practice of psychiatric nursing* (5th ed.). St. Louis: Mosby–Year Book.

Boscarino, J. A. (1995). Post-traumatic stress and associated disorders among Vietnam veterans: The significance of combat exposure and social support. *Journal of Traumatic Stress, 8,* 317–335.

Charron, H. S. (1998). Anxiety disorders. In E. M. Vararolis (Ed.). *Foundations of psychiatric mental health nursing* (3rd ed.). Philadelphia: W. B. Saunders.

DiVasto, P. (1985). Measuring the aftermath of rape. *Journal of Psychosocial Nursing and Mental Health Services, 23*(2), 33–35.

Green, B. (1990). Buffalo Creek survivors in the second decade: Stability of stress symptoms. *American Journal of Orthopsychiatry, 60*(1), 43–54.

Green, B. L., & Lindy, J. D. (1994). Post-traumatic stress disorder in victims of disasters. *Psychiatric Clinics of North America, 17,* 301–309.

Horowitz, M. J. (1986b). Stress response syndromes: A review of posttraumatic and adjustment disorders. *Hospital and Community Psychiatry, 37,* 241–248.

Pfefferbaum, B., Gurwich, R. H., McDonald, N. B., et al. (2000). Post-traumatic stress among young children after the death of a friend or acquaintance in a terrorist bombing. *Psychiatric Services, 51*(3), 386–388.

Tanaka, K. (1991). Post-trauma response. In G. K. McFarland & M. D. Thomas (Eds.). *Psychiatric mental health nursing: Application of the nursing process.* Philadelphia: J. B. Lippincott.

Tyra, P. (1993). Older woman and rape. *Journal of Gerontological Nursing, 5,* 7–12.

Rape Trauma Syndrome

Adams, C., & Fay, J. (1989). *Free of the shadows.* Oakland: New Harbinger.

Aguilera, D. C., & Messick, J. M. (1982). *Crisis intervention: Theory and methodology* (4th ed.). St. Louis: C. V. Mosby.

Anderson, C. (1981–82). Males as sexual assault victims: Multiple levels of trauma. *Journal of Homosexuality, 7,* 145–159.

Andrews, J. (1992). Sexual assault: After care instructions. *Journal of Emergency Nursing, 18,* 152.

Beckman, C., & Groetzinger, L. (1990). Treating sexual victims. *Physician Assistant, 2,* 123–130.

Brozan, N. (1985, August 10). Rape trauma: Seeking court acceptance. *The New York Times,* p. 43.

Burgess, A. W. (1995). *Occupational Health Nursing, 33*(8), 405–410.

Burgess, A. W., Dowdell, R. N., & Prentley, R. (2000). Sexual abuse of nursing home residents. *Journal of Psychosocial Nursing, 38*(6), 10–18.

Collins, G. (1982, January 18). Counseling male rape victims. *The New York Times,* p. 27.

Davis, L., & Brody, E. (1979). *Rape and older women: A guide to prevention and protection.* Rockville, MD: U.S. Department of Health, Education and Welfare, Public Health Service, Alcohol, Drug Abuse, and Mental Health Administration, National Institute of Mental Health.

DiVasto, P. (1985). Measuring the aftermath of rape. *Journal of Psychosocial Nursing and Mental Health Services, 23*(2), 33–35.

Dwyer, J. (1987). Examination and treatment of the sexual assault victim. *Physician Assistant, 11,* 110–109.

Ellis, G. M. (1994). Acquaintance rape. *Perspectives in Psychiatric Care, 30,* 11–16.

Fielo, S. (1987). How does crime affect the elderly? *Geriatric Nursing, 8*(2), 80–83.

Foley, T., & Darvies, M. (1987). *Rape: Nursing care of victims.* St. Louis: C. V. Mosby.

Foubert, J. D. (2000). The longitudinal effects of a rape-prevention program on fraternity men's attitudes, behavioral intent and behavior. *Journal of American College Health, 48*(1), 158–163.

Francis, S. (1993). Rape and sexual assault. In B. S. Johnson (Ed.). *Psychiatric–mental health nursing: Adaptation and growth.* Philadelphia: J. B. Lippincott.

Heinrich, L. (1987). Care of the female rape victim. *Nursing Practitioner, 12*(11), 9.

Holmes, M. M. (1999). Clinical management of rape in adolescent girls. *Patient Care,* (8), 41–44+.

Holmstrom, L., & Burgess, A. W. (1975). Development of diagnostic categories: Sexual trauma. *American Journal of Nursing, 75,* 1288–1291.

Jalowiec, A., & Powers, M. J. (1981). Stress and coping in hypertensive and emergency room patients. *Nursing Research, 30,* 10–15.

Kaufman, A. (1980). Male rape victims: Non-institutionalized assault. *American Journal of Medicine, 137,* 221–223.

Parker, B., & Campbell, J. C. (1995). Care of survivors of abuse and violence. In G. W. Stuart & S. J. Saudeen (Eds.). *Principles and practice of psychiatric nursing* (5th ed.). St. Louis: Mosby–Year Book.

Peter, L. & Whitehill, D. C. (1998). Management of female sexual assault. *American Family Physician, 58*(4), 920–926.

Ruckman, L. (1992). Rape: How to begin the healing. *American Journal of Nursing, 9,* 48–51.

Smith-DiJulio, K. (1998). Evidence of maladaptive responses to crisis: Rape. In E. Varcarolis (Ed.). *Foundations of psychiatric–mental health nursing* (3rd ed.). Philadelphia: W. B. Saunders.

Symes, L. (2000). Arriving at readiness to recover emotionally after sexual assault. *Archives of Psychiatric Nursing, 14*(1), 30–38.

U.S. Department of Justice, Federal Bureau of Investigation. (1989). *Uniform crime reports for the United States.* Washington, DC: U.S. Government Printing Office.

Children and Adolescents

Furniss, T. (1983). Mutual influences and interlocking professional–family process in the treatment of child sexual abuse and incest. *Child Abuse and Neglect, 7,* 207–223.

Kauffman, C. K., Neill, M. K., & Thomas, J. N. (1986). The abusive parent. In S. H. Johnson (Ed.). *High-risk parenting: Assessment and nursing strategies for families at risk.* Philadelphia: J. B. Lippincott.

Pownall, M. (1985). Health visiting: A family affair? . . . Sexual abuse of children. *Nursing Times, 81*(43), 58, 60–61.

POWERLESSNESS

Averill, J. (1973). Personal control over aversive stimuli and its relationship to stress. *Psychological Bulletin, 80,* 286.

Chang, B. (1978). Generalized expectancy, situational perception and morale among the institutionalized aged. *Nursing Research, 27,* 316–324.

Davidhizar, R., & Giger, J. N. (1994). You have power, too! Imprint, *41*(4), 64–66.

Drew, B. L. (1990). Differentiation of hopelessness, helplessness, and powerlessness using Erik Erikson's "Roots of Virtue." *Archives of Psychiatric Nursing, 4,* 322–327.

Fuller, S. (1978). Inhibiting helplessness in elderly people. *Journal of Gerontological Nursing, 4,* 18–21.

Kersten, L. (1990) Changes in self concept during pulmonary rehabilitation; Part 1 and 2. *Heart and Lung, 19,* 456–470.

Lambert, V. A., & Lambert, C. E. (1981). Role theory and the concept of powerlessness. *Journal of Psychosocial Nursing and Mental Health Services, 19*(9), 11–14.

Ledy, N. (1990). A structural model of stress, psychosocial resources and symptomatic experiences in chronic physical illness. *Nursing Research, 39,* 230–236.

Lee, R., Graydon, J., & Ross, E. (1991). Effects of psychological well being, physical status and social support on oxygen dependent COPD patient's level of functioning. *Research in Nursing and Health, 14,* 323–328.

Miller, J. (1983). *Powerlessness: Coping with chronic illness.* Philadelphia: F. A. Davis.

Miller, J. F. (1985). Concept development of powerlessness: A nursing diagnosis. In J. F. Miller (Ed.). *Coping with chronic illness, overcoming powerlessness.* Philadelphia: F. A. Davis.

Miller, J. F. (1984). Development and validation of a diagnostic label: Powerlessness. In M. J. Kim & A. McLane (Eds.). *Classification of nursing diagnoses: Proceedings of the fifth national conference.* St Louis: C. V. Mosby.

O'Heath, K. (1991). Powerlessness. In M. Maas, K. Buckwalter, & M. Hardy (Eds.). *Nursing diagnoses and interventions for the elderly.* Redwood City, CA: Addison-Wesley Nursing.

Richmond, T. S., & Metcalf, J. A. (1986). Psychosocial responses to spinal cord injury. *Journal of Neuroscience Nursing, 18,* 183–187.

Richmond, T. S., Metcalf, J., Daly, M., & Kish, J. R. (1992). Powerlessness in acute spinal cord injury patients: A descriptive study. *Journal of Neuroscience Nursing, 24*(3), 146–152.

Seeman, M. (1967). Powerlessness and knowledge: A comparative study of alienation and learning. *Sociometry, 30*(1), 105–123.

Seligman, M. (1975). *Helplessness: On depression, development, and death.* San Francisco: W. H. Freeman.

Simmons, R., & West, G. (1984–85). Life changes, coping resources and health among the elderly. *International Journal of Aging and Human Development, 20,* 173–189.

Spielman, B. J. (1986). Rethinking paradigms in geriatric ethics. *Journal of Religion and Health, 25*(2), 79–83.

Staples, P., Baruth, P., Jefferies, M., & Warder, L. (1994). Empowering the angry patient. *Canadian Nurse, 90*(4), 28–30.

Stephenson, C. A. (1979). Powerlessness and chronic illness: Implications for nursing. *Baylor Nursing Educator, 1*(1), 17–28.

Weaver, T., & Narsavage, G. (1992). Physiological and psychological variables related to functional status in chronic obstructive pulmonary disease. *Nursing Research, 41,* 286–291.

Zauszniewski, J. A. (1994). Nursing diagnosis and depressive illness. *Nursing Diagnosis, 5*(3), 106–114.

INEFFECTIVE PROTECTION

Agency for Health Care Policy and Research [AHCPR] Panel for the Prediction and Prevention of Pressure Ulcers in Adults. (1992, May). *Pressure ulcers in adults: Prediction and prevention.* Clinical Practice Guidelines Number 3, AHCPR, Bulletin No. 92-0047. Rockville, MD: Agency for Health Care Policy & Research, Public Health Services, U.S. Department of Health and Human Services.

Bates-Jensen, B. M. (1999). Chronic wound assessment. *Nursing Clinics of North America, 34*(4), 799–846.

Bennett, M. A. (1995). Report of the task force on the implications for darkly pigmented skin in the prediction and prevention of pressure ulcers. *Advances in Wound Care, 8*(6), 34–35.

Bergstrom, N., Bennett, M. A., Carlson, C. E., et al. (1994) *Treatment of pressure ulcers.* Clinical Practice Guideline, No. 15. Rockville, MD: U.S. Department of Health and Human Services. Public Health Service, Agency for Health Care Policy and Research. AHCPR Publication No. 95-0652.

Boynton, P. R., Jaworski, D., & Paustian, C. (1999). Meeting the challenges of healing chronic wounds in older adults. *Nursing Clinics of North America, 34*(4), 921–932.

Hill, M. J. (1994). *Skin disorders.* Philadelphia: Mosby-Year Book.

Maklebust, J. (1997). Pressure ulcers: Decreasing the risk for older adults. *Geriatric Nursing, 18*(6), 250–254.

Maklebust, J. (1998). Caring for homecare patients with pressure ulcers. *Home Healthcare Nurse.* Philadelphia: Lippincott-Raven.

Maklebust, J., & Sieggreen, M. (2000). *Pressure ulcers: Guidelines for prevention and nursing management* (3rd ed.). Springhouse, PA: Springhouse.

National Pressure Ulcer Advisory Panel. (1992). *Monograph on pressure ulcer prevention.* Buffalo: NPUAP.

Novotny, J. (1989). Adolescents, acne, and the side-effects of Accutane. *Pediatric Nursing, 15,* 247–248.

Parish, L. C., Witkowski, J. A., & Crissey, J. T. (1997). *The decubitis ulcer in clinical practice.* New York: Springer-Verlag.

Thomas, D. R., & Allman, R. M. (1997). Pressure ulcers. *Clinics in Geriatric Medicine, 13*(3).

Upton, L. (1989). Growth and development of the infant. In R. L. Foster, M. M. Hunsberger, & J. J. T. Anderson (Eds.). *Family-centered nursing care of children.* Philadelphia: W. B. Saunders.

Wysocki, A. (1999). Skin anatomy, physiology and pathophysiology. *Nursing Clinics of North America, 34*(4), 777–798.

Impaired Oral Mucous Membrane

Aronovitch, S. A. (1997). Oral care and its role in WOC nursing. *Journal of Wound and Ostomy Care Nursing, 24*(2), 79–85.

Beck, S. L. (2001). Mucositis. In S. L. Groenwald, M. Goodman, M. H. Frogge, C. H. Yarbro, (Eds.). *Cancer symptom management* (4th ed.). Boston: Jones & Bartlett Publishers.

Clancio, S. Kazmierczak, M., Mather, R. C., Ho, A., & Bessinger, M. (1996). *Clinical and microbiological effects of baking soda and peroxide oral care products* (poster). Presented at International Association of Dental Research. San Francisco: March 13–17.

Kemp, J., & Brackett, H. (2001). Mucositis. In R. A. Gates, R. M. Fink (Eds.). *Oncology nursing secrets* (pp. 245–249). Philadelphia: Hanley & Belfus.

Holmes, S., & Mountain, E. (1993). Assessment of oral status: Evaluation of three oral assessment guides. *Journal of Clinical Nursing, 2,* 35–40.

Tombes, M. B., & Galluci, B. (1993). The effects of hydrogen peroxide rinses on the normal mucosa. *Nursing Research, 332*–337.

Western Consortium for Cancer Nursing Research. (1991). Development of a staging system for chemotherapy induced stomatitis. *Cancer Nursing, 14*(1), 6–12.

RELOCATION STRESS

Adshead, H., Nelson, H., Gooderally, V., & Gollogly, P. (1991). Guidelines for successful relocation. *Nursing Standard, 5*(28), 32–35.

Anderzén, I., Arnetz, B. B., Söderström, T., & Söderman, E. (1997). Stress and sensitization in children: A controlled prospective psychophysiological study of children exposed to international relocation. *Journal of Psychosomatic Research, 43*(3), 259–269.

Armer, J. M. (1996). An exploration of factors influencing adjustment among relocating rural elders. *Image, 28*(1), 35–39.

Barnhouse, A. H., Brugler, C. J., & Harkulich, J. T. (1992). Relocation stress syndrome. *Nursing Diagnosis, 3*(4), 166–167.

Beirne, N. F., Patterson, M. N., Galie, M., & Goodman, P. (1995). Effects of a fast-track closing on a nursing facility population. *Health and Social Work, 20,* 117–123.

Borup, J. H., Gallego, D. T., & Heffernam, P. G. (1979). Relocation and its effect on mortality. *The Gerontologist, 19,* 135–140.

Brugler, C., Titus, M., & Nypaver, J. (1993). Relocation stress syndrome: A patient and staff approach. *Journal of Nursing Administration, 23*(1), 45–50.

Craig, C. Q. (1997). "Do not go gentle into that good night": When a psychiatric hospital closes. *Psychiatric Services, 48*(4), 541–542.

Cutler, L., & Garner, M. (1995). Reducing relocation stress after discharge from the intensive therapy unit. *Intensive and Critical Care Nursing, 11*(6), 333–335.

Flanagan, V., Slattery, M. J., Chase, N. S., Meade, S. K., & Cronenwett, L. R. (1996). Mothers' perceptions of the quality of their infants' back transfer: Pilot study results. *Neonatal Network, 15*(2), 27–33.

Fried, T. R., Gillick, M. R., & Lipsitz, L. A. (1997). Short-term functional outcomes of long-term care residents with pneumonia treated with and without hospital transfer. *Journal of American Geriatrics Society, 45*(3), 302–306.

Gass, K. A., Gaustad, G., Oberst, M. T., & Hughes, S. (1992). Relocation appraisal, functional independence, morale, and health of nursing home residents. *Issues in Mental Health Nursing, 13,* 239–253.

Haight, B. K. (1995). Suicide risk in frail elderly people relocated to nursing homes. *Geriatric Nursing, 16,* 104–107.

Harkulich, J., & Brugler, C. (1991). Relocation and the resident. *Activities, Adaptation and Aging, 15*(4), 51–60.

Harkulich, J. T., & Brugler, C. J. (1992). Relocation stress. In K. Gettrust & P. Brabec (Eds.). *Nursing diagnosis in clinical practice: Guides for care planning.* Louisville, KY: Delmar.

Houser, D. (1974). Safer care for the M.I. patient. *Nursing '74, 4*(7), 42–47.

Hulewat, P. (1996). Resettlement: A cultural and psychological crisis. *Social Work, 41*(2), 129–135.

Johnson, R. A. (1996). The meaning of relocation among elderly religious sisters. *Western Journal of Nursing Research, 18*(2), 172–185.

Johnson, R. A., & Hlava, C. (1994). Translocation of elders: Maintaining the spirit. *Geriatric Nursing, 15,* 209–212.

Kaisik, B. H. & Ceslowitz, S. B. (1996). Easing the fear of nursing home placements: The value of stress inoculation. *Geriatric Nursing, 17*(4), 182–186.

Kosasih, J. B., Borca, H. H., Wenninger, W. J., & Duthie, E. (1998). Nursing home rehabilitation after acute rehabilitation: Predictors and outcomes. *Archives of Physical Medical Rehabilitation, 79*(6), 670–673.

Lander, S. M., Brazill, A. L., & Landrigan, P. M. (1997). Intrainstitutional relocation. Effects on residents' behavior and psychosocial functioning. *Journal of Gerontological Nursing, 23*(4), 35–41.

Lee, D. T. (1997). Residential care placement: Perceptions among elderly Chinese people in Hong Kong. *Journal of Advanced Nursing, 26*(3), 602–607.

Lethbridge, B., Somboom, O. P., & Shea, H. L. (1976). The transfer process. *Canadian Nurse, 72,* 39–40.

Marsico, T., & Puskar, K. R. (1986). Family relocation: Helping children adjust. *Pediatric Nursing, 12*(2), 108–110.

Matter, D. E., & Matter, R. M. (1988). Helping young children cope with the stress of relocation: Action steps for the counselor. *Elementary School Guidance and Counseling, 23*(10), 23–29.

Maun, C. (1996). Easing the trauma of placement. *Provider, 22*(8), 25–26.

McDonald Gibbins, S. A., & Chapman, J. S. (1996). Holding on: Perceptions of premature infants' transfers. *Journal of Obstetric, Gynecologic, and Neonatal Nursing, 25*(2), 147–153.

Meacham, C. L., & Brandriet, L. M. (1997). The response of family and residents to long-term care placement. *Clinical Gerontologist, 18*(1), 63–66.

Miles, M. S. (1999). Parents who received transfer preparation had lower anxiety about their children's transfer from the pediatric intensive care unit to a general pediatric ward. *Applied Nursing Research, 12*(3), 114–120.

Miller, S. (1995). *After the boxes are unpacked.* Denver, CO: Focus on the Family.

Minckley, B. B., Burrows, D., Ehrat, K., Harper, L., Jenkin, S. A., Minckley, W. F., Page, B., Schramm, D. E., & Wood, C. (1979). Myocardial infarct stress-of-transfer inventory: Development of a research tool. *Nursing Research, 28,* 4–9.

Mitchell, M. G. (1999). The effects of relocation of elderly. *Perspectives in Gerontological Nursing, 23*(1), 2–7.

Morgan, S. (1996). Reach out and touch someone . . . elderly relocation trauma. *Journal of Gerontological Nursing, 22*(7), 5.

Najarian, L. M., Goenjian, A. K., Pelcovitz, D., Mandel, F., & Najarian, B. (1996). Relocation after a disaster: Posttraumatic stress disorder in Armenia after the earthquake. *Journal of the American Academy of Child and Adolescent Psychiatry, 35*(3), 374–383.

Nypaver, J. M., Titus, M. J., & Brugler, C. J. (1996). Patient transfer to rehabilitation: Just another move? *Rehabilitation Nursing, 21*(2), 94–97.

Oleson, M., & Shadick, K. (1993). Application of Moos and Schaefer's (1986) model to nursing care of elderly persons relocating to a nursing home. *Journal of Advanced Nursing, 18,* 479–485.

Osborne, O. H., Murphy, H. Leichman, S. S., Griffin, M., Hagerott, R. J., Ekland, E. S., & Thomas, M. D. (1990). Forced relocation of hospitalized psychiatric patients. *Archives of Psychiatric Nursing, 4,* 221–227.

Puskar, K. R. (1986). The usefulness of Mahler's phases of the separation–individuation process in providing a theoretical framework for understanding relocation. *Maternal–Child Nursing Journal, 15*(1), 15–22.

Puskar, K. R. (1990). Relocation support groups for corporate wives. *American Association of Occupational Health Nurses Journal, 38*(1), 25–31.

Puskar, K. R., & Dvorsak, K. G. (1991). Relocation stress in adolescents: Helping teenagers cope with a moving dilemma. *Pediatric Nursing, 17,* 295–298.

Puskar, K. R., & Rohay, J. M. (1999). School relocation and stress in teens. *Journal of School Nursing, 15*(1), 16–22.

Raviv, A., Keinan, G., Abazoh, Y., & Raviv, A. (1990). Moving as a stressful life event for adolescents. *Journal of Community Psychology, 18,* 130–140.

Reed, J., Roskell Payton, V., & Bond, S. (1998). The importance of place for older people moving into care homes. *Social Science in Medicine, 46*(7), 859–867.

Reinardy, J. R. (1995). Relocation to a new environment: Decisional control and the move to a nursing home. *Health and Social Work, 20*(1), 31–38.

Rodgers, B. L. (1997). Family members' experiences with the nursing home placement of an older adult. *Applied Nursing Research, 10*(2), 57–63.

Rosenkoetter, M. M. (1996). Changing life patterns of the resident in long-term care and the community-residing spouse. *Geriatric Nursing, 17*(6), 267–272.

Smider, N. A., Essex, M. J., & Ryff, C. D. (1996). Adaptation to community relocation: The interactive influence of psychological resources and contextual factors. *Psychology of Aging, 11*(2), 362–372.

Vernberg, E. M. (1990). Experiences with peers following relocation during early adolescence. *American Journal of Orthopsychiatry, 60,* 466–472.

Wilson, S. A. (1997). The transition to nursing home life: A comparison of planned and unplanned admissions. *Journal of Advanced Nursing, 26*(5), 864–871.

RISK FOR INEFFECTIVE RESPIRATORY FUNCTION

Burns, S. M. (1991). Preventing diaphragm fatigue in the ventilated patient. *Dimensions of Critical Care Nursing, 10,* 13–20.

Burns, S. (1998). Mechanical ventilation and weaning. In M. R. Kinney, S. B. Dunbar, J. A. Burns, S. M., Burns, J. E., & Truwit, J. D. (1994). Comparison of five clinical weaning indices. *American Journal of Critical Care, 3,* 342–353.

Burns, S. M., Clochesy, J. M., Goodnough Hanneman, S. K., Ingersoll, G. E., Knebel, A. R., & Shekleton, M. (1995). Weaning from long-term mechanical ventilation. *American Journal of Critical Care, 4,* 4–22.

Carrieri-Kohlman, V. (1991). Dyspnea in the weaning patient: Assessment and intervention. *AACN Clinical Issues in Critical Care Nursing, 2,* 464–473.

Chan, L. (1998). Effectiveness of a music therapy intervention on relaxation and anxiety for patients receiving ventilation assistance. *Heart and Lung, 27*(3), 169–176.

Change, V. (1995). Protocol for prevention of complications of endotracheal intubation. *Critical Care Nurse, 13*(4), 19–26.

Curley, M., & Fackler, J. (1998). Weaning from mechanical ventilation: Patterns in young children recovering from acute hypoxemic respiratory failure. *American Journal of Critical Care, 7*(5), 335–345.

Geisman, L. K. (1989). Advances in weaning from mechanical ventilation. *Critical Care Nursing Clinics of North America, 1,* 697–705.

Huckabay, L., & Daderian, A. (1989). Effect of choices on breathing exercises post open heart surgery. *Dimensions of Critical Care Nursing, 9,* 190–201.

Hunsberger, M. (1989). Nursing strategies: Altered respiratory function. In R. L. Foster, M. M. Hunsberger, & J. J. T. Anderson (Eds.). *Family-centered nursing care of children.* Philadelphia: W. B. Saunders.

Janson-Bjerklie, S., Ferketich, S., Benner, P., & Becker, G. (1992). Clinical markers of asthma severity risk: Importance of subjective as well as objective factors. *Heart and Lung, 21,* 265–272.

Janson-Bjerklie, S., Ruma, S., Stulbarg, M., & Carrieri, V. (1987). Predictors of dyspnea intensity in asthma. *Nursing Research, 36,* 179–183.

Jenny, J., & Logan, J. (1998). Caring and comfort metaphors used by critical care patients. *Image, 30*(2), 197–208.

Jenny, J., & Logan, J. (1991). Analyzing expert nursing practice to develop a new nursing diagnosis: Dysfunctional ventilatory weaning response. In R. M. Carroll-Johnson (Ed.). *Classification of nursing diagnoses: Proceedings of the ninth conference.* Philadelphia: J. B. Lippincott.

Jenny, J., & Logan, J. (1994). Promoting ventilator independence. *Dimensions of Critical Care Nursing, 13,* 29–37.

Knebel, A. R. (1991). Weaning from mechanical ventilation: Current controversies. *Heart and Lung, 20,* 321–331.

Leon, L. (1999). Smoking Cessation—Developing a Workable Program. *Nursing Spectrum, FL9*(18), 12–13.

Logan, J., & Jenny, J. (1990). Deriving a new nursing diagnosis through qualitative research: Dysfunctional ventilatory weaning response. *Nursing Diagnosis, 1*(1), 37–43.

Logan, J., & Jenny, J. (1991). Interventions for the nursing diagnosis Dysfunctional Ventilatory Weaning Response: A qualitative study. In R. M. Carroll-Johnson (Ed.). *Classification of nursing diagnosis: Proceedings of the ninth conference.* Philadelphia: J. B. Lippincott.

Mannino, D. M., Homa, D. M., Pertowski, C. A. et al. (1999). Surveillance for asthma—United States, 1960–1995. *Morbidity and Mortality Weekly Report CDC Surveillance Summaries, 47,* 1–27.

Marini, J. J. (1991). Editorials. *New England Journal of Medicine, 324,* 1496–1498.

McCarley, C. (1999). A model of chronic dyspnea. *Image, 31*(3), 231–236.

Owen, C. (1999). New directions in asthma management. *American Journal of Nursing, 99*(3), 26–34.

Schmierer, T. (2000). Prevention of allergies and asthma starts in pregnancy. Accessed from *http://www.advancefornurses.com/pastarticles/aug28_00cover.html* 10/4/00.

Slutsky, A. S. (1993). ACCP consensus conference: Mechanical ventilation. *Chest, 104,* 1833–1859.

Tobin, M. J. (1994). Mechanical ventilation. *New England Journal of Medicine, 330,* 1056–1061.

Treloar, D. M., & Stechmiller, J. K. (1995). Use of a clinical assessment tool for orally intubated patients. *American Journal of Critical Care, 4,* 355–360.

Truesdell, C. (2000). Helping patients with COPD manage episodes of acute shortness of breath. *MedSurg Nursing, 9*(4), 178–182.

Witta, K. (1990). New techniques for weaning difficult patients from mechanical ventilation. *AACN Clinical Issues, 1,* 260–266.

Yang, K. L., & Tobin, M. J. (1991). A prospective study of indexes predicting the outcome of trials of weaning from mechanical ventilation. *New England Journal of Medicine, 324,* 1445–1451.

Internet Resources

Agency for Healthcare Research and Quality (*http://www.ahrg.gov/*)

Allergy and Asthma Web Page (*http://www.cs.unc.edu/~kupstas/FAQ1.html*)

Asthma and Allergy Foundation of America (*http://www.aafa.org/*)

Asthma Management Model (*http://www.nbibisupport.com/asthma/research.html*)

Global Initiative for Obstructive Lung Disease (*http://www.coldcopd.com*)

Joint Council of Allergy, Asthma, and Immunology (*http://www.icaai.org/*)

Quitting Smoking Guidelines (*http://www.surgeon-general.gov/tobacco/default.htm*)

QuitNet (http:/www.quitnet.org/qn_main.itml)

SELF-CARE DEFICIT SYNDROME

Brody, E. (1985). Parent care as a normative family stress. *The Gerontologist, 25*(1), 19–29.

Chang, B., Uman, G., & Hirsh, M. (1998). Predictive power of clinical indicators for self-care deficit. *Nursing Diagnosis, 9*(2), 71–81.

Maher, A. B., Salmond, S. W., & Pellino, T. (1998). *Orthopedic nursing* (2nd ed.). Philadelphia: W. B. Saunders.

Mosher, R. B., & Moore, J. B. (1998). The relationship of self-concept & self-care in children with cancer. *Nursing Science Quarterly, 11*(3), 116–122.

Tracey, C. (1992). Hygiene assistance. In G. Bulechek & J. McCloskey (Eds.). *Nursing interventions: Essential nursing treatments.* Philadelphia: W. B. Saunders.

DISTURBED SELF-CONCEPT

Baumeister, R. F., Smart, L., & Boden, J. M. (1996). Relation of threatened egotism to violence and aggression: The dark side of high self-esteem. *Psychological Review, 103*(1), 5–33.

Bergamasco, E. C., Rossi, L., da Amancio C. G., & Carvalho, E. C. (2002). Body image of patients with burn sequellae. *Burns, 28,* 47–52.

Camp-Sorrell, D. (2000). Chemotherapy: toxicity management. In Yarbro, C., Frogge, M. H., Goodman, M., & Groenwald, S. *Career Nursing* (5th ed.). Boston: Jones and Bartlett.

Carscadden, J. S. *Above the cutting edge: A workbook for people who want to stop self-injury.* London. Ontario: London Psychiatric Hospital.

Cooley, M. E., Yeomans, A., & Cobb, S. (1986). Sexual and reproductive issues for women with Hodgkin's disease. *Cancer Nursing, 9,* 248–255.

Drapo, P. J. (1997). Mental retardation. In B. S. Johnson (Ed.). *Psychiatric-Mental Health Nursing: Adaptation and growth.* Philadelphia: J. B. Lippincott.

Dudas, S. (1993). Altered body image and sexuality. In S. Groenwald, M. Frogge, M. Goodman, M., & C. Yarbo (Eds.). *Cancer nursing: Principles and practices.* Boston: Jones and Bartlett.

Friedman-Campbell, M., & Hart, C. A. (1984). Theoretical strategies and nursing interventions to promote psychological adaptation to spinal cord injuries and disability. *Journal of Neurosurgical Nursing, 16,* 335–342.

Ganje-Fling, M. A., & McCarthy, P. (1996). Impact of childhood sexual abuse on client spiritual development: Counseling implications. *Journal of Counseling and Development, 74*(3), 253–258.

Grainger, R. (1990). How to feel good about being you. *American Journal of Nursing, 90*(4), 14.

Harper, J., & Marshall, E. (1992). Adolescents' problems and their relationship to self-esteem. *Adolescence, 26,* 799–807.

Hunter, K., Linn, M., & Harris, R. (1981–82). Characteristics of high and low self-esteem in the elderly. *International Journal of Aging and Human Development, 14,* 117–126.

Leuner, J., Coler, M., & Norris, J. (1994). Self esteem. In M. Rantz & P. LeMone (Eds.). *Classification of nursing diagnosis: Proceedings of the eleventh conference.* Glendale, CA: CINAHL.

Meisenhelder, J. B. (1985). Self-esteem: A closer look at clinical interventions. *International Journal of Nursing Studies, 22,* 127–135.

Miller, S. (1987). Promoting self-esteem in the hospitalized adolescent: Clinical interventions. *Issues of Comprehensive Pediatric Nursing, 10,* 187–194.

Morse, K. (1997). Responding to threats to integrity to self. *Science, 19*(4), 21–36.

Murray, M. F. (2000). Coping with change: Self-talk. *Hospital Practice, 31*(5), 118–120.

Norris, J., & Kunes-Connell, M. (1985). Self-esteem disturbance. *Nursing Clinics of North America, 20,* 745–761.

Norris, J., & Kunes-Connell, M. (1987). Self-esteem disturbance: A clinical validation study. In A. McLane (Ed.). *Classification of nursing diagnoses: Proceedings of the seventh conference.* St. Louis: C. V. Mosby.

Pierce, J., & Wardle, J. (1997), Cause and effect beliefs and self esteem of overweight children. *Journal of Child Psychology and Psychiatry and Allied Disciplines, 38*(6), 645–650.

Polatajko, H. J. (1991). The effect of a sensory integration program on academic achievement, motor performance, and self-esteem in children identified as learning disabled: Results of a clinical trial. *Occupational Therapy Journal of Research, 11,* 155–176.

Price, B. (1990). A model for body-image care. *Journal of Advanced Nursing, 5,* 585–593.

Scipien, G. M., Chard, M. A., Howe, J., & Barnard, M. U. (1990). *Pediatric nursing care.* St. Louis: C. V. Mosby.

Specht, J. A., King, G. A., & Francis, P. V. (1998). A preliminary study of strategies for maintaining self-esteem in adolescents with physical disabilities. *Canadian Journal of Rehabilitation, 11*(3), 109–116.

Swanson, B., Cronin-Stubbs, R., & Sheldon, J. (1989). The impact of psychosocial factors on adapting to physical disability: A review of the research literature. *Rehabilitation Nursing, 14*(2), 64–68.

Taylor, S. (1999). *Positive illusions.* New York: Basic Books.

Van-Dongen, C. J. (1998). Self-esteem among persons with severe mental illness. *Issues in Mental Health Nursing, 19*(1), 29–40.

Whitehead, J. R. (1991). Effects of fitness test type, teacher, and gender on exercise intrinsic motivation and physical self-worth. *Journal of School Health, 61*(1), 11–16.

Whitfield, C. (1990). *A gift of myself.* Deerfield Beach, FL: Public Health Communications.

Willoughby, C., King, G., & Polatajko, H. (1996). A therapist's guide to children's self-esteem. *American Journal of Occupational Therapy, 50*(2), 124–132.

Winkelstein, M. L. (1989). Fostering positive self-concept in the school-age child. *Pediatric Nursing, 15,* 229–233.

RISK FOR SELF-HARM

Blazer, D. G. (1982). *Depression in late life.* St. Louis: C. V. Mosby.

Boxwell, A. (1988). Geriatric suicide, the preventable death. *Nurse Practitioner, 13*(6), 10–14.

Carscadden, J. S. (1993a). *On the cutting edge: A guide for working with people who self injure.* London, Ontario: London Psychiatric Hospital.

Carscadden, J. S. (1993b). *Above the cutting edge: A workbook for people who want to stop self injury.* London, Ontario: London Psychiatric Hospital.

Carscadden, J. S. (1997). *Beyond the cutting edge: A survival kit for families of self-injurers.* London, Ontario: London Psychiatric Hospital.

Carscadden, J. S. (1998). *Premise for practice (relationship management team).* London, Ontario: London Psychiatric Hospital.

Dawson, D. F., & MacMillan, H. L. (1993). *Relationship management of the borderline patient: From understanding to treatment.* New York: Brunner/Mazel Publishers.

Dresser, J. G. (1999). Wrapping: A technique for interrupting self-mutilation. *Journal of the American Psychiatric Nurses Association, 5*(2), 67–70.

Egan, M. P., Rivera, S. G., Robillard, R. R., & Hanson, A. (1997). The no suicide contract: Helpful or harmful? *Journal of Psychosocial Nursing, 35*(3).

Fekar, C. R., & Koslap-Petraco, M. (1991). What about gay teenagers? (letter). *American Journal of Diseases of Children, 145,* 252.

Gibbs, A. (1990). Aspects of communication with people who have attempted suicide. *Journal of Advanced Nursing, 15,* 1245–1249.

Hatton, C., & Valente, S. (1977). Assessment of suicidal risk. In C. Hatton (Ed.). *Suicide: Assessment and intervention.* New York: Appleton-Century-Crofts.

Jacobs, D. (1989). Evaluation and care of suicidal behavior in emergency settings. In D. Jacobs & H. Brown (Eds.). *Suicide: Understanding and responding.* Madison, CT: International University Press.

Jennings, A. (1994). On being invisible in the mental health system. *Journal of Mental Health Administration,* 21 (Fall).

Laughrey, L., Jackson, J., Molla, P., & Wobbleton, J. (1997). Patient self-mutilation: When nursing becomes a nightmare. *Journal of Psychosocial Nursing, 35*(4).

Mallinson, R. K. (1999). The lived experiences of AIDS-related multiple losses by HIV-negative gay men. *Journal of the Association of Nurses in AIDS Care, 10*(5), 22–31.

Mellick, E., Buckwalter, & Stolley (1992). Suicide among elderly white men: Development of a profile. *Journal of Psychosocial Nursing, 30*(2), 29–34.

McIntosh, J. L. (1985). Suicide among the elderly: Levels and trends. *American Journal of Orthopsychiatry, 55*(4), 288–293.

Pallikkathayil, L., & Flood, M. (1991). Adolescent suicide. *Nursing Clinics of North America, 26,* 623–630.

Seigel, K., & Meyer, I. (1999). Hope and resilience in suicide ideation and behavior of gay and bisexual men following notification of HIV infection. *AIDS Education & Prevention, 11*(1), 53–64.

Smith, S. B. (1995). Restraints: Retraumatization for rape victims? *Journal of Psychosocial Nursing, 33*(7).

DISTURBED SENSORY PERCEPTION

Drury, J., & Akins, J. (1991). Sensory–perceptual alterations. In M. Maas, K. Buckwalter, & M. Hardy (Eds.). *Nursing diagnoses and interventions for the elderly.* Menlo Park, CA: Addison-Wesley Nursing.

Wilson, L. D. (1993). Sensory perceptual alteration: Diagnosis, prediction and intervention in the hospitalized adult. *Nursing Clinics of North America, 28,* 747–765.

INEFFECTIVE SEXUALITY PATTERNS

Alteneder, R. & Hartzekk, D. (1999). Addressing couples' sexuality concerns during the childbearing period: Use of the PLISSIT model. *Journal of Obstetric, Gynecologic, and Neonatal Nursing, 26*(6), 651–658.

Annon, J. S. (1976). The PLISS + model: A proposed conceptual scheme for the behavioral treatment of sexual problems. *Journal of Sex Education and Therapy, 2,* 211–215.

Barclay, L., Donoron, J., & Genovese, A. (1996). Men's experiences during their partner's first pregnancy:

A grounded theory analysis. *Australian Journal of Advanced Nursing, 13*(3), 12–24.

DiIorio, C., Parsons, M., Lehr, S., Adame, D., & Carlone, J. (1993). Factors associated with use of safer sex practices among college freshmen. *Research in Nursing and Health, 16,* 343–350.

Division of STD Prevention. (1997). *Sexually transmitted disease surveillance, 1996.* U.S. Department of Health and Human Services, Public Health Service, Atlanta: Centers for Disease Control & Prevention.

Donoran, J. (1995). The process of analysis during a grounded theory study of men during their partners' pregnancies. *Australian Journal of Advanced Nursing, 21*(4), 708–715.

Gilbert, E., & Harmon, J. (1998). *Manual of high risk pregnancy and delivery* (2nd ed.). St. Louis: Mosby-Year Book.

Gray, J. (1995). *Mars and Venus in the bedroom: A guide to lasting romance and passion.* New York: HarperCollins.

Horn, B. (1993). Cultural beliefs and teenage pregnancy. *Nurse Practitioner, 8*(8), 35, 39, 74.

Katzun, L. (1990). Chronic illness and sexuality. *American Journal of Nursing, 90,* 57–59.

Lion, E. (1982). *Human sexuality in nursing process.* New York: John Wiley & Sons.

Polomeno, V. (1999). Sex and babies: Pregnant couples' postnatal sexual concerns. *Journal of Prenatal Education, 8*(4), 9–18.

Smith, M. (1993). Pediatric sexuality: Promoting normal sexual development in children. *Nurse Practitioner, 18,* 37–44.

Waterhouse, J. (1993). Discussing sexual concerns with health care professionals. *Journal of Holistic Nursing, 11,* 125–134.

Waterhouse, J., & Metcalfe, M. (1991). Attitudes toward nurses discussing sexual concerns with patients. *Journal of Advanced Nursing, 16,* 1048–1054.

Wilmoth, M. C. (1993). Development and testing of the sexual behaviors questionnaire. *Dissertation Abstracts International, 54,* 6137B–6138B.

Wilmoth, M. C. (1994a). Strategies for becoming comfortable with sexual assessment. *Oncology Nursing News, 12*(2), 6–7.

Wilmoth, M. C. (1994b). Nurses' and patients' perspectives on sexuality: Bridging the gap. *Innovations in Oncology Nursing, 10,* 34–36.

World Health Organization. (1975). *Education and treatment in human sexuality: The training of health professionals.* Report of a WHO Meeting, Technical Report Series No. 572. Geneva: WHO.

DISTURBED SLEEP PATTERN

Blissit, P. (2001). Sleep, memory and learning. *Journal of Neurosurgical Nursing, 33*(4), 208–215.

Berger R. J., & Oswald, I. (1962). Effects of sleep deprivation on behavior, subsequent sleep and dreaming. *Journal of Mental Science, 108,* 457.

Cohen, F., & Merritt, S. (1992). Sleep promotion. In G. Bulechek & J. McCloskey (Eds.). *Nursing interventions: Essential nursing treatments* (2nd ed.). Philadelphia: W. B. Saunders.

Cureton-Lane, R. A., & Fontaine, D. K. (1997). Sleep in pediatric ICU. *American Journal of Critical Care, 6*(1), 56–63.

Dines-Kalinowski, C. M. (2000). Dream weaver. *33*(4), 48–49.

Hammer, B. (1991). Sleep pattern disturbance. In M. Maas, K. Buckwalter, & M. Hardy (Eds.). *Nursing diagnoses and interventions for the elderly.* Redwood City, CA: Addison-Wesley Nursing.

Haponik, E. (1994). Sleep problems. In W. Hazzard, E. Bieman, J. Bless, W. Ettinger, & J. Halter (Eds.). *Principles of geriatric medicine and gerontology.* New York: McGraw-Hill.

Hayashi, Y., & Endo, S. (1982). All-night sleep polygraphic recordings of healthy aged persons: REM and slow-wave sleep. *Sleep, 5,* 277–283.

Landis, C. & Moe, K. (2004). Sleep and menopause. *Nursing Clinics of North America, 39*(1), 97–115.

Larkin, V., & Butler, M. (2000). The implications of rest and sleep following childbirth. *British Journal of Midwifery, 8*(7), 438–442.

Rechtschaffen, A., & Kales, A. (1968). *A manual of standardized terminology, techniques and scoring system for sleep stages of human subjects.* NIHM Publication 204. Washington, DC: U.S. Government Printing Office.

Sebilia, A. (1981). Sleep deprivation and biological rhythms in the critical care unit. *Critical Care Nurse, 3,* 19.

Thelan, L. Urden, L., Lough, B., & Stacy, K. (1998). *Textbook of critical care nursing.* (3rd ed.). St Louis: C. V. Mosby.

White, M. A. (1990). Sleep onset latency and distress in hospitalized children. *Nursing Research, 39,* 134–139.

William, D. (1971). Sleep and disease. *American Journal of Nursing, 71,* 2321–2324.

Williams, R. L. & Jackson, D. (1982). Problems with sleep. *Heart and Lung, 11,* 262.

IMPAIRED SOCIAL INTERACTION

Maroni, J. (1989). Impaired social interactions. In G. McFarland & E. McFarlane (Eds.). *Nursing diagnosis and interventions.* St. Louis: C. V. Mosby.

McFarland, G., Wasli, E., & Gerety, E. (1996). *Nursing diagnoses and process in psychiatric mental health nursing* (3rd ed.). Philadelphia: J. B. Lippincott.

Parmelee, P. A., Katz, I. R., & Lawton, M. P. (1989). Depression among institutionalized aged. *Journal of Gerontology: Medical Sciences, 44*(1), 22–29.

Rawlins, R. P., Williams, S. R., & Beck, C. K. (1998). *Mental health–psychiatric nursing: A holistic life-cycle approach* (4th ed.). St. Louis: Mosby–Year Book.

CHRONIC SORROW

Burke, M. L., Hainsworth, M. A., Eakes, G. G., & Lindgren, C. L. (1992). Current knowledge and research on chronic sorrow: A foundation for inquiry. *Death Studies, 16*(3), 231–245.

Clubb, R. (1991). Chronic sorrow: Adoption patterns of parents with chronically ill children. *Pediatric Nursing, 17*(5), 41–46.

Eakes, G. G. (1995). Chronic sorrow: The lived experience of parents of chronically mentally ill individuals. *Archives of Psychiatric Nursing, 9*(2), 77–84.

Kearney, P. M., & Griffin, T. (2001). Between joy and sorrow: being a parent of a child with developmental disability. *Journal of Advanced Nursing, 34*(5), 582–592.

Lindgren, C. L., Burke, M. L., Hainsworth, M. A., & Eakes, G. G. (1992). Chronic sorrow: A lifespan concept. *Scholarly Inquiry for Nursing Practice, 24*(6), 27–42.

Mallow, G. E., & Bechtel, G. (1999). Chronic sorrow: The experience of parents with children who are developmentally disabled. *Journal of Psychosocial Nursing, 37*(7), 31–35.

Melnyk, B., Feinstein, N., Moldenhouer, Z., & Small, L. (2001). Coping of parents of children who are chronically ill. *Pediatric Nursing, 27*(6), 548–558.

Monsen, R. B. (1999). Mothers' experiences of living worried when parenting children with spina bifida. *Journal of Pediatric Nursing, 14*(3), 157–163.

Northington, L. (2000). Chronic sorrow in caregivers of school age children with sickle cell disease: A grounded theory approach. *Issues in Comprehensive Pediatric Nursing, 23*(3), 141–154.

Phillips, M. (1991). Chronic sorrow in mothers of chronically ill and disabled children. *Issues of Comprehensive Pediatric Nursing, 14*(2), 111–120.

Teel, C. (1991). Chronic sorrow: Analysis of the concept. *Journal of Advanced Nursing, 16*(11), 1311–1319.

SPIRITUAL DISTRESS

Bearon, L., & Koenig, H. (1990). Religious cognitions and use of prayer in health and illness. *The Gerontologist, 30,* 249–253.

Burkhart, L., & Solari-Twadell, A. (2001). Spirituality and religiousness: Differentiating the diagnoses through a review of the nursing diagnosis. *12*(2), 44–54.

Burkhart, M. A. (1994). Becoming and connecting: Elements of spirituality for women. *Holistic Nursing Practice, 8,* 12–21.

Cameron, M. E. (1998). Clinical sidebar. *Image, 30*(3), 275–280.

Carson, V. B. (2000). *Mental health nursing: The nurse-patient journey* (2nd ed.). Philadelphia: W.B. Saunders.

Carson, V. B., & Green, H. (1992). Spiritual well-being: A predictor of hardiness in patients with acquired immunodeficiency syndrome. *Journal of Professional Nursing, 8,* 209–220.

Corbett, K. (1998). Patterns of spirituality in persons with advanced HIV disease. *Research in Nursing and Health, 21*(2), 143–153.

DeYoung, S. (1984). Perceptions of the institutionalized elderly regarding the nurse's role in supporting spiritual well-being. In R. Fehring (Ed.). *Proceedings of the conference on spirituality.* Milwaukee, WI: Marquette University.

Emblen, J. D., & Halstead, L. (1993). Spiritual needs and interventions: Comparing the views of patients, nurses and chaplains. *Clinical Nurse Specialist, 7,* 175–182.

Giuri, A. (1980). Aging and the spiritual life. *Spiritual Life, 26,* 41–46.

Hall, C. M. (1985). Religion and aging. *Journal of Religion and Health, 24,* 70–78.

Hinton, J. (1999). The progress of awareness and acceptance of dying assessed in cancer patients and their caring relatives. *Palliative Medicine, 13*(1), 19–35.

Hungelmann, J., Kenkel-Rossi, E., Klassen, L., & Stollenwerk, R. M. (1985). Spiritual well-being in older adults, harmonious interconnectedness. *Journal of Religion and Health, 24,* 147–153.

Inlay, S. C., & Smith, D. R. (1984). Aging and religious participation. *Journal of Gerontology, 39,* 357–363.

Kendrick, K. D., & Robinson, S. (2000). Spirituality: Its relevance and purpose for clinical nursing in the new millennium. *Journal of Clinical Nursing, 9*(5), 701–705.

Millison, M. B. (1995). A review of the research on spiritual care and hospice. *The Hospice Journal, 10,* 3–17.

Mindel, C. H., & Vaughan, C. E. (1978). A multidimensional approach to religiosity and disengagement. *Journal of Gerontology, 33,* 103–108.

Moberg, D. O. (1984). Subjective measures of spiritual well-being. *Review of Religious Research, 25,* 351–364.

Nelsen, H. M. (1981). Life without afterlife: Toward a congruency of belief across generations. *Journal of Scientific Study in Religion, 20,* 109–118.

Patterson, R. A. (1984). The search for meaning: A pastoral response to suffering. *Hospital Progress, 65,* 46–49.

Piles, C. L. (1990). Providing spiritual care. *Nurse Educator, 15*(1), 36–41.

Quintero, C. (1993). Blood administration in pediatric Jehovah's Witness. *Pediatric Nursing, 19*(1), 46–48.

Ryan, E. (1985). Selecting an instrument to measure spiritual distress. *Oncology Nursing Forum, 12*(2), 93–94, 99.

Ryan, M. C., & Patterson, J. (1987). Loneliness in the elderly. *Journal of Gerontological Nursing, 13*(5), 6–12.

Shea, G. (1986). Meeting the pastoral care needs of an aging population. *Health Progress, 67*(5), 36–37, 68.

Sodestrom, K. E., & Martinson, I. M. (1987). Patients' spiritual coping strategies: A study of nurse and patient perspectives. *Oncology Nursing Forum, 14*(2), 41–46.

Stiles, M. K. (1990). The shining stranger: Nurse–family spiritual relationship. *Cancer Nursing, 13,* 235–245.

Stoll, R. I. (1984). Spiritual assessment: A nursing perspective. In R. Fehring (Ed.). *Proceedings of the conference on spirituality.* Milwaukee, WI: Marquette University.

Taylor, E. J. (2000). Spiritual and ethical end-of-life concerns. In M. Goodman, C. H. Yarbo, & S. L. Groenwald (Eds.). *Cancer nursing: Principles and practice* (5th ed.). Boston: Jones and Bartlett.

Van Heukelem, J. (1982). Assessing the spiritual needs of children and their families. In J. A. Shelley (Ed.). *The spiritual needs of children.* Downers Grove, IL: Intervarsity Press.

Wald, F. S., & Bailey, C. (1990). Nurturing the spiritual component in care for the terminally ill. *CARING Magazine, 9*(11), 64–68.

RISK FOR SUDDEN INFANT DEATH SYNDROME

American Academy of Pediatrics. (2000). Task force on infant sleep position and Sudden Infant Death Syndrome: Changing concepts of Sudden Infant Death Syndrome; Implications for infants' sleeping environment and sleep position. *Pediatrics, 105*(3), 650–656.

Anderson, J. E. (2000). Co-sleeping: Can we ever put the issue to rest? *Contemporary Pediatrics, 17*(6), 98–102, 109–110, 113–114.

Moon, R. Y. (2001). Are you talking to parents about SIDS? *Contemporary Pediatrics, 18*(3), 122–131.

O'Donnell, J. K., & Gaedeke, M. K. (1995). Sudden infant death syndrome. *Critical Care Nursing Clinics of North America, 7*(3), 473–481.

Poyser, K. (2000). Cot death: Reducing the risk and reaching out to the public. *Community Practice, 73*(12), 878–880.

Sherratt, S. (1999). The pros & cons of movement monitors. *British Journal of Midwifery, 7*(9), 569–572.

DISTURBED THOUGHT PROCESSES

Baier, M., & Murray, R. (1999). A descriptive study of insight into illness reported by persons with schizophrenia. *Journal of Psychosocial Nursing, 37*(1), 14–21.

Baker, P. (1995). Accepting the inner voices. *Nursing Times, 91*(31), 59–61.

Baltes, P. B. (1993). The aging mind: Potential and limits. *Gerontologist, 33,* 580–594.

Buccheri, R., Trystad, L., Kanas, N. & Dowling, G. (1997). Symptom management of auditory hallucinations in schizophrenia. *Journal of Psychosocial Nursing, 35*(12), 20–28.

Farrell, S. P., Harmon, R. B., & Hastings, S. (1998). Nursing management of acute psychotic episodes. *Nursing Clinics of North America, 33*(1), 187–200.

Glick, O. J. (1993). Normal thought processes: An overview. *Nursing Clinics of North America, 28,* 715–727.

Maier-Lorentz, M. (2000). Effective nursing interventions for the management of Alzheimer's disease. *Journal of Neuroscience Nursing, 32*(3), 153–157.

Rakel, B. (1991). Knowledge deficit. In M. Maas, K. Buckwalter, & M. Hardy (Eds.). *Nursing diagnoses and interventions for the elderly.* Redwood City, CA: Addison-Wesley Nursing.

Tarrier, N., Harwood, S., & Yusopoff, L. (1990). Coping strategy enhancement (CSE): A method of treating residual schizophrenic symptoms. *Behavioral Psychotherapy, 18,* 282–293.

INEFFECTIVE TISSUE PERFUSION

Baxendale, L. (1992). Pathophysiology of coronary artery disease. *Nursing Clinics of North America, 27,* 143–151.

Burch, K., Todd, K., Crosby, F., Ventura, M., Lohr, G., & Grace, M. L. (1991). PVD: Nurse patient interventions. *Journal of Vascular Nursing, 9*(4), 13–16.

Cunningham, S. (1992). The epidemiologic basis of coronary disease prevention. *Nursing Clinics of North America, 27,* 153–170.

Fahey, V. A. (1997). *Vascular nursing* (3rd ed.). Philadelphia: W. B. Saunders.

Hart, B. P. (1993). Vascular consequences of smoking and benefits of smoking cessation. *Journal of Vascular Nursing, 11*(2), 48–51.

Helt, J. (1991). Foot care and footwear to prevent amputation. *Journal of Vascular Nursing, 9*(4), 2–8.

Maves, M. (1992). Mutual goal setting. In G. Bulecheck & J. McCloskey (Eds.). *Nursing interventions.* Philadelphia: W. B. Saunders.

Patient Education Committee, Society for Vascular Nursing. (1992). *Venous disease.* Norwood, MA: Society for Vascular Nursing.

Sieggreen, M. (1987). Healing of physical wounds. *Nursing Clinics of North America, 22,* 439–448.

Sieggreen, M. (1999). Assessment of clients with vascular disorders. In S. Black, P. Hawkes, & A. Keene (Eds.). *Medical surgical nursing* (6th ed.). Philadelphia: W. B. Saunders

Skelton, N. K. (1992). Medical implications of obesity: Losing pounds and gaining years. *Postgraduate Medicine, 92,* 151–162.

UNILATERAL NEGLECT

Baggerly, J. (1992). Sensory perceptual problems following stroke. *Nursing Clinics of North America, 26,* 997–1005.

Heilman, K. M., & Valenstein, E. (1972). Frontal lobe neglect in man. *Neurology, 22,* 660–664.

Heilman, K. M., & Van Den Abell, T. (1980). Right hemisphere dominance for attention: The mechanism underlying hemispheric asymmetries of inattention (neglect). *Neurology, 30,* 327–330.

Kalbach, L. R. (1991). Unilateral neglect: Mechanisms and nursing care. *Journal of Neuroscience Nursing, 23*(2), 125–129.

Lin, K. (1996). Right-hemispheric activation approaches to neglect rehabilitation post stroke. *American Journal of Occupational Therapy, 50*(7), 504–514.

Mitchell, P. H., Hodges, L. C., Muwaswes, M., & Walleck, C. A. (1992). *AANN's neuroscience nursing* (2nd ed.). Norwalk, CT: Appleton & Lange.

IMPAIRED URINARY ELIMINATION

Carpenter, R. O. (1999). Disorders of elimination. In J. McMillan, C. D. DeAngelis, R. Feigin, & J. B. Warshaw (Eds.), *Oski's pediatrics: Principles and practice* (3rd ed.). Philadelphia: Lippincott Williams & Wilkins.

Dougherty, M. (1998). Current status of research on pelvic muscles strengthening techniques. *Journal of Wound, Ostomy and Continence, 25*(3), 75–83.

Engberg, S., McDowell, B. J., Donovan, N., Brodak, I., & Weber, E. (1997). Treatment of urinary incontinence in homebound older adults: Interface between research and practice. *Ostomy/Wound Management, 43*(10), 18–26.

Fanti, J. A., Newman, D. K., & Colling, J. (1996). *Urinary incontinence in adults: Acute and chronic management, Clinical practice guidelines No. 2.* Rockville, MD: U.S. Department of Health and Human Services.

Foye, H., & Sulkes, S. (1990). Developmental and behavioral pediatrics. In R. E. Behrman & R. Kliegman (Eds.). *Nelson essentials of pediatrics.* Philadelphia: W. B. Saunders.

Ghoniem, G. M., & Hassouna, M. (1997). Alternatives for the pharmacologic management of urge and stress urinary incontinence in the elderly. *Journal of Wound, Ostomy and Continence Nursing, 24,* 311–318.

Kelleher, R. (1997). Daytime and nighttime wetting in children: A review of management. *Journal of the Society of Pediatric Nurses, 2*(2), 73–82.

Longstaffe, S., Mofatt, M., & Whalen, J. C. (2000). Behavioral and self-concept changes after six months of enuresis treatment: A randomized, controlled trial. *Pediatrics, 105* (Suppl.), 935–940.

Macauley, M., Pettersen, L., Fader, M., Brooks, R., & Cottenden. (2004). A multicenter evaluation of absorbent products for children with incontinence and disabilities. *Journal of WOCH, 31*(4), 235–244.

Messick, G. M., & Powe, C. E. (1997). Applying behavioral research to incontinence. *Ostomy/Wound Management, 43*(10), 40–48.

Morison, M. (1998). Family attitudes to bed-wetting and their influence on treatment. *Professional Nurse, 13*(5), 321–325.

Newman, D. K., Lynch, K., Smith, D. A., & Cell, P. (1991). Restoring urinary continence. *American Journal of Nursing, 91,* 28–36.

Perkins, J. (1998). Vaginal weights for assessment and training of the pelvic floor. *Journal of Wound, Ostomy, and Continence Nursing, 25*(4), 206–216.

Sampselle, C., & DeLancey, J. (1998). Anatomy of female continence. *Journal of Wound, Ostomy and Continence Nursing, 25*(3), 63–74.

Scardillo, J., & Aronovitch, S. A. (1999). Successfully managing incontinence-related irritant dermatitis across the lifespan. *Ostomy Wound Management, 45*(4), 36–44.

Smith, D., & Newmen, D. K. (1991). Nursing management of urinary incontinence associated with Alzheimer's disease. *Journal of Home Health Care Practice, 3*(4), 25–32.

Steeman, E., & Defever, M. (1998). Urinary incontinence among elderly persons who live at home. *Nursing Clinics of North America, 33*(3), 441–455.

Urinary Incontinence Guideline Panel. (1992, March). *Urinary incontinence in adults: Clinical practice guideline.* AHCPR Pub. No. 92-0038. Rockville, MD: Agency for Health Care Policy and Research, Public Health Service, U.S. Department of Health and Human Services.

Warrady, B. A. (1991). Primary nocturnal enuresis: Current concepts about an old problem. *Pediatric Annals, 20,* 246–251.

RISK FOR VIOLENCE

Alexander, R. (1990). Incidence of impact trauma with cranial injuries ascribed to shaking. *American Journal of Diseases of Children, 144,* 724–726.

Alvarey, J. (1998). Communication with angry and aggressive clients. In E. M. Varcarolis (Ed.). *Foundations of psychiatric–mental health nursing* (3rd ed.). Philadelphia: W. B. Saunders.

Bauer, B., & Hill, S. (1994). People who defend against anxiety through aggression towards others. In E. M. Varcarolis (Ed.). *Foundations of psychiatric-mental health nursing* (2nd ed.). Philadelphia: W. B. Saunders.

Davies, W. H., & Flannery, D. (1998). Post-traumatic stress disorder in children and adolescents exposed to violence. *Pediatric Clinics of North America, 45*(2), 341–353.

Dowd, M. D. (1998). Consequences of violence. *Pediatric Clinics of North America, 45*(2), 333–339.

Edari, R., & McManus, P. (1998). Risk and resiliency factors for violence. *Pediatric Clinics of North America, 45*(2), 293–303.

Farrell, S., Harmon, R., & Hastings, S. (1998). Nursing management of acute psychotic episodes. *Nursing Clinics of North America, 33*(1), 187–200.

Harris, G. T., & Varnly, G. W. (1986). Assaults and assaulters in maximum security. *Research Reports, 3*(2), Mental Health Center, Penetanguishene, Ontario.

Hennes, H. (1998). A review of violence: Statistics among children and adolescents in the US. *Pediatric Clinics of North America, 45*(2), 269–280.

Hunter, D. S. (1989). The use of physical restraint in managing out-of-control behavior in youth: A frontline perspective. *Child and Youth Care Quarterly, 18,* 141–154.

Meddaugh, D. (1990). Reactance: Understanding aggressive behavior in long-term care. *Journal of Psychosocial Nursing, 28*(2), 28–32.

Munns, D., & Nolan L. (1991). Potential for violence. In Mass, J., Buckwalter, K., & Hardy, M. (Eds.). *Nursing diagnoses and interventions for the elderly.* Redwood City, CA: Addison-Wesley Nursing.

Norris, M., & Kennedy, C. (1992). How patients perceive the seclusion process. *Journal of Psychosocial Nursing, 30*(6), 7–13.

Ropor, J., Coutts, A., Sather, J., & Taylor, R. (1985). Restraint and seclusion. *Journal of Psychosocial Nursing, 23*(6), 18–23.

Veenema, G. (2001). Children's exposure to community violence. *Journal of Nursing Scholarship, 33*(2), 167–173.

Willis, E., & Strasburger, V. (1998). Media violence. *Pediatric Clinics of North America, 45*(2), 319–331.

WANDERING

Algase, D. L. (1999). Wandering in dementia. *Annual Review in Nursing Research, 17*(2), 185–217.

Altus, D. E., Mathews, R. M., Xaverius, P. K., Engelman, K. K., & Nolan B. D. (2000). Evaluation of an electronic monitoring system for people who wander. *American Journal of Alzheimer's Disease, 15*(2), 121–125.

Brown, J. B., Bedford, N. K. & White, S. J. (1999). *Gerontological protocols for nurse practitioners.* Philadelphia: Lippincott Williams & Wilkins.

Cohen-Mansfield, J. (1998). The effects of an enhanced environment on nursing home residents who pace. *Gerontologist, 38*(2), 199–208.

Ederly, E. S., & Donovick, P. J. (1998). Neuropsychological correlates of wandering in persons with Alzheimer's disease. *American Journal of Alzheimer's Disease, 13*(6), 317–329.

Logsdon, R. G., McCurry, T. L., Gibbons, L. E., Kukuli, W. A., & Larson, E. B. (1998). Wandering: a significant problem among community-residing individuals with Alzheimer's disease. *Journal of Gerontological Behavioral, Psychological and Social Science, 53B*(5), 294–299.

Maier-Lorentz, M. M. (2000). Effective nursing interventions for the management of Alzheimer's disease. *Journal of Neuroscience Nursing, 32*(2), 117–125.

Meiner, S. E. (2000). Wandering problems need ongoing nursing planning: a case study. *Geriatric Nursing. 21*(2), 101–106.

Pack, R. (2000). The "ins and outs" of wandering. *Nursing Homes, 49*(8), 55–59.

COLLABORATIVE PROBLEMS

Arcangelo, V., & Peters, J. (2001). *Pharmacology for nurse practitioners.* Philadelphia: Lippincott Williams & Wilkins.

Byrne, B. (2002). Deep vein thrombosis prophylaxis. *Journal of Vascular Nursing, 20*(2), 53–59

Newcombe, P. (2002). Pathophysiology of sickle cell disease crisis. *Emergency Nurse, 9*(9), 9–22.

Rausch, M., & Pollard, D. (1998). Management of the patient with sickle cell disease. *Journal of Intravenous Nursing, 21*(1), 27–40.

Tumbarello, C. (2000). Acute extremity compartmental syndrome. *Journal of Trauma Nursing, 7*(2), 30–36.

INDEX

Note: Page numbers followed by *b, f* and *t* indicate boxes, figures and tables, respectively. Capitalized entries indicate nursing diagnoses.